CLINICAL PHYSIOLOGY OF ACID-BASE AND ELECTROLYTE DISORDERS

T0198239

NOTICE

Medicine is an ever-changing science. As new research and clinical experience broaden our knowledge, changes in treatment and drug therapy are required. The authors and the publisher of this work have checked with sources believed to be reliable in their efforts to provide information that is complete and generally in accord with the standards accepted at the time of publication. However, in view of the possibility of human error or changes in medical sciences, neither the authors nor the publisher nor any other party who has been involved in the preparation or publication of this work warrants that the information contained herein is in every respect accurate or complete, and they disclaim all responsibility for any errors or omissions or for the results obtained from use of the information contained in this work. Readers are encouraged to confirm the information contained herein with other sources. For example and in particular, readers are advised to check the product information sheet included in the package of each drug they plan to administer to be certain that the information contained in this work is accurate and that changes have not been made in the recommended dose or in the contraindications for administration. This recommendation is of particular importance in connection with new or infrequently used drugs

CLINICAL PHYSIOLOGY OF ACID-BASE AND ELECTROLYTE DISORDERS

Fifth Edition

Burton David Rose, MD

Clinical Professor of Medicine
Harvard Medical School
Boston, Massachusetts
Editor-in-Chief
UpToDate
Wellesley, Massachusetts

Theodore W. Post, MD

Deputy Editor, Nephrology
UpToDate
Wellesley, Massachusetts

McGraw-Hill
MEDICAL PUBLISHING DIVISION

New York   St. Louis   San Francisco   Auckland
Bogotá   Caracas   Lisbon   London   Madrid
Mexico City   Milan   Montreal   New Delhi
San Juan   Singapore   Sydney   Tokyo   Toronto

McGraw-Hill

*A Division of The **McGraw·Hill** Companies*

CLINICAL PHYSIOLOGY OF ACID-BASE AND ELECTROLYTE DISORDERS

24 LKV 22

ISBN 0-07134682-1

This book was set in Times Roman by Keyword Publishing Services.
The editors were Marty Wonsciewicz, Kathleen McCullough, and Karen Davis.
The production supervisor was Phil Galea.
The cover designer was Mary McKeon.
The index was prepared by Kathi Unger.
LSC Communications was printer and binder.

This book is printed on acid-free paper.

Cataloging-in-Publication data is on file for this title at the Library of Congress.

To Gloria, Emily, Anne, and Daniel
and
To Claire, Garrett, and Ian

CONTENTS

PREFACE

The fifth edition of *Clinical Physiology of Acid-Base and Electrolyte Disorders* has been largely rewritten to include the many important advances that have been made and the controversies that have arisen in the past six years. As with the previous four editions, this book attempts to integrate the essentials of renal and electrolyte physiology with the common clinical disorders of acid-base and electrolyte balance. Its underlying premise is that these clinical disturbances can be best approached from an understanding of basic physiologic principles. Thus, Chapters 1 to 6 review the physiology of normal renal function and the effects of hormones on the kidney. This is followed by a discussion of the extrarenal and renal factors involved in the internal distribution of the body water and in the normal regulation of volume (sodium), water, acid-base, and potassium balance (Chapters 7 to 12). In addition to providing the foundation for understanding how disease states can overcome these regulatory processes, the initial chapters can also be used by first-year medical students studying renal physiology.

The material presented in these chapters presents the core of information that, in our opinion, the clinician should possess. Although relatively complete, it is not meant to be an exhaustive review. In those areas where controversy exists, we have chosen to note the presence of uncertainty and to refer the interested reader to appropriate references, rather than extensively reviewing each theory. Since the primary purpose of this book is to teach the reader how to approach clinical problems, the physiological discussions are correlated with situations in clinical medicine wherever possible.

The last section of the book (Chapters 13 to 28) contains a separate chapter on each major acid-base and electrolyte disturbance. In addition to discussing etiology, symptoms, diagnosis, and treatment, each chapter begins with a short summary of the pathophysiology of the specific disorder with cross-references to more complete discussions in the earlier chapters. Although this leads to a certain amount of repetition, it has the advantage of allowing each clinical chapter to be read independently of the other parts of the book, making the book easier to use by a physician dealing with an acutely ill patient.

Problems are presented at the end of most of the chapters in both the physiology and clinical sections. These problems are intended both to test understanding and to emphasize important concepts frequently misunderstood by physicians dealing with these disorders. The answers to these problems are presented in Chapter 29, and Chapter 30 contains a summary of important equations and formulas that are useful in the clinical setting.

We are extremely grateful to Colin Sieff, Donald Kohan, Philip Marsden, Evan Loh, Bruce Runyon, and Jess Mandel for contributing material to selected chapters, particularly 6, 16, 20, and 21.

PART
ONE

RENAL PHYSIOLOGY

INTRODUCTION TO
RENAL FUNCTION

The kidney normally performs a number of essential functions:

- It participates in the maintenance of the constant extracellular environment that is required for adequate functioning of the cells. This is achieved by excretion of some of the waste products of metabolism (such as urea, creatinine, and uric acid) and by specifically adjusting the urinary excretion of water and electrolytes to match net intake and endogenous production. As will be seen, the kidney is able to *regulate individually* the excretion of water and solutes such as sodium, potassium, and hydrogen largely by changes in tubular reabsorption or secretion.
- It secretes hormones that participate in the regulation of systemic and renal hemodynamics (renin, angiotensin II, prostaglandins, nitric oxide, endothelin, and bradykinin), red blood cell production (erythropoietin), and calcium, phosphorus, and bone metabolism (1,25-dihydroxyvitamin D_3 or calcitriol).
- It performs such miscellaneous functions as catabolism of peptide hormones[1,2] and synthesis of glucose (gluconeogenesis) in fasting condition.[3,4]

This chapter will review briefly the morphology of the kidney and the basic processes of reabsorption and secretion. The regulation of renal hemodynamics, the specific functions of the different nephron segments, and the relationships between hormones and the kidney will then be discussed in the ensuing chapters.

RENAL MORPHOLOGY

The basic unit of the kidney is the *nephron*, with each kidney in humans containing approximately 1.0 to 1.3 million nephrons.

Each nephron consists of a glomerulus, which is a tuft of capillaries interposed between two arterioles (the afferent and efferent arterioles), and a series of tubules lined by a continuous layer of epithelial cells (Fig. 1-1). The glomeruli are located in the outer part of the kidney, called the *cortex*, whereas the tubules are presented in both the cortex and the inner part of the kidney, the *medulla* (Figs. 1-1 and 1-2).

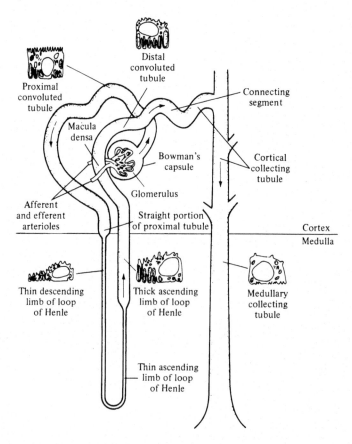

Figure 1-1 Anatomic relationships of the component parts of the nephron. (*Adapted from Vander R, Renal Physiology, 2d ed, McGraw-Hill, New York, 1980.*)

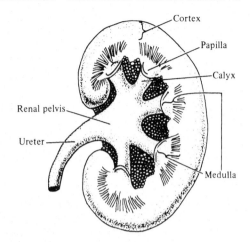

Figure 1-2 Section of a human kidney. The outer portion (the cortex) contains all the glomeruli. The tubules are located in both the cortex and the medulla, with the collecting tubules forming a large portion of the inner medulla (the papilla). Urine leaving the collecting tubules drains sequentially into the calyces, renal pelvis, ureter, and then the bladder. (*Adapted from Vander R,* Renal Physiology, *2d ed, McGraw-Hill, New York, 1980.*)

The initial step in the excretory function of the nephron is the formation of an ultrafiltrate of plasma across the glomerulus. This fluid then passes through the tubules and is modified in *two ways*: by reabsorption and by secretion. *Reabsorption* refers to the removal of a substance from the filtrate, whereas *secretion* refers to the addition of a substance to the filtrate. As will be seen, the different tubular segments make varying contributions to these processes.

Fluid filtered across the glomerulus enters Bowman's space and then the proximal tubule (Fig. 1-1). The *proximal tubule* is composed anatomically of an initial convoluted segment and a later straight segment, the pars recta, which enters the outer medulla. The *loop of Henle* begins abruptly at the end of the pars recta. It generally includes a thin descending limb and thin and thick segments of the ascending limb. The hairpin configuration of the loop of Henle plays a major role in the excretion of a hyperosmotic urine.

It is important to note that the length of the loops of Henle is not uniform (Fig. 1-3). Approximately 40 percent of nephrons have short loops that penetrate only the outer medulla or may even turn around in the cortex; these short loops lack a thin ascending limb.[5] The remaining 60 percent have long loops that course through the medulla and may extend down to the papilla (the innermost portion of the medulla). The length of the loops is largely determined by the cortical location of the glomerulus: Glomeruli in the outer cortex (about 30 percent) have only short loops; those in the juxtamedullary region (about 10 percent) have only long loops; and those in the midcortex may have either short or long loops (Fig. 1-3).

The thick ascending limb also has a cortical segment that returns to the region of the parent glomerulus. It is in this area, where the tubule approaches the afferent glomerular arteriole, that the specialized tubular cells of the *macula densa* are located (Fig. 1-4). The juxtaglomerular cells of the afferent arteriole and the macula densa compose the juxtaglomerular apparatus, which plays a central role in renin secretion (see Chap. 2).

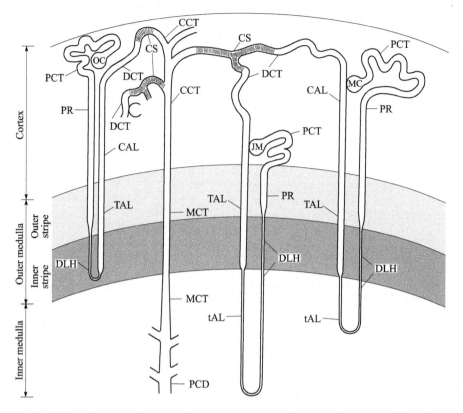

Figure 1-3 Anatomic relationships of the different nephron segments according to location of the glomeruli in the outer cortex (OC), midcortex (MC), or juxtamedullary area (JM). The major nephron segments are labeled as follows: PCT = proximal convoluted tubule; PR = pars recta, which ends in the S_3 segment at the junction of the outer and inner stripes in the outer medulla; DLH = descending limb of the loop of Henle; tAL = thin ascending limb, which is not present in outer cortical nephrons that have short loops of Henle; TAL = medullary thick ascending limb; CAL = cortical thick ascending limb, which ends in the macula densa adjacent to the parent glomerulus (see Fig. 1-4); DCT = distal convoluted tubule; CS = connecting segment; CCT = cortical collecting tubule; MCT = medullary collecting tubule; and PCD = papillary collecting duct, at the end of the medullary collecting tubule. (*Adapted from Jacobson HR*, Am J Physiol *241:F203, 1981. Used with permission.*)

After the macula densa, there are three cortical segments (Fig. 1-3): The *distal convoluted tubule*, the *connecting segment* (previously considered part of the late distal tubule), and the *cortical collecting tubule*.[6,7] The connecting segments of many nephrons drain into a single collecting tubule. Fluid leaving the cortical collecting tubule flows into the *medullary collecting tubule* and then drains sequentially into the calyces, the renal pelvis, the ureters, and the bladder (Fig. 1-2).

The segmental subdivision of the nephron is based upon different permeability and transport characteristics that translate into important differences in function.[5] In general, the proximal tubule and loop of Henle reabsorb the bulk of the filtered solutes and water, while the collecting tubules make the final small changes in

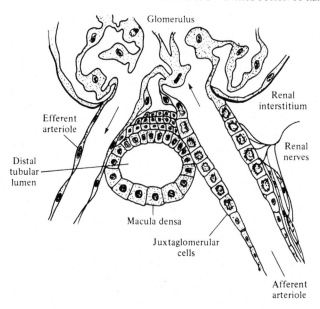

Figure 1-4   Diagram of the juxtaglomerular apparatus. The juxtaglomerular cells in the wall of the afferent arteriole secrete renin into the lumen of the afferent arteriole and the renal lymph. Stretch receptors in the afferent arteriole, the sympathetic nerves ending in the juxtaglomerular cells, and the composition of the tubular fluid reaching the macula densa all contribute to the regulation of renin secretion. (*Adapted from Davis JO, Am J Med 55:333, 1973. Used with permission.*)

urinary composition that permit solute and water excretion to vary appropriately with alterations in dietary intake.

There may also be significant heterogeneity within a given tubular segment, particularly in the proximal tubule and cortical collecting tubule. In the latter segment, for example, there are two cell types with very different functions: The *principal cells* reabsorb sodium and chloride and secrete potassium, in part under the influence of aldosterone; and the *intercalated cells* secrete hydrogen or bicarbonate and reabsorb potassium, but play no role in sodium balance.[6]

REABSORPTION AND SECRETION

The rate of glomerular filtration averages 135 to 180 L/day in a normal adult. Since this represents a volume that is more than 10 times that of the extracellular fluid and approximately 60 times that of the plasma, it is evident that almost all of this fluid must be returned to the systemic circulation. This process is called *tubular reabsorption* and can occur either across the cell or via the paracellular route between the cells. With transcellular reabsorption, the substance to be reabsorbed is first transported from the tubular lumen into the cell, usually across the luminal aspect of the cell membrane; next, it moves across the basolateral (or peritubular) aspect of the cell membrane into the interstitium and then the capillaries that surround the tubules (Fig. 1-5). With paracellular reabsorption, the substance to be reabsorbed moves from the tubular lumen across the tight junction at the luminal surface of adjacent cells (see below) into the interstitium and then into the peritubular capillaries.

Most reabsorbed solutes are returned to the systemic circulation intact. However, some are metabolized within the cell, particularly low-molecular-weight proteins in the proximal tubule.

Solutes can also move in the opposite direction, from the peritubular capillary through the cell and into the urine. This process is called *tubular secretion* (Fig. 1-5).

Filtered solutes and water may be transported by one or both of these mechanisms. For example, Na^+, Cl^-, and H_2O are reabsorbed; hydrogen ions are secreted; K^+ and uric acid are both reabsorbed and secreted; and filtered creatinine is excreted virtually unchanged, since it is not reabsorbed and only a small amount is normally added to the urine by secretion.

The transcellular reabsorption or secretion of almost all solutes is facilitated by *protein carriers* or *ion-specific channels*; these transport processes are essential, since free diffusion of ions is limited by the lipid bilayer of the cell membrane. The spatial orientation of the cells is also important, because the luminal and basolateral aspects of the cell membrane, which are separated by the *tight junction*, have different functional characteristics.

As an example, filtered sodium enters the cell passively down a favorable electrochemical gradient, since the active Na^+-K^+-ATPase pump in the basolateral membrane maintains the cell Na^+ concentration at a low level and makes the cell interior electronegative. Sodium entry occurs by a variety of mechanisms at different nephron sites, such as Na^+-H^+ exchange and Na^+-glucose cotransport in the proximal tubule, a Na^+-K^+-$2Cl^-$ carrier protein in the cortical collecting tubule and papillary collecting duct (Fig. 1-6). The sodium that enters the cells is then returned to the systemic circulation by the Na^+-K^+-ATPase pump in the basolateral membrane.[8] Removal of this Na^+ from the cell maintains the cell Na^+

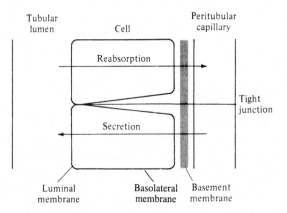

Figure 1-5 Schematic representation of reabsorption and secretion in the nephron.

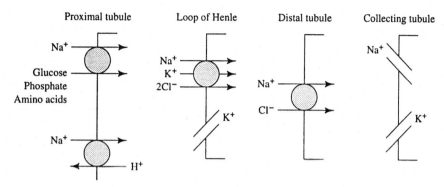

Figure 1-6 Major mechanisms of passive Na^+ entry into the cells across the luminal (apical) membrane in the different nephron segments. With the exception of the selective Na^+ channels in the collecting tubules, Na^+ reabsorption in the more proximal segments is linked to the reabsorption or secretion of other solutes. (*Adapted from Rose BD*, Kidney Int *39:336, 1991. Used with permission from* Kidney International.)

concentration at a low level, thereby promoting further diffusion of luminal Na^+ into the cell and continued Na^+ reabsorption.

This simple summary of the mechanism of Na^+ transport illustrates that reabsorption can involve both active and passive mechanisms. This is also true for tubular secretion. Potassium, for example, is secreted from the cortical collecting tubule cell into the lumen. The Na^+-K^+-ATPase pump in the basolateral membrane actively transports K^+ from the peritubular capillary into the cell; the ensuing rise in the cell K^+ concentration then promotes secretion into the lumen via K^+ channels in the luminal membrane.

The tubular cells perform these functions in an extremely efficient manner, reabsorbing almost all the filtrate to maintain the balance between intake and excretion. In an individual on a normal diet, more than 98 to 99 percent of the filtered H_2O, Na^+, Cl^-, and HCO_3^- is reabsorbed (Table 1-1). Although this process of filtration and almost complete reabsorption may seem inefficient, a high rate of filtration is required for the excretion of those waste products of metabolism (such as urea and creatinine) that enter the urine primarily by glomerular filtration.

Role of the Tight Junction

The tight junction is composed primarily of the zona occludens, which is a strand-like structure on the luminal membrane that brings adjacent cells into apposition at their luminal surface.[9,10] Within the kidney, the tight junction has two important effects on segmental function.[9,11,12]

- It serves as a relative barrier or gate to the passive diffusion of solutes and water between the cells.

Table 1-1 Summary of the net daily reabsorptive work performed by the kidney[a]

Substance	Filtered	Excreted	Percent net reabsorption
Water	180 liters	0.5–3 liters	98–99
Na^+	26,000 meq	100–250 meq	> 99
Cl^-	21,000 meq	100–250 meq	> 99
HCO_3^-	4800 meq	0	~ 100
K^+	800 meq	40–120 meq	85–95[b]
Urea	54 g	27–32 g	40–50

[a] These values are for a normal adult man on a typical Western diet. The glomerular filtration rate and therefore the filtered load of solutes and water is approximately 25 percent lower in women.

[b] The net reabsorption of K^+ reflects the interplay of two processes: the reabsorption of almost all of the filtered K^+ in the proximal tubule and loop of Henle and the secretion of K^+ into the lumen, primarily in the cortical collecting tubule under the influence of aldosterone. This latter process is the primary determinant of urinary K^+ excretion (see Chap. 12).

- It serves as a boundary or fence between the luminal (or apical) and basolateral membranes.

It has been proposed that these two functions—paracellular gate and fence for polarity—are mediated by different kinds of molecular contacts between the tight junction strands: The gate function may be due to contact between strands on apposing cells, while the fence function may be due to contact between the particles forming the strands within a single cell.[12]

The "leakiness" of the tight junction barrier to passive diffusion varies with the nephron segment. The barrier is relatively leaky in the proximal tubule, with as much as one-third of proximal Na^+ reabsorption occurring via this paracellular route. This leakiness is important, because it allows the proximal tubule to efficiently reabsorb 55 to 60 percent of the filtrate (or over 90 L/day).

In comparison, the collecting tubule is a relatively "tight" epithelium with a thicker tight junction than the proximal tubule.[9] As a result, diffusion across the tight junction is limited. This relative impermeability to passive paracellular transport allows this segment to *create and sustain* very large transepithelial concentration gradients. As an example, the medullary collecting tubule is able to lower the urine pH to 4.5, which represents a H^+ concentration that is almost 1000 times greater than that in the plasma (where the pH is about 7.40). The proximal tubule, on the other hand, can only reduce the tubular fluid pH to about 6.8, which represents a H^+ concentration only four times higher than that in the plasma.

The boundary function of the tight junction is thought to play an important role in the maintenance of the polarity of the two membranes, preventing lateral movement of transporters or channels from one membrane to the other.[9,11,12] Membrane polarity is an essential component of reabsorption or secretion in the renal tubular cells, as each component of the cell membrane plays an important role:[13]

- *Luminal membrane*: The luminal (or apical) membrane contains the channels or carriers that allow filtered solutes to enter the cells or some cellular solutes to be secreted into the lumen (Fig. 1-6).
- *Basolateral membrane*: The basolateral membrane performs two major functions. That part of the membrane adjacent to the luminal membrane (also called the lateral membrane) contains the components of the tight junction and the cell adhesion molecules that participate in cell-cell contact and communication. The more distal part of this membrane (also called the basolateral or basal-lateral membrane) plays an essential role in ion transport and hormone responsiveness, as it contains the Na^+-K^+-ATPase pumps, hormone receptors, and solute carriers and channels.
- *Basal membrane*: The basal membrane contains the basement membrane receptors that allow the cell to be anchored to the basement membrane.

As an example of transcellular transport, filtered Na^+ enters the cells across the luminal membrane via specific transporters or channels; it is then returned to the systemic circulation by the Na^+-K^+-ATPase pump to the basolateral membrane. Disruption of this normal polarity, as with opening of the tight junctions due to ischemia, is associated with an impairment in Na^+ reabsorption.[11] This may be mediated in part by the translocation of functioning Na^+-K^+-ATPase pumps onto the luminal membrane.[14]

The signals that govern the initial insertion of a protein into the luminal or basolateral membrane are incompletely understood. One signal appears to be the presence of cassettes of unique amino acids (located within the sequences of the proteins themselves) that relay localization information to cellular sorting machinery. One such amino acid motif, contiguous leucines located in the cytoplasmic tail, helps direct the vasopressin V_2 receptor to the basolateral membrane.[15]

Another mechanism may involve the type of membrane anchor: Studies in kidney cells suggest that the presence of glycosyl-phosphatidylinositol (GPI) at the C-terminal end of the protein leads to specific insertion on the luminal membrane, perhaps because this membrane is rich in glycosphingolipids.[16,17] On the other hand, the localization of the Na^+-K^+-ATPase pump to the basolateral membrane may be mediated by specific attachment to basolateral cytoskeletal proteins, such as actin microfilaments and ankyrin.[11,18] Disruption of the actin microfilaments following ischemia impairs this tethering function, allowing Na^+-K^+-ATPase pumps to diffuse onto the luminal membrane through the now open tight junctions, thereby impairing net Na^+ reabsorption.[11]

The attachment to actin and fodrin also may promote the basolateral localization of Na^+-K^+-ATPase pumps by preventing their endocytic removal. Pumps that do get inserted into the luminal membrane are removed at a rate 40 times faster than those inserted into the basolateral membrane.[19]

Aberrant localization of membrane proteins may contribute to the development of multiple disorders, such as autosomal dominant polycystic kidney disease (ADPKD). ADPKD is in most cases caused by mutations in a membrane protein termed polycystin,[20] which appears to be involved in cell adhesion.[21] Abnormal apical polarity of the Na^+-K^+-ATPase pumps in these patients may cause sodium secretion into and fluid accumulation in epithelial cysts.[22] In addition, abnormal epithelial proliferation within the cysts may be due to apical mislocation of epidermal growth factor receptors. The correlation between polycystin mutations and abnormal polarity is unclear, but may result from the dampened expression of fetal genes.

Membrane Recycling

In addition to proper polarity, normal functioning of transporting epithelia requires the delivery of newly synthesized and recycled membrane components to precise locations in the cell membrane.[23] For example, antidiuretic hormone combines with its receptor on the *basolateral membrane* of collecting tubular cells. This initiates a sequence of events in which preformed water channels (called aquaporin-2) in cytoplasmic vesicles are specifically inserted into the luminal membrane, thereby allowing the reabsorption of luminal water. The hormone-receptor complex is internalized by endocytosis in clathrin-coated pits and then enters acidic endosomes, where the hormone and receptor are split (Fig. 1-7).[23] The former is metabolized within the cell, while the receptor is returned to the basolateral membrane. Attenuation of the ADH effect is associated with endocytosis of only those areas of the luminal membrane that contain water channels, thereby restoring the relative water impermeability of the luminal membrane.

   The signaling events that control membrane recycling are incompletely understood, but activation of adenylyl cyclase appears to be involved.[24] In addition, the structure of aquaporin-2 helps dictate cellular distribution and recycling. Mutations of the aquaporin-2 gene can cause resistance to antidiuretic hormone

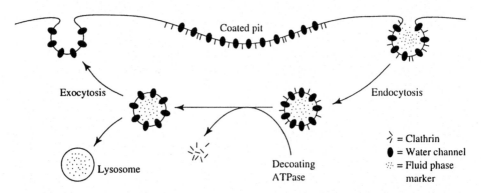

Figure 1-7   Proposed pathways of recycling of luminal membrane water channels in principal cells in the collecting tubule. Water channels are concentrated in clathrin-coated pits at the cell surface and are endocytosed in coated vesicles. These vesicles are rapidly decoated; the water channels may escape degradation and be recycled to the luminal membrane in the presence of ADH. (*From Brown D*, Kidney Int *256:F1, 1989. Used by permission from* Kidney International.)

(called nephrogenic diabetes insipidus). In the families reported thus far, the defect appears to involve misrouting and/or loss of function.[25,26]

Composition of Urine

The composition of the urine differs from that of the relatively constant extracellular fluid in two important ways. First, the quantity of solutes and water in the urine is highly variable, being dependent upon the intake of these substances. A normal subject, for example, appropriately excretes more Na^+ on a high-salt diet than on a low-salt diet. In both instances, the steady-state and therefore the extracellular volume is maintained, as output equals intake. Similarly, the urine volume is greater after a water load than after water restriction, resulting in a stable plasma Na^+ concentration.* This relation to intake means that there are *no absolute "normal" values for urinary solute or water excretion.* We can only describe a normal range which merely reflects the range of dietary intake, e.g., 100 to 250 meq/day for Na^+.

Second, ions compose 95 percent of the extracellular fluid solutes; in comparison, the urine has high concentrations of uncharged molecules, particularly urea. This allows urea and other metabolic end products to be excreted, rather than accumulating in the body.

Summary of Nephron Function

The following chapters in Part One will describe the roles of the different nephron segments in the regulation of solute and water homeostasis. These functions are summarized in Table 1-2.

As can be seen, there are marked differences in segmental function, a finding consistent with the differences in segmental histology (Fig. 1-1) and permeability and transport characteristics.[5] In addition, multiple sites participate in the regulation of the rates of excretion of the different substances in the filtrate. This diversity provides the flexibility that allows the kidney to maintain solute and water balance, even in the presence of major changes in dietary intake.

ATOMIC WEIGHT AND MOLARITY

The efficacy of regulation of solute and water balance is estimated clinically by measurement of the plasma concentrations of the appropriate substances. It is therefore important to be aware of the different ways in which solute concen-

---

* These changes in Na^+ and water excretion are relatively precise, so that increasing Na^+ intake from 100 to 200 meq/day, for example, results in a parallel rise in Na^+ excretion. If, as depicted in Table 1-1, 26,000 meq of Na^+ is filtered per day, then a 100-meq increase in excretion represents a change involving less than 0.5 percent of the filtered load. This illustrates the high degree of efficiency required to maintain salt and water balance.

Table 1-2   Contribution of the different nephron segments to solute and water homeostasis

Nephron segment	Major functions
Glomerulus	Forms an ultrafiltrate of plasma
Proximal tubule	Reabsorbs isosmotically 65 to 70 percent of the filtered NaCl and water
	Reabsorbs 90 percent of the filtered HCO_3^- (by H^+ secretion), mostly in early proximal tubule
	Major site of ammonia production in nephron
	Reabsorbs almost all of filtered glucose and amino acids
	Reabsorbs K^+, phosphate, calcium, magnesium, urea, and uric acid
	Secretes organic anions (such as urate) and cations, including many protein-bound drugs
Loop of Henle	Reabsorbs 15 to 25 percent of filtered NaCl
	Countercurrent multiplier, as NaCl reabsorbed in excess of water
	Major site of active regulation of magnesium excretion
Distal tubule	Reabsorbs a small fraction of filtered NaCl
	Major site, with connecting segment, of active regulation of calcium excretion
Connecting segment and cortical collecting tubule	Principal cells reabsorb Na^+ and Cl^- and secret K^+, in part under influence of aldosterone
	Intercalated cells secrete H^+, reabsorb K^+, and, in metabolic alkalosis, secrete HCO_3^-
	Reabsorb water in presence of antidiuretic hormone
Medullary collecting tubule	Site of final modification of the urine
	Reabsorb NaCl; urine NaCl concentration can be reduced to less than 1 meq/L
	Reabsorb water and urea relative to amount of antidiuretic hormone present, allowing a dilute or concentrated urine to be excreted
	Secrete H^+ and NH_3; urine pH can be reduced to as low as 4.5 to 5.0
	Can contribute to potassium balance by reabsorption or secretion of K^+

tration can be measured—in milligrams per deciliter (mg/dL), millimoles per liter (mmol/L), milliequivalents per liter (meq/L), or milliosmoles per liter or per kg (mosmol/L or mosmol/kg). For sodium ion (Na^+), 2.3 mg/dL (or 23 mg/L), 1 mmol/L, 1 meq/L, and 1 mosmol/kg all refer to the same concentration of Na^+.

Table 1-3 lists the atomic weights of the most important elements in the body. The atomic weight is an assigned number that allows comparison of the relative weights of the different elements. By definition, one atom of oxygen is assigned a weight of 16, and the atomic weights of the other elements are determined in relation to that of oxygen. In a molecule, i.e., a substance containing two or more atoms, the molecular weight is equal to the sum of the atomic weights of the individual atoms. As an example, the molecular weight of water (H_2O) is 18, since $[(2 \times 1) + 16] = 18$.

Table 1-3   Atomic and molecular weights of physiologically important substances

Substance	Symbol or formula	Atomic or molecular weight
Calcium ion	Ca^{2+}	40.1
Carbon	C	12.0
Chloride ion	Cl^-	35.5
Hydrogen ion	H^+	1.0
Magnesium ion	Mg^{2+}	24.3
Nitrogen	N	14.0
Oxygen	O	16.0
Phosphorus	P	31.0
Potassium ion	K^+	39.1
Sodium ion	Na^+	23.0
Sulfur	S	32.1
Ammonia	NH_3	17.0
Ammonium	NH_4^+	18.0
Bicarbonate ion	HCO_3^-	61.0
Carbon dioxide	CO_2	44.0
Glucose	$C_6H_{12}O_6$	180.0
Phosphate ion	PO_4^{3-}	95.0
Sulfate ion	SO_4^{2-}	96.1
Urea	NH_2CONH_2	60.0
Water	H_2O	18.0

One mole (mol) of any substance is defined as the molecular (or atomic) weight of that substance in grams. Similarly, one millimole (mmol) is equal to one-thousandth of a mole or the molecular (or atomic) weight in milligrams. Since the atomic weight of Na^+ is 23, 23 mg is 1 mmol and 23 mg of Na^+ in 1 liter of water represents a Na^+ concentration (written as $[Na^+]$ or 1 mmol/L. The concept of molarity is important because, from Avogadro's law, 1 mol of any nondissociable substance contains the same number of particles (approximately 6.02×10^{23}). Thus, 1 mmol of Na^+ contains the same number of atoms as 1 mmol of Cl^- even though the former weighs 23 mg and the latter weights 35.5 mg. However, 1 mmol of NaCl (58.5 mg) largely dissociates into Na^+ and Cl^- ions and therefore contains *almost twice as many particles*. As will be seen, these relationships are important in understanding electrochemical equivalence and in the measurement of osmotic pressure.

Although the concentrations of uncharged molecules, e.g., glucose and urea, also can be measured in millimoles per liter, they are more commonly measured in the clinical laboratory as milligrams per deciliter. For example, the molecular weight (mol wt) of glucose is 180. Consequently, a glucose concentration of 180 mg/L (or 18 mg/dL) is equal to 1 mmol/L. To convert from milligrams per deciliter to millimoles per liter, the following formula can be used:

$$mmol/L = \frac{mg/dL \times 10}{mol\ wt} \tag{1-1}$$

(The multiple of 10 is used to convert milligrams per deciliter into milligrams per liter.)

Electrochemical Equivalence

Positively charged particles are called *cations*, and negatively charged particles are called *anions*. When cations and anions combine, they do so according to their ionic charge (or valance), not according to their weight. Electrochemical equivalence refers to the combining power of an ion. One equivalent is defined as the weight in grams of an element that combines with or replaces 1 g of hydrogen ion (H^+). Since 1 g of H^+ is equal to 1 mol of H^+ (containing approximately 6.02×10^{23} particles), 1 mol of any univalent anion (charge equals 1^-) will combine with this H^+ and is equal to one equivalent (eq). Thus:

$$1 \, mol \, H^+ \quad + \quad 1 \, mol \, Cl^- \quad \rightarrow \quad 1 \, mol \, HCl$$
$$\text{(1 g)} \qquad\qquad \text{(35.5 g)} \qquad\qquad \text{(36.5 g)}$$

By similar reasoning, 1 mol of a univalent cation (charge equals 1^+) also is equal to 1 eq, since it can replace H^+ and combine with 1 eq of Cl^-. For example,

$$1 \, mol \, Na^+ \quad + \quad 1 \, mol \, Cl^- \quad \rightarrow \quad 1 \, mol \, NaCl$$
$$\text{(23 g)} \qquad\qquad \text{(35.5 g)} \qquad\qquad \text{(58.5 g)}$$

In contrast, ionized calcium (Ca^{2+}) is a divalent cation (charge equals 2^+). Consequently, 1 mol of Ca^{2+} will combine with 2 mol of Cl^- and is equal to 2 eq:

$$1 \, mol \, Ca^{2+} \quad + \quad 2 \, mol \, Cl^- \quad \rightarrow \quad 1 \, mol \, CaCl_2$$
$$\text{(40 g)} \qquad\qquad \text{(71 g)} \qquad\qquad \text{(111 g)}$$

The body fluids are relatively dilute, and most ions are present in milliequivalent quantities (one-thousandth of 1 eq equals 1 meq). To convert from units of millimoles per liter to milliequivalents per liter, the following formulas can be used:

$$meq/L = mmol/L \times valence \qquad\qquad (1\text{-}2)$$

or from Eq. (1-1),

$$meq/L = \frac{mg/dL \times 10}{mol \, wt} \times valence \qquad\qquad (1\text{-}3)$$

There are two advantages to measuring ionic concentrations in milliequivalents per liter. First, it emphasizes the principle that *ions combine milliequivalent for milliequivalent*, not millimole for millimole or milligram for milligram. Second, to maintain *electroneutrality*, there is an equal number of milliequivalents of cations and anions in the body fluids. As will be described in later chapters, the need to preserve electroneutrality is an important determinant of ion transport in the kidney and ion movement between the cells and the extracellular fluid. This obligatory relationship cannot be appreciated if the ionic concentrations are measured in millimoles per liter or in milligrams per deciliter (Table 1-4).

Table 1-4 Normal plasma electrolyte concentrations

Electrolyte	meq/L	mmol/L
Cations		
Na^+	142.0	142.0
K^+	4.3	4.3
Ca^{2+a}	2.5	1.25
Mg^{2+a}	1.1	0.55
Total	149.9	148.1
Anions		
Cl^-	104.0	104.0
HCO_3^-	24.0	24.0
$H_2PO_4^-$, HPO_4^{2-}	2.0	1.1
Proteins	14.0	0.9
Other[b]	5.9	5.5
Total	149.9	135.5

[a] The values of Ca^{2+} and Mg^{2+} include only the ionized (unbound) form of these ions.
[b] This includes SO_4^{2-} and organic anions such as lactate.

Despite these advantages, not all ions can be easily measured in milliequivalents per liter. The total calcium (Ca^{2+}) concentration in the blood is approximately 10 mg/dL. From Eq. (3),

$$\text{meq/L of } Ca^{2+} = \frac{10 \times 10}{40} \times 2 = 5 \, \text{meq/L}$$

However, roughly 50 to 55 percent of plasma Ca^{2+} is bound by albumin and, to a much lesser degree, citrate, so that the physiologically important *ionized* (or unbound) Ca^{2+} concentration is only 2.0 to 2.5 meq/L.

There is a different problem with phosphate, since it can exist in different ionic forms—as $H_2PO_4^-$, HPO_4^{2-}, or PO_4^{3-} and an exact valence cannot be given. We can estimate an approximate valence of minus 1.8 because roughly 80 percent of extracellular phosphate exists as HPO_4^{2-} and 20 percent as $H_2PO_4^-$. If the normal serum phosphorus concentration is 3.5 mg/dL (phosphate in the blood is measured as inorganic phosphorus), then

$$\text{meq/L of phosphate} = \frac{3.5 \times 10}{31} \times 1.8 = 2 \, \text{meq/L}$$

Similarly, only an average valence can be given for the polyvalent protein anions. If the plasma protein concentration is 0.9 mmol/L and the average valance is minus 15, then from Eq. (1-2),

$$\text{meq/L of protein} = 0.9 \times 15 = 14 \, \text{meq/L}$$

Osmotic Pressure and Osmolality

Another unit of measurement is osmotic pressure, which determines the distribution of water among the different fluid compartments, particularly between the extracellular and intracellular fluids (see Chap. 7). The osmotic pressure generated by a solution is proportional to the *number of particles* per unit volume of solvent, not to the type, valence, or weight of the particles.

The unit of measurement of osmotic pressure is the osmole. One osmole (osmol) is defined as 1 g molecular weight (1 mol) of any nondissociable substance (such as glucose) and contains 6.02×10^{23} particles. In the relatively dilute fluids in the body, the osmotic pressure is measured in milliosmoles (one-thousandth of an osmole) per kilogram of water (mosmol/kg). Since most solutes are measured in the laboratory in units of millimoles per liter, milligrams per deciliter, or milliequivalents per liter, the following formulas must be used to convert into mosmol/kg:

$$\text{mosmol/kg} = n \times \text{mmol/L}$$

or, from Eqs. (1-1) and (1-2),

$$\text{mosmol/kg} = n \times \frac{\text{mg/dL} \times 10}{\text{mol wt}} \tag{1-4}$$

$$\text{mosmol/kg} = n \times \frac{\text{meq/L}}{\text{valence}} \tag{1-5}$$

where n is the number of dissociable particles per molecule. When $n = 1$, as for Na^+, Cl^-, Ca^{2+}, urea, and glucose, 1 mmol/L will generate a potential osmotic pressure of 1 mosmol/kg. If, however, a compound dissociates into two or more particles, 1 mmol/L will generate an osmotic pressure greater than 1 mosmol/kg. At the concentrations present in the body, for example, ionic interactions reduce the random movement of NaCl so that it acts as if it were only 75 percent, rather than 100 percent, dissociated. Thus, for each 1 mmol/L of NaCl, there will be 0.75 mmol/L each of Na^+ and Cl^- and 0.25 mmol/L of NaCl, or 1.75 mosmol/kg (Table 1-5).[27]

Table 1-5   Relationship between various units of measurement

Substance	Atomic or molecular weight	mmol	meq	mosmol
Na^+	23	1	1	1
Cl^-	35.5	1	1	1
NaCl	58.5	1	2 (Na^+, Cl^-)	1.75^a
$CaCl_2$	111	1	4 (Ca^{2+}, $2Cl^-$)	$\sim 3^a$
Glucose	180	1	$\cdots$	1

[a] Both NaCl and $CaCl_2$ behave as if they are incompletely dissociated because ionic interactions limit the random movement or activity of the ions; see text for details.

In the laboratory, the osmotic concentration of a solution is measured not as an osmotic pressure but according to other properties of solutes, such as their ability to depress the freezing point or the vapor pressure of water. Solute-free water freezes at $0°C$. If 1 osmol of any solute (or combination of solutes) is added to 1 kg of water, the freezing point of this water will be depressed by $1.86°C$. This observation can be used to calculate the osmotic concentration of a solution. As an example, the freezing point of the plasma water is normally about $-0.521°C$. This represents an osmolality of 0.280 osmol/kg (0.521/1.86) or 280 mosmol/kg.

Only solutes that *cannot cross the membrane separating two compartments* generate an effective osmotic pressure. Thus, a lipid-soluble solute such as urea, which can cross the lipid bilayer of cell membranes, does not contribute to osmotic pressure but will be measured as part of the plasma osmolality by freezing point or vapor pressure depression. There is therefore a difference between the total osmolality and the effective osmolality of a solution, with the latter being determined only by osmotically active solutes (such as Na^+ and K^+ across the cell membrane) (see Chap. 7).

REFERENCES

1. Carone FA, Peterson DR. Hydrolysis and transport of small peptides by the proximal tubule. *Am J Physiol* 283:F151, 1980.
2. Madsen KM, Park CH. Lysosome distribution and cathepsin B and L activity along the rabbit proximal tubule. *Am J Physiol* 253:F1290, 1987.
3. Owen OE, Felig P, Morgan AP, et al. Liver and kidney metabolism during prolonged starvation. *J Clin Invest* 48:574, 1969.
4. Burch HB, Narins RG, Chu C, et al. Distribution along the rat nephron of three enzymes of gluconeogenesis in acidosis and starvation. *Am J Physiol* 235:F246, 1978.
5. Jacobson HR. Functional segmentation of the mammalian nephron. *Am J Physiol* 241:F203, 1981.
6. Madsen KM, Tisher CC. Structural-functional relationships along the distal nephron. *Am J Physiol* 250:F1, 1986.
7. Imai M. The connecting tubule: A functional subdivision of the rabbit distal nephron segments. *Kidney Int* 15:346, 1979.
8. Doucet A. Function and control of Na-K-ATPase in single nephron segments of the mammalian kidney. *Kidney Int* 34:749, 1988.
9. Gumbiner B. Structure, biochemistry, and assembly of tight junctions. *Am J Physiol* 253:C749, 1987.
10. Madara JL. Loosening tight junctions: Lessons from the intestine. *J Clin Invest* 83:1089, 1989.
11. Molitoris BA. Ischemia-induced loss of epithelial polarity: Potential role of the actin cytoskeleton. *Am J Physiol* 260:F769, 1991.
12. Mandel LJ, Bacallao R, Zampighi G. Uncoupling of the molecular "fence" and paracellular "gate" functions in epithelial tight junctions. *Nature* 361:552, 1993.
13. Rodriguez-Boulan E, Nelson WJ. Morphogenesis of the polarized epithelial cell phenotype. *Science* 245:718, 1989.
14. Molitoris BA. Na^+-K^+-ATPase that redistributes to apical membrane during ATP depletion remains functional. *Am J Physiol* 265:F693, 1993.
15. Brown D, Breton S. Sorting proteins to their target membranes. *Kidney Int* 57:816, 2000.
16. Brown DA, Crise B, Rose JK. Mechanism of membrane anchoring affects polarized expression of two proteins in MDCK cells. *Science* 245:1499, 1989.

17. Brown D, Waneck GL. Glycosyl-phosphatidylinositol-anchored membrane proteins. *J Am Soc Nephrol* 3:895, 1992.

18. Nelson WJ, Hammerton RW. A membrane-cytoskeletal complex containing Na^+-K^+-ATPase, ankyrin, and fodrin in Madin-Darby canine kidney (MDCK) cells: Implications for the biogenesis of epithelial cell polarity. *J Cell Biol* 108:893, 1989.

19. Hammerton RW, Krzeminski KA, Mays RW, et al. Mechanism for regulating cell surface distribution of Na^+-K^+-ATPase in polarized epithelial cells. *Science* 254:847, 1991.

20. Geng L, Segal Y, Peissel B, et al. Identification and localization of polycystin, the PKD1 gene product. *J Clin Invest* 98:2674, 1996.

21. Huan Y, van Adelsberg J. Polycystin-1, the PKD1 gene product, is in a complex containing E-cadherin and the catenins. *J Clin Invest* 104:1459, 1999.

22. Wilson PD. Epithelial cell polarity and disease. *Am J Physiol* 272:F434, 1997.

23. Brown D. Membrane recycling and epithelial cell function. *Am J Physiol* 256:F1, 1989.

24. Bichet DG, Oksche A, Rosenthal W. Congenital nephrogenic diabetes insipidus. *J Am Soc Nephrol* 8:1951, 1997.

25. Mulder SM, Knoers NV, Van Lieburg AF, et al. New mutations in the AQP2 gene in nephrogenic diabetes insipidus resulting in functional but misrouted water channels. *J Am Soc Nephrol* 8:242, 1997.

26. Hochberg Z, van Lieburg A, Even L, et al. Autosomal recessive nephrogenic diabetes insipidus caused by an aquaporin-2 mutation. *J Clin Endocrinol Metab* 82:686, 1997.

27. Edelman IS, Leibman J, O'Meara MP, Birkenfeld L. Interrelations between serum sodium concentration, serum osmolarity and total exchangeable sodium, total exchangeable potassium and total body water. *J Clin Invest* 37:1236, 1958.

RENAL CIRCULATION AND
GLOMERULAR FILTRATION RATE

The blood flow to the kidneys averages 20 percent of the cardiac output. In terms of flow per 100 g weight, the renal blood flow (RBF) is four times greater than the blood flow to the liver or exercising muscle and eight times coronary blood flow.

Blood enters the kidney through the renal arteries and passes through serial branches (interlobar, arcuate, interlobular) before entering the glomeruli via the capillary wall then leaves the glomeruli via the efferent arterioles and enters the postglomerular capillaries. In the cortex, these capillaries run in apposition to the adjacent tubules, although not necessarily to the tubule segments from the same glomerulus.[1] In addition, branches from the efferent arterioles of the juxtamedullary glomeruli enter the medulla and form the vasa recta capillaries (Fig. 2-1). Blood returns to the systemic circulation through veins similar to the arteries in name and location.

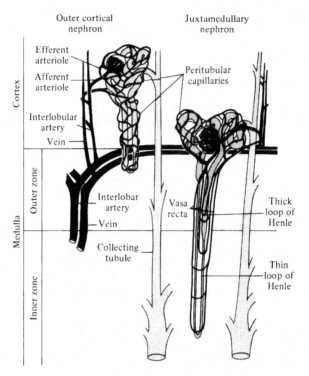

Figure 2-1 Comparison of the anatomy and blood supplies of outer cortical and juxtamedullary nephrons. Note that the efferent arterioles from the juxtamedullary nephrons not only form peritubular capillaries around the convoluted tubules but enter the medulla and form the vasa recta capillaries. (*Adapted from Pitts RF*, Physiology of the Kidney and Body Fluids, *3d ed. Copyright, 1974 by Year Book Medical Publishers, Inc, Chicago. Used by permission.*)

The renal circulation affects urine formation in the following ways:

1. The rate of glomerular filtration is an important determinant of solute and water excretion.
2. The peritubular capillaries in the cortex return reabsorbed solutes and water to the systemic circulation and can modulate the degree of proximal tubular reabsorption and secretion (see Chap. 3).
3. The vasa recta capillaries in the medulla return reabsorbed salt and water to the systemic circulation and participate in the countercurrent mechanism, permitting the conservation of water by the excretion of a hyperosmotic urine (see Chap. 4).

The remainder of this chapter will review glomerular function, the factors responsible for the regulation of the glomerular filtration rate (GFR) and renal plasma flow, and the clinical methods used to measure these parameters.

GLOMERULAR ANATOMY AND FUNCTION

The glomerulus consists of a tuft of capillaries that is interposed between the afferent and efferent arterioles. Each glomerulus is enclosed within an epithelial cell capsule (Bowman's capsule) that is continuous both with the epithelial cells that surround the glomerular capillaries and with the cells of the proximal convoluted tubule (Fig. 2-2).[2] Thus, the glomerular capillary wall, through which the filtrate must pass, consists of three layers: the fenestrated endothelial cell, the *glomerular basement membrane* (GBM), and the epithelial cell. The epithelial cells are attached to the GBM by discrete foot processes. The pores between the

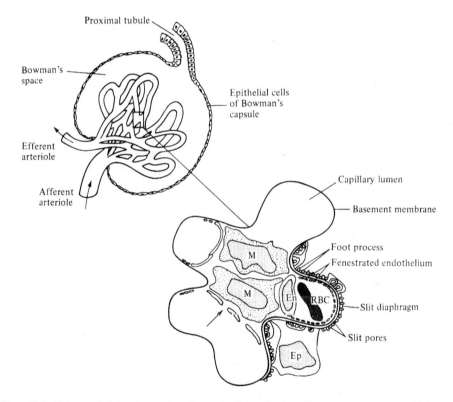

Figure 2-2   Anatomy of the glomerulus. The bottom drawing is a diagram of part of a capillary tuft with the mesangial cells (M) in the middle surrounded by capillaries. The capillary wall has three layers composed of the fenestrated endothelial cells (En), the basement membrane, and the epithelial cells (Ep), which attach to the basement membrane by discrete foot processes. Between the foot processes are slit pores which are closed by a thin membrane, the slit diaphragm. The glomerular basement surrounds the capillary loops, but most of the mesangium is separated from the capillary lumen only by the relatively permeable fenestrated endothelium (arrow). (*Adapted from Vander R*, Renal Physiology, *2d ed, McGraw-Hill, New York, 1980, and Latta H, in* Handbook of Physiology, *sec 8, Renal Physiology, vol I, Orloff J, Berliner RW, Geiger R, eds, American Physiological Society, Washington, DC, 1973. Used with permission.*)

foot processes (slit pores) are closed by a thin membrane called the *slit diaphragm*, which functions as a modified adherent junction (Fig. 2-2).[3]

The GBM is a fusion product of basement membrane material produced by the glomerular epithelial and endothelial cells.[4,5] It performs a variety of functions, including maintenance of normal glomerular architecture, anchoring of adjacent cells, and acting as a barrier to the filtration of macromolecules. It consists of the following major constituents:[4]

- Type IV collagen, which forms cords that provide the basic superstructure of the GBM.
- A variety of substances that fill the spaces between the cords, including laminin, nidogen, and heparan sulfate proteoglycans.[6] Laminin and nidogen form a tight complex, one of the major functions of which is cell adhesion to the GBM. In comparison, anionic heparan sulfate proteoglycans are largely responsible for the charge barrier to the filtration of anionic macromolecules (see below).

An abnormality in type IV collagen is responsible for the disorder hereditary nephritis (Alport's syndrome), which is a progressive form of glomerular disease (at least in males) that is often associated with hearing loss and lenticular abnormalities. The primary defect in almost all patients appears to reside in the noncollagenous domain of type IV collagen, involving the gene coding for the α_5 chain which is located on the X chromosome, the COL4A5 gene.[7,8] Abnormalities in the α_3 and α_4 chains of type IV collagen may also cause hereditary nephritis, which is not surprising, since the α_3, α_4, and α_5 chains combine to form a novel collagen that is expressed in the glomerulus and a few other tissues.[9]

Filtration Barrier and Protein Excretion

One of the major functions of the glomerulus is to allow the filtration of small solutes (such as sodium and urea) and water, while restricting the passage of larger molecules (Fig. 2-3). Solutes up to the size of inulin (mol wt 5200) are freely filtered. On the other hand, myoglobin (mol wt 17,000) is filtered less completely than inulin, while albumin (mol wt 69,000) is filtered only to a minor degree. Filtration is also limited for ions or drugs that are bound to albumin, such as roughly 40 percent of the circulating calcium.

This difference in filtration of solutes is important physiologically. The free filtration of sodium, potassium, and urea, for example, allows the kidney to maintain the steady state by excreting the load derived from dietary intake and endogenous metabolism. On the other hand, the restricted filtration of larger proteins prevents such potential problems as negative nitrogen balance, the development of hypoalbuminemia, and infection due to the loss of immunoglobulin gamma (IgG).

Figure 2-3 Fractional clearances (the ratio of the filtration of a substance to that of inulin, which is freely filtered) of anionic, neutral, and cationic dextrans as a function of effective molecular radius. Both molecular size and charge are important determinants of filtration, as smaller or cationic dextrans are more easily filtered. As a reference, the effective molecular radius of albumin (which is anionic in the physiologic pH range) is 36 Å. (*From Bohrer MP, Baylis C, Humes HD, et al, J Clin Invest 1978; 61:72, by copyright permission of the American Society for Clinical Investigation.*)

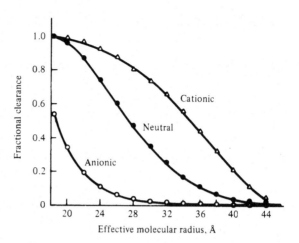

Size selectivity

As illustrated in Fig. 2-3, the GBM is both *size*- and *charge*-selective, as smaller and cationic molecules are more likely to be filtered. Both the GBM and the slit diaphragms between the foot processes of the epithelial cell contribute to size selectivity.[10,11]

The size limitation in the GBM represents functional pores in the spaces between the tightly packed cords of type IV collagen.[12] In addition, the cellular components of the glomerular capillary wall are also important determinants of glomerular permeability.[13] This is illustrated by the following observations:

- Macromolecules that pass through the GBM often accumulate below the slit diaphragms rather than passing into the urinary space.
- In vitro studies of isolated GBM indicate that the GBM is much more permeable to macromolecules than the intact glomerulus; the net effect is that the glomerular cells may be responsible for as much as 90 percent of the barrier to filtration.[14]
- Increased protein filtration in glomerular diseases may primarily occur in areas of focal foot process detachment.[15]
- A mutation in the gene for nephrin, the first protein to be specifically located at the slit diaphragm, results in congenital nephrotic syndrome.[16]

Most of the pores in the glomerular capillary wall are relatively small (mean radius about 42 Å).[17]* They partially restrict the filtration of albumin (mean radius 36 Å) but allow the passage of smaller solutes and water.[18] The endothelial

---

* The data in Fig. 2-3 used dextrans of different sizes. However, dextrans are long and pliable and may underestimate the impermeability to round macromolecules such as albumin. Studies using ficoll, which behaves as an ideal solid sphere, have estimated the pore radius to be 42 Å.[17]

cells, in comparison, do not contribute to size selectivity, since the endothelial fenestrae are relatively wide open and do not begin to restrict the passage of neutral macromolecules until their radius is larger than 375 Å.[19] These cells do, however, contribute to charge selectivity.

There is also a much less numerous second population (less than 0.5 percent) of larger pores that permit the passage of macromolecules (including IgG) as large as 70 Å.[18] In normal subjects, however, only a very small amount of filtrate passes through these pores.

Charge selectivity Molecular charge is a second major determinant of filtration across the GBM.[10,11,20] As illustrated in Fig. 2-3, cationic and neutral dextrans are filtered to a greater degree than anionic dextran sulfates of similar molecular sizes. This inhibitory effect of charge is due in part to *electrostatic repulsion* by anionic sites both in the endothelial fenestrae and in the GBM. The negative charge is primarily composed of heparan sulfate proteoglycans* (which are produced by the glomerular epithelial and endothelial cells).[2,21]

Albumin is a polyanion in the physiologic pH range. As with dextran sulfate, albumin filtration is only about 5 percent that of neutral dextran of the same molecular radius. Thus, charge as well as size limits the filtration of albumin. However, the importance of charge selectivity may not be as great as previously thought.[23,24]

Dextran infusions have also been used in humans both to assess normal function and to determine the mechanism of the increase in protein excretion that typically occurs in glomerular diseases.[20,25] As illustrated in Fig. 2-4, for example, there is an increased number of larger pores, as evidenced by a selective elevation in the clearance of neutral dextrans that are larger than 52 Å in diameter. Tunnels and cavities in the glomerular basement membrane appear to be the pathways for protein leakage.[26]

The net effect of loss of size selectivity is enhanced excretion of IgG (radius about 55 Å) as well as albumin.[27] This pattern has been demonstrated in most glomerular diseases, including membranous nephropathy, minimal change disease, focal glomerulosclerosis, and diabetic nephropathy.[20,28,29] In these conditions, however, the size defect can account for all of the increase in albumin excretion in only about one-half of cases, suggesting a concurrent defect in charge selectivity which may be most prominent in minimal change disease.[25]

Figure 2-4 also illustrates an important clinical difference between the filtration of larger proteins and that of smaller solutes and water. The reduced clearance of smaller molecules in most proteinuric states reflects a decrease in surface area (due to fewer functioning pores) induced by the glomerular disease. At the same time, there is increased clearance of large proteins due to an enhanced number of larger pores (which still represent a very small fraction of the total

---

* A different anionic compound, podocalyxin, lines the sides of the epithelial cell foot processes and is probably responsible, again by electrostatic repulsion, for maintaining the separation of adjacent foot processes.[22]

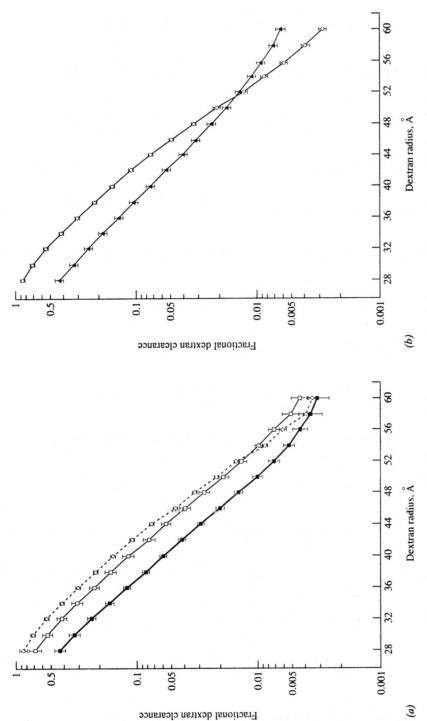

Figure 2-4 Dextran sieving profiles in patients with heavy proteinuria and the nephrotic syndrome. A fractional dextran clearance of 1 represents complete filtration. (*a*) Profiles in patients with minimal change disease when nephrotic (solid squares) and when in remission (open squares) compared to normal controls (open circles). Patients in remission are similar to controls, but during the active phase they have reduced clearance of dextrans of all sizes. Thus, the proteinuria cannot be due primarily to defective size selectivity, suggesting a primary role for loss of charge selectivity. (*b*) Profiles in patients with focal glomerulosclerosis (triangles) compared to normal controls (circles). The patients have decreased clearance of smaller dextrans but increased clearance of dextrans with a radius above 52 Å, suggesting an increased number of larger pores. (*From Guasch A, Hashimoto H, Sibley RK, et al, Am J Physiol 260:F728, 1991. Used with permission.*)

27

number of pores) and perhaps partial loss of the charge barrier (which does not affect the filtration of smaller molecules).

Other Functions

The glomerular cells also have synthetic, phagocytic, and endocrine functions. The epithelial cells, for example, are thought to be responsible for the synthesis of the GBM and for the removal of circulating macromolecules that are able to pass through the GBM and enter the subepithelial space.[2,30] The endothelial cells, on the other hand, regulate vasomotor tone, in part via the release of prostacyclin, endothelin, and nitric oxide. They may also play an important role in inflammatory disorders involving the glomerulus by expressing adhesion molecules that promote the accumulation of inflammatory cells.[31]

The mesangium, in comparison, is composed of two different types of cells. One is the mesangial cell, which has microfilaments similar to those of smooth muscle cells.[32,33] After glomerular injury or depopulation of resident mesangial cells, new mesangial cells may originate from cells that normally reside in the juxtaglomerular apparatus.[34] These cells do not appear to be macrophages or smooth muscle or endothelial cells, or to excrete renin.

The intrinsic mesangial cells can respond to angiotensin II (which is locally produced by the endothelial cells in the afferent arteriole) and can synthesize prostaglandins, both of which play an important role in the regulation of glomerular hemodynamics (see below and Chap. 6).[35] These cells also may be involved in immune-mediated glomerular diseases. They can both release a number of cytokines (including interleukin-1, interleukin-6, chemokines, and epidermal growth factor) and proliferate in response to cytokines (such as platelet-derived growth factor and epidermal growth factor).[33,36,37] These actions can contribute to the hypercellularity, mesangial matrix expansion, and glomerular injury that are often seen in these disorders.

The second cell type in the mesangium consists of circulating macrophages and monocytes that move into and out of the mesangium. These cells may have a primary phagocytic function, removing those macromolecules that enter the capillary wall but are unable to cross the basement membrane and move into the urinary space; they may also contribute to local inflammation in immune-mediated glomerular diseases.[38] Macromolecule entry into and subsequent removal from the mesangium can occur because most of the mesangium is separated from the capillary lumen only by the relatively permeable fenestrated endothelium, not by basement membrane (see Fig. 2-2).

RENIN-ANGIOTENSIN SYSTEM

Although the physiology of those hormones that importantly affect renal function is discussed in Chap. 6, antiotensin II plays such a central role in the regulation of the glomerular filtration rate that it is useful to review the renin-angiotensin system at this time.

The *afferent arteriole* of each glomerulus contains specialized cells, called the juxtaglomerular cells (see Fig. 1-4). These cells synthesize the precursor prorenin, which is cleaved into the active proteolytic enzyme renin. Active renin is then stored in and released from secretory granules.[39,40]* More proximal cells in the interlobular artery can also be recruited for renin release when the stimulus is prolonged.[41]

Renal hypoperfusion, produced by hypotension or volume depletion, and increased sympathetic activity are the major physiologic stimuli to renin secretion (Fig. 2-5). There is a gradient of response according to the location of the glomeruli: Renin release is most prominent in the outer cortical (or superficial) glomeruli, with a lesser response being seen in the midcortex and very little renin being secreted in the juxtamedullary glomeruli.[44] This pattern may reflect changes in

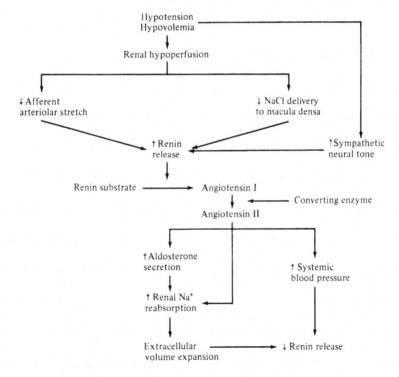

Figure 2-5   Renin-angiotensin-aldosterone system.

*Prorenin is also secreted into the systemic circulation, accounting for 50 to 90 percent of circulating renin.[40] The physiological role of prorenin is unclear, since it has no direct effect on systemic hemodynamics and does not appear to be converted into active renin in the systemic circulation.[42] There is evidence, however, that the uterus also secretes renin and prorenin, and that the latter may play a local role in the regulation of uterine function, particularly during pregnancy.[43]

glomerular perfusion pressure: The juxtamedullary glomeruli are closest to the interlobular artery (Fig. 2-1), whereas the outer cortical glomeruli are furthest away and perfused at a lower pressure. The physiologic significance of these observations is unclear.

Renin initiates a sequence of steps that begins with cleavage of a decapeptide angiotensin I from renin substrate (angiotensinogen), an α_2-globulin produced in the liver (and other organs including the kidney).[45,46] Angiotensin I is then converted into the octapeptide angiotensin II. This reaction is catalyzed by an enzyme called angiotensin converting enzyme (ACE), which is located in the lung, the luminal membrane of vascular endothelial cells, the glomerulus itself, and other organs.

Local Renin-Angiotensin Systems

The concentration of ACE is highest in the lung, and it had been thought that most angiotensin II formation occurred in the pulmonary circulation. It is now clear, however, that there are *extrarenal* renin-angiotensin systems and that angiotensin II can be synthesized at a variety of sites, including the kidney, vascular endothelium, adrenal gland, and brain.[45,47-49] These extrarenal systems may account for the persistent, although low, plasma levels of angiotensin II in anephric subjects.[50]

It is presumed that local angiotensin II production is important for the regulation of local processes. Volume depletion, for example, leads to an increase in renal messenger ribonucleic acid (RNA) expression for both renin (in the glomerulus) and angiotensinogen (in the proximal tubule).[51] Activation of the local renin system may be mediated by local factors such as prostaglandins, nitric oxide, and endothelin.[49]

The proximal tubule also contains ACE and angiotensin II receptors, suggesting that local angiotensin II formation can occur and stimulate Na^+ reabsorption.[52] The observation that the concentration of angiotensin II in the peritubular capillary and proximal tubule is approximately *1000 times* higher than that in the systemic circulation is consistent with the possibility of a local effect.[53] This can be achieved without releasing enough renin into the circulation to induce systemic vasoconstriction.

One clinical consequence of these observations is that measurement of the plasma renin activity or angiotensin II concentration may be a misleading estimate of the tissue activity of this system. In some patients with essential hypertension, for example, angiotensin II appears to be responsible for persistent renal vasoconstriction and sodium retention, even though the plasma levels of renin and angiotensin II are similar to those in hypertensives with normal renal perfusion.[54] These findings suggest a selective increase in the activity of the *intrarenal* renin-angiotensin system; the mechanism by which this occurs is not known. A similar selective activation of the intrarenal renin-angiotensin system may occur in stable congestive heart failure.[46]

Local generation of angiotensin II also can occur in vascular endothelium, where it may play an important role in the regulation of vascular tone and possibly in the development of hypertension.[45,55] Volume depletion increases angiotensinogen messenger (mRNA) levels in aortic smooth muscle. If this results in enhanced release of angiotensinogen, then either locally produced or systemic renin could initiate the sequential formation of angiotensin I and, via endothelial converting enzyme, angiotensin II.

These local effects could explain why ACE inhibitors are very useful antihypertensive agents, even in patients with low plasma renin activity and low circulating levels of angiotensin II.[47,56] Although the findings in humans are only indirect, the potential importance of local renin-angiotensin systems in the genesis of hypertension has been more convincingly demonstrated in experiments in which a mouse renin gene was inserted into rats. The presence of this extra gene for renin led to severe hypertension that was largely corrected by an ACE inhibitor or an angiotensin II receptor antagonist.[57] Despite this evidence for angiotensin-mediated hypertension, the plasma renin activity, plasma angiotensin II level, and renal renin content were all below normal, while adrenal renin content and vascular angiotensin generation were markedly elevated.[57,58] Thus, the elevation in blood pressure in this low (plasma) renin form of hypertension was mediated by local renin release in the adrenal gland and perhaps vascular endothelium.

Actions of Angiotensin II

Angiotensin II has two major systemic effects: systemic vasoconstriction and sodium and water retention. Both of these actions will tend to reverse the hypovolemia or hypotension that is usually responsible for the stimulation of renin secretion (Fig. 2-5).[59,60]

The effects of angiotensin II are mediated by binding to specific angiotensin II receptors: AT_1 and AT_2.[61] The vascular and renal tubular actions are primarily mediated by the AT_1 receptors.[61,62] The effects of the AT_2 receptors are less well understood; they may contribute to the tubular actions of angiotensin II and to the regulation of cell proliferation in the arterial wall.[61,63,64]

Renal sodium and water retention   Angiotensin II promotes renal NaCl and H_2O retention and therefore expansion of the plasma volume. This occurs by at least two mechanisms: by direct stimulation of Na^+ reabsorption in the early proximal tubule[60,65,66] and by increased secretion of aldosterone from the adrenal cortex, which enhances Na^+ transport in the cortical collecting tubule. Both systemic angiotensin II and angiotensin II generated within the adrenal gland contribute to the stimulation of aldosterone release (see Chap. 6).[51]

The proximal effect of angiotensin II appears to result at least in part from activation of the Na^+-H^+ antiporter in the luminal membrane (see page 000).[67,68,69] This enhancement of Na^+-H^+ exchange appears to be mediated by two angiotension II–dependent pathways (see Figs. 6-1 and 6-2): stimulation of an inhibitory G protein that decreases cyclic AMP generation, thereby minimizing the normally suppressive effect of cyclic AMP on Na^+-H^+ exchange,[67] and, to a lesser degree, stimulation of phosphatidylinositol turnover, resulting in the generation of protein kinase C.[68]

Studies using a highly specific AT_1 receptor antagonist suggest that angiotensin II may be responsible for as much as 40 to 50 percent of Na^+ and H_2O reabsorption in the initial S_1 segment of the proximal tubule.[64,70] The AT_2 receptors also appear to contribute to this response.[64] There is a much lesser effect in the more distal part of the proximal tubule, where there are fewer angiotensin II receptors.

Systemic vasoconstriction   Angiotensin II produces arteriolar vasoconstriction, which, by elevating systemic vascular resistance, increases the systemic blood pressure. In addition to a direct action of angiotensin II on vascular smooth muscle (which appears to be mediated primarily by protein kinase C generation[71]), experimental observations suggest that enhanced sensitivity to and facilitated release of norepinephrine may also play a contributory role.[72,73] However, the applicability of the angiotensin II–norepinephrine relationship to humans is uncertain; it may be that only high angiotensin II levels, such as those seen with advanced congestive heart failure, are sufficient to stimulate norepinephrine release.[74]

The net effect is that angiotensin II plays an *important role in the maintenance of blood pressure* in all circumstances in which renin secretion is enhanced and circulating angiotensin II levels are high. This is true in the hypertension associated with renal artery stenosis (in which renal ischemia stimulates renin release) as well as in normotensive states associated with effective circulating volume depletion,* such as true volume depletion, heart failure, and hepatic cirrhosis.[75-77] As an example, the administration of an angiotensin II inhibitor to a normotensive patient with hepatic cirrhosis can lower the blood pressure by as much as 25 mmHg, possibly leading to symptomatic hypotension.[77]

The vascular action of angiotensin II involves enhanced phosphatidylinositol turnover (see Fig. 6-2), rather than the generation of cyclic AMP, as in the proximal tubule.[78] The ensuing formation of diacylglycerol leads to the release of arachidonic acid, which can then be converted into prostaglandins or, via the lipoxygenase pathway, into metabolites of hydroxyeicosatetraenoic acid.[79] The latter compounds partially mediate angiotensin II–induced vasoconstriction (as well as aldosterone release),[79] whereas vasodilator prostaglandins tend to minimize the increase in vascular resistance.

Regulation of GFR   In addition to influencing systemic hemodynamics, angiotensin II plays an important role in the regulation of GFR and renal blood flow.[60] Although the clinical implications of these effects will be discussed below, it is helpful to review them briefly at this time. Angiotensin II can affect renal blood

---

* The concept of effective circulating volume depletion is defined in Chap. 8.

flow and the GFR by constricting the efferent and afferent glomerular arterioles and the interlobular artery.[80-82] These responses may be mediated at least in part by the local generation of the vasoconstrictor thromboxane A_2.[83]

Although both afferent and efferent arterioles are constricted, the efferent arteriole has a smaller basal diameter; as a result, the increase in efferent resistance may be as much as three times greater than that at the afferent arteriole.[84]* The net effect is a reduction in renal blood flow (due to the increase in renal vascular resistance) and an elevation in the hydraulic pressure in the glomerular capillary (P_{gc}), which tends to *maintain the GFR* when the renin-angiotensin system is activated by a fall in systemic pressure.

The likelihood of excessive renal vasoconstriction is minimized because angiotensin II also stimulates the release of vasodilator prostaglandins from the glomeruli.[86] The importance of this response can be illustrated by blocking the increase in prostaglandin synthesis with a nonsteroidal anti-inflammatory drug. In this setting, a low-sodium diet leads to more marked renal ischemia and, due to the decline in perfusion, a substantial reduction in GFR (see Fig. 2-10, below).[87] Similarly, the degree of *systemic* vasoconstriction may also be minimized by the local angiotensin II–induced release of prostacyclin.[88]

Angiotensin II has two other effects that can influence the GFR. First, it constricts the glomerular mesangium at higher concentrations, thereby lowering the surface area available for filtration. Second, angiotensin II sensitizes the afferent arteriole to the constricting signal of tubuloglomerular feedback (see "Tubuloglomerular Feedback," below).[60]

The net result is that angiotensin II has counteracting effects on the regulation of GFR: The increase in P_{gc} will tend to increase filtration, while the reduction in renal blood flow and mesangial contraction will tend to reduce filtration. The result is variable in different conditions, although how this occurs is incompletely understood. When renal perfusion pressure is reduced, as in renal artery stenosis, angiotensin II acts to maintain the GFR, and the administration of an ACE inhibitor can cause acute renal failure. In comparison, the GFR may be reduced by angiotensin II in hypertension and congestive heart failure.[60,89]

Control of Renin Secretion

In normal subjects, the major determinant of renin secretion is Na^+ intake: A high intake expands the extracellular volume and decreases renin release, whereas a low intake (or fluid loss from any site) leads to a reduction in extracellular volume and stimulation of renin secretion. Acute increases in renin secretion, as with volume depletion, primarily reflect the release of preformed renin from secretory granules.[40] More chronic stimuli lead to increased synthesis of new prorenin and renin.[40]

---

*The disparate afferent and efferent effects of angiotensin II may also be in part related to different mechanisms of constriction. Calcium channel blockers abolish the afferent response while having little or no effect on the increase in efferent tone.[85]

The associated changes in angiotensin II and aldosterone production induced by renin then allow Na^+ to be excreted with volume expansion or retained with volume depletion. Intrarenally formed angiotensin II probably plays at least a contributory role in this response, as illustrated by the rise in mRNA for both renin and angiotensin substrate in the renal cortex following a low-sodium diet.[90]

These changes in volume are primarily sensed at one or more of three sites, leading to the activation of effectors that govern the release of renin (Fig. 2-5):[39] (1) baroreceptors (or stretch receptors) in the wall of the afferent arteriole;[91] (2) the cardiac and arterial baroreceptors, which regulate sympathetic neural activity and the level of circulating catecholamines, both of which enhance renin secretion via the β_1-adrenergic receptors;[92,93] and (3) the cells of the macula densa in the early distal tubule (see Fig. 1-4), which appear to be stimulated by a reduction in chloride delivery, particularly in the Cl^- concentration in the fluid delivered to this site.[94,95]

Baroreceptors   The baroreceptors respond to changes in stretch in the afferent arteriolar wall. The ensuing alterations in renin release appear to be mediated by enhanced calcium entry into the cells when renal perfusion pressure is increased[96] and by the local release of prostanoids, particularly prostacyclin, when renal perfusion pressure is reduced.[92,97,98]

Macula densa   The macula densa dependence upon Cl^- is related to the characteristics of the Na^+-K^+-$2Cl^-$ cotransporter in the luminal membrane of the thick ascending limb and macula densa that promotes the entry of these ions into the cell (see Fig. 4-2).[94,99,100] The activity of this transporter is maximally stimulated at low concentrations of Na^+ and K^+, but is regulated within the physiologic range by alterations in the concentration of Cl^- (see Fig. 4-3).[94] As an example, the decrease in proximal NaCl reabsorption that is seen with volume expansion will enhance the Cl^- concentration at the macula densa, thereby reducing renin secretion. In comparison, the administration of Na^+ with other anions (bicarbonate, acetate) has little effect, since the tubular fluid Cl^- concentration will not rise.[94,95]

The importance of Na^+-K^+-$2Cl^-$ cotransport in the macula densa may explain the ability of loop diuretics to specifically enhance renin release. Although any diuretic can increase renin release by inducing volume depletion, the loop diuretics directly inhibit the Na^+-K^+-$2Cl^-$ transporter (see Chap. 15); as a result, less Cl^- is reabsorbed, thereby stimulating renin secretion.[94,101] The thiazide-type diuretics, on the other hand, inhibit Na^+-Cl^- cotransport primarily in the distal tubule and connecting segment; they do not directly affect the macula densa or renin release.[101]

Two factors may contribute to the mechanism by which the macula densa affects renin secretion: adenosine and PGE_2.[92,96,102,103] As an example, adenosine may mediate at least part of the suppression of renin secretion with NaCl delivery to the macula densa is increased.[102,103] The adenosine required to mediate this response may be derived from the breakdown of adenosine triphosphate (ATP) that occurs as the increase in delivery leads to enhanced local NaCl reabsorption.

On the other hand, the rise in renin release seen when NaCl delivery is reduced (as in hypovolemic states) may be mediated by increased production of PGE_2.[97,104] This effect may be related to enhanced activity of COX-2 (an isoform of cyclo-oxygenase) in epithelial cells located near the macula densa.[105]

The interaction between the renin-angiotensin system and prostaglandins may seem confusing, since each stimulates the secretion of the other[86,87,92,98] and they induce opposing vascular actions—vasoconstriction with angiotensin II and vaso-dilation with most prostaglandins. However, angiotensin II is a systemic vasocon-strictor, whereas the prostaglandins act locally, because they are rapidly metabolized when they enter the systemic circulation. Thus, the net effect of simultaneous renal secretion of angiotensin II and prostaglandins is that angio-tensin II can cause systemic vasoconstriction and raise the blood pressure, while the prostaglandins minimize the degree of renal vasoconstriction, thereby main-taining renal blood flow and GFR.[87]

The contributions of the three major factors governing renin release can be appreciated from the response to hypovolemia (see Chap. 8). The decrease in volume initially lowers the blood pressure, which diminishes the stretch in the afferent arteriole, increases sympathetic activity, and reduces NaCl delivery to the macula densa (in part by enhancing proximal reabsorption).[94] Each of these changes then promotes renin secretion. This response can be largely abolished by inhibiting its mediators with a combination of indomethacin (which inhibits prostaglandin synthesis) and propranolol (a β-adrenergic blocker).[106]

On the other hand, renin release is diminished by volume expansion (as with a high Na^+ intake). In addition to reversal of the above sequence, atrial natriuretic peptide also may contribute by directly impairing the secretion of both renin and aldosterone.[107]

DETERMINANTS OF GLOMERULAR FILTRATION RATE

The initial step in urine formation is the separation of an ultrafiltrate of plasma across the wall of the glomerular capillary. As with other capillaries, fluid move-ment across the glomerulus is governed by Starling's forces, being proportional to the permeability of the membrane and to the balance between the hydraulic and oncotic pressure gradients (see Chap. 7):

$$GFR = LpS \ (\Delta \text{ hydraulic pressure} - \Delta \text{ oncotic pressure})$$
$$= LpS \ [(P_{gc} - P_{bs}) - s(\pi_p - \pi_{bs})] \tag{2-1}$$

where Lp is the unit permeability (or porosity) of the capillary wall, S is the surface area available for filtration, P_{gc} and P_{bs} are the hydraulic pressures in the glomer-ular capillary and Bowman's space, π_p and π_{bs} are the oncotic pressures in the plasma entering the glomerulus and in Bowman's space, and s represents the reflection coefficient of proteins across the capillary wall (with values ranging from 0 if completely permeable to 1 if completely impermeable). Since the filtrate is essentially protein free, π_{bs} is 0 and s is 1. Thus,

$$GFR = LpS \left(P_{gc} - P_{bs} - \pi_p \right) \qquad (2\text{-}2)$$

The GFR in normal adults is approximately $95 \pm 20\,\text{mL/min}$ in women and $120 \pm 25\,\text{mL/min}$ in men.[108] This degree of filtration is, per weight, more than 1000 times that in muscle capillaries. Two factors account for this difference: (1) The LpS of the glomerulus is 50 to 100 times that of a muscle capillary, and (2) the capillary hydraulic pressure and therefore the mean gradient favoring filtration $(P_{gc} - P_{bs} - \pi_p)$ is much greater in the glomerulus than in a muscle capillary (Table 2-1).[109-111] Although almost all of the filtered electrolytes and water are reabsorbed, the higher GFR is required to allow the filtration and subsequent excretion of a variety of metabolic waste products such as urea and creatinine (see below).

Filtration Equilibrium

Changes in the GFR can be produced by alterations in any of the factors in Eq. (2-2) or in the rate of renal plasma flow (RPF). Before discussing the mechanisms by which these hemodynamic forces are regulated, it is important to first review how they change as fluid moves through the glomeruli. Experimental studies in rats and primates have demonstrated that the hydraulic pressures in the glomerulus and Bowman's space remain relatively constant; the capillary oncotic pressure, however, *progressively rises* due to the filtration of protein-free fluid.

Table 2-1   Approximate values for Starling's forces in muscle and glomerulus[a]

	Skeletal muscle (human)	Glomerulus (primate)	
		Afferent arteriole	Efferent arteriole
Hydraulic pressure			
Capillary	17.3	46	45
Interstitium	−3.0	10	10
Mean gradient	20.3	36	35
Oncotic pressure			
Capillary	28	23	35[b]
Interstitium	8	0	0
Mean gradient	20	23	35
Net gradient favoring filtration	+0.3	+13	0
$(\Delta P - \Delta \pi)$			
+ = filtration			
− = absorption		(Mean = +6 mmHg)	

[a] Units are mmHg. Values are from Refs. 109 and 110.
[b] The capillary oncotic pressure rises in the glomerulus because of the filtration of relatively protein-free fluid.

The net result of these changes is depicted in Fig. 2-6.[110-112] The gradient favoring filtration normally averages about 13 mmHg at the afferent arteriole but *falls to zero* before the efferent arteriole because of the elevation in plasma oncotic pressure (from 23 to 35 mmHg).

This phenomenon is called *filtration equilibrium* and, in the primate, occurs after the filtration of 20 percent of the RPF, a filtration fraction similar to that seen in humans* (where approximate normal values for the GFR and RPF are 125 and 625 mL/min, respectively). Further filtration *at the same RPF* cannot occur, i.e., the GFR cannot exceed 20 percent of the RPF, without an increase in P_{gc} or a reduction in π_p.

The presence of filtration equilibrium also means that the RPF becomes an important determinant of the GFR.[111,114] If, for example, the RPF is diminished with no alteration in P_{gc}, then filtration equilibrium will still be reached after the filtration of 20 percent of the RPF. Thus, the *GFR will fall in proportion to the decrement in RPF*, so that a 15 percent reduction in RPF will induce a 15 percent decline in GFR. Conversely, a 15 percent elevation in RPF will lead to a 15 percent rise in GFR.

Figure 2-6 Depiction of the hemodynamic forces along the length of the primate glomerular capillary. The dotted line represents the hydraulic pressure in Bowman's space, P_{bs}. The plasma oncotic pressure is added to this so that the middle solid line represents the sum of the forces retarding filtration: $P_{bs}+\pi_p$. The upper solid line represents the glomerular hydrostatic pressure (P_{gc}), and the shaded area depicts the net gradient favoring filtration, $P_{gc} - P_{bs} - \pi_p$, which is +13 mmHg at the afferent arteriole. As a result of ultrafiltration of protein-free fluid, π_p increases until the filtration gradient is abolished and filtration ceases. This is in contrast to muscle capillaries, where filtration is limited by a decline in capillary hydraulic pressure. (*Adapted from Maddox DA, Deen WM, Brenner BM*, Kidney Int *5:271, 1974, and Deen WM, Robertson CR, Brenner BM*, Am J Physiol *223:1178, 1972. Used with permission from* Kidney International.)

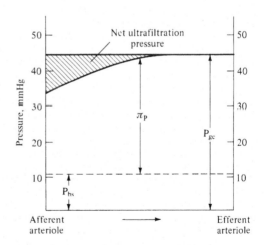

* The applicability of this model of glomerular filtration to humans is speculative, since only limited information is available.[112] Studies with glomeruli obtained from cadavers have revealed that the net permeability of the human glomerulus is higher than that in most other animals.[113] As a result, the net gradient favoring filtration has to be only about 4 mmHg, versus 6 mmHg in the primate, as in Table 2-1.

Note that the oncotic pressure of the fluid leaving the efferent arteriole and entering the peritubular capillary is determined both by the protein concentration in the plasma entering the glomerulus and by the degree to which the plasma proteins are concentrated due to the removal of the protein-free filtrate, i.e., by the filtration fraction GFR/RPF. As will be seen, the filtration fraction and the peritubular capillary oncotic pressure are important determinants of proximal tubular sodium and water reabsorption (see page 84).

Capillary Hydraulic Pressure and Arteriolar Resistance

The glomerular capillaries are uniquely interposed between two arterioles. As a result, the P_{gc} is determined by three factors: the aortic pressure, the resistance at the afferent arteriole, and the resistance at the efferent arteriole. The ability to regulate arteriolar resistances permits *rapid regulation of the GFR through changes in the P_{gc}*. Constriction of the *afferent* arteriole, for example, reduces both P_{gc} and GFR, since less of the systemic pressure is transmitted to the glomerulus; dilation of the afferent arteriole, on the other hand, enhances both of these parameters (Fig. 2-7). In comparison, constriction of the *efferent* arteriole retards fluid movement from the glomerulus into the efferent arteriole, increasing P_{gc} and GFR; dilation of the efferent arteriole facilitates fluid entry into the efferent arteriole, diminishing both of these parameters (Fig. 2-7).

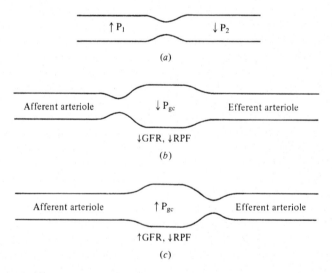

Figure 2-7 Relationship between arteriolar resistance, GFR, and RPF. (*a*) If flow is constant, constriction of a vessel results in a rise in pressure proximally (P_1) and a fall distally (P_2). (*b*) Constriction of the afferent arteriole reduces P_{gc} and GFR. (*c*) Constriction of the efferent arteriole, on the other hand, tends to increase P_{gc} and GFR. Since constriction of either arteriole also increases renal vascular resistance, RPF will fall in both (*b*) and (*c*). Arteriolar vasodilation has the opposite effects. For example, decreasing efferent arteriolar tone (as with an ACE inhibitor, which reduces the formation of angiotensin II) will lower the P_{gc}.

Arteriolar tone also affects the RPF. In the kidney, the resistance to flow across the arterioles constitutes 85 percent of renal vascular resistance, the remaining 15 percent coming from the peritubular capillaries and renal veins.[115] The relationship between RPF, the ΔP across the renal circulation, and renal vascular resistance can be expressed by the following equation:

$$RPF = \frac{\text{aortic pressure} - \text{renal venous pressure}}{\text{renal vascular resistance}} \tag{2-3}$$

This relation shows that an increase in tone at either end of the glomerulus will elevate total renal resistance and reduce RPF. Thus, GFR and RPF are regulated *in parallel* at the afferent arteriole, e.g., constriction decreases both, and *inversely* at the efferent arteriole, e.g., constriction reduces RPF but may augment P_{gc} and GFR. As a result, alterations in efferent (but not afferent) arteriolar tone affect the ratio of the GFR to the RPF (i.e., the filtration fraction), since these parameters will tend to change in opposite directions.

The opposing effects of efferent arteriolar tone on P_{gc} and RPF also mean that the direct relationship between this resistance and the GFR (Fig. 2-7) must be modified, since the RPF is an independent determinant of GFR. As an example, although efferent arteriolar constriction increases P_{gc}, the concomitant elevation in renal vascular resistance will reduce RPF, which will tend to lower the GFR. Depending upon the magnitude of efferent constriction, the net effect may be an increase, no change, or, if RPF is sufficiently reduced, even a fall in GFR.

Arteriolar resistance is partially under intrinsic myogenic control, but also can be influenced by other factors, including angiotensin II, norepinephrine, renal prostaglandins, atrial natriuretic peptide, endothelin, and tubuloglomerular feedback (see below).

Role of Other Starling's Forces

The other determinants of glomerular filtration in Eq. (2-2) are of much lesser importance in the physiologic regulation of the GFR. The permeability of the glomerular capillary wall, for example, remains relatively constant in most normal conditions.[110,111] Furthermore, *small changes in net permeability will not affect the GFR*, since the attainment of filtration equilibrium means that it is the rise in capillary oncotic pressure, not permeability, that limits the filtration of small solutes and water.[111] A variety of hormones, including angiotensin II, antidiuretic hormone, and prostaglandins, can affect the LpS.[89,116] However, the physiologic significance of these effects is uncertain, although high concentrations of angiotensin II can lead to a net decline in GFR in some settings.[89] Similarly, a reduction in LpS in disease states such as glomerulonephritis can contribute to the fall in GFR that is commonly observed; this problem is due primarily to a reduction in the surface area available for filtration.[117] The reduction in permeability becomes a limiting factor, because it is now severe enough to prevent filtration equilibrium from being reached.

Alterations in P_{bs} or the plasma oncotic pressure also affect the GFR only in disease states.[111] As an example, ureteral or intratubular obstruction leads to an increase in P_{bs}, thereby reducing the hemodynamic gradient favoring glomerular filtration.[118] On the other hand, volume depletion due to vomiting or diarrhea can result in hemoconcentration and a rise in the plasma protein concentration. This increases π_p, contributing to the decrease in GFR that may be seen in this setting.

REGULATION OF GLOMERULAR FILTRATION RATE AND RENAL PLASMA FLOW

Regulation of renal hemodynamics is primarily achieved via changes in arteriolar resistance, which can affect both RPF [from Eq. (2-3)] and GFR (by altering P_{gc} and RPF). In normal subjects, for example, changes in posture or diet can produce alterations in renal perfusion pressure. In this setting, two closely related *intrarenal* phenomena, autoregulation, and tubuloglomerular feedback, interact to maintain the GFR and RPF at a relatively constant level.[119] In comparison, pathophysiologic states, such as volume depletion, can lead to activation of systemic neurohumoral factors that can override these intrarenal effects.

Autoregulation

Since P_{gc} is an important determinant of GFR, it might be expected that small variations in arterial pressure could induce large changes in GFR. However, the GFR and RPF remain roughly constant over a wide range of arterial pressures (Fig. 2-8).[120,121] This phenomenon, which is also present in other capillaries,[122] is intrinsic to the kidney, occurring in denervated, perfused kidneys, and has been termed *autoregulation*.

Since the GFR and RPF are maintained in parallel, autoregulation must be mediated in part by changes in afferent arteriolar resistance (Fig. 2-7).[119,123] As systemic pressure rises, for example, an increase in afferent arteriolar tone prevents the elevation in pressure from being transmitted to the glomerulus, allowing P_{gc} and GFR to remain unchanged.[123] The enhanced arteriolar resistance also increases total renal vascular resistance, and, from Eq. (2-3), this increase in vascular tone balances the rise in pressure and minimizes any change in RPF.

Conversely, as blood pressure decreases, *afferent arteriolar dilation* will initially protect both GFR and RPF. However, the ability to maintain renal hemodynamics becomes impaired at mean arterial pressures below 70 mmHg. In this setting, GFR and RPF fall in proportion to the drop in blood pressure, and the GFR ceases when the systemic pressure reaches 40 to 50 mmHg.

The mechanism by which autoregulation is mediated is incompletely understood. The simplest hypothesis is that myogenic stretch receptors in the wall of the afferent arteriole are of primary importance, similar to the role of the precapillary sphincter in the muscle capillary.[122] An elevation in renal perfusion pressure, for example, will increase the degree of stretch, which will then promote arteriolar constriction;[123] this effect is mediated in part by increased cell entry of calcium.[124]

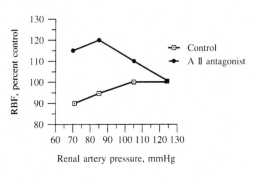

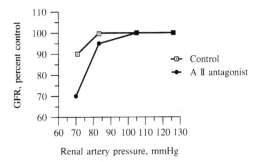

Figure 2-8 Effect of reducing renal artery pressure (from a baseline value of about 125 mmHg) on renal blood flow (RBF) and GFR, expressed as a percentage of control values in dogs fed a normal-sodium diet. The open squares represent control animals in which both RBF and GFR were maintained until the pressure was markedly reduced. The closed symbols represent animals given an intrarenal infusion of an angiotensin II antagonist; autoregulation of RBF was maintained (with an increase in the baseline level because of the fall in renal vascular resistance), but the GFR was less well regulated. Although not shown, autoregulation also applies when the renal artery pressure is initially raised. (*Adapted from Hall JE, Guyton AC, Jackson TE, et al, Am J Physiol 233:F366, 1977. Used with permission.*)

The efferent arterioles, in comparison, have different characteristics: They do not seem to respond directly to changes in stretch and therefore do not contribute directly to the myogenic response.[125] Why this occurs is not clear, but the apparent absence of voltage-gated Ca^{2+} channels in the efferent arterioles may play a contributory role.[126]

However, autoregulation of GFR is mediated by more than myogenic responses, as both angiotensin II (when the renal perfusion pressure is reduced) and tubuloglomerular feedback (especially when renal perfusion pressure is increased; see below) can play an important role.[121,127] Other regulators of renal vascular resistance, such as the vasodilator nitric oxide (endothelium-dependent relaxing factor), do not appear to participate in autoregulation.[128]

As illustrated in Fig. 2-8, for example, the administration of an angiotensin II antagonist results in the dissociation of the autoregulation of RPF and GFR.[121] As described above, the renin-angiotensin system is activated as renal perfusion pressure is lowered, resulting in both local and systemic generation of angiotensin II.[129] The preferential increase in efferent arteriolar resistance induced by angiotensin II contributes to autoregulation of GFR by preventing any fall in P_{gc}; consequently, infusion of an angiotensin II antagonist or an ACE inhibitor leads to less effective maintenance of the GFR. This *angiotensin II dependence is most prominent when the renal perfusion pressure is substantially reduced* (Fig. 2-8). Autoregulation of GFR with the initial decrease in renal artery pressure is primarily mediated by TGF and the stretch receptors.[127]

Clinical Implications   Patients with bilateral renal artery stenosis, due most often to atherosclerotic lesions, have an elevated pressure proximal to the stenosis but a normal or reduced pressure distal to the stenosis. As a result, the administration of antihypertensive therapy to lower the systemic blood pressure is likely to diminish the distal renal artery pressure (which includes that perfusing the glomeruli) to a level that is below normal. In this setting, autoregulation plays an important role in maintaining P_{gc} and GFR, a response that can be partially impaired by diminishing the production of angiotensin II with an ACE inhibitor. Up to one-half of such patients given an ACE inhibitor will have a usually mild decline in GFR, although severe (and reversible) renal failure can occur.[130,131] Diuretic-induced volume depletion appears to be an important risk factor for this problem, since it makes maintenance of the GFR even more angiotensin II–dependent.[121,132]

A similar decline in GFR can occur in the affected kidney in *unilateral* renal artery stenosis.[133] a change that can lead to eventual ischemic atrophy.[134] This is not easy to detect clinically, however, since the presence of the contralateral nonstenotic kidney prevents the development of acute renal failure (as would be evidenced by a rise in the plasma creatinine concentration; see below).

Other medications are less likely to produce this problem, since they do not interfere with autoregulation.[130,135] However, the ability of autoregulation to protect the GFR is impaired if the perfusion pressure is markedly reduced (Fig. 2-8). Thus, any antihypertensive agent can produce acute renal failure when there are *severe and bilateral* renovascular lesions (or a marked unilateral lesion in a solitary kidney).[135]

The risk of acute renal failure after ACE inhibition is not limited to renovascular disease, but can occur in any condition in which renal perfusion pressure is reduced. As an example, ACE inhibitors are standard therapy in heart failure, leading to increases in cardiac output, patient survival, and renal blood flow, as well as an improvement in functional status. Despite all of these beneficial changes, the GFR falls in about one-third of cases, presumably due to a reduction in P_{gc} induced by efferent arteriolar dilation.[136,137] This is most likely to occur in patients with a diastolic pressure below 70 mmHg who are being treated with high doses of diuretics.

Although the autoregulatory changes in arterial and arteriolar resistance are reversed when the renal perfusion pressure is elevated, angiotensin II levels are low in the basal state and it is unlikely that any further reduction is responsible for the maintenance of GFR. There is, however, substantial evidence for the role of tubuloglomerular feedback in this setting.

Tubuloglomerular Feedback

Tubuloglomerular feedback (TGF) refers to the alterations in GFR that can be induced by changes in tubular flow rate (Fig. 2-9). This phenomenon is mediated

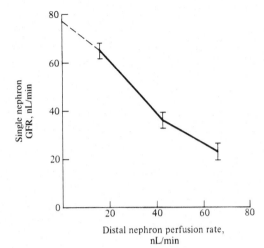

Figure 2-9   Relationship of single nephron GFR to distal nephron (macula densa) perfusion rate in dogs. As the perfusion rate increases (via the insertion of a micropipette into the late proximal tubule), there is a progressive reduction in GFR to a minimum of about one-half the basal level. (*From Navar LG, Am J Physiol 234:F357, 1978. Used with permission.*)

by the specialized cells in the *macula densa* segment at the end of the cortical thick ascending limb of the loop of Henle; these cells sense changes in the delivery and subsequent reabsorption of chloride.[94,99,100] The importance of chloride is, as described previously, probably related to the chloride dependence of the Na^+-K^+-$2Cl^-$ carrier in the luminal membrane that promotes the entry of these ions into the cell (see Fig. 4-3).[94,99,100]

TGF plays an important role in autoregulation.[127,141] An elevation in renal perfusion pressure can activate TGF via an initial rise in GFR; the ensuing increase in macula densa chloride delivery will then initiate a response that *returns both GFR and macula densa flow toward normal* (Fig. 2-9). This effect is mediated primarily by afferent arteriolar constriction, thereby decreasing the intraglomerular hydraulic pressure.[123,142]

If, on the other hand, the Na^+-K^+-$2Cl^-$ cotransporter in a single nephron is inhibited by a loop diuretic (such as furosemide), there is a marked impairment in autoregulation as renal perfusion pressure is increased.[142] That part of the autoregulatory response that persists has been thought to reflect myogenic, stretch-induced vasoconstriction.[124,142] There is, however, an alternative possibility: *cooperativity* among adjacent nephrons supplied by a common arterial branch.[143] The afferent vasoconstriction occurring in one nephron may be transmitted back up the artery and lead to vasoconstriction in adjacent nephrons. Thus, the in vivo effect of increasing distal Cl^- delivery in all nephrons will lead to a greater degree of afferent vasoconstriction in a single nephron than is induced by the macula densa in that nephron.

Mediators   The factors that mediate TGF are incompletely understood.[140] The afferent site of constriction seen with increased distal flow involves the cells of the juxtaglomerular apparatus that are responsible for renin secretion.[123] Although this observation suggests an important role for angiotensin II in tubuloglomerular feedback, this hormone appears to play a permissive role, perhaps by sensitizing the afferent arteriole to the true mediator.[144] This action of angiotensin II appears to be relatively specific, since other vasopressors such as norepinephrine and antidiuretic hormone (ADH) do not have a similar effect.[145]

The sensitizing action on TGF is essential if angiotensin II is to contribute to maintenance of the effective circulating volume by decreasing Na^+ excretion (see above).[146] The angiotensin II–mediated increase in proximal reabsorption will diminish distal flow, which should, via a decrease in the TGF signal, raise the GFR to return distal delivery to the baseline level. This response is minimized by the associated increase in sensitivity of the afferent arteriole to the mediator of TGF, thereby permitting the desired reduction in Na^+ excretion.[146]

Despite its modulating effect, angiotensin II is not the primary mediator of TGF, since changes in renin release do not correlate with TGF. As an example, increasing distal NaCl delivery will activate TGF at the same time that macula densa–mediated renin release is diminished.

There is suggestive evidence that the changes in arteriolar resistance associated with TGF may be mediated by alterations in the local release of *adenosine*,[102] which can induce the observed constriction of the afferent arteriole.[147] The TGF response to increased NaCl delivery is largely inhibited by blockade of the adenosine receptor and/or adenosine formation.[148,149] How adenosine secretion might be regulated in this setting is unknown. One possibility is that raising the GFR will increase sequentially the filtered Na^+ load, tubular sodium reabsorption, and the utilization of ATP, which results in the generation of adenosine.[102]

The adenosine hypothesis can also explain how the macula densa can concurrently perform two functions: regulating TGF and renin secretion. The increase in adenosine release with volume expansion can both activate TGF[148] and inhibit renin release.[102,103]

Another vasoconstrictor that may participate in TGF is thromboxane. Thromboxane production is increased when TGF is activated, the administration of a thromboxane mimetic increases the sensitivity of TGF, and the TGF response is blunted by a thromboxane antagonist.[151] ATP itself is also a constrictor of the afferent arteriole that may contribute to TGF.[152]

Vasodilator responses in TGF occur when macula densa flow is reduced. This may be mediated in part by reduced availability of the above vasoconstrictors.[153]

An additional significant regulator of TGF is *nitric oxide* (NO). NO, a molecular gas synthesized by cells in the macula densa, *blunts* the TGF response to increase sodium chloride delivery.[154]

NO release from the macula densa is increased in this setting, thereby countering the afferent arteriole constriction elicited in the TGF response. Thus, changes in macula densa NO production may underlie the resetting of TGF that occurs when salt intake is varied; the response is appropriately blunted with a high-salt diet, as maintenance of glomerular filtration promotes excretion of the excess salt.[155]

An alternative hypothesis suggests that changes in *interstitial Cl⁻ concentration or osmolality* constitute the signal for alterations in arteriolar resistance. The interstitial region bordered by the early distal tubule (including the macula densa) and the glomerular arterioles (see Fig. 1-4) is poorly perfused; as a result, solutes transported into this area from the luminal fluid are removed slowly, because they must diffuse over a relatively long distance before they can enter the peritubular capillaries.

Direct measurements in this region have demonstrated that, as distal flow rate and therefore macula densa Cl⁻ reabsorption are progressively increased, there is a rise in the local interstitial Cl⁻ concentration from about 150 meq/L (similar to that in plasma) to *over 600 meq/L*.[156] This increase in solute concentration or in osmolality may then directly increase afferent arteriolar tone.[150] In comparison, the interstitial Cl⁻ concentration remains relatively constant in areas that are further away from the juxtaglomerular region.[156] These sites are better perfused, and reabsorbed NaCl is rapidly removed by the peritubular capillaries.

Functions   A major function of autoregulation and TGF is to *prevent excessive salt and water losses*. To understand this concept, it is important to appreciate the differences in function between the proximal and distal segments of the nephron. The bulk of the filtrate (about 90 percent) is reabsorbed in the proximal tubule and loop of Henle, with the final *qualitative* changes in urinary excretion (such as hydrogen and potassium secretion and maximum sodium and water reabsorption) being made in the distal nephron, particularly in the collecting tubules. The collecting tubules, however, have a relatively limited *total* reabsorptive capacity. Thus, the ability of the macula densa to decrease the GFR when distal delivery is enhanced prevents distal reabsorptive capacity from being overwhelmed, which could lead to potentially life-threatening losses of sodium and water. Viewed in this light, it may be that it is *macula densa flow itself, not the GFR*, that is being maintained by autoregulation and TGF.[157]

A possible clinical example of TGF is the fall in GFR seen in acute tubular necrosis, the most common form of acute renal failure developing in the hospital. In this disorder, proximal and loop sodium reabsorption are impaired by ischemic or toxic tubular damage. Thus, the reduction of GFR (which is not easily explained by any histologic abnormality) may in part represent an *appropriate* TGF response to maintain sodium balance.[138,158] Similarly, TGF also mediates the reduction in GFR that occurs when proximal reabsorption is partially impaired by the administration of the carbonic anhydrase inhibitor acetazolamide, a proximally acting diuretic that can be useful in patients with edema and metabolic alkalosis (see page 451).[159]

On the other hand, glucosuria seems to *impair* TGF by an unknown mechanism that is in part mediated by the increase in tubular fluid glucose concentration.[138] This may play an important role in the marked fluid losses typically seen in diabetic ketoacidosis or nonketotic hyperglycemia (see Chap. 25). The osmotic diuresis induced by glucose reduces sodium and water transport in the proximal tubule and loop of Henle.[160] If TGF were normally active, the ensuing increase in delivery to the macula densa would diminish the GFR, thereby minimizing the degree of fluid loss.

Neurohumoral Influences

The intrarenal effects of autoregulation and TGF are likely to be most important in the day-to-day regulation of renal hemodynamics in normal subjects. Autoregulation also may help to maintain the GFR in patients with hypertension or with *selective* renal ischemia, as with bilateral renal artery stenosis. In fact, many of the experimental studies of autoregulation have been performed by using a suprarenal aortic clamp to selectively alter renal perfusion pressure.[121,127]

In patients, however, renal artery pressure is most often reduced because of effective circulating volume depletion (as with true volume depletion, heart failure, or cirrhosis; see Chap. 8). In these disorders, there is marked stimulation of the vasoconstrictor sympathetic nervous and renin-angiotensin systems.[76,161] As described previously, angiotensin II increases the resistance in the efferent and to a lesser degree the afferent arteriole.[80,82] In comparison, norepinephrine (either circulating or released from the renal sympathetic nerves) directly increases afferent tone and indirectly, via stimulation of the release of renin and angiotensin II, enhances efferent resistance.[80,162]

Thus, a reduction in systemic prefusion pressure is associated with renal neurohumorally mediated vasoconstriction rather than autoregulation and TGF-induced vasodilatation. The effect of these changes varies with the degree of neurohumoral activation. A relatively mild increase in renal sympathetic tone may produce no change in baseline renal perfusion, but may be sufficient to impair autoregulation (and therefore maintenance of GFR) as renal perfusion pressure is reduced.[163] In comparison, patients with advanced heart failure or severe volume depletion have more marked increments in norepinephrine and angiotensin II. In this setting, RPF is reduced at rest with a lesser fall or no change in GFR, since efferent constriction increases the P_{gc}.[80,162] This is a very effective adaptation because it preferentially shunts perfusion to the critical coronary and cerebral circulations while maintaining GFR and therefore excretory capacity.

Renal vasodilator prostaglandins play an important role in modifying these vasoconstrictive effects. Both angiotensin II and norepinephrine stimulate glomerular prostaglandin production.[86,164] The ensuing attenuation in the degree of arteriolar constriction prevents *excessive* renal ischemia, which might otherwise be induced by the high local concentration of vasoconstrictors.[87,165] To a lesser degree, increased secretion of vasodilator kinins by the kidney also may act to preserve renal perfusion in this setting.[165]

Clinical Implications   The clinical importance of these protective vasodilator responses has been amply demonstrated in humans by the administration of nonsteroidal anti-inflammatory drugs, which inhibit prostaglandin synthesis.[167] These agents, which are widely used in the treatment of arthritis and other disorders, have little effect on renal function when given to normovolemic subjects in whom the baseline level of renal prostaglandin production is relatively low.

The nonsteroidal anti-inflammatory drugs can, however, produce an acute decline in GFR and renal plasma flow when given to patients with high angiotensin II and norepinephrine levels. This most often occurs with effective circulating volume depletion due, for example, to heart failure or cirrhosis. In these conditions, prostaglandin synthesis is appropriately enhanced, and administration of a nonsteroidal anti-inflammatory drug can lead to unopposed action of the vasoconstrictors and acute renal failure (Fig. 2-10).[167,168] Studies in animals indicate that both afferent and efferent resistance are increased in this setting; the ensuing reduction in renal perfusion leads to a fall in GFR which, as mentioned above, is flow-dependent.[165]

The decrease in renal perfusion seen with effective volume depletion is also typically associated with a marked alteration in the *distribution of intrarenal blood flow*. Under normal circumstances, approximately 80 percent of renal blood flow goes to the outer cortex (where most of the glomeruli are located), 10 to 15 percent to the inner cortex (the site of the juxtamedullary nephrons; see Fig. 1-3), and the remaining 5 to 10 percent to the medulla. With hypovolemia, however, there is a marked reduction in outer cortical flow, with a preferential increase in perfusion to the inner cortex.[168-171] The mechanism by which these changes occur is unknown; angiotensin II, catecholamines, and prostaglandins have all been implicated, but their role is unproven.[171]

The physiologic significance of this intrarenal shunting of renal blood flow is also uncertain. It has been postulated that increasing inner cortical flow might promote Na^+ retention in hypovolemic states because the juxtamedullary nephrons, with their long loops of Henle, have a greater reabsorptive surface

Figure 2-10 Reduction in GFR, as estimated from the creatinine clearance, from a mean of 73 mL/min down to 32 mL/min after the administration of a nonsteroidal anti-inflammatory drug (indomethacin or ibuprofen) to 12 patients with stable hepatic cirrhosis and ascites. Urinary prostaglandin E_2 excretion was substantially greater than normal in these subjects and was markedly reduced following therapy. (*From Zipse RD, Hoefs JC, Speckhart PF, et al, J Clin Endocrinol Metab 48:895, 1979. Copyright by The Endocrine Society, 1979. Used with permission.*)

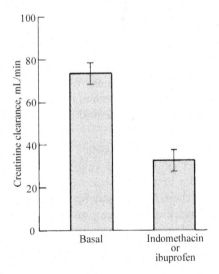

than those in the outer cortex. However, redistribution of blood flow is not necessarily associated with redistribution of glomerular filtration, making this hypothesis less likely.[172]

Volume expansion In contrast to these hormonal changes with volume depletion, volume expansion (as with a high-sodium diet) tends to be associated with increased renal perfusion and perhaps a mild rise in GFR.[54] Reduced secretion of angiotensin II and norepinephrine and enhanced release of dopamine and atrial natriuretic peptide all may contribute to this response (see Chap. 8).

- Dopamine dilates both the afferent and efferent arterioles,[119] thereby raising renal blood flow while producing a lesser increment or no change in GFR.
- Atrial natriuretic peptide, on the other hand, appears to produce the unusual combination of afferent dilation and efferent constriction, both of which will raise P_{gc} and therefore the GFR; there is a lesser alteration in RPF, since total renal vascular resistance is relatively unchanged.[173]

These hormonal alterations also facilitate excretion of the excess sodium: The release of those agents that enhance sodium reabsorption (angiotensin II, aldosterone, and norepinephrine) is diminished, whereas that of atrial natriuretic peptide and dopamine is enhanced.

Endothelin and nitric oxide Endothelin, released locally from endothelial cells, is another potent renal vasoconstrictor that affects both afferent and efferent glomerular arterioles, leading to reductions in renal blood flow and GFR.[174-176] As with the other renal vasoconstrictors, the degree of ischemia is minimized by endothelin-induced release of prostacyclin.[177]

Although endothelin is probably not an important regulator of renal hemodynamics in normal subjects, it may play a role in the reduction in GFR seen in postischemic acute renal failure. In this setting, endothelial injury may lead to the release of endothelin and subsequent renal vasoconstriction.[178] A similar mechanism may contribute to the decrease in renal perfusion induced by cyclosporine.[179,180]

Another vasoactive factor released from the endothelial cells (in addition to prostacyclin and endothelin) is nitric oxide. Nitric oxide appears to be released tonically in the renal circulation, thereby lowering renal vascular resistance (in contrast to the vasoconstrictive effect of endothelin).[174,181,182]

Glomerular hemodynamics and progressive renal failure Arteriolar resistance and renal hemodynamics also may play an important role in patients with underlying chronic renal disease. A large body of experimental and clinical evidence suggests that *intraglomerular hypertension* is partially responsible for the progression of many disorders to end-stage renal failure.[183,184]

According to this theory, the loss of nephrons (due to almost any renal disease) leads to a compensatory rise in filtration in the remaining more normal nephrons. This is an appropriate response in the short term, as it tends to maintain the total GFR. It is driven by afferent arteriolar dilatation, which leads to a rise in both P_{gc} and plasma flow. The elevation in intraglomerular pressure, however, appears to be maladaptive in the long term, since it tends to lead to progressive glomerular damage. Similar findings are seen in diabetic nephropathy, except that the renal vasodilatation is a primary event, induced in some way by hyperglycemia or insulin deficiency.[185,186]

These observations are of potentially great clinical importance, since treatment can be aimed at reversing the hemodynamic adaptations. Both dietary protein restriction and antihypertensive therapy, perhaps preferentially with an ACE inhibitor, can lower the intraglomerular pressure and diminish the degree of glomerular injury in experimental models of renal disease. Several clinical trials in chronic renal disease in humans suggest that administration of an ACE inhibitor can slow the rate of loss of GFR, particularly in diabetic nephropathy.[187-190] The efficacy of dietary protein restriction remains controversial,[191-193] with evidence of benefit being best in patients with diabetic nephropathy.[194]

The apparent preferential benefit of ACE inhibition compared to other antihypertensive drugs is thought to be related to reversal of angiotensin II–induced constriction of the efferent arteriole. Decreasing vascular resistance at this site will directly lower the intraglomerular pressure, independent of the reduction in the systemic blood pressure (Fig. 2-8).

Summary

The GFR is normally maintained within relatively narrow limits to prevent inappropriate fluctuations in solute and water excretion. Regulation of the GFR is primarily achieved by alterations in arteriolar tone that influence both the hydraulic pressure in the glomerular capillary and renal blood flow. In normal subjects, the GFR is maintained by autoregulation, a phenomenon that is mediated by at least three factors: stretch receptors in the afferent arteriole, angiotensin II, and tubuloglomerular feedback.[127] These responses, however, can be overridden by neurohumoral vasoconstiction in hypovolemic states, in an attempt to maximize coronary and cerebral perfusion.

CLINICAL EVALUATION OF RENAL CIRCULATION

Concept of Clearance and Measurement of GFR

Estimation of the GFR is an essential part of the evaluation of patients with renal disease. Since the total kidney GFR is equal to the sum of the filtration rates in each of the functioning nephrons, the total GFR can be used as an *index of functioning renal mass*. As an example, the loss of one-half of the functioning nephrons will lead to a significant decline in the GFR (which may be only 20 to

30 percent, not 50 percent, due to compensatory hyperfiltration in the remaining nephrons). At this time, fluid and electrolyte balance may still be maintained and the urinalysis may be normal. Thus, the fall in GFR may be the *earliest and only clinical sign of renal disease.*

Serial monitoring of the GFR can also be used to estimate the severity and to follow the course of kidney disease. A reduction in GFR implies either progression of the underlying disease or the development of a superimposed and potentially reversible problem, such as diminished renal perfusion due to volume depletion. An increase in GFR, on the other hand, indicates improvement or possibly hypertrophy in the remaining nephrons.

Measurement of the GFR is also helpful in determining the proper dosage of those drugs that are excreted by the kidney by glomerular filtration. When the GFR falls, drug excretion will be reduced, resulting in an increase in plasma drug levels and potential drug toxicity. To prevent this, drug dosage must be lowered in proportion to the decrease in GFR.

How can the GFR be measured? Consider a compound, such as the fructose polysaccharide inulin (not insulin), with the following properties:

1. Able to achieve a stable plasma concentration
2. Freely filtered at the glomerulus
3. Not reabsorbed, secreted, synthesized, or metabolized by the kidney

In this situation,

$$\text{Filtered inulin} = \text{excreted inulin}$$

The filtered inulin is equal to the GFR times the plasma inulin concentration (P_{in}), and the excreted inulin is equal to the product of the urine inulin concentration (U_{in}) and the urine volume (V, in milliliters per minute or liters per day). Therefore,

$$\text{GFR} \times P_{in} = U_{in} \times V \tag{2-4}$$

$$\text{GFR} = \frac{U_{in} \times V}{P_{in}} \tag{2-5}$$

The term $(U_{in} \times V)/P_{in}$ is called the clearance of inulin and is an accurate estimate of the GFR. The inulin clearance, in mL/min, refers to that volume of plasma cleared of inulin by renal excretion. If, for example, 1 mg of inulin is excreted per minute ($U_{in} \times V$) and the P_{in} is 1.0 mg/dL (or, to keep the units consistent, 0.01 mg/mL), then the clearance of inulin is 100 mL/min; that is, 100 mL of plasma has been cleared of the 1 mg of inulin that it contained.

Use and Limitations of Creatinine Clearance

Despite its accuracy, the inulin clearance is rarely performed clinically because it involves both an intravenous infusion of inulin and an assay for inulin that is not available in most laboratories. The most widely used method to estimate the GFR is the endogenous *creatinine clearance.*[108,195]

Creatinine is derived from the metabolism of creatine in skeletal muscle and is released into the plasma at a relatively constant rate. As a result, the plasma creatinine concentration (P_{cr}) is very stable, varying less than 10 percent per day in serial observations in normal subjects.

Like inulin, creatinine is freely filtered across the glomerulus and is neither reabsorbed nor metabolized by the kidney. However, some creatinine enters the urine by tubular secretion via the organic cation secretory pump in the proximal tubule, resulting in creatinine excretion exceeding the amount filtered by 10 to 20 percent.[108] Thus, the creatinine clearance (C_{cr})

$$C_{cr} = \frac{U_{cr} \times V}{P_{cr}} \tag{2-6}$$

will tend to exceed the inulin clearance by 10 to 20 percent. Fortuitously, this is balanced by an error of almost equal magnitude in the measurement of the P_{cr}. One method involves a colorimetric reaction after the addition of alkaline picrate. The plasma, but not the urine, contains noncreatinine chromogens (acetone, proteins, ascorbic acid, pyruvate), which account for approximately 10 to 20 percent of the normal P_{cr}.[108] Since both the U_{cr} and the P_{cr} are elevated to roughly the same degree, the errors tend to cancel out and the creatinine clearance is a reasonably accurate estimate of the GFR, particularly in the patient with relatively normal renal function. The normal values of the creatinine clearance are approximately $95 \pm 20\,\text{mL/min}$ in women and $120 \pm 25\,\text{mL/min}$ in men.[108]

The creatinine clearance is usually determined in the following way. The plasma creatinine concentration is measured in a venous blood sample, and the $U_{cr} \times V$ is concomitantly measured with a 24-h urine collection, since shorter collections tend to give less reliable results. Suppose, for example, that a 30-year-old woman who weighs 60 kg is being evaluated for the possible presence of renal disease and the following results are obtained:

$$P_{cr} = 1.2\,\text{mg/dL}$$

$$U_{cr} = 100\,\text{mg/dL}$$

$$V = 1080\,\text{mL/day}$$

Since

$$1080\,\text{mL/day} \div 1440\,\text{min/day} = 0.75\,\text{mL/min}$$

$$C_{cr} = \frac{100 \times 0.75}{1.2} = 63\,\text{mL/min}$$

This finding suggests that the patient has lost about one-third of her GFR.

Limitations   Although the creatinine clearance is widely used in clinical medicine, there are two major problems that limit its accuracy as an estimate of the GFR: an incomplete urine correction and increased tubular secretion of creatinine as renal function declines. The relative constancy of creatinine production and subsequent excretion can be used to assess the completeness of the urine collection. In adults under the age of 50, daily creatinine excretion should be about 20 to 25 mg/kg lean body weight in men and 15 to 20 mg/kg in women. Between the ages of 50 and 90, there is a progressive 50 percent reduction in creatinine excretion (to about 10 mg/kg in men), due primarily to a decrease in skeletal muscle mass. These relationships can be expressed by the following equations, which estimate daily creatinine excretion in mg/kg per day:[195]

$$\text{Creatinine excretion} = 28 - (\text{age in years}/6) \quad (\text{in men})$$

$$= 22 - (\text{age in years}/9) \quad (\text{in women})$$

Creatinine excretion that is much below these expected values suggests an incomplete collection. In the above 30-year-old woman, for example, creatinine excretion is 18 mg/kg per day (1080 mg ÷ 60 kg), indicating that a complete collection has probably been obtained [22 − (30/9) = 18.7].

The second major error, enhanced creatinine secretion, begins early in the course of progressive renal disease. As the GFR falls, the initial rise in the plasma creatinine concentration enhances creatinine delivery to the proximal secretory pump. This leads to an elevation in creatinine secretion, since the pump is not yet saturated.[196] At a GFR of 40 to 80 mL/min, for example, the absolute amount of creatinine secreted may have risen by *more than 50 percent* with secretion accounting for as much as 35 percent of urinary creatinine.[196] As a result, the $U_{cr} \times V$ is much higher than it would be if creatinine were excreted only by glomerular filtration, resulting in a potentially marked *overestimation* of the true GFR.[196-198]

The net effect is that the creatinine clearance may be normal (> 90 mL/min) in about one-half of patients with a true GFR (as measured by inulin clearance) of 61 to 70 mL/min and one-quarter of those with a GFR of 51 to 60 mL/min.[197] This difference may become proportionately more prominent in patients with more advanced renal disease, in whom the creatinine clearance can, in some cases, exceed the GFR by more than twofold.[198]

Thus, the creatinine clearance is not a predictably accurate measure of the GFR; all that can be concluded is that the creatinine clearance (calculated from a complete urine collection) *represents an upper limit of what the true GFR may be.* Furthermore, the degree of creatinine secretion appears to vary with time, changing the creatinine clearance independent of alterations in the GFR.[195,199,200] In some cases, the change in creatinine clearance is discordant with the change in the GFR. As an example, the degree of creatinine secretion may fall (via an unknown mechanism) at a time when the GFR is actually increasing in treated patients with lupus nephritis; this improvement, however, may be masked by no change or even a reduction in the creatinine clearance if the decrease in secretion is proportionately greater than the increase in creatinine filtration.[199,200]

The only way to determine the GFR accurately is to measure the clearance of inulin or a radiolabeled compound such as iothalamate or DTPA.[195,201] Unfortunately, determination of the inulin or iothalamate clearance is not routinely available. There are, however, two alternatives that may provide a more accurate estimate of the GFR: averaging the creatinine and urea clearances (see below) and measurement of the creatinine clearance during the administration of the H_2 blocker cimetidine, which is another organic cation that competitively inhibits creatinine secretion.

Cimetidine must be given in relatively high dose to predictably inhibit creatinine secretion in most patients.[202,203] As an example, one regimen used a single oral dose of 1200 mg plus a water load with urine collected between 3 and 6 hours for both creatinine and inulin clearance. The ratio of the creatinine to inulin clearance at baseline was about 1.5 (range 1.14 to 2.27), indicating substantial creatinine secretion. The ratio fell to 1.02 in eight patients, but remained elevated (1.33) in the remaining patients, who had more efficient urinary cimetidine excretion.[202]

It is important to appreciate, however, that *exact knowledge of the GFR is not usually required*, particularly with the ability to measure plasma levels of many of those potentially toxic drugs that are normally excreted by the kidney (such as digoxin or an aminoglycoside antibiotic). What is important to know is whether the GFR is changing (which can usually be determined from the plasma creatinine concentration alone) and whether the GFR is reduced in a patient with kidney disease who has a normal or high-normal plasma creatinine concentration (see below).

In addition to the potential errors involved in the use of the creatinine clearance, there is an additional problem: Progressive disease is not always associated with a significant reduction in GFR even if the latter is accurately measured. As noted above, nephron loss is generally associated with compensatory hypertrophy and hyperfiltration in the remaining normal or less affected nephrons. Thus, in a disease such as lupus nephritis, progressive glomerular scarring can occur during the healing phase with little reduction in the total GFR.[200,204] In this setting, the patient must also be monitored for other signs of disease progression, such as an increase in protein excretion or in the systemic blood pressure.

Plasma Creatinine and GFR

Changes in the GFR (rather than an exact measurement of the GFR) can generally be ascertained from measurement of the P_{cr}, a routine laboratory test. In a subject in the steady state,

$$\text{Creatinine excretion} = \text{creatinine production} \qquad (2\text{-}7)$$

Creatinine excretion is roughly equal to the amount of creatinine filtered (GFR $\times P_{cr}$), whereas the rate of creatinine production is relatively constant. If these substitutions are made in Eq. (2-7), then

$$\text{GFR} \times P_{cr} = \text{constant} \qquad (2\text{-}8)$$

Thus, the *plasma creatinine concentration varies inversely with the GFR*. If, for example, the GFR falls by 50 percent, creatinine excretion will also be reduced.

As a result, newly produced creatinine will accumulate in the plasma until the filtered load again equals the rate of production. Excluding changes in tubular secretion, this will occur when the P_{cr} has doubled:

$$GFR/2 \times 2P_{cr} = GFR \times P_{cr} = constant$$

In adults, the range for the normal P_{cr} is 0.8 to 1.3 mg/dL in men and 0.6 to 1.0 mg/dL in women.[108]

Creatinine production and the P_{cr} can be influenced by changes in diet. Creatinine production is determined by the total body creatine content, which itself is determined by the amount of creatine synthesized from amino acids and directly ingested in meat. As an example, creatine production can be enhanced by a high-protein or high-meat diet; this change, however, must persist over a period of weeks to months before creatinine production (and therefore the P_{cr}) is significantly enhanced, since only 1 to 2 percent of the extra creatine is converted to creatinine per day.[205] Furthermore, the increase in the P_{cr} may be less than the increment in production because a high-protein diet also tends to raise the GFR and therefore the rate of creatinine excretion.[206,207] On the other hand, switching to a meat-free diet can lower the P_{cr} by as much as 15 percent without any change in the true GFR.[208]

A more acute effect may be seen with the ingestion of cooked meat, since heating promotes the conversion of creatine to creatinine. As an example, eating a 4-oz hamburger can raise creatinine excretion by as much as 350 to 450 mg (a 20 to 30 percent increase) and can acutely elevate the P_{cr} by as much as 1 mg/dL.[205,209] Thus, the P_{cr} should optimally be measured when the patient is fasting.

The idealized reciprocal relationship between the GFR and the P_{cr} is depicted in Fig. 2-11. There are three important points to note about this relationship. First, this curve is *valid only in the steady state* when the P_{cr} is stable. If, for

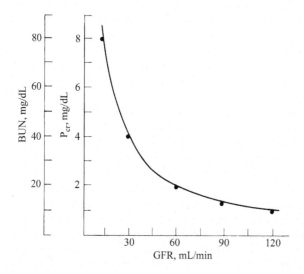

Figure 2-11 Idealized steady-state relationship between the plasma creatinine concentration (P_{cr}), blood urea nitrogen (BUN), and the GFR.

example, a patient develops acute renal failure with a sudden drop in the GFR from 120 to 12 mL/min, the P_{cr} on day 1 will be normal, since there will not have been time for creatinine to accumulate in the plasma. After 7 to 10 days, the P_{cr} will stabilize at roughly 10 mg/dL, a level consistent with the reduced GFR.

The steady state can be disturbed by changes in creatinine production as well as in urinary excretion. Thus, a malnourished patient with reduced creatinine production may have a stable P_{cr} despite a fall in GFR.

Second, it is important to appreciate the *shape* of the curve. In a patient with normal renal function, an apparently minor increase in the P_{cr} from 1.0 to 1.5 mg/dL can represent a marked fall in the GFR from 120 to 80 mL/min. In contrast, in a patient with advanced renal failure, a marked increase in the P_{cr} from 6.0 to 12.0 mg/dL reflects a relatively small reduction in the GFR from 20 to 10 mL/min. Thus, the *initial elevation in the P_{cr} represents the major loss in GFR.* Furthermore, progressive reductions in GFR in patients with advanced disease are more easy to detect by measurement of the P_{cr} (which may show a large increase) than by measurement of the GFR (which may fall by only a few mL/min, a change that may be less than the sensitivity of the assay).[195]

Third, the relationship between the GFR and the P_{cr} is dependent upon the rate of creatinine production, which is largely a function of muscle mass and meat and protein intake. In Fig. 2-11, a normal GFR of 120 mL/min is associated with a P_{cr} of 1.0 g/dL. Although this may be true for a 70-kg man, a similar GFR in a 50-kg woman might be associated with a P_{cr} of only 0.6 mg/dL. In this setting, a P_{cr} of 1.0 mg/dL is not normal and reflects a 40 percent fall in GFR.

To account for the effects of body weight, age, and sex on muscle mass, the following formula has been derived to estimate the creatinine clearance (in mL/min) from the P_{cr} in the steady state in adult men:[209,210]

$$C_{cr} = \frac{(140 - age) \times \text{lean body weight (in kg)}}{P_{cr} \times 72} \qquad (2\text{-}9)$$

This value should be multiplied by 0.85 in women, since a lower fraction of the body weight is composed of muscle.

The results obtained with this formula appear to correlate fairly well with a simultaneously measured creatinine clearance. Its usefulness can be illustrated by the observation that a P_{cr} of 1.4 mg/dL represents a creatinine clearance of 101 mL/min in an 85-kg, 20-year-old man:

$$C_{cr} = \frac{(140 - 20) \times 85}{1.4 \times 72}$$

but a creatinine clearance of only 20 mL/min in a 40-kg, 80-year-old woman:

$$C_{cr} = \frac{(140 - 80) \times 40 \times 0.85}{1.4 \times 72}$$

The latter example calls attention to the danger of overdosing elderly patients who have seriously impaired renal function despite a relatively normal P_{cr}. The use of this simple formula can help to avoid this problem but should not replace monitoring of plasma drug levels when potentially toxic agents are given.

A similar decline in creatinine production can occur in malnourished patients, such as those with cirrhosis. In addition to the loss of muscle mass, decreased meat intake and perhaps decreased hepatic production of creatine, the precursor of creatinine, can also play a contributory role. The net effect is that some cirrhotic patients with an apparently "normal" P_{cr} of 1 to 1.3 mg/dL have a GFR (as measured by inulin clearance) that can range from as low as 20 to 60 mL/min to a clearly normal value above 100 mL/min.[211,212] The low protein intake and decreased production of urea (due to the hepatic disease) also limit the rise in blood urea nitrogen (BUN) that should occur as the GFR falls (Fig. 2-11).

Thus, the presence of substantial renal dysfunction may be masked in cirrhotic patients if only the BUN and P_{cr} are measured. Calculation of the creatinine clearance will partially overcome this problem, since the reduction in creatinine production will be accounted for by a decline in creatinine excretion. However, because of increased creatinine secretion, the clearance value obtained may over-estimate the true GFR by as much as 40 percent or more in patients with renal insufficiency.[212]

In summary, the P_{cr} tends to vary inversely with the GFR in the steady state. Because of this relationship, serial measurements of the P_{cr} are typically used to monitor patients with kidney dysfunction. A rise in P_{cr} indicates disease progression, whereas a fall in P_{cr} suggests recovery of renal function (if muscle mass and meat intake are relatively constant). It is also presumed that a stable P_{cr} means stable disease, although this may not be an accurate assumption.

Limitations   It is now clear that significant disease progression can occur with *little or no change in the P_{cr}* in patients with a normal or near-normal GFR (> 60 mL/min). Three factors can contribute to this problem, two of which prevent or minimize any fall in true GFR and one of which (increased creatinine secretion) can limit the rise in P_{cr} when the GFR does fall:

1. Loss of nephrons leads to compensatory hyperfiltration in the remaining more normal nephrons, thereby maintaining the total GFR despite continued disease activity.[184] As described above, in lupus nephritis, for example, progressive glomerular scarring may be associated with no detectable change in glomerular filtration due to hypertrophy in normal or less affected glomeruli.[204]
2. Glomerular diseases damage the glomerular basement membrane, tending to lower the GFR by diminishing the effective surface area available for filtration. This effect, however, is counteracted by a rise in glomerular capillary pressure (P_{gc}) that tends to maintain the GFR despite progressive glomerular injury.[117] The mechanism by which this occurs is not well understood; an initial reduction in GFR due to the fall in surface area could lead to diminished macula densa flow and activation of TGF, which could then raise the GFR back to the baseline level.
3. When the GFR does begin to fall, the rise in the P_{cr} is lessened or prevented by an increase in tubular secretion, as described previously.[196] The potential

result of this adaption is illustrated in Fig. 2-12. Although a fall in GFR from 120 to 60 mL/min should ideally induce a doubling of the P_{cr}, many patients have only a small increase in the P_{cr} (of as little as 0.1 to 0.2 mg/dL) because of enhanced tubular secretion. With more advanced disease ($P_{cr} > 1.5$ to 2 mg/dL), the P_{cr} rises as expected, presumably due to saturation of the secretory mechanism.

The major clinical implication of these findings is that, in a patient with known renal disease, *a P_{cr} that is stable at a level under 1.5 mg/dL does not necessarily reflect stable disease.* As a result, it is important to look for other signs of disease progression, such as increased proteinuria, a more active urine sediment, or an elevation in the systemic blood pressure. In addition, variations in the degree

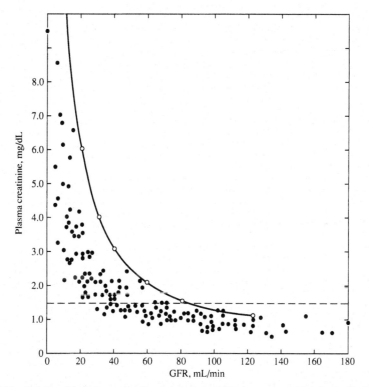

Figure 2-12   Relationship between the P_{cr} and the true GFR (as measured by the inulin clearance) in 171 patients with glomerular disease. The open circles joined by a continuous line represent the idealized relationship between these parameters if creatinine were excreted solely by glomerular filtration (see Fig. 2-11); the dotted line represents the upper limit of "normal" for the P_{cr} of 1.4 mg/dL. With the GFR varying between 120 and 60 mL/min in different patients, there is often little elevation in the P_{cr} due primarily to enhanced tubular secretion. Once the P_{cr} is above 1.5 to 2 mg/dL (132 to 176 μmol/L), tubular secretion becomes saturated and the P_{cr} rises as expected with further reductions in GFR. (*From Shemesh O, Golbetz H, Kriss JP, Myers BD*, Kidney Int *28:830, 1985. Used with permission from* Kidney International.)

of creatinine secretion can cause the P_{cr} to vary independent of the GFR.[199,200] Thus, an increase in GFR may not lead to a reduction in the P_{cr} if it is associated with a proportionate decline in creatinine secretion.[200]

Less commonly, an error arises due to an elevation in the measured P_{cr} without any change in the GFR (or BUN). This is most often due to a large meat meal,[208] ketoacidosis (in which acetoacetate can raise the P_{cr} by 0.5 to 2 mg/dL or more because it is measured as a noncreatinine chromogen),[213] or the administration of cimetidine or the antimicrobial trimethoprim (which is most often given in combination with sulfamethoxazole), both of which competitively inhibit creatinine secretion.[203,214,215]. In the last setting, the P_{cr} may increase by as much as 0.4 to 0.5 mg/dL.[215] Ranitidine, another commonly used H_2 blocker, has a less prominent effect on creatinine handling than cimetidine because it is given in much lower doses.[214]

Because of the variability in creatinine secretion and production, other endogenous markers, such as cystatin C, have been evaluated for the estimation of GFR. Cystatin C is a low-molecular-weight protein that is a member of the cystatin superfamily of cysteine protease inhibitors. It is produced by all nucleated cells, and its rate of production is relatively constant, being unaltered by inflammatory conditions or changes in diet. Preliminary studies suggest that the plasma cystatin C concentration correlates more closely with the GFR than the plasma creatinine concentration.[217] Whether the measurement of cystatin C levels will become available clinically is at present unknown.

Blood Urea Nitrogen and GFR

Changes in the GFR also can be detected by changes in the concentration of urea in the blood, measured as the BUN. Like creatinine, urea is excreted primarily by glomerular filtration, and the BUN tends to vary inversely with the GFR (Fig. 2-11).

However, two factors can alter the BUN without change in the GFR or P_{cr}: changes in urea production and tubular urea reabsorption. Urea is formed by the hepatic metabolism of amino acids that are not utilized for protein synthesis. As amino acids are deaminated, ammonia is produced. The development of toxic levels of ammonia in the blood is prevented by the conversion of ammonia (NH_3) into urea in a reaction that can be summarized by the following equation:

$$2NH_3 + CO_2 \rightarrow H_2N-CO-NH_2 + H_2O$$

Thus, urea production and the BUN are increased when more amino acids are metabolized in the liver. This may occur with a high-protein diet, enhanced tissue breakdown (due to trauma, gastrointestinal bleeding, or the administration of corticosteroids), or decreased tissue anabolism (due to tetracycline).[217] On the other hand, urea production and the BUN are reduced by severe liver disease or a low protein intake.

The second factor is that urea excretion is not determined solely by glomerular filtration. Approximately 40 to 50 percent of the filtered urea is normally reabsorbed by the tubules. This process is passive, being driven by the rise in tubular fluid urea concentration that results from the reabsorption of sodium and water. Thus, urea transport is enhanced in hypovolemic states due to the increase in sodium reabsorption. The net result is reduced urea excretion and an elevation in the BUN that is not due to a fall in GFR and therefore is not associated with a rise in the P_{cr}.[217] Under most conditions, the ratio of the BUN to the P_{cr} is 10 to 15:1. When this ratio exceeds 20:1, one of the conditions associated with enhanced urea production or effective circulating volume depletion should be suspected.[217]

In summary, a reduction in the GFR results in elevation in both the BUN and the P_{cr}. Because of the variability in urea production and reabsorption, the P_{cr} is a more reliable reflection of the GFR. For similar reasons, the urea clearance is not an accurate estimate of the GFR. Since urea is reabsorbed and the degree of reabsorption is variable, the quantity of urea excreted is much less than the amount filtered. As a result, the urea clearance is only 50 to 70 percent that of inulin.[218]

The overestimation of the GFR with the creatinine clearance and the underestimation with the urea clearance has led to the suggestion that the average of these two values should be used:

$$GFR = \frac{C_{cr} + C_{urea}}{2} \qquad (2\text{-}10)$$

This equation may be most accurate in patients with moderate to advanced renal disease ($P_{cr} > 2.5\,mg/dL$).[219]

Change in GFR with Aging

An association between age and decreasing GFR, via several hypothetical but unproven mechanisms, has been suggested by several studies.[220] In the Baltimore Longitudinal study, for example, the mean rate of decline in creatinine clearance was found to be $0.75\,mL/min$ per year.[221] However, this and other studies may be flawed because of their reliance upon endogenous creatinine clearance measurements and the presence of possible confounding conditions.

In an effort to obtain a more reliable correlation between GFR and age, another study, which examined the GFR as measured via inulin clearance, found that a majority of elderly patients with normal cardiac function had measured clearances within the normal range.[222] Thus, although the elderly appear to have lower clearance rates, comorbid conditions may significantly affect measurements of renal function among such patients, and increased age is not invariably associated with a decreased GFR.[223]

Summary

Estimation of the GFR remains an important method of monitoring patients with renal disease. There is, however, no easily available way to do this accurately. The increase in tubular secretion of creatinine as the GFR begins to fall seriously limits the validity of the creatinine clearance. Since this test can overestimate the GFR by twofold or more in patients with moderate to advanced renal disease,[198] it is best used as an *upper limit* of what the true GFR may be. The P_{cr}, on the other hand, is helpful in following the course of the disease, since the P_{cr} tends to vary inversely with the GFR (as long as muscle mass and meat intake are relatively constant). However, enhanced creatinine secretion can minimize any rise in the P_{cr} as the GFR falls from the normal level of 120 mL/min down to 60 to 80 mL/min.

Thus, a stable P_{cr} that is below 1.5 mg/dL does not necessarily mean that the renal disease is stable. In this setting, increases in systemic blood pressure and/or the activity on the urinalysis may be the only clues to progressive disease (unless an inulin or iothalamate clearance can be measured).[199] Once the P_{cr} is above 1.5 to 2 mg/dL, however, tubular secretion is saturated, and a stable P_{cr} makes it unlikely that progressive renal damage is occurring.

Variability in the production and tubular reabsorption of urea makes the BUN a less useful reflection of the GFR than the P_{cr}. The main clinical use of the BUN is in the calculation of the BUN-to-P_{cr} ratio, which, if elevated, suggests that diminished renal perfusion contributes to the renal disease (assuming that none of the causes of increased urea production is present).[217]

Measurement of Renal Plasma Flow

The principles of clearance have also been used to measure the RPF in experimental conditions; this test has little clinical utility. Paraaminohippurate (PAH) is an easily measured indicator that enters the urine by glomerular filtration and by the organic anion secretory pathway in the proximal tubule. The combination of filtration and secretion results in the almost complete removal of PAH from the plasma in a single pass through the kidney. Therefore,

$$\text{PAH delivery to kidney} = \text{PAH excretion}$$

$$\text{RPF} \times P_{PAH} = U_{PAH} \times V \tag{2-11}$$

$$\text{RPF} = \frac{U_{PAH} \times V}{P_{PAH}} = C_{PAH}$$

If the hematocrit (Hct) is known, then the renal blood flow (RBF) can be calculated from

$$\text{RBF} = \frac{C_{PAH}}{1 - \text{Hct}} \tag{2-12}$$

The normal RPF and RBF in humans are roughly 625 mL/min and 110 mL/min, respectively. Since only 85 to 90 percent of the PAH actually is removed from the circulation in a single pass, the PAH clearance will underestimate both RPF and RBF by 10 to 15 percent.

PROBLEMS

2-1   A 68-year-old man is admitted to the hospital with acute renal failure. The following plasma creatinine concentrations are obtained:

Day	Plasma creatinine, mg/dL
1	1.0
2	3.0
3	4.9

If the patient weighs 70 kg, what would you estimate the GFR to be on day 2?

2-2   Dopamine dilates both the afferent and efferent arterioles. What effect will this have on
(a) Renal blood flow
(b) GFR (in relation to the change in renal blood flow)
(c) The filtration fraction
(d) The concentration of albumin in the peritubular capillary

2-3   A patient with diabetic nephropathy has chronic renal failure (plasma creatinine concentration equals 2.1 mg/dL) and hypertension. He can be treated with an ACE inhibitor, which primarily dilates the efferent arteriole, or with other antihypertensive agents, which primarily dilate the afferent arteriole. Assuming that each form of therapy is equally effective in lowering the systemic blood pressure:
(a) Compare the likely effects of the two regimens on the glomerular capillary hydraulic pressure, P_{gc}.
(b) Could this difference be clinically important?

2-4   A creatinine clearance test is performed in an 80-kg man. The following results are obtained:

$$P_{cr} = 3.5 \text{ mg/dL}$$

$$\text{24-h urine volume} = 800 \text{ mL}$$

$$U_{cr} = 125 \text{ mg/dL}$$

(a) Calculate the creatinine clearance.
(b) Is this an accurate estimate of the GFR?

REFERENCES

1. Beeuwkes R, Bonventre JV. Tubular organization and vascular-tubular relations in the dog kidney. *Am J Physiol* 229:695, 1975.
2. Abrahamson DR. Structure and development of the glomerular capillary wall and basement membrane. *Am J Physiol* 253:F783, 1987.
3. Reiser J, Kriz W, Kretzler M, Mundel P. The glomerular slit diaphragm is a modified adherens junction. *J Am Soc Nephrol* 11:2000, 1999.
4. Weber M. Basement membrane proteins. *Kidney Int* 41:620, 1992.
5. Natori Y, O'Meara YM, Manning EC, et al. Production and polarized secretion of basement membrane components by glomerular epithelial cells. *Am J Physiol* 262:R131, 1992.
6. Groffen AJ, Veerkamp JH, Monnens LA, van den Heuvel LP. Recent insights into the structure and functions of heparan sulfate proteoglycans in the human glomerular basement membrane. *Nephrol Dial Transplant* 14:2119, 1999.
7. Kashtan CE. Alport syndrome and thin glomerular basement membrane disease. *J Am Soc Nephrol* 9:1736, 1998.
8. Harvey SJ, Zheng K, Sado Y, et al. Role of distinct type IV collagen networks in glomerular development and function. *Kidney Int* 54:1857, 1998.

9. Ding J, Stitzel J, Berry P, et al. Autosomal recessive Alport syndrome: Mutation in the COL4A3 gene in a woman with Alport syndrome and posttransplant antiglomerular basement membrane nephritis. *J Am Soc Nephrol* 5:1714, 1995.

10. Brenner BM, Hostetter TH, Humes HD. Molecular basis of proteinuria of glomerular origin. *N Engl J Med* 298:826, 1978.

11. Kanwar YS, Liu ZZ, Kashihara N, Wallner EI. Current status of the structural and functional basis of glomerular filtration and proteinuria. *Semin Nephrol* 11:390, 1991.

12. Fujigaki Y, Nagase M, Kobayasi S, et al. Intra-GBM site of the functional filtration barrier for endogenous proteins in rats. *Kidney Int* 43:567, 1993.

13. Blantz RC, Gabbai FB, Peterson O, et al. Water and protein permeability is regulated by glomerular slit diaphragm. *J Am Soc Nephrol* 4:1957, 1994.

14. Daniels BS, Deen WM, Mayer G, et al. Glomerular permeability barrier in the rat. Functional assessment by in vitro methods. *J Clin Invest* 92:929, 1993.

15. Kerjaschki D. Dysfunction of cell biological mechanisms of visceral epithelial cells (podocytes) in glomerular diseases. *Kidney Int* 45:300, 1994.

16. Ruotsalainen V, Ljungberg P, Wartiovaara J, et al. Nephrin is specifically located at the slit diaphragm of glomerular podocytes. *Proc Natl Acad Sci U S A* 96:7962, 1999.

17. Oliver JD III, Anderson S, Troy JL, et al. Determination of glomerular size-selectivity in the normal rat with ficoll. *J Am Soc Nephrol* 3:214, 1992.

18. Deen WM, Bridges CR, Brenner BM, Myers BD. Heteroporous model of glomerular size selectivity: Application to normal and nephrotic humans. *Am J Physiol* 249:F374, 1985.

19. Latta H. An approach to the structure and function of the mesangium. *J Am Soc Nephrol* 2 (suppl):S65, 1992.

20. Scandling JD, Black VM, Deen WM, Myers BD. Gomerular permselectivity in healthy and nephrotic humans. *Adv Nephrol* 21:159, 1992.

21. Groggel GC, Stevenson J, Hovingh P, et al. Changes in heparan sulfate correlate with increased glomerular permeability. *Kidney Int* 33:517, 1988.

22. Sawada H, Stukenbrok H, Kerjaschki D, Farquhar MG. Epithelial polyanion (podocalyxin) is found in the sides but not the soles of the foot processes of the glomerular epithelium. *Am J Pathol* 125:309, 1986.

23. Comper WD, Glasgow EF. Charge selectivity in kidney ultrafiltration. *Kidney Int* 47:1242, 1995.

24. Osicka TM, Comper WD. Glomerular charge selectivity for anionic and neutral horseradish peroxidase. *Kidney Int* 42:1630, 1995.

25. Guasch A, Deen WM, Myers BD. Charge selectivity of the glomerular filtration barrier in healthy and nephrotic humans. *J Clin Invest* 92:2274, 1993.

26. Ota Z, Shikata K, Ota K. Nephrotic tunnels in glomerular basement membrane as revealed by a new electron microscopic method. *J Am Soc Nephrol* 4:1965, 1994.

27. Shemesh O, Ross JC, Deen WM, et al. Nature of the glomerular capillary injury in human membranous nephropathy. *J Clin Invest* 77:868, 1986.

28. Shemesh O, Ross JC, Deen WM, et al. Nature of the glomerular capillary injury in human membranous glomerulopathy. *J Clin Invest* 77:868, 1986.

29. Golbetz H, Black V, Shemesh O, Myers BD. Mechanism of the antiproteinuric effect of indomethacin in nephrotic humans. *Am J Physiol* 256:F44, 1989.

30. Sharon Z, Schwartz MM, Pauli BU, Lewis EJ. Kinetics of glomerular visceral epithelial cell phagocytosis. *Kidney Int* 14:526, 1978.

31. Savage CO. The biology of the glomerulus: Endothelial cells. *Kidney Int* 45:314, 1994.

32. Ishino T, Kobayashi R, Wakui H, et al. Biochemical characterization of contractile proteins of rat cultured mesangial cells. *Kidney Int* 39:1118, 1991.

33. Davies M. The mesangial cell: A tissue culture view. *Kidney Int* 45:320, 1994.

34. Hugo C, Shankland SJ, Bowen-Pope DF, et al. Extraglomerular origin of the mesangial cell after injury. A new role of the juxtaglomerular apparatus. *J Clin Invest* 100:786, 1997.

35. Striker GE, Striker LJ. Glomerular cell culture. *Lab Invest* 53:122, 1985.

36. Moriyama T, Fujibayashi M, Fujiwara Y, et al. Angiotensin II stimulates interleukin-6 release from cultured mouse mesangial cells. *J Am Soc Nephrol* 6:95, 1995.

37. Kusner DJ, Luebbers EL, Nowinski RJ, et al. Cytokine- and LPS-induced synthesis of inter-leukin-8 from human mesangial cells. *Kidney Int* 39:1240, 1991.
38. Schreiner GF. The mesangial phagocyte and its regulation of contractile biology. *J Am Soc Nephrol* 2(suppl):S74, 1992.
39. Skott O, Jensen BL. Cellular and intrarenal control of renin secretion. *Clin Sci* 84:1, 1993.
40. Toffelmire EB, Slater K, Corvol P, et al. Response of prorenin and active renin to chronic and acute alterations of renin secretion in normal humans. Studies using a direct immunoradio-metric assay. *J Clin Invest* 83:679, 1989.
41. Gomez RA, Chevalier RL, Everett AD. Recruitment of renin gene-expressing cells in adult rat kidney. *Am J Physiol* 259:F660, 1990.
42. Hosoi M, Kim S, Takada T, et al. Effects of prorenin on blood pressure and plasma renin concentrations in stroke-prone spontaneously hypertensive rats. *Am J Physiol* 262:E234, 1992.
43. Shaw KJ, Do YS, Kjos S, et al. Human decidua is a major source of renin. *J Clin Invest* 83:2085, 1989.
44. Nushiro N, Ito S, Carretero OA. Renin release from microdissected superficial, midcortical, and juxtamedullary afferent arterioles in rabbits. *Kidney Int* 38:426, 1990.
45. Naftilan AJ, Zuo WM, Ingelfinger J, et al. Localization and differential regulation of angioten-sinogen mRNA expression in the vessel wall. *J Clin Invest* 88:1300, 1991.
46. Schunkert H, Ingelfinger JR, Hirsch AT, et al. Evidence for tissue specific activation of renal angiotensinogen mRNA expression in chronic stable experimental heart failure. *J Clin Invest* 90:1523, 1992.
47. Dzau, VJ. Tissue renin-angiotensin system in myocardial hypertrophy and failure. *Arch Intern Med* 153:937, 1993.
48. Kifor I, Moore TJ, Fallo F, et al. Potassium-stimulated angiotensin release from superfused adrenal capsules and enzymatically digested cells of the zona glomerulosa. *Endocrinology* 129:823, 1991.
49. Wagner C, Jensen BL, Kramer BK, Kurtz A. Control of the renal renin system by local factors. *Kidney Int* 54(suppl 67):S-78, 1998.
50. Wilkes BM, Mento PF, Pearl AR, et al. Plasma angiotensins in anephric humans: Evidence for an extrarenal angiotensin system. *J Cardiovasc Pharmacol* 17:419, 1991.
51. Ingelfinger JR, Zuo WM, Fon EA, et al. In situ hybridization evidence for angiotensinogen messenger RNA in the rat proximal tubule. An hypothesis for the intrarenal renin angiotensin system. *J Clin Invest* 85:417, 1990.
52. Yanagawa N. Potential role of local luminal angiotensin II in proximal tubule sodium trans-port. *Kidney Int* 39(suppl 32):S-33, 1991.
53. Seikaly MG, Arant BS Jr, Seney FD Jr. Endogenous angiotensin concentrations in specific intrarenal fluid compartments of the rat. *J Clin Invest* 86:1352, 1990.
54. Redgrave J, Rabinowe S, Hollenberg NK, Williams GH. Correction of abnormal renal blood flow response to angiotensin II by converting enzyme inhibition in essential hypertension. *J Clin Invest* 75:1285, 1985.
55. Oliver JA, Sciacca RR. Local generation of angiotensin II as a mechanism of regulation of peripheral vascular tone in the rat. *J Clin Invest* 74:1247, 1984.
56. Wenting GJ, DeBruyn HB, Man in't Veld AJ, et al. Hemodynamic effects of captopril in essential hypertension, renovascular hypertension and cardiac failure: Correlations with short- and long-term effects on plasma renin. *Am J Cardiol* 49:1453, 1982.
57. Bader M, Zhao Y, Sander M, et al. Role of tissue renin in the pathophysiology of hyperten-sion in TGR(mREN2) 27 rats. *Hypertension* 19:681, 1992.
58. Hilgers KF, Peters J, Veelken R, et al. Increased vascular angiotensin formation in female rats harboring the mouse *Ren-2* gene. *Hypertension* 19:687, 1992.
59. Hall JE. Intrarenal actions of converting enzyme inhibitors. *Am J Hypertens* 2:875, 1989.
60. Ischikawa I, Harris RC. Angiotensin actions in the kidney: Renewed insight into the old hormone. *Kidney Int* 40:583, 1991.
61. Goodfriend TL, Elliot ME, Catt KJ. Angiotensin receptors and their antagonists. *N Engl J Med* 334:1649, 1996.

62. Murphy TJ, Alexander RW, Griendling KK, et al. Isolation of a cDNA encoding the vascular type-1 angiotensin II receptor. *Nature* 351:233, 1991.
63. Stoll M, Steckelingd UM, Paul M, et al. The angiotensin AT_2-receptor mediates inhibition of cell proliferation in coronary endothelial cells. *J Clin Invest* 95:651, 1995.
64. Quan A, Baum M. Effect of luminal angiotensin II receptor antagonists on proximal tubule transport. *Am J Hypertens* 12:499, 1999.
65. Cogan MG. Angiotensin II: A potent controller of sodium transport in the early proximal tubule. *Hypertension* 15:451, 1990.
66. Quan A, Baum M. Regulation of proximal tubule transport by angiotensin II. *Semin Nephrol* 17:423, 1997.
67. Liu F-Y, Cogan MG. Angiotensin II stimulates early proximal bicarbonate absorption in the rat by decreasing cyclic adenosine monophosphate. *J Clin Invest* 84:83, 1989.
68. Liu-F-Y, Cogan MG. Role of protein kinase C in proximal bicarbonate absorption and angiotensin signalling. *Am J Physiol* 258:F927, 1990.
69. Geigel J, Giebisch G, Boron WF. Angiotensin II stimulates both Na^+-H^+ exchange and Na^+/HCO_3^- cotransport in the rabbit proximal tubule. *Proc Natl Acad Sci U S A* 87:7917, 1990.
70. Cogan MG, Xie M-H, Liu F-Y, et al. Effects of DuP 753 on proximal nephron and renal transport. *Am J Hypertens* 4:315s, 1991.
71. Scholz H, Kurtz A. Role of protein kinase C in renal vasoconstriction caused by angiotensin II. *Am J Physiol* 259:C421, 1990.
72. Zimmerman JB, Robertson D, Jackson EK. Angiotensin II-noradrenergic interactions in renovascular hypertensive rats. *J Clin Invest* 80:443, 1987.
73. Purdy RE, Weber MA. Angiotensin II amplification of α-adrenergic vasoconstriction: Role of receptor reserve. *Circ Res* 63:748, 1988.
74. Clemson B, Gaul L, Gubin SS, et al. Prejunctional angiotensin II receptors. Facilitation of norepinephrine release in the human forearm. *J Clin Invest* 93:684, 1994.
75. Watkins L Jr, Burton JA, Haber E, et al. The renin-angiotensin-aldosterone system in congestive failure in conscious dogs. *J Clin Invest* 57:1606, 1976.
76. Dzau VJ. Renal and circulatory mechanisms in congestive heart failure. *Kidney Int* 31:1402, 1987.
77. Schroeder ET, Anderson JH, Goldman SH, Streeten DHP. Effect of blockade of angiotensin II on blood pressure, renin and aldosterone in cirrhosis. *Kidney Int* 9:511, 1976.
78. Rasmussen H. The calcium messenger system. *N Engl J Med* 314:1164, 1986.
79. Stern N, Golub M, Novawa K, et al. Selective inhibition of angiotensin II-mediated vasoconstriction by lipoxygenase blockade. *Am J Physiol* 257:H434, 1989.
80. Myers BD, Deen WM, Brenner BM. Effects of norepinephrine and angiotensin II on the determinants of glomerular ultrafiltration and proximal tubule fluid reabsorption in the rat. *Circ Res* 37:101, 1975.
81. Yuan BH, Robinette JB, Conger JD. Effect of angiotensin II and norepinephrine on isolated rat afferent and efferent arterioles. *Am J Physiol* 258:F741, 1990.
82. Hegeraas KJ, Aukland K. Interlobular arterial resistance: Influence of renal arterial pressure and angiotensin II. *Kidney Int* 31:1291, 1987.
83. Wilcox CS, Welch WJ, Snellen H. Thromboxane mediates renal hemodynamic response to infused angiotensin II. *Kidney Int* 40:1090, 1991.
84. Denton KM, Fennessy PA, Alcorn D, Anderson WP. Morphometric analysis of the actions of angiotensin II on renal arterioles and glomeruli. *Am J Physiol* 262:F367, 1992.
85. Carmines PK, Mitchell KD, Navar LG. Effect of calcium antagonists on renal hemodynamics and glomerular function. *Kidney Int* 41(suppl 36):S-43, 1992.
86. Stahl RAK, Paravicini M, Schollmeyer P. Angiotensin II stimulation of prostaglandin E_2 and 6-keto-$F_{1\alpha}$ formation by isolated human glomeruli. *Kidney Int* 26:30, 1984.
87. Oliver JA, Pinto J, Sciacca RR, Cannon PJ. Increased renal secretion of norepinephrine and prostaglandin E2 during sodium depletion in the dog. *J Clin Invest* 66:748, 1980.
88. Vallotton M, Gerber C, Dolci W, Wüthrich RP. Interaction of vasopressin and angiotensin II in stimulation of prostacyclin synthesis in vascular smooth muscle cells. *Am J Physiol* 257:E617, 1989.

89. Ichikawa I, Pfeffer JM, Pfeffer MA, et al. Role of angiotensin II in the altered renal function of congestive heart failure. *Circ Res* 55:669, 1984.
90. Ingelfinger JR, Pratt RE, Ellison K, Dzau V. Sodium regulation of angiotensinogen mRNA expression in rat kidney cortex and medulla. *J Clin Invest* 78:1311, 1986.
91. Bock HA, Hermle M, Brunner FP, Thiel G. Pressure dependent modulation of renin release in isolated perfused glomeruli. *Kidney Int* 41:275, 1992.
92. Freeman RH, Davis JO, Villareal D. Role of renal prostaglandins in the control of renin release. *Circ Res* 54:1, 1984.
93. Kopp U, DiBona GF. Interaction of renal β_1-adrenoreceptors and prostaglandins in reflex renin release. *Am J Physiol* 244:F418, 1983.
94. Lorenz JN, Weihprecht H, Schnermann J, et al. Renin release from isolated juxtaglomerular apparatus depends on macula densa chloride transport. *Am J Physiol* 260:F486, 1991.
95. Kotchen TA, Luke RG, Ott CE, et al. Effect of chloride on renal and blood pressure responses to sodium chloride. *Ann Intern Med* 98(part 2):817, 1983.
96. Jones-Dombi T, Churchill P. The baroreceptor mechanism for controlling renin secretion: Effect of calcium channel blockers. *J Pharmacol Exp Ther* 266:274, 1993.
97. Ho S, Carretero OA, Abe K, et al. Effect of prostanoids on renin release from rabbit afferent arterioles with and without macula densa. *Kidney Int* 35:1138, 1989.
98. Data JL, Berber JG, Crump WJ, et al. The prostaglandin system: A role in canine baroreceptor control of renin release. *Circ Res* 42:454, 1978.
99. Lapointe J-Y, Bell PD, Cardinal J. Direct evidence for apical $Na^+:2Cl^-:K^+$ cotransport in macula densa cells. *Am J Physiol* 258:F1466, 1990.
100. Schlatter E, Salomonsson M, Persson AEG, Greger R. Macula densa cells sense luminal NaCl concentration via furosemide sensitive $Na^+-2Cl^--K^+$ cotransport. *Pfluegers Arch* 414:286, 1989.
101. Martinez-Maldonado M, Gely R, Tapia E, Benabe JE. Role of macula densa in diuretic-induced renin release. *Hypertension* 16:261, 1990.
102. Spielman WS, Arend JS. Adenosine receptors and signalling in the kidney. *Hypertension* 17:117, 1991.
103. Weinprecht H, Lorenz JN, Schnermann J, et al. Effect of adenosine$_1$-receptor blockade on renin release from rabbit isolated perfused juxtaglomerular apparatus. *J Clin Invest* 85:1622, 1990.
104. Greenberg SG, Lorenz JN, He X, et al. Effect of prostaglandin synthesis inhibition on macula densa-stimulated renin secretion. *Am J Physiol* 265:F578, 1993.
105. Traynor TR, Smart A, Briggs JP, Schnermann J. Inhibition of macula densa-stimulated renin secretion by pharmacological blockade of cyclooxygenase-2. *Am J Physiol* 277:F706, 1999.
106. Henrich WL, Schrier RW, Berl T. Mechanisms of renin secretion during hemorrhage in the dog. *J Clin Invest* 64:1, 1979.
107. Cuneo RC, Espiner EA, Nicholls G, et al. Effect of physiological levels of atrial natriuretic peptide on hormone secretion: Inhibition of angiotensin-induced aldosterone secretion and renin release in normal man. *J Clin Endocrinol Metab* 65:765, 1987.
108. Doolan PD, Alpen EL, Theil GB. A clinical appraisal of the plasma concentration and endogenous clearance of creatinine. *Am J Med* 32:65, 1962.
109. Guyton AC. *Textbook of Medical Physiology*, 8th ed. Saunders, Philadelphia, 1991, chap. 16.
110. Maddox DA, Deen WM, Brenner BM. Dynamics of glomerular ultrafiltration. VI. Studies in the primate. *Kidney Int* 5:271, 1974.
111. Brenner BM, Humes HD. Mechanics of glomerular ultrafiltration. *N Engl J Med* 297:148, 1977.
112. Arendshorst W, Gottschalk CW. Glomerular ultrafiltration dynamics: Historical perspective. *Am J Physiol* 248:F163, 1985.
113. Savin VJ. Ultrafiltration in single isolated human glomeruli. *Kidney Int* 24:748, 1983.
114. Brenner BM, Troy JL, Daugharty TM, et al. Dynamics of glomerular ultrafiltration in the rat. II. Plasma-flow dependence of GFR. *Am J Physiol* 223:1184, 1972.
115. Renkin E, Robinson R. Glomerular filtration. *N Engl J Med* 290:785, 1974.

116. Dworkin LD, Ichikawa I, Brenner BM. Hormonal modulation of glomerular function. *Am J Physiol* 244:F95, 1983.
117. Kaizu K, Marsh D, Zipser R, Glassock RJ. Roles of prostaglandins and angiotensin II in experimental glomerulonephritis. *Kidney Int* 28:629, 1985.
118. Yarger WE, Aynedjian HS, Bank N. A micropuncture study of postobstructive diuresis in the rat. *J Clin Invest* 51:625, 1972.
119. Steinhausen M, Endlich K, Wiegman DL. Glomerular blood flow. *Kidney Int* 38:769, 1990.
120. Navar LG. Renal autoregulation: Perspectives from whole kidney and single nephron studies. *Am J Physiol* 234:F357, 1978.
121. Hall JE, Guyton AC, Jackson TE, et al. Control of glomerular filtration rate by renin-angiotensin system. *Am J Physiol* 233:F366, 1977.
122. Johnson PC. Autoregulation of blood flow. *Circ Res* 59:483, 1986.
123. Casellas D, Moore LC. Autoregulation and tubuloglomerular feedback in juxtaglomerular arterioles. *Am J Physiol* 258:F660, 1990.
124. Harder DR, Gilbert R, Lombard JH. Vascular muscle cell depolarization and activation in renal arteries on elevation on transmural pressure. *Am J Physiol* 253:F778, 1987.
125. Hayashi K, Epstein M, Loutzenheiser R. Pressure-induced vasoconstriction of renal microvessels in normotensive and hypertensive rats: Studies in isolated perfused hydronephrotic kidney. *Circ Res* 65:1475, 1989.
126. Carmines PK, Fowler BC, Bell PD. Segmentally distinct effects of depolarization on intracellular [Ca^{2+}] in renal arterioles. *Am J Physiol* 265:F677, 1993.
127. Schnermann J, Briggs JP, Weber PC. Tubuloglomerular feedback, prostaglandins, and angiotensin in the autoregulation of glomerular filtration rate. *Kidney Int* 25:53, 1984.
128. Beierwaltes WH, Sigmon DH, Carretero OA. Endothelium modulates renal blood flow but not autoregulation. *Am J Physiol* 262:F943, 1992.
129. Kastner PR, Hall JE, Guyton AC. Control of glomerular filtration rate: Role of intrarenally formed angiotensin II. *Am J Physiol* 246:F897, 1984.
130. Hricik DE, Dunn MJ. Angiotensin-converting-enzyme inhibitor-induced renal failure: Causes, consequences, and diagnostic uses. *J Am Soc Nephrol* 1:845, 1990.
131. Jackson B, Matthews PG, McGrath BP, Johnston CI. Angiotensin converting enzyme inhibition in renovascular hypertension: Frequency of reversible renal failure. *Lancet* 1:225, 1984.
132. Hricik DE. Captopril induced renal insufficiency and the role of sodium balance. *Ann Intern Med* 103:222, 1985.
133. Wenting GJ, Tan-Tjiong HL, Derkx FHM, et al. Split renal function after captopril in unilateral renal artery stenosis. *Br Med J* 288:886, 1984.
134. Michel J-B, Dussaule J-C, Choudat L, et al. Effect of antihypertensive treatment in one-clip, two kidney hypertension in rats. *Kidney Int* 29:1011, 1986.
135. Textor SE, Novick A, Tarazi RC, et al. Critical renal perfusion pressure for renal function in patients with bilateral atherosclerotic renal vascular disease. *Ann Intern Med* 102:308, 1985.
136. Packer M, Lee WH, Medina N, et al. Functional renal insufficiency during long-term therapy with captopril and enalapril in severe chronic heart failure. *Ann Intern Med* 106:346, 1987.
137. Ljungman S, Kjekshus J, Swedberg K. Renal function in severe congestive heart failure during treatment with enalapril (the Cooperative North Scandinavian Enalapril Survival Study [CONSENSUS] trial). *Am J Cardiol* 70:492, 1992.
138. Blantz RC, Pelayo JC. A functional role for the tubuloglomerular feedback mechanism. *Kidney Int* 25:739, 1984.
139. Briggs JP, Schnermann J. The tubuloglomerular feedback mechanism: Functional and biochemical aspects. *Ann Rev Physiol* 49:251, 1987.
140. Schnermann J, Traynor T, Yang T, et al. Tubuloglomerular feedback: New concepts and developments. *Kidney Int* 54(suppl 67):S-40, 1998.
141. Moore LC. Tubuloglomerular feedback and SNGFR autoregulation in the rat. *Am J Physiol* 247:F267, 1984.
142. Moore LC, Casellas D. Tubuloglomerular feedback dependence of autoregulation in rat juxtaglomerular afferent arterioles. *Kidney Int* 37:1402, 1990.

143. Kallskog O, Marsh DJ. Tubuloglomerular feedback-initiated vascular interactions between adjacent nephrons in the rat kidney. *Am J Physiol* 259:F60, 1990.

144. Schnermann J, Briggs JP. Restoration of tubuloglomerular feedback in volume-expanded rats by angiotensin II. *Am J Physiol* 259:F565, 1990.

145. Schnermann J, Briggs JP. Effect of angiotensin and other pressor agents on tubuloglomerular feedback responses. *Kidney Int* 38(suppl 30): S-77, 1990.

146. Navar LG, Saccomani G, Mitchell KD. Synergistic intrarenal actions of angiotensin on tubular reabsorption and renal hemodynamics. *Am J Hypertens* 4:90, 1991.

147. Weihprecht H, Lorenz JN, Briggs JO, Schnermann J. Vasomotor effects of purinergic agonists in isolated rabbit afferent arterioles. *Am J Physiol* 263:F1026, 1992.

148. Schnermann J, Weihprecht H, Briggs JP. Inhibition of tubuloglomerular feedback by adenosine$_1$ receptor blockade. *Am J Physiol* 258:F553, 1990.

149. Thomson S, Bao D, Deng A, Vallon V. Adenosine formed by 5'-nucleotidase mediates tubuloglomerular feedback. *J Clin Invest* 106:289, 2000.

150. Navar LG, Inscho EW, Ibarrola M, Carmines PK. Communication between the macula densa cells and the afferent arteriole. *Kidney Int* 39(suppl 32):S-78, 1991.

151. Welch WJ, Wilcox CS. Potentiation of tubuloglomerular feedback in the rat by thromboxane mimetic. *J Clin Invest* 89:1857, 1992.

152. Navar LG. Integrating multiple paracrine regulators of renal microvascular dynamics. *Am J Physiol* 274:F433, 1998.

153. Thompson SC, Bachmann S, Bostanjoglo M, et al. Temporal adjustment of the juxtaglomerular apparatus during sustained inhibition of proximal reabsorption. *J Clin Invest* 104:1149, 1999.

154. Welch WJ, Wilcox CS, Thomson SC. Nitric oxide and tubuloglomerular feedback. *Semin Nephrol* 19:25, 1999.

155. Wilcox CS, Welch WJ. TGF and nitric oxide: Effects of salt intake and salt-sensitive hypertension. *Kidney Int* 55(suppl 55): S-9, 1996.

156. Persson B-E, Sakai T, Marsh DJ. Juxtaglomerular hypertonicity in *Amphiuma*: Tubular origin—TGF signal. *Am J Physiol* 254:F445, 1988.

157. Moore LC. Interaction of tubuloglomerular feedback and proximal nephron reabsorption in autoregulation. *Kidney Int* 22(suppl 12):S-173, 1982.

158. Thurau K. Acute renal success: The unexpected logic of oliguria in acute renal failure. *Am J Med* 61:308, 1976.

159. Leyssac PP, Karlsen FM, Skott O. Dynamics of intrarenal pressures and glomerular filtration rate after acetazolamide. *Am J Physiol* 261:F169, 1991.

160. Seely JF, Dirks JH. Micropuncture study of hypertonic mannitol diuresis in the proximal and distal tubule of the dog kidney. *J Clin Invest* 48:2330, 1969.

161. Henriksen JH, Bendtsen F, Gerbes AL, et al. Estimated central blood volume in cirrhosis: Relationship to sympathetic nervous activity, β-adrenergic blockade and atrial natriuretic factor. *Hepatology* 16:1163, 1992.

162. Tucker BJ, Mundy CA, Blantz RC. Adrenergic and angiotensin II influences on renal vascular tone in chronic sodium depletion. *Am J Physiol* 252:F811, 1987.

163. Persson PB, Ehmke H, Nafz B, Kircheim HR. Sympathetic modulation of renal autoregulation by carotid occlusion in conscious dogs. *Am J Physiol* 258:F364, 1990.

164. Bonvalet J-P, Pradelles P, Farman N. Segmental synthesis and actions of prostaglandins along the nephron. *Am J Physiol* 253:F377, 1987.

165. Schor N, Ichikawa I, Brenner BM. Glomerular adaptations to chronic dietary salt restriction or excess. *Am J Physiol* 238:F428, 1980.

166. Johnston PA, Bernard DB, Perrin NS, et al. Control of rat renal vascular resistance during alterations in sodium balance. *Circ Res* 48:728, 1981.

167. Oates JA, Fitzgerald GA, Branch RA, et al. Clinical implications of prostaglandin and thromboxane A$_2$ formation. *N Engl J Med* 319:761, 1988.

168. Patrono C, Dunn MJ. The clinical significance of inhibition of renal prostaglandin synthesis. *Kidney Int* 32:1, 1987.

68 PART ONE RENAL PHYSIOLOGY

169. Kilcoyne MM, Schmidt DH, Cannon PJ. Intrarenal blood flow in congestive heart failure. *Circulation* 47:786, 1973.
170. Epstein M, Berk DP, Hollenberg NK, et al. Renal failure in patients with cirrhosis. *Am J Med* 49:175, 1970.
171. Stein JH, Boonjarern S, Maux RC, Ferris TF. Mechanism of the redistribution of renal cortical blood flow during hemorrhagic hypotension in the dog. *J Clin Invest* 52:39, 1973.
172. Bruns FJ, Alexander EA, Riley AL, Levinsky NG. Superficial and juxtamedullary nephron function during saline loading in the dog. *J Clin Invest* 53:971, 1974.
173. Weidmann P, Hasler, L, Gnadinger MP, et al. Blood levels and renal effects of atrial natriuretic peptide in normal man. *J Clin Invest* 77:734, 1986.
174. Lüscher TF, Bock HA, Yang Z, Diederich D. Endothelium-derived relaxing and contracting factors: Perspectives in nephrology. *Kidney Int* 39:575, 1991.
175. Edwards RM, Trizna W, Ohlstein EH. Renal microvascular effects of endothelin. *Am J Physiol* 259:F217, 1990.
176. Kohan DE. Endothelins in the normal and diseased kidney. *Am J Kidney Dis* 29:2, 1997.
177. Chou S-Y, Dahnan A, Porush JG. Renal actions of endothelin: Interaction with prostacyclin. *Am J Physiol* 259:F645, 1990.
178. Kon V, Yoshioka T, Fogo A, Ichikawa I. Glomerular actions of endothelin in vivo. *J Clin Invest* 83:1762, 1989.
179. Kon V, Sugiura M, Inagami T, et al. Role of endothelin in cyclosporine-induced glomerular dysfunction. *Kidney Int* 37:1487, 1990.
180. Lanese DM, Conger JD. Effects of endothelin receptor antagonist on cyclosporine-induced vasoconstriction in isolated rat renal arterioles. *J Clin Invest* 91:2144, 1993.
181. Rademacher J, Forstermann U, Frohlich JC. Endothelium-derived relaxing factor influences renal vascular resistance. *Am J Physiol* 259:F9, 1990.
182. Berthold H, Just A, Kirchheim HR, et al. Interaction between nitric oxide and endogenous vasoconstrictors in control of blood flow. *Hypertension* 34:1254, 1999.
183. Jacobson HR, Klahr S. Chronic renal failure: Pathophysiology; Management. *Lancet* 338:419,423, 1991.
184. Olson JL, Heptinstall RM. Nonimmunologic mechanisms of glomerular injury. *Lab Invest* 1988, 59:564, 1988.
185. Anderson S, Rennke HG, Garcia DL, Brenner BM. Short and long term effects of antihypertensive therapy in the diabetic rat. *Kidney Int* 36:526, 1989.
186. Zatz R, Meyer TW, Rennke HG, Brenner BM. Predominance of hemodynamic rather than metabolic factors in the pathogenesis of diabetic nephropathy. *Proc Natl Acad Sci U S A* 82:5963, 1985.
187. Maschio G, Alberti D, Janin G, et al. Effect of the angiotensin-converting-enzyme inhibitor benazepril on the progression of chronic renal insufficiency. *N Engl J Med* 334:939, 1996.
188. Ruggenenti P, Perna A, Gherardi G, et al. Renal function and requirement for dialysis in chronic nephropathy patients on long-term ramipril: REIN follow-up trial. *Lancet* 352:1252, 1998.
189. Lewis EJ, Hunsicker LG, Bain RP, Rohde RD. The effect of angiotensin-converting enzyme inhibition on diabetic nephropathy. *N Engl J Med* 329:1456, 1993.
190. Wilmer WA, Hebert LA, Lewis EJ, et al. Remission of nephrotic syndrome in type 1 diabetes: Long-term follow-up of patients in the Captopril study. *Am J Kidney Dis* 34:308, 1999.
191. Klahr S, Levey AS, Beck GJ, et al. The effects of dietary protein restriction and blood-pressure control on the progression of chronic renal disease. *N Engl J Med* 330:877, 1994.
192. Levy AS, Greene T, Beck GJ, et al. Dietary protein restriction and the progression of chronic renal disease: What have all of the results of the MDRD study shown? Modification of Diet in Renal Disease Study Group. *J Am Soc Nephrol* 10:2426, 1999.
193. Kasiske BL, Lakatua JD, Ma JZ, Louis TA. A meta-analysis of the effects of dietary protein restriction on the rate of decline in renal function. *Am J Kidney Dis* 31:954, 1998.

194. Zeller K, Whittaker E, Sullivan L, et al. Effect of restricting dietary protein on the progression of renal failure in patients with insulin-dependent diabetes mellitus. *N Engl J Med* 324:78, 1991.
195. Levey AS. Measurement of renal function in chronic renal disease. *Kidney Int* 38:167, 1990.
196. Shemesh O, Golbetz H, Kriss JP, Myers BD. Limitations of creatinine as a filtration market in glomerulopathic patients. *Kidney Int* 28:830, 1985.
197. Kim KE, Onesti G, Ramirez O, et al. Creatinine clearance in renal disease. A reappraisal. *Br Med J* 4:11, 1969.
198. Bauer JH, Brooks CS, Burch RN. Clinical appraisal of creatinine clearance as a measurement of glomerular filtration rate. *Am J Kidney Dis* 2:337, 1982.
199. Petri M, Bockenstedt L, Colman J, et al. Serial assessment of glomerular filtration rate in lupus nephropathy. *Kidney Int* 34:832, 1988.
200. Myers BD, Chagnac A, Golbetz H, et al. Extent of glomerular injury in active and resolving lupus nephritis: A theoretical analysis. *Am J Physiol* 260:F717, 1991.
201. Perrone RD, Steinman TI, Beck GJ, et al. Utility of radioisotopic filtration markers in chronic renal insufficiency: Simultaneous comparison of ^{125}I-iothalamate, ^{169}Yb-DTPA, ^{99m}Tc-DTPA, and inulin. *Am J Kidney Dis* 16:224, 1990.
202. van Acker BAC, Koomen GCM, Koopman MG, et al. Creatinine clearance during cimetidine administration for measurement of glomerular filtration rate. *Lancet* 340:1326, 1992.
203. Hilbrands LB, Artz MA, Wetzels JFM, Koene RAP. Cimetidine improves the reliability of creatinine as a marker of glomerular filtration. *Kidney Int* 40:1171, 1991.
204. Chagnac A, Kiberd BA, Farinas MC, et al. Outcome of the acute glomerular injury in proliferative lupus nephritis. *J Clin Invest* 84:922, 1989.
205. Levey AS, Berg RL, Gassman JJ, et al. Modification of Diet in Renal Disease (MDRD) Study Group. Creatinine filtration, secretion and excretion during progressive renal disease. *Kidney Int* 36(suppl 27):S-73, 1989.
206. Castellino P, Levin R, Shohat J, DeFronzo RA. Effect of specific amino acid groups on renal hemodynamics in humans. *Am J Physiol* 258:F992, 1990.
207. Kontessis P, Jones S, Dodds R, et al. Renal, metabolic and hormonal responses to ingestion of animal and vegetable proteins. *Kidney Int* 38:136, 1990.
208. Payne RB. Creatinine clearance: A redundant clinical investigation. *Ann Clin Biochem* 23:243, 1986.
209. Cockcroft DW, Gault MH. Prediction of creatinine clearance from serum creatinine. *Nephron* 16:13, 1976.
210. Gault MH, Longerich LL, Harnett JD, Weslowski C. Predicting glomerular function from adjusted serum creatinine. *Nephron* 62:249, 1992.
211. Papadakis MA, Arieff AI. Unpredictability of clinical evaluation of renal function in cirrhosis. Prospective study. *Am J Med* 82:945, 1987.
212. Caregaro L, Menon F, Angeli P, et al. Limitation of serum creatinine level and creatinine clearance as filtration markers in cirrhosis. *Arch Intern Med* 154:201, 1994.
213. Molitch ME, Rodman E, Hirsch CA, Dubinsky E. Spurious creatinine elevations in ketoacidosis. *Ann Intern Med* 93:2800, 1980.
214. Rocci ML Jr, Vlasses PH, Ferguson RK. Creatinine serum concentrations and H_2-receptor antagonists. *Clin Nephrol* 22:814, 1984.
215. Berg KJ, Gjellestad A, Nordby G, et al. Renal effects of trimethoprim in cyclosporin- and azathioprine-treated kidney allografted patients. *Nephron* 43:218, 1989.
216. Newman DJ, Thakkar H, Edwards RG, et al. Serum cystatin C measured by automated immunoassay: A more sensitive marker of changes in GFR than serum creatinine. *Kidney Int* 47:312, 1995.
217. Dossetor JB. Creatininemia versus uremia: The relative significance of blood urea nitrogen and serum creatinine concentrations in azotemia. *Ann Intern Med* 65:1287, 1966.
218. Smith HW, Goldring W, Chasis H. The measurement of the tubular excretory mass, effective blood flow and filtration rate in the normal human kidney. *J Clin Invest* 17:263, 1938.

219. Lubowitz H, Slatopolsky E, Shankel S, et al. Glomerular filtration rate determination in patients with chronic renal disease *JAMA* 199:252, 1967.
220. Rodriguez-Puyol D. The aging kidney. *Kidney Int* 54:2247, 1998.
221. Lindeman RD, Tobin J, Shock NW. Association between blood pressure and the rate of decline in renal function with age. *Kidney Int* 26:861, 1984.
222. Fliser D, Franek E, Joest M. Renal function in the elderly: Impact of hypertension and cardiac function. *Kidney Int* 51:1196, 1997.
223. Fliser D, Franek E, Ritz E. Renal function in the elderly—Is the dogma of an inexorable decline of renal function correct (editorial)? *Nephrol Dial Transplant* 12:1553, 1997.

PROXIMAL TUBULE

Fluid filtered at the glomerulus enters the proximal tubule, where about 55 to 60 percent of the filtrate is normally reabsorbed.[1] The primary event in proximal tubular function is the active transport of Na^+, which then allows water and many of the other filtered solutes to be reabsorbed *passively* in a reabsorbate that is isosmotic to plasma. In addition, some solutes are secreted rather than reabsorbed in this segment, including hydrogen ions (H^+) and organic anions and cations.

Although the proximal tubule plays a major role in solute transport, the degree of reabsorption of individual solutes is not uniform. Almost all of the filtered glucose and amino acids are reabsorbed in this segment, but only about 90 percent of the HCO_3^-, 65 percent of the Na^+, and 55 percent of the Cl^- (Fig. 3-1).[1] This chapter will review the basic aspects of how the proximal tubule selectively performs these functions as well as some of the clinical implications of the relationship between the reabsorption of Na^+ and that of the other solutes in the filtrate.

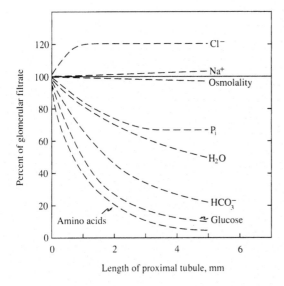

Figure 3-1 Changes in tubular fluid composition along the length of the proximal tubule. For solutes, the lines represent the solute concentration as a percent of that present in the glomerular filtrate. In comparison, the line for H_2O represents the percent of the filtered load remaining in the tubule. Some solutes, such as bicarbonate, glucose, and amino acids, are almost entirely reabsorbed in the early proximal tubule, resulting in a marked reduction in their tubular fluid concentrations. Sodium, on the other hand, is reabsorbed to the same degree as water, so that there is no change in the sodium concentration as fluid moves down the proximal tubule. However, the preferential reabsorption in the early proximal tubule of sodium with bicarbonate and glucose has an important secondary effect: The ensuing passive reabsorption of water leads to a rise in the tubular fluid chloride concentration above that in the plasma. As will be seen, this chloride gradient is sufficient to drive passive sodium chloride reabsorption in the later aspects of the proximal tubule. (*Adapted from Rector FC Jr, Am J Physiol 244:F461, 1983, and Maddox DA, Gennari JF, Am J Physiol 252:F573, 1987. Used with permission.*)

ANATOMY

The proximal tubule has a convoluted segment, which begins at the glomerulus, and then a straight segment (pars recta), which ends in the outer medulla in the descending limb of the loop of Henle (see Fig. 1-3). However, closer examination has revealed the presence of *three* distinct proximal segments with different cell types: S_1 in the early convoluted segment; S_2 in the late convoluted segment and early pars recta; and S_3 in the remainder of the pars recta (Fig. 3-2).[2] These cell types can be isolated in relative purity via the use of monoclonal antibodies directed against cell surface peptidases uniquely expressed in each type, such as leucine aminopeptidase in the S_3 segment.[3]

The cells in the different proximal segments are, to some degree, associated with different functional characteristics. The S_1 segment, for example, is a high-capacity site that plays a larger quantitative role in Na^+ and HCO_3^- reabsorption than the later segments.[1] Both an increased number of transporters in the luminal

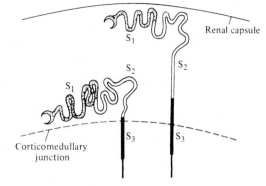

Figure 3-2 Distribution of the S_1, S_2, and S_3 segments defined by cell type in the proximal tubules from outer cortical (right) and juxtamedullary (left) nephrons. (*From Woodhall PB, Tisher CC, Simonton CA, Robinson RR, J Clin Invest 61:1320, 1978, by copyright permission of the American Society for Clinical Investigation.*)

membrane and a greater surface area available for reabsorption play a contributory role. In comparison, tubular secretion by the organic anion and cation secretory pumps is most prominent in the S_2 segment.[2]

CELL MODEL FOR PROXIMAL TRANSPORT

The anatomy of the proximal tubule is similar to that of other transporting epithelia (Fig. 3-3).[4,5] The cells have two membranes with different permeability and transport characteristics:

- The *luminal* (or apical) membrane, which separates the cell from the tubular lumen, contains a variety of transmembrane protein carriers that facilitate solute entry into the cell and, to a lesser degree, solute secretion into the lumen.[5]
- The *basolateral* (or peritubular) membrane separates the cell from the interstitium and peritubular capillary. This membrane contains the Na^+-K^+-ATPase pump as well as transporters and channels that allow reabsorbed solutes to be returned to the systemic circulation. As will be seen, the *Na^+-K^+-ATPase pump indirectly provides the energy that allows virtually all of the transport proteins to passively translocate filtered solutes.*

The proximal tubular cells are separated by an intercellular space, which is open both at the capillary end and to a lesser degree at the luminal end across the *tight junction*. The tight junction is composed of protein molecules that bring adjacent cells into apposition; it also serves as a boundary between the luminal and basolateral membranes, preventing the lateral diffusion of membrane proteins from one membrane to the other (see page 9).[6]

The proximal tubule can reabsorb more than 100 L/day in subjects with normal renal function (55 to 60 percent of a daily filtration rate of 150 to 180 liters). It is well suited for this task because of a series of adaptations, each of which facilitates net reabsorption of the filtrate:

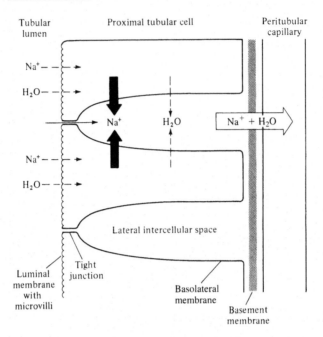

Tubular
lumen

Proximal tubular cell

Peritubular
capillary

Na⁺

H₂O

Na⁺

H₂O

Na⁺

H₂O

Na⁺ + H₂O

Lateral intercellular space

Luminal
membrane
with
microvilli

Tight
junction

Basolateral
membrane

Basement
membrane

Figure 3-3   Schematic representation of active Na^+ and H_2O reabsorption in the proximal tubule. Na^+ enters the cell passively (dashed arrows) via carrier proteins in the luminal membrane; it is then actively transported into the intercellular space (dark solid arrow) by the Na^+-K^+-ATPase pump in the basolateral membrane. Water follows the movement of Na^+ down the osmotic gradient created by solute transport out of the lumen. Some of this may occur through the tight junction as well as across the cell membranes. The Na^+ and H_2O that enter the intercellular space can either move into the peritubular capillary and be returned to the systemic circulation or leak back into the lumen across the tight junction.

- The luminal membrane has microvilli which increase the surface area available for reabsorption. In addition, the microvilli have a brush border that contains specific carrier proteins as well as an enzyme, carbonic anhydrase, which plays an important role in HCO_3^- reabsorption (see Chap. 11).
- Solute reabsorption creates an osmotic gradient that allows water to be reabsorbed in part across the cells. This process can occur because both the luminal and basolateral membranes are relatively water permeable as a result of the presence of water channels within the membrane;[7,8,9] these water channels, called aquaporin-1, appear to be similar to those in red cells.[9] Targeted disruption of the genes for these channels results in the inability to reabsorb fluid within the proximal tubules.[10] In comparison, the luminal membranes of the ascending limb of the loop of Henle and the entire distal nephron largely lack water channels and do not allow osmotic water transport in the basal state (see Chaps. 4 and 5). Antidiuretic hormone, however, can increase the water permeability of the collecting tubule cells by causing a different type of preformed water

channels, called aquaporin-2, in the cytosol to move to and fuse with the luminal membrane (see Chap. 6); this process is one of the essential steps both in distal water reabsorption and in the formation of a concentrated urine.

- The preferential reabsorption of HCO_3^- in the early proximal tubule results in osmotic water transport and a subsequent rise in the tubular fluid Cl^- concentration (Fig. 3-1). As will be discussed below, this Cl^- gradient is sufficient to allow as much as one-third of proximal NaCl and water reabsorption to occur passively through the tight junction.[11,12] This capacity for passive transport is reflected in the observation that, despite the high rate of total reabsorption, Na^+-K^+-ATPase activity in the proximal tubule is much lower than that in the thick ascending limb or distal tubule.[13]

- Substantial passive reabsorption can occur because the tight junction of the proximal tubule is relatively "leaky" in comparison to other nephron segments.[6] On freeze-fracture electron microscopy, the tight junction has a strand-like appearance. The proximal tubule has only one strand, versus up to eight in tight epithelia, such as the distal nephron.[6] Thus, transport through the paracellular pathway in the proximal tubule is a low-resistance route in comparison to having to traverse both the luminal and basolateral membranes.

In general, filtered Na^+ passively enters the cell across the luminal membrane and is then actively transported by the Na^+-K^+-ATPase pump into the intercellular space. The removal of Na^+ and other solutes from the lumen initially lowers the luminal osmolality, creating an osmotic gradient of up to 15 mmHg that promotes the reabsorption of H_2O.[14,15] Water movement is also promoted by an additional factor: The preferential reabsorption of $NaHCO_3$ in the early proximal tubule leads to an elevation in the tubular fluid Cl^- concentration; this makes the *effective* luminal osmolality even lower, since the tight junction is relatively permeable to Cl^-, which therefore functions as an ineffective osmole (see "Passive Transport" below).[15]

The reabsorbate that accumulates in the intercellular space can then enter the peritubular capillary and be returned to the systemic circulation or can leak back into the lumen across the tight junction. As will be seen, net proximal Na^+ and water reabsorption is affected by multiple factors, including filtered solutes that are reabsorbed with Na^+, peritubular capillary hemodynamics, and neurohumoral factors such as angiotensin II, norepinephrine, and dopamine.

Cell Entry

Luminal Na^+ must enter the cells before it can be reabsorbed. The primary step in this process is the *Na^+-K^+-ATPase pump in the basolateral membrane*, which has two functions that create a favorable electrochemical gradient for passive Na^+ entry into the cells (Fig. 3-4). First, the pump maintains the effective cell Na^+ concentration at about 20 to 30 meq/L by transporting Na^+ out of the cell; this is

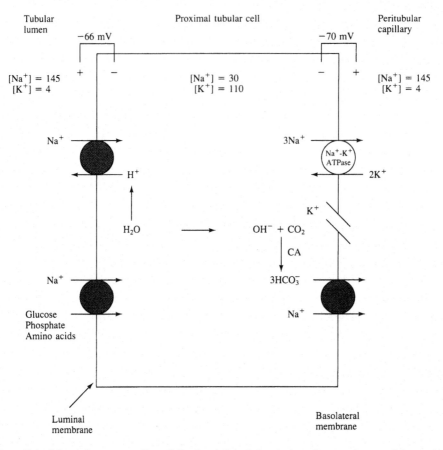

Figure 3-4 Schematic representation of the chemical and electrical gradients and some of the carrier-mediated mechanisms involved in proximal tubular solute transport. The low cell Na^+ concentration that is maintained by the Na^+-K^+-ATPase pump in the basolateral membrane permits secondary active transport in which passive Na^+ entry into the cell is coupled by specific cotransporters to the uphill reabsorption of glucose, phosphate, and amino acids, or to the secretion of H^+. Units are meq/L; CA represents carbonic anhydrase.

well below the value of 145 meq/L in the filtrate.[16] Second, the pump contributes to the development of a *cell interior negative potential* by promoting the net loss of cations; this results both from the $3Na^+$:$2K^+$ stoichiometry of the pump and from the subsequent back diffusion of this K^+ out of the cell through ATP-sensitive K^+ channels in the basolateral membrane.[17]*

---

* The activity of the Na^+-K^+-ATPase pump and the K^+ channel appropriately vary in parallel. A reduction in pump activity, due for example to decreased Na^+ reabsorption, results in ATP accumulation in the cell, which then downregulates the ATP-sensitive K^+ channels.[18] Less K^+ exit through these channels is required in this setting, since there is less K^+ entry via the Na^+-K^+-ATPase pump.

The net effect is a highly favorable electrochemical gradient that promotes passive Na^+ entry into the cells. This process, however, must occur via a transmembrane carrier or channel, since ions are unable to freely cross the lipid bilayer of the cell membranes. In the proximal tubule, Na^+ movement across the luminal membrane is partially linked to the *cotransport* of other solutes, as specific Na^+-glucose, Na^+-amino acid, and Na^+-phosphate carrier proteins are present in the brush border vesicles in the luminal membrane (Fig. 3-4).[19-21,22] Both sites must be occupied on the carrier for cotransport to occur.[19]

Na^+ entry also occurs by *countertransport* (or antiport) with H^+, as the carrier promotes both Na^+ reabsorption and H^+ secretion into the lumen (the latter step leading primarily to HCO_3^- reabsorption; see Chap. 11).[23,24]

As an example, one experiment used to document Na^+-dependent glucose reabsorption is illustrated by the study of proximal brush border vesicles in Fig. 3-5. The glucose concentration was the same in the bath and the vesicle, leading to no glucose uptake into the vesicle in the absence of a transvesicle Na^+ gradient. However, glucose uptake was markedly stimulated when the bath Na^+ concentration was elevated to 10 times that in the vesicle.

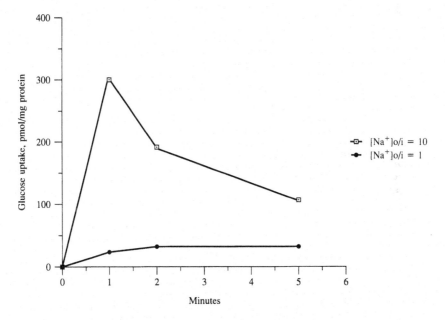

Figure 3-5   Time course of D-glucose uptake in response to changes in the electrochemical potential in proximal brush border luminal membrane vesicles. Vesicles were initially incubated so that the Na^+, K^+, and glucose concentrations were the same in the medium and the vesicle. In this setting, there was minimal glucose uptake by the vesicles (closed circles). If, however, the vesicles were bathed in a medium in which the Na^+ concentration ($[Na^+]_0$) was 10 times that inside the vesicle ($[Na^+]_i$), there was a marked stimulation of glucose uptake (open squares) despite the absence of a transvesicle glucose gradient. These findings indicate the presence of a Na^+-glucose cotransporter. Although not shown, creation of a favorable glucose gradient was able to enhance the uptake of Na^+. (*Adapted from Beck JC, Sacktor B*, J Biol Chem *253:5531, 1978. Used with permission.*)

The mechanism by which coupled transport occurs is incompletely understood. The binding of the cotransported solute (as with glucose) appears to lead to a conformational change in the transport protein that results in opening of the gate for a transmembrane Na^+ pathway. As a result, Na^+ crosses the membrane down its favorable inward gradient, and flow of the cotransported solute is in some way linked to that of Na^+;[25] the helical structure of these transporters appears to facilitate this process.[26] This passive process is called *secondary active transport*, since the energy is indirectly provided by the Na^+-K^+-ATPase pump.

In addition to this primary role for Na^+, there is also evidence that the other solutes increase the reabsorption of Na^+. As an example, the removal of glucose, amino acids, and/or bicarbonate from the luminal fluid markedly impairs proximal Na^+ reabsorption.[27,28] Two factors may contribute to this effect: (1) attachment of the cotransported solute to the carrier may increase its affinity for Na^+, and (2) glucose and bicarbonate are effective osmoles that, as they accumulate in the intercellular space, promote the passive reabsorption of NaCl and H_2O across the tight junction (see "Passive Mechanisms of Proximal Transport" below).

Movement into the Intercellular Space

At the basolateral membrane, Na^+ that has entered the cell must be transported into the intercellular space against electrical and concentration gradients (Fig. 3-4). The energy required for this process is derived from the hydrolysis of ATP by the Na^+-K^+-ATPase pump. This pump, which is also essential for Na^+ reabsorption in other nephron segments,[13] transports Na^+ out of the cell and K^+ into the cell in a $3:2$, not a $1:1$, ratio (Fig. 3-4).[29]

Solutes other than Na^+ move passively across the basolateral membrane, again by carrier-mediated transport. As depicted in Fig. 3-4, for example, carbonic acid (H_2CO_3) within the cell dissociates into H^+ and HCO_3^- ions. The former is secreted into the lumen by the Na^+-H^+ antiporter, whereas HCO_3^- is returned to the systemic circulation by a $3HCO_3^-/1Na^+$ carrier in the basolateral membrane.[30]

The energy for this process is derived from a more complex form of secondary active transport. The central step is again the Na^+-K^+-ATPase pump, which pumps K^+ into the cell, thereby raising the cell K^+ concentration. The latter change promotes passive K^+ exit from the cell via K^+ channels in the basolateral membrane, a process that makes the cell interior *negative* with respect to the interstitium; this potential then drives the net transfer of negative charge out of the cell via the $3HCO_3^-/1Na^+$ carrier.

Note that K^+ entry into the cells via the Na^+-K^+-ATPase pump and the backleak of this K^+ out of the cells varies in parallel with Na^+ transport. The link between these processes appears to be ATP, which normally inhibits the basolateral K^+ channels.[31] If, for example, Na^+ reabsorption rises, the associated elevation in Na^+-K^+-ATPase activity will lower cell ATP stores, thereby removing the inhibitory effect of ATP and increasing the number of open K^+ channels in the basolateral membrane. Thus, the extra K^+ that has been pumped into the cells can diffuse back out.

These reabsorptive processes are dependent upon the maintenance of normal membrane polarity in which the transporters, channels, and Na^+-K^+-ATPase pump are correctly located. Both experimental animals and humans often have delayed recovery of tubular Na^+ reabsorption after a period of renal ischemia.[32,33] Studies in animals suggest that this defect may result from the loss of membrane polarity, as an ischemia-induced increase in the permeability of the tight junction allows the lateral movement of Na^+-K^+-ATPase pumps from the basolateral to the luminal membrane.[34-36] Loss of Na^+-K^+-ATPase pumps from the proximal tubule basolateral membrane has also been demonstrated in renal transplant recipients in whom there is a delay in graft reperfusion.[37]

Mechanisms of Chloride Reabsorption

After Na^+, Cl^- is the most prevalent ion in the filtrate. Both active and passive processes contribute to proximal Cl^- reabsorption, each of which is indirectly linked to active Na^+ transport.[38] Active Cl^- reabsorption appears to occur via an anion exchanger in the luminal membrane, in which luminal Cl^- is exchanged at least in part for cellular *formate*. Although the formate concentration is only about 0.25 to 0.5 meq/L in the filtrate, this anion is able to promote Cl^- reabsorption because it is recycled across the luminal membrane (Fig. 3-6).[38-40] Filtered formate initially combines with H^+ secreted by the Na^+-H^+ antiporter to form formic acid (HF). The latter is uncharged and able to freely diffuse across the luminal membrane. The cell, however, has a lower H^+ concentration than the lumen, due to the secretion of H^+. As a result, the reaction

$$HF \leftrightarrow H^+ + formate$$

within the cell is driven to the right. The H^+ is then secreted again, while the formate returns to the lumen via a *formate-chloride exchanger*.[40-42] Formic acid is reformed in the lumen, and the process can be repeated. The energy for these ion exchangers is again provided indirectly by the Na^+-K^+-ATPase pump. By maintaining a low cell Na^+ concentration, this pump allows the continued Na^+-H^+ exchange that is essential for formate recycling. If, on the other hand, the proximal Na^+-H^+ exchanger is inhibited, there is a parallel inhibition of almost all of active transcellular chloride transport.[42,43]

The quantitative role of formate in Cl^- reabsorption is uncertain. As a result, it has been speculated that other anion exchangers, such as chloride-hydroxyl or chloride-oxalate exchangers, also play a contributory role.[40-42,44,45] Regardless of the mechanism, the reabsorbed Cl^- is returned to the systemic circulation across the basolateral membrane. Both a selective Cl^- channel and a KCl cotransporter appear to contribute to Cl^- exit,[40,46] but other transporters also may a role.[47] The energy of these transport processes is respectively provided by the cell interior negative potential and by the high cell K^+ concentration in relation to that in the interstitium.

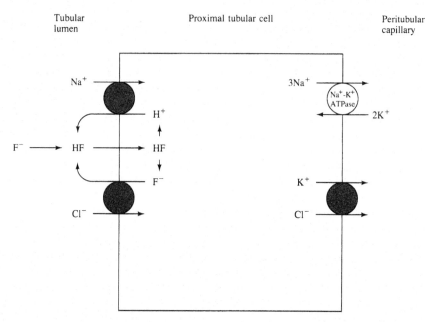

Figure 3-6 Role of filtered formate (F^-) in active Cl^- reabsorption in the proximal tubule. The essential steps are transport of uncharged formic acid (HF) into the cell, formate secretion and Cl^- reabsorption via a formate-chloride exchanger, and recycling of formate into the cell as formic acid. Reabsorbed Cl^- is returned to the peritubular capillary by a KCl cotransporter in the basolateral membrane.

Passive Mechanisms of Proximal Transport

Passive mechanisms appear to account for about *one-third* of proximal fluid reabsorption.[11,12,14] The mechanism by which this occurs is as follows: The early proximal convoluted tubule reabsorbs most of the filtered glucose, amino acids, and HCO_3^-, but a lesser amount of Cl^- (Fig. 3-1). Water is then reabsorbed down an osmotic gradient.[14]

The net effect is that the tubular fluid has an osmolality similar to that of the plasma, a *higher chloride concentration*, and relatively little glucose, bicarbonate, or amino acids. In contrast, the intercellular spaces in the later segments of the proximal tubule have solute concentrations similar to that of the plasma, since they are in equilibrium with fluid in the peritubular capillary (Fig. 3-7). If the tight junction were equally permeable to all solutes, there would be no net fluid movement, since the effective osmolalities of the two solutions would be similar. However, the permeability to Cl^- exceeds that to the other solutes, particularly HCO_3^-.[14,48]

In this setting, passive fluid reabsorption can occur across the tight junction into the intercellular space by two mechanisms*:

---

* Passive fluid reabsorption appears to occur only in the outer cortical and midcortical nephrons. In contrast, active Na^+ transport appears to account for almost all NaCl reabsorption in the juxtamedullary proximal tubules, which are not preferentially permeable to chloride.[12,48]

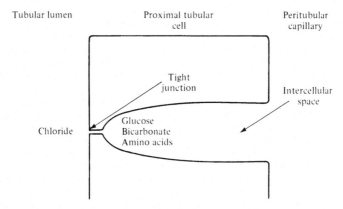

Figure 3-7   Schematic representation of the differences in solute composition between the lumen and the intercellular space in the later segments of the proximal tubule. In comparison to the plasma and intercellular space, the lumen has a very low concentration of bicarbonate, glucose, and amino acids but a relatively high chloride concentration.

- Chloride can traverse the tight junction down its concentration gradient, with sodium and water then following down respective electrical and osmotic gradients. (Bicarbonate, glucose, and amino acids do not move in the opposite direction to the same degree, since the tight junction is much less permeable to these solutes.) The presence of primary Cl^- transport has been demonstrated by the finding of a transepithelial potential difference that is *lumen-positive* (due to the reabsorption of the anion Cl^-) in the late proximal tubule.[12] The potential difference would be lumen-negative if Na^+ transport were the primary event.

- Water can move across the tight junction down an osmotic gradient, with sodium chloride following both by solvent drag and by diffusion, since the loss of water raises the solute concentrations in the lumen.[4] This movement of water occurs because the tight junction is preferentially permeable to Cl^-;[48] as a result, Cl^- is a relatively *ineffective* osmole (see Chap 1). Thus, the *effective osmolality* in the intercellular space exceeds that in the lumen (thereby promoting water reabsorption), even though the total osmolality is the same in both compartments.[15]

It is likely that HCO_3^- is the most important of the solutes that promote passive transport, since it is present in the highest concentration [24 mmol/L versus only 5 mmol/L (90 mg/dL) for glucose]. A clinical example of the effect of HCO_3^- is seen in the response to the administration of acetazolamide. This proximally acting diuretic is a carbonic anhydrase inhibitor that diminishes the reabsorption of bicarbonate. It also produces a substantial reduction in proximal NaCl reabsorption, even though it has no known direct action on Cl^- transport.[49] This chloruresis presumably reflects diminished passive reabsorption, resulting from the decrease in HCO_3^- transport.

A similar reduction in proximal NaCl reabsorption occurs in metabolic acidosis, a disorder in which the plasma HCO_3^- concentration is decreased (see Chap. 19).[50] In this setting, less HCO_3^- is filtered (because of the low plasma level), and therefore less is available for proximal reabsorption.

In summary, other than the Na^+-K^+-ATPase pump, the *Na^+-H^+ antiporter is the main determinant of proximal Na^+ and water reabsorption*. It has three major effects on proximal transport: (1) It directly promotes HCO_3^- reabsorption, particularly in the early proximal tubule; (2) the preferential reabsorption of HCO_3^- and water creates the gradient for the passive reabsorption of Cl^-; and (3) it promotes active Cl^- reabsorption by operating in parallel with the Cl^-/formate and other Cl^-/anion exchangers. It is not surprising, therefore, that activity of the Na^+-H^+ exchanger varies appropriately with salt intake, increasing on a low-salt diet (when enhanced proximal reabsorption will tend to prevent volume depletion) and decreasing on a high-salt diet.[51]

Neurohumoral influences These diet-induced changes in proximal Na^+-H^+ exchange and NaCl and water reabsorption are mediated at least in part by angiotensin II and norepinephrine.[51-54]* The secretion of these hormones varies inversely with the effective circulating volume (see Chap. 8). Thus, volume depletion increases angiotensin II and norepinephrine release, leading to enhanced proximal transport and an appropriate reduction in urinary sodium excretion.

Although angiotensin II increases the activity of the Na^+-H^+ exchanger and enhances HCO_3^- reabsorption in the early (S_1 segment) proximal tubule, it does not induce an important change in net proximal HCO_3^- transport. This finding is related to the flow dependence of HCO_3^- but not Cl^- reabsorption in the latter S_2 segment. Thus, the increase in HCO_3^- reabsorption in the initial proximal tubule leads to a reduction in HCO_3^- delivery to (and therefore a fall in HCO_3^- reabsorption in) the later proximal segments.[52,55] The net effect is no net change in delivery of HCO_3^- out of the proximal tubule. There is, however, decreased distal Cl^- delivery, since there is no adaptive decrease in late proximal Cl^- transport.[55]

Thus, angiotensin II has an overall stimulatory effect on proximal NaCl and H_2O reabsorption, but not usually on net acidification. Angiotensin II may be responsible for as much as 40 to 50 percent of NaCl and H_2O transport in the S_1 segment.[56] There is a much smaller effect in the more distal proximal tubule, where there are fewer angiotensin II receptors.

Dopamine is another hormone that regulates proximal transport, acting to *diminish* Na^+ reabsorption. This effect is associated with partial inhibition of both of the major steps involved in transtubular Na^+ transport: (1) decreased activity of the Na^+-H^+ exchanger, thereby reducing the entry of luminal Na^+ into the cell,[54,57] and (2) reduced activity of the basolateral Na^+-K^+-ATPase pump,

---

*Angiotensin II and norepinephrine also promote proximal transport by their vasoconstrictive effects, which, by increasing the filtration fraction, increases uptake of the reabsorbate by the peritubular capillary (see below).

perhaps due to phosphorylation of the pump by a dopamine-dependent phosphoprotein.[58,59]

These actions of dopamine may be physiologically important, since dopamine production is enhanced by volume expansion. Furthermore, blocking the effect of dopamine with a receptor antagonist attenuates the natriuretic response to volume expansion.[60]

Capillary Uptake

The movement of the reabsorbate from the intercellular space into the peritubular capillary (derived from the efferent arteriole) is governed by Starling's forces (Fig. 3-8):

$$\text{Capillary uptake} = \text{LpS} (\Delta \text{ oncotic pressure} - \Delta \text{ hydraulic pressure})$$

$$= \text{LpS}\left(s\left[\pi_{ptc} - \pi_{if}\right] - \left[P_{ptc} - P_{if}\right]\right)$$

where Lp is the unit porosity of the capillary wall, S is the surface area available for absorption, s is the reflection coefficient of proteins across the capillary wall (ranging from 0 if freely permeable to 1 if completely impermeable), π_{ptc} and π_{if} are the oncotic pressures in the peritubular capillary and interstitium, and P_{ptc} and P_{if} are the hydraulic pressures in the capillary and interstitium.

The approximate normal values for the hydraulic and oncotic pressures in the peritubular capillary are depicted in Fig. 3-8. The mean hydraulic pressure is much less than arterial pressure due to the resistances at the glomerular arterioles. In contrast, the oncotic pressure is higher than that in the systemic circulation because of the removal of protein-free filtrate in the glomerulus. Although the exact values are somewhat controversial, the net approximate effect is a relatively large gradient ($\pi_{ptc} - P_{ptc} = 13\,\text{mmHg}$) within the capillary that favors fluid

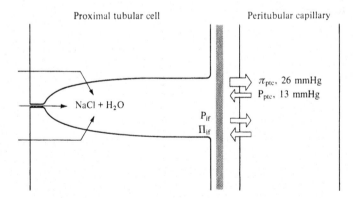

Figure 3-8   Role of Starling's forces in the uptake of the reabsorbate by the peritubular capillary. Approximate values for the capillary hydraulic and oncotic pressures are included and show a relatively large gradient favoring fluid movement into the capillary. The interstitial pressures are of lesser magnitude and tend to balance out, thereby making a smaller contribution to net fluid movement.

uptake from the intercellular space.[61] This gradient will be somewhat dissipated along the length of the proximal tubule, since uptake of the reabsorbate will lower the π_{ptc} by dilution. In comparison, the hydraulic and oncotic pressures in the interstitial fluid are of lesser magnitude (less than 5 mmHg) and generally make a smaller contribution to net fluid movement.[61]

One way that net fluid reabsorption can be regulated is by alterations in these capillary hemodynamic forces, which are influenced by glomerular arteriolar tone. As an example, the degree to which the systemic blood pressure is transmitted to the peritubular capillary is dependent upon glomerular arteriolar resistance. Arteriolar constriction increases the pressure drop across the glomerulus, thereby reducing peritubular capillary hydraulic pressure; arteriolar dilation, in comparison, allows the peritubular capillary pressure to rise toward that in the systemic circulation.

The capillary oncotic pressure, on the other hand, is determined by two factors: the baseline plasma protein concentration and the fraction of the renal plasma flow (RPF) that is filtered across the glomerulus (called the *filtration fraction*, GFR/RPF). If relatively more fluid is filtered, i.e., if the filtration fraction is increased, there will be a greater than usual elevation in the protein concentration in the fluid leaving the glomerulus and entering the peritubular capillary. Changes in the filtration fraction are primarily induced by changes in resistance at the *efferent* arteriole. Efferent arteriolar constriction will tend to raise the GFR (by increasing glomerular hydraulic pressure) and lower the RPF (because of the elevation in renal vascular resistance), thereby increasing the filtration fraction and the peritubular capillary oncotic pressure (see page 38).

Thus, alterations in peritubular capillary hemodynamics induced by efferent arteriolar constriction—increased oncotic pressure, reduced hydraulic pressure—promote capillary uptake and net proximal reabsorption. This becomes clinically important because both angiotensin II and norepinephrine, released in response to effective circulating volume depletion, increase the resistance at the efferent and, to a lesser degree, the afferent arterioles, thereby raising the filtration fraction.[62] In congestive heart failure, for example, angiotensin II and norepinephrine levels, the filtration fraction, and proximal reabsorption are all frequently elevated, thereby contributing to the low rate of Na^+ and water excretion that is commonly seen (see Chap. 16).[63] (As described above, angiotensin II and norepinephrine also promote proximal Na^+ reabsorption via stimulation of Na^+-H^+ exchange.[52,54,56])

Backflux across the Tight Junction

The mechanism by which changes in peritubular capillary hemodynamics influence proximal reabsorption is incompletely understood.[4] It has been suggested that fluid transported into the intercellular space can either move into the peritubular capillary or leak back into the lumen across the tight junction. This choice is influenced in part by the balance of Starling's forces across the capillary wall. In volume expansion, for example, enhanced movement of raffinose or sucrose from the peritubular capillary into the tubular lumen has been demonstrated.[64] Since these sugars do not enter cells, this movement must reflect increased permeability of the tight junction, and suggests that the associated reduction in proximal reabsorption may be mediated by increased backflux from the intercellular space into the lumen.

Changes in capillary hemodynamics may play an important role in this response. Both angiotensin II and norepinephrine release are diminished by hypervolemia; the ensuing efferent arteriolar dilation could lower the filtration fraction and impair capillary uptake, thereby promoting backleak across the tight junction.

There is, however, a major problem with this passive backflux theory. Microperfusion studies have demonstrated that lowering the oncotic pressure in the peritubular capillary reduces the reabsorption of NaCl, but not that of glucose or HCO_3^-.[65] Although this could be explained by the known higher permeability of the tight junction to Cl^-,[14,48] it is the active, not passive reabsorption of NaCl that is impaired.[66]

Glomerulotubular Balance

The efficiency with which proximal transport is regulated can be appreciated from the phenomenon of glomerulotubular balance. The urinary excretion of Na^+ and water is equal to the difference between the amount filtered across the glomerulus and the amount reabsorbed by the tubules. To maintain the extracellular fluid volume, it is important that tubular reabsorption varies with the spontaneous changes (some of which are diet-induced) that can occur in the GFR.

As an example, a normal adult male filters approximately 180 L/day (125 mL/min); the urine output, however, is usually only 1 to 2 liters, as over 98 percent of the filtrate is reabsorbed. If there were a slight elevation in GFR to 183 L/day but no change in tubular reabsorption, the result would be a 3-liter increase in urine output and a serious reduction in the extracellular fluid volume. Fortunately, this does not occur, since, over a wide range of spontaneous and experimental variations in the GFR, there is a proportional change in tubular reabsorption.[67-69] Thus, a 1.5 percent increase in the GFR (from 180 to 183L/day) is associated with a similar increment in tubular reabsorption, resulting in only a small elevation in the urine output.

This response, in which the absolute level of tubular reabsorption is directly related to the filtration rate, is called *glomerulotubular balance*. Notice that at all levels of GFR in Fig. 3-9, approximately 60 percent of the filtrate is reabsorbed in the proximal tubule. Similarly, the more distal nephron segments reabsorb a constant fraction of the load delivered to them from the proximal tubule.[68,69] This is another way to define glomerulotubular balance: that the fractional tubular reabsorption remains roughly constant despite changes in the GFR.

The mechanism by which glomerulotubular balance is mediated in the proximal tubule is incompletely understood, but both peritubular and luminal factors are thought to contribute.[67,70,71] If, for example, the GFR increases while RPF remains constant, the protein concentration in the plasma leaving the glomerulus will rise due to the loss of more protein-free filtrate. The ensuing elevation in the oncotic pressure in the peritubular capillary can then enhance net proximal reabsorption.[70,71]

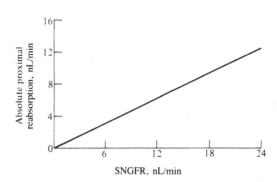

Figure 3-9   Glomerulotubular balance in the proximal tubule. Since fractional Na^+ and water reabsorption remains constant, absolute proximal reabsorption in a nephron is directly proportional to the single nephron glomerular filtration rate (SNGFR). A similar relationship between absolute Na^+ reabsorption and the amount of Na^+ delivered to the segment is present in the loop of Henle and the distal tubule. (*Adapted from Spitzer A, Brandis M, J Clin Invest 53:279, 1974, by copyright permission of the American Society for Clinical Investigation.*)

It is likely that the presence of factors in the filtrate that enhance Na^+ and H_2O reabsorption also play a major role in glomerulotubular balance in the proximal tubule.[67] As described above, bicarbonate, glucose, and amino acids augment Na^+ reabsorption both by cotransporting carriers in the luminal membrane (Fig. 3-4) and by the subsequent creation of chloride and osmotic gradients for passive reabsorption (Fig. 3-7). An elevation in GFR will augment the filtered load of these (and other) solutes, and their subsequent reabsorption can contribute to glomerulotubular balance for Na^+ and H_2O.[67]

Glomerulotubular balance in the proximal tubule, loop of Henle, and distal tubule is one of three intrarenal mechanisms that act to prevent fluid delivery from exceeding the limited total reabsorptive capacity of the collecting tubules.[69] The others are *autoregulation*, which keeps the GFR relatively constant despite variations in renal arterial pressure, and *tubuloglomerular feedback*, which lowers the GFR if the load to the macula densa segment of the early distal tubule is increased (see Chap. 2). Thus, one view of nephron function is that the proximal tubule and loop of Henle are responsible for the reabsorption of the bulk of the filtrate, with the distal nephron (particularly the collecting tubules) making small variations in electrolyte and water excretion in accordance with changes in intake.[69] This process operates most efficiently if the distal delivery of filtrate is kept at a nearly constant level.

The relationship between glomerular filtration and tubular reabsorption is not fixed, and may be reset at a different level when there are changes in the effective circulating volume (see Chap. 8). The fraction of the filtered Na^+ and water reabsorbed in the proximal tubule tends to be *increased by volume depletion and decreased by volume expansion*.[73,74] These changes are appropriate, however, since the maintenance of constant fractional Na^+ reabsorption is not desirable in these conditions. Enhanced reabsorption leading to Na^+ and water retention is a proper response to volume depletion. As mentioned previously, these changes are mediated at least in part by angiotensin II and nonrepinephrine (either circulating or released from the renal sympathetic nerves).[52,54-56]

Summary

The proximal tubule reabsorbs isosmotically about 55 to 60 percent of the filtrate. This process occurs in three steps: entry into the cell across the luminal membrane, movement across the basolateral membrane into the intercellular space, and uptake by the peritubular capillary. Despite the large amount of reabsorption that occurs, the only major active (energy-requiring) step is mediated by the Na^+-K^+-ATPase pump in the basolateral membrane. In addition to directly promoting Na^+ reabsorption, this pump maintains the low cell Na^+ concentration that allows passive Na^+ entry into the cell.

The reabsorption of many other solutes (such as glucose, phosphate, amino acids, and bicarbonate) occurs by carrier-mediated coupled transport with Na^+ across the luminal membrane. Furthermore, the preferential reabsorption of these solutes with Na^+ in the early proximal tubule creates osmotic and concentration gradients that permit about one-third of total proximal Na^+ and H_2O reabsorption to occur passively through the tight junction (see Fig. 3-7).

Uptake by the peritubular capillary of fluid transported into the intercellular space is regulated by Starling's forces. Depending upon the magnitude of these forces, which can be influenced by vasoactive hormones, the reabsorbate either enters the capillary and is returned to the systemic circulation or leaks back into the lumen across the tight junction. Modulations in net proximal tubular reabsorption appear to be influenced by luminal, peritubular capillary, and neurohumoral factors.

The data upon which the above conclusions are based were primarily obtained from studies in experimental animals. Human studies are, of course, more limited. However, the importance of luminal membrane cotransporters in humans was suggested by findings in an infant who was born without the proximal tubular brush border and presumably without the carrier proteins that it normally contains. This child had *no tubular reabsorption* of glucose, amino acids, or phosphate, as evidenced by a rate of excretion for these compounds that was essentially equal to the filtered load (determined from the GFR times the plasma concentration).[75] The plasma bicarbonate concentration was 11 meq/L (normal equals about 24 meq/L); assuming that proximal bicarbonate reabsorption by the Na^+-H^+ antiporter was also negligible, this value of 11 meq/L presumably reflects the bicarbonate reabsorptive capacity of the more distal segments. This distal contribution probably explains why patients with type 2 (or proximal) renal tubular acidosis, who have an impairment in proximal bicarbonate reabsorption, usually are able to maintain their plasma bicarbonate concentration at or above 12 meq/mL (see Chap. 19).

PRIMACY OF SODIUM TRANSPORT IN PROXIMAL TUBULAR FUNCTION

The relationship between the proximal reabsorption of sodium and that of many other filtered solutes is often important clinically. This is particularly true in hypovolemic states, in which the increase in proximal Na^+ transport is associated with a *parallel rise in the reabsorption of bicarbonate, urea, calcium, and uric acid.* The remainder of this chapter will review the different transport systems for these solutes (both in the proximal tubule and in other nephron segments) and the potential clinical relevance of their relationship to Na^+ reabsorption. In many cases, the changes that occur are at the expense of the homeostatic requirements for these solutes.

Bicarbonate

Approximately 80 percent of the filtered HCO_3^- is reabsorbed in the proximal tubule and the remainder in the distal tubule and collecting tubules. HCO_3^- reabsorption is accomplished by the active transport of H^+ from the cell into the lumen; this process is mediated primarily by the Na^+-H^+ antiporter in the proximal tubule and by a H^+-ATPase pump in the distal nephron (see Chap. 11).

Relation of $T_{mHCO_3^-}$ to sodium transport   The term $T_{mHCO_3^-}$ refers to the maximum tubular reabsorptive capacity for HCO_3^- per unit time. To measure this parameter, $NaHCO_3^-$ is infused intravenously to raise the plasma HCO_3^- concentration and, therefore, the filtered load. Tubular reabsorption, measured in milliequivalents of HCO_3^- reabsorbed per minute, can then be calculated from

Tubular reabsorption = filtered load − urinary excretion

$$= GFR \times plasma\,[HCO_3^-] - urine\,[HCO_3^-] \times volume$$

The results of such an experiment are illustrated in Fig. 3-10. There appears to be a maximum HCO_3^- reabsorption of 26 to 28 meq/L of glomerular filtrate.* This would be an appropriate mechanism by which the kidney prevents the plasma HCO_3^- concentration from exceeding the normal value of 22 to 26 meq/L, since the extra HCO_3^- would be excreted in the urine. However, the proximal reabsorption of HCO_3^- is linked (by the Na^+-H^+ antiporter) to Na^+ transport, and the infusion of $NaHCO_3$ expands the extracellular volume, a stimulus known to diminish proximal Na^+ and perhaps HCO_3^- reabsorption.[73,76]

Figure 3-11 depicts the results of two HCO_3^- titration experiments in a patient with moderate renal failure. When $NaHCO_3^-$ induced volume expansion was allowed to occur, HCO_3^- reabsorption reached a plateau when the plasma HCO_3^- concentration was 28 meq/L. In comparison, when volume expansion was minimized by prior volume depletion, HCO_3^- reabsorption continued to rise even when the plasma HCO_3^- concentration reached 36 meq/L. In the rat, a $T_{mHCO_3^-}$ cannot be demonstrated if hypervolemia is prevented, even if the plasma HCO_3^- concentration is greater than 60 meq/L.[76]

These observations demonstrate that there is *no absolute T_m for HCO_3^-*, since the reabsorptive capacity varies directly with the fractional reabsorption of

---

* Since the $T_{mHCO_3^-}$ is measured in meq reabsorbed per minute, the maximum reabsorption of 28 meq/L of glomerular filtrate must be corrected for the GFR. If the GFR were 125 mL/min (or 0.125 L/min), then the $T_{mHCO_3^-}$ would be 3.5 meq/min (28 meq/L × 0.125 L/min).

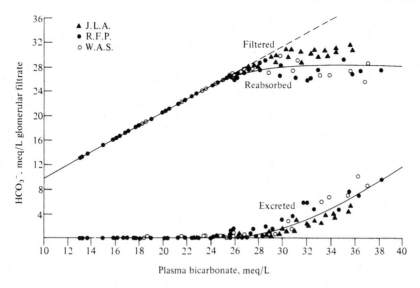

Figure 3-10 Filtration, reabsorption, and excretion of bicarbonate as a function of plasma concentration in normal humans. (*From Pitts RF, Ayer J, Shiess W,* J Clin Invest *28:35, 1949, by copyright permission of the American Society for Clinical Investigation.*)

Na^+.[76,77] This assumes clinical importance in patients with volume depletion and metabolic alkalosis (high plasma HCO_3^- concentration, elevated arterial pH). The normal response to an increase in the plasma HCO_3^- concentration is to excrete the excess HCO_3^- in the urine. However, hypovolemia and the associated hypochloremia enhance HCO_3^- reabsorption, resulting in the retention of the excess HCO_3^- and perpetuation of the alkalosis (see Chap. 18). HCO_3^- excretion will rise only if the stimulus to Na^+ and Cl^- retention is removed by the restoration of normovolemia.

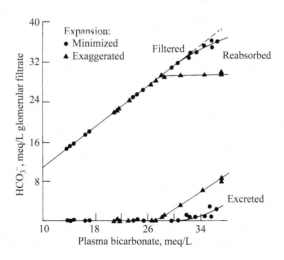

Figure 3-11 Bicarbonate titration curves obtained from a patient with a GFR of 37 mL/min studied under conditions of minimized and exaggerated expansion of extracellular fluid volume. (*From Slatopolsky E, Hoffsten P, Purkerson M, Bricker NS,* J Clin Invest *49:988, 1970, by copyright permission of the American Society for Clinical Investigation.*)

Glucose

Under normal conditions, all the filtered glucose is reabsorbed in the proximal tubule and returned to the systemic circulation via the peritubular capillaries. This process occurs in two steps. Filtered glucose enters the cell by passive cotransport with Na^+ (even though glucose moves uphill against a concentration gradient) (see Fig. 3-5);[19,20] it then leaves the cell at the basolateral membrane, probably by diffusion via specific glucose transporters that are Na^+-independent and that are limited to the basolateral membrane.[78,79]

The Na^+-glucose cotransporters have different characteristics in the different proximal segments.[20] The S_1 and S_2 segments have a high-capacity, low-affinity carrier that is able to remove most of the filtered glucose. (This glucose is largely returned to the systemic circulation, since these segments do not primarily use glucose for oxidative metabolism).[80]

The high degree of early proximal reabsorption results in relatively little glucose being delivered to the S_3 segment. To reabsorb the remaining glucose, the carrier at this site has a higher affinity and a $2:1$ binding ratio, i.e., $2Na^+:1$ glucose. Thus, the additive effect of the favorable inward gradient of two Na^+ ions is used to drive the uphill transport of glucose against an increasing concentration gradient.[19] Similar differences are present in the glucose transporters in the basolateral membrane that return reabsorbed glucose to the systemic circulation: low-affinity in the S_1 segment; and high-affinity in the later parts of the proximal tubule.[78]

The cDNAs for the high-capacity, low-affinity carrier, termed $SGLT_2$, and the low capacity high-affinity carrier, termed $SGLT_1$, have both been cloned and sequenced.[81,82] Both transporters are highly homologous at the amino acid level and are able to transport sodium and glucose via transmembrane pores. $SGLT_2$ is found exclusively in the proximal tubule, while $SGLT_1$ is also expressed in the gastrointestinal tract.

Studies in normovolemic subjects have shown a T_m for glucose of approximately 375 mg/min (Fig. 3-12). Thus, glucose should not appear in the urine until the filtered load exceeds this value. If the GFR is 125 mL/min, glucosuria should not begin until the plasma glucose concentration is greater than 300 mg/dL [125 mL/min × 3 mg/mL (or 300 mg/dL) equals 375 mg/min]. (The normal plasma glucose concentration is 60 to 100 mg/dL, fasting.)

However, glucose can usually be detected in the urine when the plasma glucose concentration exceeds 180 to 200 mg/dL. This deviation from the T_m is called *splay* and has been ascribed to heterogeneity in the relationship between glomerular size and proximal tubular length within individual nephrons.[83] A nephron with a large glomerulus (i.e., high filtered load) or a relatively short proximal tubule (i.e., low reabsorptive capacity) will spill glucose in the urine at a lower plasma glucose concentration than predicted from the T_m for the whole kidney.

Clinically, glucosuria is most commonly seen when the filtered load is increased due to hyperglycemia in uncontrolled diabetes mellitus. Less often, there is a defect in proximal reabsorption that may be selective, as in renal glucosuria,[84] or part of a generalized abnormality in proximal transport, as in

Figure 3-12 Filtration, reabsorption, and excretion of glucose as a function of plasma concentration in normal humans. The curves for reabsorption and secretion are drawn in two ways: (1) as idealized, sharply breaking curves; and (2) as rounded curves more descriptive of the true relationships. With a T_m for glucose of 375 mg/min and a GFR of 125 mL/min, glucose excretion should not begin until the plasma glucose concentration is greater than 300 mg/dL (sharply breaking curve). However, due to tubular heterogeneity (see text), there is "splay" in the glucose titration curve (rounded curves) and glucosuria beings when then the plasma glucose concentration exceeds 180 to 200 mg/dL, well before the saturation of tubular reabsorptive capacity. The relative lack of splay in the HCO_3^- titration curve (Fig. 3-10) may be due to the ability of distal HCO_3^- reabsorption to compensate for variations in proximal transport. This is in contrast to glucose, which is reabsorbed entirely in the proximal tubule. (*From Pitts RF,* Physiology of the Kidney and Body Fluids, *3d ed. Copyright © 1974 by Year Book Medical Publishers, Inc, Chicago. Used by permission. Adapted from Wright HR, Russo HF, Sheggs HR, et al,* Am J Physiol *149:130, 1947.*)

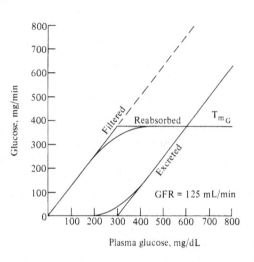

the Fanconi syndrome.[85] In renal glucosuria, the appearance of glucose in the urine at a normal plasma glucose concentration is thought to be due either to a decreased number of glucose carriers or to a reduction in the affinity of the carriers for glucose.[86]

Urea

Urea, which is an end product of protein metabolism, is lipid-soluble and able to cross most cell membranes by passive diffusion. The reabsorption of water in the proximal tubule increases the tubular fluid urea concentration, thereby allowing urea to be reabsorbed passively down a concentration gradient. This may be facilitated by a constitutive transporter. Urea also is reabsorbed in the more distal nephron segments, the importance of which will be discussed in Chap. 4. The net effect is that only 50 to 60 percent of the filtered urea is normally excreted.

The urea concentration in the blood is measured as the blood urea nitrogen (BUN). The BUN tends to vary inversely with the GFR, a reflection of the importance of glomerular filtration in urea excretion (see Chap. 2). Thus, an elevation in the BUN is often due to a fall in GFR. There are, however, two important exceptions: conditions associated with enhanced urea production, such as gastrointestinal bleeding, corticosteroid therapy, or a high-protein diet; and volume depletion, in which the increase in proximal Na^+ and H_2O reabsorption results in enhanced urea reabsorption and consequently a rise in the BUN. This is referred to as *prerenal azotemia*, since the elevation in BUN is not due to renal disease and is associated with no or a lesser elevation in the plasma creatinine concentration.[87]

Calcium

Dietary Na^+, K^+, and Cl^- are almost completely absorbed in the gastrointestinal tract, and their steady-state concentrations in the extracellular fluid are maintained primarily by changes in urinary excretion. In contrast, calcium and phosphate absorption are incomplete, and variations in intestinal absorption and calcium phosphate release from bone, as well as in urinary excretion, contribute to the regulation of calcium and phosphate balance.

Approximately 40 percent of the plasma Ca^{2+} is bound to albumin and is not filtered at the glomerulus. Of the remaining 60 percent, 50 percent is physiologically important ionic (free) Ca^{2+}, and 10 percent is bound to citrate, bicarbonate, or phosphate. The filtered Ca^{2+} is reabsorbed throughout the nephron, with about 5 percent being excreted on a regular diet.[88] Approximately 80 to 85 percent of the filtered Ca^{2+} is reabsorbed in the proximal tubule and medullary loop of Henle; most, but not all, of this transport is passive, following gradients established by NaCl and water reabsorption.[89-91] Passive calcium reabsorption in the thick ascending limb occurs via the paracellular pathway, a process that appears to be facilitated by a tight junction protein called paracellin-1.[92]

The regulation of Ca^{2+} excretion according to physiologic needs appears to occur primarily in the cortical distal nephron, including the distal tubule and the adjacent cortical thick ascending limb of the loop of Henle and the connecting segment (see Fig. 1-3).[89,91,93] In these segments, parathyroid hormone (PTH) and to a lesser degree vitamin D stimulate Ca^{2+} reabsorption. PTH activates a hormone-specific adenylate cyclase system.[93,94-98] while vitamin D induces the production of calcium-binding proteins (calbindins)[99] and by enhancing the effect of PTH.[100]

Luminal Ca^{2+} appears to enter the cells through Ca^{2+} channels in the apical membrane, down a favorable electrochemical gradient (cell interior negative, low cell Ca^{2+} concentration of less than 200 nanomol/L).[95,97] PTH increases Ca^{2+} entry, although the mechanism by which this occurs is incompletely understood. It has been suggested that the primary effect of PTH is to increase the number of open Cl^- channels in the basolateral membrane; the ensuing loss of anionic chloride from the cell will hyperpolarize the cell membrane, thereby enhancing both the activity of the voltage-dependent Ca^{2+} channels in the luminal membrane and the gradient for passive Ca^{2+} entry into the cell.[93,97] A vitamin D–dependent calcium-binding protein also appears to facilitate Ca^{2+} uptake at the luminal membrane.[99]

Extrusion of this Ca^{2+} into the peritubular interstitium may then occur at least in part via a basolateral Ca^{2+}-ATPase pump or a $3Na^{+}$-$1Ca^{2+}$ exchanger.[89,95,101] The latter transporter, which may be responsible for up to 70 percent of calcium extrusion, uses the favorable inward electrochemical gradient for Na^{+} entry (in this setting occurring at the basolateral membrane) to drive the reabsorption of Ca^{2+}.[94,101] In addition to increasing the number of open Cl^{-} channels in the basolateral membrane, PTH may also increase the number of Na^{+}-Ca^{2+} exchangers, thereby enhancing Ca^{2+} extrusion from the cell.[102,103]

Clinical Implications   The interaction between these humoral factors can be illustrated by the response to an increase in dietary calcium intake. The ensuing rise in Ca^{2+} absorption from the gut leads to a small elevation in the plasma Ca^{2+} concentration, which diminishes the release of both PTH and calcitriol (1,25-dihydroxycholecalciferol, the most active form of vitamin D; see Chap. 6). The net effect is reduced distal Ca^{2+} reabsorption and excretion of the excess Ca^{2+}.

The thick ascending limb also may contribute to the calciuric response after a calcium load. This effect appears to be mediated by the calcium-sensing receptor, which is expressed on the basolateral membrane of these cells (see "Magnesium" below).[104]

On the other hand, a reduction in the plasma Ca^{2+} concentration below 8.5 to 9 mg/dL (the lower limit of normal) usually results in a fall in urinary Ca^{2+} excretion to very low levels.[105] This response is mediated in part by hypocalcemia-induced stimulation of PTH and calcitriol secretion.

Let us now consider how these relationships are altered in patients with hypoparathyroidism.[105] Since PTH is the major stimulus to calcitriol synthesis, there is a deficiency of both hormones in this disorder. As a result, the relationship between the plasma Ca^{2+} concentration and urinary Ca^{2+} excretion is reset: The impairment in Ca^{2+} reabsorption leads to persistent calciuria even though the patient may have a plasma Ca^{2+} concentration below 7.5 mg/dL. If calcitriol is now given to correct the hypocalcemia, there will still be PTH deficiency and a persistent defect in distal Ca^{2+} transport. Consequently, an elevation in the plasma Ca^{2+} concentration to a still low level of 8 mg/dL may be associated with a significant rise in urinary Ca^{2+} excretion. Any attempt at further correction of the hypocalcemia will lead to increasing hypercalciuria and possible calcium stone formation.[105,106] Thus, the development of hypercalciuria often limits the degree to which the plasma Ca^{2+} concentration can be normalized.

The passive reabsorption of most of the filtered Ca^{2+} in the proximal tubule and loop of Henle also is important clinically, since it means that Ca^{2+} transport in these segments will be affected by changes in net NaCl transport. Thus, on a constant Ca^{2+} intake, variations in Na^{+} reabsorption (due to diet, drugs, or changes in the effective circulating volume) will alter both Na^{+} and Ca^{2+} excretion.[107]

These characteristics are useful in the therapy of hypercalcemia and of nephrolithiasis due to hypercalciuria.[88,107]

- Hypercalcemia can be corrected by increasing Ca^{2+} excretion. This can be achieved by decreasing Na^+ reabsorption in the proximal tubule with a high NaCl intake, and in the loop of Henle by the use of a diuretic that inhibits loop NaCl reabsorption, such as furosemide.
- Conversely, lowering calcium excretion may reduce the frequency of stone formation in patients with idiopathic hypercalciuria.[108] This can be achieved by increasing Na^+ and, secondarily, Ca^{2+} reabsorption in the proximal tubule and loop of Henle by inducing volume depletion with a low Na^+ intake and a diuretic.[107-109] However, the diuretic must act *distal to the medullary thick ascending limb* so that it can enhance the excretion of Na^+ without also increasing that of Ca^+. Both the thiazide diuretics, which act in the distal tubule, and amiloride, which acts in the connecting segment, are useful in this regard.

In addition to inducing volume depletion, these agents also lower Ca^{2+} excretion by directly stimulating distal Ca^{2+} reabsorption.[110,111] How this occurs is not well understood; it is likely to be indirect, since the two diuretics act by different mechanisms (see Chap. 15). One theory proposes a central role for enhanced Ca^{2+} uptake at the luminal membrane via a mechanisms similar to that noted above for parathyroid hormone.[111,112] According to this hypothesis, a diuretic-induced reduction in Cl^- entry across the luminal membrane combined with continued Cl^- exit through Cl^- channels in the basolateral membrane results in hyperpolarization of the cell.[111] The net effect is increased activity of the voltage-dependent luminal Ca^{2+} channels and an enhanced electrical gradient favoring Ca^{2+} uptake from the lumen.

The fall in the cell Na^+ concentration following diuretic-induced inhibition of Na^+ uptake also may play a contributory role.[95,103] This intracellular change will enhance the gradient for passive Na^+ entry across the basolateral membrane and therefore for Ca^{2+} extrusion from the cell via the basolateral Na^+-Ca^{2+} exchanger.

Phosphate

Eighty to ninety-five percent of the filtered phosphate is normally reabsorbed, with almost all of this occurring in the proximal tubule. Filtered phosphate initially moves from the lumen into the cell via specific Na^+-phosphate cotransporters in the luminal membrane.[22,113,114] These transporters generally have a $3Na^+ : 1HPO_4^{2-}$ stoichiometry; this allows the favorable inward gradient of three Na^+ ions to drive continued phosphate uptake despite a falling tubular fluid phosphate concentration.[115] High-affinity transporters in the late proximal tubule also contribute to the ability to reabsorb most of the filtered phosphate.[116] The phosphate that enters the cell then diffuses passively out across the basolateral membrane via an uncertain mechanism.[114]

There are three different Na^+-phosphate cotransporters.[22,117] Type II appears to be the most important Na^+-phosphate cotransporter within the proximal tubule, as evidenced by severe renal phosphate wasting in mice with targeted inactivation of this protein.[118]

Proximal phosphate transport is primarily regulated by two factors, both of which specifically affect the activity of the Na^+-phosphate carrier: the *plasma phosphate concentration* and *parathyroid hormone*.[114,119-121] A low-phosphate diet or hypophosphatemia, for example, leads to virtual abolition of phosphate excretion in the urine, an effect that is primarily mediated by increased activity of the type II cotransporter.[22,113,114] In mice without type II transporter genes, proximal phosphate transport with chronic phosphate deprivation is only 15 percent that of wild-type mice.[83]

In contrast, Na^+-phosphate carrier activity is diminished after a phosphate load,[120] resulting in an appropriate increase in urinary excretion. Although this in part represents a direct effect of the rise in plasma phosphate concentration,[120] increased secretion of PTH also plays a contributory role.[113,123] Enhanced PTH release in this setting occurs because phosphate loading can reduce the plasma Ca^{2+} concentration by driving the following reaction to the right

$$Ca^{2+} + HPO_4^{2-} \leftrightarrow CaHPO_4$$

and can decrease the renal production of calcitriol, thereby removing the normal inhibitory effect of this hormone on the parathyroid gland.[124,125]

Another factor that can affect proximal phosphate reabsorption is metabolic acidosis. In this setting, transporter activity is diminished, leading to an increase in phosphate excretion.[114] The phosphaturia is in part beneficial in that it enhances buffer excretion, thereby allowing more acid to be excreted. Two factors may be involved in this response: direct inhibition of the Na^+-phosphate cotransporter as the affinity for the Na^+ interaction is reduced,[115] and, due to the fall in tubular fluid pH, conversion of HPO_4^{2-} to $H_2PO_4^-$, which has a lower affinity for the phosphate binding site on the cotransporter.[114,126]

Magnesium

Circulating Mg^{2+} is partially protein-bound, so that only about 70 to 80 percent is filtered across the glomerulus. In general, about 3 percent of the filtered Mg^{2+} escapes reabsorption in humans and is excreted.[127,128] This value is appropriately increased after a Mg^{2+} load and falls to very low levels with Mg^{2+} depletion. In contrast to other solutes, however, most of the filtered Mg^{2+} (50 to 60 percent) is reabsorbed in the cortical thick ascending limb of the loop of Henle and distal convoluted tubule, not in the proximal tubule (20 to 30 percent).[127] Furthermore, alterations in Mg^{2+} excretion are primarily due to changes in loop transport. As an example, a low-Mg^{2+} diet leads to a rapid fall in Mg^{2+} excretion that is due to enhanced loop Mg^{2+} reabsorption and that may occur even before there is a fall in the plasma Mg^{2+} concentration or in the filtered Mg^{2+} load.[129]

The cellular mechanisms of Mg^{2+} transport in the thick ascending limb are incompletely understood. The bulk of Mg^{2+} transport appears to be passive, occurring by paracellular diffusion between the cells and being driven by the favorable electrical gradient resulting from the reabsorption of sodium chloride (see Fig. 4–2).[127,128,130] Paracellular magnesium reabsorption at this site appears to be facilitated by a tight junction protein called paracellin-1.[92]

Factors controlling Mg^{2+} transport act through changes on the voltage and/or permeability of the paracellular pathway. Thus, decreased reabsorption and Mg^{2+} wasting can be induced by the administration of a loop diuretic, which inhibits sodium and chloride reabsorption, or by mutations in the paracellin-1 gene.[92] Since paracellin-1 appears to mediate the passive reabsorption of calcium as well as magnesium, patients with mutations present with renal magnesium and calcium wasting.[92]

Magnesium transport in the cortical thick ascending limb is also influenced by variations in the plasma magnesium and/or calcium concentrations in a manner that permits Mg^{2+} reabsorption to vary appropriately with Mg^{2+} intake. This regulatory process is mediated in part by a calcium (and magnesium) sensing receptor located in the basolateral membrane of thick ascending limb cells.[104] Binding of calcium or magnesium to the extracellular domain of the receptor initiates a series of intracellular signals, which result in the inhibition of apical (luminal) potassium channels.[104,131] The latter effect will inhibit sodium chloride reabsorption, thereby increasing Mg^{2+} excretion by preventing the generation of passive gradients for Mg^{2+} reabsorption. This process is reversed by hypomagnesemia, resulting in a marked increase in loop reabsorption and a reduction in urinary excretion.

In addition to paracellular transport in the thick ascending limb, Mg^{2+} handling also involves an active transcellular process in the distal convoluted tubule.[127,132] This process may be activated by changes in the plasma Mg^{2+} concentration and may occur via a Na^+/Mg^{2+} exchanger.

A number of hormones, including ADH, parathyroid hormone, glucagon, calcitonin, and β-adrenergic agonists, can stimulate Mg^{2+} reabsorption in the cortical thick ascending limb and distal convoluted tubule via the generation of cyclic AMP.[133,134] It is not likely, however, that these responses play an important role in Mg^{2+} regulation, since the secretion of these hormones is not affected by alterations in Mg^{2+} balance.

Uric Acid

Uric acid is formed from metabolism of purine nucleotides. With a pK_a of about 5.35, the reaction

$$Uric\ acid \leftrightarrow Urate^- + H^+$$

is shifted far to the right at the normal arterial pH of 7.40. As a result, most uric acid circulates as the urate anion. Filtered urate is handled entirely in the proximal tubule, where three separate processes are involved.[135-137]

- Reabsorption of most of the filtered urate in the early proximal tubule
- Tubular secretion by the organic anion secretory pathway in the mid-proximal tubule of an amount normally equal to about 50 percent of the filtered load
- Postsecretory reabsorption of most of the secreted urate in the late proximal tubule.

The net effect is the excretion of 6 to 12 percent of the amount filtered. Alterations in excretion according to urate homeostasis are thought to be mediated primarily by changes in the rate of tubular secretion.

The mechanisms by which these processes occur is incompletely understood, but *anion exchangers* appear to play an important role. Urate *reabsorption*, for example, may be mediated by a urate$^-$-OH$^-$ (or urate$^-$-HCO$_3^-$) countertransporter in the luminal membrane that operates in parallel with the Na$^+$-H$^+$ exchanger (Fig. 3-13a).[136,137] The latter, which is driven by the low cell Na$^+$ concentration, creates a gradient in which the cell is more alkaline [and therefore has a higher OH$^-$ (and HCO$_3^-$ concentration) than the lumen. This favorable gradient for OH$^-$ exit can then drive urate reabsorption.

The subsequent exit of reabsorbed urate across the basolateral membrane may occur by facilitated diffusion down a favorable electrochemical gradient. Exchange with an interstitial anion, such as Cl$^-$ (which has a much higher concentration in the interstitium than in the cell), could also play a contributory role.[136] A urate transporter has been cloned that may play a role in urate excretion.[138]

The steps involved in urate *secretion* are less clear.[135,136] Urate may enter the cell at the basolateral membrane in exchange for a cell anion (see "Secretory Pathways," below) (Fig. 3-13b). Secretion across the luminal membrane could then occur by simple diffusion or in exchange for an anion such as Cl$^-$, which has a high luminal concentration and therefore a favorable gradient for entry into the cell.[135]

Although these models explain how urate can be transported, it still remains uncertain why urate is reabsorbed in the early and late portions of the proximal tubule and is secreted in the midportion. The current prevailing hypothesis is that net urate reabsorption or secretion within an anatomic segment is determined by the absolute number of reabsorption or secretion transporters located within the membranes of these segments.[135]

Net urate reabsorption also varies directly with proximal Na$^+$ transport, and in the presence of volume depletion, both Na$^+$ and urate excretion are reduced.[139] The mechanism by which urate handling is affected in this setting is incompletely understood, although angiotensin II may play a role. This hormone, the release of which is enhanced by hypovolemia, increases proximal Na$^+$-H$^+$ antiporter activity,[53,54] a change that could promote a parallel rise in urate$^-$-OH$^-$ exchange. In addition, increased proximal water reabsorption will enhance the tubular fluid urate concentration, thereby promoting urate entry into the cell.

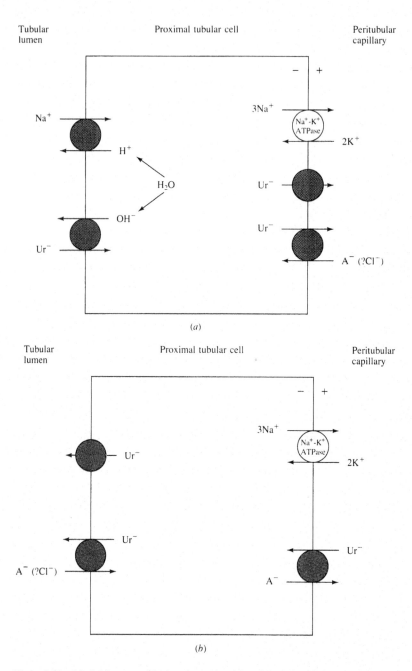

Figure 3-13 Model for urate (Ur⁻) reabsorption (*a*) and secretion (*b*) in the proximal tubule. (*a*) Urate reabsorption begins with entry into the cell via a urate⁻-OH⁻-exchanger that is driven by the pH gradient created by the Na⁺-H⁺ antiporter. The reabsorbed urate then leaves the cell by carrier-mediated diffusion or possibly by anion exchange with an anion such as Cl⁻. (*b*) Urate secretion, on the other hand, begins with urate entry into the cell across the basolateral membrane, probably in exchange for cell anions (A⁻), such as citric acid intermediates. Movement from cell to lumen can then occur by simple diffusion or by exchange with an anion which has a relatively high luminal concentration, such as Cl⁻.

Regardless of the mechanism, increased net proximal reabsorption is responsible for the elevation in the plasma urate concentration (hyperuricemia) frequently seen in patients on diuretic therapy. If, however, the diuretic-induced Na^+ and water losses are replaced, hyperuricemia does not develop, since there is no stimulus to Na^+ retention.[140]

Proteins

Filtered proteins are almost entirely reabsorbed in the proximal tubule. Several mechanisms are involved in this process, as proteins of different sizes have different transport systems.[141,142,143]

Amino acids primarily enter the cell by cotransport with sodium and then are returned to the systemic circulation by facilitated diffusion across the basolateral membrane.[21] There are several different sodium-dependent amino acid carriers, each of which recognizes different groups of amino acids.

There are also sodium-independent transporters for neutral amino acids (such as leucine, isoleucine, and phenylalanine) and for cystine and other dibasic amino acids (ornithine, arginine, and lysine).[144,145] Mutations in the gene named SCL3A1, which encodes a protein that mediates sodium-independent transport of cystine and dibasic acids in the proximal tubule and small intestine, are responsible for "classic" cystinuria.[146,147] This disorder is characterized by diminished reabsorption of cystine and the formation of cystine stones, since cystine is poorly soluble in urine.

There are also Na^+-dependent cotransporters in the basolateral membrane that allow some amino acids (such as glycine and glutamine) to enter the cell at both membranes. The physiologic importance of this effect is incompletely understood. The increased entry of glutamine may play a role in acid-base balance, since this amino acid is the primary source of ammonium production in the proximal tubule (see Chap. 11).

Larger proteins are handled differently.[141,142] Small peptides, such as angiotensin II, are hydrolyzed by brush border peptidases, and the amino acids are then reabsorbed. Larger compounds, such as insulin and lysozyme, enter the cell by carrier-mediated endocytosis and are then transported into lysosomes, where they are metabolized to amino acids.[141,148] The efficiency of endocytosis is in part dependent upon molecular change, with proteins that are cationic (that is, proteins that have an isoelectric point above that of the urine pH) being reabsorbed more completely than those that are anionic.[141,148,149] This charge dependence may reflect more avid binding of cationic proteins to anionic phospholipids in the luminal membrane.

In addition, albumin can be reabsorbed by a second, low-affinity, high-capacity endocytic process, when it is filtered in greater than normal amounts.[150] This most commonly occurs in the nephrotic syndrome, in which enhanced reabsorption and subsequent catabolism of filtered albumin may contribute to the associated hypoalbuminemia.

   The net effect of proximal reabsorption and catabolism of proteins is twofold: (1) the preservation of nitrogen balance by minimizing urinary losses and (2) participation in hormonal homeostasis, since the kidney is a major site of metabolism for polypeptide hormones such as insulin, gastrin, and glucagon.[141]

Citrate

In normal subjects, 65 to 90 percent of the filtered citrate is reabsorbed by, and then mostly metabolized in, the proximal tubule.[151] As with the uptake of most of the solutes, the entry of filtered citrate into the proximal tubular cells is dependent upon the favorable electrochemical gradient for Na^+ being mediated by a $3Na^+ : 1$ citrate^2-cotransporter in the luminal membrane, also called the Na^+/dicarboxylate cotransporter.[151-153]

   An important determinant of net citrate reabsorption is the state of acid-base balance.[151,154] Acidemia is associated with increased proximal citrate reabsorption. This change may be appropriate from the viewpoint of acid-base balance. The metabolism of each milliequivalent of citrate generates 3 meq of bicarbonate; thus, increasing citrate reabsorption with acidemia is beneficial in that it prevents the loss of alkali in the urine, a change that would further lower the extracellular pH.

   The relationship between acid-base balance and citrate handling is in part due to the fall in luminal pH, which promotes the conversion of citrate^{3-}, the major circulating form, into citrate^{2-}, which appears to be more easily reabsorbed.[154] The associated intracellular acidosis also enhances citrate entry into the mitochondria (via an unknown mechanism); the ensuing reduction in the cytosolic citrate concentration creates a more favorable gradient for citrate reabsorption from the tubular lumen.[151] These changes are reversed by alkalemia, which diminishes citrate reabsorption and therefore increases urinary citrate excretion.

   In addition to metabolic acidosis, hypokalemia is another condition in which proximal citrate reabsorption is enhanced.[155] A somewhat similar mechanism may be involved, since the loss of K^+ leads to a transcellular cation exchange in which K^+ leaves the cells to replete the extracellular stores and, to maintain electroneutrality, H^+ and Na^+ enter the cells. The ensuing intracellular acidosis may be responsible for the increased citrate reabsorption.

   Citrate handling becomes clinically important in some patients who form calcium stones. Citrate is a potent inhibitor of calcium oxalate and calcium phosphate precipitation by combining with free Ca^{2+} to form a nondissociable but soluble complex. Hypocitraturia is a risk factor for stone disease[108,156,157] and can be corrected by the administration of alkali. Potassium citrate has most often been used in this setting because it has two advantages.[157,158] First, citrate (which is rapidly metabolized to bicarbonate) is generally better tolerated than bicarbonate, which can cause gastrointestinal symptoms due to local gas formation. Second, the potassium salt is preferred because sodium citrate will produce volume expansion, which, as described above, will increase Na^+ and secondarily

Ca^{2+} excretion.[158] The latter effect could negate any stone-preventing benefit derived from the rise in citrate excretion.

SECRETORY PATHWAYS

In addition to their reabsorptive functions, the proximal tubular cells secrete hydrogen ions (see Chap. 11) and organic cations and anions.[159-161] The last two processes occur primarily in the S_2 segment (see Fig. 3-1), which has the highest number of secretory pumps.[2,162] In general, tubular secretion occurs in three steps: movement of the organic solute from the peritubular capillary into the interstitium by diffusion; transport of the solute into the cell across the basolateral membrane; and secretion from the cell into the lumen across the luminal membrane.[161]

Organic Cation Secretion

The mechanism by which these processes may occur can be illustrated from studies with organic cations, examples of which include creatinine and drugs such as cimetidine, trimethoprim, and quinidine (Fig. 3-14).[163,164] It is likely that passive forces play a primary role in cell entry across the basolateral membrane, since the cation concentration in the extracellular fluid is higher than that in the cell and there is a cell interior negative potential. This process appears to occur by facilitated diffusion via cation-cation countertransport proteins, with substantial intracellular sequestration of organic cations.[161,165]

A large number of specific transporters expressed on the basolateral membrane have been isolated and cloned. These include a polyspecific cation transporter, named OCT1.[166] This transporter is sodium-independent and can transport a wide variety of cations, including choline, dopamine, and acetylcholine.

For most organic cations, subsequent secretion across the luminal membrane appears to occur in parallel with the Na^+-H^+ antiporter.[163] The latter leads to a rise in the tubular fluid hydrogen concentration that allows secretion of the organic cation to be linked to the favorable inward H^+ gradient by different *H^+-cation exchangers* (Fig. 3-14).[164,167,168] Notice that the energy for each of these steps is again provided indirectly by the Na^+-K^+-ATPase pump. The low cell Na^+ concentration drive the Na^+-H^+ antiporter, and the high cell K^+ concentration results in passive K^+ diffusion out of the cell and the generation of cell negativity.

P-glycoprotein, a plasma membrane constituent that mediates outward active transport of toxic and nontoxic substances, also may play a role in proximal organic cation secretion. It is localized to the luminal membrane of the proximal tubule, and increased expression leads to enhanced cation secretion.[169]

The organic cations tend to compete for common secretory mechanisms.[167,168] As a result, the presence of cimetidine, for example, can diminish the secretion of creatinine, reversibly raising the plasma creatinine concentration without any

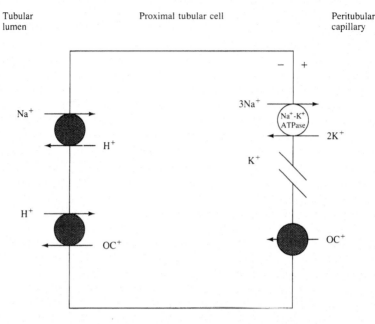

Figure 3-14 Model for organic cation (OC^+) secretion in the proximal tubule. Entry into the cell occurs in part by passive carrier-mediated diffusion across the basolateral membrane down favorable concentration and electrical gradients. Secretion into the lumen occurs by a H^+-OC^+ exchanger that is driven by the H^+ gradient created by the Na^+-H^+ antiporter.

decline in the glomerular filtration rate.[170] This effect may also be useful clinically by making the creatinine clearance a more accurate estimate of the glomerular filtration rate.[171,172]

Organic Anion Secretion

Organic anions, both endogenous (urate, hippurate, ketoacid anions) and exogenous (penicillins, cephalosporins, salicylates, diuretics, radiocontrast media) compete for different secretory pathways. The mechanism by which this occurs is not well understood, but, as described above for urate, anion exchangers at the basolateral membrane and perhaps the luminal membrane appear to play an essential role (Fig. 3-13b).[160,161,163,173]

Citric acid cycle intermediates (particularly α-ketoglutarate) appear to be important at the basolateral membrane. These compounds can enter the cell by cotransport with sodium across the basolateral membrane and also are produced within the cell; this intracellular accumulation creates a favorable outward gradient that can then be used to drive the uptake of organic anions via an intermediate-organic anion exchanger.[160,163] The number and distribution of negative charges seems to be a major determinant of the degree of binding to the anion exchanger.[173]

A large number of organic anion transporters in the basolateral membrane have been characterized and/or cloned. As an example, the organic anion transporter 1 has specificity for organic anions, including para-aminohippurate and α-ketoglutarate.[174] Additional basolateral transporters include the multidrug resistance transport-associated protein. Secretion of the organic anion into the lumen may then occur by facilitated diffusion, since the cell interior negative potential creates a favorable electrical gradient.[163]

Competition for these pathways can be important clinically. As an example, fasting subjects frequently develop hyperuricemia. It is thought that this is secondary to the ketonemia of fasting, which could diminish urate secretion. Organic anion secretion can also be inhibited by the drug probenecid.[173] This property is useful in selected patients, as probenecid has been given in conjunction with penicillin therapy. By reducing penicillin secretion (and excretion), higher blood levels of the antibiotic can be achieved.

The fact that these pathways are relatively nonspecific and are able to secrete foreign substances make them well adapted for a *major role in the elimination of drugs and chemicals from the body*. This is particularly important for those agents that are highly albumin-bound and therefore cannot be excreted by glomerular filtration. Albumin binding promotes proximal secretion in two ways. First, binding appears to be required for secretion, which does not occur with free organic anions.[175] Second, binding facilitates the urinary excretion of these compounds by maximizing their *rate of delivery to the secretory sites in the kidney*. Albumin and other large proteins cannot easily cross the peripheral capillary membranes; as a result, protein-bound compounds are largely restricted to the vascular space, with limited access to the interstitium or the cells.[176]

Other transport processes may be involved in the renal handling of organic solutes. In particular, these substances can undergo passive reabsorption or secretion depending upon the urine pH. Salicylic acid, for example, exists both as the intact acid and the organic anion:

$$\text{Salicylic acid} \leftrightarrow \text{H}^+ + \text{salicylate}^-$$

The intact acid, but not the organic anion, can freely diffuse across cell membranes because it is nonpolar. This difference makes salicylate excretion *pH-dependent*. Raising the urine pH (which lowers the free H^+ concentration) will shift the above reaction to the right. The ensuing fall in the urinary salicylic acid concentration will minimize the back-diffusion of secreted salicylic acid out of the tubular lumen, thereby increasing total drug excretion.[177] Thus, elevating the urine pH is an important component of the treatment of salicylate intoxication.

PROBLEMS

3-1 If there is no change in the extracellular volume, what effect will an increase in the GFR have on the following?

(*a*) Fractional Na^+ reabsorption

(*b*) Absolute Na^+ reabsorption

3-2 Parathyroid hormone acts in part by decreasing the activity of the Na^+-H^+ antiporter in the proximal tubule. What effect should this have on the proximal reabsorption of the following?
(a) Bicarbonate
(b) Chloride
(c) Water

3-3 A subject with a previous BUN of 10 mg/dL and plasma creatinine concentration of 1.0 mg/dL reports 3 days of diarrhea and poor appetite. On physical examination, the patient appears to be volume-depleted. Blood tests at this time reveal a BUN of 40 mg/dL, creatinine concentration of 1.0 mg/dL, and plasma urate concentration of 10.1 mg/dL (normal is 4 to 8 mg/dL). Ketones (such as β-hydroxybutyrate) are noted in the urine and are believed to reflect the ketosis associated with fasting.
(a) Why has the BUN increased?
(b) Has there been a substantial change in the GFR?
(c) What factors are responsible for the hyperuricemia?

3-4 Patients with the distal form of renal tubular acidosis have a low plasma HCO_3^- concentration and a relatively high urine pH (see Chap. 21). What effect should this have on the following?
(a) Proximal NaCl reabsorption
(b) Proximal citrate reabsorption
(c) The likelihood of calcium phosphate stone formation

REFERENCES

1. Maddox DA, Gennari JF. The early proximal tubule: A high-capacity delivery-responsive reabsorptive site. *Am J Physiol* 252:F573, 1987.
2. Woodhall PB, Tisher CC, Simonton CA, Robinson RR. Relationship between para-amino-hippurate secretion and cellular morphology in rabbit proximal tubules. *J Clin Invest* 61:1320, 1978.
3. Helbert MJ, Dauwe SE, Van der Biest I, et al. Immunodissection of the human proximal nephron: Flow sorting of $S_1S_2S_3$, S_1S_2, and S_3 proximal tubular cells. *Kidney Int* 52:414, 1997.
4. Rector FC Jr. Sodium, bicarbonate, and chloride absorption by the proximal tubule. *Am J Physiol* 244:F461, 1983.
5. Kinne RKH. Selectivity and direction: Plasma membranes in renal transport. *Am J Physiol* 260:F153, 1991.
6. Gumbiner B. Structure, biochemistry, and assembly of tight junctions. *Am J Physiol* 253:C749, 1987.
7. Sabolic I, Valenti G, Verbavatz J, et al. Localization of the CHIP 28 water channel in rat kidney. *Am J Physiol* 263:C1225, 1992.
8. Nielsen S, Kwon T-H, Christensen BM, et al. Physiology and pathophysiology of renal aquaporins. *J Am Soc Nephrol* 10:647, 1999.
9. Lee MD, King LS, Agre P. The aquaporin family of water channel proteins in clinical medicine. *Medicine (Baltimore)* 76:141, 1997.
10. Schnermann J, Chou CL, Ma T, et al. Defective proximal tubule reabsorptive capacity in transgenic aquaporin-1 null mice. *Proc Natl Acad Sci U S A* 95:9660, 1998.
11. Neumann KH, Rector FC Jr. Mechanism of NaCl and water reabsorption in the proximal convoluted tubule of rat kidney: Role of chloride concentration gradients. *J Clin Invest* 58:1110, 1976.
12. Jacobson HR. Characteristics of volume reabsorption in rabbit superficial and juxtamedullary proximal convoluted tubules. *J Clin Invest* 63:410, 1979.
13. Katz AI. Distribution and function of classes of ATPases along the nephron. *Kidney Int* 29:21, 1986.
14. Schafer JA. Mechanism coupling the absorption of solutes and water in the proximal nephron. *Kidney Int* 25:708, 1984.

15. Green R, Giebisch G. Osmotic forces determining water reabsorption in the proximal tubule of rat kidney. *Am J Physiol* 257:F669, 1989.
16. Gullans SR, Avison MJ, Ogino T, et al. NMR measurements of intracellular sodium in the mammalian proximal tubule. *Am J Physiol* 249:F160, 1985.
17. Kone BC, Brady HR, Gullans SR. Coordinated regulation of intracellular K^+ in the proximal tubule: Ba^{2+} blockade down-regulates Na^+-K^+-ATPase and upregulates two K^+ permeable pathways. *Proc Natl Acad Sci U S A* 86:6431, 1989.
18. Hurst AM, Beck JS, Laprade R, Lapointe J-Y. Na^+ pump inhibition downregulates an ATP-sensitive K^+ channel in rabbit proximal convoluted tubule. *Am J Physiol* 264:F760, 1993.
19. Sacktor B. Sodium-coupled hexose transport. *Kidney Int* 36:342, 1989.
20. Turner RJ, Moran A. Heterogeneity of sodium dependent D-glucose transport sites along the proximal tubule: Evidence from vesicle studies. *Am J Physiol* 242:F406, 1982.
21. Zelikovic I, Chesney RW. Sodium-coupled amino acid transport in renal tubule. *Kidney Int* 36:351, 1989.
22. Murer H, Lotscher M, Kaissling B, et al. Renal brush border membrane Na/Pi-cotransport: Molecular aspects in PTH-dependent and dietary regulation. *Kidney Int* 49:1769, 1996.
23. Malnic G. Hydrogen secretion in renal cortical tubules: Kinetic aspects. *Kidney Int* 32:136, 1987.
24. Alpern RJ, Moe OW, Preisig PA. Chronic regulation of the proximal tubular Na/H antiporter: From HCO_3 to SRC (editorial). *Kidney Int* 48:1386, 1995.
25. Hoshi T. Electrophysiology of *Triturus* nephron: Cable properties and electrogenic transport systems. *Kidney Int* 37:157, 1990.
26. Williams KA. Three-dimensional structure of the ion-coupled transport protein NhaA. *Nature* 403:112, 2000.
27. Burg M, Patlak C, Green N, Villey D. Organic solutes in fluid absorption by renal proximal convoluted tubules. *Am J Physiol* 231:627, 1976.
28. Barfuss DW, Schafer JA. Rate of formation and composition of absorbate from proximal nephron segments. *Am J Physiol* 247:F117, 1984.
29. Avison MJ, Gullans SR, Ogino T, et al. Measurement of Na^+-K^+ coupling ratio of Na^+-K^+-ATPase in rabbit proximal tubules. *Am J Physiol* 253:C126, 1987.
30. Soleimani M, Grassi SM, Aronson PS. Stoichiometry of Na^+-HCO_3^- cotransport in basolateral membrane vesicles isolated from the rabbit renal cortex. *J Clin Invest* 79:1276, 1987.
31. Beck JS, Breton S, Mairbaurl H, et al. Relationship between sodium transport and intracellular ATP in isolated professed rabbit proximal convoluted tubule. *Am J Physiol* 261:F634, 1991.
32. Hanley MJ. Isolated nephron segments in a rabbit model of ischemic acute renal failure. *Am J Physiol* 239:F17, 1980.
33. Myers BD, Miller C, Mehigan JT, et al. Nature of the renal injury following total renal ischemia in man. *J Clin Invest* 73:329, 1984.
34. Molitoris BA, Falk SA, Dahl RH. Ischemia-induced loss of epithelial polarity. Role of the tight junction. *J Clin Invest* 84:1334, 1989.
35. Molitoris BA. Ischemia-induced loss of epithelial polarity: Potential role of the actin cytoskeleton. *Am J Physiol* 260:F769, 1991.
36. Sutton TA, Molitoris BA. Mechanisms of cellular injury in ischemic acute renal failure. *Semin Nephrol* 18:490, 1998.
37. Kwon O, Corrigan G, Myers BD, et al. Sodium reabsorption and distribution of Na^+/K^+-ATPase during postischemic injury to the renal allograft. *Kidney Int* 55:963, 1999.
38. Berry CA, Rector FC Jr. Electroneutral NaCl absorption in the proximal tubule: Mechanisms of apical Na-coupled transport. *Kidney Int* 36:403, 1989.
39. Schild L, Giebisch G, Karniski LP, Aronson PS. Effect of formate on volume reabsorption in the rabbit proximal tubule. *J Clin Invest* 79:32, 1987.
40. Wang T, Giebisch G, Aronson PS. Effects of formate and oxalate on volume absorption in rat proximal tubule. *Am J Physiol* 263:F37, 1992.

41. Preisig PA, Alpern RJ. Contributions of cellular leak pathways to net NaHCO$_3$ and NaCl absorption. *J Clin Invest* 83:1859, 1989.

42. Wang T, Egbert AL Jr, Abbiati T, et al. Mechanisms of stimulation of proximal tubule chloride transport by formate and oxalate. *Am J Physiol* 271:F446, 1996.

43. Preisig PA, Rector FC Jr. Role of Na$^+$-H$^+$ antiport in rat on proximal tubule NaCl absorption. *Am J Physiol* 255:F461, 1988.

44. Kurtz I, Nagami G, Yanagawa N, et al. Mechanism of apical and basolateral Na$^+$-independent Cl$^-$/base exchange in rabbit superficial proximal straight tubule. *J Clin Invest* 94:173, 1994.

45. Aronson PS. Ion exchangers mediating NaCl transport in the proximal tubule. *Wien Klin Wochenschr* 109:435, 1997.

46. Sasaki S, Ishibashi K, Yoshiyama N, Shiigai T. KCl cotransport across the basolateral membrane of rabbit renal proximal straight tubules. *J Clin Invest* 81:194, 1988.

47. Ullrich KJ, Capasso G, Rumrich G, et al. Coupling between proximal tubular transport processes: Studies with ouabain, SITS, and HCO$_3$ free solutions. *Pflugers Arch* 348:245, 1977.

48. Green R, Giebisch G. Reflection coefficients and water permeability in rat proximal tubule. *Am J Physiol* 257:F658, 1989.

49. Mathisen O, Monclair T, Holdaas H, Kiil F. Bicarbonate as mediator of proximal tubular NaCl reabsorption and glomerulotubular balance. *Scand J Lab Clin Invest* 38:7, 1978.

50. Cogan MG, Rector FC. Proximal reabsorption during metabolic acidosis in the rat. *Am J Physiol* 242:F499, 1982.

51. Moe OW, Tejedor A, Levi M, et al. Dietary NaCl modulates Na$^+$-H$^+$ antiporter activity in renal cortical apical membrane vesicles. *Am J Physiol* 260:F130, 1991.

52. Cogan MG, Angiotensin II: A potent controller of sodium transport in the early proximal tubule. *Hypertension* 15:451, 1990.

53. Liu F-Y, Cogan MG. Antiotensin II stimulates early proximal bicarbonate absorption in the rat by decreasing cyclic adenosine monophosphate. *J Clin Invest* 84:83, 1989.

54. Gesek FA, Schoolwerth AC. Hormonal interactions with the proximal Na$^+$-H$^+$ exchanger. *Am J Physiol* 258:F514, 1990.

55. Liu F-Y, Cogan MG. Role of angiotensin II in glomerulotubular balance. *Am J Physiol* 259:F72, 1990.

56. Cogan MG, Xie M-H, Liu F-Y, et al. Effects of DuP 753 on proximal nephron and renal transport. *Am J Hypertens* 4:315s, 1991.

57. Felder CC, Campbell T, Albrecht F, Jose PA. Dopamine inhibits Na$^+$-H$^+$ exchanger activity in renal BBMV by stimulation of adenylate cyclase. *Am J Physiol* 259:F297, 1990.

58. Aperia A, Fryckstedt J, Svensson L, et al. Phosphorylated Mr 32,000 dopamine- and cAMP-regulated phosphoprotein inhibits Na$^+$-K$^+$-ATPase activity in renal tubule cells. *Proc Natl Acad Sci U S A* 88:2798, 1991.

59. Bertorello A, Aperia A. Regulation of Na$^+$-K$^+$-ATPase activity in kidney proximal tubules: Involvement of GTP binding proteins. *Am J Physiol* 256:F57, 1989.

60. Hansell P, Fasching A. The effect of dopamine receptor blockade on natriuresis is dependent on the degree of hypervolemia. *Kidney Int* 93:253, 1991.

61. Ichikawa I, Brenner BM. Mechanism of inhibition of proximal tubule fluid reabsorption after exposure of the rat kidney to the physical effects of expansion of extracellular fluid volume. *J Clin Invest* 64:1466, 1979.

62. Tucker BJ, Mundy CA, Blantz RC. Adrenergic and angiotensin II influences on renal vascular tone in chronic sodium depletion. *Am J Physiol* 252:F811, 1987.

63. Dzau VJ. Renal and circulatory mechanisms in congestive heart failure. *Kidney Int* 31:1402, 1987.

64. Boulpaep EL. Permeability changes of the proximal tubule of Necturus during saline loading. *Am J Physiol* 222:517, 1971.

65. Berry CA, Cogan MG. Influence of peritubular protein on solute absorption in the rabbit proximal tubule. A specific effect on NaCl transport. *J Clin Invest* 68:506, 1982.

66. Baum M, Berry CA. Peritubular protein modulates neutral active NaCl absorption in rabbit proximal convoluted tubule. *Am J Physiol* 248:F790, 1985.
67. Häberle DA, Von Baeyer H. Characteristics of glomerulotubular balance. *Am J Physiol* 244:F355, 1983.
68. Wright FS. Flow-dependent transport processes: Filtration, absorption, secretion. *Am J Physiol* 243:F1, 1982.
69. Kunau RT Jr, Webb HL, Borman SC. Characteristics of sodium reabsorption in the loop of Henle and distal tubule. *Am J Physiol* 227:1181, 1974.
70. Brenner BM, Troy JL. Postglomerular vascular protein concentration: Evidence for a causal role in governing fluid reabsorption and glomerulotubular balance by the renal proximal tubule. *J Clin Invest* 50:336, 1971.
71. Ichikawa I, Hoyer JR, Seiler MW, Brenner BM. Mechanism of glomerulotubular balance in the setting of heterogeneous glomerular injury. Preservation of a close functional linkage between individual nephrons and surrounding microvasculature. *J Clin Invest* 69:185, 1982.
72. Moore LC. Interaction of tubuloglomerular feedback and proximal nephron reabsorption in autoregulation. *Kidney Int* 22(suppl 12):S-173, 1982.
73. Dirks JH, Cirksena WJ, Berliner RW. The effect of saline infusion on sodium reabsorption by the proximal tubule of the dog. *J Clin Invest* 44:1160, 1965.
74. Stein JH, Osgood RW, Boonjarern S, et al. Segmental sodium reabsorption in rats with mild and severe volume depletion. *Am J Physiol* 227:351, 1974.
75. Manz F, Waldherr R, Fritz HP, et al. Idiopathic de-Toni-Debre-Fanconi syndrome with absence of proximal tubular brush border. *Clin Nephrol* 22:149, 1984.
76. Purkerson M, Lubowitz H, White R, Bricker NS. On the influence of extracellular fluid volume expansion on bicarbonate reabsorption in the rat. *J Clin Invest* 48:1754, 1969.
77. Kurtzman NA. Regulation of renal bicarbonate reabsorption by extracellular volume. *J Clin Invest* 49:586, 1970.
78. Thorens B, Lodish HJ, Brown D. Differential localization of two glucose transporter isoforms in rat kidney. *Am J Physiol* 259:C286, 1990.
79. Dominguez JH, Camp K, Malanu L, Garvey WT. Glucose transporters of rat proximal tubule: Differential expression and subcellular distribution. *Am J Physiol* 262:F807, 1992.
80. Ruegg CE, Mandel LJ. Bulk isolation of renal PCT and PST. I. Glucose-dependent metabolic differences. *Am J Physiol* 259:F164, 1990.
81. Wells RG, Pajor AM, Kanai Y, et al. Cloning of a human kidney cDNA with similarity to the sodium-glucose cotransporter. *Am J Physiol* 263:F459, 1992.
82. Kanai Y, Lee WS, You G, et al. The human kidney low affinity Na^+/glucose cotransporter SGLT2. Delineating of the major renal reabsorptive mechanism for D-glucose. *J Clin Invest* 93:397, 1994.
83. Oliver J, MacDowell M. The structural and functional aspects of the handling of glucose by the nephrons and the kidney and their correlation by means of structural-functional equivalents. *J Clin Invest* 40:1093, 1961.
84. Elsas LJ, Rosenberg LE. Familial renal glycosuria: A genetic reappraisal of hexose transport by kidney and intestine. *J Clin Invest* 48:1845, 1969.
85. Roth KS, Foreman JW, Segal S. The Fanconi syndrome and mechanisms of tubular transport dysfunction. *Kidney Int* 20:705, 1981.
86. Wolff LI, Goodwin BL, Phelps CE. T_m-limited renal tubular reabsorption and the genetics of renal glucosuria. *J Theor Biol* 11:10, 1966.
87. Dossetor JB. Creatininemia versus uremia: The relative significance of blood urea nitrogen and serum creatinine concentrations in azotemia. *Ann Intern Med* 65:1287, 1966.
88. Sutton RAL. Disorders of renal calcium excretion. *Kidney Int* 23:665, 1983.
89. Friedman PA, Gesek FA. Calcium transport in renal epithelial cells. *Am J Physiol* 264:F181, 1993.
90. Ng RCK, Rouse D, Suki WN. Calcium transport in the rabbit superficial proximal convoluted tubule. *J Clin Invest* 74:834, 1984.

91. Friedman PA. Basal and hormone-activated calcium absorption in mouse renal thick ascending limbs. *Am J Physiol* 254:F62, 1988.
92. Simon DB, Lu Y, Choate KA, et al. Paracellin-1, a renal tight junction protein required for paracellular Mg^{2+} reabsorption. *Science* 285:103, 1999.
93. Friedman PA, Gesek FA. Hormone-responsive Ca^{2+} entry in distal convoluted tubules. *J Am Soc Nephrol* 4:1396, 1994.
94. Shimizu T, Yoshitomi K, Nakamura M, Imai M. Effects of PTH, calcitonin, and cAMP on calcium transport in rabbit distal nephron segments. *Am J Physiol* 259:F408, 1990.
95. Bourdeau JE, Lau K. Regulation of cytosolic free calcium concentration in the rabbit connecting tubule: A calcium-reabsorbing epithelium. *J Lab Clin Med* 119:650, 1992.
96. Costanzo LS, Windhager EE. Effects of PTH, ADH, and cyclic AMP on distal tubular Ca and Na reabsorption. *Am J Physiol* 239:F478, 1980.
97. Gesek FA, Friedman PA. On the mechanism of parathyroid hormone stimulation of calcium uptake by mouse distal convoluted tubule cells. *J Clin Invest* 90:749, 1992.
98. Bacskai BJ, Friedman PA. Activation of latent Ca^{2+} channels in renal epithelial cells by parathyroid hormone. *Nature* 347:388, 1990.
99. Bouhtiauy I, Lajeunesse D, Christakos S, Lajeunesse MG. Two vitamin D_3-dependent calcium binding proteins increase calcium reabsorption by different mechanisms I. Effect of CaBP 28K. *Kidney Int* 45:461, 1994.
100. Friedman PA, Gesek FA. Vitamin D_3 accelerates PTH-dependent calcium transport in distal convoluted tubule cells. *Am J Physiol* 265:F300, 1993.
101. Bindels RJM, Ramakers PLM, Dempster JA, et al. Role of Na^+/Ca^{2+} exchange in transcellular Ca^{2+} transport across primary cultures of rabbit kidney collecting system. *Pflugers Arch* 420:566, 1992.
102. Bouhtiauy I, Lajeunesse D, Brunette MG. The mechanism of parathyroid hormone action on calcium reabsorption by the distal tubule. *Endocrinology* 128:251, 1991.
103. Shimizu T, Nakamura M, Yoshitomi K, Imai M. Interaction of trichlormethiazide or amiloride with PTH in stimulating Ca^{2+} absorption in rabbit CNT. *Am J Physiol* 261:F36, 1991.
104. Hebert SC. Extracellular calcium-sensing receptor: Implications of calcium and magnesium handling in the kidney. *Kidney Int* 50:2129, 1996.
105. Kurokawa K. Calcium-regulating hormones and the kidney. *Kidney Int* 32:760, 1987.
106. Winer KK, Yanovski JA, Cutler GB Jr. Synthetic human parathyroid hormone 1-34 versus calcitriol and calcium in the treatment of hypoparathyroidism. Results of a short-term randomized crossover trial. *JAMA* 276:631, 1996.
107. Martinez-Maldonado M, Eknoyan G, Suki WN. Diuretics in nonedematous states. *Arch Intern Med* 131:797, 1973.
108. Coe FL, Parks JH, Asplin JR. The pathogenesis and treatment of kidney stones. *N Engl J Med* 327:1141, 1992.
109. Breslau N, Moses AM, Weiner IM. The role of volume contraction in the hypocalciuric action of chlorothiazide. *Kidney Int* 10:164, 1976.
110. Costanzo LS. Localization of diuretic action in microperfused rat distal tubules: Ca and Na transport. *Am J Physiol* 248:F527, 1985.
111. Gesek FA, Friedman PA. Mechanism of calcium transport stimulation by chlorothiazide in mouse distal collecting tubule cells. *J Clin Invest* 90:429, 1992.
112. Brunette MG, Mailloux J, Lajeunesse D. Calcium transport through the luminal membrane of the distal tubule: Inter-relationship with sodium. *Kidney Int* 41:281, 1992.
113. Biber J, Custer M, Magagnin S, et al. Renal Na/Pi-cotransporters. *Kidney Int* 49:981, 1996.
114. Murer H. Cellular mechanisms in proximal tubular Pi reabsorption: Some answers and more questions. *J Am Soc Nephrol* 2:1649, 1992.
115. Busch A, Waldegger S, Herzer T, et al. Electrophysiological analysis of Na^+/Pi cotransport mediated by a transporter cloned from rat kidney and expressed in *Xenopus* oocytes. *Proc Natl Acad Sci U S A* 91:8205, 1994.
116. Walker JJ, Yan TS, Quamme GA. Presence of multiple sodium-dependent phosphate transport processes in proximal brush-border membranes. *Am J Physiol* 252:F226, 1987.

117. Tenenhouse HS. Recent advances in epithelial sodium-coupled phosphate transport. *Curr Opin Nephrol Hypertens* 8:407, 1999.

118. Beck L, Karaplis AC, Amizuka N, et al. Targeted inactivation of Npt2 in mice leads to severe renal phosphate wasting, hypercalciuria, and skeletal abnormalities. *Proc Natl Acad Sci U S A* 95:5372, 1998.

119. Kempson SA, Shah SV, Werness PG, et al. Renal brush border membrane adaptation to phosphorus deprivation: Effects of fasting versus low phosphorus diet. *Kidney Int* 18:36, 1980.

120. Cheng L, Dersch C, Kraus E, et al. Renal adaptation to phosphate load in the acute thyroparathyroidectomized rat: Rapid alteration in brush border membrane phosphate transport. *Am J Physiol* 246:F488, 1984.

121. Hammerman MR, Karl IE, Hruska KA. Regulation of canine renal vesicle Pi transport by growth hormone and parathyroid hormone. *Biochim Biophys Acta* 603:322, 1980.

122. Hoag HM, Martel J, Gauthier C, Tenenhouse HS. Effects of Npt2 gene ablation and low-phosphate diet on renal Na(+)/phosphate cotransport and cotransport gene expression. *J Clin Invest* 104:679, 1999.

123. Hruska KA, Klahr S, Hammerman MR. Decreased luminal membrane transport of phosphate in chronic renal failure. *Am J Physiol* 242:F17, 1982.

124. Reiss E, Canterbury JM, Bercovitz MA, Kaplan EL. The role of phosphate in the secretion of parathyroid hormone in man. *J Clin Invest* 49:2146, 1970.

125. Portale AA, Halloran BP, Morris RC Jr. Dietary intake of phosphorus modulates the circadian rhythm of serum concentrations of phosphorus. Implications for the renal production of 1,25-dihydroxyvitamin D. *J Clin Invest* 80:1147, 1987.

126. Quamme GA. Effect of pH on Na^+-dependent phosphate transport in renal outer cortical and outer medullary BBMV. *Am J Physiol* 258:F356, 1990.

127. Quamme GA. Renal magnesium handling: New insights in understanding old problems. *Kidney Int* 52:1180, 1997.

128. DeRouffignac C, Quammer GA. Renal magnesium handling and its hormonal control. *Physiol Rev* 74:305, 1994.

129. Shafik IM, Quamme GA. Early adaptation of renal magnesium reabsorption in response to magnesium restriction. *Am J Physiol* 257:F974, 1989.

130. Shareghi GR, Agus ZA. Magnesium transport in the cortical thick ascending limb of Henle's loop in the rabbit. *J Clin Invest* 69:759, 1982.

131. Wang WH, La M, Hebert SC. Cytochrome P-450 metabolites mediate extracellular Ca^{2+}-induced inhibition of apical K channels in the TAL. *Am J Physiol* 271:C103, 1996.

132. Bapty BW, Dai LJ, Ritchie G, et al. Extracellular $Mg^{2(+)}$- and $Ca^{2(+)}$-sensing in mouse distal convoluted tubule cells. *Kidney Int* 53:583, 1998.

133. de Rouffignac C, Di Stefano A, Wittner M, et al. Consequences of differential effects of ADH and other peptide hormones on thick ascending limb of mammalian kidney. *Am J Physiol* 260:R1023, 1991.

134. Dai LJ, Bapty B, Ritchie G, et al. Glucagon and arginine vasopressin stimulate Mg^{2+} uptake in mouse distal convoluted tubule cells. *Am J Physiol* 274:F328, 1998.

135. Kahn AM. Effect of diuretics on the renal handling of urate. *Semin Nephrol* 8:305, 1988.

136. Kahn AM. Indirect coupling between sodium and urate transport in the proximal tubule. *Kidney Int* 36:378, 1989.

137. Guggino SE, Martin GJ, Aronson PS. Specificity and modes of the anion exchanger in dog renal microvillus membranes. *Am J Physiol* 244:F612, 1982.

138. Leal-Pinto E, Tao W, Rappaport J, et al. Molecular cloning and functional reconstitution of a urate transporter/channel. *J Biol Chem* 27:617, 1997.

139. Weinman EJ, Eknoyan G, Suki WN. The influence of the extracellular fluid volume on the tubular reabsorption of uric acid. *J Clin Invest* 55:283, 1975.

140. Steele TH, Oppenheimer S. Factors affecting urate excretion following diuretic administration in man. *Am J Med* 47:564, 1969.

141. Carone FA, Peterson DR. Hydrolysis and transport of small peptides by the proximal tubule. *Am J Physiol* 238:F151, 1980.

142. Daniel H, Herget M. Cellular and molecular mechanisms of renal peptide transport. *Am J Physiol* 273:F1, 1997.

143. Palacin M, Estevez R, Bertran J, Zorzano A. Molecular biology of mammalian plasma membrane amino acid transporters. *Physiol Rev* 78:969, 1998.

144. Tate SS, Yan N, Udenfriend S. Expression-cloning of a Na-independent neutral amino acid transporter in rat kidney. *Proc Natl Acad Sci U S A* 89:1, 1992.

145. Kanai Y, Stelzner MG, Lee W, et al. Expression of mRNA (D2) encoding a protein involved in amino acid transport in S3 proximal tubule. *Am J Physiol* 263:F1087, 1992.

146. Calonge MJ, Gasparini P, Chillaron J, et al. Cystinuria caused by mutation in rBAT, a gene involved in the transport of cystine. *Nat Genet* 6:420, 1994.

147. Palacin M, Estevez R, Zorzano A. Cystinuria calls for heteromultimeric amino acid transporters. *Curr Opin Cell Biol* 10:455, 1998.

148. Ulbricht CJ, Gutjahr E, Cannon JK, et al. Effect of low molecular weight proteins and dextran on renal cathpsin B and L activity. *Kidney Int* 37:918, 1990.

149. Christensen EI, Rennke HG, Carone FA. Renal tubular uptake of protein: Effect of molecular change. *Am J Physiol* 244:F436, 1983.

150. Park CH, Maack T. Albumin absorption and catabolism by isolated perfused proximal convoluted tubules of the rabbit. *J Clin Invest* 73:767, 1984.

151. Hamm LL. Renal handling of citrate. *Kidney Int* 38:728, 1990.

152. Jorgensen KE, Kragh-Hansen U, Roigaard-Petersen H, Sheikh MI. Citrate uptake by basolateral and luminal membrane vesicles from rabbit kidney cortex. *Am J Physiol* 244:F686, 1983.

153. Pajor AM. Citrate transport by the kidney and intestine. *Semin Nephrol* 19:195, 1999.

154. Brennan S, Hering-Smith K, Hamm LL. Effect of pH on citrate reabsorption in the proximal tubule. *Am J Physiol* 255:F301, 1988.

155. Levi M, McDonald LA, Preisig PA, Alpern RJ. Chronic K depletion stimulates rat renal brush-border membrane Na-citrate cotransporter. *Am J Physiol* 261:F767, 1991.

156. Parks JH, Coe FL. A urinary calcium-citrate index for the evaluation of nephrolithiasis. *Kidney Int* 30:85, 1986.

157. Pak CYC, Peterson R, Sakhaee K, et al. Correction of hypocitraturia and prevention of stone formation by combined thiazide and potassium citrate therapy in thiazide-unresponsive hypercalciuric nephrolithiasis. *Am J Med* 79:284, 1985.

158. Sakhaee K, Nicar M, Hill K, Pak CYC. Contrasting effects of potassium citrate and sodium citrate therapies on urinary chemistries and crystallization of stone-forming salts. *Kidney Int* 24:348, 1983.

159. Grantham JJ. Studies of organic anion and cation transport in isolated segments of proximal tubules. *Kidney Int* 22:519, 1982.

160. Burckhardt G, Ullrich KJ. Organic anion transport across the contraluminal membrane—dependence on sodium. *Kidney Int* 36:370, 1989.

161. Pritchard JB, Miller DS. Renal secretion of organic anions and cations. *Kidney Int* 49:1649, 1996.

162. Shimomura A, Chonko AM, Grantham JJ. Basis for heterogeneity of *para*-aminohippurate secretion in rabbit proximal tubules. *Am J Physiol* 240:F430, 1981.

163. Pritchard JB, Miller DS. Comparative insights into the mechanisms of renal organic anion and cation secretion. *Am J Physiol* 261:F1329, 1991.

164. McKinney TD, Kunnemann ME. Cimetidine transport in rabbit renal cortical brush border membrane vesicles. *Am J Physiol* 252:F525, 1987.

165. Dantzler WH, Wright SH, Catsudthipong V, Brokl OH. Basolateral tetraethylammonium transport in intact tubules: Specificity and *trans*-stimulation by electroneutral organic cation exchange. *Am J Physiol* 261:F386, 1991.

166. Zhang L, Dressner MJ, Chun JK, et al. Cloning and functional characterization of a rat renal organic cation transporter isoform (rOCT1A). *J Biol Chem* 272:16548, 1997.

167. Miyamoto Y, Tiruppathi C, Ganapathy V, Leibach FH. Multiple transport systems for organic cations in renal brush-border membrane vesicles. *Am J Physiol* 256:F541, 1989.

168. Ott RJ, Hui AC, Yuan G, Giacomini KM. Organic cation transport in human renal brush-border membrane vesicles. *Am J Physiol* 261:F443, 1991.

169. Pan BF, Dutt A, Nelson JA. Enhanced transepithelial flux of cimetidine by Madin-Darby canine kidney cells overexpressing human P-glycoprotein. *J Pharmacol Exp Ther* 270:1, 1994.

170. Rocci ML Jr, Vlasses PH, Ferguson RK. Creatinine serum concentrations and H$_2$-receptor antagonists. *Clin Nephrol* 22:814, 1984.

171. Hilbrands LB, Artz MA, Wetzels JFM, Koene RAP. Cimetidine improves the reliability of creatinine as a marker of glomerular filtration. *Kidney Int* 40:1171, 1991.

172. van Acker BA, Koomen GC, Koopman MG, et al. Creatinine clearance during cimetidine administration for measurement of glomerular filtration rate. *Lancet* 340:1326, 1992.

173. Ullrich KJ, Rumrich G. Contraluminal transport systems in the proximal renal tubule involved in secretion of organic anions. *Am J Physiol* 254:F453, 1988.

174. Sekine T, Watanabe N, Hosoyamada M, et al. Expression cloning and characterization of a novel multispecific organic anion transporter. *J Biol Chem* 272:18526, 1997.

175. Besseghir K, Mosig D, Roch-Ramel F. Facilitation by serum albumin of renal tubular secretion of organic anions. *Am J Physiol* 256:F475, 1989.

176. Inoue M, Koyama H, Nagase S, Morino Y. Renal secretion of phenolsulfonphthalein: Analysis of its vectorial transport in normal and mutant analbuminemic rats. *J Lab Clin Med* 105:484, 1985.

177. Chatton JY, Besseghir K, Roch-Ramel F. Salicyclic acid permeability properties of the rabbit cortical collecting duct. *Am J Physiol* 259:F613, 1990.

LOOP OF HENLE AND THE
COUNTERCURRENT MECHANISM

The 40 to 45 percent of the filtrate that is not reabsorbed in the proximal tubule enters the loop of Henle, which has a characteristic hairpin configuration in the medulla. The loop of Henle consists of four different segments: the *descending* limb; the *thin ascending* limb; the *medullary thick ascending* limb; and the *cortical thick ascending* limb, which ends at the macula densa adjacent to the parent glomerulus (Fig. 4-1). These segments perform two major functions: (1) They reabsorb approximately 25 to 35 percent of the filtered NaCl, primarily in the thick ascending limb, and (2) they reabsorb NaCl *in excess of water*, an effect that is essential for the excretion of urine with an osmolality different from that of the plasma. As will be seen, this latter characteristic of loop function is dependent upon the varying transport and permeability properties of the different loop segments.

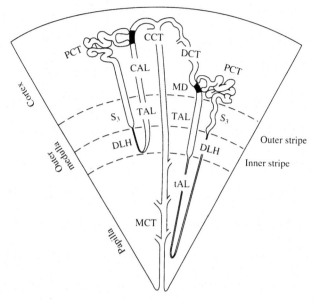

Figure 4-1 Representation of the anatomic relationships of the outer cortical and juxtamedullary nephrons. PCT = proximal convoluted tubule (S_1 and S_2 segments); S_3 = last segment of the proximal tubule, which ends at the junction of the outer and inner stripes in the outer medulla; DLH = descending limb of the loop of Henle; tAL = thin ascending limb; TAL = medullary thick ascending limb; CAL = cortical thick ascending limb, which ends in the macula densa (MD, depicted as the shaded area adjacent to the glomerulus); DCT = distal convoluted tubule; CCT = cortical collecting tubule; and MCT = medullary collecting tubule. Note that the outer cortical nephrons have no thin ascending limb, a short loop that turns around in the outer medulla, and a relatively long cortical aspect of the thick ascending limb. The latter segment is very short in juxtamedullary nephrons, which have glomeruli that are near the corticomedullary junction. (*From Hogg RJ, Kokko JP*, Rev Physiol Biochem Pharmacol *86:95, 1979. Used with permission.*)

CELL MODEL FOR SODIUM CHLORIDE TRANSPORT

Active NaCl transport in the thick ascending limb is driven by the basolateral Na^+-K^+-ATPase pump. The activity of this transporter is higher in the thick ascending limb than in other nephron segments, indicating the importance of active Na^+ reabsorption at the site.[1-3] The Na^+-K^+-ATPase pump has two major effects on Na^+ handling: It actively transports reabsorbed Na^+ out of the cell and back into the systemic circulation via the peritubular capillaries, and it maintains a low cell Na^+ concentration that allows luminal Na^+ to continue to enter the cell down a concentration gradient.[1]

Mechanism of NaCl Entry

Sodium chloride entry into the medullary and cortical aspects of the thick ascending limb (including the macula densa) primarily occurs via an electroneutral Na^+-K^+-$2Cl^-$ carrier in the luminal membrane (Fig. 4–2)[4-9]. Net transport into

Tubular
lumen

Thick ascending limb cell

Peritubular
capillary

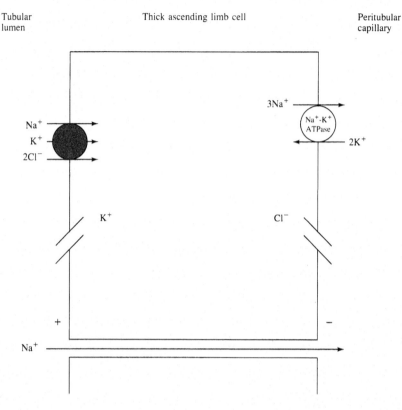

Figure 4-2 Schematic model of the major steps involved in NaCl transport in the medullary thick ascending limb of the loop of Henle. Entry into the cell occurs via a passive Na^+-K^+-$2Cl^-$ carrier in the luminal membrane. The energy for this process is indirectly provided by the Na^+-K^+-ATPase pump in the basolateral membrane that maintains a relatively low cell Na^+ concentration. The return of reabsorbed Na^+ and Cl^- to the systemic circulation occurs via the Na^+-K^+-ATPase pump and a Cl^- channel, respectively. Recycling of K^+ across the luminal membrane creates a lumen-positive potential that allows one-half of loop Na^+ reabsorption, as well as Ca^{2+} and Mg^{2+} reabsorption, to occur passively via the paracellular route.

the cell is seen only when all four sites on the carrier are occupied. Confirmation of the $1:1:2$ stoichiometry for this transporter in the thick ascending limb has come from the following observations:

- Na^+ is required, since removal of Na^+ from the lumen abolishes the reabsorption of Cl^-.
- Cl^- is required, since removal of Cl^- abolishes the reabsorption of Na^+.
- K^+ is required, since removal of K^+ prevents the reabsorption of both Na^+ and Cl^-.
- The process is electroneutral, since changing the transepithelial electrical potential is without effect on NaCl reabsorption.

A number of Na^+-K^+-$2Cl^-$ cotransporters have been cloned and characterized. The cotransporter termed NKCC2 is principally responsible for Na^+-K^+-$2Cl^-$ transport in the apical membrane of the thick ascending limb.[10] Mutations in this transporter cause classic Bartter's syndrome;[11] this disorder has clinical features (hypokalemia, metabolic alkalosis, and hypercalciuria) similar to those seen in patients given a loop diuretic, which inhibits the Na^+-K^+-$2Cl^-$ cotransporter of the thick ascending limb.

Sodium that enters the cells via Na^+-K^+-$2Cl^-$ cotransport is returned to the systemic circulation by the active Na^+-K^+-ATPase pump in the basolateral membrane; chloride, on the other hand, exits through selective Cl^- channels (Fig. 4-2).[12] Mutations in the gene for these channels result in the same manifestations as classic Bartter's syndrome.[13] In comparison, solute transport in the descending and thin ascending limbs is passive, occurring down favorable concentration and osmotic gradients (see below).

Loop transport is very different from that in the proximal tubule. Filtered glucose, amino acids, and phosphate are almost entirely removed in the proximal tubule by coupled transport with Na^+ (see Fig. 3-4). Thus, loop Na^+ reabsorption is not linked to organic solutes and must occur by coupled transport with Cl^- or by Na^+-H^+ exchange, leading to HCO_3^- reabsorption.

Several important characteristics of the loop NaCl reabsorption deserve emphasis:

- The affinity of the carrier for Na^+ and K^+ is very high, reaching near maximum activity at concentrations under 5 to 10 meq/L (Fig. 4-3).[8] In comparison, it is *Cl^- delivery that is rate-limiting*, as net NaCl transport increases directly with the tubular fluid Cl^- concentration. The loop diuretics, such as furosemide, appear to inhibit loop NaCl reabsorption by competing for the Cl^- site on the carrier (see Chap. 15).

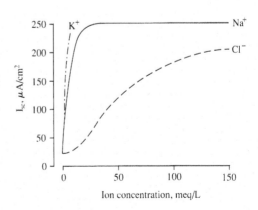

Figure 4-3 The dependence of the equivalent short circuit current (I_{sc}, a measure of active NaCl transport) on the luminal concentrations of K^+, Na^+, and Cl^- in the cortical thick ascending limb of the loop of Henle in the rabbit. The carrier has a very high affinity for Na^+ and K^+, reaching near maximum activity at concentrations under 10 meq/L; as a result, the luminal Cl^- concentration is normally the rate-limiting step in NaCl entry into the cell. A similar process occurs in the medullary thick ascending limb. (*From Greger R, Velazquez H,* Kidney Int *31:590, 1987. Reprinted by permission from* Kidney International.)

- It might appear that K^+ should also be limiting, since its concentration is so much lower than that of Na^+ or Cl^-. This problem is overcome, however, by *recycling* of K^+ across the luminal membrane via specific K^+ channels.[6,15,16] Thus, reabsorbed K^+ is returned to the lumen for continued activation of the Na^+-K^+-$2Cl^-$ carrier. The activity of the K^+ channels is inhibited by adenosine triphosphate (ATP), which allows it to be appropriately linked to the level of Na^+ reabsorption. As more Na^+ enters the cell, for example, transport of this Na^+ out of the cell by the Na^+-K^+-ATPase pump lowers cell ATP levels. The latter change increases the activity of the luminal membrane K^+ channels, permitting the return of reabsorbed K^+ into the lumen and further Na^+ reabsorption. Mutations in this channel cause another variant of Bartter's syndrome,[16] illustrating the requirement for the integrated function of multiple channels for normal loop transport.
- The backleak of cationic K^+ plus the movement of reabsorbed anionic Cl^- (via a Cl^- channel) into the peritubular capillary generates a net positive current from capillary to lumen, thereby creating a lumen-positive potential difference (Fig. 4-2). This potential is important because it can drive the *passive paracellular reabsorption* of cations, such as Na^+, Ca^{2+}, and Mg^{2+}.[6,17,18]

Role in Acid-Base Balance

In addition to the reabsorption of NaCl, the medullary thick limb also contributes to the regulation of acid-base balance. It reabsorbs most of the HCO_3^- that is delivered out of the proximal tubule.[19] This process is primarily mediated by a Na^+-H^+ exchanger in the luminal membrane (see Fig. 20,21).[19,20] Loop HCO_3^- reabsorption is appropriately stimulated by acidemia[20,21] and inhibited by alkalemia,[21] thereby promoting the desired changes in HCO_3^- excretion.

The medullary thick limb also reabsorbs luminal NH_4^+ as NH_4^+ substitutes for K^+ on the Na^+-K^+-$2Cl^-$ cotransporter.[22-24] The net effect is recycling of ammonia within the medulla, thereby maximizing urinary NH_4^+ excretion in the presence of an acid load.[20] The physiologic significance of ammonia recycling is reviewed on page 341.

Role in Urine Calcium Excretion

Although calcium is passively reabsorbed in the thick ascending limb, following the lumen-positive gradient created by sodium reabsorption, the loop of Henle may still participate in the regulation of calcium excretion with changes in calcium intake. Cacium-sensing receptors expressed on the basolateral membrane on the cells of the thick ascending limb appear to mediate this process.[25,26]

When calcium intake is increased, some of the excess calcium is absorbed, enters the systemic circulation, and slightly raises the plasma calcium concentration. Binding of calcium to the calcium-sensing receptor leads to the generation of an arachidonic acid metabolite (which may be 20-HETE[24]) that inhibits the potassium channel in the luminal membrane.[27] Inhibition of potassium recycling via the potassium channel reduces sodium chloride reabsorption via the Na^+-K^+- $2Cl^-$ cotransporter, thereby diminishing the generation of the lumen-positive electrical gradient and the subsequent passive reabsorption of calcium.

Passive Na^+ Reabsorption and Medullary Hypoxia

Almost one-half of oxygen utilization by the thick ascending limb is involved in active NaCl transport.[28] It is important to note in this regard that the $2Cl^-$-to-$1Na^+$ stoichiometry of the luminal Na^+-K^+-$2Cl^-$ carrier *reduces the energy requirement for net Na^+ transport by 50 percent*: For every two Cl^- ions that are reabsorbed, one Na^+ ion is actively transported out of the cell by the Na^+-K^+-ATPase pump and one Na^+ ion is passively reabsorbed between the cells down the lumen-positive electrical gradient (Fig. 4-2).[6]

This increase in efficiency is physiologically important because the renal medulla is relatively poorly oxygenated. The medulla usually receives less than 10 percent of the renal blood flow. Furthermore, the hairpin configuration of the vasa recta capillaries results in the exchange of oxygen between the oxygen-rich blood leaving the cortex and entering the descending capillary limb and the oxygen-poor blood draining the inner medulla in the ascending capillary limb (Fig. 4-4). The net effect is that the P_{O_2} bathing the thick limb cells in the outer medulla is as low as 10 to 20 mmHg.[29] Thus, the ability of the Na^+-K^+-$2Cl^-$ carrier to lower the energy requirement for Na^+ reabsorption may help to preserve the functional integrity of the tubular cells. A similar adaptation is present in the *thin* ascending limb, where Na^+ reabsorption appears to be entirely passive, occurring down a concentration gradient between the tubular fluid and the medullary interstitium (see "NaCl Reabsorption in the Thin Ascending Limb," below).

Clinical Implications   Hypoperfusion-induced acute tubular necrosis is one of the most common causes of acute renal failure developing in the hospital. This finding is somewhat surprising, since the kidney is more highly perfused than most other organs yet cellular injury is usually limited to the kidney.

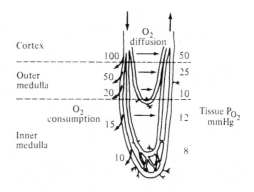

Figure 4-4 Development of medullary hypoxia due to the exchange of oxygen between the descending and ascending limbs of the vasa recta capillaries (straight arrows) and to oxygen consumption by the medullary cells (curved arrows). (*From Brezis M, Rosen S, Silva P, Epstein FH*, Kidney Int 26:375, 1984. *Reprinted by permission from* Kidney International.)

Experimental evidence suggests that this apparent paradox can be explained in part by preferential injury to the thick ascending limb and the S_3 segment of the proximal tubule, which ends in the outer medulla (Fig. 4-1). These cells normally function in a borderline ischemic environment and are therefore particularly susceptible to injury when renal perfusion is impaired.[29]

It is of potential interest in this regard that, in response to renal ischemia, the thick ascending limb cells produce nonprostaglandin, cytochrome P450 arachidonic acid metabolites that diminish NaCl transport;[30,31] this response is mediated at least in part by reduced activity of the luminal Na^+-K^+-$2Cl^-$ transporter.[31] The inhibitory effect of ischemia could represent an appropriate *protective* response, since reducing cellular transport and therefore energy requirement may preserve cell viability when there is inadequate energy delivery.[29,30] Adenosine, a breakdown product of ATP, also may contribute to this local adaptation. The release of adenosine from the thick limb is increased when renal perfusion is reduced; as with the arachidonic acid metabolites, adenosine also reduces active NaCl reabsorption.[32]

Concentration and Flow Dependence of Loop Reabsorption

The loop of Henle, like the proximal tubule, tends to reabsorb a relatively constant fraction of the load delivered to it (this is the phenomenon of glomerulotubular balance; see page 85).[33] In the proximal tubule, total reabsorption is ultimately limited by the availability of luminal solutes (such as bicarbonate, glucose, and amino acids) to be cotransported with Na^+ and by the balance of hemodynamic forces in the peritubular capillary that promotes or retards fluid uptake.

In comparison, *solute concentration* is the limiting factor in the thick ascending limb.[8,33,34] The ascending limb is essentially impermeable to water. As a result, NaCl reabsorption leads to a reduction in the luminal concentration of these ions. In this setting, two factors combine to restrict the level of net reabsorption:

- The fall in the tubular fluid Cl^- concentration progressively decreases the activity of the Na^+-K^+-$2Cl^-$ carrier, thereby diminishing NaCl entry into the cell (Fig. 4-3).
- The reduction in NaCl concentration below that in the plasma promotes the backleak of NaCl into the lumen across the tight junction.

Eventually, the reduced reabsorptive flux will be balanced by a backflux of equal magnitude. This steady state appears to occur at a minimum Cl^- concentration of 50 to 75 meq/L in the cortical aspect of the thick ascending limb.[8,34]

The limiting concentration gradient can explain the flow dependence of loop reabsorption. Suppose, for example, that more fluid is delivered to the ascending limb because of an increase in glomerular filtration rate. If NaCl reabsorption remains constant in the early part of the medullary thick ascending limb, there will be less of a reduction in the tubular fluid Cl^- concentration. Thus, the fluid in the more distal parts of the ascending limb will have a *higher* Cl^- concentration, which will promote increased entry into the cell.[33]

Flow dependence also influences the *distribution* of NaCl reabsorption between the medullary and cortical aspects of the thick limb. As will be described below, antidiuretic hormone (ADH) stimulates NaCl reabsorption in the medullary thick limb by increasing entry via the Na^+-K^+-$2Cl^-$ carrier; this effect is mediated at least in part by enhanced generation of cyclic AMP.[6] The increase in reabsorption will reduce the Cl^- concentration, thereby limiting reabsorption in the cortical thick limb, which can reabsorb Cl^- only until the limiting gradient of 50 to 75 meq/L is reached. The net effect is that NaCl reabsorption is increased in the medullary portion but not in the thick limb as a whole; this response permits increased efficiency of the countercurrent system and subsequent urinary concentration without affecting overall loop NaCl transport.[6]

Other peptide hormones also act to increase cyclic AMP generation and NaCl transport in the thick ascending limb.[35] These include glucagon in the medullary segment and glucagon, calcitonin, parathyroid hormone, and β-adrenergic agonists in the cortical segment. The function of these responses is not clear. They are not likely to be important regulators of NaCl balance, but parathyroid hormone and perhaps calcitonin do contribute to the local regulation of Ca^{2+} and Mg^{2+} reabsorption, particularly in the cortical thick ascending limb (see Chap. 3).[35]

Transport in Cortical Thick Ascending Limb

The cortical aspect of the thick ascending limb makes a variable contribution to nephronal NaCl reabsorption. The juxtamedullary nephrons have long medullary loops (which are essential for concentrating ability; see below) but short cortical segments. In comparison, the cortical aspect is more prominent in the outer cortical nephrons, which are relatively far from the corticomedullary junction (Fig. 4-1).

The Na^+-K^+-$2Cl^-$ carrier appears to mediate most of NaCl reabsorption in the cortex, as it does in the medullary thick limb.[8,36] In addition, the cortical thick ascending limb also plays a major role in Ca^{2+} and Mg^{2+} reabsorption. This segment is the site at which more than 50 percent of the filtered Mg^{2+} is reabsorbed, a level that changes appropriately with alterations in Mg^{2+}-free in states of magnesium depletion due primarily to increased reabsorption in the thick ascending limb and distal convoluted tubule. Some of this Mg^{2+} transport is passive, occurring between the cells down the lumen positive gradient created by the Na^+-K^+-$2Cl^-$ carrier (see Fig. 4-2) and being regulated in part by the calcium-sensing receptor as described above for calcium.[25] In addition, specific changes in Mg^{2+} handling are mediated by an active transcellular process in the distal convoluted tubule that may be activated by changes in the plasma Mg^{2+} concentration.[17,37]

The cortical thick ascending limb is also one of the sites (with the distal tubule and connecting segment) at which Ca^{2+} reabsorption is actively regulated according to the physiologic needs (see Chap. 3). Parathyroid hormone plays an important role in this process, increasing Ca^{2+} reabsorption by activating a hormone-specific adenylate cyclase.[38]

COUNTERCURRENT MECHANISM

Fluid leaving the proximal tubule is isosmotic to plasma. However, the excretion of an isosmotic urine is usually not adequate to meet the homeostatic requirements of the body. After a water load, for example, water must be excreted in excess of solute. This requires the excretion of urine that is hypoosmotic to plasma. Conversely, water must be retained and a hyperosmotic urine excreted after a period of water restriction. The formation of a dilute (hypoosmotic to plasma) or concentrated (hyperosmotic to plasma) urine is achieved via the *countercurrent mechanism*, which includes the loop of Henle, the cortical and medullary collecting tubules, and the blood supply to these segments.

Before discussing these processes in detail, it is useful to summarize their basic aspects. The excretion of a *concentrated* urine involves two major steps:

- The medullary interstitium is made hyperosmotic by the reabsorption of NaCl without water in the medullary ascending limb of the loop of Henle. Urea entry into the interstitium from the medullary collecting tubule also contributes to this process.
- As the urine enters the medullary collecting tubule, it equilibrates osmotically with the interstitium, resulting in the formation of a concentrated urine. ADH, released from the posterior pituitary, plays an essential role in this process by increasing collecting tubule permeability to water, which is very low in the basal state. ADH appears to act by inserting aquaporin-2 *water channels* into the luminal membrane, thereby allowing transcellular water reabsorption to occur down an osmotic gradient (see Chap. 6).

In addition, two modifying factors are important for the *maintenance* of medullary hyperosmolality:

- Water equilibrating in the medullary collecting tubule dilutes the interstitium, a change that would decrease maximum concentrating ability. To minimize this effect, the volume of urine presented to this segment is markedly reduced in the cortex by ADH-sensitive water reabsorption in the cortical collecting tubule.
- Medullary blood flow in the vasa recta is arranged in a hairpin configuration to minimize removal of the excess interstitial solute.

Urinary *dilution* also has two basic steps, the first of which is the same as in urinary concentration:

- NaCl reabsorption without water in the ascending limb of the loop of Henle decreases the osmolality of the tubular fluid at the same time as it increases the osmolality of the interstitium.
- The urine remains dilute if water reabsorption in the collecting tubules is minimized by keeping these segments poorly permeable to water. This requires the relative absence of ADH.

Countercurrent Multiplication: Loops of Henle

In humans, the maximum urine osmolality that can be attained is 900 to 1400 mosmol/kg; the normal plasma osmolality is much lower, at about 285 mosmol/kg. Since the urine becomes concentrated by equilibrating with the medullary interstitium, this means that a similar high osmolality must be achieved in the interstitium. The process by which the interstitial osmolality in the medulla is increased from 285 mosmol/kg (isosmotic to plasma) to 900 to 1400 mosmol/kg is called *countercurrent multiplication*. (*Countercurrent* refers to the opposite directions of flow in the descending and ascending limbs that result from the hairpin configuration of the loop.)

The exact mechanism of countercurrent multiplication is incompletely understood.[39-41] The following discussion has been simplified by emphasizing the generation of an interstitial osmotic gradient from the corticomedullary junction to the inner medulla. At any level, however, there are also likely to be variations in the interstitial osmolality with increasing distance from the vasa recta capillary bundles.[41]

One essential factor in countercurrent multiplication is the different permeability and transport characteristics of the descending and ascending limbs of the loop of Henle. The descending limb is permeable to water and to a lesser degree NaCl and urea, whereas both the thin and thick segments of the ascending limb are *impermeable to water*, but are able to transport NaCl into the interstitium (Table 4-1). These differences in water permeability are related to the presence (thin descending limb) or absence (ascending limb) of water channels in the luminal membrane.[42,43] The water channels in the thin descending limb are called aquaporin-1;[43,44] they are similar to those in the luminal membrane of the proximal tubule but different from the ADH-sensitive water channels (called aquaporin-2) in the collecting tubules (see Chap. 6).[45]

As will be seen, the *only active step* in countercurrent multiplication is NaCl reabsorption in the thick ascending limb, the mechanism for which is depicted in Fig. 4-2. In contrast, only passive solute transport appears to occur in the descending and *thin* ascending limbs.[39,41] The mechanism by which the thin ascending limb might reabsorb NaCl will be reviewed below; for the sake of simplicity, the following discussion on the generation of the interstitial osmotic gradient will assume that the thin and thick ascending limbs function in a homogeneous manner.

The efficiency of countercurrent multiplication varies directly with the *length* of the thick ascending limb. Thus, this process primarily occurs in the 30 to 40

Table 4-1   Passive permeability of the loop of Henle and distal nephron segments to NaCl, urea, and water[a]

Segment	NaCl	Urea	Water	
			Basal	ADH
Descending limb	± to ++	± to +	++	++
Ascending limb				
Thin segment	++	+	0	0
Thick segment	0	0	0	0
Distal tubule and connecting segment	0	0	0	0
Cortical collecting tubule	0	0	0	++
Medullary collecting tubule				
Outer	0	0	0	++
Inner	0	±[b]	±	++

[a] Data from Refs. 38 and 41. Symbols include: ++, highly permeable; +, moderately permeable; ±, less permeable; 0, relatively impermeable.

[b] The urea permeability in the innermost part of the medullary collecting tubule is increased in the presence of ADH.

percent of nephrons that have long loops of Henle that descend into the inner medulla (Fig. 4-1). The glomeruli of these nephrons are located in the juxtamedullary area and the midcortex. In contrast, there is little direct contribution from the outer cortical nephrons, which have short loops that turn around in the outer medulla or even the inner cortex (Fig. 4-1).

Generation of Medullary Interstitial Hyperosmolality

If one could start at a hypothetical time zero, the fluid in the descending and ascending limbs and in the interstitium would be isosmotic to plasma, similar to that delivered into the descending limb from the proximal tubule (Fig. 4-5). The first and primary step in countercurrent multiplication is the transport of NaCl from the ascending limb of the loop of Henle into the interstitium; this process is limited by the maximum transtubular gradient that can be achieved, which in this example is 200 mosmol/kg. Since the ascending limb is impermeable to water, this results in an increase in interstitial osmolality from 285 to 385 mosmol/kg. The fluid in the descending limb then equilibrates osmotically with the interstitium, primarily by water movement out of the tubule. As water enters the interstitium, interstitial osmolality is maintained by continued NaCl transport out of the ascending limb. The net effect is the establishment of a 200-mosmol/kg gradient between the fluid in the ascending limb (185 mosmol/kg) and that in the interstitium and descending limb (385 mosmol/kg).

As urine flows through the tubules, and NaCl transport in the ascending limb continues, the initial step in Fig. 4-5 is *multiplied*, resulting in the generation of a

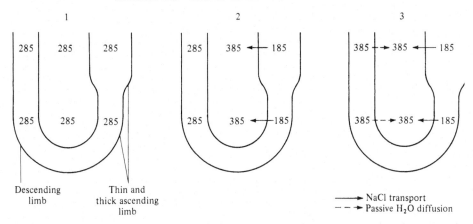

Figure 4-5 Role of active NaCl transport in initiating countercurrent multiplication. In step 1, at time zero, the fluid in the descending and ascending limbs and the interstitium is isosmotic to plasma. In step 2, NaCl is transported out of the ascending limb into the interstitium to a gradient of 200 mosmol/kg. In step 3, the fluid in the descending limb equilibrates osmotically with the hyperosmotic interstitium, primarily by water movement out of the tubule. Dilution of the interstitium by this water movement is prevented by continued NaCl transport out of the ascending limb. The result is the creation of an osmotic gradient between the ascending limb and the relatively hyperosmotic descending limb and interstitium.

much higher interstitial osmolality. An example of how this might occur is shown in Fig. 4-6. For the sake of simplicity, steps 1 to 8 are depicted as discrete instants in time, even though ion transport and urine flow occur simultaneously in the intact kidney. In steps 1 and 2, a gradient of 200 mosmol/kg is established between the fluid in the ascending limb and that in the descending limb and interstitium. In step 3, urine moves through the tubules, with the hyperosmotic fluid in the descending limb flowing into the ascending limb. As NaCl is again pumped into the interstitium to a gradient of 200 mosmol/kg in step 4, the osmolality of the inner medullary interstitium is now 485 mosmol/kg, as compared with 385 mosmol/kg in step 2.

These steps illustrate the basic aspects of countercurrent multiplication: NaCl transport out of the ascending limb makes the interstitium and descending limb hyperosmotic; the hyperosmotic fluid in the descending limb then flows in a countercurrent fashion into the ascending limb; the combination of a higher tubular fluid osmolality in the inner medullary ascending limb (385 mosmol/kg in step 3 versus 285 mosmol/kg in step 1) and reestablishment of the 200 mosmol/kg gradient between the ascending limb and interstitium results in a further elevation in interstitial osmolality.

As the sequence in Fig. 4-6 goes on (steps 5 to 8), the osmolality continues to rise, being highest in the tubule at the hairpin turn and in the interstitium at the papillary tip (the inner medulla). The osmolality at these sites is directly proportional both to the length of the loops and to the gradient achieved between the ascending limb and the interstitium. In humans, the maximum osmolality at the

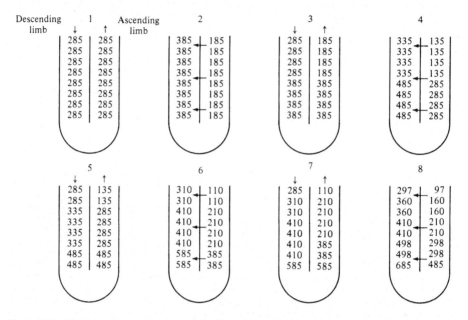

Figure 4-6 Principle of countercurrent multiplication based upon the assumption that, at any level along the loop of Henle, a concentration gradient of 200 mosmol/kg can be established between ascending and descending limbs of the loop of Henle by the transport of NaCl. The osmolality of the interstitium is the same as that in the descending limb and has been omitted from the diagram. (*Adapted from Pitts RF*, Physiology of the Kidney and Body Fluids, *3d ed. Copyright ©1974 by Year Book Medical Publishers, Inc, Chicago. Used by permission.*)

papillary tip can reach 900 to 1400 mosmol/kg (Fig. 4-7).* This is relatively ineffi-cient in comparison with other mammals. As an example, the desert rat, which infrequently comes in contact with water, has relatively long loops of Henle and can attain interstitial and urine osmolalities in the range of 5000 mosmol/kg.

In addition to increased length of the loop of Henle, more efficient urinary concentration in some species is also due to stimulation of NaCl reabsorption in the medullary thick ascending limb by ADH.[6,46,47] A cyclic adenosine mono-phosphate (AMP)–mediated rise in activity of the luminal Na^+-K^+-$2Cl^-$ carrier seems to be responsible for this effect.[46] The applicability of these findings to humans is uncertain, since studies in isolated human tubules have not demonstrated an ADH-induced increase in cyclic AMP activity in the thick ascending limb.[48]

Notice also that the osmolality of the tubular fluid leaving the ascending limb is hypoosmotic to plasma (Fig. 4-7). This fluid is further diluted by NaCl reab-sorption without water in the cortical aspect of the thick ascending limb. As a result, the osmolality of the urine leaving the loop of Henle is approximately 100 mosmol/kg.[8] If the collecting tubules are impermeable to water (ADH

---

*Only about one-half of the papillary solute is NaCl, with urea accounting for most of the remainder (see "Role of Urea" below).

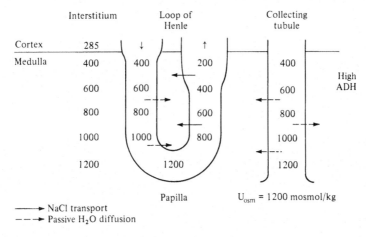

Figure 4-7 Countercurrent multiplication and the excretion of a concentrated urine. The transport of NaCl from the ascending limb results in the formation of an interstitial osmolal gradient from 285 mosmol/kg in the cortex to 1200 mosmol/kg at the papillary tip. In the presence of ADH, the urine becomes concentrated as it equilibrates with the interstitium in the medullary collecting tubule. The contribution of urea to the concentrating process is discussed in the text and has been omitted from the diagram. The collecting tubule is also the site of active Na^+ transport, the importance of which is discussed in Chap. 5.

absent), this dilute urine will be excreted relatively unchanged. In contrast, if the collecting tubules are permeable to water (ADH present), the urine will equilibrate with the interstitium and a concentrated urine will be excreted (Fig. 4-7). Thus, the *final osmolality of the urine is mostly determined by the water permeability of the collecting tubules, not by events in the loop of Henle.**

Collecting Tubules

As with the loops of Henle, the cortical and medullary collecting tubules possess distinct permeability characteristics, being in the basal state relatively impermeable to the passive movement of NaCl, and, with the exception of the innermost part of the medullary collecting tubule, to urea and water (Table 4-1).[49,50] The impermeability to NaCl is essential, since it permits the high NaCl concentration in the interstitium to act as an effective osmotic gradient between the tubular fluid and interstitium.

ADH promotes urinary concentration primarily by increasing the water permeability of the collecting tubules[40,49,50] via the insertion of unique water channels (called aquaporin-2) into the luminal membrane (see Chap. 6).[45,51] In the medullary collecting tubule, this allows the tubular fluid to reach osmotic equilibrium with the hyperosmotic interstitium.[40,52] The reabsorbed water then returns to the systemic circulation via the capillaries of the vasa recta.

---

* Although the interstitial osmolal gradient is primarily created by those nephrons with long loops, urine from all nephrons drains into the collecting tubules (see Fig. 4-1) and equilibrates osmotically with the interstitium in the presence of ADH.

The *cortical* collecting tubule plays an equally important role in the concentrating process. The maximum urine osmolality attained in the medulla cannot exceed that in the interstitium at the papillary tip. As water leaves the medullary collecting tubule, it decreases the interstitial osmolality by dilution, thereby reducing the maximum urine osmolality that can be achieved. This effect is minimized *because the volume of fluid present to the medullary collecting tubule is markedly reduced by ADH-induced water reabsorption in the cortical collecting tubule.*[49,52]* In the presence of ADH, the hypoosmotic fluid entering the cortical collecting tubule equilibrates with the cortical interstitium, which is isosmotic to plasma (Fig. 4-8).

If, for example, the osmolality of the tubular fluid entering the cortical collecting tubule is 100 mosmol/kg, then osmotic equilibration will result in the reabsorption of almost two-thirds of the water that has been delivered. Furthermore, additional water will be reabsorbed, down the osmotic gradient established by aldosterone-induced NaCl reabsorption in this segment (see Chap. 8). This marked reduction in tubular fluid volume permits concentration of the urine to proceed in the medulla with minimum dilution of the medullary interstitium. Since cortical blood flow is more than 10 times the maximum rate of urine flow, the water reabsorbed in the cortex is rapidly returned to the systemic circulation without dilution of the cortical interstitium.

In the absence of ADH, the collecting tubules remain poorly permeable to water. As a result, much less water is reabsorbed and a dilute urine is excreted. Since active NaCl transport continues in these segments, the minimum urine osmolality may be reduced from 100 mosmol/kg in the distal tubule to 50 to 75 mosmol/kg in the final urine.

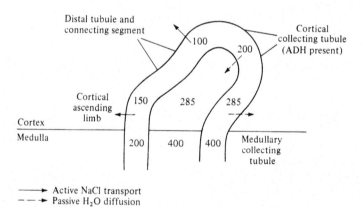

Figure 4-8   Representation of the role of the cortical collecting tubule in the concentrating process. As a result of water reabsorption in this segment, the hypoosmotic urine formed in the ascending limb of the loop of Henle is made isosmotic to plasma and is much reduced in volume.

---

* Water reabsorption is probably minimal in the distal tubule and connecting segment, which, like the ascending limb, are relatively impermeable to water both in the basal state and in the presence of ADH.[53,54]

ADH is able to play this central role in the regulation of water excretion because its release *varies directly with the plasma osmolality* (Fig. 4-9). Thus, a water load sequentially lowers the plasma osmolality, ADH secretion, collecting tubule permeability to water, and the urine osmolality. The net effect is excretion of the excess water. These steps are reversed with water loss, as the increase in plasma osmolality stimulates the release of ADH, resulting in a rise in urine osmolality and a marked reduction in further water loss. Increased water intake due to a concurrent stimulation of thirst then returns water balance to normal.

Role of Urea

The discussion thus far has emphasized the importance of NaCl accumulation in the medullary interstitium in the concentrating process. However, almost one-half of the approximately 1200 mosmol of solute per kilogram present at the papillary tip during antidiuresis is *urea*.[39] The high interstitial concentration of urea is produced by diffusion down a favorable concentration gradient from the inner medullary collecting tubule into the interstitium (Fig. 4-10).[43,55]

ADH, acting in both the cortex and the medulla, plays a central role in this process by increasing the water permeability of the collecting tubules. As water is reabsorbed in the cortex and outer medulla, the *urea concentration in the tubular fluid rises markedly*, since these segments are essentially impermeable to urea.[49,50] In contrast, permeability to urea in the innermost part of the medullary collecting tubule is relatively high in the basal state (mediated by specific luminal membrane urea carriers[56,57]) and is increased further by ADH, apparently by insertion of new urea transporters into the luminal membrane.[50,58,59] These effects allow urea to passively diffuse into the interstitium at this site.

The ADH-regulated urea transporter, UT1, that is responsible for urea transport in the medullary collecting tubule has been identified and cloned.[57] As

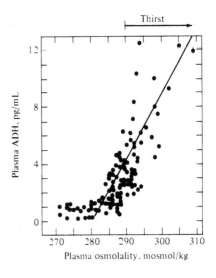

Figure 4-9 Relationship of plasma ADH concentration to plasma osmolality in normal humans in whom the plasma osmolality was changed by varying the state of hydration. Notice that the osmotic threshold for thirst is a few mosmol/kg higher than that for ADH. (*Adapted from Robertson GL, Aycinena P, Zerbe RL, Am J Med 72:339, 1982. Used with permission.*)

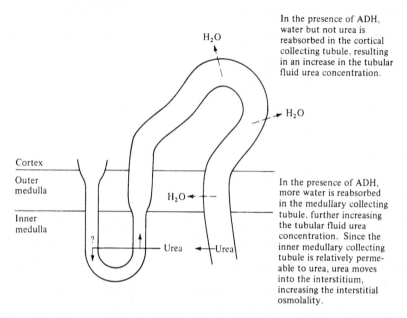

In the presence of ADH, water but not urea is reabsorbed in the cortical collecting tubule, resulting in an increase in the tubular fluid urea concentration.

In the presence of ADH, more water is reabsorbed in the medullary collecting tubule, further increasing the tubular fluid urea concentration. Since the inner medullary collecting tubule is relatively permeable to urea, urea moves into the interstitium, increasing the interstitial osmolality.

Figure 4-10 Mechanism by which urea achieves high concentrations in the medullary interstitium.

expected, UT1 is principally expressed in the innermost part of the medullary collecting tubule.

In addition to ADH, urea accumulation in the medulla is also indirectly dependent upon active NaCl transport in the ascending limb. The ensuing increase in interstitial osmolality affects urea transport in two ways. First, it directly increases the activity of the inner medullary urea transporter via an effect that is independent of ADH.[60] Second, loop NaCl reabsorption makes the tubular fluid dilute and the interstitium concentrated, thereby creating the osmotic gradients that allow water reabsorption to occur in the collecting tubules; the increase in water reabsorption raises the tubular fluid urea concentration, enhancing the gradient for urea entry into the interstitium.

Some of the urea that accumulates in the interstitium *reenters* the tubule in the thin ascending limb and the descending limb.[39,40,55] This recirculation of urea occurs via a second urea transporter, UT2.[57] The net effect of this *urea recycling* is that the quantity of urea in the early distal tubule is the same as or slightly exceeds the amount filtered, even though 60 to 65 percent of the filtered urea has been reabsorbed in the proximal tubule.[61] Thus, both urinary and interstitial urea concentrations are maintained at high levels in the presence of ADH.*

---

*The volume of the medullary interstitium is relatively small. The weight of both kidneys in humans is approximately 350 g, most of which is composed of nephron segments, tubular fluid, and blood vessels. Thus, the attainment of high concentrations of urea in the medullary interstitium requires only small amounts of urea. Since approximately 27 to 32 g (about 500 mmol) of urea is excreted per day, the interstitial accumulation of urea does not importantly affect total urea excretion.

The rise in medullary interstitial osmolality produced by urea allows the concentrating process to be more efficient in several ways. The most evident is that the higher interstitial osmolality maximizes concentrating ability and allows the excretion of large quantities of urea without obligating concurrent water loss.[58] The interstitial accumulation of urea also promotes osmotic water movement out of the descending limb of the loop of Henle. This water flux leads to an elevation in the tubular fluid Na^+ concentration entering the *thin* ascending limb and to a reduction (by dilution) in the interstitial Na^+ concentration. Both of these changes promote passive Na^+ reabsorption in the thin ascending limb (see below). Thus, urea indirectly plays an important role in primary step in the countercurrent mechanism: the transport of Na^+ out of the ascending limb into the medullary interstitium.

The overall importance of urea in the concentrating process can be appreciated from experimental studies in which ADH secretion is minimal because of a large water load or hereditary diabetes insipidus.[62,63] In the absence of ADH, urea accumulation in the interstitium is virtually abolished, since the decline in water reabsorption in the cortical and outer medullary collecting tubules prevents the increase in the tubular fluid urea concentration that is necessary for urea diffusion (Fig. 4-11). NaCl accumulation is also reduced because, as just described, urea accumulation indirectly promotes NaCl reabsorption in the thin ascending limb.

These findings demonstrate that *papillary osmolality is not constant but varies with the availability of ADH*. It is likely that a similar situation exists in humans. In

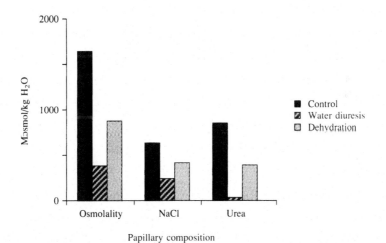

Papillary composition

Figure 4-11 Simultaneous measurement of renal papillary osmolality, sodium concentration, and urea concentration in rats in the control state, after a water load, and 2 h after the reinstitution of fluid restriction plus the administration of ADH. Water loading, which is associated with the inhibition of ADH release, led to a marked reduction in papillary osmolality that was mostly due to the virtual abolition of urea accumulation. These changes rapidly returned toward normal when ADH was given. (*Data from Levitin H, Goodman A, Pigeon G, Epstein FH*, J Clin Invest *41:1145, 1962, by permission from the American Society for Clinical Investigation.*)

patients with central diabetes insipidus or those who shut off ADH secretion by chronic water loading (see Chap. 24), the ability to concentrate the urine after the administration of ADH is impaired.[64] In one study, maintaining a high fluid intake in normal subjects for only 3 days was sufficient to lower the maximum ADH-induced urine osmolality by over 400 mosmol/kg (from approximately 1180 mosmol/kg to 760 mosmol/kg).[65] Washout of medullary urea and NaCl was probably responsible for this effect.

NaCl Reabsorption in Thin Ascending Limb

NaCl reabsorption in the thin ascending limb appears to be primarily passive, not active as in the thick ascending limb.[41,66] How a favorable concentration gradient for NaCl diffusion might be created can be appreciated if we review the aspects of countercurrent multiplication that have been discussed thus far (Fig. 4-12).[39,40] Active NaCl reabsorption without water in the thick ascending limb makes the

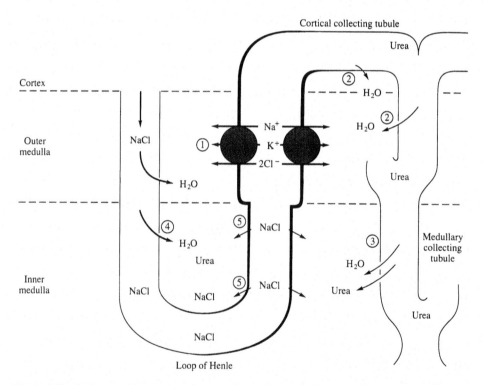

Figure 4-12 Summary of the steps involved in countercurrent multiplication in which a concentration gradient is established that permits passive NaCl reabsorption in the thin ascending limb in the inner medulla. The thickened lines represent the water impermeability of the ascending limb. See text for details. (*From Jamison RL, Maffly RH,* N Engl J Med *295:1059, 1976. By permission from the* New England Journal of Medicine.)

tubular fluid dilute and the interstitium concentrated (step 1). This dilute fluid, in the presence of ADH, equilibrates osmotically with the isosmotic interstitium in the cortical collecting tubule (step 2) and then with the hyperosmotic interstitium in the medullary collecting tubule (step 3). The removal of water (but not urea) from the tubular fluid in these segments results in a marked elevation in the urea concentration, which diffuses into the interstitium in the inner medullary collecting tubule (step 3).[50]

At this point, let us suppose that the interstitial osmolality at the papillary tip is 1200 mosmol/kg, half of which is NaCl (300 meq/L of both Na^+ and Cl^-) and half of which is urea. The fluid entering the descending limb from the proximal tubule has an osmolality of about 300 mosmol/kg, a Na^+ concentration of 150 meq/L, and a urea concentration below 10 mmol/L, similar to that in the plasma. If we assume that equilibration with the hyperosmotic interstitium occurs entirely by water movement out of the tubule (step 4), then three-quarters of this fluid must be reabsorbed to raise the tubular fluid osmolality to 1200 mosmol/kg, the value at the hairpin turn in the interstitium (Fig. 4-7). If, however, osmotic equilibration is impaired because of the absence of aquaporin-1, then concentrating ability is reduced.[44]

This elevation in osmolality will be accompanied by a fourfold increase in the tubular fluid Na^+ concentration to about 600 meq/L, well above that in the interstitium. This will promote passive NaCl diffusion out of the thin ascending limb, which is relatively permeable to these ions (step 5).[41] Although there is a similar inward gradient for urea in this segment (since the interstitial concentration is so high), the degree of urea entry into the tubule is much less because of a lower urea permeability (Table 4-1).[41] Thus, the net effect is NaCl reabsorption without water and a reduction in the tubular fluid osmolality, both of which are required for countercurrent multiplication.

The major problem with this model is that it is dependent upon osmotic equilibration in the descending limb occurring almost entirely by water removal, thereby leading to a marked elevation in the transtubular NaCl concentration gradient. It is possible, however, that the high interstitial concentration of urea could lead to passive diffusion of this solute into the tubule. This is likely to occur, since parts of the descending limb have a relatively high urea permeability (Table 4-1).[40,41] To the degree that osmotic equilibration occurs by urea entry, there will be a lesser rise in the tubular fluid NaCl concentration.

The net effect is that there does not appear to be a sufficient transtubular NaCl gradient established to support the degree of passive transport required for countercurrent multiplication to proceed. Thus, the exact mechanism by which thin ascending limb reabsorption occurs is at present incompletely understood.[40,41,66] It is possible that some component of active transport may be required in the later part of the thin ascending limb.[67]

This model also does not explain the mechanisms of transcellular NaCl reabsorption in the thin ascending limb. Evidence suggests that Na^+ reabsorption primarily occurs via the paracellular pathway between the cells,[68] while Cl^- reabsorption occurs via a kidney-specific Cl⁻ channel called CLC-K1.[69] How these processes are linked is not clear, but the importance of the Cl⁻ channel in urinary concentration has been demonstrated by the finding of polyuria due to ADH resistance in mice that lack this channel.[69]

Countercurrent Exchange: Vasa Recta

The capillaries of the vasa recta are derived from the efferent arterioles of the juxtamedullary glomeruli and have a hairpin configuration, similar to the loops of Henle (Fig. 4-13) They play an important role in the *maintenance of mass balance in the medulla* by returning the NaCl and water reabsorbed in the loop of Henle and medullary collecting tubule to the systemic circulation. The ascending vasa recta are well adapted for such a role, since Starling's forces in these vessels are much in favor of fluid uptake: The oncotic pressure which promotes uptake is approximately 26 mmHg, whereas the hydraulic pressure which pushes fluid out of the capillary is only about 9 mmHg at the papillary tip.[70,71] The net effect is that

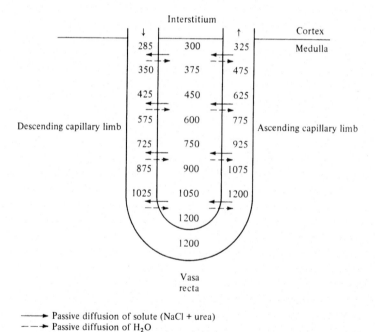

Figure 4-13 Principle of countercurrent exchange in the vasa recta capillaries. In the descending capillary limb, solute enters and water leaves the capillary down concentration gradients, tending to reduce interstitial osmolality. These processes are reversed in the ascending capillary limb, thereby preserving the interstitial osmolal gradient. (*Adapted from Pitts RF*, Physiology of the Kidney and Body Fluids, *3d ed. Copyright © 1974 by Year Book Medical Publishers, Inc, Chicago. Used by permission.*)

the flow rate leaving the medulla in the ascending vasa recta is almost twice that entering the medulla in the descending vasa recta.[72]

The vasa recta also play an integral role in the *maintenance* of the medullary osmotic gradient.[70] The vasa recta reach osmotic equilibrium with the interstitium, since they are permeable to solutes and water. In the descending vasa recta, solute enters and water leaves as the plasma osmolality reaches a value similar to that in the interstitium at the papillary tip (Fig. 4-13). The very high interstitial sodium chloride and urea concentrations generate a sufficient osmotic pressure to promote free water loss, even though the direct effect of the intracapillary Starling's forces is to promote water and solute movement into the capillary.[73]

If the vasa recta left the kidney at the papilla, the combination of solute removal and water addition would reduce medullary osmolality. However, the medullary osmotic gradient is maintained because the vasa recta turn around at the papillary tip and return to the cortex. As a result, the solute removed from the interstitium in the descending limb is returned to the interstitium, i.e., exchanged, in the ascending limb down a favorable concentration gradient from the lumen to the interstitium. Similarly, water added to the interstitium in the descending limb reenters the capillary in the ascending limb. Allowing for a lag in equilibration, the blood returning to the cortex is only slightly hyperosmotic to plasma (325 mosmol/ kg).

Notice that this process of *countercurrent exchange* is driven by the preexisting transcapillary osmotic and concentration gradients. It is not dependent upon Starling's forces, which, as described above, are more important in the net removal of the solutes and water that have entered the interstitium by tubular reabsorption.

The low rate of medullary blood flow (6 percent of renal blood flow), which is partially under neurohumoral control,[74] also contributes to the maintenance of interstitial hyperosmolality. If medullary blood flow is increased, more blood at 325 mosmol/kg will leave the medulla, and a significant washout of medullary solute can occur, with a reduction in interstitial osmolality.[70]

Washout of medullary solute can alter loop NaCl and water handling via the following sequence. It will diminish water reabsorption in the descending limb of the loop of Henle, since there is now a lesser osmotic gradient between the tubular fluid and the interstitium (step 4 in Fig. 4-12). This reduction in water removal will result in a lesser rise in the tubular fluid Na^+ concentration, thereby decreasing passive NaCl reabsorption in the thin ascending limb (step 5 in Fig. 4-12).

A clinical example in which each of these changes in loop function occurs is during an *osmotic diuresis* in which a large amount of nonreabsorbed solute is present in the urine. This may be seen with glucosuria in uncontrolled diabetes mellitus (see Chap. 25) or after an intravenous infusion of mannitol. In these settings, medullary blood flow is enhanced by an unknown mechanism,[75] resulting sequentially in a decrease in papillary osmolality,[76] and an elevation in both urine volume and Na^+ excretion, primarily due to a fall in descending limb water reabsorption and ascending limb Na^+ reabsorption.[77]

Summary

The countercurrent mechanism permits the kidney to excrete urine with an osmolality that varies in humans from a minimum of 50 mosmol/kg to a maximum of 900 to 1400 mosmol/kg. The primary event in this process is active NaCl transport out of the thick ascending limb of the loop of Henle into the medullary interstitium, producing dilution of the tubular fluid and concentration of the interstitium. Because of the different permeability characteristics of the descending and ascending limbs, this first step results in countercurrent multiplication in which a medullary osmotic gradient is created that reaches its maximum at the papillary tip.

The osmolal changes that may occur as the tubular fluid moves through the nephron are summarized in Fig. 4-14. The isosmotic urine delivered from the proximal tubule becomes hyperosmotic in the descending limb as it equilibrates with the medullary interstitium and then becomes hypoosmotic in the ascending limb as NaCl is reabsorbed without water. The *final osmolality of the urine is determined in the collecting tubules in a manner dependent upon ADH*:

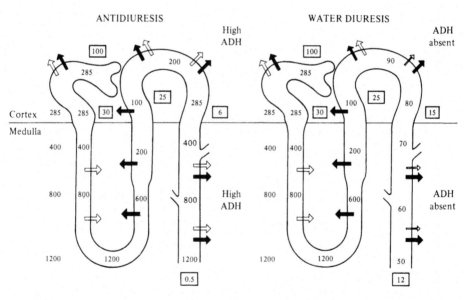

→ NaCl transport
⇨ Passive H₂O diffusion

Figure 4-14   Summary of NaCl and H_2O transport throughout the nephron during an antidiuresis and a water diuresis. The tubular fluid and interstitial concentrations are expressed in milliosmoles per kilogram (mosmol/kg); the large, boxed numbers represent the percentage of the glomerular filtrate remaining in the tubule at each site. Note that the composition and volume of the tubular fluid are essentially the same at the end of the loop of Henle as the excretion of a concentrated or dilute urine is determined primarily in the collecting tubules.

- In the presence of ADH, collecting tubule water permeability is increased, allowing osmotic equilibration of the tubular fluid with the isosmotic interstitium in the cortex and then the hyperosmotic interstitium in the medulla. The result is the excretion of a concentrated urine. ADH also contributes to the high medullary osmolality by permitting urea entry into the interstitium and, in some species, by promoting NaCl reabsorption in the medullary thick ascending limb.
- In the absence of ADH, the hypoosmotic urine leaving the loop of Henle does not equilibrate with the interstitium, and a dilute urine is excreted.

These effects of ADH are dose-related. This is important because normal daily needs usually do not require maximal dilution or concentration of the urine. A normal subject, for example, may need to excrete 800 mosmol of solute and 2 liters of water per day to remain in the steady state. The excretion of urine with an average osmolality of 400 mosmol/kg requires a submaximal ADH response.

Clinical Example

This chapter has emphasized the importance of ADH in the production of a concentrated urine. However, other factors also can contribute, including the effective circulating volume (i.e., the rate of effective tissue perfusion). As an example, the absence of ADH, as after a water load or with impaired production due to central diabetes insipidus, is generally associated with a urine osmolality below 100 mosmol/kg and a urine output that can exceed 10 L/day.

If, however, effective volume depletion is superimposed, the urine osmolality can rise to as high as 400 mosmol/kg or more.[78,79] In this setting, the associated reduction in glomerular filtration rate and increment in proximal Na^+ and water reabsorption can markedly diminish water delivery to the collecting tubules. The inner medullary collecting tubule is mildly permeable to water even in the absence of ADH.[50] As a result, the combination of a very lower rate of delivery and a small amount of water reabsorption at this site can substantially raise the urine osmolality.[79] The net effect is that the presence of diabetes insipidus may be masked, since neither marked polyuria nor a very dilute urine is present. Volume repletion will reverse these changes and allow the correct diagnosis to be suspected.

MAINTENANCE OF CELL VOLUME

Maintenance of protein function within the cells generally requires a relatively constant cell volume, although it is possible that it is the concentration of intracellular proteins rather than volume itself that is being regulated.[80] This is an important issue for the cells in the medulla, such as those in the thick ascending limb and inner medullary collecting tubule, since the interstitial milieu in which they reside may undergo wide changes in osmolality, as illustrated in Fig. 4-12.

Although the luminal membrane of ascending limb cells is impermeable to water, osmotic equilibration with the interstitium can occur across the basolateral membrane. As a result, the rise in interstitial osmolality induced by ADH will cause water movement out of the tubular cells and cell shrinkage. This effect is transient, however, because the cells are able to adapt by increasing their osmolality, thereby holding water within the cells.[81,82] This protective response is, at least acutely, mediated by ADH. Acting on the *basolateral* membrane, ADH promotes the entry of interstitial NaCl into the cells, apparently by activating parallel Na^+-H^+ and Cl^--HCO_3^- exchangers.[82] A similar process occurs in the inner medullary collecting tubule, which is exposed to the same changes in interstitial osmolality[83] and which has aquaporin-3 and aquaporin-4 water channels in the basolateral membrane.[84]

Another defense mechanism in the response to hypertonicity is the generation or uptake of new organic solutes, which leads to the osmotic movement of water into the cell and the restoration of cell volume. These solutes include sorbitol, inositol, betaine, taurine, and glycerophosphocholine.[85-89] These solutes, which have been called *osmolytes*, have the advantage that changes in their concentration within the cells do not appear to interfere with enzyme activity. In comparison, an elevation in the cell Na^+ or K^+ concentration may preserve cell volume at the expense of normal protein function.[85,86]

The mechanism by which osmolyte net production or uptake is enhanced in the thick ascending limb and inner medullary collecting tubule is becoming better understood.[90] One possible signal is the cellular ionic strength ($Na^+ + K^+$ concentration).[87,91] With hyperosmolality, for example, the osmotic movement of fluid out of the cells plus the initial Na^+ and K^+ uptake raises the cellular ionic strength. This appears to activate osmotic response elements on the genes that regulate the activity of aldose reductase and the transporters for betaine and inositol.[90,92]

- The activity of aldose reductase, the enzyme that catalyzes the formation of sorbitol from glucose, is increased;[90,91,93] this change may be accompanied by reduced activity of sorbitol dehydrogenase, thereby diminishing sorbitol conversion to fructose.[93]

- There is also enhanced activity of Na^+-inositol and Na^+-betaine cotransporters, changes that will promote the cellular uptake of these solutes.[90,94] This increase in transport appears to occur across the basolateral membrane; this is appropriate since the interstitial fluid (which is in equilibrium with the plasma) is likely to have a higher concentration of inositol and betaine than the lumen (due to proximal reabsorption of most of the filtered osmolytes).[95]

- The accumulation of glycerophosphocholine (GPC) appears to result from reduced degradation (a change that is mediated by diminished activity of the enzyme GPC:choline phosphodiesterase)[96] as well as increased synthesis (from phosphatidycholine, the precursor of GPC).[97]

The total osmolyte concentration within the cells is another important determinant of osmolyte accumulation. The administration of an aldose reductase inhibitor, for example, will prevent the generation of sorbitol; however, the net response to hyperosmolality is not impaired since the reduction in sorbitol is balanced by an increase in other osmolytes, particularly enhanced uptake of betaine.[98]

If, on the other hand, the interstitial osmolality falls (as with a water load), there will be a tendency for water to move into the cells, leading to cell swelling. In this setting, the cell volume is maintained by reversing the above responses. Aldose reductase activity is reduced[93] and the excess intracellular sorbitol and other osmolytes rapidly leak out of the cell due to the expression of specific carriers or channels in the cell membrane.[85,95,99] Loss of ions, particularly K^+ and Cl^-, also occurs through specific channels in the luminal and peritubular membrane, respectively (see Fig. 4-2).[81]

TAMM-HORSFALL MUCOPROTEIN

The thick ascending limb secretes a protein called Tamm-Horsfall mucoprotein (THMP) or uromodulin.[100,101] THMP is a membrane protein that is principally located on the luminal surface of the cell membrane.[102]

The function of THMP is unclear. It may have some immunodulatory activity[100,101] and is important clinically because it represents the *matrix of all urinary casts*.[103] The casts may contain only the matrix (hyaline casts) or can include degenerated cells or filtered proteins (granular casts), or intact cells that are present in the tubular fluid (red, white, or epithelial cell casts).[104] The type of cast that is present often has important diagnostic implications, e.g., red cell casts are virtually pathognomonic of glomerulonephritis or vasculitis. In contrast, hyaline or granular cast formation is not necessarily indicative of renal disease, since it can be seen in physiologic states such as exercise or fever.[104]

THMP has been implicated in the pathogenesis of cast nephropathy, a form of renal failure associated with multiple myeloma in which dense intratubular casts occlude the flow of urine. Only some light chains appear to have this property, which seems to require coaggregation with THMP.[105]

It has also been suggested that THMP plays an etiologic role in other disease states, such as the inflammatory response in interstitial nephritis. Tubular injury in this setting may lead to the release of THMP, which can then attract neutrophils by binding to specific receptors on the cell surface.[106]

PROBLEMS

4-1 Explain the roles of the following in the production and maintenance of the hypertonicity of the medullary interstitium:
   (a) NaCl reabsorption in the medullary ascending limb
   (b) Urea accumulation

(c) Flow in the vasa recta capillaries

4-2   What is the role of NaCl reabsorption without water in the medullary ascending limb on:
(a) The excretion of a concentrated urine?
(b) The excretion of a dilute urine?
What is the contribution of NaCl reabsorption without water in the cortical ascending limb and distal tubule to these processes?

4-3   In some species, ADH stimulates NaCl reabsorption in the medullary thick ascending limb. What effect would this have on:
(a) Concentrating ability?
(b) NaCl delivery out of the *cortical* thick ascending limb into the distal tubule?

4-4   In addition to osmotic diuretics, other diuretics are available which increase the urine output by inhibiting active NaCl reabsorption (see Chap. 17). What would be the likely site of action of a nonosmotic diuretic if it:
(a) Inhibited both concentration and dilution?
(b) Inhibited dilution but not concentration?

4-5   What is the mechanism by which water is reabsorbed in the descending limb of the loop of Henle? How might this change during:
(a) An osmotic diuresis?
(b) A water diuresis due to central diabetes insipidus (absence of ADH)?

4-6   What effect will a low-protein diet (urea is an end product of protein metabolism) have on concentrating ability?

REFERENCES

1. Katz AI. Distribution and function of classes of ATPases along the nephron. *Kidney Int* 29:21, 1986.
2. Farman N, Corthesy-Theulaz I, Bonvalet JP, Rossier BC. Localization of α-isoforms of Na^+-K^+-ATPase in rat kidney by in situ hybridization. *Am J Physiol* 260:C468, 1991.
3. Gamba G. Molecular biology of distal nephron sodium transport mechanisms. *Kidney Int* 56:1606, 1999.
4. Xu JC, Lytle C, Zhu TT, et al. Molecular cloning and functional expression of the bumetanide-sensitive Na-K-Cl cotransporter. *Proc Natl Acad Sci U S A* 91:2201, 1994.
5. Haas M. The Na-K-Cl cotransporters. *Am J Physiol* 267:C869, 1994.
6. Molony DA, Reeves WB, Andreoli TB. Na^+-K^+2Cl^- cotransport and the thick ascending limb. *Kidney Int* 36:418, 1989.
7. Lapointe J-Y, Bell PD, Cardinal J. Direct evidence for apical Na^+:Cl^-:K^+ cotransport in macula densa cells. *Am J Physiol* 258:F1466, 1990.
8. Greger R, Velazquez H. The cortical thick ascending limb and early distal convoluted tubule in the urine concentrating mechanism. *Kidney Int* 31:590, 1987.
9. Obermuller N, Kunchaparty S, Ellison DH, Bachmann S. Expression of the Na-K-2Cl cotransporter by macula densa and thick ascending limb cells of rat and rabbit nephron. *J Clin Invest* 98:635, 1996.
10. Gamba G, Miyanoshita A, Lombardi M, et al. Molecular cloning, primary structure, and characterization of two members of the mammalian electroneutral sodium-(potassium)-chloride cotransporter family expressed in kidney. *J Biol Chem* 269:17713, 1994.
11. Simon DB, Karet FE, Handam JB, et al. Bartter's syndrome, hypokalemic alkalosis with hypercalciuria is caused by mutations in the Na-K-2Cl cotransporter NKCC2. *Nat Genet* 13:183, 1996.
12. Winters CJ, Reeves WB, Andreoli TE. Cl^- channels in basolateral renal medullary vesicles. VIII. Partial purification and functional reconstitution of basolateral mTAL Cl^- channels. *Kidney Int* 45:803, 1994.

13. Simon DB, Bindra RS, Mansfield TA, et al. Mutations in the chloride channel gene, CLCNKB, cause Bartter's syndrome type III. *Nat Genet* 17:171, 1997.

14. Wang W, White S, Geibel J, Giebisch G. A potassium channel in the apical membrane of rabbit thick ascending limb of Henle's loop. *Am J Physiol* 248:F244, 1990.

15. Gamba G. Molecular biology of distal nephron sodium transport mechanisms. *Kidney Int* 56:1606, 1999.

16. Simon DB, Karet FE, Rodriguez-Soriano J, et al. Genetic heterogeneity of Bartter's syndrome revealed by mutations in the K^+ channel, ROMK. *Nat Genet* 14:152, 1996.

17. Quamme GA. Renal magnesium handling: New insights in understanding old problems. *Kidney Int* 52:1180, 1997.

18. Friedman PA. Basal and hormone-activated calcium absorption in mouse renal thick ascending limbs. *Am J Physiol* 254:F62, 1988.

19. Capasso G, Unwin R, Agulian S, Giebisch G. Bicarbonate transport along the loop of Henle. I. Microperfusion studies of load and inhibitor sensitivity. *J Clin Invest* 88:430, 1991.

20. Good DW. Adaptation of HCO_3^- and NH_4^+ transport in rat MTAL: Effects of chronic metabolic acidosis and Na^+ intake. *Am J Physiol* 258:F1345, 1990.

21. Capasso G, Unwin R, Ciani F, et al. Bicarbonate transport along the loop of Henle. II. Effects of acid-base, dietary, and neurohumoral determinants. *J Clin Invest* 94:830, 1994.

22. DuBose TD Jr, Good DW, Hamm LL, Wall SM. Ammonium transport in the kidney: New physiological concepts and their clinical applications. *J Am Soc Nephrol* 1:1193, 1991.

23. Garvin JL, Burg MB, Knepper MA. Active NH_4^+ reabsorption by the medullary thick ascending limb. *Am J Physiol* 255:F57, 1988.

24. Amlal H, Legoff C, Vernimmen C, et al. $Na^{(+)}$-K^+(NH_4^+)-$2Cl^-$ cotransport in medullary thick ascending limb: Control by PKA, PKC, and 20-HETE. *Am J Physiol* 271:C455, 1996.

25. Hebert SC. Extracellular calcium-sensing receptor: Implications for calcium and magnesium handling in the kidney. *Kidney Int* 50:2129, 1996.

26. Riccardi D, Lee WS, Lee K, et al. Localization of the extracellular Ca^{2+}-sensing receptor and PTH/PTHrP receptor in rat kidney. *Am J Physiol* 271:F951, 1996.

27. Wang WH, Lu M, Hebert SC. Cytochrome P-450 metabolites mediate extracellular Ca^{2+}-induced inhibition of apical K^+ channels in the TAL. *Am J Physiol* 271:C103, 1996.

28. Chamberlin ME, LeFurgey A, Mandel LJ. Suspension of medullary thick ascending limb tubules from the rabbit kidney. *Am J Physiol* 247:F955, 1984.

29. Brezis M, Rosen S, Silva P, Epstein FH. Renal ischemia: A new perspective. *Kidney Int* 26:375, 1984.

30. Carroll MA, Schwartzman M, Baba M, et al. Renal cytochrome *P*-450-related arachidonate metabolism in rabbit aortic coarctation. *Am J Physiol* 255:F151, 1988.

31. Escalante B, Erlij D, Falck JR, McGiff JC. Effect of cytochrome P450 arachidonate metabolites on ion transport in rabbit kidney loop of Henle. *Science* 251:799, 1991

32. Beach RE, Good DW. Effects of adenosine on ion transport in rat medullary thick ascending limb. *Am J Physiol* 263:F482, 1992.

33. Wright FS. Flow-dependent transport processes: Filtration, absorption, secretion. *Am J Physiol* 243:F1, 1982.

34. Reeves WB, et al. Diluting power of thick limbs of Henle. III. Modulation of in vitro diluting power. *Am J Physiol* 255:F1145, 1988.

35. de Rouffignac C, Di Stefano A, Wittner M, et al. Consequences of differential effects of ADH and other peptide hormones on thick ascending limb of mammalian kidney. *Am J Physiol* 260:R1023, 1991.

36. Di Stefano A, Greger R, de Rouffignac C, Wittner M. Active NaCl transport in the cortical thick ascending limb of Henle's loop of the mouse does not require the presence of bicarbonate. *Pflugers Arch* 420:290, 1992.

37. Bapty BW, Dai LJ, Ritchie G, et al. Extracellular Mg^{2+}- and Ca^{2+}-sensing in mouse distal convoluted tubule cells. *Kidney Int* 53:583, 1998.

38. Gesek FA, Friedman PA. On the mechanism of parathyroid hormone stimulation of a calcium uptake by mouse distal convoluted tubule cells. *J Clin Invest* 90:749, 1992.

39. Jamison RL, Maffly RH. The urinary concentrating mechanism. *N Engl J Med* 295:1059, 1976.
40. Sands JM, Kokko JP. Current concepts of the countercurrent multiplication system. *Kidney Int* 57(suppl): S93, 1996.
41. Wexler AS, Kalaba RE, Marsh DJ. Three-dimensional anatomy and renal concentrating mechanisms. I. Modeling results. *Am J Physiol* 260:F368, 1991.
42. Chou CL, Nielsen S, Knepper MA. Structural functional correlation in chinchilla long loop of Henle thin limbs: A novel papillary subsegment. *Am J Physiol* 265:F863, 1993.
43. Nielsen S, Pallone T, Smith BL, et al. Aquaporin-1 water channels in short and long loop descending thin limbs and in descending vasa recta in rat kidney. *Am J Physiol* 268:F1023, 1995.
44. Chou CL, Knepper MA, van Hoek AN, et al. Reduced water permeability and altered ultrastructure in thin descending limb of Henle in aquaporin-1 null mice. *J Clin Invest* 103:491, 1999.
45. Nielsen S, Kwon T-H, Christensen BM, et al. Physiology and pathophysiology of renal aquaporins. *J Am Soc Nephrol* 10:647, 1999.
46. Molony DA, Reeves WB, Hebert SC, Andreoli TE. ADH increases apical Na^+, K^+, $2Cl^-$ entry into mouse medullary thick ascending limbs of Henle. *Am J Physiol* 252:F177, 1987.
47. Kim GH, Ecelbarger CA, Mitchell C, et al. Vasopressin increases Na-K-2Cl cotransporter expression in thick ascending limb of Henle's loop. *Am J Physiol* 276:F96, 1999.
48. Morel F, Imbert-Teboul M, Chabardes D. Receptors to vasopressin and other hormones in the mammalian kidney. *Kidney Int* 31:512, 1987.
49. Kokko JP. The role of the collecting duct in urinary concentration. *Kidney Int* 31:606, 1987.
50. Sands JM, Nonoguchi H, Knepper MA. Vasopressin effects on urea and H_2O transport in inner medullary collecting duct subsegments. *Am J Physiol* 253:F823, 1987.
51. Deen PM, Verdijk MA, Knoers NV, et al. Requirement for human renal water channel aquaporin-2 for vasopressin-dependent concentration of urine. *Science* 264:92, 1994.
52. Gottschalk CW, Mylle M. Micropuncture study of the mammalian urinary concentrating mechanism: Evidence for the countercurrent hypothesis. *Am J Physiol* 196:927, 1959.
53. Woodhall PB, Tisher CC. Response of the distal tubule and cortical collecting duct to vasopressin in the rat. *J Clin Invest* 52:3095, 1973.
54. Imai M. The connecting tubule: A functional subdivision of the rabbit distal nephron segments. *Kidney Int* 15:346, 1979.
55. Knepper MA, Roch-Ramel F. Pathways of urea transport in the mammalian kidney. *Kidney Int* 31:629, 1987.
56. You G, Smith CP, Kanai Y, et al. Cloning and expression of the vasopressin-regulated urea transporter. *Nature* 365:844, 1993.
57. Shayakul C, Steel A, Hediger MA. Molecular cloning and characterization of the vasopressin-regulated urea transporter of rat kidney collecting ducts. *J Clin Invest* 98:2580, 1996.
58. Knepper MA, Star RA. The vasopressin-regulated urea transporter in rat inner medullary collecting duct. *Am J Physiol* 259:F393, 1990.
59. Nielsen S, Knepper MA. Vasopressin activates collecting duct urea transporters and water channels by distinct physical processes. *Am J Physiol* 265:F204, 1993.
60. Sands JM, Schrader DC. An independent effect of osmolality on urea transport in rat terminal inner medullary collecting ducts. *J Clin Invest* 88:137, 1991.
61. Lassiter W, Mylle M, Gottschalk CW. Net transtubular movement of water and urea in saline diuresis. *Am J Physiol* 206:669, 1964.
62. Levitin H, Goodman A, Pigeon G, Epstein FH. Composition of the renal medulla during water diuresis. *J Clin Invest* 41:1145, 1962.
63. Harrington AR, Valtin H. Impaired urinary concentration after vasopressin and its gradual correction in hypothalamic diabetes insipidus. *J Clin Invest* 47:502, 1968.
64. Miller M, Kalkos T, Moses AM, et al. Recognition of partial defects in antidiuretic hormone secretion. *Ann Intern Med* 73:721, 1970.

65. Epstein FH, Kleeman CR, Hendrikx A. The influence of bodily hydration on the renal concentrating process. *J Clin Invest* 36:629, 1957.

66. Kondo Y, Abe K, Igarashi Y, et al. Direct evidence for the absence of active Na^+ reabsorption in hamster ascending thin limb of Henle's loop. *J Clin Invest* 91:5, 1993.

67. Stephenson JL, Zhang Y, Tewarson R. Electrolyte, urea, and water transport in a two-nephron central core model of the renal medulla. *Am J Physiol* 257:F399, 1989.

68. Koyama S, Yoshitomi K, Imai M. Effect of protamine on ion conductance of ascending thin limb of Henle's loop from hamsters. *Am J Physiol* 261:F593, 1991.

69. Matsumura Y, Uchida S, Kondo Y, et al. Overt nephrogenic diabetes insidipus in mice lacking the CLC-K1 chloride channel. *Nat Genet* 21:95, 1999.

70. Zimmerhackl BL, Robertson CR, Jamison RL. The medullary microcirculation. *Kidney Int* 31:641, 1987.

71. Sanjana VM, Johnston PA, Deen WM, et al. Hydraulic and oncotic pressure measurements in inner medulla of mammalian kidney. *Am J Physiol* 228:1921, 1975.

72. Zimmerhackl B, Robertson CR, Jamison RL. Fluid uptake in the renal papilla by vasa recta estimated by two methods simultaneously. *Am J Physiol* 248:F347, 1985.

73. Pallone TL. Effect of sodium chloride gradients on water flux in rat descending vasa recta. *J Clin Invest* 87:12, 1991.

74. Chou S-Y, Porush JG, Faubert PF. Renal medullary circulation: Hormonal control. *Kidney Int* 37:1, 1990.

75. Thurau K. Renal hemodynamics. *Am J Med* 36:698, 1964.

76. Goldberg M, Ramirez MA. Effects of saline and mannitol diuresis on the renal concentrating mechanism in dogs: Alterations in renal tissue solutes and water. *Clin Sci* 32:475, 1967.

77. Seely JF, Dirks JH. Micropuncture study of hypertonic mannitol diuresis in the proximal and distal tubule of the dog kidney. *J Clin Invest* 48:2330, 1969.

78. Berliner RW, Davidson DG. Production of hypertonic urine in the absence of pituitary antidiuretic hormone. *J Clin Invest* 36:1416, 1957.

79. Valtin HV, Edwards BR. GFR and the concentration of urine in the absence of vasopressin: Berliner-Davidson re-explored. *Kidney Int* 31:634, 1987.

80. Parker JC. In defense of cell volume. *Am J Physiol* 265:C1191, 1993.

81. Sun AM, Saltzberg SN, Kikeri D, Herbert SC. Mechanisms of cell volume regulation by the mouse thick ascending limb of Henle. *Kidney Int* 38:1019, 1990.

82. Blumenfeld JD, Grossman EB, Sun AM, Hebert SC. Sodium-coupled ion cotransport and the volume regulatory increase response. *Kidney Int* 36:434, 1989.

83. Sun A, Hebert SC. Rapid hypertonic cell volume regulation in the perfused inner medullary collecting duct. *Kidney Int* 36:831, 1989.

84. Murillo-Carretero MI, Ilundain AA, Echevarria M. Regulation of aquaporin mRNA expression in rat kidney by water intake. *J Am Soc Nephrol* 10:696, 1999.

85. Garcia-Perez A, Burg MB. Importance of organic osmolytes for osmoregulation by renal medullary cells. *Hypertension* 16:595, 1990.

86. Chamberlin ME, Strange K. Anisosmotic cell volume regulation: A comparative view. *Am J Physiol* 257:C159, 1989.

87. Yancey PH, Burg MB. Distribution of major organic osmolytes in rabbit kidney in diuresis and antidiuresis. *Am J Physiol* 257:F602, 1989.

88. Yamauchi A, Miyai A, Shimada S, et al. Localization and rapid regulation of Na^+/myo-inositol cotransporter in rat kidney. *J Clin Invest* 96:1195, 1995.

89. Nakanishi T, Uyama O, Sugita M. Osmotically regulated taurine content in rat renal inner medulla. *Am J Physiol* 261:F957, 1991.

90. Burg MB. Molecular basis of osmotic regulation. *Am J Physiol* 268:F983, 1995.

91. Uchida S, Garcia-Perez A, Murphy H, Burg M. Signal for induction of aldose reductase in renal medullary cells by high external NaCl. *Am J Physiol* 256:C614, 1989.

92. Ferraris J, Williams CK, Jung K-Y, et al. ORE, a eukaryotic minimal essential osmotic response element: The aldose reductase gene in hyperosmotic stress. *J Biol Chem* 271:18318, 1996.

93. Sands JM, Schroder DC. Coordinated response of renal medullary enzymes regulating net sorbitol production in diuresis and antidiuresis. *J Am Soc Nephrol* 1:58, 1990.
94. Mockel GW, Lai LW, Guder WG, et al. Kinetics and osmoregulation of Na^+- and Cl^--dependent betaine transporter in rat renal medulla. *Am J Physiol* 272:F100, 1997.
95. Yamauchi A, Kwon HM, Uchida S, et al. Myo-inositol and betaine transporters regulated by tonicity are basolateral in MDCK cells. *Am J Physiol* 261:F197, 1991.
96. Zablocki K, Miller SPF, Garcia-Perez A, Murg MB. Accumulation of glycerophosphocholine (GPC) by renal cells: Osmotic regulation of GPC:choline phosphodiesterase. *Proc Natl Acad Sci U S A* 88:7820, 1991.
97. Kwon E, Jung K, Edsall L, et al. Osmotic regulation of synthesis of glycerophosphocholine from phosphatidylcholine in MDCK cells. *Am J Physiol* 268:C402, 1995.
98. Moriyama T, Garcia-Perez A, Olson AD, Burg MB. Intracellular betaine substitutes for sorbitol in protecting renal medullary cells from hypertonicity. *Am J Physiol* 260:F494, 1991.
99. Siebens AW, Spring KR. A novel sorbitol transport mechanism in cultured renal papillary epithelial cells. *Am J Physiol* 257:F937, 1989.
100. Kumar S, Muchmore A. Tamm-Horsfall mucoprotein—uromodulin (1950–1990). *Kidney Int* 37:1395, 1990.
101. Hession C, Decker JM, Sherblom AP. Uromodulin (Tamm-Horsfall glycoprotein): A renal ligand for lymphokines. *Science* 237:1479, 1987.
102. Malagolini N, Cavallone D, Serafini-Cessi F. Intracellular transport, cell-surface exposure and release of recombinant Tamm-Horsfall glycoprotein. *Kidney Int* 52:1340, 1997.
103. Rutecki GJ, Goldsmith C, Schreiner GE. Characterization of proteins in urinary casts: Fluorescent antibody identification of Tamm-Horsfall mucoprotein in matrix and serum proteins in granules. *N Engl J Med* 284:1049, 1971.
104. Rose BD. *Pathophysiology of Renal Disease*, 2d ed. McGraw-Hill, New York, 1987, p. 82.
105. Huang ZQ, Sanders PW. Localization of a single binding site for immunoglobulin light chains on human Tamm-Horsfall glycoprotein. *J Clin Invest* 99:732, 1997.
106. Thomas DB, Davies M, Peters JR, Williams JD. Tamm Horsfall protein binds to a single class of carbohydrate specific receptors on human neutrophils. *Kidney Int* 44:423, 1993.

FIVE

FUNCTIONS OF THE DISTAL NEPHRON

INTRODUCTION

The distal nephron begins at the macula densa at the end of the cortical thick ascending limb and consists of four segments, each of which has one or more distinct cell types: the distal tubule, the connecting segment (previously considered part of the late distal tubule), the cortical collecting tubule, and the medullary collecting tubule (see Fig. 1-3). These segments perform different functions and can be separated both by histologic appearance and by hormone responsiveness (Table 5-1).[1-4]

The distal nephron, particularly the collecting tubules, is the site at which the *final qualitative changes in urinary excretion* are made. Thus, maximal concentration of the urine, potassium secretion (which accounts for most of urinary potassium excretion), maximal acidification of the urine, and sodium conservation all occur in the collecting tubules. As an example, the Na^+ concentration is about 75 meq/L in the fluid leaving the loop of Henle but can be appropriately reduced to less than 1 meq/L by the end of the medullary collecting tubule in states of volume depletion.

This steep concentration gradient between the tubular fluid and the plasma can be maintained because the distal nephron is relatively impermeable to the

Table 5-1   Hormone responsiveness of distal nephron segments

Segment	Antidiuretic hormone	Aldosterone	Parathyroid hormone	Calcitriol	Atrial natriuretic peptide
Distal convoluted tubule	0	0	+	+	0
Connecting segment	0	+	+	+	0
Cortical collecting tubule					
Principal cells	+	+	±	±	0
Intercalated cells	?	+	0	0	0
Medullary collecting tubule					
Outer	+	+	0	0	0
Inner	+	+	0	0	+

passive transcellular or paracellular movement of both water (in the absence of antidiuretic hormone) and Na^+. Consequently, the gradient generated by active Na^+ transport is less likely to be dissipated by passive back-diffusion from the plasma into the tubular fluid. This impermeability to Na^+ and water movement is probably related to the thickness of the tight junction, which, on electron microscopy, is composed of up to eight strands in the distal nephron.[5] In comparison, the proximal tubule is a highly permeable epithelium, with only one strand demonstrable on electron microscopy.[5] As a result, the proximal tubular fluid Na^+ concentration does not normally fall below that in the plasma, since backflux of Na^+ down its concentration gradient can occur through the tight junction (see Chap. 3).

Although the collecting tubules can generate and maintain large concentration gradients, their *total* reabsorptive capacity is limited. In terms of active Na^+ transport, this is exemplified by a lower level of Na^+-K^+-ATPase activity than is present in other nephron segments (except for the descending and thin ascending limbs of the loop of Henle, where transport is essentially passive).[6] As a result, the collecting tubules function most efficiently when the bulk of the filtrate is reabsorbed in the proximal tubule and loop of Henle, and distal delivery is held relatively constant. As described in Chaps. 2, 3, and 4, three intrarenal processes minimize changes in distal delivery in normal subjects:

- *Autoregulation*, which maintains the glomerular filtration rate (GFR) in the presence of variations in renal arterial pressure
- *Glomerulotubular balance*, in which proximal and loop reabsorption increase if there is an elevation in the GFR
- *Tubuloglomerular feedback*, which lowers the GFR in the load to the macula densa is enhanced

These processes are important, since an inappropriate increase in distal delivery could overwhelm reabsorptive capacity, leading to potentially serious losses of NaCl and water.

This chapter will briefly review the major functions of different cell types in the distal nephron. In general, *cellular function correlations closely with hormonal responsiveness* (Table 5-1). As examples, Na^+ reabsorption and K^+ secretion occur in those Na^+-reabsorbing cells that respond to aldosterone; water reabsorption occurs primarily when antidiuretic hormone (ADH) is present, and then only in those cells that respond to ADH; and calcium reabsorption is seen only in those cells that respond to parathyroid hormone (PTH) and calcitriol. In addition, the intercalated cells in the cortical collecting tubule plus the tubular cells in the outer medulla primarily secrete H^+, a response that is affected by changes in the extracellular pH and to a lesser degree by aldosterone. The role of each of these processes in the maintenance of ion and water balance will be discussed in detail in Chaps. 8 to 12.

DISTAL TUBULE

Sodium and Water

The distal tubule normally reabsorbs about 5 percent of the filtered NaCl.[7] The mechanism by which this appears to occur is depicted in Fig. 5-1. Na^+ entry into the cell is primarily mediated by electroneutral Na^+-Cl^- cotransport.[8-10] Two mechanisms contribute to this response: a Na^+-Cl^- cotransporter;[9,11,12] and, to a lesser degree, parallel Na^+-H^+ and Cl^--HCO_3^- exchangers.[13]

With the Na^+-Cl^- cotransporter, the attachment of Na^+ to its site increases the affinity of the Cl^- site for its ligand; the transporter then undergoes a conformational change that translocates both Na^+ and Cl^- across the apical (or luminal) membrane.[9] The energy for this process is, as in other nephron segments, indirectly provided by the basolateral Na^+-K^+-ATPase pump. This pump maintains a low cell Na^+ concentration, which promotes passive NaCl entry into the cell (see page 75). It also creates a cell interior negative potential, which is important for electrogenic transport (e.g., Na^+ reabsorption through the Na^+ channels in the cortical collecting tubule; see below) but not for electroneutral NaCl transport.

With parallel exchangers, on the other hand, intracellular water and CO_2 combine to form H^+ and HCO_3^- ions (see Fig. 3-3), which are then secreted into the lumen in exchange for Na^+ and Cl^-, respectively. The secreted H^+ and HCO_3^- then combine in the lumen to form carbonic acid, which, since it is uncharged and therefore lipid-soluble, can recycle into the cell and dissociate into H^+ and HCO_3^- to promote further NaCl reabsorption.

Notice that the mechanisms of entry in the distal tubule are different from those in the loop of Henle, where there is also a requirement for K^+ by the Na^+-K^+-$2Cl^-$ carrier in the apical membrane (see Fig. 4-2). This difference has some clinical implications, since the latter carrier is inhibited by the loop diuretics, such

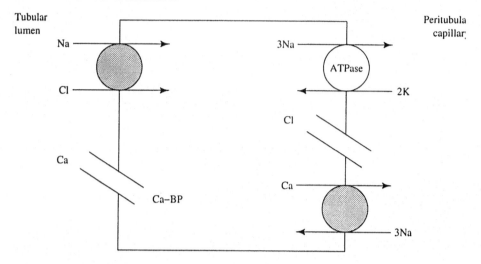

Figure 5-1 Schematic representation of the mechanisms of sodium chloride and calcium reabsorption in the distal tubule. The entry of filtered sodium chloride into the cell is mediated by a neutral Na-Cl cotransporter in the luminal (apical) membrane; the energy for this process is provided by the favorable electrochemical gradient for sodium (low cell sodium concentration and cell interior electronegative). At the basolateral membrane, reabsorbed sodium is pumped out of the cell by the Na^+-K^+-ATPase pump, while reabsorbed chloride exits via a chloride channel. Thiazide diuretics inhibit sodium chloride reabsorption by competing for the chloride site on apical Na-Cl cotransporter. The distal tubule is also the major site of active calcium reabsorption. Calcium enters the cell via a calcium transporter that is probably a voltage-dependent calcium channel. Reabsorbed calcium combines with a vitamin D-induced calcium binding protein (Ca-BP), moves across the cell, and is then extruded at the basolateral membrane by a Ca-ATPase (now shown) and, to a greater degree, a 3Na:1Ca exchanger which again uses the energy provided by the favorable inward gradient for sodium.

as furosemide.[7] The Na^+-Cl^- cotransporter in the distal tubule, on the other hand, is relatively unresponsive to the loop diuretics but is impaired by the thiazide-type diuretics, which produce their effect primarily by reducing NaCl reabsorption in this segment.[7,8,10,14] Mutations in the Na^+-Cl^- cotransporter gene produce Gitelman's syndrome, a disorder characterized by hypokalemia, metabolic alkalosis, and hypocalciuria, findings similar to those induced by chronic thiazide therapy.[15]

Like that in the loop of Henle, *distal tubular Na^+ reabsorption varies directly with Na^+ delivery* and therefore participates in glomerulotubular balance.[16] Thus, an increase in delivery results in a proportionate rise in segmental Na^+ reabsorption. This effect is independent of hormones such as aldosterone[17] and, as in the loop of Henle, is probably related to changes in the Na^+ concentration in the tubular fluid.[18,19] If more Na^+ is delivered to the distal tubule, the associated elevation in the luminal Na^+ concentration favors continued passive Na^+ entry into the tubular cell. The degree to which this occurs is ultimately limited by the Na^+ concentration gradient between the tubular fluid and the plasma that the distal tubule can maintain. The fluid entering the distal tubule normally has a Na^+ concentration of about 75 meq/L; when this value is lowered to approximately 40 meq/L by tubular reabsorption, further Na^+ transport essentially ceases as a result of both decreased binding to the Na^+-Cl^- cotransporter and backflux down a now very favorable concentration gradient through the tight junction.[8,9]

A common clinical example of this flow dependence occurs when distal delivery is enhanced by the use of a loop diuretic. In this setting, distal tubular Na^+ reabsorption rises substantially,[7,20] a change that is accompanied by tubular hypertrophy[19,20] and by a necessary increase in Na^+-K^+-ATPase activity to return the extra Na^+ to the systemic circulation.[20,21] This distal adaptation can, in some edematous patients, severely limit the natriuretic response to a loop diuretic. This problem can often be overcome by the addition of a thiazide diuretic to block Na^+ transport in both segments (see page 437). If, on the other hand, distal Na^+ reabsorption is chronically diminished by the administration of a thiazide diuretic that inhibits the Na^+-Cl^- cotransporter, then tubular reabsorptive capacity and the Na^+-K^+-ATPase activity are reduced.[22]

These observations suggest that the cell Na^+ concentration is an important *chronic* determinant of transport capacity.[22] Reducing cell entry and therefore the cell Na^+ concentration with a thiazide diuretic diminishes NaCl reabsorptive capacity, while enhancing these parameters with a loop diuretic increases transport capacity.

A similar distal tubular adaptation occurs when NaCl delivery is increased chronically by a high-salt diet.[23] This additional illustration shows that flow dependence does not necessarily result in appropriate changes in Na^+ excretion. At a time when tubular Na^+ reabsorption should be diminished to allow excretion of the excess intake, the distal tubule actually has a higher rate of Na^+ reabsorption. The proximal and collecting tubules, under the influence of angiotensin II, aldosterone, and atrial natriuretic peptide, are the major sites at which Na^+ excretion is regulated in relation to needs (see Chap. 8).

In contrast to its role in NaCl handling, the distal tubule reabsorbs a minimal quantity of water. The water permeability of this segment is low in the basal state and does not appear to increase after the administration of ADH.[17] As a result, the distal tubule contributes to urinary dilution, since the reabsorption of NaCl without water will lower the tubular fluid osmolality.

Calcium

The early cortical distal nephron, including the cortical thick ascending limb as well as the distal tubule and connecting segment, is one major site at which urinary Ca^{2+} excretion is actively regulated (Fig. 5-1).[24-26] This process appears to be regulated primarily by parathyroid hormone and perhaps calcitriol (which induces the production of a calcium-binding protein), both of which promote Ca^{2+} reabsorption.[27-29] The mechanism by which this occurs is reviewed in Chap. 3 (see page 92).

When calcium intake is increased, some of the excess calcium is absorbed, enters the systemic circulation, and slightly raises the serum calcium concentration. It has traditionally been taught that suppression of PTH release with a subsequent reduction in distal tubular calcium reabsorption is responsible for the ensuing increase in calcium excretion. This appropriate change may be augmented by the effects of hypercalcemia on the calcium-sensing receptor in the basolateral membrane of the ascending limb of Henle's loop.[30]

One characteristic of distal tubular function is that the reabsorption of Ca^{2+} can be dissociated from that of Na^+. PTH, for example, promotes the reabsorption of Ca^{2+} in this segment without changing that of Na^+, an effect that is mediated by the activation of adenylyl cyclase[31] and may involve facilitated entry of luminal Ca^{2+} into the cells.[28]

This ability to dissociate distal tubular Ca^{2+} and Na^+ handling may be important clinically in the treatment of recurrent calcium stone formation due to hypercalciuria. The thiazide diuretics are often beneficial in this setting because they impair the reabsorption of NaCl but *increase that of Ca^{2+}*, leading to a desired reduction in Ca^{2+} excretion[32] and a lower rate of new stone formation.[33,34] How this might occur is discussed on page 92.[32]

Hydrogen and Potassium

The distal tubule may contribute to H^+ secretion and the reabsorption of HCO_3^-, although the collecting tubules are quantitatively much more important.[35,36] Some potassium secretion also may occur at this site, the physiologic significance of which is uncertain (see Chap. 12).[37,38]

CONNECTING SEGMENT

The connecting segment lies between the distal tubule and the initial portion of the cortical collecting tubule and shares characteristics of both segments. Like the distal tubule, it is impermeable to water, even in the presence of ADH; it participates in active Ca^{2+} reabsorption, being responsive to both PTH and calcitriol;[27,39] and it partially reabsorbs Na^+ by a thiazide-sensitive Na^+-Cl^- cotransporter in the apical membrane (in rabbits but apparently not in rats).[22,40,41] Like the cortical collecting tubule, however, it also reabsorbs Na^+ (via a Na^+ channel) and secretes K^+ in response to aldosterone.[1,41,42]

CORTICAL COLLECTING TUBULE

The cortical collecting tubule has two cell types with very different functions: principal cells (about 65 percent) and intercalated cells.[1,43,44] The types of transport that occur in these cells are depicted in Figs. 5-2 and 5-3. The principal cells have Na^+ and K^+ channels in the luminal membrane[45-47] and, as in all Na^+-

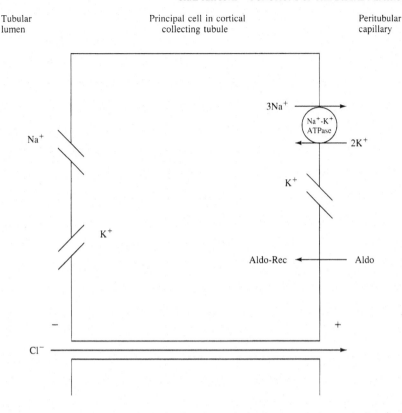

Tubular
lumen

Principal cell in cortical
collecting tubule

Peritubular
capillary

Figure 5-2   Ion transport in the principal cell in the cortical collecting tubule. Luminal Na^+ enters the cell through a Na^+ channel in the luminal membrane. The lumen-negative voltage created by this movement of Na^+ then promotes either the secretion of K^+ or the reabsorption of Cl^- via the paracellular route. These processes are promoted by aldosterone (Aldo), which enters the cell and combines with its cytoslic receptor (Rec). These cells also can reabsorb water in the presence of ADH.

reabsorbing cells, Na^+-K^+-ATPase pumps in the basolateral membrane. The intercalated cells, in comparison, do not transport NaCl, since they have a lower level of Na^+-K^+-ATPase activity and have few if any apical membrane Na^+ channels, which are required for the entry of luminal Na^+ into the cell.[1,6,46] These cells appear to play an important role in H^+ and HCO_3^- handling and in K^+ reabsorption in states of K^+ depletion.

Principal Cells

Sodium and potassium   The principal cells contribute to net Na^+ reabsorption and are the primary site of K^+ secretion. The entry of luminal Na^+ into these cells primarily occurs down a concentration gradient through ion-specific Na^+ channels[48,49] in the apical membrane.[45,46]

Tubular
lumen

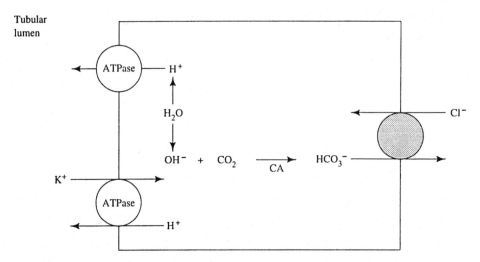

Figure 5-3   Transport mechanisms involved in hydrogen secretion and bicarbonate and potassium reabsorption in type A intercalated cells in the cortical collecting tubule and in the medullary collecting tubule cells. Water within the cell dissociates into hydrogen and hydroxyl anions. The former are secreted into the lumen by H^+-ATPase pumps in the luminal membrane; chloride may be cosecreted with hydrogen to maintain electroneutrality. The hydroxyl anions in the cell combine with carbon dioxide to form bicarbonate in a reaction catalyzed by carbonic anhydrase (CA). Bicarbonate is then returned to the systemic circulation via chloride-bicarbonate exchangers in the basolateral membrane. The favorable inward concentration gradient for chloride (plasma and interstitial concentration greater than that in the cell) provides the energy for bicarbonate reabsorption H^+-K^+-ATPase pumps, which lead to both hydrogen secretion and potassium reabsorption, may also be present in the luminal membrane. The number of these pumps increases with potassium depletion, suggesting that their main function is to promote potassium conservation.

In comparison to the *electroneutral* Na^+-K^+-$2Cl^-$ and Na^+-Cl^- entry mechanisms in the thick ascending limb and distal tubule, movement through the Na^+ channel is electrogenic in that it creates a lumen-negative potential difference. It is important to consider why a Na^+ channel rather than a cotransporter *must be present* in the later part of the collecting tubules. These segments can lower the urine Na^+ concentration to below 5 meq/L in states of volume depletion. This value is less than that in the cells; thus, an electroneutral cotransporter that depends upon a favorable concentration gradient for Na^+ entry would not work in this setting. Rather, it is the cell electronegativity (generated largely by the Na^+-K^+-ATPase pump and subsequent leakage of K^+ back out of the cell; see page 92) that provides the entry into the cell; this negative potential can affect only *electrogenic* Na^+ transport.

The relative lumen-negative potential created by Na^+ reabsorption then promotes either passive Cl^- reabsorption via the paracellular pathway (the major route of Cl^- transport in this segment)[43,50] or K^+ secretion from the cell into the lumen[51,52] through aldosterone-sensitive K^+ channels in the apical membrane.[47]

Na^+ reabsorption in this segment also enhances K^+ secretion by a second mechanism: The transport of reabsorbed Na^+ out of the cell by the Na^+-K^+-ATPase pump increases K^+ entry across the basolateral membrane. The ensuing rise in cell K^+ concentration and therefore in the K^+ transport pool permits continued K^+ secretion, which is the *primary determinant of urinary K^+ excretion* (see Chap. 12).

Aldosterone plays a central role in these transport processes, primarily by increasing the number of open Na^+ channels in the apical membrane (see page 179).[52-55] As an example, going from a high- to a low-sodium diet (which is associated with enhanced aldosterone release and increased Na^+ reabsorption in the cortical collecting tubule) can increase the number of open Na^+ channels per cell from less than 100 to approximately 3000.[45]

There is also a later increase in Na^+-K^+-ATPase activity and in the number of open luminal K^+ channels. These changes can at least initially be prevented by blocking the Na^+ channel with the diuretic amiloride, suggesting that they are in part secondary to enhanced Na^+ flux through the cell.[52] As an example, increasing cell Na^+ concentration directly and rapidly stimulates Na^+-K^+-ATPase activity.[56] This initial response may be then sustained by a later increase in Na^+-K^+-ATPase synthesis mediated by aldosterone.[57]

Two different types of mutations in the luminal Na^+ channel have been described. The first is an activating mutation in Liddle's syndrome, a disorder with clinical characteristics similar to those of a high-aldosterone state: excessive sodium reabsorption and potassium secretion.[58] The second is an inactivating mutation in the autosomal recessive form of pseudohypoaldosteronism that produces signs of a low-aldosterone state: hyperkalemia and a tendency to hypovolemia due to Na^+ wasting.[59]

The cortical and medullary collecting tubules usually reabsorb 5 to 7 percent of the filtered Na^+, and variations in Na^+ reabsorption in these segments are probably the *major determinant of diet-induced fluctuations in daily Na^+ excretion.*[60,61] For example, a reduction in Na^+ intake enhances aldosterone release via activation of the renin-angiotensin system (see Chap. 6). This results in increased Na^+ reabsorption both in the cortical collecting tubule and, to a lesser degree, in the papillary (or innermost) segment of the medullary collecting tubule (see below),[43,62] leading to an appropriate fall in Na^+ excretion. The opposite sequence occurs with a Na^+ load as aldosterone secretion is diminished. Enhanced release of atrial natriuretic peptide also may contribute to the natriuresis in this setting, in part by diminishing Na^+ reabsorption (via a reduction in the number of open Na^+ channels) in the papillary and perhaps the cortical segment of the collecting tubule (see Chap. 6).[63]

In addition to these effects of Na^+ regulating hormones, Na^+ reabsorption in the cortical collecting tubule may also be influenced by alterations in Na^+ delivery, locally produced prostaglandin E_2, and perhaps antidiuretic hormone:

- Decreasing Na^+ delivery, as might occur with volume depletion, leads to an increase in the number of open Na^+ channels in the apical membrane.[64]

This response appears to be mediated by an initial fall in cell Na^+ concentration (due to the decline in delivery) and a subsequent reduction in the cell levels of protein kinase C (see Fig. 6-2). This enzyme normally diminishes Na^+ reabsorption; thus, a decrease in its activity is associated with an increased number of open Na^+ channels in an appropriate effort to conserve volume by preventing further Na^+ loss. The physiologic role of this effect remains to be determined.

- By activating the EP1 receptor, prostaglandin E_2 inhibits Na^+ transport in the cortical collecting tubule.[65-67] ADH, on the other hand, may increase Na^+ reabsorption, perhaps by inserting new Na^+ channels in the apical membrane.[53] The importance of these hormonal effects in the regulation of Na^+ balance is uncertain, particularly since they appear to be present in only some species.[53,66]

Water   The water permeability of the apical membrane of the principal cells is relatively low in the basal state (in contrast to the highly permeable proximal tubule, which has water channels in both the apical and basolateral membranes).[68] However, collecting tubule water permeability can be increased substantially by ADH, which inserts cytosolic vesicles containing preformed water channels into the apical membrane (see Chap. 6).[68-71] These water channels, termed *aquaporin-2*, are different from those in the proximal tubule, which are called aquaporin-1.[68,72]

The increase in luminal membrane water permeability induced by the insertion of these water channels allows the dilute fluid entering the cortical collecting tubule (about 100 mosmol/kg) to equilibrate osmotically with the isosmotic cortical interstitium. As described in the preceding chapter, this ADH-mediated water reabsorption plays an important role in urinary concentration by markedly diminishing the volume of fluid delivered to the hyperosmotic medulla (see Fig. 4-8).

The increase in water reabsorption induced by ADH might also be expected to diminish K^+ secretion, since the latter process varies directly with urinary flow (see Chap. 12).[42] This does not occur, however, because the inhibitory effect of the decline in flow is counterbalanced by direct stimulation of K^+ secretion by ADH.[73] This response may be mediated by insertion of new K^+ channels into the apical membrane[74,75] or by stimulation of local Na^+ reabsorption, which will enhance the electrical gradient favoring K^+ secretion.[76]

Clinical Implications   Lithium therapy can lead to polyuria and polydipsia in 20 to 30 percent of patients.[77] This toxic effect results from interference with the ability of ADH to increase the water permeability of the collecting tubules, thereby reducing water reabsorption (see Chap. 24). For this problem to occur, filtered lithium must first gain access to the collecting tubular cells, apparently by entering the cell through the apical membrane Na^+ channels. This observation is important clinically, since blocking the Na^+ channel with the potassium-sparing diuretic amiloride can minimize the severity and possibly prevent the development of this defect in urinary concentration.[78]

Intercalated Cells

Hydrogen and bicarbonate   The intercalated cells are primarily involved in the Na^+-independent regulation of acid-base balance.[1,35,79,80] As depicted in Fig. 5-3, intracellular water and carbon dioxide can, in the presence of carbonic anhydrase, lead to the formation of H^+ and HCO_3^- ions. The former is then secreted into the lumen by a H^+-ATPase pump[81] or a H^+-K^+-ATPase pump,[82] whereas the latter returns to the systemic circulation across the basolateral membrane via a Cl^--HCO_3^- exchanger.[79,83] The Cl^--HCO_3^- exchanger is structurally similar to, but not identical with, the band 3 exchanger found on red cells. The bicarbonate exchanger is the product of transcription initiation on a *kidney-specific* site of the AE1 gene. Mutations in this gene can impair urinary acidification and produce a picture of distal renal tubular acidosis (see below).[84]

The net effect of these processes is H^+ loss in the urine and an elevation in the plasma bicarbonate concentration. This process is appropriately stimulated by acidemia, since the ensuing urinary changes will result in an increase in the extracellular pH toward normal (see Chap. 11).[85]

Aldosterone appears to contribute to this process by enhancing the activity of the H^+-ATPase pump.[86] In normal subjects, this effect is probably permissive, since there is little evidence that changes in acid-base balance alter the release of aldosterone. However, changes in aldosterone secretion can affect acid-base balance. Disease states associated with hyperaldosteronism usually lead to increased urinary H^+ loss and metabolitic alkalosis, while hypoaldosteronism is often associated with H^+ retention and metabolic acidosis (see pages 846 and 900).

The homeostatic needs are reversed in the presence of an alkaline load. In this setting, loss of HCO_3^- in the urine is required. Although this can be achieved by reabsorbing less of the filtered HCO_3^- in the proximal and distal nephron, the cortical collecting tubule contributes to this process by *secreting* HCO_3^- form the cell into the lumen.[87-89] This is achieved by *reversing the polarity* of the transporters in Fig. 5-3 in a second population of intercalated cells, called the type B intercalated cells as opposite to the hydrogen-secreting type A intercalated cells (Fig. 5-4).[87,88]

In the type B intercalated cells, H^+ and HCO_3^- ions are again formed within the cell; however, the H^+ ions are now secreted into the peritubular capillary by the H^+-ATPase pump, which is located in the basolateral, rather than the apical, membrane. The HCO_3^- ions, on the other hand, are secreted into the lumen by an anion exchanger in the apical membrane. The identity of this transporter is uncertain, however, as it does not appear to represent the same Cl^--HCO_3^- exchanger that is present in the basolateral membrane of the H^+-secreting intercalated cells.[85]

The importance of these proteins in the maintenance of acid balance is illustrated by the observation that mutations in the H^+-ATPase proton pump result in distal renal tubular acidosis, a disorder characterized by diminished acid

Tubular
lumen

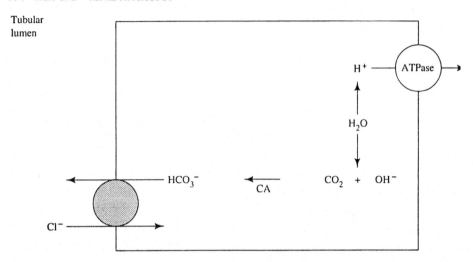

Figure 5-4 Transport mechanisms involved in the secretion of bicarbonate into the tubular lumen in the type B intercalated cells in the cortical collecting tubule. Water within the cell dissociates into hydrogen and hydroxyl anions. The former are secreted into the peritubular capillary by H^+-ATPase pumps in the basolateral membrane. The hydroxyl anions combine with carbon dioxide to form bicarbonate in a reaction catalyzed by carbonic anhydrase (CA). Bicarbonate is then secreted into the tubular lumen via chloride-bicarbonate exchangers in the luminal membrane. The favorable inward concentration gradient for chloride (lumen concentration greater than that in the cell) provides the energy for bicarbonate secretion.

secretion.[90] These individuals also have sensorineural deafness, suggesting that the proton pump also maintains the proper concentration of H^+ in the inner ear.

Potassium   Although the cortical collecting tubule normally secretes K^+, there can be *net reabsorption* in this segment in the presence of K^+ depletion.[91] This process occurs in the types A and B intercalated cells and appears to be mediated by an active H^+-K^+-ATPase pump in the apical membrane that reabsorbs K^+ and secretes H^+ (Fig. 5-3).[92,93] The activity of this transporter is increased with hypokalemia, an effect that may be mediated by the associated reduction in the cell K^+ concentration. In addition to maintenance of K^+ balance, this transporter also contributes to the increase in acid secretion in metabolic acidosis.[92,94]

Within the type B intercalated cell, potassium reabsorption is also linked with Cl^- reabsorption via the luminal Cl^--HCO_3^- exchanger.[93] Concurrent activity of this exchanger and the H^+-K^+-ATPase pump may result in active KCl reabsorption.[95]

Water   The intercalated cells are relatively impermeable to water in the basal state and appear to be minimally responsive to ADH, which primarily affects the adjacent principal cells.[96,97]

MEDULLARY COLLECTING TUBULE

The distinction between the outer and inner medullary collecting tubules is arbitrarily based upon location, with the dividing point being the level at which the thick ascending limbs of the loop of Henle begin (see Fig. 1-3). Nevertheless, this differentiation is physiologically appropriate because the cells in these segments have some important differences in function and hormone responsiveness (Table 5-1).

Outer Medulla

Hydrogen   The transition between the cortical and outer medullary collecting tubules is not abrupt; as a result, the early portion of the medullary segment has cells that contribute to Na^+ reabsorption and K^+ secretion, similar to that seen in the cortical *principal* cells.[43,98] However, the majority of cells in the outer medullary collecting tubule are comparable to the cortical *intercalated* cells (although there are variations between species), being involved in active H^+ secretion by H^+-ATPase and H^+-K^+-ATPase pumps in the apical membrane (Fig. 5-3).[94,98,99] The activity of these pumps, which is much greater than that in the cortex,[35] is stimulated in part by acidemia and by aldosterone.[86,100] The net effect is that this segment plays an important role in acidifying the urine (i.e., in lowering the urine pH to its minimum level) and in the excretion of ammonium, the major mechanism by which the kidney excretes the dietary acid load (see Chap. 11).[101,102]

Potassium   The outer medullary cells are also capable of reabsorbing K^+,[103] perhaps via an apical membrane H^+-K^+-ATPase, similar to that in the cortical intercalated cells. This response can contribute to K^+ conservation in the states of K^+ depletion and also is essential for the recycling of K^+ within the medulla (see page 357).[103]

Water   The other major function of the outer medullary collecting tubule is its role in urinary concentration. This segment is impermeable to water in the basal state.[3] In the presence of ADH, however, water permeability rises markedly due to insertion of aquaporin-2 water channels into the luminal membrane,[68] allowing equilibration with the hyperosmotic medullary interstitium (see Chap. 4).

Inner Medulla

The inner medulla is composed of several cell types:[104] The initial one-third has cells similar in function to those of the principal and intercalated cells in the cortex and outer medulla, while the inner two-thirds contains a decreasing number of principal cells and is composed primarily of a distinct cell type that contributes to Na^+ reabsorption and the production of a concentrated urine[1,105,106] but plays a lesser role in urinary acidification.[107]

Sodium Na^+ entry into the inner medullary cells primarily occurs through an amiloride-sensitive cation-selective channel.[108-110] The lumen-negative potential created by this movement of Na^+ may then promote passive Cl^- reabsorption via the paracellular route, similar to that in the cortical collecting tubule (see Fig. 5-2).

The factors that stimulate this reabsorptive process are incompletely understood, but aldosterone plays a contributory role.[43,62,106,108] The net effect is that the urine Na^+ concentration can be reduced to 5 meq/L or less in the presence of volume depletion, a setting in which aldosterone release is enhanced. As mentioned at the beginning of this chapter, passive Na^+ entry into the cells cannot be driven by a concentration gradient in this setting, since the lumen now has a lower Na^+ concentration than the cell. Rather the cell interior negative potential provides the electrical gradient that promotes Na^+ movement into the cell.

In contrast, Na^+ reabsorption in the inner medulla falls with volume expansion, a response that may be mediated both by the reduction in aldosterone secretion and by increased release of atrial natriuretic peptide. The latter hormone activates guanylate cyclase, leading to the production of cyclic guanosine monophosphate (GMP); this compound then appears to diminish Na^+ reabsorption by decreasing the number of open Na^+ channels in the apical membrane.[111-113]

Water   The inner medullary collecting tubule plays an important role in water reabsorption and the excretion of a concentrated urine. As in the other aspects of the collecting tubule, the water permeability of the inner medullary segment is increased by ADH, allowing osmotic equilibration with the hyperosmotic medullary interstitium.[3]

There is, however, one important difference from the response seen in the cortex and outer medulla. The latter segments are impermeable to urea, both in the basal state and in the presence of ADH. The inner medulla, on the other hand, has a relatively high basal urea permeability that is mediated by specific urea transporters in the basolateral and, to a lesser degree, the apical membrane.[114,115] Furthermore, the net urea permeability is increased approximately fourfold by ADH, primarily by increasing the number of luminal transporters.[114,116] These characteristics allow urea to accumulate in the medullary interstitium, where it accounts for about one-half of the interstitial solute and therefore limits urinary water loss by contributing to the excretion of a maximally concentrated urine (see Fig. 4-10).

Potassium   The inner medullary collecting tubule can contribute to the maintenance of K^+ balance. This segment usually reabsorbs K^+, an effect that is more pronounced with K^+ depletion. On the other hand, it can secrete K^+ after a K^+ load.[106] Tubular secretion presumably occurs through the cation-selective channels in the apical membrane.[109] These channels also may have a role in limiting the degree of maximum K^+ conservation. K^+-depleted subjects can only lower the urine K^+ concentration to a minimum of 5 to 15 meq/L; it may be that a lower luminal K^+ level is prevented by passive leakage of K^+ out of the cells through these channels.

Hydrogen   The inner medullary cells secrete hydrogen ions,[107,117] a response that is enhanced by stimuli similar to those in the other acid-secreting cells in the collecting tubule: acidemia and aldosterone.[107]

Cell volume regulation   In addition to their transport functions, the inner medullary collecting tubule cells (as well as those in the thick ascending limb) must maintain their cell volume in the face of constantly changing osmotic pressure in the interstitium. Fluid restriction, for example, will sequentially raise ADH levels, increase interstitial osmolality, and cause cell shrinkage by osmotic water movement out of the cells across the water-permeable basolateral membrane, which contains both aquaporin-3 and aquaporin-4 water channels.[118] Fluid loading, on the other hand, will produce the opposite changes, leading to cell swelling.

Despite this changing environment, the tubular cells are able to maintain their volume by altering the concentration both of ions (sodium and potassium) and of organic solutes (called osmolytes) that have the advantage of not interfering with the protein function.[119] These processes are reviewed on page 135.

RENAL PELVIS, URETERS, AND BLADDER

Minor modifications in the composition of the urine can occur after the urine has left the tubules. The renal pelvis is modestly permeable to urea and water. As a result, urea may diffuse out of and water into the pelvis from the inner medulla.[120,121] Similar compositional changes of as much as 7 to 15 percent can occur in the ureters and bladder, particularly in low-flow states when contact time is prolonged.[122,123]

REFERENCES

1. Madsen KM, Tisher CC. Structural-functional relationships along the distal nephron. *Am J Physiol* 250:F1, 1986.
2. Imai M, Nakamura R. Function of distal convoluted and connecting tubules studied by isolated nephron fragments. *Kidney Int* 22:465, 1982.
3. Kokko JP. The role of the collecting duct in urinary concentration. *Kidney Int* 31:606, 1987.
4. Morel F, Imbert-Teboul M, Chabardes D. Receptors to vasopressin and other hormones in the mammalian kidney. *Kidney Int* 32:512, 1987.
5. Gumbiner B. Structure, biochemistry, and assembly of tight junctions. *Am J Physiol* 253:C749, 1987.
6. Katz AI. Distribution and function of classes of ATPases along the nephron. *Kidney Int* 29:21, 1986.
7. Hropot M, Fowler N, Karlmark B, Giebisch G. Tubular action of diuretics: Distal effects on electrolyte transport and acidification. *Kidney Int* 28:477, 1985.
8. Stokes JB. Electroneutral NaCl transport in the distal tubule. *Kidney Int* 36:427, 1989.

9. Gamba G, Saltzberg SN, Lombardi M, et al. Primary structure and functional expression of a cDNA encoding the thiazide-sensitive electroneutral sodium-chloride cotransporter. *Proc Natl Acad Sci U S A* 90:2749, 1993.

10. Stanton BA. Cellular actions of thiazide diuretics in the distal tubule. *J Am Soc Nephrol* 1:836, 1990.

11. Gamba G. Molecular biology of distal nephron sodium transport mechanisms. *Kidney Int* 56:1606, 1999.

12. Gamba G, Miyanoshita A, Lombardi M, et al. Molecular cloning, primary structure, and characterization of two members of the mammalian electroneutral sodium-(potassium)-chloride cotransporter family expressed in kidney. *J Biol Chem* 269:17713, 1994.

13. Stanton BA. Electroneutral NaCl transport by distal tubule: Evidence for Na^+/H^+-Cl^-/HCO_3^- exchange. *Am J Physiol* 254:F80, 1988.

14. Bachman S, Velazquez H, Obermuller N, et al. Expression of the thiazide-sensitive Na-Cl cotransporter by rabbit distal convoluted tubule cells. *J Clin Invest* 96:2510, 1995.

15. Simon DB, Nelson-Williams C, Bia MJ, et al. Gitelman's variant of Bartter's syndrome, inherited hypokalemic alkalosis, is caused by mutations in the thiazide-sensitive Na-Cl cotransporter. *Nat Genet* 12:24, 1996.

16. Kunau RT Jr, Webb HL, Borman SC. Characteristics of sodium reabsorption in the loop of Henle and distal tubule. *Am J Physiol* 227:1181, 1974.

17. Gross JB, Imai M, Kokko JP. A functional comparison of the cortical collecting tubule and the distal convoluted tubule. *J Clin Invest* 55:1284, 1975.

18. Wright FS. Flow-dependent transport processes: Filtration, absorption, secretion. *Am J Physiol* 243:F1, 1982.

19. Stanton BA, Kaissling B. Regulation of renal ion transport and cell growth by sodium. *Am J Physiol* 257:F1, 1989.

20. Ellison DH, Velasquez H, Wright FS. Adaptation of the distal convoluted tubule of the rat. Structural and functional effects of dietary salt intake and chronic diuretic infusion. *J Clin Invest* 83:113, 1989.

21. Scherzer P, Wald H, Popovtzer MM. Enhanced glomerular filtration and Na^+-K^+-ATPase with furosemide administration. *Am J Physiol* 252:F910, 1987.

22. Morsing P, Velazques H, Wright FS, Ellison DH. Adaptation of distal convoluted tubule of rats. II. Effects of chronic thiazide infusion. *Am J Physiol* 261:F137, 1991.

23. Shimizu T, Yoshitomi K, Taniguchi J, Imai M. Effect of high NaCl intake on Na^+ and K^+ transport in the rabbit distal convoluted tubule. *Pfluegers Arch* 414:500, 1989.

24. Broner F. Renal calcium transport: Mechanisms and regulation—an overview. *Am J Physiol* 257:F707, 1989.

25. Friedman PA, Gesek FA. Calcium transport in renal epithelial cells. *Am J Physiol* 264:F181, 1993.

26. Poujeol P, Bidet M, Tauc M. Calcium transport in rabbit distal cells. *Kidney Int* 48:1102, 1995.

27. Shimizu T, Yoshitomi K, Nakamura M, Imai M. Effects of PTH, calcitonin, and cAMP on calcium transport in rabbit distal nephron segments. *Am J Physiol* 259:F408, 1992.

28. Gesek FA, Friedman PA. On the mechanism of parathyroid hormone stimulation of calcium uptake by mouse distal convoluted tubule cells. *J Clin Invest* 90:749, 1992.

29. Friedman PA, Gesek FA. Vitamin D_3 accelerates PTH-dependent calcium transport in distal convoluted tubule cells. *Am J Physiol* 265:F300, 1993.

30. Herbert SC. Extracellular calcium-sensing receptor: Implications for calcium and magnesium handling in the kidney. *Kidney Int* 50:2129, 1996.

31. Costanzo LS, Windhager EE. Effects of PTH, ADH, and cyclic AMP on distal tubular Ca and Na reabsorption. *Am J Physiol* 239:F478, 1980.

32. Gesek FA, Friedman PA. Mechanism of calcium transport stimulation by chlorothiazide in mouse distal collecting tubule cells. *J Clin Invest* 90:429, 1992.

33. Coe FL, Parks JH, Asplin JR. The pathogenesis and treatment of kidney stones. *N Engl J Med* 327:1141, 1992.

34. Ettinger B, Citrov JT, Livermore B, Dolman LI. Chlorthalidone reduces calcium oxalate calculus recurrence but magnesium hydroxide does not. *J Urol* 139:679, 1988.

35. Levine DZ, Jacobson HR. The regulation of renal acid excretion: New observations from studies of distal nephron segments. *Kidney Int* 29:1099, 1986.

36. Chan YL, Malnic G, Giebisch G. Renal bicarbonate reabsorption in the rat. III. Distal tubule perfusion study of load dependence and bicarbonate permeability. *J Clin Invest* 84:931, 1989.

37. Schnermann J, Steipe B, Briggs JP. In situ studies of distal convoluted tubule in rat: II. Potassium secretion. *Am J Physiol* 252:F970, 1987.

38. Velazquez H, Ellison DH, Wright FS. Chloride-dependent potassium secretion in early and late distal tubules. *Am J Physiol* 253:F555, 1987.

39. Bourdeau JE, Lau K. Regulation of cytosolic free calcium concentration in the rabbit connecting tubule: A calcium-reabsorbing epithelium. *J Lab Clin Med* 119:650, 1992.

40. Shimizu T, Yoshitomi K, Nakamura M, Imai M. Site and mechanism of action of trichlormethazide in rabbit distal nephron segments perfused in vitro. *J Clin Invest* 82:721, 1988.

41. Shimizu T, Nakamura M. Ouabain-induced cell swelling in rabbit connecting tubule: Evidence for a thiazide-sensitive Na^+-Cl^- cotransporter. *Pflugers Arch* 421:314, 1992.

42. Wright FS. Renal potassium handling. *Semin Nephrol* 7:174, 1987.

43. Stokes JB. Sodium and potassium transport by the collecting duct. *Kidney Int* 38:679, 1990.

44. Muto S, Muto S, Giebisch G. Na-dependent effects of DOCA on cellular transport properties of CCDs from ADX rabbits. *Am J Physiol* 253:F753, 1987.

45. Frindt G, Sackin H, Palmer LG. Whole-cell currents in rat cortical collecting tubule: Low-Na diet increases amiloride-sensitive conductance. *Am J Physiol* 258:F502, 1990.

46. Sauer M, Flemmer A, Thurau K, Beck F-X. Sodium entry in principal and intercalated cells of the isolated perfused cortical collecting duct. *Pflugers Arch* 416:88, 1990.

47. Wong W, Schwab A, Giebisch G. Regulation of small-conductance K^+ channel in apical membrane of rat cortical collecting tubule. *Am J Physiol* 259:F494, 1990.

48. Canessa CM, Schild L, Buell G, et al. Amiloride-sensitive epithelial cell Na^+ channel is made of three homoglous subunits. *Nature* 367:463, 1994.

49. Horisberger JD. Amiloride-sensitive Na channels. *Curr Opin Cell Biol* 10:443, 1998.

50. Dietl P, Schwiebert E, Stanton BA. Cellular mechanism of chloride transport in the cortical collecting duct. *Kidney Int* 40(suppl 33):S-125, 1991.

51. Sansom SC, O'Neil RG. Mineralocorticoid requirement of apical cell membrane Na^+ and K^+ transport of the cortical collecting duct. *Am J Physiol* 248:F858, 1985.

52. Sansom S, Muto S, Giebisch G. Na-dependent effects of DOCA on cellular transport properties of CCDs from ADX rabbits. *Am J Physiol* 253:F753, 1987.

53. Schafer JA, Hawk CT. Regulation of Na^+ channels in the cortical collecting duct by AVP and mineralocorticoids. *Kidney Int* 41:255, 1992.

54. Chen SY, Bhargava A, Mastroberardino L, et al. Epithelial sodium channel regulated by aldosterone-induced protein sgk. *Proc Natl Acad Sci U S A* 96:2514, 1999.

55. Masilamani S, Kim G-H, Mitchell C, et al. Aldosterone-mediated regulation of EnaC alpha, beta, and gamma subunit proteins in rat kidney. *J Clin Invest* 104:R19, 1999.

56. Coutry N, Blot-Chabaud M, Mateo P, et al. Time course of sodium-induced Na^+-K^+-ATPase recruitment in rabbit cortical collecting tubule. *Am J Physiol* 263:C61, 1992.

57. Horisberger J-D, Rossier BC. Aldosterone regulation of gene transcription leading to control of ion transport. *Hypertension* 19:221, 1992.

58. Shimketa RA, Warnock DG, Bositis CM, et al. Liddle's syndrome: Heritable human hypertension caused by mutations in the beta subunit of the epithelial Na channel. *Cell* 79:407, 1994.

59. Chang SS, Grunder S, Hanukoglu A, et al. Mutations in the subunits of the epithelial sodium channel cause salt wasting with hyperkalaemic acidosis, pseudohypoaldosteronism type 1. *Nat Genet* 12:248, 1996.

60. Stein JH, Osgood RW, Boonjarern S, et al. Segmental sodium reabsorption in rats with mild and severe volume depletion. *Am J Physiol* 227:351, 1974.

61. Stein JH, Osgood RW, Boonjarern S, Ferris TF. A comparison of the segmental analysis of sodium reabsorption during Ringer's and hyperoncotic albumin infusion in the rat. *J Clin Invest* 52:2313, 1973.
62. Husted RF, Laplace JR, Stokes JB. Enhancement of electrogenic Na^+ transport across rat inner medullary collecting duct by glucocorticoid and by mineralocorticoid hormones. *J Clin Invest* 86:498, 1990.
63. de Zeeuw D, Janssen WMT, de Jong PE. Atrial natriuretic factor: Its (patho)physiological significance in humans. *Kidney Int* 41:1115, 1992.
64. Ling BN, Eaton DC. Effects of luminal Na^+ on single Na^+ channels in A6 cells, a regulatory role for protein kinase C. *Am J Physiol* 256:F1094, 1989.
65. Hebert RL, Jacobson HR, Breyer MD. Prostaglandin E_2 inhibits sodium transport in rabbit cortical collecting duct by increasing intracellular calcium. *J Clin Invest* 87:1992, 1991.
66. Chen L, Reif MC, Schafer J. Clonidine and PGE_2 have different effects on Na^+ and water transport in rat and rabbit CCD. *Am J Physiol* 261:F123, 1991.
67. Guan Y, Zhang Y, Breyer RM, et al. Prostaglandin E_2 inhibits renal collecting duct Na^+ absorption by activating the EP1 receptor. *J Clin Invest* 102:194, 1998.
68. Nielsen S, Kwon T-H, Christensen BM, et al. Physiology and pathophysiology of renal aquaporins. *J Am Soc Nephrol* 10:647, 1999.
69. Sasaki S, Fushimi K, Saito H, et al. Cloning, characterization, and chromosomal mapping of human aquaporin of collecting duct. *J Clin Invest* 93:1250, 1994.
70. Deen PM, Verdijk MA, Knoers NV, et al. Requirement for human renal water channel aquaporin-2 for vasopressin-dependent concentration of urine. *Science* 264:92, 1994.
71. Fushimi K, Uchida S, Hara Y, et al. Cloning and expression of apical membrane water channel of rat kidney collecting tubule. *Nature* 361:549, 1993.
72. Schnermann J, Chou CL, Ma T, et al. Defective proximal tubule reabsorptive capacity in transgenic aquaporin-1 null mice. *Proc Natl Acad Sci U S A* 95:9660, 1998.
73. Field MJ, Stanton BA, Giebisch G. Influence of ADH on renal potassium handling: A micropuncture and microperfusion study. *Kidney Int* 25:502, 1984.
74. Guggino SE, Suarez-Isla BA, Guggino WB, Sacktor B. Forskolin and antidiuretic hormone stimulate a Ca^{2+}-activated K^+ channel in cultured kidney cells. *Am J Physiol* 249:F448, 1985.
75. Wang WH. View of K^+ secretion through the apical K channel of cortical collecting duct. *Kidney Int* 48:1024, 1995.
76. Schlatter E, Schafer JA. Electrophysiological studies of principal cells of rat collecting tubules. Antidiuretic hormone increases the apical membrane Na^+ conductance. *Pflugers Arch* 409:81, 1987.
77. Boton R, Gaviria M, Batlle DC. Prevalence, pathogenesis, and treatment of renal dysfunction associated with chronic lithium therapy. *Am J Kidney Dis* 10:329, 1987.
78. Batlle DC, von Riotte AB, Gaviria M, Grupp M. Amelioration of polyuria by amiloride in patients receiving long-term lithium therapy. *N Engl J Med* 312:408, 1985.
79. Steinmetz PR. Cellular organization of urinary acidification. *Am J Physiol* 251:F173, 1986.
80. Kim J, Kim Y-H, Cha J-H, et al. Intercalated cell subtypes in connecting tubule and cortical collecting duct of rat and mouse. *J Am Soc Nephrol* 10:1, 1999.
81. Nelson RD, Guo XL, Masood K, et al. Selectively amplified expression of an isoform of the vascular H-APTase 56-kilodalton subunit in renal intercalated cells. *Proc Natl Acad Sci U S A* 89:3541, 1992.
82. Tsuchiya K, Giebisch G, Welling PA. Molecular characterization and distribution of H/K ATPase catalytic subunit gene products in the kidney. *J Am Soc Nephrol* 4:881, 1993.
83. Kudrycki KE, Schull GE. Primary structure of the rat kidney band 3 anion exchange protein deduced from a cDNA. *J Biol Chem* 264:8185, 1989.
84. Karet FE, Gainza FJ, Gyory AZ, et al. Mutations in the chloride-bicarbonate distal renal tubular acidosis. *Proc Natl Acad Sci U S A* 94:6337, 1998.
85. Verlander JW, Madsen KM, Tisher CC. Effect of acute respiratory acidosis on two populations of intercalated cells in the rabbit cortical collecting duct. *Am J Physiol* 253:F1142, 1987.

86. Garg LC, Narang N. Effects of aldosterone on NEM-sensitive ATPases in rabbit nephron segments. *Kidney Int* 34:13, 1988.
87. Bastani B, Purcell H, Hemken P, et al. Expression and distribution of renal vascular proton-translocating adenosine triphosphatase in response to chronic acid and alkali loads in the rat. *J Clin Invest* 88:126, 1991.
88. Schuster VL. Cortical collecting duct bicarbonate secretion. *Kidney Int* 40(suppl 33): S-47, 1991.
89. Star RA, Burg MB, Knepper MA. Bicarbonate secretion and chloride absorption by rabbit cortical collecting ducts. Role of chloride/bicarbonate exchange. *J Clin Invest* 76:1123, 1985.
90. Karet FE, Finberg KE, Nelson RD, et al. Mutations in the gene encoding B1 subunit of H^+-ATPase cause renal tubular acidosis with sensorineural deafness. *Nat Genet* 21:84, 1999.
91. Stanton BA, Biemesderfer D, Wade JB, Giebisch G. Structural and functional study of the rat distal nephron: Effects of potassium adaptation and depletion. *Kidney Int* 19:36, 1981.
92. Garg LC. Respective roles of H-ATPase and H-K-ATPase in ion transport in the kidney. *J Am Soc Nephrol* 2:949, 1991.
93. Weigner ID, Wingo CS. Hyperkalemia: A potential silent killer. *J Am Soc Nephrol* 9:1535, 1998.
94. Armitage FE, Wingo CS. Luminal acidification in K-replete OMCDi: Contributions of H-K-ATPase and bafilomycin-A1-sensitive H-ATPase. *Am J Physiol* 267:F450, 1994.
95. Zhou X, Xia SL, Wingo CS. Chloride transport by the rabbit cortical collecting duct: Dependence on H, K-ATPase. *J Am Soc Nephrol* 9:2194, 1998.
96. Fejes-Toth G, Fejes-Toth A. Isolated principal and intercalated cells hormone responsiveness and Na^+-K^+-ATPase activity. *Am J Physiol* 256:F742, 1989.
97. Lencer WI, Brown D, Ausiello D, Verkman AS. Endocytosis of water channels in rat kidney: Cell specificity and correlation with in vivo antidiuresis. *Am J Physiol* 259:C920, 1990.
98. Koeppen B. Electrophysiological identification of principal and intercalated cells in the rabbit outer medullary collecting duct. *Pflugers Arch* 409:138, 1987.
99. Brown D, Hirsch S, Gluck S. Localization of a proton-pumping ATPase in rat kidney. *J Clin Invest* 82:2114, 1988.
100. Stone DK, Seldin DW, Kokko JP, Jacobson HR. Mineralocorticoid modulation of rabbit kidney medullary collecting duct acidification. A sodium-independent effect. *J Clin Invest* 72:77, 1983.
101. DuBose TD Jr, Good DW, Hamm LL, Wall SM. Ammonium transport in the kidney: New physiological concepts and their clinical applications. *J Am Soc Nephrol* 1:1193, 1991.
102. Flessner MF, Wall SM, Knepper MA. Permeability of rat collecting duct segments to NH_3 and NH_4^+. *Am J Physiol* 260:F264, 1991.
103. Jamison RL. Potassium recycling. *Kidney Int* 31:695, 1987.
104. Clapp WL, Madsen KM, Verlander JW, Tisher CC. Morphologic heterogeneity along the rat inner medullary collecting duct. *Lab Invest* 60:219, 1989.
105. Rocha AS, Kudo LH. Water, urea, sodium, chloride, and potassium transport in the in vitro isolated perfused papillary collecting duct. *Kidney Int* 22:485, 1982.
106. Diezi J, Michaud P, Aceves J, Giebisch G. Micropuncture study of electrolyte transport across papillary collecting duct of the rat. *Am J Physiol* 224:623, 1973.
107. Wall SM, Sands JM, Flessner MF, et al. Net acid transport by isolated perfused inner medullary collecting ducts. *Am J Physiol* 258:F75, 1990.
108. Zeidel ML. Hormonal regulation of inner medullary collecting duct sodium transport. *Am J Physiol* 265:F159, 1993.
109. Light DB, McCann FV, Keller TM, Stanton BA. Amiloride-sensitive cation channel in apical membrane of inner medullary collecting duct. *Am J Physiol* 255:F278, 1988.
110. Benos DJ, Awayda MS, Berdiev BK, et al. Diversity and regulation of amiloride-sensitive Na^+ channels. *Kidney Int* 49:1632, 1996.
111. Zeidel M, Kikeri D, Silva P, et al. Atrial natriuretic peptides inhibit conductive sodium uptake by rabbit inner medullary collecting duct cells. *J Clin Invest* 82:1067, 1988.

112. Ujiie K, Nonoguchi H, Tomita K, Marumo F. Effects of ANP and cGMP synthesis in inner medullary collecting duct subsegments of rats. *Am J Physiol* 259:F535, 1990.

113. Ciampolillo F, McCoy DE, Green RB, et al. Cell-specific expression of amiloride-sensitive Na-conducting ion channels in the kidney. *Am J Physiol* 274:C1303, 1996.

114. Knepper MA, Star RA. The vasopressin-regulated urea transporter in rat inner medullary collecting duct. *Am J Physiol* 259:F393, 1990.

115. Sands JM, Timmer RT, Gunn RB. Urea transporters in kidney and erythrocytes. *Am J Physiol* 273:F321, 1997.

116. Sands JM, Nonoguchi H, Knepper MA. Vasopressin effects on urea and H_2O transport in inner medullary collecting duct subsegments. *Am J Physiol* 253:F823, 1987.

117. Ishibashi K, Sasaki S, Yoshiyama N, et al. Generation of pH gradient across the rabbit collecting duct segments perfused in vitro. *Kidney Int* 31:930, 1987.

118. Murillo-Carretero MI, Ilundain AA, Echevarria M. Regulation of aquaporin mRNA expression in rat kidney by water intake. *J Am Soc Nephrol* 10:696, 1999.

119. Garcia-Perez A, Burg MB. Importance of organic osmolytes for osmoregulation by renal medullary cells. *Hypertension* 16:595, 1990.

120. Bonventre JV, Roman RJ, Lechene C. Effect of urea concentration of pelvic fluid on renal concentrating ability. *Am J Physiol* 239:F609, 1980.

121. Bargman J, Leonard SL, McNeely E, et al. Examination of transepithelial exchange of water and solute in the rat renal pelvis. *J Clin Invest* 74:1860, 1984.

122. Levinsky NG, Berliner RW. Changes in composition of urine in ureter and bladder at low urine flow. *Am J Physiol* 196:549, 1959.

123. Walser BL, Yagil Y, Jamison RL. Urea flux in the ureter. *Am J Physiol* 255:F244, 1988.

EFFECTS OF HORMONES ON RENAL FUNCTION

The preceding chapters discussed the reabsorptive and secretory functions of the individual nephron segments. These processes are affected by a variety of hormones, some of which are synthesized within the kidney, such as renin (see Chap. 2), calcitriol (the most active metabolite of vitamin D), protaglandins, and kinins. As will be seen, these hormones play an important role in the maintenance of fluid and electrolyte balance, since they allow the *individual regulation* of the rate of excretion of the different solutes and water. The kidney also secretes erythropoietin, a hormone that promotes red cell production by the bone marrow.

This chapter reviews the major mechanisms of action and the regulation of secretion of those hormones that have important effects on renal function. How these hormones interact with other factors to permit the maintenance of fluid and electrolyte balance will then be discussed in Chaps. 8 to 12.

MECHANISMS OF HORMONE ACTION

The hormones that influence renal function generally work by activating specific cellular proteins via phosphorylation or by inducing the synthesis of new proteins. A hormone can initiate these events by affecting adenylyl cyclase, guanylyl cyclase, phosphatidylinositol turnover, or, with steroid hormones, ribonucleic acid (RNA) transcription (Table 6-1).[1-9]

Adenylyl Cyclase

Some of the responses mediated by adenylyl cyclase begin by attachment of the hormone to its specific receptor on the basolateral membrane of the tubular cell. This hormone-receptor complex then affects the activation state of a guanine nucleotide regulatory protein, such as the stimulatory (G_s) or inhibitory (G_i) proteins (Fig. 6-1).[1,2,7,8] G_s, for example, has three components, alpha (α), beta (β), and gamma (γ), with the α subunit normally binding guanosine diphosphate (GDP) in the inactive state. Binding of hormone to its receptor causes the α subunit to release GDP, take up intracellular guanosine triphosphate (GTP), and at least partially dissociate from the β-γ subunit. This G_α-GTP complex is able to activate adenylyl cyclase, leading to the conversion of adenosine triphosphates (ATP) into cyclic adenosine monophosphate (AMP).

The generation of cyclic AMP is followed sequentially by activation of a protein kinase (due to binding of cyclic AMP to a regulatory subunit on the kinase[10]), phosphorylation of specific cell proteins (by the transfer of phosphate from intracellular ATP to the protein), and the physiologic effects of the hormone. Hormone activity is eventually shut off by a GTPase intrinsic to the α molecule

Table 6-1 Mechanism of action of major hormones affecting renal function

Adenylyl cyclase		Prosphatidylinositol	RNA transcription
Stimulate	Inhibit	turnover	(steroid hormones)
Vasopressin (V_2)	Prostaglandins	Vasopressin (V_1)	Aldosterone
Parathyroid hormone	α_2-Adrenergic	Angiotensin II	Calcitriol
β-Adrenergic	Angiotensin II	Norepinephrine	
Prostaglandins	(tubular effect)	(α_1-adrenergic)	
(vascular effect)		Parathyroid hormone	

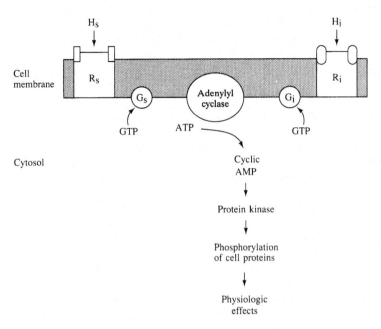

Figure 6-1   Schematic representation of the adenylyl cyclase–cyclic AMP system. Activation begins when a stimulatory hormone (H_s) combines with its receptor (R_s). The hormone-receptor complex interacts with the regulatory protein G_2, allowing it to take up guanosine triphosphate (GTP). This activated form of G_s then stimulates adenylyl cyclase. This step is followed sequentially by the formation of cyclic AMP, activation of a protein kinase, phosphorylation of cell proteins, and the physiologic effects of the hormone. Other hormones (H_i) inhibit adenylyl cyclase by binding to their receptor (R_i) and then activating an inhibitory regulatory protein (G_i).

that hydrolyzes bound GTP.[1] The β-γ subunit may also be an important regulator of these processes.[11]

On the other hand, activation of G_i results in diminished adenylyl cyclase activity and a reduction in cellular cyclic AMP levels.[1,2] Like G_x, G_i also dissociates into α, β, and γ subunits.

Guanylyl cyclase   An analogous but separate intracellular pathway involves the activation of *guanylyl cyclase*, leading to the subsequent formation of cyclic guanosine monophosphate (GMP) and phosphorylation of specific cell proteins.[3,9] This pathway appears to mediate the actions of atrial natriuretic peptide (ANP; see below) and of direct vasodilators, such as nitroprusside and nitroglycerine.

The initial event in this system is, for ANP, attachment to its extracellular receptor on the cell membrane. This transmembrane protein has a conserved intracellular regulatory and cyclase catalytic domain.[9,12] Stimulatory and inhibitory regulatory proteins, as with adenylyl cyclase, do not seem to be involved.

Binding of ANP to its receptor appears to induce a conformational change (such as dimerization) in the kinase domain, leading to activation of guanylyl cyclase activity and the generation of cyclic GMP.[3] In the kidney, this process leads to closing of Na^+ channels in the luminal membrane in the inner medullary collecting duct (see below), which is not well understood.[13]

Phosphatidylinositol Turnover

Another mechanism of hormone action involves the turnover of membrane lipids. This process is again initiated by binding of the hormone (e.g., angiotensin II and norepinephrine) to its cell receptor, leading to the activation of a G protein (called G_q, as compared to G_s, which stimulates adenylyl cyclase) and the formation of $G\alpha$-GTP (Fig. 6-2).[1,4] In this setting, however, membrane-bound phospholipase C, rather than adenylyl cyclase, is activated.

Phospholipase C then promotes the breakdown of a membrane lipid, phosphatidylinositol 4,5-biphosphate, into two compounds: inositol 1,4,5-triphosphate (IP_3) and diacylglycerol. IP_3 mediates the acute effect of the hormone by increasing the release of calcium from stores in endoplasmic reticulum and by enhancing the uptake of extracellular calcium. The net effect is an elevation in the cytosolic calcium concentration. This calcium binds to calmodulin, leading to the phosphor-

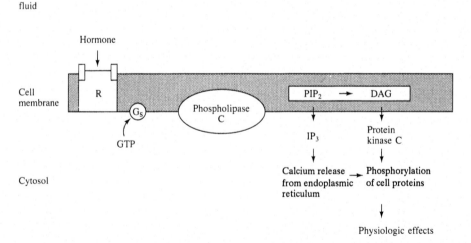

Figure 6-2 Schematic representation of the phosphatidylinositol pathway. The combination of a hormone with its receptor (R) leads to activation of a stimulatory regulatory protein (G_s) with a subsequent increase in activity of membrane-bound phospholipase C. This enzyme results in the breakdown of a membrane lipid, phosphatidylinositol 4,5-biphosphate (PIP_2), into two compounds: inositol 1,4,5-triphosphate (IP_3) and diacylglycerol (DAG). The former mediates the acute action of the hormone by inducing the release of calcium from stores in endoplasmic reticulum; the latter is responsible for the sustained hormone effect by activating protein kinase C, leading to the phosphorylation of cell proteins.

ylation of specific cell proteins and the physiologic effects of the hormone. The calcium effect, however, is short-lived, and sustained action of the hormone is mediated by diacylglycerol, which activates protein kinase C. The latter compound then causes the desired changes in cell activity.

The formation of diacylglycerol may also play an additional role, since the fatty acid at position 2 is arachidonic acid, the precursor of the prostaglandins. Arachidonic acid can be released from diacylglycerol by phospholipase A_2, an enzyme that can be hormonally activated. This may explain, for example, how antidiuretic hormone (ADH) increases local prostaglandin production and, in part, how prostaglandins then modulate the actions of ADH (see below).[14,15]

RNA Transcription

Steroid hormones, such as aldosterone, calcitriol, and cortisol, have a different mechanism of action, involving new protein synthesis (Fig. 6-3). These hormones are lipid-soluble and therefore are able to diffuse across the cell membrane and combine with specific receptors that are located in the cytosol rather than the cell

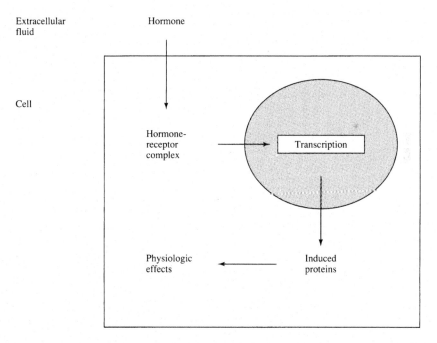

Figure 6-3   Model for the mechanism of action of steroid hormones, such as aldosterone and calcitriol. The hormone enters the cell by diffusion and combines with a specific receptor in the cytosol. The active hormone-receptor complex, which unmasks the DNA binding site on the receptor, then migrates to the nucleus where it interacts with specific genes, leading to RNA transcription and the eventual production of new proteins that are responsible for the physiologic actions of the hormone.

membrane.[5,6] Attachment of hormone to its receptor results in unmasking of the DNA-binding site on the receptor.[5,6,16] As a result, the hormone-receptor complex is able to migrate into the nucleus and to bind to specific sites near the genes that are responsible for the physiologic actions of the hormone. Subsequent steps include messenger RNA and ribosomal RNA transcription and the eventual synthesis of new proteins.

The discovery of analogs of steroid hormones, which have receptor complex binding properties different from those of the endogenous hormones, may permit the administration of agents that possess the desirable properties of these hormones but circumvent their adverse effects. As an example, oxacalcitriol, a vitamin D or calcitriol analog, has a low affinity for vitamin D–binding protein; as a result, more of the drug circulates in the free (unbound) form, allowing it to be metabolized more rapidly than calcitriol.[17] This leads to a shorter half-life, which could explain the small and transient stimulation of intestinal calcium absorption and a lower likelihood of inducing hypercalcemia than with calcitriol itself. The ability to minimize the risk of hypercalcemia with a vitamin D analog may be important clinically when the drug is given to suppress secondary hyperparathyroidism in patients with chronic renal failure (see page 207).

A more important clinical example of tissue-selective activity occurs with selective estrogen receptor modulators, such as raloxifene. In vitro experiments suggest that raloxifene has different effects from estradiol at the estrogen receptor, including differential modulation of DNA response elements,[18] causing a different conformational change in the transactivation domain of the ligand-binding domain.[19] In patients, raloxifene preserves the beneficial effects of estrogen on bone and apparently the heart[20] without promoting endometrial hyperplasia or increasing the risk of breast cancer.[21]

ANTIDIURETIC HORMONE AND WATER BALANCE

Antidiuretic hormone (the human form is called arginine vasopressin) is a polypeptide synthesized in the supraoptic and paraventricular nuclei in the hypothalamus (Fig. 6-4).[22] Secretory granules containing ADH migrate down the axons of the supraopticohypophyseal tract into the posterior lobe of the pituitary, where they are stored and subsequently released after appropriate stimuli. In addition, some of the secretory granules produced in the paraventricular nuclei enter the cerebrospinal fluid or the portal capillaries in the median eminence (Fig. 6-4).[22] The latter effect probably accounts for the observation that lesions of the posterior pituitary or supraopticohypophyseal tract below the median eminence do not usually lead to permanent diabetes insipidus (ADH lack), since ADH produced in the hypothalamus still has access to the systemic circulation.

ADH is rapidly metabolized in the liver and kidney, with a half-life in the circulation of only 15 to 20 min.

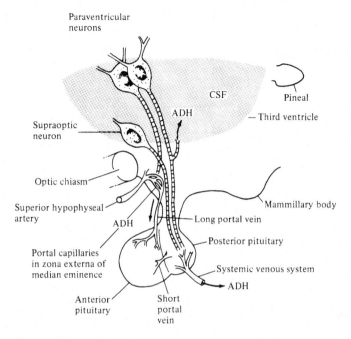

Paraventricular
neurons

Supraoptic
neuron

CSF

Pineal

ADH

— Third ventricle

Optic chiasm

Superior hypophyseal
artery

Mammillary body

ADH

—Long portal vein

Portal capillaries
in zona externa of
median eminence

—Posterior pituitary

—Systemic venous system

→ ADH

Anterior
pituitary

Short
portal
vein

Figure 6-4   Diagram of the mammalian hypothalamus and pituitary gland showing pathways for the secretion of antidiuretic hormone (ADH). The hormone is formed in the supraoptic and paraventricular nuclei, transported in granules along their axons, and then secreted at three sites: the posterior pituitary gland, the portal capillaries of the median eminence, and the cerebrospinal fluid (CSF) of the third ventricle. (*Adapted from Zimmerman EA, Robinson AG,* Kidney Int 10:12, 1976. Reprinted by permission from Kidney International.)

Actions

ADH is the primary physiologic determinant of the rate of free water excretion. Its major renal effect is to augment the water permeability of the luminal membranes of the cortical and medullary collecting tubules, thereby promoting water reabsorption via osmotic equilibration with the hypertonic interstitium (see Chap. 4 for a review of the countercurrent mechanism and of the other tubular mechanisms by which ADH can promote urinary concentration). The ADH-induced increase in collecting tubule water permeability occurs primarily in the principal cells, as the adjacent intercalated cells are mostly involved in acid or bicarbonate secretion (see Chap. 5).[23,24]

There are two major receptors for ADH: the V_1 and V_2 receptors. Activation of the V_1 receptors induces vasoconstriction and enhancement of prostaglandin release (see below), while the V_2 receptors mediate the antidiuretic response as well as other functions (see Fig. 6-5).[25] A third receptor, the V_3 or V_{1b} receptor, appears to mediate the effect of ADH on the pituitary, facilitating the release of ACTH.[26]

Activation of adenylyl cyclase by ADH via the V_2 receptor initiates a sequence of events in which a protein kinase is activated, leading to preformed cytoplasmic

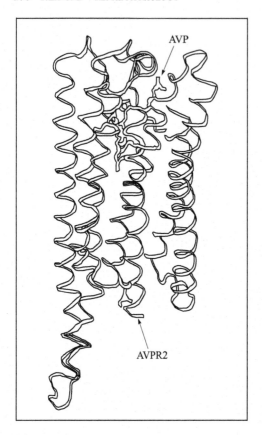

Figure 6-5 Interaction between AVP and its receptor. Schematic representation of the relation between arginine vasopressin (AVP, antidiuretic hormone) and the AVP receptor 2 (AVPR2). The receptor is depicted as seven coiled red ribbons. AVP is nestled within a pocket formed by the transmembrane domains of AVPR2. (*Adapted from Bochet DG, Oksche A, Rosenthal E,* J Am Soc Nephrol *8:1951, 1997. Used with permission.*)

vesicles that contain unique *water channels*.[27-29] The principal ADH-sensitive water channel, called *aquaporin-2*, is normally stored in the cytosol;[29-30] under the influence of ADH, it moves to and fuses with the luminal membrane,[24,31] thereby allowing water to be reabsorbed down the favorable osmotic gradient.[32,33] This process results in the formation of intramembranous particle aggregates that are visible on electron microscopy (see Fig. 6-6).[31,34]

Once the water channels span the luminal membrane and permit osmotic water movement into the cells,[34] water is rapidly returned to the systemic circulation across the basolateral membrane, which both is water permeable (even in the absence of ADH) and has a much greater surface area than the luminal membrane.[35] When the ADH effect has worn off, the water channels aggregate within clathrin-coated pits, from which they are removed from the luminal membrane by endocytosis and returned to the cytoplasm.[31,34]

A defect in any step in this pathway, such as attachment of ADH to its receptor or the function of the water channel, can cause resistance to the action of ADH and an increase in urine output. This disorder is called nephrogenic diabetes insipidus (DI) (see page 754). As examples:

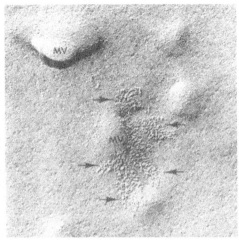

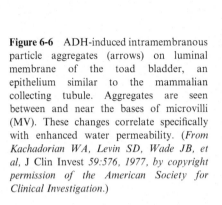

Figure 6-6 ADH-induced intramembranous particle aggregates (arrows) on luminal membrane of the toad bladder, an epithelium similar to the mammalian collecting tubule. Aggregates are seen between and near the bases of microvilli (MV). These changes correlate specifically with enhanced water permeability. (*From Kachadorian WA, Levin SD, Wade JB, et al, J Clin Invest 59:576, 1977, by copyright permission of the American Society for Clinical Investigation.*)

- Hereditary nephrogenic DI is usually transmitted in an X-linked fashion, with the genetic defect involving a number of different mutations (or deletions) in the V_2 receptor gene that can lead to decreased hormone binding, impaired intracellular transport or coupling to the adenylyl cyclase system, or diminished synthesis or accelerated degradation of the receptor.[36,37]
- A second, autosomal recessive form of hereditary nephrogenic DI has been described in which there appears to be mutations in the aquaporin-2 gene.[30,38,39,40] These mutations may lead to impaired trafficking of the water channels with lack of fusion with the luminal membrane and/or decreased channel function.[30,39]

Electrolyte handling   In addition to increasing water permeability, ADH appears to affect a variety of other processes in the cortical collecting tubule, enhancing the reabsorption of Na^+ and the secretion of K^+.[23-25] The physiologic role of these effects is uncertain, since ADH does not appear to be important in the maintenance of electrolyte or acid-base balance. However, the stimulation of K^+ secretion allows ADH to *regulate water transport without interfering with that of K^+*. The rate of distal urinary flow is normally an important determinant of the rate of K^+ secretion and subsequent excretion (see Chap. 12). ADH-stimulated water reabsorption should, by lowering distal flow, inappropriately diminish K^+ secretion; this is prevented by the direct stimulatory effect of ADH on K^+ handling.[42]

Vascular resistance   As mentioned above, the antidiuretic effects of ADH are mediated by the V_2 receptors, which, in the kidney, stimulate adenylyl cyclase activity.[14] In comparison, the V_1 receptors promote phosphatidylinositol turnover and primarily act to increase vascular resistance (hence the name *vasopressin*).[44] ADH release is markedly stimulated in the presence of effective circulating volume depletion (see below). In general, the vasopressor role of ADH is relatively minor, as the blood pressure is maintained primarily by the renin-angiotensin and sympathetic nervous systems (see Chap. 8).[44]

Renal prostaglandins ADH stimulates the production of prostaglandins (particularly prostaglandin E_2 and prostacyclin) in a variety of cells within the kidney, including those in the thick ascending limb, collecting tubules, medullary interstitium, and glomerular mesangium.[45-47] The prostaglandins that are produced then impair both the antidiuretic and vascular actions of ADH.[15,48-50] The former effect is in part due to a reduction in ADH-induced generation of cyclic AMP; stimulation of the inhibitory regulatory protein G_i (see Fig. 6-1) and of protein kinase C formation (see Fig. 6-2) appears to contribute to this response.[15,48]

These findings have suggested that a short *negative feedback loop* may be present in which ADH enhances local prostaglandin production, thereby preventing an excessive antidiuretic response. It is of interest, however, that the effect of ADH on prostaglandin synthesis is mediated by the V_1, not the antidiuretic V_2, receptors.[45,47] Activation of the V_1 receptors promotes phosphatidylinositol turnover, leading to the formation of diacylglycerol, from which arachidonic acid, the precursor of the prostaglandins, can be released via activation of phospholipase A_2 (see Fig. 6-2).[8,51]

The renal site of V_1-receptor stimulation of prostaglandin synthesis is uncertain. The collecting tubular cells have both V_1 (20 percent of the total ADH receptors in the cortical collecting tubule) and V_2 receptors,[52,53] and it is possible that a local negative feedback system is in place.[45] However, stimulation of these V_1 receptors appears to occur only at supraphysiologic concentrations of ADH.[54]

Alternatively, the major function of the ADH-prostaglandin relationship may involve the regulation of renal hemodynamics. ADH, acting via the V_1 receptors, is a systemic and renal vasoconstrictor.[50] The local production of prostaglandins by the kidney (particularly the glomeruli) minimizes the increase in renal vascular resistance, thereby maintaining renal perfusion.[50]

Other extrarenal effects ADH has other renal effects of potential clinical importance, including a role in the regulation of cortisol release and of factor VIII and von Willebrand's factor from vascular endothelium.[25] ADH is cosecreted with corticotropin releasing hormone (CRH) from single neurons in the paraventricular nuclei[22] and promotes the secretion of ACTH by corticotropes in the pituitary via activation of V_3 receptors.[26] Cortisol has an inhibitory effect on the secretion of both CRH and ADH from the paraventricular nuclei. Adrenal insufficiency (in which cortisol secretion is reduced) removes this inhibitory effect, leading to a persistent rise in ADH release.[22,55] The associated impairment in water excretion can result in water retention and hyponatremia, a common electrolyte disorder in patients with cortisol deficiency (see page 710).

ADH, acting through the V_2 receptors, also can stimulate the release of factor VIII and von Willebrand factor from vascular endothelium.[25] Although this response is of uncertain significance in normal subjects, the administration of ADH has been effective in transiently improving the bleeding tendencies in a variety of disorders, including hemophilia, von Willebrand's disease, and advanced renal failure.[25,56]

Control of ADH Secretion

The major stimuli to ADH secretion are hyperosmolality and effective circulating volume depletion (Figs. 6-7 and 6-8).[57,58] These responses are appropriate, since the water retention induced by ADH will both lower the plasma osmolality (P_{osm}) and raise the extracellular volume toward normal. Conversely, lowering the P_{osm} by water loading will diminish ADH release. The ensuing reduction in collecting tubule water reabsorption will decrease the urine osmolality (U_{osm}), thereby allowing the excess water to be excreted. Since the half-life of ADH in the circulation is 15 to 20 min, the maximum diuresis after a water load is delayed for 90 to 120 min, the time required for the metabolism of the previously circulating ADH.

Osmoreceptors   The location of the osmoreceptors governing ADH release was demonstrated by the classic experiments of Verney.[59] These experiments utilized local infusions of hypertonic saline, which raised the local P_{osm} without affecting the systemic P_{osm}. Such an infusion into the carotid artery, but not the femoral artery, resulted in enhanced ADH secretion and an antidiuresis. These findings indicated that the osmoreceptors, which are separate from the hormone-producing cells, are located in the brain, not in the periphery.[55]

Studies in rats suggest that separate osmoreceptors are located in the upper small bowel.[60] Thus, ingestion of a hypertonic NaCl solution leads to a rapid increase in ADH release that is prevented by lesions in the splanchnic nerves. The physiologic role of these osmoreceptors is unclear; they may contribute to the regulation of water balance or participate in the sensation of satiety.

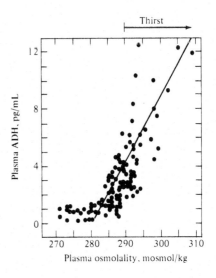

Figure   6-7 Relationship   of   plasma   ADH concentration   to   plasma   osmolality   in   normal humans in whom the plasma osmolality was changed by varying the state of hydration. Notice that the osmotic threshold for thirst is a few mosmol/kg higher than that for ADH. (*Adapted from Robertson GL, Aycinena P, Zerbe RL, Am J Med 72:339, 1982. Used with permission.*)

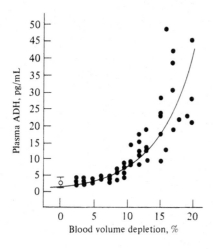

Figure 6-8 Relationship of ADH levels to isosmotic changes in blood volume in the rat. Notice that much higher ADH levels can occur with hypovolemia than with hyperosmolality, although a relatively large fall in blood volume is required before this response is initiated. (*From Dunn FL, Brennan TJ, Nelson AE, Robertson GL, J Clin Invest 52:3212, 1973, by copyright permission of the American Society for Clinical Investigation.*)

The increment in P_{osm} is perceived by the hypothalamic osmoreceptors as an effective osmotic gradient between the plasma and the receptor cell. It is postulated that the osmoreceptor is activated by changes in intracellular water content, thereby altering intracellular osmolality. Water channels make the osmoreceptor cell membrane permeable to water, permitting water movement out of the cell with hypernatremia (or other causes of hyperosmolality) and into the cell with hyponatremia. The ensuing reduction in cell volume in hypernatremia increases the activity of stretch-inactivated cation channels,[61,62] leading to depolarization of the cell, which in some way stimulates ADH secretion and synthesis. These steps are reversed with hyponatremia.

In general, the *plasma sodium concentration is the primary osmotic determinant of ADH release*, since Na^+ salts are the major effective extracellular solutes (see page 246).[58] In contrast, increments in the plasma urea concentration (measured as the blood urea nitrogen, or BUN) do not affect ADH secretion, because urea is an ineffective osmole that readily crosses cell membranes and will not induce water movement out of the osmoreceptor cells.

The contribution of glucose, the other major extracellular solute, to ADH regulation is somewhat more complicated.[63] In normal subjects, a rise in the plasma glucose concentration increases the release of insulin. Insulin can then promote glucose entry into the osmoreceptor cells, making glucose an ineffective osmole that will not affect the secretion of ADH. In uncontrolled diabetes mellitus, however, hyperglycemia is associated with insulin deficiency. In this setting, glucose acts as an effective osmole that can promote ADH release.[63]

The osmoreceptors are extremely sensitive, responding to alterations in the P_{osm} of as little as 1 percent.[57,58,64] In humans, the osmotic threshold for ADH release is about 280 to 290 mosmol/kg (Fig. 6-7).[57,58] Below this level, there is little if any circulating ADH, and the urine should be maximally dilute, with an osmolality below 100 mosmol/kg. Above the osmotic threshold, there is a progressive and relatively linear rise in ADH secretion. This system is so efficient that the P_{osm}

usually does not vary by more than 1 to 2 percent, despite wide fluctuations in water intake. As an example, a large water load will lower the P_{osm} and essentially shut off the release of ADH. The net effect is the excretion of more than 80 percent of the excess water within 4 h.

Role of thirst   The response to hyperosmolality, as can occur with water loss due to exercise-induced sweating on a hot day, includes a second factor, as thirst as well as ADH release is stimulated (Fig. 6-9). The net effect is that both increased water intake and reduced water excretion combine to return the P_{osm} to normal (Fig. 6-9).[57] The osmotic threshold for thirst (which can be estimated only indirectly) has been reported to be either 2 to 5 mosmol/kg higher than or roughly equivalent to that for ADH release.[65,66] It is not clear whether these parameters are controlled by the same or by two different osmoreceptors.

Even though thirst is regulated centrally (including cortical areas that influence nonessential or social drinking), it is sensed peripherally as the sensation of a dry mouth.[55,67] The cessation of thirst (satiety) is also mediated initially in the periphery by *oropharyngeal mechanoreceptors*[68,69] that are stimulated by swallowing relatively large volumes of fluid.[70]

It might be expected, for example, that the hyperosmotic stimulus to thirst and ADH release would be attenuated as the P_{osm} returns toward normal. However, studies in experimental animals and humans have demonstrated that drinking leads to a marked, but transient, suppression of thirst and ADH within 10 to 20 min, *before there has been any appreciable reduction in the* P_{osm}.[68-70] This

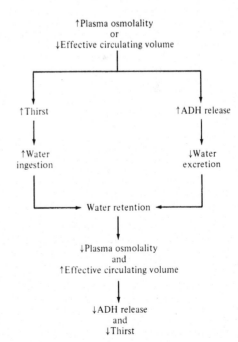

Figure 6-9   Feedback loop for the stimulation of ADH release and thirst.

response can be considered to be appropriate, since there is a 30- to 60-min delay before ingested water is completely absorbed. Thus, water intake would be markedly excessive if it continued until the P_{osm} were normalized, since there would still be a substantial volume of nonabsorbed water remaining in the gastrointestinal tract. The oropharyngeal receptors allow *slow repletion of the water deficit* to occur in discrete steps, as the suppression of thirst and ADH release will be transient as long as the P_{osm} remains elevated.

Like ADH, thirst is also stimulated by volume depletion.[67] How this occurs is incompletely understood.

Volume receptors   Patients with effective circulating volume depletion—as with vomiting, cirrhosis, or heart failure (see Chap. 8)—may secrete ADH, even in the presence of a low plasma osmolality.[57,71-73] These findings indicate the existence of nonosmolal, volume-sensitive receptors for ADH release (Fig. 6-8). Parasympathetic afferents in the carotid sinus baroreceptors are of primary importance in this response. Changes in the rate of afferent discharge from these neurons affect the activity of the vasomotor center in the medulla and subsequently the rate of ADH secretion by the cells in the paraventricular nuclei.[14] (The supraoptic nuclei, in comparison, are important for osmoregulation but do not appear to participate in this volume-sensitive response.[14])

Although low-pressure receptors in the left atrium play a contributory role in some animal species, they appear to be less important in humans, in whom a moderate reduction in intracardiac filling pressure does not stimulate ADH release unless there is a concomitant decline in systemic blood pressure.[74,75]

The carotid sinus baroreceptors, like other "volume" receptors, are actually pressure receptors. However, they are able to function indirectly as volume receptors. How this occurs can be appreciated from the formula relating pressure, cardiac output, and vascular resistance:

$$\text{Mean arterial pressure} = \text{cardiac output} \times \text{systemic vascular resistance}$$

Thus, a fall in cardiac output due to volume depletion or primary cardiac disease will lead to an initial decline in mean arterial pressure, which can be sensed by the carotid sinus baroreceptors. In experimental models of heart failure, for example, there is a fall in urine output and a rise in urine osmolality. These changes can be prevented by carotid baroreceptor denervation, indicating that the increment in ADH release is governed by baroreceptor afferents.[76]

This product of cardiac output and systemic vascular resistance actually equals the pressure drop across the circulation, i.e., mean arterial pressure minus mean venous pressure. However, the latter is normally so much lower (1 to 7 mmHg) than the former that ignoring the venous pressure produces only a small error.

The sensitivity of the volume receptors is different from that of the osmoreceptors. The latter respond to alterations in P_{osm} of as little as 1 percent (Fig. 6-7); in comparison, small, acute reductions in volume that are sufficient to increase the secretion of renin and norepinephrine *have little effect on the release of ADH*.

Acutely, ADH is secreted nonosmotically in humans only if there is a large enough change in the effective volume to produce a reduction in the systemic blood pressure.[75,76] Once hypotension occurs, there may be a marked rise in ADH secretion, resulting in circulating hormone levels that can substantially exceed those induced by hyperosmolality (compare Figs. 6-7 and 6-8).[57,75] Acute mild volume expansion generally has little effect on ADH release in humans.[77]

Interactions of the osmotic and volume stimuli   The hormone-producing cells in the supraoptic and paraventricular nuclei receive input from both the osmotic and the volume receptors, resulting in positive or negative interactions.[57,58] Thus, volume depletion potentiates the ADH response to hyperosmolality but can prevent the inhibition of ADH release normally induced by a fall in the P_{osm} (Fig. 6-10).[57,73,78]

These relationships are often clinically relevant. As an example, hypovolemic states are a common cause of water retention and hyponatremia (see Chap. 23). This occurs in part because the nonosmotic stimulation of ADH release prevents the normal excretion of ingested water. On the other hand, chronic volume expansion, as in primary hyperaldosteronism, can shift the osmotic threshold upward, leading to a mild elevation in the P_{osm} and plasma Na^+ concentration.[58]

Other factors affecting ADH secretion   ADH release can also be influenced by a variety of other factors that are not directly related to osmolal or volume balance (Table 6-2). Nausea is probably the most potent, potentially leading to as much as 500-fold rise in circulating ADH levels; neither the physiologic role of this response nor the mechanism by which it occurs is well understood.[79]

In some circumstances, these additional stimuli to ADH release can become clinically important. In surgical patients, for example, elevated levels of ADH may persist for several days after the operation,[80] a stress response that appears to be mediated by pain afferents.[81] If a large amount of free water is given in this setting,

Figure 6-10 The influence of hemodynamic status on the osmoregulation of ADH in otherwise healthy humans. The numbers in the center circles refer to the percentage change in volume or pressure; N refers to the normovolemic normotensive subject. Notice that the hemodynamic status affects both the slope of the relationship between the plasma ADH and osmolality and the osmotic threshold for ADH release. (*Adapted from Robertson GL, Shelton RL, Athar S,* Kidney Int *10:25, 1976, Reprinted by permission from* Kidney International.)

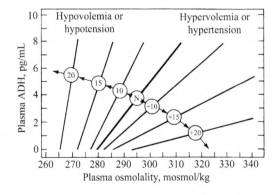

Table 6-2   Factors influencing ADH secretion

Stimuli	Inhibitors
Hyperosmolality	Hypoosmolality
Hypovolemia	Hypervolemia
Stress, e.g., pain	Ethanol
Nausea	Phenytoin
Pregnancy	
Hypoglycemia	
Nicotine	
Morphine	
Other drugs (see Table 23-3)	

water retention, severe hyponatremia, and potentially irreversible neurologic damage may ensue.[82]

Pregnancy, on the other hand, lowers the osmoregulatory threshold for ADH release and thirst.[65] As a result, there is a downward resetting of the osmostat, leading to a fall in the normal plasma Na^+ concentration by about 5 meq/L. This change, which is rapidly reversed after delivery, may be mediated by increased release of human chorionic gonadotropin (hCG).[83] hCG may act indirectly via the release of relaxin.[84]

ALDOSTERONE

The steps involved in adrenal cortical steroid synthesis are illustrated in Fig. 6-11. The major adrenal hormones are synthesized in different areas of the adrenal cortex: aldosterone in the zona glomerulosa, and glucocorticoids (particularly cortisol), androgens, and estrogens in the zona fasciculata and reticularis. The zona glomerulosa is well adapted for the production of aldosterone.[85,86] It has a low concentration of 17α-hydroxylase, the enzyme necessary for cortisol and androgen synthesis. More importantly, the final steps in the conversion of corticosterone to aldosterone, the addition of an hydroxyl group at the 18-carbon position and its subsequent oxidation to an aldehyde, occur only in the zona glomerulosa.[85,86] These two reactions are mediated by a single multifunctional cytochrome P450 enzyme called aldosterone synthase (or corticosterone methyl oxidase),[86-88] the activity of which is normally suppressed in the zona fasciculata. This suppression is important physiologically because it prevents aldosterone secretion from being inappropriately regulated by ACTH.

Aldosterone synthase has over 95 percent homology with 11-hydroxylase (which converts deoxycortisol to cortisol in the zona fasciculata), and their genes are located in the same region on chromosome 8.[89] This relationship becomes clinically important in the familial disorder glucocorticoid-remediable hyperaldosteronism. A chimeric gene, containing the regulator portion of 11β-

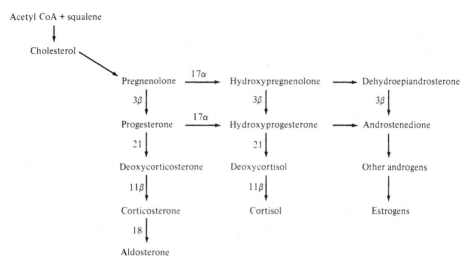

Acetyl CoA + squalene

Cholesterol

Figure 6-11   Schematic pathways of adrenal steroid biosynthesis. The numbers at the arrows refer to specific enzymes: 17α equals 17α-hydroxylase; 3β equals 3β-hydroxysteroid dehydrogenase; 21 equals 21-hydroxylase; 11β equals 11β-hydroxylase; 18 refers to a two-step process resulting in the addition of an aldehyde at the 18-carbon position. The last reactions occur only in the zona glomerulosa, which is the site of aldosterone secretion.

hydroxylase and the synthetic region of aldosterone synthase, is formed in this condition, in which the regulator portion of 11β-hydroxylase makes aldosterone synthesis ACTH-dependent.[90]

Actions

Aldosterone acts primarily in the distal nephron to increase the reasbsorption of Na^+ and Cl^- and the secretion of K^+ and H^+ (Fig. 6-12). Like other steroid hormones, aldosterone acts by diffusing into the tubular cell and then attaching to a specific cytosolic receptor (see Fig. 6-3).[5,91] The hormone-receptor complex then migrates to the nucleus, where it interacts with specific sites on the nuclear chromatin to enhance messenger RNA and ribosomal RNA transcription. This in turn is translated into the synthesis of new proteins called aldosterone-induced proteins (AIPs).[92,93] The time required for these processes to occur accounts for the 90-min latent period before electrolyte excretion is affected.

How these proteins act is not well understood. Aldosterone increases the abundance of the α subunit and promotes the phosphorylation of the β and γ subunits of the luminal membrane Na^+ channel through which luminal Na^+ enters the cells.[94,95] One early AIP is a serine kinase that appears to regulate Na^+ channel activity.[96,97] Another AIP is a K-ras2, but its actions are not known.[98]

Cortisol as a mineralocorticoid   Cortisol, which circulates in much higher concentrations than aldosterone, binds with equal affinity to the aldosterone receptor.[99]

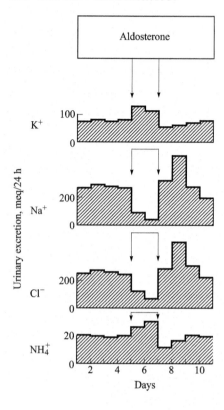

Figure 6-12 Effect of aldosterone on the daily urinary excretion of K^+, Na^+, Cl^-, and H^+ (as NH_4^+) in a normal subject maintained on a constant dietary intake. Note that the quantitatively most prominent effect is the marked reduction in NaCl excretion. (*From Liddle GW1, Arch Intern Med 102:998, 1958. By permission of the American Medical Association, copyright 1958.*)

However, cortisol does not act as a major mineralocorticoid because target tissues, such as the aldosterone-sensitive cells in the collecting tubules and salivary glands, possess enzymes, such as 11β-hydroxysteroid dehydrogenase, that convert cortisol to cortisone and other inactive metabolites.[6,100,101] Thus, only aldosterone physiologically activates the receptor. If, however, 11β-hydroxysteroid dehydrogenase is inactivated, then cortisol can act as the primary endogenous mineralocorticoid, leading to manifestations of primary hyperaldosteronism such as hypertension, hypokalemia, and metabolic alkalosis (see Chap. 27). One example is the chronic ingestion of licorice, which contains glycyrrhetinic acid, an inhibitor of 11β-hydroxysteroid dehydrogenase.[101,102]

NaCl and potassium The primary sites of action of aldosterone are in the connecting segment and the collecting tubules.[103,104] Its effects vary with the specific cell type that is affected. Perhaps most important, aldosterone promotes the reabsorption of NaCl and the secretion of K^+ in the connecting segment and in the principal cells in the cortical collecting tubule;[105-107] it also appears to enhance Na^+ reabsorption but not K^+ secretion in the papillary (inner medullary) collecting tubule.[108]

The cell model for how these processes occur is shown in Fig. 5-2. Aldosterone stimulates ionic transport in these cells by increasing the number of open Na^+ and K^+ channels in the luminal membrane as well as the activity of the Na^+-K^+-ATPase pump in the basolateral membrane.[5,91,94,106] As an example, going from a high- to a low-sodium diet (which is associated with enhanced aldosterone release) can increase the number of open Na^+ channels per cell from less than 100 to approximately 3000.[109] Both opening of previously silent channels and insertion of new channels in the luminal membrane appear to contribute to this response.[94,110]

The aldosterone-induced elevation in luminal Na^+ permeability promotes Na^+ diffusion into the tubular cell; this Na^+ is then returned to the systemic circulation by the Na^+-K^+-ATPase pump.[5] The movement of Na^+ through its channel is electrogenic in that it creates a lumen-negative potential difference. Electroneutrality is maintained in this setting either by passive Cl^- reabsorption via the paracellular pathway or by K^+ secretion from the cell into the lumen. Na^+ reabsorption also enhances K^+ secretion by a second mechanism: The transport of reabsorbed Na^+ out of the cell by the Na^+-K^+-ATPase pump increases K^+ entry across the basolateral membrane. The ensuing rise in cell K^+ concentration permits continued K^+ secretion, which is the primary determinant of urinary K^+ excretion (see Chap. 12).

The increase in luminal Na^+ permeability represents a primary hormonal action, since blocking these channels with the diuretic amiloride at least transiently prevents the aldosterone-induced increases in K^+ secretion, luminal K^+ permeability, and Na^+-K^+-ATPase activity.[106,111] Thus, the latter effects are in part secondary to the rise in Na^+ entry; as an example, an elevation in cell Na^+ concentration directly and rapidly increases the number of active Na^+-K^+-ATPase pumps in the basolateral membrane.[112] However, the later increase in Na^+-K^+-ATPase activity is probably induced in part by aldosterone, as some aldosterone-induced proteins may be subunits on the Na^+-K^+-ATPase pump.[5,113]

Hydrogen   The stimulatory effect of aldosterone on H^+ secretion occurs in different collecting tubular cells from those that transport Na^+: in the intercalated cells in the cortex and in the tubular cells in the outer medulla.[114,115] These cells, like the principal cells that reabsorb Na^+, are able to respond to aldosterone because they contain mineralocorticoid receptors.[116] Their main function in normal conditions is H^+ secretion via H^+-ATPase pumps in the apical membrane; they do not contribute to net Na^+ reabsorption (see Fig. 5-3).

Aldosterone also indirectly stimulates H^+ secretion in the cortex via its effect on Na^+ reabsorption in the principal cells. The associated generation of a lumen-negative potential creates a favorable electrical gradient for H^+ accumulation in the lumen.[117] These effects of aldosterone are probably permissive, since there is little evidence that acid-base balance directly influences aldosterone release.

Extrarenal effects   Aldosterone reduces the concentration of Na^+ and raises that of K^+ in colonic and salivary secretions and in sweat.[5,118] These changes are generally of limited physiologic importance, although colonic secretion of K^+ can become an important route of K^+ elimination in patients with end-stage renal disease.[119]

Control of Aldosterone Secretion

Aldosterone plays an important role in the maintenance of volume and K^+ balance via its effects on NaCl and K^+ excretion.[120] Thus, it is appropriate that angiotensin II (the production of which varies inversely with volume) and an elevation in the plasma K^+ concentration are the major stimuli of aldosterone secretion.

Angiotensin II and hyperkalemia act on the zona glomerulosa, promoting the conversion of cholesterol to pregnenolone and, more importantly, of corticosterone to aldosterone via stimulation of aldosterone synthase (Fig. 6-11).[121,122] As an example, chronic sodium restriction leads to a tenfold increase in messenger RNA for aldosterone synthase and in aldosterone synthase activity (as estimated from enhanced conversion of corticosterone to aldosterone).[122]

Aldosterone release can also be affected by other factors, being enhanced by adrenocorticotropic hormone (ACTH) and hyponatremia, and suppressed by ANP (see "Atrial Natriuretic Peptide," below).

Renin-angiotensin system   The volume stimulus to aldosterone secretion is primarily mediated by the reinin-angiotensin system (see Chap. 2).[123,124] In normal subjects, both the plasma renin activity and aldosterone release vary inversely with dietary Na^+ intake (Fig. 6-13). An increase in Na^+ intake, for example, initially expands the extracellular volume, resulting in reductions in renin and aldosterone production. These changes allow the excess Na^+ to be excreted by reducing Na^+ reabsorption in the proximal tubule (the site of action of angiotensin II) and in the cortical and papillary collecting tubules (the sites of action of aldosterone).[106,108,125] ANP, the secretion of which is increased by volume expansion, can contribute to the suppression of the aldosterone release in this setting (see below).

Conversely, a reduction in the effective circulating volume will enhance the secretion of renin and therefore that of aldosterone. The ensuing Na^+ retention returns the volume toward normal. The importance of renin in this sequence has been demonstrated by the loss of the hypovolemic stimulus to aldosterone release in nephrectomized patients.[126]

Plasma K^+ concentration   Aldosterone secretion is stimulated by K^+, increasing linearly as the plasma K^+ concentration rises above 3.5 meq/L.[127,128] This represents a direct effect on the zona glomerulosal[129] and is extremely sensitive, as increments in the plasma K^+ concentration of as little as 0.1 to 0.2 meq/L can induce a significant elevation in aldosterone release.[127] The resultant increase in K^+

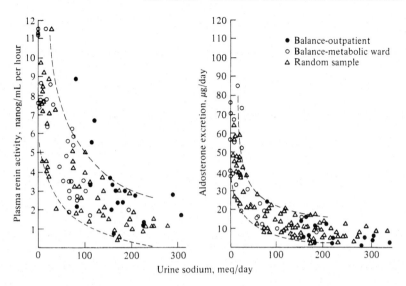

Figure 6-13   Relation of both plasma renin activity and 24-h urinary excretion of aldosterone to the concurrent daily rate of sodium excretion, used as an estimate of daily Na^+ intake. For these normal subjects, the data indicate an inverse relationship between dietary Na^+ intake and renin and aldosterone secretion. (*From Laragh JH, Baer I, Brunner HR, et al, Am J Med 52:633, 1972. Used with permission.*)

excretion then returns the plasma K^+ concentration toward normal (Fig. 6-14).[107,120]

There appears to be a positive interaction between K^+ and angiotensin II, in that the presence of one stimulus to aldosterone production increases the response to the other.[128,130] This synergism may in part involve activation of a local *intra-adrenal* renin-angiotensin system. In isolated zona glomerulosa cells, for example, a rise in extracellular K^+ concentration enhances adrenal renin and angiotensin II release.[131,132] Furthermore, the associated increase in aldosterone secretion in this setting is impaired by the presence of an angiotensin converting enzyme (ACE) inhibitor that reduces the local production of angiotensin II.[131,132]

ACTH   ACTH, released from the anterior pituitary, enhances adrenal glucocorticoid and androgen synthesis and release by increasing the gene expression for a number of adrenal enzymes, including 17α-hydroxylase, 21-hydroxylase, and 11β-hydroxylase.[86] It also causes a transient rise in aldosterone secretion that is mediated both by activation of adenylyl cyclase and by a small increase in Ca^{2+} entry.[133] The limitation in the ACTH response may be due to two factors:

- Overproduction of deoxycorticosterone (Fig. 6-11), an ACTH-dependent steroid with relatively potent mineralocorticoid activity. The ensuing fluid retention will diminish the secretion of renin and secondarily that of aldosterone.

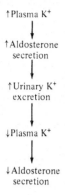

↑Plasma K⁺

↑Aldosterone
  secretion

↑Urinary K⁺
  excretion

↓Plasma K⁺

↓Aldosterone
  secretion   **Figure 6-14**   Role of aldosterone in potassium homeostasis.

- The induction by ACTH of 17α-hydroxylase activity in the *zona glomerulosa*, thereby converting this segment to cortisol production; this is an appropriate response when ACTH production is chronically stimulated in critically ill patients.[134]

Plasma sodium concentration   Aldosterone secretion may be increased by hyponatremia and reduced by hypernatremia.[135,136] These changes can be seen with as little as a 4- to 5-meq/L change in the plasma Na^+ concentration. However, the plasma Na^+ concentration does not play an important role in modulating aldosterone release in normal subjects, since it is normally held relatively constant (±1 to 2 percent) by the effects of ADH and thirst (see above). Even when hyponatremia is present, its effect on aldosterone is frequently *overridden by concomitant changes in the effective circulating volume*. As an example, aldosterone secretion is increased in the hyponatremic patient who is volume-depleted but may be reduced in a patient who is volume-expanded, as in the syndrome of inappropriate ADH secretion.[137]

Maintenance of Sodium and Potassium Balance

Since aldosterone affects both Na^+ and K^+ handling, it might be expected that regulation of the excretion of one ion would interfere with that of the other. This does not occur because of two additional effects: (1) K^+ secretion is highly dependent upon the rate of sodium and water delivery to the cortical collecting tubule (see Chap. 12), and (2) K^+ balance can influence Na^+ reabsorption in the thick ascending limb of the loop of Henle (and perhaps the proximal tubule).[138,139]

How these factors interact to allow Na^+ and K^+ excretion to be regulated independently is summarized in Table 6-3. Effective circulating volume depletion, for example, activates the renin-angiotensin-aldosterone system. This response appropriately reduces Na^+ excretion by increasing reabsorption both in the proximal tubule (via angiotensin II) and in the distal nephron (via aldosterone). K^+ excretion, on the other hand, is not importantly affected in this setting;[140] the increase in proximal reabsorption reduces distal fluid delivery, thereby counter-

Table 6-3   Interrelationships between aldosterone and Na^+ and K^+ balance

Clinical state	Aldosterone secretion	Proximal or loop reabsorption	Distal Na^+ delivery	Δ Urinary excretion Na^+	K^+
Na^+ depletion	↑	↑	↓	↓	0
Na^+ load	↓	↓	↑	↑	0
K^+	↑	↓	↑	0	↑
K^+ depletion	↓	↑	↓	0	↓

acting the stimulatory effect of aldosterone. This explains why untreated patients with heart failure or cirrhosis (who are effectively volume-depleted due to systemic vasodilatation; see Chap. 16) do not spontaneously develop K^+ wasting and hypokalemia, even though aldosterone secretion is frequently elevated.

Sodium loading reverses this sequence, as Na^+ excretion is increased, while K^+ balance is maintained due to the offsetting effects of increased distal delivery and reduced aldosterone secretion.[141] If, however, aldosterone release is not diminished because of a nonsuppressible adrenal adenoma, K^+ wasting and hypokalemia will ensue.[141] Thus, administration of a high-Na^+ diet has been used as a screening test to unmask primary hyperaldosteronism.

A K^+ load, on the other hand, enhances aldosterone secretion and may reduce loop Na^+ transport.[139] As a result, the aldosterone-induced increase in cortical collecting tubule Na^+ reabsorption is counteracted by the elevation in Na^+ delivery from the more proximal segments. The net effect is an appropriate increase in the excretion of K^+ with little change in that of Na^+.

Aldosterone Escape

If aldosterone is given to a normal subject on an adequate salt intake, NaCl and water retention and K^+ loss are seen initially, leading to a rise in blood pressure, weight gain, and potassium depletion. However, after a weight gain of approximately 3 kg, a spontaneous diuresis ensues, returning the plasma volume toward normal (Fig. 6-15).[142,143]

This phenomenon has been called *aldosterone escape*.[144] It does not, however, represent aldosterone resistance, since urinary K^+ loss continues[142] and the cortical collecting tubule remains responsive to aldosterone.[145] Rather, the escape phenomenon appears to be due to decreased Na^+ reabsorption in some other nephron segment, perhaps the loop of Henle or the papillary collecting tubule.[143] Two factors, which are induced by the initial volume expansion, are thought to play a major role in this response: increased secretion of ANP, which acts both by increasing the glomerular filtration rate and by diminishing Na^+ reabsorption in the inner medullary collecting duct (see "Atrial Natriuretic Peptide," below), and an elevation in systemic blood pressure (Fig. 6-15).[144] Both animals and humans demonstrate a close temporal relationship in which the rise in plasma ANP levels

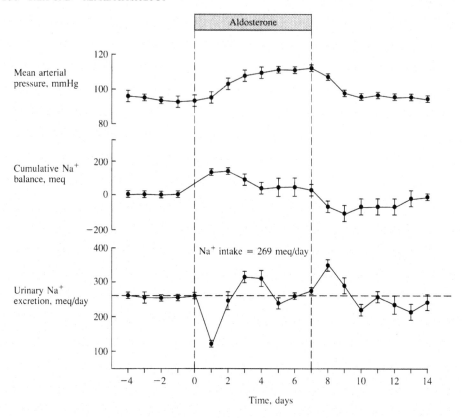

Figure 6-15 The phenomenon of aldosterone escape in dogs. The combination of aldosterone administration and the ingestion of a high-Na$^+$ diet leads initially to Na$^+$ retention, volume expansion, and a rise in systemic blood pressure. After several days, however, there is a spontaneous diuresis, resulting in the return of Na$^+$ balance toward normal but persistent hypertension. Although it is not shown, prevention of the rise in renal arterial pressure by use of a suprarenal clamp prevents the natriuresis and is associated with progressive fluid retention and hypertension. [*From Hall JE, Granger JP, Smith MJ Jr, Premen AJ*, Hypertension *6(suppl I):I-183, 1983. By permission of the American Heart Association, Inc.*]

precedes the onset of the natriuresis by 1 to 2 days.[146,147] The role of ANP, however, remains uncertain. Studies in animals made ANP-deficient by immunization reveal no impairment in the escape phenomenon, indicating that ANP may contribute to the natriuresis but is not essential for it to occur.[148]

On the other hand, escape can be prevented if a clamp is placed around the suprarenal aorta *to maintain renal arterial pressure at the baseline level* (see Fig. 8-9).[149] Furthermore, the continued volume expansion in this setting can lead to pulmonary edema and a much more marked degree of hypertension.[149] This ability of the rise in renal perfusion pressure to limit the degree of Na$^+$ retention is called a *pressure natriuresis*. The site of action of this hemodynamic effect is unclear, as a variety of nephron segments may be involved (see page 272).[144,150]

The clinical correlate of aldosterone escape occurs in patients with primary hyperaldosteronism, who have autonomous overproduction of aldosterone (see Chap. 27).[151] Hypokalemia and hypertension are typically seen in this setting, but not edema, since continued fluid retention is prevented.

ATRIAL NATRIURETIC PEPTIDE

Expansion of the extracellular volume with a Na^+ load results in an appropriate increase in Na^+ excretion. It was initially felt that this response could be explained by an increase in glomerular filtration rate (GFR) or a reduction in aldosterone secretion. However, preventing a rise in GFR and administering high doses of aldosterone may not impair the excretion of the Na^+ load.[152] Furthermore, cross-circulation experiments between volume-expanded and euvolemic animals suggest that the natriuretic response is mediated at least in part by some humoral factor or factors,[152] one of which is ANP.

ANP is released from myocardial cells in the atria and in some cases the ventricles, and circulates primarily as a 28-amino-acid polypeptide consisting of amino acids 99–126 from the C-terminal end of pro-ANP.[153-155] Most of the physiologic actions of ANP appear to be mediated by attachment to specific receptors on the cell membrane, with subsequent activation of guanylyl cyclase[3,12] and the formation of cyclic GMP.[3,156-158,159]

Actions

ANP has two major actions: It is a direct vasodilator, lowering the systemic blood pressure and it increases urinary Na^+ and water excretion.[154,157,159] The natriuretic and diuretic effects of this hormone may be mediated by a variety of renal and extrarenal changes. In the kidney, for example, ANP directly increases the GFR and reduces Na^+ reabsorption; the natriuretic action appears to be primarily due to the inhibition of sodium reabsorption in the medullary collecting tubule.[156,160-162] In comparison, the outer medullary collecting tubule appears to be unaffected.[162]

Although this action is controversial, ANP also may diminish Na^+ reabsorption in the proximal tubule (primarily in the deep juxtaglomerular nephrons). This response may be mediated by an increase in peritubular capillary hydraulic pressure (see Chap. 3) and/or by the local release of dopamine.[163] There is indirect evidence in humans that ANP may have a proximal action, in that the excretion of phosphate and lithium (which are almost entirely reabsorbed in the proximal tubule) is increased by ANP.[164]

The relative roles of the increased filtration and decreased reabsorption in the natriuresis induced by ANP is uncertain. Some investigators believe that the decline in collecting tubule Na^+ reabsorption is the initial response, since the concentration of ANP required to achieve this effect is significantly lower than that required to affect the glomeruli.[165] With more marked volume expansion and higher ANP levels, the increment in GFR may then contribute to the natriuresis. On the other hand, two lines of evidence suggest that the increase in filtered load may be essential: (1) The natriuresis can be prevented if there is no rise in GFR, and (2) simply blocking collecting tubule Na^+ channels without increasing the GFR (with the potassium-sparing diuretic amiloride) produces only a modest natriuresis.[166]

The rise in glomerular filtration rate induced by ANP is associated with little or no change in renal blood flow, suggesting that ANP produces both afferent arteriolar dilation and efferent arteriolar constriction (see page 38).[157,167] The direct tubular effect, in comparison, appears to be mediated by a cyclic GMP-dependent protein kinase, which closes the Na^+ channels through which luminal Na^+ normally enters the cell (see Fig. 5-4).[13,156]

In addition to these tubular and glomerular effects, ANP has a variety of other actions that also promote increased secretion of Na^+ and water. It can reduce basal renin release, inhibit angiotensin II- and potassium-induced aldosterone secretion (the latter primarily via a direct action on the adrenal gland), inhibit the increases in proximal Na^+ reabsorption and aldosterone release induced by angiotensin II, and diminish the collecting tubular response to ADH.[168-171] Thus, the fall in activity of the renin-angiotensin-aldosterone system seen with volume expansion may be mediated in part by ANP.

Other actions ANP can be synthesized by a variety of tissues other than the atria, suggesting local autocrine or paracrine effects. As an example, ANP is produced in the vascular wall, where it may diminish endothelial and vascular smooth muscle growth.[172]

Control of ANP Secretion

ANP is primarily released from the atria in response to volume expansion, which is sensed as an increase in atrial stretch.[173,174] Although both atria appear to contribute,[175,176] there is suggestive evidence that the right atrium may be quantitatively more important.[176] Furthermore, chronic cardiac overload, as occurs in congestive heart failure, can lead to recruitment of hormone production by myocardial cells in the ventricles[177,178] and, at least in animals, by the lungs.[179] There is also evidence that the carotid and renal baroreceptors contribute to ANP release by sending afferent signals back to the brain.[180]

Studies in humans and experimental animals have generally revealed that the release of ANP is increased in any hypervolemic state. This includes heart failure,[175,177] aldosterone escape,[146,147] renal failure,[181] and a salt-containing snack.[182] Furthermore, the rise in ANP secretion can be reversed by successful treatment of heart failure or, in renal failure, by removal of the excess fluid via dialysis or restriction of Na^+ intake.[181,183]

Physiologic role Despite the multiple sites at which ANP can affect Na^+ excretion and its appropriate release in response to changes in volume, the *physiologic* *role of ANP as a natriuretic agent remains uncertain.*[166,184,185] Infusion studies in humans have revealed that ANP generally produces only a modest diuresis, perhaps because the concomitant fall in blood pressure induced by ANP counteracts its natriuretic effects.[154,186] The following observations are compatible with a permissive role of hemodynamics in the renal response to ANP:

- Lowering the renal arterial pressure blocks the natriuretic effect of ANP, while only slightly reducing that of the loop diuretic furosemide.[187]
- Transgenic mice given an extra ANP gene have plasma ANP levels that are 10 times normal.[186] These animals have a reduced blood pressure and remain in normal sodium balance. If, however, the blood pressure is elevated by volume expansion, the natriuretic effect of ANP is unmasked resulting in a marked increase in sodium excretion.
- Patients with heart failure and cirrhosis have high ANP levels, but avidly retain Na^+ (see Chap. 16). In experimental animals, this apparent resistance to ANP can be reversed by increasing the renal perfusion pressure to normal.[188,189]

In summary, the exact role of ANP as a natriuretic agent is unproven, and it is possible that urodilatin and brain natriuretic peptide are more important natriuretic hormones (see below). The physiologic importance of most hormones has been demonstrated in part by removal of their site of production; unfortunately, the cardiac source of ANP limits the feasibility of this approach.

More complete definition of the role of ANP requires the availability of antagonists to this hormone or its receptor. Injection of an antibody directed against ANP significantly diminishes baseline sodium excretion, attenuates the natriuretic response to acute volume expansion, and further decreases the already low rate of sodium excretion in congestive heart failure.[190,191] Similar observations have been made in animals made ANP-resistant by immunization.[148] Thus, ANP may play a contributory role in the day-to-day regulation of Na^+ excretion, although it is likely that changes in angiotensin II and aldosterone are of greater importance.[166]

Despite this acute role, *ANP resistance does not interfere with the response to chronic volume expansion*, as induced by oral salt loading or by mineralocorticoid escape (see "Aldosterone," above).[148] This finding, which is similar to the maintenance of Na^+ balance with aldosterone excess or deficiency, indicates that other factors (such as pressure natriuresis) can compensate if the normally important role of ANP is impaired (see page 272).

Although of uncertain importance physiologically, ANP-induced diuresis may be useful pharmacologically if its duration of action is prolonged. In both animals and humans, the administration of an endopeptidase inhibitor (which slows the degradation of ANP) and/or a cyclic GMP phosphodiesterase inhibitor (which slows the degradation of the second messenger) produces a relatively large natriuresis with little effect on the systemic blood pressure.[184,192-194]

The natriuretic response to endopeptidase inhibition can be enhanced by the concurrent administration of an angiotensin converting enzyme (ACE) inhibitor, which reverses both the vasoconstriction and increased proximal reabsorption induced by angiotensin II.[195] This interaction could be important in the treatment of edema in patients with heart failure, since most patients are treated with an ACE inhibitor to reduce systemic afterload (see Chap. 16).[196]

Urodilatin   A separate ANP-like hormone has been identified in human urine and called urodilatin.[197,198] ANP is a 28-amino-acid peptide consisting of amino acids 99–126 from the C-terminal end of pro-ANP; urodilatin, in comparison, consists of amino acids 95–126.

Urodilatin appears to be produced within the kidney, since plasma levels are negligible. The distal tubule produces an ANP-like prohormone which, via a processing pathway that may be unique to the kidney, may be the precursor of urodilatin.[199] Urodilatin does not seem to be catabolized by the endopeptidase that metabolizes ANP.

The characteristics of urodilatin make it well adapted to regulate sodium excretion, since, unlike that of ANP, the effect of urodilatin is not limited by systemic hypotension or local catabolism. Its lack of catabolism by endopeptidases may result in more urodilatin reaching its site of action in the distal nephron when compared to ANP.

Initial studies suggested that sodium excretion varies more closely with changes in urodilatin excretion than with plasma ANP levels.[197,198] When given as an infusion, urodilatin appears to have natriuretic potency similar to that of ANP.[200] How urodilatin release might be regulated is uncertain.

Brain natriuretic peptide   Brain natriuretic peptide (BNP) is a natriuretic hormone that is homologous to ANP. It was initially identified in the brain but is also present in the heart, particularly the ventricles.[201] The circulating concentration of BNP is less than 20 percent of that of ANP in normal subjects but can equal or exceed that of ANP in patients with congestive heart failure.

The physiologic role of this hormone remains to be determined. The infusion of BNP to normal volunteers suggests that the compound has natriuretic activity similar to that of ANP.[202] In addition, it may be responsible for the cerebral salt-wasting syndrome that can accompany severe neurologic injury, as with subarachnoid hemorrhage.[203]

C-type natriuretic peptide   C-type natriuretic peptide (CNP) is structurally similar to the other natriuretic peptides. It activates cyclic GMP via a different receptor from ANP and BNP. CNP is produced by vascular endothelial cells and in the kidney.[204,205] Initial studies have suggested that its major function may involve regulation of local blood flow.[204] However, its pathophysiologic role in humans is unclear, as the administration of low doses has little effect on systemic hemodynamics, renal function, or the renin-angiotensin system.[206]

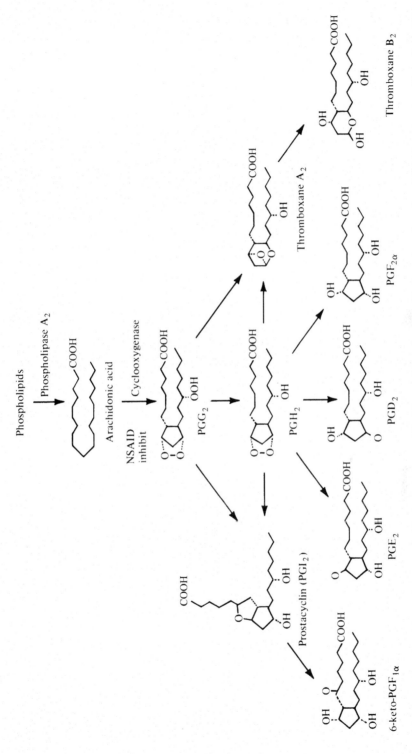

Figure 6-16 Biosynthesis of prostaglandins and thromboxane. All of the products shown in this figure have been found in kidney or urine. (*From Dunn MJ, Zambraski EJ, Kidney Int 18:609, 1980. Reprinted by permission from Kidney International.*)

Marker for left ventricular dysfunction   Plasma levels of ANP and BNP may be useful as a marker for asymptomatic left ventricular dysfunction in patients with heart disease.[207-209] The increase in cardiac filling pressure in this setting is the stimulus for the release of these natriuretic hormones.

PROSTAGLANDINS

Prostaglandins are derived from the metabolism of arachidonic acid, with the initial step being catalyzed by the cyclooxygenase (COX) enzyme (Fig. 6-16). These hormones are produced at a variety of sites within the kidney, including glomerular and vascular endothelium, the medullary and to a lesser degree the cortical collecting tubule cells, and the renomedullary interstitial cells.[45,210] In general, the tubules primarily synthesize PGE_2, while the glomeruli produce both PGE_2 and prostacyclin.[45,210,211] The renal prostaglandins have important local functions but little systemic activity, since they are rapidly metabolized in the pulmonary circulation.

Two related isoforms of the COX enzyme have been described: COX-1, which is expressed in most tissues, but variably; and COX-2, which is usually undetectable in most tissues but is increased during states of inflammation.[212]

This section will primarily review the known renal actions of PGE_2 and prostacyclin. Other arachidonic acid derivatives, such as thromboxane B_2, the leukotrienes (which are formed via the lipoxygenase pathway), and the epoxyeicosatrienoic acids (which are cytochrome P450-dependent) also can affect renal function, but their clinical significance is at present incompletely understood.[61,213-215] Thromboxane is similar to the prostaglandins in that its rate of production is relatively low in normal subjects and inhibition of its synthesis has little effect on renal functions.[213] Thromboxane can, however, cause vasoconstriction and mesangial contraction, and may contribute to the fall in glomerular filtration rate and increase in protein excretion frequently seen in glomerular disease.[213]

The intrarenal effects have important clinical implications because of the widespread use of nonsteroidal anti-inflammatory drugs (NSAIDs) (Table 6-4).[216,217] Most traditional NSAIDs are nonselective inhibitors of both COX-1 and COX-2, and most of the renal toxicities described below have been associated with these agents. Selective COX-2 inhibitors are also available. Compared to the nonselective agents, they provide similar analgesic and anti-inflammatory activity, but markedly lower gastroduodenal toxicity.[218,219]

COX-2 is constitutively expressed at low levels in the kidney.[220] Its effect on renal function in adults is unclear; however, it appears to have a major role in renal development, as animals with deletion of the COX-2 gene have dysplastic tubules and immature glomeruli.[221] By comparison, mice without the COX-1 enzyme gene have minimal renal abnormalities.

Table 6-4   Renal actions of the prostaglandins and possible complications with nonsteroidal anti-inflammatory drugs

Effect of prostaglandins	Possible drug complication
Maintain renal blood flow and glomerular filtration rate by ameliorating angiotensin II and norepinephrine-induced renal vasoconstriction	Acute renal failure in conditions associated with increased release of renal vasoconstrictors (Table 6-5)
Antagonize systemic vasoconstriction	May raise the blood pressure in hypertensive patients treated with a diuretic or β-adrenergic blocker; can worsen cardiac output in heart failure due to increased afterload
Increase the secretion of renin	Hyperkalemia due to hyporeninemic hypoaldosteronism, primarily in patients with renal insufficiency
Antagonize water-retaining effect of antidiuretic hormone (ADH)	Can potentiate effect of ADH, possibly promoting the development of hyponatremia
May increase sodium excretion in states of effective volume depletion	May promote more intense sodium retention; can impair response to diuretics

Actions

The renal prostaglandins have both vascular and tubular actions (Table 6-4). These effects result from the activation of distinct cell surface receptors, which are all members of the G-protein-coupled family of seven-transmembrane receptors.[222] Different subtypes of these receptors exist, resulting in the varied actions of a particular prostaglandin.[222]

Renal hemodynamics   Renal prostaglandins are primarily vasodilators (except for PGF_{2a} and thromboxane). They appear to play no role in the regulation of renal perfusion in the basal state when their secretion rate is relatively low. However, prostaglandin synthesis is increased (mostly within the glomeruli) by vasoconstrictors such as angiotensin II, norepinephrine, vasopressin (acting via the V_1 receptor), and endothelin.[47,50,223,224] Each of these hormones activates phosphatidylinositol turnover (see Fig. 6-2), leading to the formation of diacylglycerol, which contains arachidonic acid at position 2.[51] The latter can then be released from diacylglycerol by the action of phospholipase A_2. The ensuing prostaglandin-induced vasodilation partially counteracts the neurohumoral vasoconstriction, thereby minimizing the degree of renal ischemia (see page 45).[223,225]

The net clinical effect is that nonselective NSAIDs do not impair renal perfusion in normal subjects, but can lead to *reversible renal ischemia and renal insufficiency* in a variety of disease states, particularly hypovolemic disorders in which angiotensin II and norepinephrine secretion are increased (Table 6-5). These include true volume depletion and edematous states associated with effective cir-

Table 6-5 Conditions associated with nonsteroidal anti-inflammatory drug–induced, hemodynamically mediated acute renal failure

True volume depletion (vomiting, diarrhea, diuretic therapy)
Congestive heart failure
Hepatic cirrhosis
Glomerular diseases, including the nephotic syndrome and lupus nephritis
Hypercalcemia, which directly induces renal vasoconstriction

culating volume depletion, such as cirrhosis and congestive heart failure (Fig. 6-17).[216,217,226] In both of the last two disorders, for example, increasing severity of the underlying disease is associated with increased secretion of the three "hypovolemic" hormones—angiotensin II, norepinephrine, and ADH—and, at least initially, of the renal prostaglandins.[72,73,227]

The likelihood of inducing acute renal failure with an NSAID is related to the intensity of the underlying renal vasoconstriction. Patients with marked sodium retention (and higher levels of angiotensin II, norepinephrine, ADH, and renal prostaglandins) often have a relatively large reduction in the glomerular filtration rate if NSAIDs are given.[228,229] This deleterious effect is usually rapidly reversible with discontinuation of the offending drug.

It is unclear whether the selective COX-2 inhibitors have a similar adverse effect. Preliminary clinical trials did not demonstrate significant changes in renal function, but most patients were not at risk for this complication.

Systemic hemodynamics The vasodilator activity of the renal prostaglandins also acts to lower systemic vascular resistance. Thus, the administration of a non-

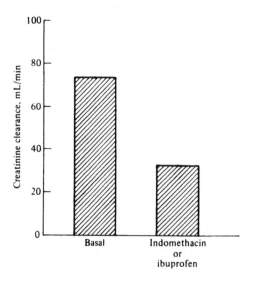

Figure 6-17 Reduction in GFR, as estimated from the creatinine clearance from a mean of 73 mL/min down to 32 mL/min, after the administration of a nonsteroidal anti-inflammatory drug (indomethacin or ibuprofen) to 12 patients with stable hepatic cirrhosis and ascites. Urinary prostaglandin E_2 excretion was substantially greater than normal in these subjects and was markedly reduced following therapy. (*From Zipser RD, Hoefs JC, Speckhart PF, et al,* J Clin Endocrinol Metab *48:895, 1979. Copyright © 1979 by The Endocrine Society.*)

selective NSAID to a hypertensive patient treated with a diuretic, β-adrenergic blocker, or ACE inhibitor can raise the systemic blood pressure by an average of 3 to 5 mmHg and by as much as 5 to 10 mmHg in some patients.[230-232] The NSAID-induced increment in vascular resistance can have an additional detrimental effect in patients with advanced heart failure. The associated increase in afterload in this setting can lead to a further reduction in cardiac contractibility and cardiac output.[233]

Renin secretion   The stimulation of renin secretion induced by baroreceptors in the afferent glomerular arteriole and by the macula densa cells in the early distal tubule appears to be mediated in part by locally produced prostaglandins.[234,235] These responses are blocked by an NSAID; as a result, prostaglandin synthesis inhibition can lead to *hyporeninemic hypoaldosteronism* (since angiotensin II is the major stimulus to aldosterone secretion) and an impairment in urinary K^+ excretion (see Chap. 28). The net effect is that the plasma K^+ concentration rises by a mean of 0.2 meq/L in normal subjects[236] and 0.6 meq/L in patients with renal insufficiency,[237] with the occasional development of overt hyperkalemia in the latter setting.[238]

Antagonism of ADH effect   ADH increases the production of renal prostaglandins, which then antagonize both its hydroosmotic and vascular effects (see "Antidiuretic Hormone," above).[11,15,50] The clinical relevance of this relationship is uncertain. The administration of NSAID to humans removes the inhibitory prostaglandin effect, possibly leading to increased ADH-induced water reabsorption and an elevation in urine osmolality to a level that can exceed 200 mosmol/kg.[239,240] The associated water retention can then cause a reduction in the plasma Na^+ concentration. This is most likely to occur when there is nonsuppressible ADH release, as a result of volume depletion or the syndrome of inappropriate ADH secretion (see Chap. 25). In normal subjects, however, the initial fall in the plasma Na^+ concentration will diminish ADH secretion, thereby minimizing the likelihood of water retention.

Sodium excretion   The renal prostaglandins also may have a natriuretic effect, via reduced Na^+ reabsorption in the thick ascending limb and in the collecting tubules.[216,241-243] It is unclear how applicable these findings are to humans, since there are major species differences in animals: As an example, prostaglandin E_2 inhibits cortical collecting tubule Na^+ reabsorption in rabbits but not in rats.[244]

If prostaglandins do promote Na^+ excretion, they will do so only when their rate of production is increased. Thus, prostaglandins have little effect in the basal state but may play a role in hypovolemic states, where they may modulate the Na^+-retaining as well as the renal vasoconstrictive effects of angiotensin II, norepinephrine, and possibly endothelin.[245] Consequently, inhibiting prostaglandin synthesis with an NSAID can promote further sodium retention in this setting, both by reducing glomerular filtration rate and by increasing tubular reabsorption.[216] These effects also can *limit the responsiveness of edematous patients to diuretic therapy*.[236,246]

In addition to regulating net Na^+ excretion, the prostaglandins produced in the medulla may help to protect the thick ascending limb cells against ischemic injury when the patient is volume-depleted. The medulla normally has a very low P_{O_2}, due in part to countercurrent exchange of oxygen (see page 117). This relative hypoxia is exacerbated when renal perfusion is diminished in hypovolemic states. By diminishing NaCl reabsorption in the thick ascending limb, prostaglandins reduce the energy requirement of these cells, thereby allowing them to better tolerate the decrease in oxygen delivery.[247]

HORMONAL REGULATION OF CALCIUM AND PHOSPHATE BALANCE

The maintenance of calcium and phosphate homeostasis involves changes in intestinal, bone, and renal function. Regulation of intestinal function is important because, in contrast to the complete absorption of dietary NaCl and KCl, the absorption of Ca^{2+} and phosphate is incomplete. This limitation is due both to the requirement for vitamin D and to the formation of insoluble salts such as calcium phosphate, calcium oxalate, and magnesium phosphate in the intestinal lumen. As an example, a normal adult may ingest 1000 mg of Ca^{2+} per day, of which roughly 400 to 500 mg may be absorbed. However, 300 mg of calcium from digestive secretions is lost in the stool, resulting in the net absorption of only 100 to 200 mg.[248] In the steady state, this quantity of calcium is excreted in the urine.

Most of the body Ca^{2+} and much of the phosphate exist as hydroxyapatite, $Ca_{10}(PO_4)_6(OH)_2$, the main mineral component of bone. Phosphate also is present in high concentration in the cells. Within the plasma, both Ca^{2+} and phosphate circulate in different forms. Of the plasma Ca^{2+}, roughly 40 percent is bound to albumin; 15 percent is complexed with citrate, sulfate, or phosphate; and 45 percent exist as the physiologically important ionized (or free) Ca^{2+}. Plasma phosphorus, in comparison, consists of phospholipids, ester phosphates, and inorganic phosphates. The latter are completely ionized, circulating primarily as HPO_4^{2-} or $H_2PO_4^-$ in a ratio of $4:1$ at a plasma pH of 7.40 (see page 305).

Although only a small fraction of the total body calcium and phosphate is located in the plasma, it is the *plasma concentrations of ionized Ca^{2+}* and *inorganic phosphate* that are under hormonal control. This function is mediated primarily by parathyroid hormone and vitamin D, which affect intestinal absorption, bone formation and resorption, and urinary excretion.[248-253] The physiologic roles of other hormones, such as calcitonin and estrogens, in the regulation of Ca^{2+} and phosphate balance are incompletely understood and will not be discussed further.[254]

Parathyroid Hormone

Parathyroid hormone (PTH) is a polypeptide secreted from the parathyroid glands in response to a decrease in the plasma concentration of ionized Ca^{2+}.[251] This change is sensed by a specific Ca^{2+}-sensing protein in the cell membrane of the parathyroid cells.[252,255] The receptor permits variations in the plasma Ca^{2+} concentration to be sensed by the parathyroid gland, leading to the desired changes in PTH secretion. Polymorphisms of this receptor may underlie a significant portion of the variability observed in the serum calcium concentrations in normal individuals,[256] while inactivating mutations lead to hypercalcemia because a higher plasma Ca^{2+} concentration is required to activate the receptor and suppress PTH release.[257-259]

PTH acts to increase the plasma Ca^{2+} concentration in three ways (Fig. 6-18):

1. In the presence of permissive amounts of vitamin D, it stimulates bone resorption, resulting in the release of calcium phosphate.
2. It enhances intestinal Ca^{2+} and phosphate absorption by promoting the formation within the kidney of calcitriol (1,25-dihydroxycholecalciferol), the major active metabolite of vitamin D (see below).
3. It augments active renal Ca^{2+} reabsorption.

These effects are reversed by a small elevation in the plasma Ca^{2+} concentration, which lowers PTH secretion.

PTH also influences phosphate balance, although its actions may be offsetting (Fig. 6-18). It tends to increase phosphate entry into the extracellular fluid by its effects on bone and intestinal absorption. However, PTH also reduces proximal tubular phosphate reabsorption, resulting in enhanced excretion. The urinary effect usually predominates in patients with relatively normal renal function, as PTH tends to lower the plasma phosphate concentration.

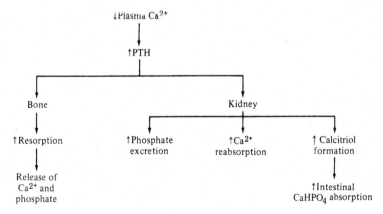

Figure 6-18   Effect of PTH on Ca^{2+} and phosphate metabolism. The net effect is an increase in the plasma Ca^{2+} concentration with no change or a decrease in the plasma phosphate concentration.

Renal calcium and phosphate handling   The renal effects of PTH are in part mediated by activation of specific adenylyl cyclase systems (see Fig. 6-2) in the proximal tubule and the early cortical distal nephron, including the cortical thick ascending limb, the distal tubule, and the connecting segment.[254,260] Activation of phospholipases C and A_2 and the subsequent breakdown of phosphatidylinositol also mediates some of the actions of PTH, particularly the reduction in proximal phosphate reabsorption.[261-263] Stimulation of phospholipase C in the proximal tubule occurs at a lower and more physiologic concentration of PTH than stimulation of adenylyl cyclase.[264]

PTH diminishes the proximal reabsorption of phosphate by decreasing the activity of the type II Na^+-*phosphate cotransporter* in the luminal membrane;[261,265,266] as a result, luminal phosphate is less able to enter the cells and be returned to the systemic circulation (see Chap. 3).

In comparison, the stimulatory effect of PTH on Ca^{2+} reabsorption occurs primarily in the early cortical distal nephron, particularly the distal tubule and connecting segment.[267-269] The mechanism by which PTH may enhance distal Ca^{2+} transport is reviewed on page 92.

A clinical example of the importance of the interaction between PTH and calcitriol for renal Ca^{2+} handling occurs in hypoparathyroidism, a disorder in which both PTH and calcitriol levels are reduced.[254] The ensuing decrease in distal Ca^{2+} reabsorption results in persistent Ca^{2+} excretion, despite the presence of a plasma Ca^{2+} concentration that may be below 7.5 mg/dL (normal equals 8.5 to 10.5 mg/dL). If calcitriol is given in this setting to raise the plasma Ca^{2+} concentration, there will still be PTH deficiency and a persistent partial defect in distal Ca^{2+} reabsorption. As a result, it may not be possible to safely raise the plasma Ca^{2+} concentration much above 8 mg/dL without inducing marked hypercalciuria, which can predispose to calcium stone formation.

Acid-base balance   PTH also may contribute to the regulation of acid-base balance in the presence of an acid load. A fall in extracellular pH stimulates PTH secretion, and the ensuing increase in phosphate excretion can appropriately enhance net acid excretion by buffering secreted H^+ ions.[43,270] PTH also minimizes the fall in pH by a second mechanism, promoting bone buffering of the excess acid (see page 313).

Vitamin D

Vitamin D_3 (cholecalciferol) is a fat-soluble steroid that is present in the diet and also can be synthesized in the skin from 7-dehydrocholesterol in the presence of ultraviolet light (Fig. 6-19).[248,253,271] The hepatic enzyme 25-hydroxylase places a hydroxyl group in the 25 position of the vitamin D molecule, resulting in the formation of 25-hydroxyvitamin D or calcidiol.

Calcidiol produced by the liver enters the circulation and travels to the kidney, bound to vitamin D-binding protein. In the kidney, tubular cells contain two enzymes (1α-hydroxylase and 24α-hydroxylase) that can further hydroxylate cal-

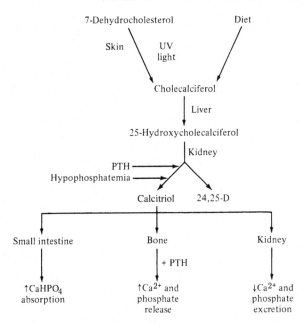

Figure 6-19   Metabolic activation of vitamin D and its effects on calcium and phosphate homeostasis. The result is an increase in the plasma Ca^{2+} and phosphate concentrations.

cidiol, producing 1,25-dihydroxyvitamin D (calcitriol), the most active form of vitamin D, or 24,25-dihydroxyvitamin D, an inactive metabolite.[248,250,253,272] Studies in vitamin D-deficient animals suggest that the proximal tubule is the important site of calcitriol synthesis. In contrast, studies in the normal human kidney under conditions of vitamin D sufficiency indicate that the distal nephron is the predominant site of 1α-hydroxylase expression.[273]

Calcitriol can also be synthesized in activated macrophages and thymic-derived lymphocytes.[274-276] This assumes importance in granulomatous diseases, such as active pulmonary sarcoidosis and tuberculosis, and in lymphoma, in which overproduction of calcitriol can lead to increased intestinal calcium absorption, hypercalciuria, and hypercalcemia.[277-281] This effect appears to be mediated by interferon gamma[282] and, in tuberculosis, may have a physiologic role in promoting the ingestion and elimination of the tuberculous bacilli by macrophages and minimizing tissue destruction.[274]

The formation of calcitriol is primarily stimulated by *PTH* and *hypophosphatemia* in an attempt to maintain Ca^{2+} and phosphate balance.[248,283] In comparison, the hepatic production of calcifediol is largely substrate-dependent and is not hormonally regulated.[249,250] The responsiveness of this system can be modulated by changes in the plasma Ca^{2+} concentration in that hypercalcemia impairs and hypocalcemia promotes PTH-induced calcitriol production.[284] This interaction is appropriate for the maintenance of Ca^{2+} balance; the facilitory action of hypocalcemia, for example, results in a greater increment in calcitriol release, thereby promoting return of the plasma Ca^{2+} concentration toward normal. Excessive stimulation is prevented by the rise in plasma Ca^{2+} itself and by negative feedback regulation of the 1α-hydroxylase via binding of calcitriol to the vitamin D receptor.[272]

The regulatory role of phosphate is also important, since calcitriol is the primary hormone that responds to changes in phosphate balance. Phosphate depletion tends to raise and phosphate loading to lower renal calcitriol production.[283] The fall in calcitriol levels after a phosphate load protects against hyperphosphatemia by limiting further intestinal phosphate absorption. On the other hand, markedly increased levels of 1α-hydroxylase messenger RNA are found in mice with renal phosphate wasting and hypophosphatemia due to the targeted inactivation of the sodium-phosphate wasting and hypophosphatemia due to the targeted inactivation of the sodium-phosphate cotransporter gene.[285]

Calcitriol is degraded in part by being hydroxylated at the 24-position by a 24-hydroxylase. The activity of the 24-hydroxylase gene is increased by calcitriol (which therefore promotes its own inactivation) and reduced by PTH (thereby allowing more active hormone to be formed).

Actions   The main action of calcitriol is to enhance the availability of calcium and phosphate both for new bone formation and for the *prevention of symptomatic hypocalcemia and hypophosphatemia*. This is primarily achieved by increases in bone resorption, intestinal absorption, and renal tubular Ca^{2+} reabsorption (Fig. 6-19).[249,250,254] Some of the bone and renal actions of calcitriol are mediated by PTH, as calcitriol enhances the PTH-induced stimulation of both bone resorption and distal reabsorption.[254,267,286]

Calcitriol regulates the plasma Ca^{2+} concentration in one other way—by binding to receptors in the parathyroid gland, leading to a diminution in further PTH production and release.[264,270,271,283,284,286-290] This modulating effect prevents the development of an excessive PTH response. Its physiologic role in normal subjects is uncertain. In patients with chronic renal failure, however, calcitriol deficiency appears to be an important determinant of the associated secondary hyperparathyroidism (see below).[289,290]

Regulation of Plasma Calcium and Phosphate Concentrations

Figures 6-20 and 6-21 depict a model for the role of PTH and vitamin D in the maintenance of the plasma Ca^{2+} and phosphate concentrations. The plasma Ca^{2+} concentration, as routinely measured in the laboratory, includes all the Ca^{2+} in the plasma, of which only about 45 percent circulates in the physiologically important ionized or unbound state. In general, measuring the total plasma Ca^{2+} concentrations is sufficient, since changes in this parameter usually are associated with parallel changes in the ionized concentration. A common exception occurs in patients with hypoalbuminemia, in whom the concomitant decrease in ion binding leads to a reduction in the total plasma Ca^{2+} concentration without change in the ionized form. To correct for this, the measured plasma Ca^{2+} concentration should

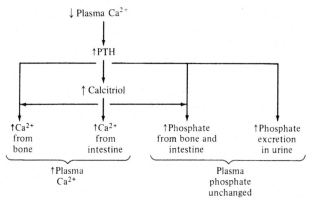

Figure 6-20 Physiologic sequence of events following the development of hypocalcemia. Because of the PTH interaction with vitamin D, the end result is a rise in the plasma Ca^{2+} concentration, with little or no change in the plasma phosphate concentration. (*Redrawn from deLuca H*, Am J Med *58:39, 1975. Used with permission.*)

be increased by 0.8 mg/dL for each 1.0 g/dL fall in the plasma albumin concentration (normal plasma albumin concentration equals 4.0 to 5.0 g/dL). If, for example, the plasma concentration of Ca^{2+} is 7.5 mg/dL and that of albumin is 2.0 g/dL (roughly 2.0 g/L less than normal), then the corrected plasma Ca^{2+} concentration would be 7.5 + (2 × 0.8) or 9.1 mg/dL, which is normal.

PTH and calcitriol are essential for the maintenance of the plasma Ca^{2+} concentration, since their absence is associated with *progressive hypocalcemia* due to decreases in bone resorption and intestinal absorption and an increase in

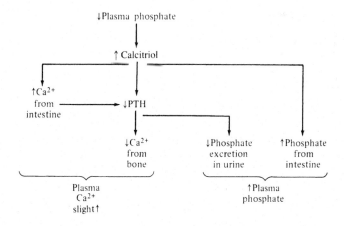

Figure 6-21 Sequence of events following the stimulation of calcitriol formation by hypophosphatemia. The net effect is an increase in the plasma phosphate concentration with only a slight increase in the plasma Ca^{2+} concentration. Both the latter change and a direct inhibitory effect of calcitriol probably contribute to the decline in PTH release in this setting. (*Redrawn from DeLuca H*, Am J Med *58:39, 1975. Used with permission.*)

urinary Ca^{2+} excretion.[254] In addition to their individual effects, both hormones are able to interact so that *Ca^{2+} and phosphate balance can be independently regulated.*

If, for example, hypocalcemia does occur, there is a direct stimulus to PTH secretion and the subsequent formation of calcitriol (Fig. 6-20). PTH increases calcium phosphate release from bone and urinary phosphate excretion, whereas calcitriol augments intestinal calcium phosphate absorption. Both hormones also reduce urinary Ca^{2+} excretion.[254] The net effect is an increase in the plasma Ca^{2+} concentration with little change in the plasma phosphate concentration. This sequence is reversed with hypercalcemia or a high-Ca^{2+} diet, as both PTH secretion and calcitriol production are diminished.

The normal plasma phosphate concentration, measured in the laboratory as the plasma inorganic phosphorus concentration (i.e., the concentration of phosphorus contained in the inorganic phosphates), is 2.5 to 4.5 mg/dL. In the presence of dietary phosphate restriction or hypophosphatemia, there is increased gene expression and synthesis of new Na^+-phosphate cotransporters, thereby enhancing proximal phosphate reabsorption.[291] In addition, calcitriol synthesis is directly enhanced,[283] increasing intestinal calcium phosphate absorption (Fig. 6-21). The ensuing small rise in the plasma Ca^{2+} concentration and perhaps a direct inhibitory effect of calcitriol suppress PTH secretion, reducing calcium phosphate release from bone and further lowering urinary phosphate excretion. The net effect of these adaptations is virtual abolition of phosphate excretion in the urine (unless hypophosphatemia is due to phosphate wasting) and an increase in the plasma phosphate concentration toward normal. This response is achieved with only a slight increment in the plasma Ca^{2+} concentration.

The hormonal response to hyperphosphatemia, which most often occurs in renal failure, is discussed in the next section. The direct changes in proximal function are the opposite of those induced by phosphate depletion: decreased proximal phosphate reabsorption, due in part to reduced expression of the gene for the Na^+-phosphate cotransporter,[291] and diminished calcitriol synthesis.

Calcium and Phosphate Metabolism in Renal Failure

Although a complete discussion of the abnormalities in mineral metabolism that occur in patients with chronic renal failure is beyond the scope of this chapter, it is useful to review briefly how the homeostatic mechanisms governing calcium and phosphate balance can be impaired in this setting due to alterations in phosphate excretion and in PTH and calcitriol release.[292-294]

Phosphate balance and secondary hyperparathyroidism   Renal failure is characterized by a decrease in the functioning renal mass and, therefore, in the total GFR. With the initial fall in GFR, there is a reduction in the filtered phosphate load and consequently in phosphate excretion. If intake remains constant, the net effect will be phosphate retention and a small increase in the plasma phosphate concentration. This mild *phosphate retention is intimately related to the common development* *of secondary hyperparathyroidism.* As illustrated in Fig. 6-22, progressive renal failure is associated with a marked increase in circulating PTH levels that correlates roughly with the degree of decline in GFR. If, however, phosphate retention is prevented by restricting phosphate intake, *secondary hyperparathyroidism does not occur.*[295,296]

The mechanism by which phosphate retention leads to hyperparathyroidism is incompletely understood. It was initially thought that excess phosphate will drive the following reaction to the right:[297]

$$Ca^{2+} + HPO_4^{2-} \leftrightarrow CaHPO_4$$

The ensuing reduction in the plasma Ca^{2+} concentration can then stimulate the secretion of PTH, which, by increasing Ca^{2+} release from bone and phosphate excretion in the urine, will *return both the plasma Ca^{2+} and phosphate concentrations to normal* (Fig. 6-23).

However, several observations are not compatible with this hypothesis. First, the initial minor degree of hyperphosphatemia may not be sufficient to cause a large enough reduction in the plasma Ca^{2+} concentration to enhance PTH release.[298] Second, maintenance of normocalcemia by the administration of Ca^{2+} does not prevent the development of hyperparathyroidism.[299]

An alternative and not mutually exclusive theory is that phosphate retention acts by *diminishing the renal production of calcitriol.*[289,292] This will then lead to

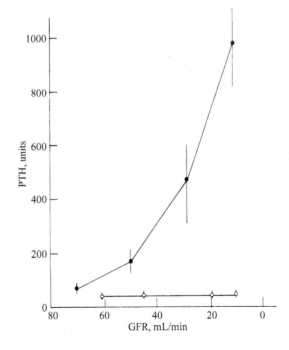

Figure 6-22   The relationship between PTH levels and GFR in two groups of dogs: those maintained on a 1200-mg/day phosphorus diet (closed circles) and those maintained on a diet containing less than 100 mg of phosphorus per day (open circles). (*From Slatopolsky E, Caglar S, Pennell JP, et al, J Clin Invest 50:492, 1971, by copyright permission of the American Society for Clinical Investigation.*)

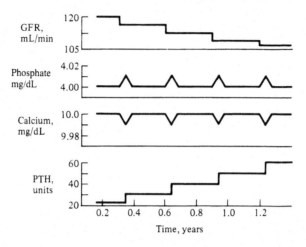

Figure 6-23   Hypothetical model for the development of secondary hyperparathyroidism in advancing chronic renal failure. Each decrement in GFR promotes phosphate retention and a small reduction in the plasma Ca^{2+} concentration. The latter change, plus a possible decline in calcitriol levels, stimulates PTH secretion, which, at least initially, is able to return the plasma Ca^{2+} and phosphate concentrations to normal. (*From Slatopolsky E, Bricker NS,* Kidney Int *4:14, 1973. Reprinted by permission from* Kidney International.)

hyperparathyroidism both by lowering the plasma Ca^{2+} concentration and by removing the inhibitory effect of calcitriol on PTH secretion.[289,290] The following observations are compatible with this hypothesis:

- Plasma calcitriol levels are often reduced in patients with mild to moderate renal insufficiency, not elevated as would be expected from the presence of hyperparathyroidism.[300,301] Even the finding of normal or near-normal calcitriol levels does not necessarily preclude a role for initial calcitriol deficiency, since the secondary hyperparathyroidism will increase calcitriol synthesis.

- The institution of dietary phosphate restriction is able to reverse many of the abnormalities in mineral metabolism: The plasma level of calcitriol is increased, while that of PTH is diminished;[302,303] and intestinal Ca^{2+} absorption is markedly improved.[302] In advanced renal failure, the decline in PTH secretion can occur without change in the plasma levels of calcitriol (presumably due to the marked reduction in functioning renal mass) or of Ca^{2+}. This observation suggests that hyperphosphatemia itself may contribute to the hyperparathyroidism, a theory that has been confirmed in both experimental and human studies.[304-306]

- The administration of calcitriol to normalize the plasma calcitriol can prevent[299] or reverse secondary hyperparathyroidism,[290,307] an effect that cannot be achieved by raising the plasma Ca^{2+} concentration with Ca^{2+} supplementation.[290,299]

Partial resistance to the action of calcitriol also may play an important role in the pathogenesis of hyperparathyroidism. In particular, normal concentration of calcitriol may be unable to suppress PTH secretion, perhaps due to a decreased number of calcitriol receptors in the parathyroid gland.[308] This change can be demonstrated relatively early (when the plasma creatinine concentration has only doubled) in experimental animals; at a later stage, retained uremic toxins may contribute by decreasing both receptor synthesis and hormone-receptor function.[309,310] This defect may also explain why supraphysiological levels of calcitriol (via intravenous or intraperitoneal administration) can markedly diminish PTH release in patients on maintenance dialysis, while physiologic oral doses are relatively ineffective.[290,311,312]

Regardless of the exact mechanism, the hypersecretion of PTH is initially appropriate, since it tends to normalize both the plasma Ca^{2+} and phosphate concentrations. This effect is not complete, as some patients may have a mild elevation in the plasma phosphate concentration of less than 1 mg/dL; this minor degree of hyperphosphatemia may be sufficient to cause the persistent impairment in calcitriol release and therefore the continued drive to PTH secretion.[301] In addition, each succeeding decrement in GFR will enhance the tendency toward phosphate retention, thereby requiring a further rise in PTH release (Fig. 6-23).[295]

In the long term, however, the development of hyperparathyroidism is in part *maladaptive*, because chronic exposure to high levels of PTH can lead to potentially serious bone disease, called osteitis fibrosa.[292-294] Furthermore, PTH loses its ability to maintain normophosphatemia when the GFR falls below 30 mL/min. Because of the inhibitory effect of PTH on proximal phosphate reabsorption, the fraction of the filtered phosphate that is reabsorbed can fall from the normal value of 80 to 95 percent to as low as 15 percent in severe renal failure.[313] At this point, PTH is unable to further increase phosphate excretion but continues to promote phosphate release from bone, resulting in persistent hyperphosphatemia if intake is not diminished. This may lead to the development of a vicious cycle, since, as noted above, hyperphosphatemia in advanced renal failure can directly stimulate further PTH release.[304-306]

The combination of marked hyperphosphatemia and a normal or low-normal plasma Ca^{2+} concentration will result in a very high calcium-phosphate product and a tendency for calcium phosphate precipitation into arteries, joints, soft tissues, and the viscera; this process is called *metastatic calcification*.[314] Total parathyroidectomy (usually with autotransplantation of some parathyroid tissue into the forearm) may be performed in this setting, since it will lower PTH levels as well as the plasma *calcium and phosphate* concentrations (Fig. 6-24).[314-317] The latter changes are due to diminished bone resorption and to the deposition of calcium phosphate in bones previously demineralized by chronic hyperparathyroidism.

Prevention of secondary hyperparathyroidism   In view of the deleterious consequences of prolonged hypersecretion of PTH, a variety of modalities have been tried in an attempt to prevent this complication. The most obvious is limiting net

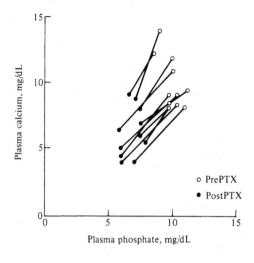

Figure 6-24 Changes in total plasma calcium and phosphate levels observed in 11 uremic patients before and following subtotal parathyroidectomy (PTX) for severe secondary hyperparathyroidism. (*From Massry SG, Coburn JW, Popovtzer MM*, Arch Intern Med *124:431, 1969. Copyright 1969, American Medical Association.*)

phosphate absorption. Dietary restriction can be attempted, but compliance is often a major problem. Furthermore, urinary phosphate excretion falls to such low levels in end-stage renal disease that limiting intake is not sufficient to prevent phosphate accumulation. In this setting, phosphate balance can be maintained only by binding dietary phosphate in the intestine, most frequently by using a phosphate binder such as calcium carbonate or calcium acetate.[318-321] This will lead to the formation of insoluble calcium phosphate precipitates in the gut and decreased intestinal phosphate absorption. Absorption of some of this calcium can also raise the plasma Ca^{2+} concentration, which may further lower PTH levels.

Aluminum-containing antacids were once widely used but created a major new problem: *aluminum intoxication* due to the gradual tissue accumulation of absorbed aluminum, particularly in bone and the brain. The clinical manifestations of this syndrome include osteomalacia, bone and muscle pain, microcytic anemia, and in selected cases dementia.[322] There is no safe dose that is also effective as a phosphate binder.[323]

Calcium citrate has also been used; however, this preparation is contraindicated in renal failure, since citrate can markedly increase intestinal aluminum absorption and predispose to aluminum toxicity.[321,324] Citrate appears to act in two ways: It combines with aluminum to form the soluble and absorbable aluminum citrate salt, and it complexes with intestinal calcium. The ensuing decrease in free calcium then leads to increased permeability of the tight junctions between the cells, a change that can markedly enhance passive aluminum absorption.[324] Similar considerations apply to the concurrent administration of aluminum with sodium citrate (Bicitra), which has been used to treat uremic acidosis.

The main problem with calcium carbonate or calcium acetate therapy is that hypercalcemia is a not infrequent complication with this therapy.[318,320] As a result, close monitoring is essential, particularly in patients who are also being treated with a vitamin D metabolite such as calcitriol.[320] An aluminum-containing antacid or preferably sevelamer (RenaGel, see below) can be added if hyperphosphatemia persists or hypercalcemia limits the use of calcium.

Any phosphate binder should be *given with meals* to impair the absorption of dietary phosphate.[325] Administration between meals, in comparison, binds only the phosphate in intestinal secretions, leading to a much lesser inhibition of net phosphate uptake. The increased binding of calcium or aluminum to phosphate has a second advantage in that cation absorption is also impaired. As a result, the risks of both hypercalcemia and aluminum intoxication are reduced.[325]

The problems with phosphate binders containing calcium, aluminum, or magnesium has led to a search for different compounds that could bind phosphate. One such compound is the nonabsorbable agent sevelamer (RenaGel), which contains neither calcium nor aluminum. It is a cationic polymer that binds phosphate through ion exchange. It is as effective as calcium antacids but, because of its expense, is currently used primarily in patients who develop hypercalcemia.[326-328]

Correction of calcitriol deficiency is another important component of therapy in patients with hyperparathyroidism. In patients already on dialysis, for example, the intravenous or intraperitoneal administration of calcitriol can lead to a marked suppression in PTH release[290,311,312] and improvement in PTH-induced osteitis fibrosa.[312,329]

Calcitriol should not be given unless the plasma phosphate concentration has been controlled, since the calcitriol-induced increase in intestinal phosphate absorption can exacerbate underlying hyperphosphatemia. Careful monitoring for the development of hypercalcemia is also required. The risk of hypercalcemia may be circumvented in the future by the administration of synthetic vitamin D analogs (such as 22-oxacalcitriol, 1α-hydroxyvitamin D_2, or 19-nor) that have no or less calcemic or phosphatemic effect but are still able to suppress PTH secretion.[330-334] The factors responsible for the selective actions of these analogs are incompletely understood.

Another factor that may be beneficial is correction of the metabolic acidosis that commonly accompanies chronic renal failure. Buffering of the excess acid in bone leads to loss of bone mineral, possibly contributing to the development of hyperparathyroid bone disease.[335]

CATECHOLAMINES

Catecholamines, released from the sympathetic nerves and the adrenal medulla (norepinephrine and epinephrine), play a central role in circulatory homeostasis via their cardiac and vascular effects (see Chap. 8). They also can importantly influence renal function, as adrenergic innervation has been identified in the renal vasculature and in the proximal tubule, loop of Henle, and distal tubule.[336-338] Renal sympathetic activity tends to be increased in states of effective circulating volume depletion. In this setting, norepinephrine is a potent vasoconstrictor, acting to reduce renal blood flow and therefore to preserve perfusion to the critical coronary and cerebral circulations.[336,337,339]

Enhanced sympathetic activity also increases Na^+ reabsorption, an effect that may contribute to the compensatory renal Na^+ retention seen with volume depletion.[337,340] At least three factors may participate in this response: (1) direct stimulation of proximal and loop Na^+ transport,[340-343] which is primarily mediated by stimulation of the α_1-adrenergic receptors;[341] (2) altered peritubular capillary hemodynamics, resulting from the increase in arteriolar resistance (see page 83); and (3) activation of the renin-angiotensin-aldosterone system by the β_1-adrenergic receptors (see page 33).[341]

The α_2-adrenergic receptors produce an opposite response, increasing Na^+ and water excretion. These actions reflect at least in part a decrease in proximal Na^+ transport and in collecting tubule water reabsorption.[343-345] The diuretic effect appears to be mediated by activation of an inhibitory G_i regulatory protein, which impairs the ability of ADH to increase adenylyl cyclase activity and subsequent water reabsorption (see Fig. 6-1).[344,345]

The ability of norepinephrine to increase Na^+ reabsorption at the same time that it tends to elevate the systemic blood pressure is important physiologically because it prevents inappropriate urinary Na^+ wasting. The sympathetic nervous system is activated in states of volume depletion; the ensuing rise in blood pressure would tend, via pressure natriuresis (see page 272), to increase Na^+ excretion if it were not for the concomitant stimulation of Na^+ reabsorption.[346] (Similar considerations apply to angiotensin II, which is also both a vasoconstrictor and a stimulator of proximal Na^+ reabsorption; see Chap. 2.)

Dopamine

Another catecholamine, dopamine, is primarily synthesized in the proximal tubule from circulating L-dopa, via the enzyme L-amino acid decarboxylase;[347-349] dopaminergic nerves are also present in the kidney, but their physiologic significance is unclear.[350] Dopamine generally has renal effects opposite to those of norepinephrine and epinephrine. At lower concentrations, it is a renal vasodilator that acts at the interlobular arteries and both the afferent and efferent arterioles.[351,352] Both a direct effect of dopamine and increased release of prostacyclin may contribute to this decrease in vascular resistance.[353]

The combined afferent and efferent dilation results in a marked increase in renal blood flow with a *much lesser or no elevation in GFR*, since the reduction in efferent tone will tend to diminish the intraglomerular pressure (see page 38).[354,355] At higher concentrations, however, dopamine can induce vasoconstriction, a response that may be mediated by activation of α-adrenergic receptors.[351]

Dopamine also tends to reduce proximal Na^+ reabsorption,[356] an effect that is mediated by partial inhibition of both of the major steps involved in transtubular Na^+ reabsorption (see Chap. 3): (1) The activity of the Na^+-H^+ exchanger in the luminal membrane is diminished via the formation of cyclic AMP, thereby reducing the entry of luminal Na^+ into the cell,[357] and (2) the activity of the Na^+-K^+-

ATPase pump is decreased, thereby reducing the transport of Na^+ out of the cell into the peritubular interstitium and then the peritubular capillary.[348,358]

The net effect is that the administration of dopamine to patients can lead to a natriuresis as well as an increase in renal perfusion.[355,356] It is not clear, however, whether endogenous dopamine is a physiologically important natriuretic hormone. The local production of dopamine in the proximal tubule is appropriately enhanced by volume expansion,[348,359] a response that is mediated at least in part by increased activity of L-amino acid decarboxylase.[348] This may contribute to the ensuing natriuresis, since the administration of a dopamine receptor inhibitor to experimental animals impairs the response to modest volume expansion.[360]

The vasodilator and natriuretic properties of dopamine have led to the frequent use of low-dose, "renal-dose" dopamine (0.5 to 3 g/kg per minute) both to increase the urine output and to preserve renal function in oliguric patients at risk for postischemic acute tubular necrosis.[349] Unfortunately, several clinical trials have failed to document the efficacy of dopamine in these settings.[361-363]

KININS

Kinins are another set of hormones produced in the kidney.[364,365] The process begins with the secretion of the enzyme kallikrein by the cells in the distal tubule and connecting segment (Fig. 6-25). This enzyme catalyzes the conversion of inactive kininogen (a plasma protein that may also be produced locally) into lysyl-bradykinin and then, in the presence of an aminopeptidase, into bradykinin. Kinin generation probably occurs both in the tubular lumen and, since secreted kallikrein appears to reach the vascular compartment, in the vascular space. On the other hand, filtered kinins are rapidly metabolized by kininases in the proximal tubule and therefore are not likely to have any intratubular effect.[364]

The physiologic role of the renal kinins is incompletely understood. Like the prostaglandins, they are vasodilators that may act to minimize renal ischemia in hypovolemic states in which angiotensin II and norepinephrine secretion are

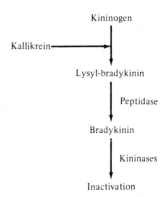

Figure 6-25 Kallikrein-kinin system.

increased.[366,367] Their site of production in the distal nephron also suggests that they may have an intraluminal effect on Na^+ and water handling in the collecting tubules. Compatible with this hypothesis are the observations that kinins diminish Na^+ reabsorption in the inner medulla (by closing Na^+ channels in the luminal membrane)[368] and impair the ability of ADH to increase local water reabsorption.[11] The latter effect appears to be indirect, being mediated by kinin-induced prostaglandin production.

Renal kinins appear to have a significant role in the developing kidney. The expression of bradykinin receptor mRNA is elevated 10- to 30-fold in neonatal kidney as compared with adult kidney.[369] How kinins act in the maturing kidney is unknown.

The kinins are probably not important circulating hormones, since they are rapidly metabolized in the circulation by kininases, one of which is angiotensin converting enzyme. This is the same enzyme that catalyzes the conversion of angiotensin I into angiotensin II.

ERYTHROPOIETIN

Erythropoietin (EPO) is a glycoprotein growth factor that is the primary stimulus to erythropoiesis, promoting the terminal differentiation of erythroid colony-forming units (CFU-E) into normoblasts and then erythrocytes.[370] Mice with homozygous null mutations of EPO or the EPO receptor (EPOR) genes form erythroid burst-forming units (BFU-E) and CFU-E normally but fail to differentiate into mature erythrocytes.[371]

Erythropoietin is produced by the kidney and to a much lesser degree (less than 10 percent) by the liver. A population of interstitial fibroblasts appears to be a major source of renal EPO synthesis,[372,373] although some studies have suggested an important role for the proximal tubular cells.[374] Interstitial cells positive for EPO mRNA are limited to the deep cortex and outer medulla in the unstimulated kidney. With increasing anemia, the number of positive cells increases in number and spreads into the superficial cortex.[373]

Decreased oxygen delivery, most often due to anemia or hypoxemia, is the primary stimulus to erythropoietin release.[370] The oxygen sensor is probably a heme protein[375] that may be a cytochrome *b*-like flavohemoprotein (see Fig. 6-26).[376,377]

The following model has been proposed to explain the action of this sensor. Binding of oxygen to the sensor shifts its conformation from a deoxygenated (off) set to an oxygenated (on) state; the oxy form activates a series of events leading to repression of EPO gene transcription.[378,379] This sequence is reversed with decreased oxygen delivery; activation as the deoxygenated state leads to synthesis of a protein that binds to the active site on the enhancer region of the EPO gene, resulting in increased EPO production.[380] The ensuing rise in red cell production will tend to return oxygen-carrying capacity toward normal.

Events downstream from the oxygen sensor involved in activation of EPO gene expression require de novo protein synthesis, including the production of

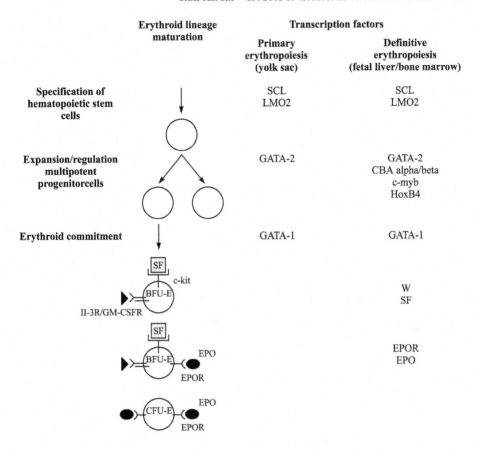

Figure 6-26 Formation of erythroid progenitors. Schematic representation of the formation of erythroid progenitors (BFU-E and CFU-E) from hematopoietic stem cells and multipotent progenitor cells. The transcription factors important for the maturation and differentiation of hematopoietic stem cells (HSC) and expansion of the stem/progenitor compartment are indicated on the right, according to whether they are important for primary erythropoiesis in the yolk sac and/or definitive erythropoiesis in the fetal liver and/or bone marrow. Certain growth factors and their receptors, such as Steel factor (SF)/c-kit and erythropoietin (EPO/EPOR), are important or essential for erythropoiesis, respectively; by comparison, other growth factors, such as IL-3 or GM-CSF, act synergistically but are not essential. Abbreviations include EPO and EPOR = erythropoietin and its receptor, respectively; SF and W (c-kit) = Steel factor and its receptor, respectively; IL-3R = interleukin-3 receptor; BFU-E = erythroid blast-forming units; and CFU-E = erythroid colony-forming units.

specific transcription factors.[381] One of these is hypoxia-inducible factor-1, the activity of which is essential for enhanced EPO production.[382,383] Mice that lack this factor die at midgestation, while heterozygotes, although developmentally normal, fail to respond adequately to chronic hypoxia.[384]

The kidney is well suited to be the site of EPO production because it is able to dissociate changes in blood flow alone from those in oxygenation. Reducing renal blood flow, for example, will also tend to diminish both the glomerular filtration rate and total tubular Na^+ reabsorption. Since active transport is responsible for most of renal oxygen consumption, the relation between oxygen delivery (reduced by hypoperfusion) and oxygen utilization (reduced by decreased reabsorption) is relatively well maintained, thereby preventing an inappropriate increase in EPO synthesis.[373]

EPO in Chronic Renal Failure

The importance of erythropoietin has been demonstrated in patients with chronic renal failure. Anemia is common in this setting and is due primarily to reduced renal EPO production, a presumed reflection of the reduction in functioning renal mass.[370,385] This relationship has been convincingly demonstrated in studies in which recombinant human EPO has been administered intravenously, subcutaneously, or intraperitoneally to anemic patients undergoing chronic dialysis (see Fig. 6-27).[370,386,387] Elevation of the hematocrit to the desired goal of 33 to 36 percent can be achieved in the majority of patients if an adequate dose of EPO is given. Both lower and higher hematocrits have been associated with increased mortality.[388,389]

Correction of anemia with EPO in patients with end-stage renal disease is typically associated with an often marked improvement in the sense of well-being.[370,386,387] This observation demonstrated that many symptoms previously

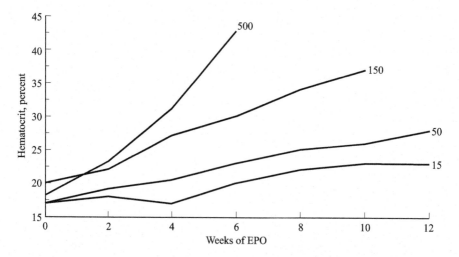

Figure 6-27   Dose response of EPO-induced correction of uremic anemia. Slope of the rate of increase in the hematocrit in patients on maintenance dialysis given various doses (15 to 500 units/kg) of erythropoietin (EPO) three times per week. The response is fastest at the highest dose, but a gradual and adequate rise in hematocrit is achieved in most patients with 50 units/kg. (*Data from Eschbach JW, Egrie JC, Downing MR, et al, N Engl J Med 316:73, 1987. Used with permission.*)

attributed to toxins retained because of the renal failure were due to anemia (or possibly to EPO deficiency).

ENDOTHELIN

The endothelin (ET) family consists of three 21-amino-acid peptides (ET-1, ET-2, and ET-3).[391] Each ET is formed as a propeptide known as big ET, which is converted to the mature peptide by endothelin converting enzymes located both inside and outside of cells.[392,393]

Once secreted, ETs bind to two general classes of receptors: endothelin A (ETA) and endothelin B (ETB).[394,395] Two important features of ET-receptor interaction help explain the actions of ET:

- ET remains bound to the receptor for several hours, imparting a sustained effect.
- ET generally binds to receptors located on the same cell as, or on cells immediately adjacent to, the cells that secreted the peptide.

ETs are produced by most cell types in the kidney and have a wide variety of biologic actions. The most important are:

- Regulation of vascular resistance
- Modulation of fluid and electrolyte transport
- Regulation of cell proliferation and extracellular matrix accumulation.

Regulation of Vascular Tone

ETs, via stimulation of the ETA receptor, are extremely powerful vaso-constrictors;[396] their effect is an order of magnitude greater than that of any other known vasoconstrictor. The renal vasculature is approximately an order of magnitude more sensitive to ET than any other vascular bed.[397] Studies with nonselective ET receptor antagonists suggest that ET mediates part of the systemic and renal vasoconstrictive effects of angiotensin II.[398]

The use of selective receptor antagonists has helped clarify the individual roles of the ETA and ETB receptors.[399] Administration of an ETA receptor antagonists produces local vasodilation that can be almost totally abolished by inhibition of nitric oxide synthesis. In comparison, vascular resistance rises when an ETB receptor antagonist is given, either alone or after ETA receptor antagonism. Thus, the ETB receptor appears to mediate vasodilation.

Most ETs in the renal vasculature are released by endothelial cells and act on neighboring vascular smooth muscle. Endothelial cell ET-1 release is stimulated by other vasoconstrictors, thrombogenic agents, and inflammatory cytokines, and is reduced by vasodilators (particularly nitric oxide) and anticoagulants.[400]

It is unlikely that ETs are involved in the minute-to-minute regulation of renal vascular resistance. Rather, ETs are released in substantial amounts by renal endothelial cells when a prolonged and severe decrease in renal blood flow occurs. This may be appropriate, as in marked prerenal states, in an attempt to maintain coronary and cerebral perfusion. However, ET-induced vasoconstriction can also be injurious, as with prolonged ET-mediated renal vasoconstriction following ischemic renal injury or after renal exposure to nephrotoxins (such as cyclosporine, radiocontrast media, endotoxin, amphotericin B, and other agents).[400,401]

Modulation of Fluid and Electrolyte Transport

ETs are produced by most tubule segments, with the collecting duct being the predominant nephron site of synthesis. Once released, ETs bind to ETB receptors, found in most nephron segments.

Like that of the vasculature, the ET modulation of fluid and electrolyte transport involves the long-term, rather than instantaneous, regulation of fluid and electrolyte homeostasis. In general, ETs have an inhibitory effect (and may function as autocrine inhibitors) on tubular sodium and water reabsorption. At peptide concentrations most likely to be present in the proximal tubule, ETs can suppress Na-K-ATPase[402,403] and Na-H antiporter activity. This effect is mediated, at least in part, via increased levels of arachidonate metabolites.[404]

ETs also inhibit sodium and water reabsorption by the cortical collecting tubule, antagonizing the actions of ADH and aldosterone. These effects are mediated in part by reductions in cAMP accumulation and apical sodium channel activity.[405,406] ETs are potent inhibitors of ADH-stimulated cAMP accumulation in the inner medullary collecting duct; they also reduce Na-K-ATPase activity via stimulation of prostaglandin E_2 production.[404]

Enhanced nephron ET production may result in either physiologically appropriate or toxic effects.[404] As an example, a prolonged increase in water intake enhances the production of ET-1, which inhibits collecting duct water reabsorption, appropriately increasing water excretion. On the other hand, a sustained decrease in nephron ET-1 production, as has been suggested to occur in essential hypertension, could enhance salt and water retention and contribute to the hypertensive state.

At first glance, it may appear confusing that ET raises blood pressure by constricting the renal vasculature, but also lowers blood pressure by promoting renal sodium and water excretion. However, the actions of ET must be viewed in the context of the target cell and the activated receptor. Thus, the apparent paradox is explained by the observation that the activation of ETA and ETB receptors raises and lowers systemic blood pressure, respectively.

Regulation of Cell Proliferation and Extracellular Matrix Accumulation

Cell proliferation and extracellular matrix accumulation are altered by the endothelins, with ET-1 increasing the following parameters:[405,406]

- The release of tissue inhibitor of metalloproteinase
- The release of cytokines that stimulate matrix accumulation
- The production of renal cell fibronectin and collagen

These peptides can also stimulate proliferation of a variety of renal cell types.

Although these effects may be important during normal development, they are more relevant clinically in the development of pathophysiologic processes. In particular, ETs have a role in the gradual progression of glomerular sclerosis and interstitial fibrosis that occurs with irreversible renal injury. Inhibiting ET substantially reduces renal scarring in models of chronic renal failure, while humans with a variety of renal diseases have increased renal ET-1 production.[400,407-411]

NITRIC OXIDE

Nitric oxide (NO) has a major role as a messenger molecule in most human organ systems.[412] In the blood vessel wall, basal and calcium-agonist-stimulated release of NO largely accounts for the bioactivity of endothelium-derived relaxing factor (EDRF).[413] In the kidney, as well as in other solid organs, physiologic concentrations of NO function as a tonic vasodilator, working essentially instantaneously.[414] However, higher concentrations can be toxic, including damaging cellular constituents (such as DNA), and inducing hypotension in those with sepsis.[415]

Basic Physiology

NO, a molecular gas, is formed by the action of one of three isoforms of nitric oxide synthase (NOS). The isoforms were named based upon the cell types in which they were first isolated: neuronal NOS (nNOS or NOS1), inducible or macrophage NOS (iNOS, NOS2), and endothelial NOS (eNOS, NOS3). All three enzymes, which are cytochrome P450-like proteins, facilitate the addition of the guanidino nitrogen of the amino acid arginine to molecular oxygen, producing NO and water.

The expression of the three NOS isoforms differs, resulting in varying amounts of NO production. In general, eNOS and nNOS are constitutively active, producing relatively low levels of NO, with the output varying with changes in the intracellular calcium concentration. By comparison, the transcriptional regulation of iNOS can be markedly induced, particularly by inflammatory cytokines, resulting in extremely large amounts of NO.

NO is a paracrine mediator that works differently from endocrine mediators, such as angiotensin II and ADH. NO, which is produced and released by individual cells, readily penetrates the biological membranes of neighboring cells, modulating a number of signaling cascades. Since it has an extremely short half-life, it exerts its effects locally and transiently.

The most recognized cellular target of NO is heme-containing soluble guanylate cyclase. The stimulation of this compound enhances the synthesis of cyclic GMP (cGMP) from guanosine triphosphate (GTP), increasing the cytosolic levels of cGMP. The effects of NO can be enhanced by inhibiting the breakdown of cGMP, a process catalyzed by a family of phosphodiesterases.

Other cellular targets for NO also exist:

- NO interacts with thiol groups on proteins and small molecules, resulting in the formation of S-nitrosothiols.
- NO can target Fe/S groups at the catalytic centers of proteins, including hemoglobin.[416]
- The formation of peroxynitrite from NO and superoxide radical has been implicated in cellular toxicity via the propensity of peroxynitrite to induce posttranslational changes in the tyrosine residues of proteins.[417]

Thus, the biologic effects of NO depend upon the concentration of NO produced as well as upon features specific to the local environment, particularly the presence and production of thiols and superoxide.

Expression of nitric oxide in the kidney All three NOS isoforms can be expressed in the kidney. The renal pattern of isoform expression (whether in normal individuals or in certain disorders) may be clinically important, as perturbations in NO bioactivity have been described in a number of kidney-dependent pathologic states.[418]

Inconsistencies and controversies concerning the expression of NOS isoforms are due in part to variations in the methods of detection and/or the product being detected (such as mRNA and/or protein)[419,420]:

- nNOS is principally expressed in the macula densa and the inner medullary collecting duct.
- Although this is somewhat controversial, iNOS has been localized to several tubule segments (principally the thick medullary ascending limb but also the distal convoluted tubule and proximal tubule), the glomerulus, and the interlobular and arcuate arteries.
- eNOS is expressed in the endothelium of glomerular capillaries, afferent and efferent arterioles, and intrarenal arteries.

The greatest enzymatic activity for NO production in the kidney is found in the inner medullary collecting duct (IMCD). IMCD NOS activity is three- to sixfold higher than that observed in the glomeruli.[421]

Nitric Oxide and the Kidney

Insight into the role of NO in the kidney is primarily derived from experiments examining the altered expression of the NOS isoforms, the effects of inhibiting

NOS (thereby lowering levels of NO), or the administration of NO donors. The most important actions of NO in the kidney are

- Regulation of renal hemodynamics
- Modulation of fluid and electrolyte transport
- Regulation of damage in response to injury

Renal hemodynamics As mentioned above, eNOS is expressed to a variable extent in endothelial cells of the afferent arteriole, glomerulus, and efferent arteriole.[422] Endothelial-derived NO plays a major role in maintaining arteriolar dilation by participating in the paracrine control of renal glomerular vascular resistance and mesangial cell tone. In the rat, acute systemic NOS inhibition causes marked increases in afferent and efferent arteriolar resistances and a fall in glomerular capillary ultrafiltration coefficient.[423] In addition, chronic systemic blockade of NO bioactivity in rats induced by pharmacologic inhibition of NOS enzyme activity results in significant glomerular capillary hypertension.[424] In these models, the marked increases in efferent arteriolar resistance also reflected important contributions from both angiotensin II and endothelin-1.[425]

The systemic blood pressure is significantly affected by NO. In animal models, hypertension results from deletion of the genes for eNOS[426,427] or from chronic inhibition of NO synthesis,[424,428] while hypotension occurs in transgenic mice that overexpress eNOS.[429] With inhibition of NO synthesis or deletion of eNOS genes, significant reductions in renal plasma flow and glomerular filtration rate parallel the development of the hypertension.[426,428]

In some clinical settings, enhanced eNOS activity may be deleterious; it may, for example, contribute to the renal vasodilation and glomerular hyperfiltration observed in diabetic nephropathy. In a diabetic rat model, enhanced glomerular filtration and renal plasma were blocked by the administration of a nonselective NOS blocker.[430] Increased protein levels of eNOS, but not of iNOS, were observed in the glomeruli of these animals, suggesting that the hemodynamic effects were due to enhanced eNOS activity.[430]

Solute and water transport Although many renal responses to NOS blockade are mediated by actions on the microcirculation, NO also affects solute and water transport by directly altering the function of specific segments of the nephron. In particular, NO appears to play a role in the moment-to-moment homeostatic control of renal sodium excretion and extracellular fluid volume.

- Intrarenal NO synthesis is increased during periods of enhanced salt intake, thereby facilitating renal sodium excretion. The administration of NO donors also augments sodium elimination.
- By comparison, acute or chronic blockade of NO synthesis (with NOS inhibitors) impairs urinary sodium excretion, even at concentrations that do not affect renal glomerular or systemic hemodynamics. As an example,

chronic administration of a NOS inhibitor in humans results in a 40 percent reduction in the fractional excretion of sodium.[431]

Thus, increased and decreased levels of NO enhance and impair the urinary excretion of sodium, respectively. This is due to effects on epithelial transporters located in specific nephronal segments. Specifically, NO inhibits sodium entry in the cortical collecting duct, Na-H exchange in the proximal tubule, and Na-K-ATPase activity in varied nephronal segments.[432,433] NO also impairs the responsiveness of the collecting tubule to ADH, facilitating the excretion of water.[434]

Tubuloglomerular feedback   Some of the effects of NOS inhibition on body fluid homeostasis are thought to be mediated by changes in nNOS function expressed in the macula densa. NO synthesized by nNOS in the macula densa blunts the tubuloglomerular feedback (TGF) response in which increasing sodium chloride delivery to the macula densa lowers the glomerular filtration rate to maintain distal flow at a relatively constant level.[435]

However, micropuncture experiments using NOS antagonists indicate that NO does not mediate TGF. Rather, NO release from the macula densa is a modulating factor that is augmented during increased sodium chloride delivery, thereby countering the afferent arteriole constriction elicited in the TGF response. Thus, changes in macula densa NO production may underlie the resetting of TGF that occurs when salt intake is varied; the response is appropriately blunted with a high-salt diet, as maintenance of glomerular filtration promotes excretion of the excess salt.[436]

Role in renal injury   The role of NO in the response to renal injury varies based upon the cell type and NO isoform. The function of endothelial-derived NO as a tonic vasodilator as well as its ability to inhibit platelet activation and adhesion may help minimize injury in glomerulonephritis. This has been illustrated in studies in mice in which targeted inactivation of the eNOS gene increases the sensitivity to glomerular injury.[426,437]

However, NO generated by mesangial and tubular epithelial cells may exacerbate damage, due in part to the ability of these cells to induce the expression of iNOS in response to inflammatory stimuli.[438] Although mesangial cells do not express appreciable amounts of any of the NOS isoforms under basal conditions, they can be induced to express iNOS, a feature that has been documented in human glomerulonephritis, animal models of glomerular injury, and in vitro experiments using inflammatory cytokines.[439-441] As an example, exposure of mesangial cells to tumor necrosis factor-α (TNF-α) causes a 30-fold increase in cGMP content that is first evident at 8 h and is maximal by 24 h.[442]

With inflammatory stimuli, increased levels of NO may enhance injury by suppressing eNOS (resulting in vasoconstriction) and directly causing epithelial cell damage.[439] Cellular injury is most likely due to the formation of peroxynitrite from NO and superoxide radical.

SUMMARY

Variations in hormone secretion are referred to as primary, i.e., nonphysiologic, or secondary, i.e., physiologic. As an example, aldosterone release is appropriately increased by volume depletion; this is called secondary hyperaldosteronism. Conversely, the autonomous hypersecretion of aldosterone due to an adrenal adenoma is referred to as primary hyperaldosteronism. A brief review of the clinical characteristics of these primary disorders can be helpful at this time by illustrating the role of the particular hormone in the regulation of water and electrolyte homeostasis. Most of these conditions will be discussed in detail in the relevant clinical chapters in Part Two.

Primary excessive secretion of ADH results in increased water reabsorption in the collecting tubules. This is called the *syndrome of inappropriate ADH secretion* and is characterized by water retention, hypoosmolality, and hyponatremia. Volume expansion and edema do not occur in this disorder because, similar to the findings in aldosterone escape, the initial fluid retention leads to a spontaneous diuresis that may be mediated in part by a rise in renal perfusion pressure and perhaps by increased release of ANP (see Fig. 6-15).

In contrast, water reabsorption is reduced in the absence of ADH, as large volumes (up to 10 to 20 L/day) of dilute urine are produced. This may be due to deficient hormone secretion (central diabetes insipidus) or to renal resistance to the effects of ADH (nephrogenic diabetes insipidus). Despite the polyuria, patients with either form of diabetes insipidus tend to remain in near normal water balance, because stimulation of thirst leads to an increase in fluid intake to match the higher urine output.

Primary hyperaldosteronism is associated with enhanced K^+ and H^+ secretion in the cortical collecting tubule, resulting in hypokalemia and metabolic alkalosis. The initial Na^+ and water retention also promote the development of hypertension; however, fluid retention lasts for only a few days, due to aldosterone escape.

Hypoaldosteronism, in comparison, is characterized by variable degrees of hyperkalemia, metabolic acidosis, and Na^+ wasting. The most prominent change is the rise in the plasma K^+ concentration, since aldosterone is the primary hormone affecting urinary K^+ excretion. Marked loss of Na^+, on the other hand, is usually not a major feature of this disorder in adults, because other antinatriuretic factors (such as angiotensin II and a reduction in renal perfusion pressure) are activated by the initial volume depletion (see Chap. 8).

PTH increases bone resorption, the urinary excretion of phosphate, and renal calcitriol synthesis. As a result, hypercalcemia and a normal or diminished plasma phosphate concentration are produced by the primary hypersecretion of PTH. In contrast, hypoparathyroidism leads to hypocalcemia (which is in part due to the associated calcitriol deficiency) and hyperphosphatemia.

Calcitriol increases the availability of calcium and phosphate primarily by increasing their rate of intestinal absorption and their release from bone. Consequently, calcitriol deficiency is characterized by hypocalcemia and hypophosphatemia; lack of calcitriol may also be associated with rickets in children and osteomalacia in adults, since adequate levels of calcitriol, calcium, and phosphate are necessary for normal bone mineralization.

Vitamin D excess (due to the chronic intake of high doses of vitamin D or to a granulomatous disease such as sarcoidosis) typically leads to increased intestinal Ca^{2+} absorption, enhanced bone resorption, hypercalciuria, and, in some cases, hypercalcemia.[277,278,281,390] The changes in Ca^{2+} balance induced by prolonged ingestion of vitamin D are primarily due to calcifediol, the 25-hydroxylated precursor of calcitriol. The hepatic synthesis of calcifediol is substrate-dependent and not physiologically regulated;[249] as a result, increased vitamin D intake can lead to a marked increase in calcifediol production.[390] This compound is less active but, in this setting, is able to promote the development of hypercalcemia. In comparison, there is no large increase in calcitriol synthesis, because of the inhibitory effects of the rise in the plasma Ca^{2+} concentration and the associated reduction in PTH release.[390]

PROBLEMS

6-1   Aldosterone secretion can be increased by an autonomous adrenal adenoma or in the presence of volume depletion. What will the plasma renin activity be in these two conditions?

6-2   Patients with renal failure have an elevated plasma osmolality due to the increase in the BUN, but do not have persistent ADH release. Why?

6-3   Thirst protects against the development of hypernatremia. Why doesn't the ability to shut off osmotic thirst protect against hyponatremia?

6-4   What effect will the following have on renal calcitriol synthesis?
  (a) Ingestion of a high-phosphate diet
  (b) Hypoparathyroidism
  (c) Ingestion of a high-calcium diet
  (d) Renal disease in which phosphate intake is restricted to prevent phosphate retention

6-5   What effect will each of the following have on the release of aldosterone, ANP, and ADH?
  (a) Ingestion of a Na^+ load (potato chips, for example) without water
  (b) Ingestion of a water load, which is normally rapidly excreted without change in extracellular volume
  (c) An intravenous infusion of isotonic saline
  (d) Marked diarrhea in which the plasma Na^+ concentration remains normal

6-6   Loop diuretics cause hypercalciuria by diminishing Ca^{2+} reabsorption in the thick ascending limb of the loop of Henle. They do not, however, cause hypocalcemia. Why?

6-7   Aldosterone increases Na^+ reabsorption. Why doesn't the retained Na^+ result in an elevation in the plasma Na^+ concentration?

6-8   Patients with which of the following conditions are likely to develop a decline in renal function following the administration of a nonsteroidal anti-inflammatory drug?
  (a) Low-salt diet
  (b) High-salt diet
  (c) Untreated hypertension
  (d) Heart failure
  (e) Severe vomiting

REFERENCES

1. Speigel AM, Weinstein LS, Shenker A. Abnormalities in G-protein coupled signal transduction pathways in human disease. *J Clin Invest* 92:1119, 1993.
2. Miller RT. Transmembrane signalling through G proteins. *Kidney Int* 39:421, 1991.
3. Wong SK-F, Garbers D. Receptor guanylyl cyclases. *J Clin Invest* 90:299, 1992.
4. Berridge MJ. Inositol triphosphate and calcium signalling. *Nature* 361:315, 1993.
5. Bastl CP, Hayslett JP. The cellular action of aldosterone in target epithelia. *Kidney Int* 42:250, 1992.
6. Funder JW. Mineralocorticoids, glucocorticoids, receptors and response elements. *Science* 259:1132, 1993.
7. Vaughan M. Signaling by heterotrimeric G proteins minireview series. *J Biol Chem* 273:667, 1998.
8. Neer EJ. Heterotrimeric G proteins: Organizers of transmembrane signals. *Cell* 80:249, 1995.
9. Schulz S, Waldman SA. The guanylyl cyclase family of natriuretic peptide receptors. *Vitam Horm* 57:123, 1999.
10. Snyder HM, Noland TD, Breyer MD. cAMP-dependent protein kinase mediates hydrosmotic effect of vasopressin in collecting duct. *Am J Physiol* 263:C147, 1992.
11. Clapham DE, Neer EJ. New role of G-protein beta-gamma-dimers in transmembrane signalling. *Nature* 365:403, 1993.
12. Duda T, Goraczniak RM, Sharma RK. Site-directed mutational analysis of a guanylate cyclase cDNA reveals the atrial natriuretic factor signaling site. *Proc Natl Acad Sci U S A* 88:7882, 1991.
13. Light DB, Corbin JD, Stanton BA. Dual ion-channel regulation by cyclic GMP and cyclic GMP-dependent protein kinase. *Nature* 344:336, 1990.
14. Abramow M, Beauwens R, Cogan E. Cellular events in ADH action. *Kidney Int* 32(suppl 21):S-56, 1987.
15. Hebert RL, Jacobson HR, Breyer MD. PGE_2 inhibits AVP-induced water flow in cortical collecting ducts by protein kinase C activation. *Am J Physiol* 259:F318, 1990.
16. Denis M, Poellinger L, Wikstrom A-C. Requirement of hormone for thermal conversion of the glucocorticoid receptor to a DNA-binding site. *Nature* 333:686, 1988.
17. Brown AJ, Finch J, Grieff M, et al. The mechanism for the disparate actions of calcitriol and 22-oxacalcitriol in the intestine. *Endocrinology* 133:1158, 1993.
18. Yang NN, Venugopalan M, Hardikar S, Glasebrook A. Identification of an estrogen response element activated by metabolites of 17β-estradiol and raloxifene. *Science* 273:1222, 1996.
19. Brzozowski AM, Pike AC, Dauter Z, et al. Molecular basis of agonism and antagonism in the oestrogen receptor. *Nature* 389:753, 1997.
20. Delmas PD, Bjarnason NH, Mitlak BH, et al. Effects of raloxifene on bone mineral density, serum cholesterol concentrations, and uterine endometrium in postmenopausal women. *N Engl J Med* 337:1641, 1997.
21. Chlebowski RT, Collyar DE, Somerfield MR, Pfister DG for the American Society of Clinical Oncology Working Group on Breast Cancer Risk Reduction Strategies. Tamoxifen and raloxifene. *J Clin Oncol* 17:1939, 1999.
22. Zimmerman EA, Nilaver G, Hou-Yu A, Silverman AJ. Vasopressinergic and oxytocinergic pathways in central nervous system. *Fed Proc* 43:91, 1984.
23. Lencer WI, Brown D, Ausiello D, Verkman AS. Endocytosis of water channels in rat kidney: Cell specificity and correlation with in vivo antidiuresis. *Am J Physiol* 259:C920, 1990.
24. Nielsen S, DiGiovanni SR, Christensen EI, et al. Cellular and subcellular immunolocalization of vasopressin-regulated water channels in rat kidney. *Proc Natl Acad Sci U S A* 90:1163, 1993.
25. Bichet DG, Razi M, Lonergan M, et al. Hemodynamic and coagulation responses to 1-desamino [6-D-arginine] vasopressin in patients with congential nephrogenic diabetes insipidus. *N Engl J Med* 318:881, 1988.

26. Sugimoto T, Saito M, Mochizuki S, et al. Molecular cloning and functional expression of a cDNA encoding the human V1b vasopressin receptor. *J Biol Chem* 269:27088, 1994.

27. Sasaki S, Fushimi K, Saito H, et al. Cloning, characterization, and chromosomal mapping of human aquaporin of collecting duct. *J Clin Invest* 93:1250, 1994.

28. Hayashi M, Sasaki S, Tsuganazawa H, et al. Expression and distribution of aquaporin of collecting duct are related by vasopressin V_2 receptors in rat kidney. *J Clin Invest* 94:1778, 1994.

29. Deen PM, Verdijk MA, Knoers NV, et al. Requirement for human renal water channel aquaporin-2 for vasopressin-dependent concentration of urine. *Science* 264:92, 1994.

30. Deen PM, Croes H, van Aubel RA, et al. Water channels encoded by mutant aquaporin-2 genes in nephrogenic diabetes insipidus are impaired in their cellular trafficking. *J Clin Invest* 95:2291, 1995.

31. Harris HW Jr, Strange K, Zeidel M. Current understanding of the cellular biology and molecular structure of antidiuretic hormone-stimulated water transport pathway. *J Clin Invest* 88:1, 1991.

32. Yamamoto T, Sasaki S. Aquaporins in the kidney: Emerging new aspects. *Kidney Int* 54:1041, 1998.

33. Nielsen S, Kwon T-H, Christensen BM, et al. Physiology and pathophysiology of renal aquaporins. *J Am Soc Nephrol* 10:647, 1999.

34. Brown D. Membrane recycling and epithelial cell function. *Am J Physiol* 256:F1, 1989.

35. Strange K, Spring KR. Absence of significant cellular dilution during ADH-stimulated water reabsorption. *Science* 235:1068, 1987.

36. Bichet DG, Oksche A, Rosenthal W. Congenital nephrogenic diabetes insipidus. *J Am Soc Nephrol* 8:1951, 1997.

37. Ala Y, Morin D, Mouillac B, et al. Functional studies of twelve mutant V_2 vasopressin receptors related to nephrogenic diabetes insipidus: Molecular basis of a mild clinical phenotype. *J Am Soc Nephrol* 9:1861, 1998.

38. Oksche A, Moller A, Dickson J, et al. Two novel mutations in the aquaporin-2 and the vasopressin V_2 receptor genes in patients with congenital nephrogenic diabetes insipidus. *Hum Genet* 98:5, 1996.

39. Hochberg Z, van Lieburg A, Even L, et al. Autosomal recessive nephrogenic diabetes insipidus caused by an aquaporin-2 mutation *J Clin Endocrinol Metab* 82:686, 1997.

40. Tamarappoo BK, Verkman AS. Defective aquaporin-2 trafficking in nephrogenic diabetes insipidus and correction by chemical chaperones. *J Clin Invest* 101:2257, 1998.

41. Schafer JA, Hawk CT. Regulation of Na^+ channels in the cortical collecting duct by AVP and mineralocorticoids. *Kidney Int* 41:255, 1992.

42. Field MJ, Stanton BA, Giebisch G. Influence of ADH on renal potassium handling: A micropuncture and microperfusion study. *Kidney Int* 25:502, 1984.

43. Cassola AC, Giebisch G, Wong W. Vasopressin increases density of apical low-conductive K^+ channels in rat CCD. *Am J Physiol* 264:F502, 1993.

44. Goldsmith SR. Vasopressin as a vasopressor. *Am J Med* 82:1213, 1987.

45. Bonvalet J-P, Pradelles P, Farman N. Segmental synthesis and actions of prostaglandins along the nephron. *Am J Physiol* 253:F377, 1987.

46. Kirschenbaum MA, Lowe AG, Trizna W, Fine LG. Regulation of vasopressin action by prostaglandins. Evidence for prostaglandin synthesis in the rabbit cortical collecting tubule. *J Clin Invest* 70:1193, 1982.

47. Scharschmidt LA, Dunn MJ. Prostaglandin synthesis by rat glomerular mesangial cells in culture. Effects of angiotensin II and arginine vasopressin. *J Clin Invest* 71:1756, 1983.

48. Breyer MD, Jacobson HR, Hebert RL. Cellular mechanisms of prostaglandin E_2 and vasopressin interactions in the collecting duct. *Kidney Int* 38:618, 1990.

49. Stokes JB. Integrated actions of renal medullary prostaglandins in the control of water excretion. *Am J Physiol* 240:F471, 1981.

50. Yared A, Kon V, Ichikawa I. Mechanism of preservation of glomerular perfusion and filtration during acute extracellular fluid volume depletion. Importance of intrarenal vasopressin-

prostaglandin interaction for protecting kidneys from constrictor action of vasopressin. *J Clin Invest* 75:1477, 1985.

51. Exton JH. Calcium-signalling in cells' molecular mechanisms. *Kidney Int* (suppl 23):S-68, 1987.
52. Terada Y, Tomita K, Nonoguchi H, et al. Differential localization and regulation of two types of vasopressin receptor messenger RNA in microdissected rat nephron segments using reverse transcription polymerase chain reaction. *J Clin Invest* 92:2339, 1993.
53. Ammar A, Roseau S, Butlen D. Pharmacological characterization of V1α vasopressin receptor in the rat cortical collecting duct. *Am J Physiol* 262:F456, 1992.
54. Ando Y, Breyer MD, Jacobson HR. Dose-dependent heterogeneous actions of vasopressin in rabbit cortical collecting tubules. *Am J Physiol* 256:F556, 1989.
55. Zimmerman EA, Ma L-Y, Nilaver G. Anatomical basis of thirst and vasopressin secretion. *Kidney Int* 32(suppl 21):S-14, 1987.
56. Zeigler ZR, Megaludis A, Fraley DS. Desmopressin (d-DAVP) effects on platelet rheology and von Willebrand factor activities in uremia. *Am J Hematol* 39:90, 1992.
57. Baylis PH. Osmoregulation and control of vasopressin secretion in healthy humans. *Am J Physiol* 253:R671, 1987.
58. Robertson GL. Physiology of ADH secretion. *Kidney Int* 32(suppl 21):S-20, 1987.
59. Verney EB. Absorption and excretion of water: The antidiuretic hormone. *Lancet* 2:781, 1946.
60. Choi-Kwon S, Baertschi AJ. Splanchnic osmosensation and vasopressin: Mechanisms and neural pathways. *Am J Physiol* 261:E18, 1991.
61. Oliet SH, Bourque CW. Mechanosensitive channels transduce osmosensitivity in supraoptic neurons. *Nature* 364:341, 1993.
62. Voisin DL, Chakfe Y, Bourque CW. Coincident detection of CSF Na$^+$ and osmotic pressure in osmoregulatory neurons of the supraoptic nucleus. *Neuron* 24:253, 1999.
63. Vokes TP, Aycinena PR, Robertson GL. Effects of insulin on osmoregulation of vasopressin. *Am J Physiol* 252:E538, 1987.
64. Leaf A, Mamby AR. The normal antidiuretic mechanism in man and dog: Its regulation by extracellular fluid tonicity. *J Clin Invest* 31:54, 1952.
65. Lindheimer MD, Marron WM, Davison JM. Osmoregulation of thirst and vasopressin release in pregnancy. *Am J Physiol* 257:F1598, 1989.
66. Thompson CJ, Selby P, Baylis PH. Reproducibility of osmotic and nonosmotic tests of vasopressin secretion in men. *Am J Physiol* 260:R533, 1991.
67. Mann JFE, Johnson AK, Ritz E, Ganten D. Thirst and the renin-angiotensin system. *Kidney Int* 32(suppl 21):S-27, 1987.
68. Williams TDM, Lightman SL. Oral hypertonic saline causes transient fall of vasopressin in humans. *Am J Physiol* 251:R214, 1986.
69. Thompson CJ, Burd JM, Baylis PH. Acute suppression of plasma vasopressin and thirst after drinking in hypernatremic humans. *Am J Physiol* 252:R1138, 1987.
70. Appelgren BH, Thrasher TN, Keil LC, Ramsay DJ. Mechanism of drinking-induced inhibition of vasopressin secretion in dehydrated dogs. *Am J Physiol* 261:R1226, 1991.
71. Leaf A, Mamby AR. An antidiuretic mechanism not regulated by extracellular fluid tonicity. *J Clin Invest* 31:60, 1952.
72. Perez-Ayuso RM, Arroyo V, Campos J, et al. Evidence that renal prostraglandins are involved in renal water metabolism in cirrhosis. *Kidney Int* 26:72, 1984.
73. Mettauer B, Rouleua J-L, Bichet D, et al. Sodium and water excretion abnormalities in congestive heart failure. *Ann Intern Med* 105:161, 1986.
74. Bie P, Secher NH, Astrup A, Warberg J. Cardiovascular and endocrine responses to head-up tilt and vasopressin infusions in humans. *Am J Physiol* 251:R735, 1986.
75. Goldsmith SR, Francis GS, Cowley AW, Cohn JN. Response of vasopressin and norepinephrine to lower body negative pressure in humans. *Am J Physiol* 243:H970, 1982.
76. Anderson RJ, Cadnapaphornchai P, Harbottle JA, et al. Mechanism of effect of thoracic inferior vena cava constriction on renal water excretion. *J Clin Invest* 54:1473, 1974.

77. Goldsmith SR, Cowley AJ Jr, Francis GS, Cohn JN. Effect of increased intracardiac and arterial pressure on plasma vasopressin in humans. *Am J Physiol* 246:H647, 1984.

78. Dunn FL, Brennan TJ, Nelson AE, Robertson GL. The role of blood osmolality and volume in regulating vasopressin secretion in the rat. *J Clin Invest* 52:3212, 1973.

79. Editorial. Nausea and vasopressin. *Lancet* 337:1133, 1991.

80. Moore FD. Common patterns of water and electrolyte change in injury, surgery, and disease. *N Engl J Med* 258:277, 1958.

81. Ukai M, Moran W Jr, Zimmerman B. The role of visceral afferent pathways on vasopressin secretion and urinary excretory patterns during surgical stress. *Ann Surg* 168:16, 1968.

82. Arieff AI. Hyponatremia, convulsions, respiratory arrest, and permanent brain damage after elective surgery in healthy women. *N Engl J Med* 314:1529, 1986.

83. Davison JM, Shiells EA, Philips PR, Lindheimer MD. Serial evaluation of vasopressin release and thirst in human pregnancy. Role of human chorionic gonadotropin in the osmoregulatory changes of gestation. *J Clin Invest* 81:798, 1988.

84. Danielson LA, Sherwood OD, Conrad KP. Relaxin is a potent renal vasodilator in conscious rats. *J Clin Invest* 103:525, 1999.

85. White PC, New MI, Dupont B. Congenital adrenal hyperplasia. *N Engl J Med* 316:1519, 1987.

86. White PC. Disorders of aldosterone biosynthesis and action. *N Engl J Med* 331:250, 1994.

87. Ulick S, Wang JZ, Morton DH. The biochemical phenotypes of two inborn errors in the biosynthesis of aldosterone. *J Clin Endocrinol Metab* 74:1415, 1992.

88. Holland OB, Carr B. Modulation of aldosterone synthase messenger ribonucleic acid levels by dietary sodium and potassium and by adrenocorticotropin. *Endocrinology* 132:2666, 1993.

89. Taymans SE, Pack S, Pak E, et al. Human CYP11B2 (aldosterone synthase) maps to chromosome 8q24.3. *J Clin Endocrinol Metab* 83:1033, 1998.

90. Lifton RP, Dluhy RG, Powers M, et al. A chimeric 11-hydroxylase/aldosterone synthase gene causes glucocorticoid-remediable aldosteronism and human hypertension. *Nature* 355:262, 1992.

91. Horisberger J-D, Rossier BC. Aldosterone regulation of gene transcription leading to control of ion transport. *Hypertension* 19:221, 1992.

92. Minuth WW, Steckelings U, Gross P. Appearance of specific proteins in the apical plasma membrane of cultured renal collecting duct principal cell epithelium after chronic administration of aldosterone and arginine vasopressin. *Differentiation* 38:194, 1988.

93. Verrey F. Early aldosterone action: Toward filling the gap between transcription and transport. *Am J Physiol* 277:F319, 1999.

94. Masilamani S, Kim GH, Mitchel C, et al. Aldosterone-mediated regulation of ENaC alpha, beta, and gamma subunit proteins in rat kidney. *J Clin Invest* 104:R19, 1999.

95. Shimkets RA, Lifton R, Canessa CM. In vivo phosphorylation of the epithelial sodium channel. *Proc Natl Acad Sci U S A* 95:3301, 1998.

96. Chen SY, Bhargava A, Mastroberardino L, et al. Epithelial sodium channel regulated by aldosterone-induced protein sgk. *Proc Natl Acad Sci USA* 86:2514, 1999.

97. Naray-Fejes-Toth A, Canessa C, Cleaveland ES, et al. sgk is an aldosterone-induced kinase in the renal collecting duct. Effects on epithelial Na^+ channels. *J Biol Chem* 274:16973, 1999.

98. Spindler B, Verrey F. Aldosterone action: Induction of p21 (ras) and fra-2 and transcription-independent decrease in myc, jun, and fos. *Am J Physiol* 276:C1154, 1999.

99. Funder J. Enzymes and the regulation of sodium balance. *Kidney Int* 41(suppl 37):S114, 1992.

100. Kenouch S, Coutry N, Farman N, Bonvalet J-P. Multiple patterns of 11-hydroxysteroid dehydrogenase catalytic activity along the mammalian nephron. *Kidney Int* 42:56, 1992.

101. Funder JW. 11-β-hydroxysteroid dehydrogenase: New answers, new questions. *Eur J Endocrinol* 134:267, 1996.

102. Farese RV Jr, Biglieri EG, Shackleton CHL, et al. Licorice-induced hypermineralocorticoidism. *N Engl J Med* 325:1223, 1991.

103. Stanton B, Pan L, Deetjen H, et al. Independent effects of aldosterone and potassium on induction of potassium adaptation in rat kidney. *J Clin Invest* 79:198, 1987.

104. Garg LC, Knepper MA, Burg MB. Mineralocorticoid effects on Na-K-ATPase in individual nephron segments. *Am J Physiol* 240:F536, 1981.
105. Muto S, Muto S, Giebisch G. Na-dependent effects of DOCA on cellular transport properties of CCDs from ADX rabbits. *Am J Physiol* 253:F753, 1987.
106. Sansom S, Muto S, Giebisch G. Na-dependent effects of DOCA on cellular transport properties of CCDs from ADX rabbits. *Am J Physiol* 253:F753, 1987.
107. Rabinowitz L. Aldosterone and potassium homeostasis. *Kidney Int* 49:1738, 1996.
108. Husted RF, Laplace JR, Stokes JB. Enhancement of electrogenic Na^+ transport across rat inner medullary collecting duct by glucocorticoid and by mineralocorticoid hormones. *J Clin Invest* 86:498, 1990.
109. Frindt G, Sackin H, Palmer LG. Whole-cell currents in rat cortical collecting tubule: Low-Na diet increases amiloride-sensitive conductance. *Am J Physiol* 258:F502, 1990.
110. Kemendy AD, Kleyman TR, Eaton DC. Aldosterone alters the open probability of amiloride-blockable sodium channels in A6 epithelia. *Am J Physiol* 263:C825, 1992.
111. Hayhurst RA, O'Neil RG. Time-dependent actions of aldosterone and amiloride on Na^+-K^+-ATPase of cortical collecting duct. *Am J Physiol* 254:F689, 1988.
112. Coutry N, Blot-Chabaud M, Mateo P, et al. Time course of sodium-induced Na^+-K^+-ATPase recruitment in rabbit cortical collecting tubule. *Am J Physiol* 263:C61, 1992.
113. Fujii Y, Takemoto F, Katz AI. Early effects of aldosterone on Na-K pump in rat cortical collecting tubules. *Am J Physiol* 259:F40, 1990.
114. Garg LC, Narang N. Effects of aldosterone on NEM-sensitive ATPases in rabbit nephron segments. *Kidney Int* 34:13, 1988.
115. Hays SR. Mineralocorticoid modulation of apical and basolateral membrane H^+/OH^-/HCO_3^- transport process in rabbit inner stripe of outer medullary collecting duct. *J Clin Invest* 90:180, 1992.
116. Naray-Fejes-Toth A, Rusvai E, Fejes-Toth G. Mineralocorticoid receptors and 11-hydroxysteroid dehydrogenase activity in renal principal and intercalated cells. *Am J Physiol* 266:F76, 1994.
117. Batlle DC. Segmental characterization of defects in colleting tubule acidification. *Kidney Int* 30:546, 1986.
118. Lauler D, Hickler RB, Thorn G. The salivary sodium-potassium ratio. A useful "screening" test for aldosteronism in hypertension. *N Engl J Med* 267:1136, 1962.
119. Panese S, Martin RS, Virginillo M, et al. Mechanism of enhanced transcellular potassium-secretion in man with chronic renal failure. *Kidney Int* 31:1377, 1987.
120. Young DB. Quantitative analysis of aldosterone's role in potassium regulation. *Am J Physiol* 255:F811, 1988.
121. Shibata H, Ogishima T, Mitani F, et al. Regulation of aldosterone synthase cytochrome P450 in rat adrenals by angiotensin II and potassium. *Endocrinology* 128:2534, 1991.
122. Adler GK, Chen R, Menachery AI, et al. Sodium restriction increases aldosterone synthesis by increased late pathway, not early pathway, messenger ribonucleic acid levels and enzyme activity in normal rats. *Endocrinology* 133:2235, 1993.
123. Aguilera G, Catt KJ. Regulation of aldosterone secretion by the renin-angiotensin system during sodium restriction in rats. *Proc Natl Acad Sci U S A* 75:4057, 1978.
124. Ames R, Borkowski A, Sicinski A, Laragh J. Prolonged infusions of angiotensin II and norepinephrine on blood pressure, electrolyte balance, and aldosterone and cortisol secretion in normal man and in cirrhosis with ascites. *J Clin Invest* 44:1171, 1965.
125. Sansom SC, O'Neil RG. Mineralocorticoid requirement of apical cell membrane Na^+ and K^+ transport of the cortical collecting duct. *Am J Physiol* 248:F858, 1985.
126. Cooke CR, Gann DS, Whelton PK, et al. Hormonal responses to acute volume changes in anephric subjects. *Kidney Int* 23:71, 1983.
127. Himathongam T, Dluhy R, Williams GH. Potassium-aldosterone-renin interrelationships. *J Clin Endocrinol Metab* 41:153, 1975.
128. Young DB, Smith MJ Jr, Jackson TE, Scott RE. Multiplicative interaction between angiotensin II and K concentration in stimulation of aldosterone. *Am J Physiol* 247:E328, 1984.

129. Williams GH, Braley LM. Effects of dietary sodium and potassium intake on acute stimulation of aldosterone output by isolated human adrenal cells. *J Clin Endocrinol Metab* 45:55, 1977.
130. Pratt JH, Rothrock JK, Dominguez JH. Evidence that angiotensin-II and potassium collaborate to increase cytosolic calcium and stimulate the secretion of aldosterone. *Endocrinology* 125:2463, 1989.
131. Shier DN, Kusano E, Stoner GD, et al. Production of renin, angiotensin II, and aldosterone by adrenal explant cultures: Response to potassium and converting enzyme inhibition. *Endocrinology* 125:486, 1989.
132. Kifor I, Moore TJ, Fallo F, et al. Potassium-stimulated angiotensin release from superfused adrenal capsules and enzymatically digested cells of the zona glomerulosa. *Endocrinology* 129:823, 1991.
133. Rasmussen H. The calcium messenger system. *N Engl J Med* 31:1164, 1986.
134. Braley LM, Adler GK, Mortensen RM, et al. Dose effect of adrenocorticotropin on aldosterone and cortisol biosynthesis in cultured bovine adrenal glomerulosa cells. In vitro correlate of hyperreninemic hypoaldosteronism. *Endocrinology* 131:187, 1992.
135. Taylor RE Jr, Glass GT, Radke KJ, Schneider EG. Specificity of effect of osmolality on aldosterone secretion. *Am J Physiol* 252:E118, 1987.
136. Merrill DC, Ebert TJ, Skelton MM, Cowley AW Jr. Effect of plasma sodium on aldosterone secretion during angiotensin II stimulation in normal humans. *Hypertension* 14:164, 1989.
137. Bartter FC, Liddle GW, Duncan LE Jr, et al. The regulation of aldosterone secretion in man: The role of fluid volume. *J Clin Invest.* 35:1306, 1956.
138. Good DW, Wright FS. Luminal influences on potassium secretion: Sodium concentration and fluid flow rate. *Am J Physiol* 236:F192, 1979.
139. Jamison RL. Potassium recycling. *Kidney Int* 31:695, 1987.
140. Finn A, Welt L. Effect of aldosterone administration on electrolyte excretion and GFR in the rat. *Am J Physiol* 204:243, 1963.
141. George JM, Wright L, Bell NH, Bartter FC. The syndrome of primary aldosteronism. *Am J Med* 48:343, 1970.
142. August JT, Nelson DH, Thorn GW. Response of normal subjects to large amounts of aldosterone. *J Clin Invest* 37:1549, 1958.
143. Knox FG, Burnett JC Jr, Kohan DE, et al. Escape from the sodium-retaining effects of mineralocorticoids. *Kidney Int* 17:263, 1980.
144. Gonzalez-Campoy JM, Romero JC, Knox FG. Escape from the sodium-retaining effects of mineralcorticoids: Role of ANF and intrarenal hormone systems. *Kidney Int* 35:767, 1989.
145. Schwartz GJ, Burg MB. Mineralocorticoid effects on cation transport by cortical collecting tubules in vitro. *Am J Physiol* 235:F576, 1978.
146. Ballerman BJ, Bloch KD, Seidman JG, Brenner BM. Atrial natriuretic peptide transcription, secretion, and glomerular receptor activity during mineralocorticoid escape in the rat. *J Clin Invest* 78:840, 1986.
147. Capuccio FP, Markandu ND, Buckley MG, et al. Changes in the plasma levels of atrial natriuretic peptides during mineralocorticoid escape in man. *Clin Sci* 72:531, 1987.
148. Grunwald JE, Sakata M, Michener ML, et al. Is atriopeptin a physiological or pathophysiological substance? *J Clin Invest* 81:1036, 1988.
149. Hall JE, Granger JP, Smith MJ Jr, Premen AJ. Role of renal hemodynamics and arterial pressure in aldosterone "escape." *Hypertension* 6(suppl I): I-183, 1984.
150. Cowley AW. Role of the renal medulla in volume and arterial pressure regulation. *Am J Physiol* 273:R1, 1997.
151. Melby JC. Primary aldosteronism. *Kidney Int* 26:769, 1984.
152. de Wardener HE, Mills IH, Clapham WF, Hayter CJ. Studies on the efferent mechanism of the sodium diuresis which follows the administration of intravenous saline in the dog. *Clin Sci* 21:249, 1961.
153. DeBold AJ, Borenstein HB, Veress AT, Sonnenberg H. A rapid and potent natriuretic response to intravenous injection of atrial myocardial extract in rats. *Life Sci* 28:89, 1981.
154. Goetz KL. Physiology and pathophysiology of atrial peptides. *Am J Physiol* 254:E1, 1988.

155. Espiner EA, Richards AM, Yandle TG, et al. Natriuretic hormones. *Endocrinol Metab Clin North Am* 24:481, 1995.
156. Zeidel M, Kikeri D, Silva P, et al. Atrial natriuretic peptides inhibit conductive sodium uptake by rabbit inner medullary collecting duct cells. *J Clin Invest* 82:1067, 1988.
157. Weidmann P, Hasler L, Gnadinger MP, et al. Blood levels and renal effects of atrial natriuretic peptide in normal man. *J Clin Invest* 77:734, 1986.
158. Nonoguchi H, Knepper MA, Manganiello VC. Effects of atrial natriuretic peptide on cyclic guanosine monophosphate and cyclic adenosine monophosphate accumulation in microdissected nephron segments in rats. *J Clin Invest* 79:500, 1987.
159. Wilkins MR, Redondo J, Brown LA. The natriuretic peptide family. *Lancet* 349:1307, 1997.
160. Gunning ME, Brady HR, Otuechere G, et al. Atrial natriuretic peptide (31–67) inhibits Na$^+$ transport in rabbit inner medullary collecting duct. Role of prostaglandin E2. *J Clin Invest* 89:1411, 1992.
161. van de Stolpe A, Jamison RL. Micropuncture study of the effect of ANP on the papillary collecting duct in the rat. *Am J Physiol* 254:F477, 1988.
162. Ujiie K, Nonoguchi H, Tomita K, Marumo F. Effects of ANP and cGMP synthesis in inner medullary collecting duct subsegments of rats. *Am J Physiol* 259:F535, 1990.
163. Winaver J, Burnett JC, Tyce GM, Dousa TP. ANP inhibits Na$^+$-H$^+$ antiport in proximal tubular brush border membrane: Role of dopamine. *Kidney Int* 38:1133, 1990.
164. Brown J, O'Flynn MA. Acute effects of physiological increments of atrial natriuretic peptide. *Kidney Int* 36:645, 1989.
165. Mejia R, Sands JM, Stephenson JL, Knepper MA. Renal actions of atrial natriuretic factor: A mathematical modeling study. *Am J Physiol* 257:F1146, 1989.
166. Cogan MG. Atrial natriuretic peptide. *Kidney Int* 37:1148, 1990.
167. Fried TA, McCoy RN, Osgood RW, Stein JH. Effects of atriopeptin-II on determinants of glomerular filtration rate in the in vitro perfused dog glomerulus. *Am J Physiol* 250:F1119, 1986.
168. Ganguly A. Atrial natriuretic peptide–induced inhibition of aldosterone secretion: A quest for mediators. *Am J Physiol* 263:E181, 1992.
169. Cuneo RC, Espiner EA, Nicholls G, et al. Effect of physiological levels of atrial natriuretic peptide on hormone secretion: Inhibition of angiotensin-induced aldosterone secretion and renin release in normal man. *J Clin Endocrinol Metab* 65:765, 1987.
170. Harris PJ, Thomas D, Morgan TO. Atrial natriuretic peptide inhibits angiotensin-stimulated proximal tubular salt and water reabsorption. *Nature* 326:697, 1987.
171. Nonoguchi H, Sands JM, Knepper MA. Atrial natriuretic factor inhibits vasopressin-stimulated water permeability in rabbit inner medullary collecting duct. *J Clin Invest* 82:1383, 1988.
172. Morishita R, Gibbons G, Pratt RE, et al. Autocrine and paracrine effects of atrial natriuretic peptide gene transfer on vascular smooth muscle and endothelial cell growth. *J Clin Invest* 94:824, 1994.
173. Espiner WA, Richards AM, Yandle TG, et al. Natriuretic hormones. *Endocrinol Metab Clin North Am* 24:481, 1995.
174. Edwards BS, Zimmerman RS, Schwab TR. Atrial stretch, not pressure, is the principal determinant controlling the acute release of atrial natriuretic peptide. *Circ Res* 62:191, 1988.
175. Raine AEG, Erne P, Burgisser E, et al. Atrial natriuretic peptide and atrial pressure in patients with congestive heart failure. *N Engl J Med* 315:533, 1986.
176. Garcia R, Cantin M, Thibault G. Role of right and left atria in natriuresis and atrial natriuretic factor release during blood volume changes in the conscious rat. *Circ Res* 61:99, 1987.
177. Yasue H, Obata K, Okamura K, et al. Increased secretion of atrial natriuretic polypeptide from the left ventricle in patients with dilated cardiomyopathy. *J Clin Invest* 83:46, 1989.
178. Saito Y, Nakao K, Arai H, et al. Augmented expression of atrial natriuretic polypeptide gene in ventricle of human failing heart. *J Clin Invest* 83:298, 1989.
179. Gutkowska J, Nemer M, Sole MJ, et al. Lung is an important source of atrial natriuretic factor in experimental cardiomyopathy. *J Clin Invest* 83:1500, 1989.

180. Antunes-Rodrigues J, Machado BH, Andrade HA, et al. Carotid-aortic and renal barorecep-tors mediate the atrial natriuretic peptide release induced by blood volume expansion. *Proc Natl Acad Sci U S A* 89:6828, 1992.

181. Saxenhoffer H, Gnadinger MP, Weidmann P, et al. Plasma levels and dialysance of atrial natriuretic peptide in terminal renal failure. *Kidney Int* 32:554, 1987.

182. Homcy C, Gaivin R, Zisfein J, Graham RM. Snack-induced release of atrial natriuretic pep-tide (letter). *N Engl J Med* 313:1484, 1984.

183. Katoh Y, Kurosawa T, Takeda S, et al. Atrial natriuretic peptide levels in treated congestive heart failure. *Lancet* 1:851, 1986.

184. de Zeeuw D, Janssen WMT, de Jong PE. Atrial natriuretic factor: Its (patho)physiological significance in humans. *Kidney Int* 41:1115, 1992.

185. Goetz KL. Evidence that atriopeptin is not a physiological regulatory of sodium excretion. *Hypertension* 15:9, 1990.

186. Field LJ, Veress PT, Steinhelper ME, et al. Kidney function in ANF-transgenic mice: Effect of blood volume expanders. *Am J Physiol* 260:R1, 1991.

187. Davis CL, Briggs JP. Effect of reduction in renal arterial pressure on atrial natriuretic peptide–induced natriuresis. *Am J Physiol* 252:F146, 1987.

188. Redfield MM, Edwards BS, Heublein DM, Burnett JC Jr. Restoration of renal response to atrial natriuretic factor in experimental low-output heart failure. *Am J Physiol* 257:R917, 1989.

189. López C, Jiménez W, Arroyo V, et al. Role of altered systemic hemodynamics in the blunted renal response to atrial natriuretic peptide in rats with cirrhosis and ascites. *J Hepatol* 9:217, 1989.

190. Rudd MA, Plavin S, Hirsch AT, et al. Atrial natriuretic factor-specific antibody as a tool for physiological studies. Evidence for role of atrial natriuretic factor in aldosterone and renal elec-trolyte regulation. *Circ Res* 65:1324, 1989.

191. Awazu M, Imada T, Kon V, et al. Role of endogenous atrial natriuretic peptide in congestive heart failure. *Am J Physiol* 257:R641, 1989.

192. Northridge DB, Newby DE, Rooney E, et al. Comparison of the short-term effects of candox-atril, an orally active neutral endopeptidase inhibitor, and frusemide in the treatment of patients with chronic heart failure. *Am Heart J* 138:1149, 1999.

193. Wilkins MR, Unwin RJ, Kenny AJ. Endopeptidase-24.11 and its inhibitors: Potential thera-peutic agents for edematous disorders and hypertension. *Kidney Int* 43:273, 1993.

194. Chen HH, Schirger JA, Chau WL, et al. Renal response to acute neutral endopeptidase inhibi-tion in mild and severe experimental heart failure. *Circulation* 100:2443, 1999.

195. Margulies KB, Perella MA, McKinley LJ, Burnett JC Jr. Angiotensin inhibition potentiates the renal responses to neutral endopeptidase inhibition in dogs with congestive heart failure. *J Clin Invest* 88:1636, 1991.

196. Rouleau JL, Pfeffer MA, Stewart DJ, et al. Vasopeptidase inhibition or angiotensin converting enzyme in heart failure? Results of the IMPRESS trial. Presented at 72nd Annual Scientific Sessions of the American Heart Association, Atlanta, 1999.

197. Goetz KL. Renal natriuretic peptide (urodilatin?) and atriopeptin. Evolving concepts. *Am J Physiol* 261:F921, 1991.

198. Hildebrandt DA, Mizelle HL, Brands MW, Hall JE. Comparison of renal actions of urodilatin and atrial natriuretic peptide. *Am J Physiol* 262:R395, 1992.

199. Ritter D, Chao J, Needleman P, et al. Localization, synthetic regulation, and biology of renal atriopeptin-like prohormone. *Am J Physiol* 263:F503, 1992.

200. Endlich K, Forssman WG, Steinhausen M. Effects of urodilatin in the rat kidney: Comparison with ANF and interaction with vasoactive substances. *Kidney Int* 47:1558, 1995.

201. Mukoyama M, Nakao K, Hosada K, et al. Brain natriuretic peptide as a novel cardiac hor-mone in humans. Evidence for an exquisite dual natriuretic peptide system, atrial natriuretic peptide and brain natriuretic peptide. *J Clin Invest* 88:1402, 1991.

202. Davidson NC, Struthers AD. Brain natriuretic peptide. *J Hypertens* 12:329, 1994.

203. Berendes E, Walter M, Cullen P, et al. Secretion of brain natriuretic peptide in patients with aneurysmal subarachnoid hemorrhage. *Lancet* 349:245, 1997.

204. Vesely DL, Douglas MA, Dietz JR, et al. Three peptides from the atrial natriuretic factor prohormone amino terminus lower blood pressure and produce diuresis, natriuresis, and/or kaliuresis in humans. *Circulation* 90:1129, 1994.
205. Mattingly MT, Brandt RR, Heublein DM, et al. Presence of C-type natriuretic peptide in human kidney and urine. *Kidney Int* 46:744, 1994.
206. Barletta G, Lazzeri C, Vecchiarino S, et al. Low-dose C-type natriuretic peptide does not affect cardiac and renal function in humans. *Hypertension* 31:802, 1998.
207. Lerman A, Gibbons RJ, Rodeheffer RJ, et al. Circulating N-terminal atrial natriuretic peptide as a marker for symptomless left ventricular dysfunction. *Lancet* 341:1105, 1993.
208. Motwani JG, McAlpine H, Kennedy N, Struthers AD. Plasma brain natriuretic peptide as an indicator for angiotensin-converting-enzyme inhibition after myocardial infarction. *Lancet* 341:1109, 1993.
209. McDonagh TA, Robb SD, Murdoch DR, et al. Biochemical detection of left-ventricular systolic dysfunction. *Lancet* 351:9, 1998.
210. Farman N, Fradelles P, Bonvalet J-P. PGE_2, $PGF_{2\alpha}$, 6-keto-$PGF_{1\alpha}$, and TxB_2 synthesis along the rabbit nephron. *Am J Physiol* 252:F53, 1987.
211. Stahl RAK, Paravicini M, Schollmeyer P. Angiotensin II stimulation of prostaglandin E_2 and 6-keto-$F_{1\alpha}$ formation by isolated human glomeruli. *Kidney Int* 26:30, 1984.
212. DeWitt DL, Meade EA, Smith WL. PGH synthase isoenzyme selectivity: The potential for safer nonsteroidal antiinflammatory drugs. *Am J Med* 95:40S, 1993.
213. Remuzzi F, FitzGerald GA, Patrono C. Thromboxane synthesis and action within the kidney. *Kidney Int* 41:1483, 1992.
214. Badr KF, Brenner BM, Ichikawa I. Effects of leukotriene D_4 on glomerular dynamics in the art. *Am J Physiol* 253:F239, 1987.
215. Carroll MA, Balazy M, Huang DD, et al. Cytochrome P450-derived renal HETES: Storage and release. *Kidney Int* 51:1696, 1997.
216. Patrono C, Dunn MJ. The clinical significance of inhibition of renal prostaglandin synthesis. *Kidney Int* 32:1, 1987.
217. Oates JA, Fitzgerald GA, Branch RA, et al. Clinical implications of prostaglandin and thromboxane A_2 formation. *N Engl J Med* 319:761, 1988.
218. Simon LS, Weaver AL, Graham DY, et al. Anti-inflammatory and upper gastrointestinal effects of celecoxib in rheumatoid arthritis: A randomized controlled trial [see comments]. *JAMA* 282:1921, 1999.
219. Langman MJ, Jensen DM, Watson DJ, et al. Adverse upper gastrointestinal effects of rofecoxib compared with NSAIDs. *JAMA* 282:1929, 1999.
220. Dubois RN, Abramson SB, Crofford L, et al. Cyclooxygenase in biology and disease. *FASEB J* 12:1063, 1998.
221. Morhan SG, Langenbach R, Loftin CD, et al. Prostaglandin syntase 2 gene disruption causes severe renal pathology in the mouse. *Cell* 83:473, 1995.
222. Bryer MD, Jacobson HR, Breyer RM. Functional and molecular aspects of renal prostaglandin receptors. *J Am Soc Nephrol* 7:8, 1996.
223. Oliver JA, Pinto J, Sciacca RR, Cannon PJ. Increased renal secretion of norepinephrine and prostaglandin E2 during sodium depletion in the dog. *J Clin Invest* 66:748, 1980.
224. Chou S-Y, Dahnan A, Porush JG. Renal actions of endothelin: Interaction with prostacyclin. *Am J Physiol* 259:F645, 1990.
225. Schor N, Ichikawa I, Brenner BM. Glomerular adaptations to chronic dietary salt restriction or excess. *Am J Physiol* 238:F428, 1980.
226. Clive DM, Stoff JS. Renal syndromes associated with nonsteroidal anti-inflammatory drugs. *N Engl J Med* 310:563, 1984.
227. Dzau VJ, Packer M, Lilly LS, et al. Prostaglandins in severe congestive heart failure. Relation to activation of the renin-angiotensin system and hyponatremia. *N Engl J Med* 310:347, 1984.

228. Laffi G, Daskalopoulos G, Kronberg I, et al. Effects of sulindac and ibuprofen in patients with cirrhosis and ascites. An explanation for the renal-sparing effect of sulindac. *Gastroenterology* 90:182, 1986.

229. Zipser RD, Hoefs JC, Speckart PF, et al. Prostaglandins: Modulators of renal function and pressor resistance in chronic liver disease. *J Clin Endocrinol Metab* 48:895, 1979.

230. Pope JE, Anderson JJ, Felson DT. A meta-analysis of the effects of nonsteroidal anti-inflammatory drugs on blood pressure. *Arch Intern Med* 153:477, 1993.

231. Wong DG, Spence JD, Lamki L, et al. Effect of non-steroidal anti-inflammatory drugs on control of hypertension by β-blockers and diuretics. *Lancet* 1:997, 1986.

232. Sahloul MZ, al-Kiek R, Ivanovich P, Mujais SK. Nonsteroidal anti-inflammatory drugs and antihypertensives. Cooperative malfeasance. *Nephron* 56:345, 1990.

233. Dzau VJ. Renal and circulatory mechanisms in congestive heart failure. *Kidney Int* 31:1402, 1987.

234. Freeman RH, Davis JO, Villareal D. Role of renal prostaglandins in the control of renin release. *Circ Res* 54:1, 1984.

235. Ho S, Carretero OA, Abe K, et al. Effect of prostanoids on renin release from rabbit afferent arterioles with and without macula densa. *Kidney Int* 35:1138, 1989.

236. Ruilope LM, Robles RG, Paya C, et al. Effects of long-term treatment with indomethacin on renal function. *Hypertension* 8:677, 1986.

237. Whelton A, Stout RL, Spilman PS, Klassen DK. Renal effects of ibuprofen, piroxicam, and sulindac in patients with asymptomatic renal failure. A prospective, randomized, crossover comparison. *Ann Intern Med* 112:568, 1990.

238. Zimran A, Dramer M, Plaskin M, Hershko C. Incidence of hyperkalaemia induced by indomethacin in a hospital population. *Br Med J* 291:107, 1985.

239. Kramer HJ, Glanzer K, Dusing R. Role of prostaglandins in the regulation of renal water excretion. *Kidney Int* 19:851, 1981.

240. Berl T, Raz A, Wald H, et al. Prostaglandin synthesis inhibition and the action of vasopressin: Studies in man and rat. *Am J Physiol* 232:F529, 1977.

241. Herbert RL, Jacobson HR, Breyer MD. Prostaglandin E_2 inhibits sodium transport in rabbit cortical collecting duct by increasing intracellular calcium. *J Clin Invest* 87:1992, 1991.

242. Satoh T, Cohen HT, Katz AI. Intracellular signalling in the regulation of renal Na-K-ATPase. I. Role of cyclic AMP. *J Clin Invest* 89:1496, 1992.

243. Ling BN, Kokko KE, Eaton DC. Inhibition of apical Na^+ channels in rabbit cortical collecting tubules by basolateral prostaglandin E_2 is modulated by protein kinase C. *J Clin Invest* 90:1328, 1992.

244. Chen L, Reif MC, Schafer J. Clonidine and PGE_2 have different effects on Na^+ and water transport in rat and rabbit CCD. *Am J Physiol* 261:F123, 1991.

245. Zeidel ML, Brady HR, Kone BC, et al. Endothelin, a peptide inhibitor of Na^+-K^+-ATPase in intact renal tubular epithelial cells. *Am J Physiol* 257:C1101, 1989.

246. Brater DC. Analysis of the effect of indomethacin on the response to furosemide in man: Effect of dose of furosemide. *J Pharmacol Exp Ther* 210:386, 1979.

247. Silva P, Rosen S, Spokes K, et al. Influence of endogenous prostaglandins on mTAL injury. *J Am Soc Nephrol* 1:808, 1990.

248. Kumar R. Vitamin D and calcium transport. *Kidney Int* 40:1177, 1991.

249. Holick MF. Vitamin D and the kidney. *Kidney Int* 32:912, 1987.

250. Reichel H, Koeffler HP, Norman AW. The role of the vitamin D endocrine system in health and disease. *N Engl J Med* 320:980, 1989.

251. Brown EM. PTH secretion in vivo and in vitro. Regulation by calcium and other secretagogues. *Miner Electrolyte Metab* 8:130, 1982.

252. Brown EM, Herbert SC. Calcium-receptor-regulated parathyroid and renal function. *Bone* 20:303, 1997.

253. Brown AJ, Dusso A, Slatopolsky E. Vitamin D. *Am J Physiol* 277:F157, 1999.

254. Kurokawa K. Calcium-regulating hormones and the kidney. *Kidney Int* 32:760, 1987.

255. Brown EM, Herbert SC. A cloned extracellular Ca^{2+}-sensing receptor: Molecular mediator of the actions of extracellular Ca^{2+} on parathyroid and kidney cells? *Kidney Int* 49:1042, 1996.
256. Cole DE, Peltekova VD, Rubin LA, et al. A986S polymorphism of the calcium-sensing receptor and circulating calcium concentrations. *Lancet* 353:112, 1999.
257. Pollak MR, Brown EM, Chou YH, et al. Mutations in the human Ca^{2+}-sensing receptor gene causes familial hypocalciuric hypercalcemia and neonatal severe hyperparathyroidism. *Cell* 75:1297, 1993.
258. Pollak MR, Chou YH, Marx SJ, et al. Familial hypocalciuric hypercalcemia and neonatal severe hyperparathyroidism. Effects of mutant gene dosage on phenotype. *J Clin Invest* 93:1108, 1994.
259. Rose BD, Hebert SC. Disorders of the calcium-sensing receptor: Familial hypocalciuric hypercalcemia and autosomal dominant hypocalcemia. In Rose BD (ed): *UpToDate in Medicine* Wellesley, MA, UpToDate, 2000
260. Chabardes D, Gagnan-Brunette M, Imbert-Teboul M, et al. Adenylate cyclase responsiveness to hormones in various portions of the human nephron. *J Clin Invest* 65:439, 1980.
261. Biber J, Custer M, Magagnin S, et al. Renal Na/Pi-cotransporters. *Kidney Int* 49:981, 1996.
262. Dunlay R, Hruska K. PTH receptor coupling to phospholipase C is an alternate pathway of signal transduction in bone and kidney. *Am J Physiol* 258:F223, 1990.
263. Sheu JN, Baum M, Harkins EW, Quigley R. Maturational changes in rabbit renal cortical phospholipase A_2 activity. *Kidney Int* 52:71, 1997.
264. Murer H, Werner A, Reshkin S, et al. Cellular mechanisms in proximal tubular reabsorption of inorganic phosphate. *Am J Physiol* 260:C885, 1991.
265. Murer H, Lotscher M, Kaissling B, et al. Renal brush border membrane Na/Pi-cotransport: Molecular aspects in PTH-dependent and dietary regulation. *Kidney Int* 49:1769, 1996.
266. Pfister M, Lederer E, Forgo J, et al. Downregulation of the Na/Pi cotransporter type II by parathyroid hormone (PTH) in OK cells. *J Biol Chem* 272:20125, 1997.
267. Friedman PA, Gesek FA. Calcium transport in renal epithelial cells. *Am J Physiol* 264:F181, 1993.
268. Gesek GA, Friedman PA. On the mechanism of parathyroid hormone stimulation of calcium uptake by mouse distal convoluted tubule cells. *J Clin Invest* 90:749, 1992.
269. Bouhtiauy I, Lajeunessè D, Brunette MG. The mechanisms of parathyroid hormone action on calcium reabsorption by the distal tubule. *Endocrinology* 128:251, 1991.
270. Bichara M, Mercier O, Borensztein P, Paillard M. Acute metabolic acidosis enhances circulating parathyroid hormone which contributes to the renal response against acidosis in the rat. *J Clin Invest* 86:430, 1990.
271. Kawashima H, Kurokawa K. Metabolism and sites of action of vitamin D in the kidney. *Kidney Int* 29:98, 1986.
272. Takeyama K, Kitanaka S, Sato T, et al. 25-hydroxyvitamin D_2 1α-hydroxylase and vitamin D synthesis. *Science* 277:1827, 1997.
273. Zehnder D, Bland R, Walker EA, et al. Expression of 25-hydroxyvitamin D3-1α-hydroxylase in the human kidney. *J Am Soc Nephrol* 10:2465, 1999.
274. Cadranel J, Garabedian M, Milleron B, et al. 1,25$(OH)_2D_3$ production by T lymphocytes and alveolar macrophages recovered by lavage from normocalcemic patients with tuberculosis. *J Clin Invest* 85:1588, 1990.
275. Dusso A, Finch J, Delmez J, et al. Extrarenal production of calcitriol. *Kidney Int* 38(suppl 29):S-36, 1990.
276. Reichel H, Koeffler HP, Barbers R, Norman AW. Regulation of 1,25-dihydroxyvitamin D3 production by cultured alveolar macrophages from normal donors and from patients with pulmonary sarcoidosis. *J Clin Endocrinol Metab* 65:1201, 1987.
277. Sharma OP. Vitamin D, calcium, and sarcoidosis. *Chest* 109:535, 1996.
278. Sandler LM, Winearls CG, Fraher LJ, et al. Studies of the hypercalcemia of sarcoidosis: Effects of steroids and exogenous vitamin D_3 on the circulating concentration of 1,25-dihydroxy vitamin D_3. *Q J Med* 53:165, 1984.

279. Kozeny GA, Barbato AL, Bansal VK, et al. Hypercalcemia associated with silicone-induced granulomas. *N Engl J Med* 311:1103, 1984.

280. Seymour JF, Gagel RF. Calcitriol: the major humoral mediator of hypercalcemia in Hodgkin's disease and non-Hodgkin's lymphomas. *Blood* 82:1383, 1993.

281. Adams JS. Vitamin D metabolite-related hypercalcemia. *Endocrinol Clin North Am* 18:765, 1989.

282. Dusso AS, Kamimura S, Gallieni M, et al. Gamma-interferon-induced resistance to 1.25-$(OH)_2D_3$ in human monocytes and macrophages: A mechanism for the hypercalcemia of various granulomatoses. *J Clin Endocrinol Metab* 82:2222, 1997.

283. Portale AA, Halloran PP, Morris RC Jr. Physiologic regulation of the serum concentration of 1,25-dihydroxyvitamin D by phosphorus in normal men. *J Clin Invest* 83:1494, 1989.

284. Matsumoto T, Ikeda K, Morita K, et al. Blood Ca^{2+} modulates responsiveness of renal 25(OH)D3-1a-hydroxylase to PTH in rats. *Am J Physiol* 253:E503, 1987.

285. Tenenhouse HS, Hoag HM, Gauthier C, et al. Effect of Na^+-phosphate cotransporter (NPT2) gene knock-out on renal 25-hydroxyvitamin D-1α- and 24-hydroxylase gene expression (abstract). *J Am Soc Nephrol* 9:571A, 1998.

286. Gerblich AA, Genuth SM, Haddad JG. A case of idiopathic hypoparathyroidism and dietary vitamin D deficiency: The requirement for calcium and vitamin D for bone, but not renal responsiveness to PTH. *J Clin Endocrinol Metab* 44:507, 1977.

287. Bouhtiauy I, Lajeunessé D, Brunnette MG. Effect of vitamin D depletion on calcium transport by the luminal and basolateral membrane of the proximal and distal nephrons. *Endocrinology* 132:115, 1993.

288. Russell J, Lettieri D, Sherwood LM. Suppression by $1,25(OH)_2D_3$ of transcription of preproparathyroid hormone gene. *Endocrinology* 119:2864, 1986.

289. Slatopolsky E, Lopez-Hilker S, Delmez J, et al. The parathyroid-calcitriol axis in health and chronic renal failure. *Kidney Int* 38(suppl 29):S-41, 1990.

290. Slatopolsky E, Weerts C, Thielan J, et al. Marked suppression of secondary hyperarathyroidism by intravenous administration of 1,25-dihydroxycholecalciferol in uremic patients. *J Clin Invest* 74:2136, 1984.

291. Levi M, Lotscher M, Sorribas V, et al. Cellular mechanisms of acute and chronic adaptation of rat renal Pi transporter to alterations in dietary Pi. *Am J Physiol* 267:F900, 1994.

292. Hruska KA, Teitelbaum SL. Mechanisms of disease: Renal osteodystrophy. *N Engl J Med* 333:166, 1995.

293. Malluche H, Faugere M-C. Renal bone disease 1990: An unmet challenge for the nephrologist. *Kidney Int* 38:193, 1990.

294. Rose BD, Henrich WL. Pathogenesis of renal osteodystrophy. In Rose BD (ed): *UpToDate in Medicine*. Wellesley, MA, UpToDate, 2000.

295. Slatopolsky E, Bricker NS. The role of phosphorus restriction in the prevention of secondary hyperparathyroidism in chronic renal disease. *Kidney Int* 4:141, 1973.

296. Rutherford WE, Bordier P, Marie P, et al. Phosphate control and 25-hydroxycholecalciferol administration in preventing experimental renal osteodystrophy in the dog. *J Clin Invest* 60:332, 1977.

297. Herbert LA, Lemann J Jr, Petersen JR, Lennon EJ. Studies of the mechanism by which phosphate infusion lowers serum calcium concentration. *J Clin Invest* 45:1886, 1966.

298. Adler AJ, Ferran N, Berlyne GM. Effects of inorganic phosphate on serum ionized calcium concentration in vitro: A reassessment of the trade-off hypothesis. *Kidney Int* 28:932, 1985.

299. Lopez-Hilker S, Galceran T, Chan Y-L, et al. Hypocalcemia may not be essential for the development of secondary hyperparathyroidism in chronic renal failure. *J Clin Invest* 78:1097, 1986.

300. Koenig KG, Lindberg JS, Zerwekh JE, et al. Free and total 1,25-dihydroxyvitamin D levels in subjects with renal disease. *Kidney Int* 41:161, 1992.

301. Prince RL, Hutchinson BG, Kent JC. Calcitriol deficiency with retained synthetic reserve in chronic renal failure. *Kidney Int* 33:722, 1988.

302. Llach F, Massry SG. On the mechanism of secondary hyperparathyroidism in moderate renal insufficiency. *J Clin Endocrinol Metab* 61:601, 1985.
303. Portale AA, Booth BE, Halloran BP, Morris RC Jr. Effect of dietary phosphate on circulating concentrations on 1,25-dihydroxyvitamin D and immunoreactive parathyroid hormone in children with moderate renal insufficiency. *J Clin Invest* 73:1580, 1984.
304. Slatopolsky E, Finch J, Denda M, et al. Phosphorus restriction prevents parathyroid gland growth. High prosphorus directly stimulates PTH secretion in vitro. *J Clin Invest* 97:2534, 1996.
305. Fine A, Cox D, Fontaine B. Elevation of serum phosphate levels affects parathyroid hormone levels in only 50% of hemodialysis patients, which is unrelated to changes in serum calcium. *J Am Soc Nephrol* 3:1947, 1993.
306. Almaden Y, Hernandex A, Torregrosa V, et al. High phosphate level directly stimulates parathyroid hormone secretion and synthesis by human parathyroid tissue in vitro. *J Am Soc Nephrol* 9:1845, 1998.
307. Quarles LD, Davidai GA, Schwab SJ, et al. Oral calcitriol and calcium: Efficient therapy for uremic hyperparathyroidism. *Kidney Int* 34:840, 1988.
308. Fukuda N, Tanaka H, Tominaga Y, et al. Decreased 1,25-dihydroxyvitamin D3 receptor density is associated with a more severe form of parathyroid hyperplasia in chronic uremic patients. *J Clin Invest* 92:1436, 1993.
309. Hsu CH, Patel SR, Vanholder R. Mechanism of decreased intestinal calcitriol receptor concentration in renal failure. *Am J Physiol* 264:F662, 1993.
310. Hsu CH, Patel SR, Young EW, Vanholder R. The biological action of calcitriol in renal failure. *Kidney Int* 46:605, 1994.
311. Delmez JA, Dougan S, Gearing BK, et al. The effects of intraperitoneal calcitriol on calcium and parathyroid hormone. *Kidney Int* 31:795, 1987.
312. Andress DL, Coburn JW, et al. Intravenous calcitriol in the treatment of refractory osteitis fibrosa of chronic renal failure. *N Engl J Med* 321:274, 1989.
313. Slatopolsky E, Robson AM, Elkan I, Bricker NS. Control of phosphate excretion in uremic man. *J Clin Invest* 47:1865, 1968.
314. Katz AI, Hampers CL, Merill JP. Secondary hyperparathyroidism and renal osteodystrophy in chronic renal failure: Analysis of 195 patients with observations on the effects of chronic dialysis, kidney transplantation and subtotal parathyroidectomy. *Medicine* 48:333, 1969.
315. Llach F. Parathyroidectomy in chronic renal failure: Indications, surgical approach and the use of calcitriol. *Kidney Int* 38(suppl 29):S-62, 1990.
316. Gagne ER, Urena P, Leite-Silva S, et al. Short- and long-term efficacy of total parathyroidectomy with immediate autografting compared with subtotal parathyroidectomy in hemodialysis patients. *J Am Soc Nephrol* 3:1008, 1992.
317. Stracke S, Jehle PM, Sturm D, et al. Clinical course after total parathyroidectomy without autotransplantation in patients with end-stage renal failure. *Am J Kidney Dis* 33:304, 1999.
318. Fournier A, Moriniere P, Ben Hamida F, et al. Use of alkaline calcium salts as phosphate binder in uremic patients. *Kidney Int* 42(suppl 38):S-50, 1992.
319. Slatopolsky E, Weerts C, Lopez-Hilker S, et al. Calcium carbonate as a phosphate binder in patients with chronic renal failure undergoing dialysis. *N Engl J Med* 315:157, 1986.
320. Delmez JA, Tindira CA, Windus DW, et al. Calcium acetate as a phosphorus binder in hemodialysis patients. *J Am Soc Nephrol* 3:96, 1992.
321. Mai ML, Emmett M, Sheikh MS, et al. Calcium acetate, an effective phosphate binder in patients with chronic renal failure. *Kidney Int* 36:690, 1989.
322. Slatopolsky E. The interaction of parathyroid hormone and aluminum on renal osteodystrophy. *Kidney Int* 31:842, 1987.
323. Salusky TB, Foley J, Nelson P, Goodman WG. Aluminum accumulation during treatment with aluminum hydroxide and dialysis in children and young adults with chronic renal disease. *N Engl J Med* 324:527, 1991.
324. Molitoris BA, Froment DH, Mackenzie TA, et al. Citrate: A major factor in the toxicity of orally administered aluminum compounds. *Kidney Int* 36:949, 1989.

325. Schiller LR, Santa Ana CA, Shiekh MS, et al. Effect of the time of administration of calcium acetate on phosphorus binding. *N Engl J Med* 320:1110, 1989.

326. Slatopolsky EA, Burke SK, Dillon MA, and the RenaGel study group. RenaGel, a nonabsorbed calcium- and aluminium-free phosphate binder, lowers serum phosphorus and parathyroid hormone. *Kidney Int* 55:299, 1999.

327. Bleyer AJ, Burke SK, Dillon M, et al. A comparison of the calcium-free phosphate binder sevelamer hydrochloride with calcium acetate in the treatment of hyperphosphatemia in hemodialysis patients. *Am J Kidney Dis* 33:694, 1999.

328. Chertow GM, Dillon M, Burke SK, et al. A randomized trial of sevelamer hydrochloride (RenaGel) with and without supplemental calcium: Strategies for the control of hyperphosphatemia and hyperparathyroidism in hemodialysis patients. *Clin Nephrol* 51:18, 1999.

329. Coburn JW. Use of oral and parenteral calcitriol in the treatment of renal osteodystrophy. *Kidney Int* 38(suppl 29):S-54, 1990.

330. Slatopolsky E, Berkoben M, Kelber J, et al. Effects of calcitriol and non-calcemic vitamin D analogs on secondary hyperparathyroidism. *Kidney Int* 42(suppl 38):S-43, 1992.

331. Finch JL, Brown AJ, Kubodera N, et al. Differential effects of $1,25\text{-}(OH)_2D_3$ and 22-oxacalcitriol on phosphate and calcium metabolism. *Kidney Int* 43:561, 1993.

332. Tan AU, Levin BS, Mazess RB, et al. Effective suppression of parathyroid hormone by 1α-hydroxy-vitamin D2 in hemodialysis patients with moderate to severe secondary hyperparathyroidism. *Kidney Int* 51:317, 1997.

333. Monier-Faugeree M-C, Geng Z, Friedler RM, et al. 22-Oxacalcitriol suppresses secondary hyperparathyroidism without inducing low bone turnover in dogs with renal failure. *Kidney Int* 55:821, 1999.

334. Martin KJ, Gonzalez E, Gellens M, et al. 19-Nor-1α-25-dihydroxyvitamin D2 (Paricalcitol) safely and effectively reduces the levels of intact parathyroid hormone in patients on hemodialysis. *J Am Soc Nephrol* 9:1427, 1998.

335. Lefebvre A, de Vernejoul MC, Gueris J, et al. Optimal correction of acidosis changes progression of dialysis osteodystrophy. *Kidney Int* 36:1112, 1989.

336. Moss NG. Renal function and renal afferent and efferent nerve activity. *Am J Physiol* 243:F425, 1982.

337. DiBona GF. Neural control of renal function: Cardiovascular implications. *Hypertension* 13:539, 1989.

338. Barajas L, Powers K, Wang P. Innervation of the renal cortical tubules: A quantitative study. *Am J Physiol* 247:F50, 1984.

339. Tucker BJ, Mundy CA, Blantz RC. Adrenergic and angiotensin II influences on renal vascular tone in chronic sodium depletion. *Am J Physiol* 252:F811, 1987.

340. DiBona GF, Herman PJ, Sawin LL. Neural control of renal function in edema-forming states. *Am J Physiol* 254:R1017, 1988.

341. Osborn JL, Holdaas H, Thames MD, DiBona GF. Renal adrenoreceptor mediation of antinatriuretic and renin secretion responses to low frequency renal nerve stimulation in the dog. *Circ Res* 53:298, 1983.

342. Bello-Reuss E. Effect of catecholamines on fluid reabsorption by the isolated proximal convoluted tubule. *Am J Physiol* 238:F347, 1980.

343. Rouse D, Williams S, Suki WN. Clonidine inhibits fluid absorption in the rabbit proximal convoluted tubule. *Kidney Int* 38:80, 1990.

344. Pedrosa Ribeiro C, Ribeiro-Neto F, Field JB, Suki WN. Prevention of α_2-adrenergic inhibition of ADH action by pertussis toxin in rabbit cortical collecting tubule. *Am J Physiol* 253:C105, 1987.

345. Gellai M. Modulation of vasopressin antidiuretic action by renal α_2-adrenoceptors. *Am J Physiol* 259:F1, 1990.

346. Ehmke, Persson PB, Seyfarth M, Kirchheim HR. Neurogenic control of pressure natriuresis in conscious dogs. *Am J Physiol* 259:F466, 1990.

347. Jose PA, Raymond JR, Bates MD, et al. The renal dopamine receptors. *J Am Soc Nephrol* 2:1265, 1992.

348. Seri I, Cone BC, Gullans SR, et al. Influence of Na$^+$ intake on dopamine-induced inhibition of renal cortical Na$^+$– K$^+$–ATPase. *Am J Physiol* 258:F52, 1990.
349. Denton MD, Chertow GM, Brady HR. "Renal-dose" dopamine for the treatment of acute renal failure: Scientific rationale, experimental studies and clinical trials. *Kidney Int* 49:4, 1996.
350. DiBona GF. Renal dopamine containing nerves. What is their functional significance? *Am J Hypertens* 3:64s, 1990.
351. Steinhausen M, Weis S, Fleming J, et al. Response of in vivo renal microvessels to dopamine. *Kidney Int* 30:361, 1986.
352. Edwards RM. Response of isolated renal arterioles to acetylcholine, dopamine, and bradykinin. *Am J Physiol* 248:F183, 1985.
353. Bughi S, Horton R, Antonpillai I, et al. Comparison of dopamine and fenoldopam effects on renal blood flow and prostacyclin excretion in normal and essential hypertensive subjects. *J Clin Endocrinol Metab* 69:1116, 1989.
354. Olsen NV, Hansen JM, Ladefoged SD, et al. Renal tubular reabsorption of sodium and water during infusion of low-dose dopamine in normal man. *Clin Sci* 78:503, 1990.
355. Felder RA, Felder CC, Eisner GM, Jose PA. The dopamine receptor in adult and maturing kidney. *Am J Physiol* 257:F315, 1989.
356. Bello-Reuss E, Higashi Y, Kaneda Y. Dopamine decreases fluid reabsorption in straight potions of rabbit proximal tubule. *Am J Physiol* 242:F634, 1982.
357. Felder CC, Campbell T, Albrecht F, Jose PA. Dopamine inhibits Na$^+$-H$^+$ exchanger activity in renal BBMV by stimulation of adenylate cyclase. *Am J Physiol* 259:F297, 1990.
358. Aperia A, Fryckstedt J, Svensson L, et al. Phosphorylated Mr 32,000 dopamine- and cAMP-regulated phosphoprotein inhibits Na$^+$-K$^+$-ATPase activity in renal tubule cells. *Proc Natl Acad Sci U S A* 88:2798, 1991.
359. Alexander RW, Gill JR Jr, Yamabe H, et al. Effects of dietary sodium and of acute saline infusion on the interrelationship between dopamine excretion and adrenergic activity in man. *J Clin Invest* 54:194, 1974.
360. Hansell P, Fasching A. The effect of dopamine receptor blockade on natriuresis is dependent on the degree of hypervolemia. *Kidney Int* 93:253, 1991.
361. Lassnigg A, Donner E, Grubhofer G, et al. Lack of renoprotective effects of dopamine and furosemide during cardiac surgery. *J Am Soc Nephrol* 11:97, 2000.
362. Marik PE, Iglesias J. Low-dose dopamine does not prevent acute renal failure in patients with septic shock and oliguria. NORASEPT II Study Investigators [In Process Citation]. *Am J Med* 107:387, 1999.
363. Vargo DL, Brater DC, Rudy DW, Swan SK. Dopamine does not enhance furosemide-induced natriuresis in patients with congestive heart failure. *J Am Soc Nephrol* 7:1032, 1996.
364. Scicli AG, Carretero OA. Renal kallikrein-kinin system. *Kidney Int* 29:120, 1986.
365. Fuller PJ, Funder JW. The cellular physiology of glandular kallikrein. *Kidney Int* 29:953, 1986.
366. Johnston PA, Bernard DB, Perrin NS, et al. Control of rat renal vascular resistance during alterations in sodium balance. *Circ Res* 48:728, 1981.
367. Margolius HS. Kallikreins and kinins: Some unanswered questions about system characteristics and roles in human disease. *Hypertension* 26:221, 1995.
368. Zeidel ML, Jabs K, Kikeri D, Silva P. Kinins inhibit conductive Na$^+$ uptake by rabbit inner medullary collecting duct cells. *Am J Physiol* 258:F1584, 1990.
369. el-Dahr SS, Figueroa CD, Gonzalez CB, Muller-Esterl W. Ontogeny of bradykinin B2 receptors in the rat kidney: Implications for segmental nephron maturation. *Kidney Int* 51:739, 1997.
370. Erslev AJ. Erythropoietin. *N Engl J Med* 324:1339, 1991.
371. Wu H, Liu X, Jaenisch R, et al. Generation of committed erythroid BFU-E and CFU-E progenitors does not require erythropoietin or the erythropoietin receptor. *Cell* 83:59, 1995.
372. Maxwell PH, Osmond MK, Pugh CW, et al. Identification of the renal erythropoietin-producing cells using transgenic mice. *Kidney Int* 44:1149, 1993.
373. Ratcliffe PJ. Molecular biology of erythropoietin. *Kidney Int* 44:887, 1993.

374. Loya F, Yang Y, Lin H, et al. Transgenic mice carrying the erythropoietin gene promoter linked to lacZ express the reporter in proximal convoluted tubule cells after hypoxia. *Blood* 84:1831, 1994.
375. Goldberg MA, Dunning SP, Bunn HF. Regulation of the erythropoietin gene: Evidence that the oxygen sensor is a heme protein. *Science* 242:1412, 1988.
376. Acker H. Mechanisms and meaning of cellular oxygen sensing in the organism. *Respir Physiol* 95:1, 1994.
377. Ebert BL, Bunn HF. Regulation of the erythropoietin gene. *Blood* 94:1864, 1999.
378. Blanchard KT, Fandrey J, Goldberg MA, et al. Regulation of the erythropoietin gene. *Stem Cells* 11(suppl 1):1, 1993.
379. Porter DL, Goldberg MA. Regulation of erythropoietin production. *Exp Hematol* 21:399, 1993.
380. Beck I, Weinmann R, Caro J. Characterization of the hypoxia-responsive enhancer in the human erythropoietin gene shows presence of hypoxia-inducible 120 Kd nuclear DNA-binding protein in erythropoietin-producing and nonproducing cells. *Blood* 82:704, 1993.
381. Semenza GL. Regulation of erythropoietin production. New insights into molecular mechanisms of oxygen homeostasis. *Hematol Oncol Clin North Am* 8:863, 1994.
382. Wang GL, Jiang BH, Rue EA, et al. Hypoxia-inducible factor 1 is a basic-helix-loop-helix-PAS heterodimer regulated by cellular C_2 tension. *Proc Natl Acad Sci U S A* 92:5510, 1995.
383. Wang GL, Semenza GL. Purification and characterization of hypoxia-inducible factor 1. *J Biol Chem* 270:1230, 1995.
384. Yu AY, Shimoda LA, Iyer NV, et al. Impaired physiological responses to chronic hypoxia in mice partially deficient for hypoxia-inducible factor 1α. *J Clin Invest* 103:691, 1999.
385. Besarab A, Caro J, Jarrell BE, et al. Dynamics of erythropoiesis following renal transplantation. *Kidney Int* 32:526, 1987.
386. Eschbach JW, Egrie JC, Downing MR, et al. Correction of anemia of end-stage renal disease with recombinant human erythropoietin: Results of a combined phase I and II clinical trial. *N Engl J Med* 316:73, 1987.
387. Cronin RE, Henrich WL. Erythropoietin for the anemia of chronic renal failure. In Rose BD (ed): *UpToDate in Medicine*. Wellesley, MA, UpToDate, 2000.
388. Besarab A, Bolton WK, Browne JK, et al. The effects of normal as compared with low hematocrit values in patients with cardiac disease who are receiving hemodialysis and epoetin. *N Engl J Med* 339:584, 1998.
389. Ma Jz, Ebben J, Xia H, Collins AJ. Hematocrit level and associated mortality in hemodialysis patients. *J Am Soc Nephrol* 10:610, 1999.
390. Hughes MR, Baylink DJ, Jones PG, Haussler MR. Radioligand receptor assay for 25-hydroxyvitamin D_2/D_3 and 1a-25-hydroxyvitamin D_2/D_3: Application to hypervitaminosis D. *J Clin Invest* 58:61, 1976.
391. Inoue A, Yanagisawa M, Kimura S, et al. The human endothelin family: Three structurally and pharamcologically distinct isopeptides predicted by three separate genes. *Proc Natl Acad Sci U S A* 86:2863, 1989.
392. Emoto N, Yanagisawa M. Endothelin-converting enzyme-2 is a membrane-bound phosphoramidon-sensitive metalloprotease with acidic pH optimum. *J Biol Chem* 270:15262, 1995.
393. Xu D, Emoto N, Giaid A, et al. ECE-1: A membrane-bound metalloprotease that catalyzes the proteolytic activation of big endothelin-1. *Cell* 78:473, 1994.
394. Hosoda K, Nakao K, Tamura N, et al. Organization, structure, chromosmal assignment, and expression of the gene encoding the human endothelin-A receptor. *J Biol Chem* 267:18797, 1992.
395. Sakamoto A, Yanagisawa M, Sakurai T, et al. Cloning and functional expression of human cDNA for the ETB endothelin receptor. *Biochem Biophys Res Commun* 178:656, 1991.
396. Yanagisawa M, Jurihara H, Kimura S, et al. A novel potent vasoconstrictor peptide produced by vascular endothelial cells. *Nature* 332:411, 1988.
397. Madeddu P, Troffa C, Glorioso N, et al. Effect of endothelin on regional hemodynamics and renal function in awake normotensive rats. *J Cardiovasc Pharmacol* 14:818, 1989.

398. Herizi A, Jover B, Bouriquet N, Mimran A. Prevention of the cardiovascular and renal effects of angiotensin II by endothelin blockade. *Hypertension* 31:10, 1998.

399. Verhaar MC, Strachan FE, Newby DE, et al. Endothelin-A receptor antagonist-mediated vasodilatation is attenuated by inhibition of nitric oxide synthesis and by endothelin-B receptor blockade. *Circulation* 97:752, 1998.

400. Kohan D. Endothelins in the normal and diseased kidney. *Am J Kidney Dis* 29:2, 1997.

401. Lanese DM, Conger JD. Effects of endothelin receptor antagonist on cyclosporine-induced vasoconstriciton in isolated rat renal arterioles. *J Clin Invest* 91:2144, 1993.

402. Garvin J, Sanders K. Endothelin inhibits fluid and bicarbonate transport in part by reducing Na^+/K^+ ATPase activity in the rat proximal straight tubule. *J Am Soc Nephrol* 2:976, 1991.

403. Ominato M, Satoh T, Katz AI. Endothelins inhibit Na-K-ATPase activity in proximal tubules: Studies of mechanisms. *J Am Soc Nephrol* 5:588, 1994.

404. Kohan D. Endothelins: Renal tubule synthesis and actions. *Clin Exp Pharmacol Physiol* 23:337, 1996.

405. Tomita K, Nonoguchi H, Marumo F. Effects of endothelin on peptide-dependent cyclic adenosine monophosphate accumulation along the nephron segments of the rat. *J Clin Invest* 85:2014, 1990.

406. Tomita K, Nonguchi H, Terada Y, et al. Effects of ET-1 on water and chloride transport in cortical collecting ducts of the rat. *Am J Physiol* 264:F690, 1993.

407. Ong ACM, Jowett TP, Firth JD, et al. An endothelin-1 mediated autocrine growth loop involved in human renal tubular regeneration. *Kidney Int* 48:390, 1995.

408. Ruiz-Ortega M, Gomez-Garre D, Alcazar R, et al. Involvement of angiotensin II and endothelin in matrix protein production and renal sclerosis. *J Hypertens Suppl* 12:S51, 1994.

409. Orisio S, Benigni A, Bruzzi I, et al. Renal endothelin gene expression is increased in remnant kidney and correlates with disease progression. *Kidney Int* 43:354, 1993.

410. Chatziantoniou C, Dussaule JC. Endothelial and renal vascular fibrosis: Of mice and men. *Curr Opin Nephrol Hypertens* 9:31, 2000.

411. Benigni A, Corna D, Maffi R, et al. Renoprotective effect of contemporary blocking of angiotensin II and endothelin-1 in rats with membranous nephropathy. *Kidney Int* 54:353, 1998.

412. Kone BC, Baylis C. Biosynthesis and homeostatic roles of nitric oxide in the normal kidney. *Am J Physiol* 272:F561, 1997.

413. Lane P, Gross SS. Cell signaling by nitric oxide. *Semin Nephrol* 19:215, 1999.

414. Bredt DS. Endogenous nitric oxide synthesis: Biological functions and pathophysiology. *Free Radic Res* 31:577, 1999.

415. Marsden PA, Brenner BM. Nitric oxide and endothelins: Novel autocrine/paracrine regulators of the circulation. *Semin Nephrol* 11:169, 1991.

416. Gow AJ, Stamler JS. Reactions between nitric oxide and haemoglobin under physiological conditions. *Nature* 391:169, 1998.

417. Ronson RS, Nakamura M, Vinten-Johansen J. The cardiovascular effects and implications of peroxynitrite. *Cardiovasc Res* 44:47, 1999.

418. Bankir L, Kriz W, Goligorsky M, et al. Vascular contributions to pathogenesis of acute renal failure. *Ren Fail* 20:663, 1998.

419. Kone BC, Higham S. Nitric oxide inhibits transcription of the Na^+-K^+-ATPase alpha1-subunit gene in an MTAL cell line. *Am J Physiol* 276:F614, 1999.

420. Kone BS. Localization and regulation of nitric oxide synthase isoforms in the kidney. *Semin Nephrol* 19:230, 1999.

421. Wu F, Park F, Cowley AW Jr, Mattson DL. Quantification of nitric oxide synthase activity in microdissected segments of the rat kidney. *Am J Physiol* 276:F874, 1999.

422. Marsden PA, Brock TA, Ballerman BJ. Glomerular endothelial cells respond to calcium-mobilizing agonists with release of EDRF. *Am J Physiol* 258:F1295, 1990.

423. Baylis C, Qiu C. Importance of nitric oxide in the control of renal hemodynamics. *Kidney Int* 49:1727, 1996.

424. Baylis C, Mitruka B, Deng A. Chronic blockade of nitric oxide synthesis in the rat produces systemic hypertension and glomerular damage. *J Clin Invest* 90:278, 1992.

425. Qiu C, Baylis C. Endothelin and angiotensin mediate most glomerular responses to nitric oxide inhibition. *Kidney Int* 55:2390, 1999.

426. Knowles JW, Reddick RL, Jennette JC, et al. Enhanced atherosclerosis and kidney dysfunction in eNOS[-/-]Apoe[-/-] mice are ameliorated by enalapril treatment. *J Clin Invest* 105:451, 2000.

427. Huang PL, Huang Z, Mashimo H, et al. Hypertension in mice lacking the gene for endothelial nitric oxide synthase. *Nature* 377:239, 1995.

428. Qiu C, Muchant D, Beierwaltes WH, et al. Evolution of chronic nitric oxide inhibition hypertension. Relationship to renal function. *Hypertension* 31:21, 1998.

429. Ohashi Y, Kawashima S, Hirata KI, et al. Hypotension and reduced nitric oxide–elicited vasorelaxation in transgenic mice overexpressing endothelial nitric oxide synthase. *J Clin Invest* 102:2061, 1998.

430. Veelken R, Hilgers KF, Hartner A, et al. Nitric oxide synthase isoforms and glomerular hyperfiltration in early diabetic nephropathy. *J Am Soc Nephrol* 11:71, 2000.

431. Bech JN, Nielsen CB, Ivarsen P, et al. Dietary sodium affects systemic and renal hemodynamic response to NO inhibition in healthy humans. *Am J Physiol* 274:F914, 1998.

432. Stoos BA, Garcia NH, Garvin JL. Nitric oxide inhibits sodium reabsorption in the isolated perfused cortical collecting duct. *J Am Soc Nephrol* 6:89, 1995.

433. Kang DG, Kim JW, Lee J. Effects of nitric oxide synthesis inhibition on the Na,K-ATPase activity in the kidney. *Pharmacol Res* 41:121, 2000.

434. Garcia NH, Pomposiello SI, Garvin JL. Nitric oxide inhibits ADH-stimulated osmotic water permeability in cortical collecting ducts. *Am J Physiol* 270:F206, 1996.

435. Welch WJ, Wilcox CS, Thomson SC. Nitric oxide and tubuloglomerular feedback. *Semin Nephrol* 19:251, 1999.

436. Wilcox CS, Welch WJ. TGF and nitric oxide: Effects of salt intake and salt-sensitive hypertension. *Kidney Int* (suppl 55):S-9, 1996.

437. Heeringa P, van Goor H, Itoh-Lindstrom Y, et al. Lack of endothelial nitric oxide synthase aggravates murine accelerated anti-glomerular basement membrane glomerulonephritis. *Am J Pathol* 156:879, 2000.

438. Goligorsky MS, Noiri E. Duality of nitric oxide in acute renal injury. *Semin Nephrol* 19:263, 1999.

439. Cattell V. Nitric oxide in glomerulonephritis. *Semin Nephrol* 19:277, 1999.

440. Jansen A, Cook T, Taylor GM, et al. Induction of nitric oxide synthase in rat immune complex glomerulonephritis. *Kidney Int* 45:1215, 1994.

441. Furusu A, Miyazaki M, Abe K, et al. Expression of endothelial and inducible nitric oxide synthase in human glomerulonephritis. *Kidney Int* 53:1760, 1998.

442. Marsden PA, Ballermann BJ. Tumor necrosis factor alpha activates soluble guanylate cyclase in bovine glomerular mesangial cells via an L-arginine-dependent mechanism. *J Exp Med* 172:1843, 1990.

REGULATION OF WATER
AND ELECTROLYTE BALANCE

CHAPTER

SEVEN

THE TOTAL BODY WATER AND
THE PLASMA SODIUM
CONCENTRATION

The body water is distributed among three major compartments: the intracellular space; the interstitium, which constitutes the extracellular environment of the cells; and the vascular space. Regulation of the intracellular volume, which is essential for normal cellular function, is achieved in part by regulation of the plasma osmolality through changes in *water* balance. In comparison, maintenance of the plasma volume, which is essential for adequate tissue perfusion, is closely related to the regulation of *sodium* balance. Sodium and water homeostasis will be reviewed in detail in the following two chapters. It is useful, however, to first discuss the factors involved in the distribution of water across the cell membrane (between the intracellular and extracellular fluids) and across the capillary wall (between the vascular space and the interstitium).

EXCHANGE OF WATER BETWEEN CELLULAR AND EXTRACELLULAR FLUIDS

Osmotic forces are the prime determinant of water distribution in the body. Water can freely cross almost all cell membranes; as a result, the body fluids are in osmotic equilibrium, as the osmolalities of the intracellular and extracellular fluids are the same.[1]

The concept of osmotic pressure can be easily understood from the simple experiment in Fig. 7-1. Suppose distilled water in a beaker is separated into two compartments by a membrane that is permeable to water but not to solutes, and glucose is added to the fluid on one side of the membrane. Water molecules exhibit

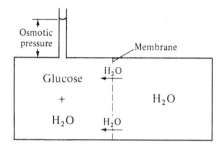

Figure 7-1   Effect of adding an impermeable solute such as glucose to the fluid on one side of a membrane. As water moves into the glucose compartment, a hydraulic pressure is generated (measured by the height of the column of water above the glucose compartment) which at equilibrium will be equal to the osmotic pressure of the solution.

random motion and can diffuse across a membrane by a mechanism similar to that for diffusion of solutes. When solutes are added to water, however, the intermolecular cohesive forces lead to a reduction in the random movement (or activity) of the water molecules.[2,3] Since water moves from an area of high activity to one of low activity, water will flow into the compartment containing glucose.

In theory, this movement of water, called *osmosis*, should continue indefinitely, because the activity of water will always be lower in the glucose compartment. However, since the compartment is rigid, the increase in volume will result in an elevation in hydrostatic pressure, causing the fluid column above the compartment to rise. This hydrostatic pressure tends to push water back into the solute-free compartment. Equilibrium will be reached when the hydrostatic pressure (as measured by the height of the column) is equal to the forces pulling water across the membrane. This hydrostatic pressure that opposes the osmotic movement of water is called the *osmotic pressure* of the solution.

The osmotic pressure that is generated is proportional to the *number of particles* per unit volume of solvent, not to the type, valence, or weight of the particles. The solute, however, must be unable to cross the cell membrane. Let us now consider what would happen in a beaker similar to that in Fig. 7-1 if a lipid-soluble and freely diffusible solute such as urea were added to one compartment (Fig. 7-2). The added urea would move down a concentration gradient into the solute-free compartment. The new equilibrium state would be characterized by equal urea concentrations in each compartment, not by water movement into the urea compartment. As a result, no osmotic pressure is generated by urea at equilibrium and urea is considered to be an *ineffective osmole*.

Osmotic pressure is important in vivo because it determines the distribution of water between the extracellular and intracellular spaces. Each of these compartments has one solute that is primarily limited to that compartment and therefore is the major determinant of its osmotic pressure: Na^+ salts are the principal extracellular osmoles and act to hold water in the extracellular space; conversely, K^+ salts account for almost all the intracellular osmoles (most of the other major cell cation, Mg^{2+}, is bound and osmotically inactive) and act to hold water within the cells.

Although the cell membrane is permeable to both Na^+ and K^+, these ions are able to act as effective osmoles because they are restricted to their respective

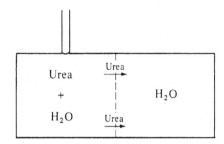

Figure 7-2 Effect of adding a permeable solute such as urea to the fluid on one side of a membrane. In this setting, equilibrium is reached by urea equilibration across the membrane rather than by water movement into the urea compartment. Consequently, no osmotic pressure is generated.

compartments by the Na^+-K^+-ATPase pump in the cell membrane. The net effect is that the volumes of the extracellular and intracellular fluids are determined by the amount of water present and by the ratio of *exchangeable* Na^+ to *exchangeable* K^+.*

Under normal circumstances, the water and electrolyte content in the body is maintained within relatively narrow limits, as variations in dietary intake are matched by appropriate changes in urinary excretion. Nevertheless, it is important to understand the potential physiologic effects of alterations in solute or water balance, since these disturbances often occur in the clinical setting.

If, for example, the osmolality of one fluid compartment is changed, water will move across the cell membrane to reestablish osmotic equilibrium. How this affects water distribution and solute concentration can be appreciated from the following examples (Fig. 7-3). For the sake of simplicity, let us assume that the osmolality of the body fluids is 280 mosmol/kg and is due entirely to 140 meq/L of Na^+ salts in the extracellular fluid and to 140 meq/L of K^+ salts in the cells; i.e., we are assuming that Na^+ and K^+ salts dissociate completely into cations and anions. As depicted in Fig. 7-3a, an average 70-kg man might have a total body water (TBW) of 42 liters (or 42 kg) of which 25 liters (60 percent) is intracellular and 17 liters (40 percent) is extracellular.

What will happen if 420 meq of NaCl (420 mosmol) without water is added to the extracellular fluid (Fig. 7-3b)? Since the NaCl remains extracellular, there will be an increase in the extracellular fluid osmolality, resulting in *water movement out of the cells* down an osmotic gradient. The following calculations can be used to estimate the characteristics of the total body water in the new equilibrium state:

1. Initial total body solute = 280 mosmol/kg × 42 kg = 11,760 mosmol
2. Initial extracellular solute = 280 mosmol/kg × 17 kg = 4760 mosmol
3. New total body solute = 11,760 + 420 = 12,180 mosmol

---

* The exchangeable portion is used because about 30 percent of the body Na^+ and a smaller fraction of the body K^+ are bound in areas such as bone, where they are "nonexchangeable" and therefore osmotically inactive. These ions also may be partially bound in intracellular organelles such as the nucleus and lysosomes.[4]

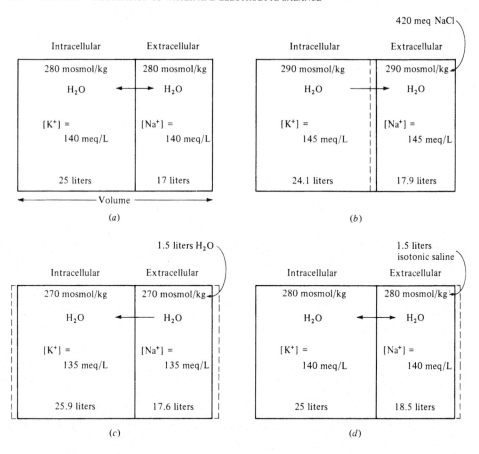

Figure 7-3 Osmolality of the body fluids and the distribution of the total body water between the intracellular and extracellular fluids (*a*) in the control state and after the addition of (*b*) NaCl, (*c*) H_2O, or (*d*) isotonic NaCl and H_2O to the extracellular fluid. For simplicity, it is assumed that Na^+ salts account for all the extracellular osmoles and K^+ salts for all the intracellular osmoles. See text for details. (*Adapted from Earley LE, in Maxwell MH, Kleeman CR (eds.):* Clinical Disorders of Fluid and Electrolyte Metabolism, *2d ed. New York: McGraw-Hill, 1972. Used with permission.*)

4. New body water osmolality = 12,180 mosmol ÷ 42 kg = 290 mosmol/kg
5. New extracellular solute = 4760 + 420 = 5180 mosmol
6. New extracellular volume = 5180 mosmol ÷ 290 mosmol/kg = 17.9 kg
7. New intracellular volume = 42 − 17.9 = 24.1 kg
8. New extracellular or plasma $[Na^+]$ = osmolality ÷ 2 = 145 meq/L

Thus, increasing the quantity of extracellular solute results in the movement of 900 mL of water from the cells into the extracellular fluid. The net effect is an *increase in the osmolality of both compartments*, even though the added solute is restricted to the extracellular space. This illustrates why the total body water (50 to

60 percent of lean body weight) must be used when calculating the volume of distribution of changes in plasma osmolality.

A different sequence occurs if 1.5 liters of solute-free water is added to the extracellular fluid, e.g., by ingestion. This reduces the extracellular fluid osmolality, creating an osmotic gradient favoring the *entry of water into the cells* (Fig. 7-3c). In estimating the new steady state, steps 1 and 2 are the same as those above:

1. Initial total body solute $= 11,760$ mosmol
2. Initial extracellular solute $= 4760$ mosmol
3. Initial intracellular solute $= 11,760 - 4760 = 7000$ mosmol
4. New total body water $= 42 + 1.5 = 43.5$ kg
5. New body water osmolality $= 11,760$ mosmol $\div 43.5$ kg $= 270$ mosmol/kg
6. New extracellular volume $= 4760$ mosmol $\div 270$ mosmol/kg $= 17.6$ kg
7. New intracellular volume $= 7000$ mosmol $\div 270$ mosmol/kg $= 25.9$ kg
8. Ratio of intracellular volume to TBW $= 25.9 \div 43.5 = 60$ percent
9. New extracellular or plasma $[Na^+]$ = osmolality $\div 2 = 135$ meq/L

Since there is no change in the ratio of intracellular to extracellular solute in this example, the fractional composition of the TBW is unchanged (cell water is still 60 percent of TBW). However, the TBW is increased, resulting in *expansion* and *dilution* of both compartments.*

Finally, if both NaCl and water are given as 1.5 liters of isotonic NaCl, there will be no change in osmolality and consequently no water movement across the cell membrane (Fig. 7-3d). Since the administered NaCl remains in the extracellular space, the *only effect* is a 1.5-liter increase in the extracellular fluid volume.

The results of these experiments are summarized in Table 7-1 and illustrate an important and often misunderstood concept, that the *plasma Na^+ concentration is a measure of concentration and not of volume*. In each instance, the extracellular fluid volume is increased because of an elevation in the TBW and/or the total exchangeable Na^+; despite this uniform change in volume, however, the plasma Na^+ concentration is, respectively, increased, decreased, and unchanged. This occurs because the plasma Na^+ concentration reflects the *ratio* of the amounts of solute and water present, not the absolute amount of either solute or water. Thus, there is *no necessary correlation between the plasma Na^+ concentration and the extracellular fluid volume*. These parameters change in a parallel direction when Na^+ is administered (Fig. 7-3b) but in an opposite direction (low plasma Na^+ concentration, high extracellular fluid volume) when water retention occurs (Fig. 7-3c). Furthermore, since the extracellular volume is the primary determinant of

---

* In this example, it is assumed that the administered water is retained. In normal subjects, however, excess water is excreted so rapidly that there is little change in volume or sodium excretion (see Chap. 9). Increases in extracellular volume and sodium excretion after a water load occur only if there is some defect in water excretion, as with persistent secretion of antidiuretic hormone (see Chap. 23).

Table 7-1 Osmotic and volume effects of addition of NaCl, water, and isotonic saline

Substance added	Plasma osmolality	Plasma sodium	Extracellular volume	Intracellular volume	Urine sodium
NaCl	↑	↑	↑	↓	↓
Water	↓	↓	↑	↑	↑
Isotonic NaCl	0	0	↑	0	↑

urinary sodium excretion (see Chap. 8), there is also *no relationship* between the plasma Na^+ concentration and the rate of sodium excretion (Table 7-1). When water is retained, for example, the plasma Na^+ concentration falls by dilution, but urinary sodium excretion will rise because of the increase in extracellular volume.

One final point deserves emphasis in these experiments. The intracellular volume varies inversely with the plasma Na^+ concentration, decreasing with hypernatremia and increasing with hyponatremia. These changes are important clinically because the neurologic symptoms associated with acute changes in the plasma Na^+ concentration are primarily related to these alterations in cell volume in the brain (see Chaps. 23 and 24).

Relation of Plasma Sodium Concentration to Osmolality

The osmolality of the plasma (P_{osm}) is equal to the sum of the osmolalities of the individual solutes in the plasma.* Most of the plasma osmoles are Na^+ salts, with lesser contributions from other ions, glucose, and urea. The osmotic effect of the plasma ions can usually be estimated from $2 \times$ *plasma Na^+ concentration*. The validity of this approximation results from the interplay of several factors:

- Ionic interactions in plasma *reduce the random movement* of NaCl so that it acts osmotically as if it were only 75 percent, not 100 percent, dissociated. As a result, 1 mmol of NaCl behaves as if it dissociates into roughly 1.75 particles (0.75 Na^+, 0.75 Cl^-, and 0.25 NaCl);[5] thus, the plasma Na^+ concentration must be multiplied by 1.75 to estimate the osmotic effect of sodium salts.
- Only 93 percent of the plasma is normally composed of water, with fat and proteins making up the remaining 7 percent. In most laboratories, the plasma Na^+ concentration is measured per liter of plasma. This value must be divided by 0.93 to arrive at the physiologically important Na^+ concentration in the plasma water (Na^+ being present only in the aqueous phase of plasma). Thus,

---

* The units and the methods used to measure the plasma osmolality are reviewed in Chap. 1.

$$\text{Osmolality of } Na^+ \text{ salts} = (1.75 \div 0.93) \times \text{plasma } [Na^+]$$

$$= 1.88 \times \text{plasma } [Na^+]$$

- The remaining $0.12 \times$ plasma Na^+ concentration is equal to $17 \, mosmol/kg$ (0.12×140), which happens to be the approximate osmotic pressure generated by K^+, Ca^{2+}, and Mg^{2+} salts.

The osmotic contributions of glucose and urea, both of which are measured in milligrams per deciliter, can be calculated from Eq. (7-1):

$$mosmol/kg = (mg/dL \times 10) \div mol \ wt \qquad (7\text{-}1)$$

The molecular weight of glucose is 180 and that of the two nitrogen atoms in urea (since urea is measured as the blood urea nitrogen, or BUN) is 28. Therefore, the P_{osm} can be estimated from

$$P_{osm} \cong 2 \times \text{plasma } [Na^+] + \frac{[glucose]}{18} + \frac{BUN}{2.8} \qquad (7\text{-}2)$$

The *effective* plasma (and extracellular fluid) osmolality is determined by those osmoles that act to hold water within the extracellular space. Since urea is an ineffective osmole,

$$\text{Effective } P_{osm} \cong 2 \times \text{plasma } [Na^+] + \frac{[glucose]}{18} \qquad (7\text{-}3)$$

The normal values for these parameters are

$$\text{Plasma } [Na^+] = 137\text{--}145 \, meq/L$$

$$[Glucose] = 60\text{--}100 \, mg/dL, \ \text{fasting}$$

$$BUN = 10\text{--}20 \, mg/dL$$

$$P_{osm} = 275\text{--}290 \, mosmol/kg$$

$$\text{Effective } P_{osm} = 270\text{--}285 \, mosmol/kg$$

Under normal circumstances, glucose accounts for only $5 \, mosmol/kg$, and Eq. (7-3) can be simplified to

$$\text{Effective } P_{osm} = 2 \times \text{plasma } [Na^+] \qquad (7\text{-}4)$$

Thus, in most conditions, the plasma Na^+ concentration is a reflection of the P_{osm}, a finding consistent with the fact that Na^+ salts are the principal extracellular osmoles.

Determinants of the Plasma Sodium Concentration

Since the body fluids are in osmotic equilibrium,

$$\text{Effective } P_{osm} = \text{effective osmolality of total body water}$$

$$= \frac{\text{extracellular solute} + \text{intracellular solute}}{\text{total body water}}$$

As described above, exchangeable Na^+ (Na_e^+) salts are the primary effective extracellular solutes, and exchangeable K^+ (K_e^+) salts are the primary effective intracellular solutes. Thus

$$\text{Effective } P_{osm} \cong \frac{2 \times Na_e^+ + 2 \times K_e^+}{\text{TBW}} \qquad (7\text{-}5)$$

(The multiple 2 is used to account for the osmotic contribution of the anions accompanying Na^+ and K^+.) If we now combine Eqs. (7-4) and (7-5), both of which are formulas for the effective P_{osm}, we get[5]

$$\text{Plasma } [Na^+] \cong \frac{Na_e^+ + K_e^+}{\text{TBW}} \qquad (7\text{-}6)$$

As illustrated in Fig. 7-4, this relationship holds over a wide range of plasma Na^+ concentrations in humans.

The importance of these variables for the plasma Na^+ concentration can be appreciated from the examples in Fig. 7-3. Increasing the Na_e^+ elevates the plasma Na^+ concentration (Fig. 7-3b); increasing the TBW decreases the plasma Na^+

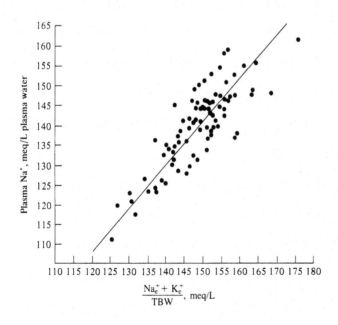

Figure 7-4
Relation between the plasma water Na^+ concentration and the ratio of ($Na_e^+ + K_e^+$)/TBW. (*Adapted from Edelman I, Leibman J, O'Meara MP, Birkenfeld L, J Clin Invest 37:1236, 1958, by copyright permission of The American Society for Clinical Investigation.*)

concentration (Fig. 7-3c); and increasing the Na_e^+ and TBW proportionately has no effect on the plasma Na^+ concentration (Fig. 7-3d).

The effect of changes in potassium balance is less apparent but can be important clinically.[6,7] Suppose, for example, that K^+ is lost from the extracellular fluid because of diarrhea, leading to a fall in the plasma K^+ concentration. This will create a concentration gradient favoring the movement of K^+ from the cells into the extracellular fluid. Since large proteins and organic phosphates are the major intracellular anions and cannot easily leave the cells, electroneutrality is preserved by Na^+ (and H^+) entry into the cells, thereby lowering the plasma Na^+ concentration.

The major clinical application of these concepts occurs in patients with hyponatremia (low plasma Na^+ concentration) or hypernatremia (high plasma Na^+ concentration) (see Chaps. 22 to 24). From the relationship in Eqs. (7-4) and (7-6) we can see that hyponatremia usually represents hypoosmolality and can be produced by Na^+ and K^+ loss or, most commonly, by water retention. Excretion of the excess water in the urine is normally a very effective defense against the development of hyponatremia. Thus, a fall in the plasma Na^+ concentration is almost always associated with a defect in urinary water excretion, due most often to the presence of antidiuretic hormone.

On the other hand, hypernatremia represents hyperosmolality and can be produced by Na^+ gain or water loss. The toxicity of hyperkalemia (high plasma K^+ concentration) prevents the retention of enough K^+ to cause an important elevation in the plasma Na^+ concentration. The primary protective mechanism against hypernatremia is the stimulation of thirst, thereby increasing water intake and lowering the plasma Na^+ concentration to normal. Thus, hypernatremia generally occurs in infants or comatose adults who cannot express a normal thirst response.

Notice that the regulation of the plasma Na^+ concentration and therefore the plasma osmolality occurs by changes in *water balance* (see Chap. 9). Although it is tempting to assume that maintenance of the plasma Na^+ concentration must be related to Na^+ balance, this is not the case. Alterations in sodium balance are used to maintain the plasma volume and tissue perfusion, not the plasma Na^+ concentration (see Chap. 8). Too much sodium is manifested as edema, and too little sodium results in hypovolemia.

EXCHANGE OF WATER BETWEEN PLASMA AND INTERSTITIAL FLUID

The supply of nutrients to the cells and the removal of waste products from the cells occur in the capillaries and postcapillary venules by the diffusion of solutes and gases (O_2 and CO_2) between the plasma and the interstitial fluid. Equally important is the maintenance of a proper distribution of water between these compartments.

Although osmotic forces contribute to the distribution of water across the capillary wall, the situation differs from that across the cell membrane. Since the capillary is permeable to Na⁺ salts and glucose, these substances do not behave as effective osmoles. It is only the *plasma proteins*, which move across the capillary wall to a limited degree, that act as effective osmoles and therefore hold water in the vascular space. This osmotic pressure generated by the plasma proteins is called the colloid osmotic pressure or the *plasma oncotic pressure*.

Fluid does not continuously move into the capillary because the oncotic pressure is largely balanced by the capillary hydraulic (or hydrostatic) pressure. This pressure is generated by the propulsion of blood from the heart and tends to push water out of the vessels into the interstitium. Although less important, oncotic and hydraulic pressures present in the interstitium also contribute to the regulation of fluid exchange between the plasma and the interstitial fluid (Fig. 7-5).

The relationship between net filtration from the vascular space into the interstitium and the hydraulic and oncotic pressure gradients across the capillary wall can be expressed by Starling's law[8-11]:

$$\text{Net filtration} = \text{LpS} \ (\Delta \text{ hydraulic pressure} - \Delta \text{ oncotic pressure})$$

$$= \text{LpS} \left[\left(P_{cap} - P_{if} \right) - s\left(\pi_{cap} - \pi_{if} \right) \right] \tag{7-7}$$

where Lp is the unit permeability (or porosity) of the capillary wall, S is the surface area available for fluid movement, P_{cap} and P_{if} are the capillary and interstitial fluid hydraulic pressures, π_{cap} and π_{if} are the capillary and interstitial fluid oncotic pressures, and s represents the reflection coefficient of proteins across the capillary wall (with values ranging from 0 if completely permeable to 1 if completely impermeable). The interstitial oncotic pressure is derived primarily from filtered plasma proteins and to a lesser degree from proteoglycans in the interstitium.

The normal values for these parameters in experimental animals and humans in the resting state is uncertain, largely because of difficulties in measurement of each of the parameters, with the exception of the capillary oncotic pressure. Furthermore, capillary hemodynamics are not necessarily uniform within an organ, as both open and closed capillaries may be present.

What is clear, however, is that capillaries in different organs have different hemodynamic and permeability characteristics (Table 7-2). In skeletal muscle, for example, capillary pressure is much lower than systemic pressure (because of the high precapillary resistance) and the capillary wall is relatively impermeable to

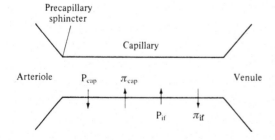

Figure 7-5 Schematic representation of the factors controlling fluid movement across the capillary wall between the plasma and the interstitial fluid.

Table 7-2   Approximate values for Starling's forces in muscle, lung, and kidney[a]

	Skeletal muscle	Alveoli	Glomeruli
Hydraulic pressure			
Capillary (mean)	17.3	8	45
Interstitium	−3.0	−2	10
Mean gradient	20.3	10	35
Oncotic pressure			
Capillary (mean)	28	26	29[b]
Interstitium	8	18	0
Mean gradient	20	8	29
Net gradient favoring filtration ($\Delta P - \Delta\pi$)	0.3	2	6

[a]Units are mmHg. Values are from Refs. 9, 10, 12, and 13.
[b]The mean capillary oncotic pressure rises in the glomerulus because of the filtration of relatively protein-free fluid.

proteins;[9,10] the interstitial hydraulic pressure, in comparison, has a negative value that appears to be generated by the lymphatic removal of interstitial fluid.

The net effect is a 0.3- to 0.5-mmHg gradient favoring filtration, with the filtrate being returned to the systemic circulation by the lymphatic vessels. This gradient is not uniform within the capillary circulation. Although the *mean* hydraulic pressure is about 17 mmHg, the pressure within most of the capillary is higher at 25 to 30 mmHg;[9,11,12] thus, filtration occurs throughout the capillary.[11] Most of this filtrate then reenters the vascular space in the highly permeable *postcapillary venules*, where the hydraulic pressure falls to 10 mmHg, a level below the oncotic pressure gradient.[11]

In comparison to those in skeletal muscle, the alveolar capillaries have both a lower capillary hydraulic pressure (due to perfusion from the low-pressure right ventricle) and a lower transcapillary oncotic pressure gradient (because of a higher permeability to proteins).[10,13] The result is a small gradient favoring filtration, which is slightly larger than that in skeletal muscle. Once again, the fluid that is filtered is normally removed by the lymphatic vessels.[10]

The smaller transcapillary oncotic pressure gradient across the alveolar capillary wall has important clinical implications, because it means that the rate of filtration is relatively unaffected by changes in the plasma oncotic pressures. As an example, a fall in the plasma albumin concentration (called hypoalbuminemia) might be expected to promote fluid movement into the interstitium as a result of the associated reduction in the plasma oncotic pressure. However, the interstitial oncotic pressure will undergo a *parallel decline*, due in part to less albumin movement from the vascular space into the interstitium. The net effect with mild to moderate hypoalbuminemia is *no change in the transcapillary oncotic pressure gradient*; as a result, a low plasma albumin concentration alone is not likely to produce pulmonary edema, which is a potentially life-threatening condition (see "Safety Factors," below).[14]

Finally, the glomerular capillaries are unique in that they have a much higher hydraulic pressure, due in part to a *lower* precapillary resistance.[15] This is physiologically important because the high pressure gradient plus a 50- to 100-fold increase in net permeability allow the glomeruli to maintain a very high rate of filtration (see Chap. 2).

Capillary Hydraulic Pressure and Autoregulation

The average capillary hydraulic pressure is determined by the interplay of three factors: the arterial pressure, which has a normal mean value of 85 to 95 mmHg in humans; the resistance at the precapillary sphincter (Fig. 7-5); and the postcapillary resistance in the venules and veins. The precapillary sphincter resistance determines the degree to which the arterial pressure is transmitted to the capillary. This is important physiologically because the ability to vary sphincter tone allows the capillary hydraulic pressure and therefore the rate of capillary filtration to be held *relatively constant in the presence of changes in arterial pressure*.[16] How this occurs can be appreciated from the relationship between resistance (R), the pressure drop across the resistance (ΔP), and the blood flow (Q):

$$\Delta P = Q \times R \tag{7-8}$$

Thus, an increase in resistance elevates the ΔP, and a decrease in resistance reduces the ΔP. If, for example, the arterial pressure is increased, a rise in precapillary resistance by constriction of the sphincter will increase the ΔP, thereby preventing an increment in the capillary pressure (and in capillary blood flow, since the elevations in pressure and resistance balance out). If this did not occur, then every patient with high blood pressure would tend to develop edema (defined as a palpable swelling due to expansion of the interstitial fluid volume), since the increase in capillary hydraulic pressure would act to push water out of the vascular space into the interstitium. Although neural and humoral factors may contribute, capillary resistance is largely under local control, e.g., by stretch receptors in the sphincter wall and local metabolic factors, a process that is called *autoregulation*.[16] (Autoregulation of the glomerular filtration rate is a more complex process that also involves the efferent glomerular arteriole.)

In contrast to these events at the arterial end of the capillary, the resistance at the venous end is less well regulated by local factors. Consequently, alterations in venous pressure produce parallel changes in capillary hydraulic pressure (see below).

Plasma Oncotic Pressure

The relationship between the protein concentration and the oncotic pressure it generates can be estimated from van't Hoff's law:

$$\text{Oncotic pressure} = cRT \tag{7-9}$$

where c is the solute concentration in moles per unit volume of water, R is a constant with the same value as the gas constant per mole, and T is the absolute temperature in kelvins. Since R and T are constants, the oncotic pressure should be a linear function of protein concentration.

This expectation, however, does not hold true. As depicted in Fig. 7-6, the oncotic pressure generated by the plasma proteins is greater than that predicted on the basis of protein concentration from van't Hoff's law. This difference is due in part to the Gibbs-Donnan equilibrium, since more particles are present in the protein-containing compartment. According to the Gibbs-Donnan equilibrium, the product of the concentrations of the major cations and anions in one compartment is equal to the product in the other compartment, assuming free diffusibility across the membrane. If, for example, Na^+ and Cl^- are the only diffusable ions in the plasma and interstitial fluid, then

$$[Na^+]_p \times [Cl^-]_p = [Na^+]_{if} \times [Cl^-]_{if}$$

The Na^+ and Cl^- concentrations in the interstitium will be equal at about 145 meq/L. In comparison, the plasma water Na^+ concentration will exceed that of Cl^- by about 15 meq/L ($[Na^+] = [Cl^-] + 15$]), which is the approximate negative charge on the plasma proteins. Thus

$$\left([Cl^-]_p + 15\right) \times [Cl^-]_p = 145 \times 145$$

$$[Cl^-]_p = 137.7 \, meq/L$$

$$[Na^+]_p = 152.7 \, meq/L$$

The net effect is that the total number of milliequivalents of Na^+ and Cl^- per liter in the plasma water ($137.7 + 152.7 = 290.4$) exceeds that in the interstitial fluid ($145 + 145 = 290$) by 0.4 meq/L or 0.4 mmol/L. Although this difference appears small, the normal plasma protein concentration is only 0.9 to 1 mmol/L.

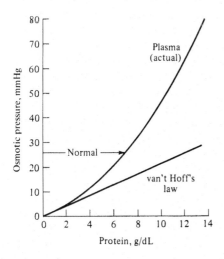

Figure 7-6 Relationship between protein concentration and osmotic pressure as predicted from van't Hoff's law and as actually occurs with plasma. (*Adapted from Landis E, Pappenheimer JR, in Hamilton WF, Dow P (eds.):* Handbook of Physiology, *sec 2,* Circulation, *vol II. American Physiological Society, Washington, D.C., 1963. Used with permission.*)

Consequently, the total osmotic effect of the plasma proteins is increased from 0.9 mosmol/kg (0.9 mmol/L equals 0.9 mosmol/kg)) to 1.3 mosmol/kg by the Gibbs-Donnan effect. Since 1 mosmol/kg generates an osmotic pressure of 19.3 mmHg, this effect increases the capillary oncotic pressure from 17.4 mmHg (0.9×19.3) by concentration alone to 25 to 26 mmHg (1.3×19.3). (Other, poorly understood factors also contribute to this discrepancy between the predicted and actual values for the oncotic pressure produced by the plasma proteins).[17]

Safety Factors

Since the mean gradient only slightly favors filtration, it might be assumed that a small increase in capillary hydraulic pressure (due to an elevated venous pressure) or a small decrease in plasma oncotic pressure (due to hypoproteinemia) would lead to fluid movement into the interstitium and ultimately to clinically apparent edema. However, experimental and clinical observations indicate that edema does not occur until there is a relatively large change in one or both of these parameters.

Three factors contribute to this protective response[9,10]:

- Lymphatic flow is able to increase, so that the excess filtrate can initially be carried away.
- As fluid initially moves into the interstitium, the oncotic pressure will fall (both by dilution and by the lymphatic removal of interstitial proteins), thereby minimizing the gradient for further entry into the interstitium.
- The increase in interstitial fluid volume will cause the interstitial hydraulic pressure to rise; edema cannot occur until the normally negative value becomes positive.[9]

The importance of these safety factors varies from organ to organ. In skeletal muscle, for example, all three contribute. In comparison, the hepatic sinusoids are relatively open and freely permeable to proteins.[10] As a result, there is normally *no oncotic pressure* gradient across the sinusoids, since the plasma and interstitial oncotic pressures are roughly equal. Thus, the hydraulic pressure gradient is unopposed, although the intrasinusoidal pressure is relatively low because most of the hepatic perfusion derives from the low-pressure portal venous system. In this setting, it is hepatic lymph flow that is primarily responsible for preventing the accumulation of excess interstitial fluid.

Although estimated values for Starling's forces in different organs are listed in Table 7-2, methodologic difficulties make the accuracy of these measurements uncertain. In subcutaneous tissue, for example, where clinically evident peripheral edema is usually detected, studies in humans suggest that the interstitial oncotic pressure may be as high as 12 to 15 mmHg, rather than only 8 mmHg.[18,19]

The potential clinical relevance of this issue can be appreciated from the mechanism of edema formation in patients who have hypoalbuminemia due to urinary protein losses in the nephrotic syndrome.[20,21] In this setting, the fall in the plasma albumin concentration leads to less entry of albumin into the interstitium and a parallel decline in the interstitial protein concentration. This change *maintains the transcapillary oncotic pressure gradient* at a near normal value and therefore minimizes the degree of fluid loss into the interstitium* (Fig. 7-7). If, for example, the respective plasma and interstitial oncotic pressures were 28 and 8 mmHg (as in Table 7-2), then loss of interstitial proteins to balance the decrease in plasma oncotic pressure could account for a maximum safety factor of only 8 mmHg. In comparison, protection against fluid movement into the interstitium would be increased up to twofold if the true interstitial value were 12 to 15 mmHg; as a result, hypoalbuminemia would be less likely to produce edema.

Studies in both humans and experimental animals with the nephrotic syndrome are consistent with the latter hypothesis, since primary renal sodium retention (induced by the underlying renal disease) often plays a major role in edema formation.[20,22] In animals with the unilateral nephrotic syndrome, for example, there is unilateral Na^+ retention, indicating that intrarenal rather than systemic factors are of primary importance (see page 484).[22] Increased collecting tubule reabsorption appears to be responsible for the Na^+ retention in this setting, although how this occurs is not well understood.[21,23,24]

The relative importance of underfilling (due to hypoalbuminemia-induced plasma volume depletion) and overflow (due to primary renal sodium retention) in the generation of edema associated with hypoalbuminemia appears to be variable in different patients.[20,25,26] Two settings have been identified in which underfilling clearly occurs: acute hypoalbuminemia, in which there is not time for the

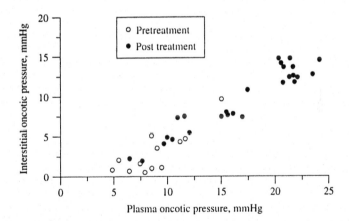

Figure 7-7 Relationship between plasma and interstitial oncotic pressures in nephrotic patients with minimal change disease before (open circles) and after (closed circles) corticosteroid-induced remission of the proteinuria. These values are reduced in parallel during active disease with little change in the transcapillary oncotic pressure gradient and therefore little tendency to promote edema formation. (*Adapted from Koomans HA, Kortlandt W, Geers AB, Dorhout Mees EJ, Nephron 40:391, 1985. Used with permission.*)

* This response is similar to that described above for the alveolar capillaries, where the protection is even more prominent because the interstitial oncotic pressure is higher, at 18 mmHg (Table 7-2).

interstitial oncotic pressure to fall; and severe hypoalbuminemia (plasma albumin concentration less than 1.0 g/dL), in which the transcapillary oncotic gradient cannot be maintained because the interstitial value cannot be further reduced.[27] An example of underfilling edema due to acute hypoalbuminemia is saline resuscitation for massive bleeding, lowering the plasma albumin concentration by dilution. It may also be present in acute onset nephrotic syndrome[26] but is less common in stable disease.[27]

PROBLEMS

7-1 What is the relationship between the plasma Na^+ concentration and the plasma osmolality? Between the plasma Na^+ concentration and the extracellular volume?

7-2 If glucose is added to the extracellular fluid, what will happen to the following?

(a) The plasma osmolality
(b) The extracellular volume
(c) The intracellular volume
(d) The plasma Na^+ concentration

7-3 Laboratory tests for a patient provide the following plasma values:

$$\text{Osmolality} = 290 \text{ mosmol/kg}$$

$$\text{Sodium} = 125 \text{ meq/L}$$

$$\text{Urea nitrogen} = 28 \text{ mg/dL}$$

If glucose is the only other osmole in the extracellular fluid, calculate the plasma glucose concentration in mg/dL.

7-4 What effect will the following have on the plasma volume?

(a) An elevation in arterial blood pressure
(b) A decrease in venous pressure
(c) A reduction in the plasma albumin concentration to 3 g/dL (normal equals 4 to 5 g/dL)

REFERENCES

1. Maffly RH, Leaf A. The potential of water in mammalian tissues. *J Gen Physiol* 42:1257, 1959.
2. Kiil F. Molecular mechanisms of osmosis. *Am J Physiol* 256:R801, 1989.
3. Wright E, Schulman G. Principles of epithelial transport. In Maxwell MH, Kleeman CR, Narins RG (eds): *Clinical Disorders of Fluid and Electrolyte Metabolism*, 4th ed. New York, McGraw-Hill, 1987.
4. LeFurgey A, Spencer AJ, Jacobs W, et al. Elemental microanalysis of organelles in proximal tubules. I. Alterations in transport and metabolism. *J Am Soc Nephrol* 1:1305, 1991.
5. Edelman IS, Leibman J, O'Meara MP, Birkenfield L. Interrelations between serum sodium concentration, serum osmolarity and total exchangeable sodium, total exchangeable potassium and total body water. *J Clin Invest* 37:1236, 1958.
6. Laragh JH. The effect of potassium chloride on hyponatremia. *J Clin Invest* 33:807, 1954.
7. Fichman MP, Vorherr H, Kleeman CR, Telfer N. Diuretic-induced hyponatremia. *Ann Intern Med* 75:853, 1971.
8. Starling E. On the absorption of fluids from the connective tissue spaces. *J Physiol (Lond)* 19:312, 1896.
9. Guyton AC. *Textbook of Medical Physiology*, 8th ed. Philadelphia, Saunders, 1991, chap. 16.
10. Taylor AE. Capillary fluid filtration: Starling forces and lymph flow. *Circ Res* 49:557, 1981.

11. Renkin EM. Regulation of the microcirculation. *Microvasc Res* 30:251, 1985.
12. Davis MJ. Control of bat wing capillary pressure and blood flow during reduced renal perfusion pressure. *Am J Physiol* 255:H1114, 1988.
13. Murray JF. The lung and heart failure. *Hosp Prac* 20(4):55, 1985.
14. Zarins CK, Rice CL, Peters RM, Virgilio RW. Lymph and pulmonary response to isobaric reduction in plasma oncotic pressure in baboons. *Circ Res* 43:925, 1978.
15. Maddox DA, Deen WM, Brenner BM. Dynamics of glomerular ultrafiltration. VI. Studies in the primate. *Kidney Int* 5:271, 1974.
16. Johnson PC. Autoregulation of blood flow. *Circ Res* 59:483, 1986.
17. Curry F-R. Mechanics and thermodynamics of transcapillary exchange. In Renkin EM, Michel CC (eds): *Handbook of Physiology*, sec. 2, The cardiovascular system, vol. IV, microcirculation, Part 1. American Physiological Society, Washington, DC, 1984.
18. Fauchald PF. Transcapillary colloid osmotic pressure gradient and body fluid volumes in renal failure. *Kidney Int* 29:895, 1986.
19. Bernard DB. Extrarenal complications of the nephrotic syndrome. *Kidney Int* 33:1184, 1988.
20. Humphreys MH. Mechanisms and management of nephrotic edema. *Kidney Int* 45:266, 1994.
21. Perico N, Remuzzi G. Edema of the nephrotic syndrome: The role of the atrial peptide system. *Am J Kidney Dis* 22:355, 1993.
22. Ichikawa I, Rennke HG, Hoyer JR, et al. Role for intrarenal mechanisms in the impaired salt excretion of experimental nephrotic syndrome. *J Clin Invest* 71:91, 1983.
23. Valentin J, Qiu C, Muldowney WP, et al. Cellular basis for blunted volume expansion natriuresis in experimental nephrotic syndrome. *J Clin Invest* 90:1302, 1992.
24. Feraille E, Vogt B, Rousselot M, et al. Mechanism of enhanced Na-K-ATPase activity in cortical collecting duct from rats with nephrotic syndrome. *J Clin Invest* 91:1295, 1993.
25. Schrier RW, Fassett RG. A critique of the overfill hypothesis of sodium and water retention in the nephrotic syndrome. *Kidney Int* 53:1111, 1998.
26. Vande Walle JG, Donckerwolcke RA, van Isselt JW, et al. Volume regulation in children with early relapse of minimal change nephrosis with or without hypovolaemic symptoms. *Lancet* 36:148, 1995.
27. Vande Walle JG, Donckerwolcke RA, Koomans HA. Pathophysiology of edema formation in children with nephrotic syndrome not due to minimal change disease. *J Am Soc Nephrol* 10:323, 1999.

REGULATION OF THE EFFECTIVE
CIRCULATING VOLUME

The maintenance of adequate tissue perfusion is essential for normal cellular metabolism by providing nutrients and by removing waste products. It is not surprising, therefore, that multiple sensors and multiple effectors are involved in this process. The presence of several levels of control illustrates an important difference between the regulation of volume and the regulation of osmolality or the concentration of a particular solute. Maintenance of concentration can often be achieved with only a single sensor (such as the hypothalamic osmoreceptors), since all tissues are perfused by the same arterial blood. In comparison, there may be marked variability in regional perfusion, necessitating the presence of local sensors.

A simple example is changing from the sitting to the standing position, which, by gravity, tends to result in hyperperfusion of and fluid accumulation in the lower extremities and hypoperfusion of the brain.[1] In this setting, activation of the carotid sinus baroreceptors with a subsequent increase in sympathetic activity helps to preserve cerebral perfusion (see below).

This chapter will review how the effective circulating volume is regulated, both in the face of changes in dietary Na^+ intake and in disease states in which tissue perfusion is altered. In particular, it will show how the neurohumoral influences and the reabsorptive characteristics of the different nephron segments that have been discussed in Chaps. 2 to 6 are integrated in an appropriate fashion to maintain the steady state. The physiologic and clinical importance of the steady state will also be reviewed.

DEFINITION

The *effective circulating volume* refers to that part of the extracellular fluid (ECF) that is in the arterial system (normally about 700 mL in a 70-kg man) and is effectively perfusing the tissues.[2] However, a better physiological definition is the *pressure perfusing the arterial baroreceptors* in the carotid sinus and glomerular afferent arterioles, since it is changes in pressure (or stretch) rather than volume or flow that is generally sensed at these sites.

The effective circulating volume usually varies directly with the ECF volume. Both of these parameters are typically proportional to total body Na^+ stores, since Na^+ salts are the primary extracellular solutes that act to hold water within the extracellular space (see page 241). As a result, the *regulation of Na^+ balance (by alterations in urinary Na^+ excretion) and the maintenance of the effective circulating volume are closely related functions.* Na^+ loading will tend to produce volume expansion, whereas Na^+ loss will lead to volume depletion.

In some settings, however, the effective circulating volume may be *independent of the ECF volume, the plasma volume, or even the cardiac output* (Table 8-1). In congestive heart failure, for example, the effective circulating volume is reduced because a primary decrease in cardiac output lowers the pressure at the baroreceptors.[2,3] As will be discussed below, this decline in pressure and flow induces compensatory fluid retention by the kidney, leading to expansion of the extracellular fluid. The net result is effective volume depletion in association with increases in both the plasma and total ECF volumes.

The increase in volume in this setting is in part *appropriate* because the associated rise in intracardiac filling pressure can, by increasing cardiac stretch, improve cardiac contractibility and raise the cardiac output and systemic blood pressure toward normal (see Chap. 16). On the other hand, the elevation in intravascular pressure can also be maladaptive in that it promotes fluid movement out of the vascular space, potentially leading to both pulmonary and peripheral edema.

The effective circulating volume may also, in some cases, be *independent of the cardiac output.* As well as in connection with a reduction in cardiac output, effective volume depletion can occur when perfusion pressure is reduced by a fall in

Table 8-1 Potential independence of effective circulating volume from other measurable hemodynamic parameters

Clinical condition	Effective circulating volume	ECF volume	Plasma volume	Cardiac output
Na^+-depleted normal subjects	↓	↓	↓	↓
Heart failure	↓	↑	↑	↓
Arteriovenous fistula	0	↑	↑	↑
Advanced hepatic cirrhosis	↓	↑	↑	N/↑

systemic vascular resistance (peripheral vasodilatation).[2] In the presence of an arteriovenous fistula, for example, the cardiac output is elevated by an amount equal to the flow through the fistula.[4] However, this fluid can be considered to be circulating *ineffectively*, since it bypasses the capillary circulation. Thus, the patient is normovolemic, despite the presence of a cardiac output that may be substantially elevated.

The potential dissociation between the effective circulating volume and the cardiac output can also be illustrated by the hemodynamic volume and the cardiac output can also be illustrated by the hemodynamic changes seen in patients with advanced cirrhosis and ascites (Table 8-1).[2,3] In this disorder, the ECF volume is expanded because of the ascites; the plasma volume is increased, in part as a result of fluid accumulation in the markedly dilated but slowly circulating splanchnic venous circulation;[5] and the cardiac output is often elevated because of multiple arteriovenous fistulas throughout the body, such as the spider angiomas on the skin.[6]

Despite all of these signs suggesting volume expansion, most of the excess fluid is hemodynamically ineffective, and these patients *behave as if they were volume-depleted* as a result of marked peripheral vasodilatation. This is exemplified by reductions in systemic vascular resistance and blood pressure, a very low rate of urinary Na^+ excretion (often below 10 meq/day),[7] a reduction in the blood volume in the cardiopulmonary circulation,[8] and a progressive increase in the secretion of the hormones typically released in response to hypovolemia: renin, norepineph-rine, and antidiuretic hormone (ADH).[7-9] (The hemodynamic changes in cirrhosis are discussed in more detail in Chap. 16.)

In summary, the effective circulating volume is an unmeasured entity that reflects tissue perfusion and may be independent of other hemodynamic para-meters.[2] The diagnosis of effective volume depletion is usually made by demon-strating renal Na^+ retention, as evidenced by a *urine Na^+ concentration below 15 to 20 meq/L*. This relationship is generally true as long as there is neither renal Na^+ wasting (most often due to diuretic therapy or underlying renal disease) nor selec-tive renal or glomerular ischemia (as with bilateral renovascular disease or acute glomerular disease). In the latter setting, urinary Na^+ excretion may be low with-out systemic hypoperfusion, whereas obligatory Na^+ wasting can prevent the renal Na^+ retention that is normally associated with volume depletion.[10]

EFFECTIVE CIRCULATING VOLUME, RENAL SODIUM EXCRETION, AND THE STEADY STATE

The kidney is the primary regulatory of Na^+ and volume balance, as urinary Na^+ excretion responds in an appropriate manner to changes in the effective circulating volume. When there is an increase in volume, as after a Na^+ load[11] or closure of an arteriovenous fistula,[4] Na^+ excretion rises in an attempt to lower the volume toward normal. Conversely, the kidney retains Na^+ in the presence of effective volume depletion. This system of volume regulation must be very efficient, since small alterations in Na^+ intake necessitate parallel changes in Na^+ excretion that involve less than 1 percent of the filtered Na^+ load (see "Day-to-Day Regulation," below).

The time course of the response to variations in Na^+ intake is illustrated in Fig. 8-1.[11] If dietary intake is abruptly increased in a patient on a low-sodium diet, only about one-half of the excess intake is excreted on the first day. The remainder is retained, augmenting body Na^+ stores. This elevates the plasma osmolality, which stimulates both thirst and the secretion of ADH (see page 173). The increments in water intake and renal water reabsorption produce water retention, resulting in increases in the effective circulating volume and body weight and the return of the plasma osmolality to normal. (This process of osmoregulation is discussed in detail in Chap. 9.)

On subsequent days, a progressively greater fraction of the excess intake is excreted (and less retained) until by 3 to 4 days, a new steady state is achieved in which renal Na^+ excretion matches intake.[12] This new steady state is characterized by a mild increase in the effective circulating volume resulting from the Na^+ and water retained on the first 4 days.[12-15] The total quantity of Na^+ retained is directly related to the increment in Na^+ intake above the previous baseline. Thus, *the greater the increase in intake, the greater the increase in steady-state extracellular volume* (Fig. 8-2).

The same sequence occurs in reverse if Na^+ intake is reduced. Negative Na^+ balance occurs until there has been enough loss of volume to lower Na^+ excretion to the reduced level of intake.

Thus, a high-sodium diet is characterized by increases in volume and Na^+ excretion and a low-sodium diet by decrease in volume and Na^+ excretion. The changes in volume are essential, since they *constitute the signal that allows urinary Na^+ excretion to vary appropriately with fluctuations in Na^+ intake*. Let us assume, for the sake of simplicity, that Na^+ excretion in normal subjects is primarily determined by the Na^+-retaining hormone aldosterone and the Na^+-losing hormone atrial natriuretic peptide (ANP). As Na^+ intake rises from 10 to a higher

Figure 8-1 Effect of abrupt changes in Na^+ intake on body weight and renal Na^+ excretion in a normal human. The shaded areas refer to changes in total body Na^+ stores due to the difference between intake and excretion. See text for details. (*From Earley LE, in Maxwell MH, Kleeman CR (eds): Clinical Disorders of Fluid and Electrolyte Metabolism. New York, McGraw-Hill, 1972. Used with permission.*)

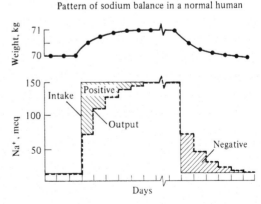

Pattern of sodium balance in a normal human

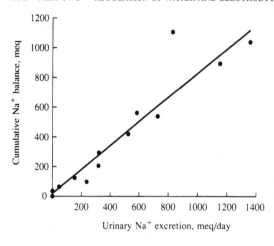

Figure 8-2 Urinary Na^+ excretion (an indicator of dietary intake in the steady state) as a function of cumulative Na^+ balance in 14 normal subjects studied at different levels of Na^+ intake. As can be seen, net Na^+ balance increases in proportion to the rise in intake, resulting in a progressively greater degree of volume expansion. (*From Walser M*, Kidney Int *27:837, 1985. Reprinted by permission from* Kidney International.)

than normal value of 350 meq/day, there must be a fall in the secretion of aldosterone and a rise in that of ANP to result in the necessary reduction in tubular Na^+ reabsorption.[15] Furthermore, the rate of release of these hormones must *stay at this new level* if Na^+ excretion is to remain at 350 meq/day (Fig. 8-3). The signal for the continued suppression of aldosterone and stimulation of ANP is the persistent volume expansion.

Clinical Implications   In addition to its role in volume regulation in normal subjects, the steady state also has important implications in the pathogenesis

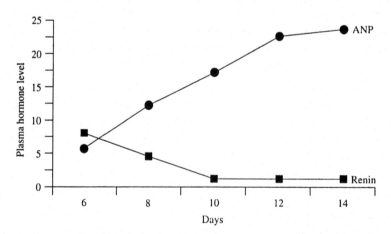

Figure 8-3 Increasing plasma levels of atrial natriuretic peptide (ANP) and falling plasma renin activity in normal subjects given a progressively increasing sodium intake from 10 to 350 meq/day after a 5-day equilibration period. These hormonal responses promote urinary excretion of the excess sodium. (*Data from Sagnella GA, Markandu ND, Buckley MG, et al*, Am J Physiol *256:R1171, 1989. Used with permission.*)

and treatment of disease states. As an example, diuretics inhibit Na^+ reabsorption at different sites in the nephron; they are most often given to patients with edema or hypertension to lower the ECF volume. The initial volume loss activates Na^+-retaining mechanisms, such as the renin-angiotensin system, which act to limit further losses. These counterregulatory forces are so efficient that, assuming the diuretic dose is constant, all of the fluid and electrolyte losses occur in the first 7 to 14 days of therapy, with the *maximum* natriuretic response being induced by the first dose (see page 455).

A steady state is also achieved with changes in intake of other electrolytes. If, for example, K^+ intake is increased, the new steady state will be characterized by a limited elevation in body K^+ stores and a small rise in the plasma K^+ concentration.[16] The latter change will be the stimulus to maintain an increased rate of K^+ excretion, a response that is mediated in part by enhanced secretion of aldosterone (see Chap. 12).

These observations have important implications for the development of many fluid and electrolyte disorders. The capacity to excrete Na^+, K^+, HCO_3^-, and H_2O is so great in normal subjects that too much Na^+ (edema), too much K^+ (hyperkalemia), too much HCO_3^- (metabolic alkalosis), or too much H_2O (hyponatremia) will *not persist unless there is an abnormality in the renal excretion of that substance*. The excretion of H_2O, for example, occurs via the suppression of the release of antidiuretic hormone, resulting in the formation of a dilute urine (see "Volume Regulation versus Osmoregulation," below). Thus, the differential diagnosis of hyponatremia primarily consists of those disorders in which ingested water cannot be excreted normally, usually because of an inability to suppress the release of antidiuretic hormone (see Chap. 23).

REGULATION OF THE EFFECTIVE CIRCULATING VOLUME

The body responds to variations in the effective circulating volume in two steps: (1) The change is sensed by the volume receptors, and (2) these receptors then activate a series of effectors that restore normovolemia by varying vascular resistance, cardiac output, and renal Na^+ and water excretion.

Volume Receptors

The primary volume receptors are in the cardiopulmonary circulation, the carotid sinuses and aortic arch, and the afferent glomerular arterioles in the kidney.[2,17,18] Although it is volume that is being regulated, it is difficult to conceive of receptors that sense total extracellular, plasma, or capillary volume. What is actually being sensed at most of the renal and extrarenal volume receptors is pressure (or stretch).[18] This allows effective volume control, since pressure and volume are usually directly related. For example, volume depletion induced by vomiting is sequentially associated with reductions in venous return to the heart, intracardiac filling pressures, cardiac output, and systemic blood pressure.

In the kidney, the major volume receptors are the stretch receptors in the juxtaglomerular apparatus of the afferent arteriole and, to a lesser degree, the macula densa cells in the early distal tubule. These receptors affect volume balance by influencing the activity of the renin-angiotensin-aldosterone system and endothelin and nitric oxide (see Chaps. 2 and 6).

In contrast, the extrarenal receptors (such as those in the atria and the carotid sinus) primarily govern the activity of the sympathetic nervous system and ANP.[2,17] Volume depletion, for example, can diminish both the intracardiac and systemic blood pressures, resulting in an increase in sympathetic tone and a reduction in the release of ANP, the consequences of which will be discussed below. These changes are reversed with volume expansion.

The role of cardiopulmonary receptors has been demonstrated in humans by the response to immersion to the neck in warm water.[19,20] In this setting, the hydrostatic pressure of the water on the lower extremities results in the redistribution of intravascular fluid from the legs to the chest. The ensuing increase in central blood volume (and subsequently in cardiac output) is associated with a marked increase in Na^+ and water excretion in an attempt to restore normovolemia (Fig. 8-4a). Although aldosterone secretion is decreased in this setting, the natriuretic response shows a better temporal correlation with the associated increase in ANP release.[19,20]

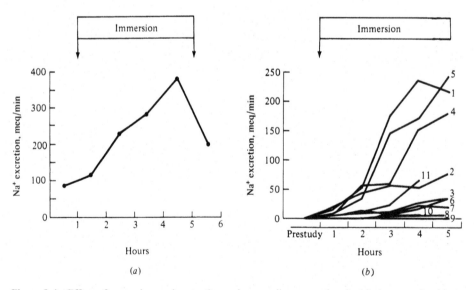

Figure 8-4 Effect of water immersion to the neck on sodium excretion in (a) six normal subjects ingesting 150 meq of Na^+ power day and (b) eleven patients with cirrhosis who excrete little Na^+ in the basal state. Sodium excretion tends to be increased in both settings, mediated at least in part by cardiopulmonary receptors sensing the associated expansion of the central blood volume. (*Adapted from Epstein M*, Circ Res *39:619, 1976, and Epstein M, Pins DS, Schneider N, Levinson R,* J Lab Clin Med *87:822, 1976. By permission of the American Heart Association, Inc.*)

A similar natriuretic response to immersion to the neck can be demonstrated in many patients with cirrhosis and ascites who excrete little Na^+ in the basal state (Fig. 8-4*b*).[3,21] This observation supports the view that the reduced Na^+ excretion in cirrhosis is due to effective volume depletion, even though these patients have, as described above, elevations in the plasma volume and cardiac output.[2]

Although multiple receptors are involved in the regulation of the effective circulating volume, *no single receptor appears to be of primary importance.* For example, Na^+ balance is generally well maintained in the presence of cardiac or renal denervation or the chronic administration of aldosterone (see below),[22-25] indicating that although these factors may be important in normal subjects, other receptors are capable of maintaining volume homeostasis. As an example, volume changes have direct mechanical effects on cardiac output and blood pressure, and the latter can influence NaCl and water excretion when other regulatory systems have failed (see "Pressure Natriuresis," below).[24]

Effectors

Multiple effectors are involved in volume control, influencing both systemic hemodynamics and urinary Na^+ excretion (Table 8-2). Since these regulatory systems (except for the sympathetic nervous system) have been discussed previously in Chaps. 2 and 6, their effects will be only briefly reviewed in this section.

Sympathetic nervous system   Sympathetic neural tone and the secretion of catecholamines (norepinephrine and epinephrine) from the adrenal medulla are reduced by volume expansion and enhanced by volume depletion.[26-28] Thus, effective volume depletion, due to fluid losses or to reduced tissue perfusion in cirrhosis or heart failure, is associated with increased systemic and renal sympathetic activity.[2,8,9,29]

Table 8-2   Principal effectors involved in volume regulation

Systemic hemodynamics
Sympathetic nervous system
Angiotensin II
Renal Na^+ excretion
Glomerular filtration rate
Angiotensin II
Peritubular capillary hemodynamics
Aldosterone
Sympathetic nervous system
Atrial natriuretic peptide
Pressure natriuresis
Plasma Na^+ concentration

Activation of sympathetic function in this setting is presumably related to an initial fall in effective cardiac output, due to decreased venous return, vasodilatation (as in cirrhosis), or primary cardiac disease. From the formula relating pressure, output, and resistance,*

Mean arterial pressure = cardiac output × systemic vascular resistance

the reduction in cardiac output lowers the systemic blood pressure. This decrease in pressure is sensed by the cardiac and arterial baroreceptors, resulting in a change in baroreceptor afferent discharge to the vasomotor centers in the brainstem.[18,26] These centers then induce an increase in peripheral sympathetic tone, initiating a series of events that act to restore normal tissue perfusion (Fig. 8-5):

- Venous constriction increases blood delivery to the heart, since about 70 percent of the vascular volume is normally contained within the venous system.
- Myocardial contractility and heart rate are increased, which, in combination with the enhanced venous return, raises the cardiac output.
- Direct arteriolar constriction increases systemic vascular resistance, thereby elevating the systemic blood pressure toward normal.
- Renin secretion is enhanced, resulting in the generation of angiotensin II, which contributes to the systemic vasoconstriction (see Chap. 1).[30]
- Renal tubular Na^+ reabsorption is enhanced because of both a direct adrenergic effect (see Chap. 6) and increases in angiotensin II and aldosterone secretion.[26,31,32]

These cardiovascular changes are reversed by volume expansion, as sympathetic activity is reduced, thereby minimizing the elevations in cardiac output and blood pressure and facilitating the excretion of the excess Na^+.[27]

The importance of this regulatory system is illustrated in Fig. 8-6. Although normal subjects easily tolerate the removal of 500 mL of blood (the equivalent of donating one unit of blood), patients with autonomic insufficiency can develop severe hypotension. These patients also have both postural hypotension, since they cannot compensate for the pooling of blood in the legs that occurs when one assumes the erect position, and an impaired ability to maximally conserve Na^+, presumably due to removal of the adrenergic stimulus to tubular Na^+ reabsorption.[26,33,34]

Angiotensin II   The physiology of the renin-angiotensin system is discussed in detail in Chap. 2. To review briefly, renin secretion is enhanced in hypovolemic disorders, resulting in the generation of angiotensin II, which has two major

---

* The product of cardiac output and systemic vascular resistance actually equals the change in pressure across the circulation, i.e., mean arterial pressure minus mean venous pressure. However, since the venous pressure is so much lower (normal equals 1 to 7 mmHg) than the mean arterial pressure, only a small error results from ignoring it.

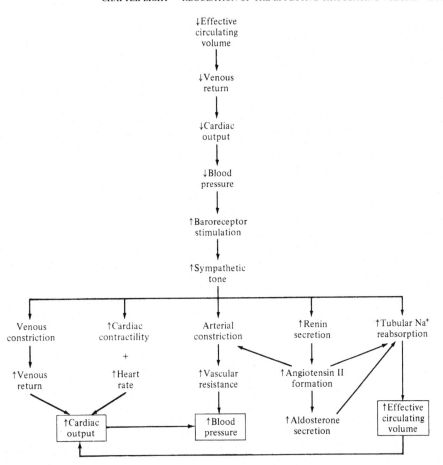

Figure 8-5 Hemodynamic responses induced by the sympathetic nervous system after effective circulating volume depletion.

actions: It raises the blood pressure by arterial vasoconstriction, both directly and by enhancing the release and effect of norepinephrine, and it induces renal Na^+ retention, both directly and by increasing the secretion of aldosterone.[35,36] Like sympathetic blockade, inhibition of the renin-angiotensin system in hypovolemic subjects can lead to marked hypotension.[37,38]

The vasoconstriction induced by angiotensin II and norepinephrine in the presence of hypovolemia is compensatory in that it tends to maintain the systemic blood pressure; however, *renal Na^+ retention is usually required for the restoration of normovolemia.* As an example, a decrease in volume due to fluid loss can be corrected only by the ingestion and subsequent retention of exogenous Na^+ and water.

The situation is different when effective volume depletion is due to heart failure or to cirrhosis with ascites. In this setting, the effect of the fluid retention

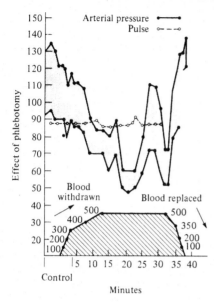

Figure 8-6   Effect of rapid removal and replacement of whole blood on the arterial blood pressure during recumbency in a patient with idiopathic autonomic insufficiency. (*From Wagner HN Jr, J Clin Invest 36:1319, 1967, by copyright permission of the American Society for Clinical Investigation.*)

is dependent upon the severity of the underlying disorder. This concept is illustrated in Fig. 8-7, which depicts the response to decreasing venous return as a result of partial constriction of the thoracic inferior vena cava.[37] There is an initial rapid decline in mean aortic pressure that is returned toward normal within 1 day, primarily by activation of the renin-angiotensin-aldosterone system. This is accompanied by a marked reduction in Na^+ excretion, leading to a progressive increase in the plasma volume and the development of ascites due to an elevation in hepatic venous pressure. By day 7, however, the degree of volume expansion is sufficient to normalize venous return. As a result, a *new steady state* is achieved in which systemic hemodynamics are normal and the plasma renin activity and aldosterone level fall and urinary Na^+ excretion rises toward the level of intake.

However, it is not always possible to reach a new steady state. If the vena caval constriction is very severe, then marked Na^+ retention and activation of the renin-angiotensin system persist, because fluid retention is unable to sufficiently enhance venous return. A similar sequence can occur in humans with heart failure. Patients who are clinically stable may have a normal blood pressure and a normal plasma renin activity, whereas patients with decompensated heart failure tend to be relatively hypotensive with high plasma renin levels.[39] Even those with relatively normal plasma renin activity may still have increased activity of the *intrarenal* renin-angiotensin system.[40]

Regulation of renal Na^+ excretion   Renal Na^+ excretion varies directly with the effective circulating volume. When the effective volume is expanded, the urine Na^+ concentration can exceed 100 meq/L. In contrast, the urine can be rendered vir-

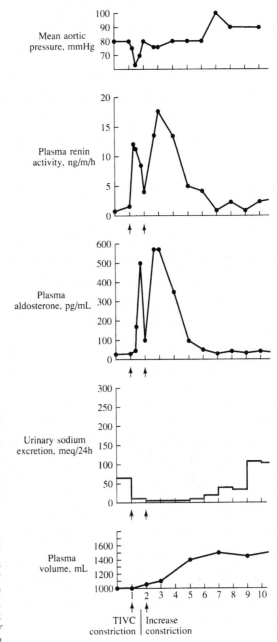

Figure 8-7 Sequential changes in mean aortic pressure, plasma renin activity, plasma aldosterone concentration, urinary sodium excretion, and plasma volume in a dog with moderate thoracic inferior vena cava constriction. There is initial hypotension, activation of the renin-angiotensin-aldosterone system, and a marked reduction in urinary Na$^+$ excretion. By day 7, however, a new steady state is achieved in which renin and aldosterone levels and Na$^+$ excretion have returned to baseline levels. The associated plasma volume expansion is responsible for restoring venous return to the heart, thereby allowing systemic hemodynamics to be normalized. (*From Watkins L Jr, Burton JA, Haber E, et al,* J Clin Invest *57:1606, 1976, by copyright permission of the American Society for Clinical Investigation.*)

tually Na^+-free (urine Na^+ concentration as low as 1 meq/L*) in the presence of volume depletion and normal renal function. These homeostatic changes in Na^+ excretion can result from alterations both in the filtered load, determined primarily by the glomerular filtration rate (GFR), and in tubular reabsorption, which is affected by multiple factors. As will be seen, *an abnormality in any one factor does not preclude the maintenance of Na^+ balance*, a finding indicative of the substantial overlap involved in volume regulation.

Glomerular filtration rate   The GFR tends to increase with volume expansion and to fall with volume depletion, both of which can contribute to the associated changes in Na^+ excretion.[41] However, alterations in the GFR are not required for the maintenance of Na^+ balance. As an example, patients with less than end-stage renal disease may have a substantial reduction in GFR. Nevertheless, they are usually able (in the absence of the nephrotic syndrome) to adjust Na^+ excretion to match intake by decreasing the rate of tubular reabsorption.[42] The importance of tubular reabsorption is also illustrated by the phenomenon of *glomerulotubular balance*, in which a primary alteration in GFR leads to a parallel change in tubular reabsorption and, therefore, relatively little variation in urinary Na^+ excretion (see page 85).[41]

Tubular reabsorption   In general, it is changes in tubular reabsorption that constitute the main adaptive response to fluctuations in the effective circulating volume. How this occurs can be appreciated from Table 8-3, which gives the sites and determinants of segmental Na^+ reabsorption. Although the loop of Henle and the distal tubule make an important overall contribution to net Na^+ handling, transport in these segments primarily varies with the amount of Na^+ delivered, i.e., reabsorption is flow-dependent (see page 118).[43,44] In comparison, the *neurohumoral regulation of Na^+ reabsorption according to body needs occurs primarily in the proximal and collecting tubules.*

As an example, mild volume depletion in the rat results in a decrease in Na^+ excretion that is mostly due to enhanced collecting tubule reabsorption;[45] this effect is mediated at least in part by an increase in the secretion of aldosterone. Proximal reabsorption may also be enhanced, especially with greater degrees of hypovolemia.[45,46] This response is associated with increased activity of the luminal membrane Na^+-H^+ exchanger that is responsible for both $NaHCO_3$ and NaCl reabsorption (see page 118).[47] Increased secretion of angiotensin II and norepinephrine probably plays an important role in this stimulation of proximal transport.[47] Reabsorption in the loop of Henle may also be increased in this setting, an effect that may be mediated by a reduction in medullary interstitial pressure (see "Pressure Natriuresis," below).[48,49]

These changes are reversed with volume expansion, as collecting tubule and, if necessary, proximal and loop NaCl and water reabsorption all may be

---

* How Na^+ can enter the cell to be reabsorbed when its luminal concentration falls below that of the cell is described on page 147.

Table 8-3   Anatomic distribution and determinants of segmental NaCl reabsorption[a]

Tubule segment	Percent filtered NaCl reabsorbed	Determinants of reabsorption
Proximal tubule	60–65	Na^+-H^+ exchange Na^+-glucose cotransport Angiotensin II Norepinephrine Peritubular capillary hemodynamics
Loop of Henle	25–30	Flow-dependent
Distal tubule	5	Flow-dependent
Collecting tubules	4	Aldosterone Atrial natriuretic peptide

[a] Data from Bennett CM, Brenner BM, Berliner R, *J Clin Invest* 47:203, 1968, by copyright permission of the American Society for Clinical Investigation.

reduced.[50-52] Decreased activity of the renin-angiotensin-aldosterone system and increased secretion of ANP (which can also raise the GFR) may be particularly important in this setting.[14,53,54]

Day-to-day regulation   The above findings were obtained from experiments in which relatively large changes in volume were induced. In normal humans, however, variations in daily Na^+ intake require very small percentage changes in Na^+ excretion for balance to be maintained. Suppose, for example, that an adult man has a GFR of 160 L/day and a plasma water Na^+ concentration of 150 meq/L. The daily filtered load of Na^+ in this setting is 24,000 meq. If intake is normally 120 meq per day, then only 0.5 percent of the filtered load has to be excreted. An increase in intake to 180 meq will require a minimal rise in fractional excretion to only 0.67 percent.

It is likely that aldosterone plays an important role as the fine modular of Na^+ excretion.[15] As illustrated in Fig. 6-13, renin and aldosterone release vary inversely with relatively minor changes in Na^+ intake. There is also evidence that the natriuretic response to a relatively small increase in Na^+ intake is associated with a rise in ANP release,[15,55] although the physiologic role of ANP remains to be proven (see page 173).[56,57] Since aldosterone and ANP affect Na^+ reabsorption in the collecting tubules, this segment may be the primary site at which volume regulation is achieved in normal humans.

Although proximal function cannot be measured directly in humans, studies monitoring changes in urate excretion suggest that changes in volume may be associated with alterations in proximal reabsorption. Net urate reabsorption occurs in the proximal tubule by a process that appears to be mediated by parallel Na^+-H^+ and urate-anion exchangers (see Fig. 3-13). Volume depletion, as occurs with diuretic therapy, for example, is often associated with decreased urate excretion and hyperuricemia, suggesting that there has been an increase in overall proximal Na^+ and urate transport.[58] On the other hand, the urate wasting and hypouricemia commonly seen in the syndrome of inappropriate ADH secretion are related in part to the associated water retention and volume expansion.[59]

Redundancy of control systems Despite the probable importance of aldosterone in Na^+ excretion, abnormalities in the secretion of this hormone are not usually associated with disturbances in Na^+ balance because other factors are able to compensate. As an example, adrenalectomized patients treated with replacement doses of a mineralocorticoid are able to maintain Na^+ balance, even though they are unable to vary the level of mineralocorticoid secretion.[60] Similarly, subjects given aldosterone or patients with an autonomous, aldosterone-secreting adrenal adenoma retain fluid for only a few days and then undergo a spontaneous diuresis that returns the volume status toward normal. This phenomenon of *aldosterone escape* (see Fig. 6-15) is due to decreased Na^+ reabsorption at some other site in the nephron, a response that may be mediated in part by ANP[25,61] and by a direct effect of the rise in renal perfusion pressure.[24]

Similar considerations in terms of the redundant regulation of Na^+ balance appear to apply to ANP. Studies in animals made ANP-deficient by immunization or by blocking of the renal action of ANP have demonstrated an impairment in the natriuretic response to acute volume expansion but not to chronic hypervolemia as induced by a high salt intake with or without a mineralocorticoid.[57,61] On the other hand, transgenic mice given an extra ANP gene have plasma ANP levels that are 10 times normal.[62] Nevertheless, Na^+ excretion is still equal to intake, perhaps due in part to the concurrent fall in blood pressure that limits the natriuretic response to ANP. Thus, ANP may contribute to but is not necessary for the maintenance of Na^+ balance.

Pressure natriuresis An essential "backup" feature of the volume regulatory system that can compensate for an abnormality in the humoral control of Na^+ excretion is the phenomenon of *pressure natriuresis* (Fig. 8-8). In normal subjects, a small elevation in blood pressure results in a relatively large increase in the urinary excretion of Na^+ and water.[63-65] In contrast to the other mediators of tubular Na^+ transport, this *pressure natriuresis* phenomenon does not require neurally or humorally mediated sensor mechanisms, since changes in volume directly affect the cardiac output and therefore the systemic blood pressure.[63]

The mechanism by which pressure natriuresis occurs is incompletely understood, as decreased reabsorption appears to occur in the proximal tubule and loop of Henle.[49,66-68] It is possible, for example, that the increase in systemic pressure is transmitted, via the vasa recta capillaries, to the medullary interstitium.[49-68] This rise in interstitial pressure can impair NaCl transport in at least two ways[67,68]:

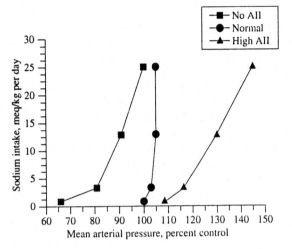

Figure 8-8 Relationship between increasing sodium intake and mean arterial pressure in normals, in the absence of angiotensin II (AII), and with an angiotensin II infusion. The inability to regulate angiotensin II and aldosterone in the last two settings necessitates an elevation in blood pressure to excrete the extra sodium. (*From Guyton AC*, Science *252:1813, 1991. Used with permission.*)

- The increase in capillary pressure can diminish the movement of reabsorbed solutes and water from the interstitium into the capillary, thereby preventing their return to the systemic circulation.
- The elevation in interstitial pressure will tend to push fluid into the water-permeable *descending* limb of the loop of Henle, counteracting the osmotic gradient favoring water movement out of this segment into the hyperosmotic interstitium. The ensuring decline in descending limb water reabsorption will *minimize the rise in the tubular fluid Na^+ concentration* that is required for subsequent passive NaCl transport in the *thin* ascending limb (see page 130). The net effect is decreased loop NaCl reabsorption.

Increased release of renal prostaglandins and, more importantly, nitric oxide may contribute to pressure natriuresis.[66,69-71] It is unclear whether this represents a direct hormonal effect on tubular transport* or is mediated by renal vasodilatation with a subsequent increase in intracapillary pressure. These changes are reversed with a fall in renal perfusion pressure, as tubular sodium and water reabsorption are enhanced.[67,72]

Nitric oxide (NO) release from the macula densa is a modulating factor that is augmented during increased sodium chloride delivery, thereby countering the afferent arteriole constriction elicited in the tubuloglomerular feedback (TGF) response. It has been suggested that enhanced macula densa NO production

---

* As described in Chap. 6, prostaglandins appear to inhibit Na^+ reabsorption in the thick ascending limb and in the cortical collecting tubule. This effect is not important in the day-to-day regulation of Na^+ excretion, since there is a low basal rate of prostaglandin production. The major stimuli to renal prostaglandin synthesis are the vasoconstrictors angiotensin II and norepinephrine, which are released in states of effective volume depletion. In this setting, the prostaglandins minimize both the renal ischemia and the associated Na^+ retention.

may underlie the resetting of TGF that occurs when salt intake is increased; the response is appropriately blunted in this setting, as maintenance of glomerular filtration promotes excretion of the excess salt.[73]

Regardless of the mechanism, pressure natriuresis can, in certain circumstances, play an important role in the maintenance of volume balance. It is not likely to contribute significantly to the day-to-day regulation of Na^+ excretion, since changes in aldosterone and perhaps ANP release are sufficient to accomplish this goal. For example, a 50-fold increase in Na^+ intake and subsequent excretion (from very low to high levels) is associated with only a 4-mmHg elevation in systemic blood pressure in normal subjects (as shown in the middle curve in Fig. 8-8).[63] In this setting, the decline in angiotensin II and aldosterone and the increase in ANP are sufficient to markedly increase Na^+ excretion without requiring a large rise in blood pressure.

If, however, there is an impairment in one or more of the neurohumoral mediators of volume regulation, then pressure natriuresis may be required to maintain Na^+ balance. This concept can be illustrated by the changes induced by increasing sodium intake when the ability to regulate angiotensin II and aldosterone according to Na^+ intake is impaired, either by very low or by very high angiotensin II levels (left and right curves in Fig. 8-8). In both cases, tubular Na^+ reabsorption cannot be decreased by diminishing the production of angiotensin II and aldosterone; as a result, a greater than normal increase in blood pressure is required to maintain Na^+ balance as intake is increased.

These experiments illustrate the role of pressure natriuresis in the regulation of blood pressure as well as that of Na^+ excretion. This can also be illustrated by the phenomenon of aldosterone escape.[25] The initial Na^+ retention and elevation in systemic blood pressure induced by aldosterone are followed by a spontaneous natriuresis that minimizes the degree of volume expansion and hypertension (see Fig. 6-15). Although the diuresis in this setting may in part be mediated by increased release of ANP,[74,75] pressure natriuresis also appears to play an important role. As shown in Fig. 8-9, use of a suprarenal aortic clamp to maintain a constant renal perfusion pressure prevents aldosterone escape from occurring. The net effect is continued Na^+ retention and the eventual development of pulmonary edema or malignant hypertension. Release of the clamp is rapidly followed by increased urinary Na^+ loss and a reduction in the systemic blood pressure.

This observation can be extended to any form of hypertension: The rise in blood pressure, whether induced by aldosterone, norepinephrine, or underlying renal disease, is eventually limited by fluid loss induced by pressure natriuresis.[63,64] In terms of Fig. 8-8, the pressure natriuresis curve is shifted to the right in hypertensive patients; that is, Na^+ balance is maintained, but at a higher than normal systemic blood pressure to overcome, for example, the Na^+-retaining effect of aldosterone.

Pressure natriuresis can also limit Na^+ excretion when renal perfusion pressure is reduced by effective volume depletion due, for example, to diuretic therapy.[65] The sodium-retaining effect in this setting is normally mediated by

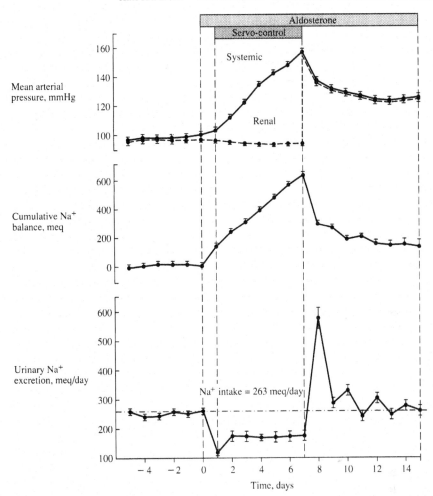

Figure 8-9 The effect of the administration of aldosterone and a high-Na$^+$ diet on mean arterial pressure, cumulative Na$^+$ balance, and urinary Na$^+$ excretion in dogs. If renal perfusion pressure is held constant by use of a suprarenal aortic clamp, Na$^+$ excretion remains at low levels and aldosterone escape does not occur. The net result is progressive Na$^+$ retention and a marked elevation in systemic blood pressure. When, however, renal perfusion pressure is allowed to rise by release of the clamp, there is a spontaneous diuresis, leading to a return in Na$^+$ balance toward normal and much less severe hypertension. (*From Hall JE, Granger JP, Smith MJ Jr, Premen AJ,* Hypertension *6(suppl 1):I-183, 1984. By permission of the American Heart Association, Inc.*)

angiotensin II and norepinephrine as described above. If, however, both systems are blocked, sodium retention still occurs in association with a fall in blood pressure (see Fig. 15-1).[76] This fall in blood pressure, which can enhance Na$^+$ reabsorption by pressure natriuresis, is due to the absence of angiotensin II– and norepinephrine-mediated vasoconstriction, which maintains the blood pressure in hypovolemic subjects.

Sympathetic nervous system   Pressure natriuresis can also explain the variable effects of sympathetic blockade on renal Na^+ handling. As described above, increased sympathetic activity raises the systemic blood pressure and enhances proximal Na^+ reabsorption.[26,31,32] The net effect on Na^+ excretion, however, is not predictable, since the elevation in renal perfusion pressure will tend to counteract the direct tubular effect.[77] In effective volume depletion, for example, the increase in adrenergic tone appropriately raises the systemic blood pressure; this would also lead to inappropriate urinary Na^+ wasting if it were not for the concurrent increase in Na^+ reabsorption.[77]

The interaction between the pressure and reabsorptive effective of the sympathetic nervous system can also be illustrated by the response to the sympatholytic agent guanethidine (a now rarely used antihypertensive drug). When given in doses that do not reduce the systemic pressure, guanethidine can inhibit the adrenergic action on the kidney, resulting in an increase in Na^+ excretion.[34] However, when guanethidine is used to lower the blood pressure in patients with hypertension, the hypotensive effect predominates and Na^+ retention is likely to occur.[78,79] This constitutes the rationale for the use of diuretics in combination with sympathetic blockers in the treatment of hypertension, since the increase in volume produced by the latter tends to minimize the hypotensive response.[78]

Also complicating the evaluation of the sympathetic effect on Na^+ excretion is the demonstration that renal sympathetic tone may occasionally be regulated independent of that in other organs. This phenomenon appears to be mediated by volume receptors in the left side of the heart, as an increase in left-sided pressure results in a *reduction in renal sympathetic tone,*[80-82] even though total sympathetic activity may be enhanced.[82]

The potential importance of this cardiorenal reflex is illustrated by the following animal experiment.[82] The induction of hypotensive hemorrhage (which lowers left-sided pressures) resulted in a decrease in renal blood flow of as much as 90 percent and a cessation of urine output, both of which were due in large part to a hypotension-induced increase in sympathetic activity and subsequent marked renal vasoconstriction. In contrast, a similar reduction in systemic blood pressure due to an acute myocardial infarction (which raises left-sided pressures) was associated with only a 25 percent fall in renal blood flow and persistence of an adequate urine output. This relative maintenance of renal perfusion and urine flow presumably was due in part to reduced renal sympathetic tone, resulting from the evaluation in left-sided intracardiac pressure. It is also possible that increased secretion of ANP contributed to the relative renal vasodilation in this setting.

Although it is uncertain how important the left-sided cardiac receptors are in humans,[83] a cardiorenal reflex can explain the clinical observation that postischemic acute tubular necrosis frequently follows hypotension due to sepsis, surgery, or hemorrhage, but is rare when renal hypoperfusion is due to heart failure.[84]

Plasma Na^+ concentrations   Urinary Na^+ excretion also may be affected by the plasma Na^+ concentration, tending to increase with hypernatremia and to fall with hyponatremia.[85-87] This effect may be mediated by changes in both the filtered Na^+ load (GFR times plasma Na^+ concentration) and the rate of tubular reabsorption. These responses can be viewed as appropriate from the viewpoint of maintenance of the plasma Na^+ concentration. Increasing Na^+ excretion with hypernatremia, for example, will tend to lower the plasma Na^+ concentration toward normal.

However, the *plasma Na^+ concentration does not play an important role in the daily regulation of Na^+ excretion*, since it is normally maintained within narrow limits by ADH and thirst (see Chap. 9). Furthermore, even in patients who are hyponatremic or hypernatremic, the effective circulating volume is a *more important determinant* of Na^+ excretion than the plasma Na^+ concentration (see "Volume Regulation versus Osmoregulation," below). For example, the syndrome of inappropriate ADH secretion is characterized by water retention, which leads to both hyponatremia and volume expansion. As a result, this disorder is initially associated with enhanced Na^+ excretion, although the increase may be somewhat less than that seen with an equivalent degree of volume expansion in a patient with a normal plasma Na^+ concentration.[88] Similarly, urinary Na^+ excretion is reduced in hypernatremic patients who are volume-depleted due, for example, to lack of replacement of insensible water losses from the skin and respiratory tract (see Chap. 24).

Summary

It is clear that multiple factors affect renal Na^+ excretion and therefore the regulation of the effective circulating volume. It seems likely that aldosterone and possibly atrial natriuretic peptide (or related peptides such as urodilatin) are responsible for day-to-day variations in Na^+ excretion through their respective ability to augment and diminish Na^+ reabsorption in the collecting tubules. As Na^+ intake is reduced, for example, the ensuing decrease in volume enhances the activity of the renin-angiotensin-aldosterone system and reduces the secretion of ANP. The net effect is enhanced Na^+ reabsorption in the collecting tubules, which seems to account for the appropriate fall in Na^+ excretion in this setting. With more marked hypovolemia, a decrease in GFR and an increase in proximal and thin ascending limb Na^+ reabsorption also contribute to Na^+ retention. Both angiotensin II and norepinephrine may contribute to this response, which is clinically important because the stimulation of proximal transport also increases the reabsorption of bicarbonate and urate (see Chap. 3). Consequently, hypovolemia can lead to the maintenance of metabolic alkalosis (because the excess bicarbonate cannot be excreted) and to hyperuricemia and gout, all of which commonly occur in patients receiving diuretic therapy.

This sequence is reversed with volume expansion, as an increase in the secretion of ANP and a reduction in that of aldosterone (Fig. 8-3) allow excretion of the excess Na^+ by diminishing collecting tubule Na^+ reabsorption. With more pronounced hypervolemia, reabsorption may also fall in the proximal tubule, often leading to enhanced urate secretion and hypouricemia.[59]

The pressure natriuresis phenomenon may be the *final defense* against changes in the effective circulating volume.[63,64] In normal subjects, it probably plays a relatively minor role, because the other regulatory systems are sufficiently sensitive to maintain Na^+ balance without a large change in extracellular volume or blood pressure.[63] If, however, there is an abnormality in one of more of these factors (as with renal disease or excess angiotensin II or aldosterone), the degree of Na^+ retention that will occur is ultimately limited, since the ensuing volume expansion raises the blood pressure, which then enhances Na^+ excretion. Eventually, a new steady state is reestablished in which intake and excretion are equal and the blood pressure is higher than normal.

Sodium reabsorption in the distal tubule and the *thick* ascending limb of the loop of Henle is primarily flow-dependent and not influenced by hormones involved in volume regulation (see Chaps. 4 and 5). As a result, changes in transport in these segments usually do not play an important role in regulating Na^+ excretion. One exception to this general rule occurs in patients treated with a loop diuretic, such as furosemide. The reduction in loop reabsorption in this setting increases fluid delivery to the distal tubule, leading to an enhanced rate of distal Na^+ reabsorption (and the requisite rise in activity of the Na^+-K^+-ATPase pump that returns reabsorbed Na^+ to the systemic circulation; see Fig. 5-1).[89-91] Similarly, blocking distal tubule Na^+ reabsorption with a thiazide-type diuretic leads to increased downstream Na^+ transport in the cortical collecting tubule, which also can respond to changes in flow.[92]

These compensatory adaptations may be important because they limit the net response to the diuretic. In most cases, an adequate diuresis is still obtained. However, increased distal reabsorption can induce *diuretic resistance* in some patients, who may require combined therapy with a loop and a thiazide diuretic to inhibit transport at several sites in the nephron (see Chap. 15).

VOLUME REGULATION VERSUS OSMOREGULATION

This chapter has dealt with the factors involved in the maintenance of the effective circulating volume. It is important, however, to be aware that these homeostatic mechanisms are very different from those involved in the maintenance of the plasma osmolality (Table 8-4). The plasma osmolality is determined by the *ratio* of solutes (primarily Na^+ and K^+ salts) and water, whereas the extracellular volume is determined by the *absolute amounts* of Na^+ and water that are present (see page 248). A few simple examples can illustrate the difference between these parameters.

- Exercising on a hot day leads to the loss of dilute fluid as sweat. The net effect is a *rise* in the plasma osmolality and Na^+ concentration but a *fall* in the extracellular volume. Similar changes can be seen in a nursing home patient who develops viral gastroenteritis, characterized by fever, profuse diarrhea, and decreased fluid intake.

Table 8-4   Difference between osmoregulation and volume regulation

	Osmoregulation	Volume regulation
What is being sensed	Plasma osmolality	Effective circulating volume
Sensors	Hypothalamic osmoreceptors	Carotid sinus
		Afferent arteriole
		Atria
Effectors	Antidiuretic hormone	Renin-angiotensin-aldosterone
	Thirst	system
		Sympathetic nervous system
		Atrial natriuretic peptide
		Pressure natriuresis
		Antidiuretic hormone
What is affected	Water excretion and, via thirst, water intake	Urine sodium excretion

- An infusion of isotonic saline will cause volume expansion, with no alteration in the plasma osmolality.
- The administration of one-half isotonic saline will initially lower the plasma sodium concentration by dilution and raise the extracellular fluid volume.

Changes in the plasma osmolality, which is primarily determined by the plasma Na^+ concentration, are sensed by osmoreceptors in the hypothalamus (see Chap. 6). These receptors affect both water intake and water excretion by influencing thirst and the release of ADH, respectively (Table 8-4). The latter increases the urine osmolality and causes water retention by enhancing the permeability of the collecting tubules to water. Notice that osmoregulation is achieved by *alterations in water balance; Na^+ handling is not directly affected unless there are concurrent changes in volume.* Although it is tempting to assume that regulation of the plasma Na^+ concentration has something to do with Na^+, it is actually water intake and excretion that are affected.

Volume regulation, on the other hand, attempts to maintain tissue perfusion. Different sensors and effectors are involved in this process, as it is urinary Na^+ excretion, not osmolality, that is primarily modified (Table 8-4). The only major area of overlap involves the hypovolemic stimulus to ADH release; the ensuing water retention will then help to restore normovolemia.

The independent roles of the osmoregulatory and volume regulatory pathways can be appreciated by returning to the examples described above.

- The rise in plasma osmolality following exercise on a hot day will stimulate both ADH release and thirst; the ensuing increase in urine osmolality and subsequent water retention will eventually return the plasma Na^+ concentration toward normal. This subject is also volume-depleted; consequently,

there will be activation of the renin-angiotensin-aldosterone system, resulting in a fall in urinary Na^+ excretion. The net effect is that the urine will
initially be highly concentrated and contain relatively little Na^+.

- Similar hormonal changes occur in the nursing home patient with gastroenteritis. However, the degree of extracellular fluid volume depletion is
likely to be greater as a result of salt loss in the diarrheal fluid.
- ADH release and thirst are not altered with an infusion of isotonic saline,
since there is no change in the plasma osmolality. In this setting, only
volume regulation is activated, as the associated volume expansion
diminishes the release of aldosterone and increases that of ANP. The net
effect is excretion of the excess Na^+ and water in a relatively isosmotic
urine.
- Half-isotonic saline causes both hypoosmolality and volume expansion.
Thus, ADH and renin release will be reduced and ANP secretion enhanced,
thereby allowing the excess NaCl to be excreted in an appropriately dilute
fluid.

Thus, the person who exercises on a hot day is dehydrated with a small degree of
volume depletion, the nursing home patient with gastroenteritis is also dehydrated
with a greater degree of volume depletion, and a patient with diarrhea who maintains a normal plasma Na^+ concentration is volume-depleted but not dehydrated.

Dehydration versus Volume Depletion

The preceding observations permit an understanding of the difference between two
terms that are often used synonymously but actually refer to different phenomena:
dehydration and volume depletion (also called hypovolemia).[93] *Dehydration* refers
to water loss that leads to an elevation in plasma sodium concentration and an
intracellular water deficit as a result of the osmotic movement of water from the
cells into the extracellular fluid. In comparison, *volume depletion* refers to a
decrease in the extracellular fluid volume as a result of the loss of sodium and
water. It can be produced by salt and water loss (as with vomitting, diarrhea,
diuretics, bleeding, or third space sequestration) or by water loss alone (i.e., dehydration).

PROBLEMS

8-1   In what direction would the plasma volume, the total extracellular fluid volume, the effective
circulating volume, and urinary Na^+ excretion change in the following conditions?
(a) An acute myocardial infarction producing a decrease in the cardiac output
(b) A high-Na^+ diet
(c) The retention of ingested water due to inappropriate secretion of ADH

8-2   What effect would you expect the administration of diuretics (which increase urinary NaCl and
water loss) to have on the secretion of renin? Diuretics are used in the treatment of hypertension.
Would this effect on renin secretion influence the degree to which the blood pressure is lowered?

8-3 Assuming that renal function is normal and that there is no obstruction to renal blood flow, which of the following offers the most accurate assessment of the effective circulating volume?

(a) Cardiac output

(b) Plasma volume

(c) Systemic blood pressure

(d) Urinary Na^+ excretion

8-4 In a stable patient chronically taking diuretics for hypertension, what will be the relationship between Na^+ intake and urinary Na^+ excretion?

8-5 What effect will each of the following have on the secretion of aldosterone, ANP, and ADH and on the urine osmolality and Na^+ excretion?

(a) An infusion of isotonic saline

(b) The intake of 1000 mL of water, which is normally excreted very rapidly, so that there is little change in extracellular volume

(c) Eating potato chips (which are very salty) while ingesting no water

(d) An infusion of half-isotonic saline

REFERENCES

1. Epstein FH, Goodyer AN, Laurason FD, Relman AS. Studies of the antidiuresis of quiet standing: The importance of changes in plasma volume and glomerular filtration rate. *J Clin Invest* 30:62, 1951.
2. Schrier RW. An odyssey into the milieu intérieur: Pondering the enigmas. *J Am Soc Nephrol* 2:1549, 1992.
3. Schrier RW. Pathogenesis of sodium and water retention in high-output and low-output cardiac failure, nephrotic syndrome, cirrhosis, and pregnancy. *N Engl J Med* 319:1065,1127, 1988.
4. Epstein FH, Post RS, McDowell M. The effect of an arteriovenous fistula on renal hemodynamics and electrolyte excretion. *J Clin Invest* 32:233, 1953.
5. Lieberman FL, Reynolds TB. Plasma volume in cirrhosis of the liver: Its relation to portal hypertension, ascites, and renal failure. *J Clin Invest* 46:1297, 1967.
6. Kowalski HJ, Abelmann WH. The cardiac output at rest in Laennec"s cirrhosis. *J Clin Invest* 32:1025, 1953.
7. Arroyo V, Bosch J, Gaya-Beltran J, et al. Plasma renin activity and urinary sodium excretion as prognostic indicators in nonazotemic cirrhosis with ascites. *Ann Intern Med* 94:198, 1981.
8. Henriksen JH, Bendtsen F, Gerbes AL, et al. Estimated central blood volume in cirrhosis: Relationship to sympathetic nervous activity, β-adrenergic blockade and atrial natriuretic factor. *Hepatology* 16:1163, 1992.
9. Perez-Ayuso RM, Arroyo V, Campos J, et al. Evidence that renal prostaglandins are involved in renal water metabolism in cirrhosis. *Kidney Int* 26:72, 1984.
10. Miller TR, Anderson RJ, Linas SL, et al. Urinary diagnostic indices in acute renal failure: A prospective study. *Ann Intern Med* 89:47, 1978.
11. Strauss MB, Lamdin E, Smith WP, Bleifer DJ. Surfeit and deficit of sodium: A kinetic concept of sodium excretion. *Arch Intern Med* 102:527, 1958.
12. Walser M. Phenomenological analysis of renal regulation of sodium and potassium balance. *Kidney Int* 27:837, 1985.
13. Bonventre JV, Leaf A. Sodium homeostasis: Steady states without a set point. *Kidney Int* 21:880, 1982.
14. Simpson FO. Sodium intake, body sodium, and sodium excretion. *Lancet* 2:25, 1988.
15. Sagnella GA, Markandu ND, Buckley MG, et al. Hormonal responses to gradual changes in dietary sodium intake in humans. *Am J Physiol* 256:R1171, 1989.
16. Rabelink TJ, Koomans HA, Hené RJ, Dorhout Mees EJ. Early and late adjustment to potassium loading in humans. *Kidney Int* 38:942, 1990.
17. Skorecki KL, Brenner BM. Body fluid homeostasis in man. *Am J Med* 70:77, 1981.

18. Kimani JK. Elastin and mechanoreceptor mechanisms with special reference to the mammalian carotid sinus. *Ciba Found Symp* 192:215, 1995.
19. Epstein M. Cardiovascular and renal effects of head-out water immersion in man. *Circ Res* 39:619, 1976.
20. Epstein M, Loutzenhemier R, Friedland E, et al. Relationship of increased plasma atrial natriuretic factor and renal sodium handling during immersion-induced central hypervolemia in normal humans. *J Clin Invest* 79:738, 1987.
21. Epstein M, Pins DS, Schneider N, Levinson R. Determinants of deranged sodium and water homeostasis in decompensated cirrhosis. *J Lab Clin Med* 87:822, 1976.
22. Peterson TV, Jones CE. Renal responses of the cardiac-denervated nonhuman primate to blood volume expansion. *Circ Res* 53:24, 1983.
23. Peterson TV, Chase NL, Gray DK. Renal effects of volume expansion in the renal-denervated nonhuman primate. *Am J Physiol* 247:H960, 1984.
24. Hall JE, Granger JP, Smith MJ Jr, Premen AJ. Role of renal hemodynamics and arterial pressure in aldosterone "escape" *Hypertension* 6(suppl 1):1–183, 1984.
25. Gonzalez-Campoy JM, Romero JC, Knox FG. Escape from the sodium-retaining effects of mineralcorticoids: Role of ANF and intrarenal hormone systems. *Kidney Int* 35:767, 1989.
26. DiBona GF. Renal neural activity in hepatorenal syndrome. *Kidney Int* 25:841, 1984.
27. Frye RL, Braunwald E. Studies of Starling's law of the heart. I. The circulatory response to acute hypervolemia and its modification by ganglionic blockade. *J Clin Invest* 39:1043, 1960.
28. Freis ED, Stanton JR, Finnerty FA Jr, et al. The collapse produced by venous congestion of the extremities or by venesection following certain hypotensive agents. *J Clin Invest* 30:435, 1951.
29. Dzau VJ. Renal and circulatory mechanisms in congestive heart failure. *Kidney Int* 31:1402, 1987.
30. Gordon RD, Kuchel O, Liddle GW, Island DP. Role of the sympathetic nervous system in regulating renin and aldosterone production in man. *J Clin Invest* 46:599, 1967.
31. Osborn JL, Holdaas H, Thames MD, DiBona GF. Renal adrenoreceptor mediation of antinatriuretic and renin secretion responses to low frequency renal nerve stimulation in the dog. *Circ Res* 53:298, 1983.
32. Gill JR Jr, Casper AGT. Role of the sympathetic nervous system in the renal response to hemorrhage. *J Clin Invest* 48:915, 1969.
33. Wilcox CS, Puritz R, Lightman SL, et al. Plasma volume regulation in patients with progressive autonomic failure during changes in salt intake or posture. *J Lab Clin Med* 104:331, 1984.
34. Gill JR Jr, Mason DT, Bartter FC. Adrenergic nervous systems in sodium metabolism: Effects of guanethidine and sodium-retaining steroids in normal man. *J Clin Invest* 43:177, 1964.
35. Cogan MG. Angiotensin II: A potent controller of sodium transport in the early proximal tubule. *Hypertension* 15:451, 1990.
36. Seidelin PH, McMurray JJ, Struthers AD. Mechanisms of the antinatriuretic action of physiological doses of angiotensin II in man. *Clin Sci* 76:653, 1989.
37. Watkins L Jr, Burton JA, Haber E, et al. The renin-angiotensin-aldosterone system in congestive failure in conscious dogs. *J Clin Invest* 57:1606, 1976.
38. Schroeder ET, Anderson JH, Goldman SH, Streeten DHP. Effect of blockade of angiotensin II on blood pressure, renin and aldosterone in cirrhosis. *Kidney Int* 9:511, 1976.
39. Dzau VJ, Colucci WS, Hollenberg NK, Williams GH. Relation of the renin-angiotensin-aldosterone system to clinical state in congestive heart failure. *Circulation* 63:645, 1981.
40. Schunkert H, Ingelfinger JR, Hirsch AT, et al. Evidence for tissue specific activation of renal angiotensinogen mRNA expression in chronic stable experimental heart failure. *J Clin Invest* 90:1523, 1992.
41. Lindheimer MD, Lalone RC, Levinsky NG. Evidence that an acute increase in glomerular filtration has little effect on sodium excretion in the dog unless extracellular volume is expanded. *J Clin Invest* 46:256, 1974.
42. Bricker NS, Fine LG, Kaplan M, et al. "Magnification phenomenon" in chronic renal disease. *N Engl J Med* 299:1287, 1978.

43. Wright FS. Flow-dependent transport processes: Filtration, absorption, secretion. *Am J Physiol* 243:F1, 1982.
44. Gregor R, Velazquez H. The cortical thick ascending limb and early distal convoluted tubule in the urine concentrating mechanism. *Kidney Int* 31:590, 1987.
45. Stein JH, Osgood RW, Boonjarern S, et al. Segmental sodium reabsorption in rats with mild and severe volume depletion. *Am J Physiol* 227:351, 1974.
46. Weiner MW, Weinman EJ, Kashgarian M, Hayslett JP. Accelerated reabsorption in the proximal tubule produced by volume depletion. *J Clin Invest* 50:1379, 1971.
47. Moe OW, Tejedor A, Levi M, et al. Dietary NaCl modulates Na^+-H^+ antiporter activity in renal cortical apical membrane vesicles. *Am J Physiol* 260:F130, 1991.
48. Faubert PF, Chou S-Y, Porush JG, et al. Papillary plasma flow and tissue osmolality in chronic caval dogs. *Am J Physiol* 242:F370, 1982.
49. Cowley AW. Role of the renal medulla in volume and arterial pressure regulation. *Am J Physiol* 273:R1, 1997.
50. Osgood RW, Reineck HJ, Stein JH. Further studies on segmental sodium transport in the rat kidney during expansion of the extracellular fluid volume. *J Clin Invest* 62:311, 1978.
51. Dirks JH, Cirksena WJ, Berliner RW. The effect of saline infusion on sodium reabsorption by the proximal tubule of the dog. *J Clin Invest* 44:1160, 1965.
52. Knox FG, Burnett JC Jr, Kohan DE, et al. Escape from the sodium-retaining effects of mineralocorticoids. *Kidney Int* 17:263, 1980.
53. Hansell P, Fasching A. The effect of dopamine receptor blockade on natriuresis is dependent on the degree of hypervolemia. *Kidney Int* 93:253, 1991.
54. Seri I, Cone BC, Gullans SR, et al. Influence of Na^+ intake on dopamine-induced inhibition of renal cortical Na^+-K^+-ATPase. *Am J Physiol* 258:F52, 1990.
55. Homcy C, Gaivin R, Zisfein J, Graham RM. Snack-induced release of atrial natriuretic peptide (letter). *N Engl J Med* 313:1484, 1984.
56. de Zeeuw D, Janssen WMT, de Jong PE. Atrial natriuretic factor: Its (patho)physiological significance in humans. *Kidney Int* 41:1115, 1992.
57. Goetz KL. Evidence that atriopeptin is not a physiological regulatory of sodium excretion. *Hypertension* 15:9, 1990.
58. Steele TH, Oppenheimer S. Factors affecting urate excretion following diuretic administration in man. *Am J Med* 47:564, 1969.
59. Beck LH. Hypouricemia in the syndrome of inappropriate secretion of antidiuretic hormone. *N Engl J Med* 301:528, 1979.
60. Rosenbaum JD, Papper S, Ashley MM. Variations in renal excretion of sodium independent of change in adrenocortical hormone dosage in patients with Addison's disease. *J Clin Endocrinol Metab* 15:1549, 1955.
61. Yokota N, Bruneau BG, Kuroski de Bold ML, de Bold AJ. Atrial natriuretic factor contributes to mineralocorticoid escape phenomenon. Evidence for a guanylate cyclase-mediated pathway. *J Clin Invest* 94:1938, 1994.
62. Field LJ, Veress PT, Steinhelper ME, et al. Kidney function in ANF-transgenic mice: Effect of blood volume expanders. *Am J Physiol* 260:R1, 1991.
63. Guyton AC. Blood pressure control—Special role of the kidneys and body fluids. *Science* 252:1813, 1991.
64. Hall JE, Mizelle L, Hildebrandt DA, Brands MW. Abnormal pressure natriuresis. A cause or consequence of hypertension. *Hypertension* 15:547, 1990.
65. Mizelle HL, Montani J-P, Hester RL, et al. Role of pressure natriuresis in long-term control of renal electrolyte excretion. *Hypertension* 22:102, 1993.
66. Roman RJ. Pressure-diuresis in volume expanded rats. Tubular reabsorption in superficial and deep nephrons. *Hypertension* 12:177, 1988.
67. Kinoshita Y, Knox FG. Role of prostaglandins in proximal tubular sodium reabsorption: Response to elevated renal interstitial hydrostatic pressure. *Circ Res* 64:1013, 1989.
68. Granger JP. Pressure natriuresis: Role of renal interstitial hydrostatic pressure. *Hypertension* 19(suppl 1):I-9, 1992.

69. Carmines PK, Bell PD, Roman RJ, et al. Prostaglandins in the sodium excretory response to altered renal arterial pressure in dogs. *Am J Physiol* 248:F8, 1985.

70. Salom HG, Lahera V, Miranda-Guardiola F, Romero JC. Blockade of pressure natriuresis induced by inhibition of renal synthesis of nitric oxide in dogs. *Am J Physiol* 262:F718, 1992.

71. Guarasci G, Line RL. Pressure-natriuresis following acute and chronic inhibition of nitric oxide synthase in rats. *Am J Physiol* 270:R469, 1996.

72. Levy M. Effects of acute volume expansion and altered hemodynamics on renal tubular function in chronic caval dogs. *J Clin Invest* 51:922, 1972.

73. Wilcox CS, Welch WJ. TGF and nitric oxide: Effects of salt intake and salt-sensitive hypertension. *Kidney Int* (suppl 55):S9, 1996.

74. Capuccio FP, Markandu ND, Buckley MG, et al. Changes in the plasma levels of atrial natriuretic peptides during mineralocorticoid escape in man. *Clin Sci* 72:531, 1987.

75. Ballerman BJ, Bloch KD, Seidman JG, Brenner BM. Atrial natriuretic peptide transcription, secretion, and glomerular receptor activity during mineralocorticoid escape in the rat. *J Clin Invest* 78:840, 1986.

76. Wilcox CS, Guzman NJ, Mitch WE, et al. Na^+, K^+, and BP homeostasis in man during furosemide: Effects of parazosin and captopril. *Kidney Int* 31:135, 1987.

77. Ehmke, Persson PB, Seyfarth M, Kirchheim HR. Neurogenic control of pressure natriuresis in conscious dogs. *Am J Physiol* 259:F466, 1990.

78. Dustan H, Tarazi RC, Bravo EL. Dependence of arterial pressure on intravascular volume in treated hypertensive patients. *N Engl J Med* 286:861, 1972.

79. Smith AJ. Fluid retention produced by guanethidine: Changes in body exchangeable sodium, blood volume, and creatinine clearance. *Circulation* 31:490, 1965.

80. Thames MD, Abboud FM. Reflex inhibition of renal sympathetic nerve activity during myocardial ischemia mediated by left ventricular receptors with vagal afferents in dogs. *J Clin Invest* 63:395, 1979.

81. Thames MD, Miller BD, Abboud FM. Baroreflex regulation of renal nerve activity during volume expansion. *Am J Physiol* 243:H810, 1982.

82. Gorfinkel HJ, Szidon JP, Hirsch LJ, Fishman AP. Renal performance in experimental cardiogenic shock. *Am J Physiol* 222:1260, 1972.

83. Cornish KG, Gilmore JP. Increased left atrial pressure does not alter renal function in the conscious primate. *Am J Physiol* 243:R119, 1982.

84. Schrier RW. Acute renal failure. *Kidney Int* 15:205, 1979.

85. Metzler CH, Thrasher TN, Keil LC, Ramsay DJ. Endocrine mechanisms regulating sodium excretion during water deprivation in dogs. *Am J Physiol* 251:R560, 1986.

86. Langberg H, Hartmann A, Ostensen J, et al. Hypernatremia inhibits $NaHCO_3$ reabsorption and associated NaCl reabsorption in dogs. *Kidney Int* 29:820, 1986.

87. Schrier RW, de Wardener HE. Tubular reabsorption of sodium ion: Influence of factors other than aldosterone and glomerular filtration rate. *N Engl J Med* 285:1231, 1971.

88. Schrier RW, Fein RL, McNeil JS, Cirksena WJ. Influence of interstitial fluid volume expansion and plasma sodium concentration on the natriuretic response to volume expansion in dogs. *Clin Sci* 36:371, 1969.

89. Scherzer P, Wald H, Popovtzer MM. Enhanced glomerular filtration and Na^+-K^+-ATPase with furosemide administration. *Am J Physiol* 252:F910, 1987.

90. Hropot M, Fowler N, Karlmark B, Giebisch G. Tubular action of diuretics: Distal effects on electrolyte transport and acidification. *Kidney Int* 28:477, 1985.

91. Loon NR, Wilcox CS, Unwin RJ. Mechanism of impaired natriuretic response to furosemide during prolonged therapy. *Kidney Int* 36:682, 1989.

92. Garg LC, Narang N. Effects of hydrochlorothiazide on Na^+-K^+-ATPase activity along the rat nephron. *Kidney Int* 31:918, 1985.

93. Mange K, Matsuura D, Cizman B, et al. Language guiding therapy: The case of dehydration versus volume depletion. *Ann Intern Med* 127:848, 1997.

REGULATION OF PLASMA OSMOLALITY

Hypoosmolality and hyperosmolality can produce serious neurologic symptoms and death, primarily as a result of water movement into and out of the brain, respectively (see Chaps. 23 and 24).[1-5] To prevent this, the plasma osmolality (P_{osm}), which is primarily determined by the plasma Na^+ concentration (see Chap. 7), is normally maintained within narrow limits by appropriate variations in *water intake* and *water excretion*. This regulatory system is governed by osmoreceptors in the hypothalamus that influence both thirst and the secretion of antidiuretic hormone (ADH).

Although it may seem that regulation of the plasma Na^+ concentration must have something to do with Na^+ balance, osmoregulation is almost entirely mediated by changes in *water balance*. Thus, the effectors for osmoregulation (ADH and thirst, affecting water excretion and water intake) are very different from those involved in volume regulation (the renin-angiotensin-aldosterone system and atrial natriuretic peptide, affecting Na^+ excretion) (see Table 8-4). This chapter will describe the sources of water intake, the sites of water loss from the body, and the roles of ADH, thirst, and renal water excretion in the maintenance of the P_{osm}.

WATER BALANCE

Obligatory Water Output

In the steady state, water intake (including that generated from endogenous metabolism) must equal water output (Table 9-1). Much of the water output involves obligatory losses in the urine and stool, and, by evaporation, from the moist surfaces of the skin and respiratory tract. The evaporative losses play an important role in *thermoregulation*; the heat required for evaporation, 0.58 kcal/1.0 mL of water, normally accounts for 20 to 25 percent of the heat lost from the body, with the remainder occurring by radiation and convection.[6] The net effect is the elimination of the heat produced by body metabolism, thereby preventing the development of hyperthermia.

In contrast to these *insensible* losses, sweat can be called a *sensible* loss. Sweat is a hypotonic fluid (Na^+ concentration equals 30 to 65 meq/L) secreted by the sweat glands in the skin. It also contributes to thermoregulation, as the secretion and subsequent evaporation of sweat result in the loss of heat from the body. In the basal state, sweat production is low, but it can increase markedly in the presence of high external temperatures or when endogenous heat production is enhanced, as with exercise, fever, or hyperthyroidism.[6] As an example, a subject exercising in a hot, dry climate can lose as much as 1500 mL/h as sweat.[7]

The obligatory renal water loss is directly related to solute excretion. If a subject has to excrete 800 mosmol of solute per day (mostly Na^+ and K^+ salts and urea) to remain in the steady state, and the maximum U_{osm} is 1200 mosmol/kg, then the excretion of the 800 mosmol will require a minimum urine volume of 670 mL/day.

Only small amounts of water, averaging 100 to 200 mL/day, are normally lost in the stool. However, gastrointestinal losses are increased to a variable degree in patients with vomiting or diarrhea. The effect of these losses on the plasma Na^+ concentration depends on the sum of the Na^+ and K^+ concentrations in the fluid that is lost (see "Measurement of Renal Water Excretion," below).

Table 9-1 Typically daily water balance in a normal human[a]

	Water intake, mL/day			Water output, mL/day	
Source	Obligatory	Elective	Source	Obligatory	Elective
Ingested water	400	1000	Urine	500	1000
Water content of food	850		Skin	500	
Water of oxidation	350		Respiratory tract	400	
			Stool	200	
Total	1600	1000		1600	1000

[a] These values assume a low rate of sweat production. When exercise and/or hot weather stimulates sweat production, water losses from the skin can increase markedly, occasionally exceeding 5 L/day. In this setting, the ensuing rise in plasma osmolality enhances thirst, resulting in an appropriate increase in water intake.

Water Intake

To maintain water balance, water must be taken in (or generated) to replace these losses (Table 9-1). Net water intake is derived from three sources: (1) ingested water, (2) water contained in foods (e.g., meat is roughly 70 percent water and certain fruits and vegetables are almost 100 percent water, and (3) water produced from the oxidation of carbohydrates, proteins, and fats. If the latter two sources account for 1200 mL/day and the obligatory water loss (from the skin, from the gastrointestinal tract, and in the urine) is 1600 mL/day, then at least 400 mL must be ingested by drinking to maintain balance. Humans drink more than this minimum requirement for social and cultural reasons, and the extra water is excreted in the urine.

REGULATION OF PLASMA OSMOLALITY

The normal plasma osmolality (P_{osm}) is 275 to 290 mosmol/kg. It usually is held within narrow limits, as variations of only 1 to 2 percent initiate mechanisms to return the P_{osm} to normal. These alterations in osmolality are sensed by receptor cells in the hypothalamus that affect water intake (via thirst) and water excretion (via ADH, which increases water reabsorption in the collecting tubules).*

In terms of water balance, a water load decreases the P_{osm}, and water loss (as with exercise on a hot day) increases the P_{osm}. In both of these settings, there is a parallel change in the plasma Na^+ concentration. These alterations in water balance must be differentiated from conditions of *isosmotic* fluid loss (such as bleeding or some cases of diarrhea), in which solute and water may be lost proportionately, producing no direct change in the P_{osm} or the plasma Na^+ concentration.

The body responds to a water load by suppressing ADH secretion, resulting in decreased collecting tubule water reabsorption and excretion of the excess water. The peak diuresis is delayed for 90 to 120 min, the time necessary for the metabolism of previously circulating ADH. As will be seen, the kidneys can excrete up to 10 to 20 L/day of water, well above any normal level of water intake. *Therefore, water retention resulting in hypoosmolality and hyponatremia occurs, with rare exceptions, only in patients with an impairment in renal water excretion* (see Chap. 23).

The correction of a water deficit (hyperosmolality) requires the intake and retention of exogenous water. This is achieved by increases in thirst and ADH release, which are induced by the elevation in the P_{osm}. In contrast to the response to hypoosmolality, in which renal water excretion is of primary importance,

---

* The physiology of the release and actions of ADH are discussed in detail in Chap. 8.

increased thirst is the major defense against hyperosmolality and hypernatremia. Although the kidney can minimize water excretion via the effect of ADH, a water deficit can be corrected only by increased dietary intake.

An example of the efficiency of the thirst mechanism occurs in patients with complete central diabetes insipidus, who, because they secrete little or no ADH, may excrete more than 10 L/day or urine. Despite this, the P_{osm} remains near normal because the thirst mechanism augments water intake to match output. Thus, *symptomatic hypernatremia generally will not occur in a patient with a normal thirst mechanism and access to water* (see Chap. 24).

Excretion of a water load generally occurs so rapidly that there is little change in volume and no activation of the volume regulatory pathways. There are, however, settings in which both the volume and osmoregulatory systems come into play. As a example, the intake of NaCl without water (as with a large quantity of potato chips) results in an elevation in the P_{osm} and, because of the rise in extracellular Na^+ stores, expansion of the effective circulating volume. The latter change promotes the renal excretion of the excess Na^+, via a response that is mediated at least in part by a reduction in the release of aldosterone and an increase in that of atrial natriuretic peptide (ANP). ADH secretion and thirst also are stimulated (by the rise in P_{osm}); the ensuing increment in water intake both lowers the P_{osm} toward normal and further expands the volume, thereby enhancing the stimulus to renal Na^+ excretion. The end result is that the urine has a high osmolality and a relatively high concentration of Na^+, a composition that is similar to net intake.

In comparison, an infusion of isotonic saline causes volume expansion but does not change the P_{osm}. Consequently, ADH release and thirst are not directly affected, and the steady state is restored by the volume regulatory pathways.

RENAL WATER EXCRETION AND REABSORPTION

In the kidney, the bulk of the filtered water is reabsorbed passively in the proximal tubule and descending limb of the loop of Henle down an osmotic gradient created by NaCl transport (see Chaps. 3 and 4). This serves to maintain the volume of the extracellular fluid. In addition, the kidney contributes to the stability of the P_{osm} by excreting or reabsorbing water without solute. This function is primarily mediated by the presence [water conservation, high urine osmolality (U_{osm})] or absence (water excretion, low U_{osm}) of ADH. In normal adults, the U_{osm} can vary from a minimum of 40 to 100 mosmol/kg[8] to a maximum of 900 to 1400 mosmol/kg.[9]*

The quantitative importance of ADH for water excretion is depicted in Table 9-2. In a subject excreting 800 mosmol of solute per day, the urine volume can vary 15-fold, depending upon the availability of ADH. In the absence of ADH, for

---

* Concentrating ability tends to fall with age, and so the maximum U_{osm} in an elderly patient may be only 500 to 700 mosmol/kg.[9,10] Why this occurs is not well understood.

Table 9-2   Effect of ADH on urine volume in a subject excreting 800 mosmol of solute per day

ADH	U_{osm}, mosmol/kg	Urine volume, L/day
0	80	10
++	400	2
+++	1200	0.67

example, the minimum U_{osm} may be 80 mosmol/kg, resulting in the excretion of the 800 mosmol of solute in 10 liters of water. In a normal subject, this degree of polyuria is rarely seen and occurs only after a massive water load. More commonly, there is a moderate amount of ADH present, and the U_{osm} is somewhere between the extremes of 80 mosmol/kg (no ADH) and 1200 mosmol/kg (maximum ADH). If this subject had to excrete 2000 mL of water to remain in water balance, the average U_{osm} would be 400 mosmol/kg, that is, 800 mosmol of solute in 2000 mL. This would require a submaximal ADH effect.

The *urine output is also affected by solute excretion*, which is equal to net solute intake in the steady state. This is particularly important in disorders in which the rate of ADH secretion is relatively constant (Fig. 9-1). In a patient with complete central diabetes insipidus, for example, there is little or no ADH and the maximum U_{osm} may be only 80 mosmol/kg. In this setting, the daily urine volume will be 10 liters if 800 mosmol of solute is excreted, but only 5 liters if 400 mosmol of solute is excreted (400 mosmol of solutes at 80 mosmol/kg equals 5 liters of urine). Thus, one form of therapy is to restrict the intake of sodium and protein (which is metabolized to urea); the ensuing reduction in solute excretion will then limit the degree of polyuria. Dietary modification may be especially important in patients

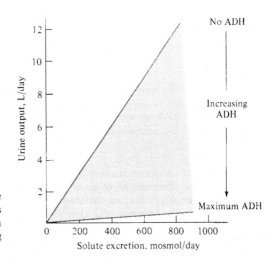

Figure 9-1 Effects of ADH and solute excretion on water excretion. It is assumed that the U_{osm} is 70 mosmol/kg in the absence of ADH and 1400 mosmol/kg with maximum ADH effect.

with *nephrogenic* diabetes insipidus, who are resistant to the action of **ADH** and who therefore will not respond to hormone administration (see Chap. 24).

Measurement of Renal Water Excretion

This simple example of the effect of solute excretion demonstrates that water excretion can vary widely without changes in the U_{osm}. Thus, *the U_{osm} which reflects the kidney's ability to dilute or concentrate the urine, is not an accurate estimate of its quantitative ability to excrete or retain water.*

To measure the amount of solute-free water that the kidney can excrete per unit time, one can calculate the *free-water clearance*, C_{H_2O}. If the urine is hypoosmotic to plasma, the total urine volume (V, in milliliters per minute or liters per day) can be viewed as having two components: one that contains all the urinary solute in a solution that is isosmotic to plasma (the osmolal clearance, or C_{osm}); and one that contains the solute-free water that makes the urine dilute (the free-water clearance); (Fig. 9-2a)[11]:

$$V = C_{osm} + C_{H_2O} \qquad (9\text{-}1)$$

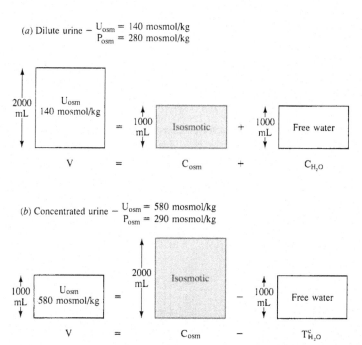

Figure 9-2 Block diagrams showing the relationship between the urine volume (V) and its two components: one containing all of the urinary solute in a solution that is isosmotic to plasma (the osmolal clearance, C_{osm}) and one consisting of free water that has either been (*a*) generated in a dilute urine (the free-water clearance, C_{H_2O}) or (*b*) reabsorbed in a concentrated urine (the free water reabsorption, $T^c_{H_2O}$). In these simple examples, the urine osmolality is one-half and twice the plasma osmolality, respectively. (*From Rose BD, Am J Med 81:1033, 1986. Used with permission.*)

The C_{osm} can be calculated from the general formula for clearance, $C = UV/P$ (see page 49):

$$C_{osm} = \frac{U_{osm} \times V}{P_{osm}} \tag{9-2}$$

If Eq. (9-1) is now solved for C_{H_2O},

$$C_{H_2O} = V - C_{osm}$$

$$= V\left(1 - \frac{U_{osm}}{P_{osm}}\right) \tag{9-3}$$

The manner in which this formula is used can be illustrated if we return to the patient with central diabetes insipidus who is excreting a maximally dilute urine. If

$$P_{osm} = 280\,mosmol/kg$$

$$U_{osm} = 80\,mosmol/kg$$

$$V = 10\,L/day$$

then

$$C_{H_2O} = 10\left(1 - \frac{80}{280}\right)$$

$$= 7.2\,L/day$$

Thus, of the 10 liters of urine being excreted, 7.2 liters exists as free water (C_{H_2O}) and 2.8 liters as an isosmotic solution containing all of the urinary solute (C_{osm}).

In the clinical setting, the excretion of large volumes of dilute urine may be *appropriate* if it follows a water load or *inappropriate* if it is due to a primary deficiency of ADH or renal resistance to its effects. In either case, the loss of solute-free water tends to raise the P_{osm} and plasma Na^+ concentration unless it is accompanied by an equivalent increase in water intake.

Physiologic factors affecting C_{H_2O}   The excretion of free water by the kidney occurs in two basic steps (see Chap. 4):

- Solute-free water is generated by NaCl reabsorption without water in the medullary and cortical aspects of the ascending limb of the loop of Henle and to a lesser degree in the distal nephron.
- This water is then excreted by keeping the collecting tubules relatively impermeable to water.

In normal subjects, the volume of free water generated in the loop of Henle (step 1) is primarily dependent upon the volume of water presented to that segment. Collecting tubular impermeability to water (step 2), on the other hand, requires the absence of ADH.

An understanding of the factors that influence C_{H_2O} has important clinical implications in patients with hyponatremia and hypoosmolality. Since the capacity for water excretion is normally so great (as much as 10 to 20 L/day), water retention leading to hyponatremia will occur only if there is a defect in water excretion or rarely if the amount of water ingested exceeds excretory capacity (see Chap. 23).* Diminished water excretion requires that one or both of the steps described above be impaired. This can occur in three settings:

- If less free water is generated because the rate of fluid delivery to the loop of Henle is reduced, as with renal failure (where less water is filtered) or volume depletion (where less water may be filtered and more is reabsorbed in the proximal tubule)
- If less free water is generated because NaCl reabsorption is inhibited by diuretics, particularly the thiazide-type diuretics (see page 702)
- If ADH is present, as with effective volume depletion, the syndrome of inappropriate ADH secretion, or adreneal insufficiency

These disorders, along with primary polydipsia, in which there is a primary increase in water intake, constitute the *entire differential diagnosis of true hyponatremia* (see Chap. 23).

Measurement of Renal Water Reabsorption

In addition to the formation of a dilute urine, the kidney is also able to excrete urine with an osmolality exceeding that of the plasma. If the urine is hyperosmotic, the urine volume can again be viewed as having two components: one containing all the urinary solute in an isosmotic solution and one containing the amount of free water that must have been removed from the urine by tubular reabsorption to raise the U_{osm} to the observed hyperosmotic value (the free-water reabsorption; $T^c_{H_2O}$). In this setting (Fig. 9-2b),

$$V = C_{osm} - T^c_{H_2O}$$

$$T^c_{H_2O} = C_{osm} - V$$

$$= V\left(\frac{U_{osm}}{P_{osm}} - 1\right) \tag{9-4}$$

In contrast to the C_{H_2O}, which is equal to the volume of free water *excreted* per unit time, the $T^c_{H_2O}$ is equal to the volume of free water *reabsorbed* per unit time.

---

* It is important to emphasize again that *hyponatremia is a disorder of water imbalance, not Na^+ imbalance.* It is usually characterized by impaired water excretion, which lowers the plasma Na^+ concentration by dilution. Urinary Na^+ loss, on the other hand, directly causes effective circulating volume depletion. It can also be associated with hyponatremia if there is both a hypovolemic stimulus to ADH release and some water intake to allow water retention to occur.

Suppose, for example, that a subject who has developed a mild water deficit puts out a concentrated urine and has the following values (similar to Fig. 9-2b):

$$P_{osm} = 290\,mosmol/kg$$

$$U_{osm} = 580\,mosmol/kg$$

$$V = 1\,L/day$$

In this setting,

$$T^c_{H_2O} = 1\left(\frac{580}{290} - 1\right)$$

$$= 1\,L/day^*$$

(9-5)

These results suggest that 1 L of free water is being added to plasma, which is appropriate in that it tends to lower the plasma osmolality back toward normal. The net effect, however, is different if the elevation in ADH release responsible for the high U_{osm} is due to the syndrome of inappropriate ADH secretion. In this setting, the retention of 1 liter of water that *would normally have been excreted* will lead to hypoosmolality and hyponatremia. This illustrates the importance of thinking in terms of $T^c_{H_2O}$ rather than of only the U_{osm}. The latter merely indicates the presence of a concentrated urine; the former tells exactly how much water is being retained by the kidney.

Electrolyte–free-water reabsorption   The formulas presented above described urinary water excretion in relation to total urinary solutes. This concept, however, must be amended when it is viewed in terms of the plasma Na^+ concentration.[11] As described in Chap. 7, the plasma Na^+ concentration is usually determined by the relationship between total exchangeable extracellular solutes (primarily Na^+ salts), total exchangeable intracellular solutes (primarily K^+ salts), and the total body water:

$$\text{Plasma } [Na^+] \cong \frac{Na^+_e + K^+_e}{TBW}$$

(9-6)

Urea does not contribute to this relationship because it freely equilibrates across the cell membrane and therefore does not influence the effective P_{osm} or the dis-

---

* These values can also be used to calculate the C_{H_2O}:

$$C_{H_2O} = 1\left(1 - \frac{580}{290}\right)$$

$$= -1\,L/day$$

Thus, $-1\,L/day$ of free water is being excreted; this is another way of stating that $1\,L/day$ is being reabsorbed. This illustrates the inverse relationship between the C_{H_2O}, which measures free-water excretion, and the $T^c_{H_2O}$, which represents free-water reabsorption:

$$C_{H_2O} = -T^c_{H_2O}$$

tribution of water between the cells and the extracellular fluid. However, urea is one of the major urinary solutes that can account for a large part of the U_{osm}. The loss of urea in the urine will cause the plasma urea concentration to fall but will not affect the plasma Na^+ concentration. Similar considerations apply to the urinary excretion of ammonium.

To more accurately assess the effect of the urine output on osmoregulation, the above formula for the $T^c_{H_2O}$ must be amended in the following ways: (1) $U_{Na^++K^+}$ is substituted for the total U_{osm}, and (2) the plasma Na^+ concentration is substituted for the P_{osm} (see page 246).[11,12] This new quantity is called the *electrolyte–free-water reabsorption* or $T^e_{CH_2O}$:*

$$T^e_{CH_2O} = V\left(\frac{U_{Na^++K^+}}{P_{Na^+}} - 1\right) \tag{9-7}$$

Suppose that the above patient with a fluid deficit and a urine osmolality of 580 mosmol/kg had 5 meq/L of Na^+ and 43 meq/L of K^+ in the urine and had a plasma Na^+ concentration of 144 meq/L. In this setting,

$$T^e_{CH_2O} = 1\left(\frac{48}{144} - 1\right)$$
$$= -670\,\text{mL/day} \tag{9-8}$$

Thus, instead of retaining 1 L of free water as calculated in Eq. (9-5), this subject actually has a negative value for the $T^e_{CH_2O}$ and is *losing 670 mL of free water per day*.

This concept is extremely important, because it illustrates again the difference between the U_{osm} and exact measurement of how much water is actually being excreted or reabsorbed. The U_{osm} of 580 mosmol/kg in this patient indicates that ADH is present and is producing a relatively concentrated urine. This response is appropriate, since it limits further water loss, which would aggravate the already present water deficit. Use of the traditional formula for free-water reabsorption in Eq. (9-5) suggests that this concentrated urine also results in the addition of 1 liter of free water to the body, directly correcting the mildly hyperosmolal state. However, the sum of Na^+ plus K^+ in the urine is less than that in the plasma. Thus, from the viewpoint of regulation of the plasma Na^+ concentration, the urine output in this patient leads to the loss of 670 mL of free water [from Eq. (9-8)], producing a *further tendency to hypernatremia*. This finding should not suggest that ADH is ineffective, since the U_{osm} would be under 100 mosmol/kg and the urine volume above 5 L/day in its absence.

Clinical Example

A 78-year-old partially demented man is admitted to the hospital because of pneumonia. Hyperalimentation with high-protein supplements (containing 30

---

* This correction should also be applied to the formula for free-water clearance in Eq. (9-3) to calculate the electrolyte–free-water clearance, $C^e_{H_2O}$.

meq/L each of Na^+ and K^+) is begun in an attempt to improve the patient's somewhat poor nutritional status. Over the ensuing 5 days, it is noted that the urine output is averaging 4 L/day, the blood urea nitrogen (BUN) has risen from 20 mg/dL to 88 mg/dL, the plasma creatinine concentration is relatively stable at 1.4 mg/dL, and the plasma Na^+ concentration has risen from 140 meq/L up to 156 meq/L despite a relatively high fluid intake. The following additional findings are obtained:

$$P_{osm} = 342 \, \text{mosmol/kg}$$

$$U_{osm} = 510 \, \text{mosmol/kg}$$

$$U_{Na^+} = 10 \, \text{meq/L}$$

$$U_{K^+} = 42 \, \text{meq/L}$$

Comment   It is not initially clear how the hypernatremia developed in this patient, since the intake was relatively dilute and the urine concentrated. Using the traditional formula for free-water reabsorption in Eq. (9-4), it appears that the kidney in this polyuric patient is actually adding 2 L/day of free water to the body, thereby protecting against the development of hypernatremia:

$$T^c_{H_2O} = 4\left(\frac{510}{342} - 1\right)$$

$$= 2 \, \text{L/day}$$

However, this patient is polyuric because of a urea osmotic diuresis, in which the excretion of large quantities of urea (derived from the catabolism of the extra dietary protein) both raises the BUN and obligates the excretion of a large volume of urine. Once again, the urine contains relatively little Na^+ and K^+. From the formula for the electrolyte–free-water reabsorption,

$$T^e_{C_{H_2O}} = 4\left(\frac{52}{156} - 1\right)$$

$$= -2.7 \, \text{L/day}$$

The etiology of the hypernatremia is now apparent: The patient is losing approximately 2.7 L of free water per day in the urine.

Physiologic factors affecting free-water reabsorption   Renal water conservation is dependent upon two basic steps (see Chap. 4):

- The formation and maintenance of the medulllary osmotic gradient
- Equilibration of the urine in the collecting tubules with the hyperosmotic medullary interstitium

ADH plays an important role in both steps by promoting the medullary accumulation of urea and by increasing the water permeability of the collecting tubules. Medullary hyperosmolality is also dependent upon NaCl reabsorption without water in the ascending limb of the loop of Henle, a process that in humans is probably independent of ADH.

The concentrating process can be impaired by a defect in ADH release, decreased responsiveness of the collecting tubule epithelium to ADH (most often due to lithium use or hypercalcemia in adults), or a primary abnormality in countercurrent function, preventing the maintenance of the hyperosmotic interstitium. When one of these disturbances is present, water excretion increases and the patient may complain of polyuria and polydipsia (see page 767). Stimulation of thirst is an important protective response, since it can counteract the increased urinary losses, thereby preventing negative water balance and the eventual development of hypernatremia.

Summary and Clinical Implications

The ability to excrete urine with an osmolality different from that of the plasma plays a central role in the regulation of water balance and maintenance of the P_{osm} and the plasma Na^+ concentration. If the P_{osm} is decreased—e.g., after a water load—ADH secretion is inhibited. This results in the excretion of a dilute urine, which permits excretion of the excess water and return of the P_{osm} to normal. If the P_{osm} is elevated—e.g., because of sweat loss—both ADH release and thirst are stimulated. The combination of diminished urinary water loss and enhanced water intake results in water retention and a decrease in the P_{osm} to normal.

In addition to the urine osmolality, solute excretion also determines how much water can be excreted (Fig. 9-1). Thus, the quantity of free water excreted or reabsorbed is best measured directly as $C^e_{H_2O}$ or $T^e_{CH_2O}$, rather than being inferred from the urine osmolality.

Although the role of solute excretion may at first glance appear to be of interest only to the physiologist, it becomes clinically important in several situations. In normal subjects, water intake is the major determinant of the urine volume through its effect on ADH release. However, when ADH secretion or responsiveness is relatively fixed (as in the syndrome of inappropriate ADH secretion or diabetes insipidus), *water intake no longer directly affects the urine volume* and the rate of solute excretion assumes primary importance. As described above, restricting dietary NaCl and protein intake is one way to diminish the urine output and the secondary polydipsia in patients with nephrogenic diabetes insipidus, who are resistant to the effects of ADH.

On the other hand, the syndrome of inappropriate ADH secretion is characterized by a reduction in the urine output and a tendency to water retention and hyponatremia (see Chap. 23). In this setting, a high-sodium, high-protein diet or the direct administration of urea in refractory cases can increase the urine output and raise the plasma Na^+ concentration toward normal.[13]

PROBLEMS

9-1   Diarrheal fluid usually is isosmotic to plasma even though its ionic composition differs from that of the plasma. Assuming that all of the diarrheal solute consists of Na^+ and K^+ salts, what effect will the loss of 2 liters of this fluid have on the following:
   (a) Effective circulating volume
   (b) Urinary Na^+ excretion
   (c) Plasma osmolality
   (d) Plasma Na^+ concentration
   (e) ADH release
   (f) Urine osmolality
If this patient drank a large quantity of water to prevent volume depletion, what would happen to the plasma Na^+ concentration?

9-2   Although secretory diarrheas, such as cholera, result in the loss of mostly Na^+ and K^+ salts, an osmotic diarrhea (as with malabsorption or the administration of lactulose for hepatic encephalopathy) may be associated with the loss of isosmotic fluid with a $Na^+ + K^+$ concentration of under 100 meq/L. What direct effect would the loss of this fluid have on the plasma Na^+ concentration?

9-3   What is the relationship between the plasma Na^+ concentration and urinary Na^+ excretion?

9-4   A patient with volume depletion due to vomiting has hyponatremia and hypoosmolality. What are the factors that may contribute to the inability to restore normal osmolality by excreting the excess water in the urine?

9-5   A subject switches from a regular diet to one consisting primarily of beer (which contains little or no Na^+, K^+, or protein) and is then given a water load. What will be the effect of this dietary change on the minimum U_{osm} that can be achieved and on the maximum C_{H_2O}

9-6   Two patients, one with heart failure via the hypovolemic stimulus and one with the syndrome of inappropriate ADH secretion, have an elevation in ADH release. Both patients have a U_{osm} of 540 mosmol/kg, a urine output of 1 L/day, and, because of water retention, a low plasma Na^+ concentration of 130 meq/L. However, the patient with inappropriate ADH secretion has no defect in Na^+ handling (since volume regulation is intact) and has urine Na^+ and K^+ concentrations of 80 and 50 meq/L, respectively. The comparable values in the patient with heart failure are 10 and 50 meq/L because of the avid Na^+ retention induced by the low cardiac output.
   (a) Is there a difference between the amount of free water excreted or reabsorbed by these two patients?
   (b) Can this difference affect the tendency to become hyponatremic?

REFERENCES

1. Pollock AS, Arieff AI. Abnormalities of cell volume regulation and their functional consequences. *Am J Physiol* 239:F195, 1980.
2. Arieff AI, Llach F, Massry SG. Neurological manifestations and morbidity of hyponatremia: Correlation with brain water and electrolytes. *Medicine* 55:121, 1976.
3. Ayus JC, Wheeler JM, Arieff AI. Postoperative hyponatremic encephalopathy in menstruant women. *Ann Intern Med* 117:891, 1992.
4. Laureno R, Karp BI. Myelinolysis after correction of hyponatremia. *Ann Intern Med* 126:57, 1997.
5. Ellis SJ. Severe hyponatraemia: Complications and treatment. *Q J Med* 88:905, 1995.
6. Guyton AC. *Textbook of Medical Physiology*, 7th ed. Philadelphia, Saunders, 1986, chap. 30.
7. Knochel JP, Dotin LN, Hamburger RJ. Pathophysiology of intense physical conditioning in hot climate: I. Mechanism of potassium depletion. *J Clin Invest* 51:242, 1972.

 8. Schoen EJ. Minimum urine total solute concentration in response to water loading in normal men. *J Appl Physiol* 10:267, 1957.
 9. Lindeman RD, van Buren HC, Raisz LG. Osmolar renal concentrating ability in healthy young men and hospitalized patients without renal disease. *N Engl J Med* 262:1306, 1960.
10. Sporn IN, Lancestremere RG, Papper S. Differential diagnosis of oliguria in aged patients. *N Engl J Med* 267:130, 1962.
11. Rose BD. New approach to disturbances in the plasma sodium concentration. *Am J Med* 81:1033, 1986.
12. Goldberg M. Hyponatremia. *Med Clin North Am* 65:251, 1981.
13. Decaux G, Genette F. Urea for long-term treatment of syndrome of inappropriate secretion of antidiuretic hormone. *Br Med J* 2:1081, 1981.

ACID-BASE PHYSIOLOGY

INTRODUCTION

Like the other components of the extracellular fluid, the H^+ concentration is maintained within narrow limits. The normal extracellular H^+ concentration is approximately 40 nanomol/L (1 nanomol/L equals 10^{-6} mmol/L), roughly *one-millionth* the millimole per liter concentrations of Na^+, K^+, Cl^-, and HCO_3^-.

Regulation of the H^+ concentration at this low level is essential for normal cellular function because of the high reactivity of H^+ ions, particularly with proteins.[1,2] This property is related to the relatively small size of hydronium ions, the hydrated form of H^+,* in comparison with that of Na^+ and K^+ ions. As a result, H^+ ions are more strongly attracted to negatively charged portions of molecules and are more tightly bound than Na^+ or K^+

When there is a change in the H^+ concentration, proteins gain or lose H^+ ions, resulting in alterations in charge distribution, molecular configuration, and consequently protein function. As an example, the rate of glycolysis (as measured by the rate of lactate production) varies inversely with the H^+ concentration, increasing as the latter is reduced (Fig. 10-1). This change in cellular

---

*In the aqueous environment in the body, H^+ ions combine with H_2O and exist primarily as hydronium ions, H_3O^+. For simplicity, H^+ will be used in place of H_3O^+ for the remainder of this discussion.

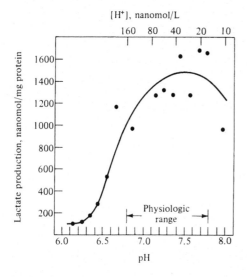

Figure 10-1 Influence of H^+ concentration and pH on lactate production by leukocytes. (*From Halperin ML, Connors HP, Relman AS, Karnovsky ML, J Biol Chem, 244:384, 1969, with permission.*)

metabolism is mediated by a similar inverse relationship between the H^+ concentration and the activity of several glycolytic enzymes, particularly phosphofructokinase.[1]

Under normal conditions, the H^+ concentration varies little from the normal value of approximately 40 nanomol/L.[3] This occurs even though acids and bases are continually being added to the extracellular fluid. The process of H^+ regulation involves three basic steps:

- Chemical buffering by the extracellular and intracellular buffers
- Control of the partial pressure of carbon dioxide in the blood by alterations in the rate of alveolar ventilation
- Control of the plasma bicarbonate concentration by changes in renal H^+ excretion

This chapter will review the basic principles of acid-base physiology, including the efficacy of buffers in preventing large changes in the H^+ concentration. The roles of ventilation and renal H^+ excretion in acid-base homeostasis are discussed in Chap. 11.

ACIDS AND BASES

Using the definitions proposed by Bronsted, an acid is a substance that can donate H^+ ions and a base is a substance that can accept H^+ ions.[4,5] These properties are independent of charge. Thus H_2CO_3, HCl, NH_4^+, and $H_2PO_4^-$ all can act as acids:

$$H_2CO_3 \quad \leftrightarrow \quad H^+ + HCO_3^-$$
$$HCl \quad \leftrightarrow \quad H^+ + Cl^-$$
$$NH_4^+ \quad \leftrightarrow \quad H^+ + NH_3$$
$$H_2PO_4^- \quad \leftrightarrow \quad H^+ + HPO_4^{2-}$$

Acid   Base

There are two classes of acids that are physiologically important: carbonic acid (H_2CO_3) and noncarbonic acids. This distinction is important because of the different rates of production and routes of elimination of these acids. Each day, the metabolism of carbohydrates and fats results in the generation of approximately 15,000 mmol of CO_2. Although CO_2 is not an acid, it combines with water to form H_2CO_3 (see below). Thus, there would be progressive accumulation of acid if the endogenously produced CO_2 were not excreted. This is prevented by the loss of CO_2 via respiration.

Noncarbonic acids, in comparison, are primarily derived from the metabolism of proteins. As an example, the oxidation of sulfur-containing amino acids results in the generation of H_2SO_4.[6] Only 50 to 100 meq/day of acid is produced from these sources;[3,6] these H^+ ions are then excreted in the urine.

Law of Mass Action

The law of mass action states that the velocity of a reaction is proportional to the product of the concentrations of the reactants. For example, water can dissociate into hydrogen and hydroxyl ions*:

$$H_2O \quad \leftrightarrow \quad H^+ + OH^-$$

The velocity with which this reaction moves to the right is equal to

$$v_1 = k_1[H_2O]$$

where K_1 is the rate constant for this reaction. Similarly, the velocity with which the reaction moves to the left can be expressed by

$$v_2 = k_2[H^+][OH^-]$$

At equilibrium, $v_1 = v_2$. Therefore,

$$k_1[H_2O] = k_2[H^+][OH^-]$$
$$K' = \frac{k_1}{k_2} = \frac{[H^+][OH^-]}{[H_2O]} \tag{10-1}$$

Since the H_2O concentration is relatively constant in the body fluids, this equation can be rearranged, so that

* This reaction actually should be written

$$H_2O + H_2O \quad \leftrightarrow \quad H_3O^+ + OH^-$$

$$K_w = [H^+] [OH^-] \tag{10-2}$$

where k_w is equal to the product of the two constants, K' and $[H_2O]$. At body temperature, $K_w = 2.4 \times 10^{-14}$. Thus, for distilled water,

$$[H^+] [OH^-] = 2.4 \times 10^{-14}$$

$$[H^+] = 1.55 \times 10^{-7} \, mol/L$$

$$[OH^-] = 1.55 \times 10^{-7} \, mol/L$$

Since the normal H^+ concentration in the extracellular fluid is 40 nanomol/L, we can see that the extracellular fluid is slightly less acid than water (where the H^+ concentration is 155 nanomol/L).

The law of mass action can be written for the dissociation of all the acids and bases in the body. For example, for the dissociation of an acid HA into H^+ and A^-,

$$K_a = \frac{[H^+] [A^-]}{[HA]} \tag{10-3}$$

where K_a is the apparent *ionization* or *dissociation constant* for this acid. In the body, K_a has a single value for the dissociation of each acid. Although K_a can vary slightly with changes in temperature, solute concentration, and H^+ concentration,[7,8] these parameters are held relatively constant under normal conditions.[8,9] Since the same principles can be applied to the dissociation of a base,

$$BOH \quad \leftrightarrow \quad B^+ + OH^-$$

the behavior of bases will not be discussed separately.[10]

Acids and bases may be strong or weak. Strong acids are those that are essentially completely ionized in the body. Since most of the acid exists as H^+ and A^-, a strong acid, from Eq. (10-3), has a relatively high K_a. HCl and NaOH are examples of a strong acid and a strong base, respectively. In comparison, $H_2PO_4^-$ is only 80 percent dissociated at the normal extracellular H^+ concentration and is considered a weak acid. As we will see, weak acids are the principal buffers in the body.

pH

The pH of a solution can be defined by the following relationship:

$$pH = -\log [H^+] \tag{10-4}$$

In the laboratory, the H^+ concentration of the blood can be measured with a glass membrane electrode that is permeable only to H^+. The diffusion of H^+ ions between the blood and the fluid in the electrode results in the generation of a measurable electrical potential (E_m) across the membrane.[9] The magnitude of this potential is proportional to the logarithm of the ratio of the H^+ concentration in the two compartments according to the Nernst equation:

$$E_m = 61 \log \frac{[H^+]_e}{[H^+]_b}$$

where the subscripts e and b refer to the fluid within the electrode and the blood, respectively. Since $[H^+]_e$ is a known value,

$$E_m \sim \log \frac{1}{[H^+]_b}$$

The $\log(1/a)$ is equal to $-\log a$. Thus,

$$E_m \sim -\log[H^+]_b$$

Since $pH = -\log[H^+]$,

$$E_m \sim pH^*$$

Since the *pH varies inversely with the H^+ concentration*, an increase in the H^+ concentration reduces the pH, and a decrease in the H^+ concentration elevates the pH. The relationship between the H^+ concentration and the pH within the physiologic range is depicted in Table 10-1. In general, the range of H^+ concentration that is compatible with life is 16 to 160 nanomol/L (pH equals 7.80 to 6.80). The normal arterial pH is approximately 7.40; thus, the normal H^+ concentration can be calculated from

$$pH = -\log[H^+]$$

$$\log[H^+] = -7.40$$

Taking the antilogarithm of both sides,

$$[H^+] = \text{antilog}(-7.40)$$

$$= \text{antilog}(0.60 - 8)$$

The antilogarithm of 0.60 is 4, and that of -8 is 10^{-8}. Thus,

$$[H^+] = 4 \times 10^{-8} \, \text{mol/L}$$

$$= 40 \, \text{nanomol/L}$$

---

* The membrane potential and the pH are actually proportional to the *activity* of H^+, that is, to the random movement of H^+ across the membrane, not to its molar concentration. Although the activity of H^+ (a_{H^+}) is directly proportional to the H^+ concentration,

$$a_{H^+} = \gamma[H^+]$$

the value of γ is dependent upon the ionic strength of the solution. In concentrated ionic solutions, ionic interaction between H^+ and anions can retard the random movement of H^+ so that its activity is significantly less than its concentration. However, the body fluids are relatively dilute, and it can be assumed without much error that γ is equal to 1 and therefore that the a_{H^+} is equal to the H^+ concentration.[5]

Table 10-1 Relationship between the arterial pH and H^+ concentration in the physiologic range

pH	$[H^+]$, nanomol/L
7.80	16
7.70	20
7.60	26
7.50	32
7.40	40
7.30	50
7.20	63
7.10	80
7.00	100
6.90	125
6.80	160

The relative merits of measuring the acidity of a solution in terms of pH or H^+ concentration have been the subject of much debate.[11] Since this issue is not likely to be important in the clinical setting, the following discussion will use both pH and H^+ concentration to familiarize the reader with these concepts.

Henderson-Hasselbalch Equation

Equation (10-3) can be rearranged in the following manner:

$$[H^+] = K_a \frac{[HA]}{[A^-]} \tag{10-5}$$

If we take the negative logarithm of both sides,

$$- \log [H^+] = - \log K_a - \log \frac{[HA]}{[A^-]}$$

Substituting pH for $- \log [H^+]$ and $+ \log ([A^-]/[HA])$ for $- \log ([HA]/[A^-])$, and defining pK_a as $- \log K_a$ (the H^+ concentration and K_a being expressed in units of moles per liter),

$$pH = pK_a + \log \frac{[A^-]}{[HA]} \tag{10-6}$$

This is the Henderson-Hasselbalch equation, which can be written for the dissociation of any weak acid. Using the Bronsted definition, in which A^- acts as a base and HA as an acid, this equation becomes

$$pH = pK_a + \log \frac{\text{base}}{\text{acid}} \tag{10-7}$$

For example, for the reaction

$$H_2PO_4^- \quad \leftrightarrow \quad H^+ + HPO_4^{2-}$$

the relationship between the concentrations of the reactants can be expressed either by the law of mass action or by the Henderson-Hasselbalch equation:

$$[H^+] = K_a \frac{[H_2PO_4^-]}{[HPO_4^{2-}]} \tag{10-8}$$

$$pH = pK_a + \log\frac{[HPO_4^{2-}]}{[H_2PO_4^-]} \tag{10-9}$$

The K_a for this reaction is 1.6×10^{-7} mol/L (or 160 nanomol/L), and the pK_a is 6.80.

To show how these equations can be used, let us calculate the HPO_4^{2-} and $H_2PO_4^-$ concentrations in the extracellular fluid if the total phosphate concentration is 1 mmol/L and the H^+ concentration equals 40 nanomol/L (pH is 7.40). From the law of mass action,

$$40 = 160\frac{[H_2PO_4^-]}{[HPO_4^{2-}]}$$

or

$$\frac{[HPO_4^{2-}]}{[H_2PO_4^-]} = 4$$

Since the total phosphate concentration is 1 mmol/L,

$$[HPO_4^{2-}] = 0.8\,\text{mmol/L}$$

$$[H_2PO_4^-] = 0.2\,\text{mmol/L}$$

The same results can be obtained from the Henderson-Hasselbalch equation:

$$7.40 = 6.80 + \log\frac{[HPO_4^{2-}]}{[H_2PO_4^-]}$$

Since the antilogarithm of 0.60 (7.40 − 6.80) is 4,

$$\frac{[HPO_4^{2-}]}{[H_2PO_4^-]} = 4$$

The phosphate system is somewhat more complicated, since phosphate also can exist as PO_4^{3-} and H_3PO_4:

$$PO_4^{3-} + H^+ \overset{1}{\leftrightarrow} HPO_4^{2-} + H^+ \overset{2}{\leftrightarrow} H_2PO_4^- + H^+ \overset{3}{\leftrightarrow} H_3PO_4$$

However, only trace amounts of PO_4^{3-} and H_3PO_4 are present in the body, since the pK_a of reaction 1 ($pK_{a1} = 12.4$) is much higher than that of reaction 3 ($pK_{a3} = 2.0$) is much lower than the extracellular pH of 7.40. For example, for reaction 1,

$$7.40 = 12.40 + \log\frac{[PO_4^{3-}]}{[HPO_4^{2-}]}$$

$$\frac{[PO_4^{3-}]}{[HPO_4^{2-}]} = \text{antilog}(-5) = 10^{-5}$$

Thus, at a pH of 7.40, there is only one molecule of PO_4^{3-} present for every 10^5 molecules of HPO_4^{2-}.

BUFFERS

One of the major ways in which large changes in H^+ concentration are prevented is by *buffering*. The body buffers, which are primarily weak acids, are able to take up or release H^+ so that changes in the free H^+ concentration are minimized. As an example, phosphate is an effective buffer, via the following reaction:

$$HPO_4^{2-} + H^+ \quad \leftrightarrow \quad H_2PO_4^-$$

If H^+ ions are added to the extracellular fluid, they will drive this reaction to the right by combining with HPO_4^{2-} to form $H_2PO_4^-$. Conversely, if H^+ ions are lost from the extracellular fluid, the reaction will move to the left as H^+ ions are released from $H_2PO_4^-$. In contrast, strong acids, such as HCl, are poor buffers at the body pH, since they are *almost completely ionized and cannot bind H^+ ions*.

The efficiency of phosphate buffering can be appreciated from the following example. Let us assume that in 1 liter of solution there are 10 mmol each of HPO_4^{2-} and $H_2PO_4^-$ as the Na^+ salts. From Eq. (10-8),

$$[H^+] = K_a \frac{H_2PO_4^-}{HPO_4^{2-}}$$

$$= 160 \times \frac{10}{10}$$

$$= 160 \text{ nanomol/L} \quad (\text{pH} = 6.80)$$

Note that when the concentrations of acid ($H_2PO_4^-$) and base (HPO_4^{2-}) are the same, the H^+ concentration equals K_a and the pH equals pK_a.

If 2 mmol of HCl is added to this solution, the excess H^+ ions can combine with HPO_4^{2-}:

$$HCl + Na_2HPO_4 \quad \rightarrow \quad NaCl + NaH_2PO_4$$

If we assume that virtually all the added H^+ is taken up by HPO_4^{2-}, then the HPO_4^{2-} concentration will fall to 8 mmol/L and the $H_2PO_4^-$ concentration will rise to 12 mmol/L. The new H^+ concentration will be

$$[H^+] = 160 \times \frac{12}{8}$$

$$= 240 \, \text{nanomol/L} \qquad (pH = 6.62)$$

Thus, even though 2 mmol/L or 2 million nanomol/L of H^+ has been added to the solution, the H^+ concentration has increased by only 80 nanomol/L. As a result, *more than 99.99 percent of the excess H^+ ions has been taken up or buffered by* HPO_4^{2-}. If no buffers had been present, the H^+ concentration would have been 2 million nanomol/L, with a pH of 2.70.

If more H^+ ions are added or if H^+ ions are removed by adding NaOH,

$$NaOH + NaH_2PO_4 \quad \rightarrow \quad Na_2HPO_4 + H_2O$$

the change in pH (or H^+ concentration) can be calculated in a similar manner. If the new pH is plotted against the amount of acid or base added, the result is the buffer curve in Fig. 10-2. Although the shape of the curve is sigmoidal, there is a linear midregion (pH equals 5.80 to 7.80) in which relatively large amounts of acid or base can be added without much change in pH. Thus, a *buffer is most efficient when the pH of the solution is within ± 1.0 pH unit of its pK_a*. If the pH is outside these limits, buffering will still occur, but a small amount of acid or base can produce a relatively large change in pH.

Bicarbonate/Carbon Dioxide Buffer System

Carbonic acid can dissociate into a hydrogen ion and a bicarbonate ion:

$$H_2CO_3 \quad \leftrightarrow \quad H^+ + HCO_3^-$$

the pK_a of this reaction is 3.57 (K_a equals 2.72×10^{-4}).[12] Since this is far from the normal pH of 7.40, it seems as if HCO_3^- would be an ineffective buffer in the body. However, H_2CO_3 is formed from the hydration of carbon dioxide (CO_2), and this

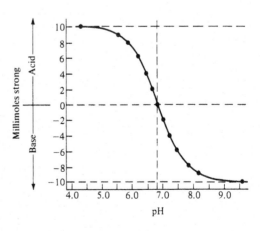

Figure 10-2 Titration curve of 1 liter of a 20 mmol/L $NaH_2PO_4^-$, Na_2HPO_4 solution. Initially, the concentration of HPO_4^{2-} equals that of $H_2PO_4^-$ at 10 mmol/L, and the concentration of H^+ equals 160 nanomol/L (pH equals 6.80). The different points represent the effects on the pH of the solution of the addition of a strong acid or base. (*From Woodbury JW, in Ruch TC, Patton HC (eds): Physiology and Biophysics, 20th ed. Philadelphia, Saunders, 1974, with permission.*)

buffer system can be more accurately described by the following series of reactions:[*]

$$CO_2 \quad \leftrightarrow \quad CO_2 + H_2O \quad \leftrightarrow \quad H_2CO_3 \quad \leftrightarrow \quad H^+ + HCO_3^-$$

gas   aqueous   (10-10)

phase   phase

Dissolved carbon dioxide   All gases partially dissolve in water (that is, they enter the aqueous phase), The degree to which this occurs is proportional to the partial pressure of the gas in the solution. In humans, the partial pressure of CO_2 (P_{CO_2}) in the arterial blood is in equilibrium with that in the alveolar air and normally is approximately 40 mmHg. At 37°C (normal body temperature), the amount of CO_2 dissolved in the plasma is

$$[CO_2]_{dis} = 0.03 \, P_{CO_2}$$
$$= 0.03 \times 40 = 1.2 \, mmol/L$$

(10-11)

where 0.03 is the solubility constant for CO_2 in the plasma.

Hydration of carbon dioxide   The equilibrium of the reaction

$$[CO_2]_{dis} + H_2O \quad \leftrightarrow \quad H_2CO_3$$

normally is far to the left, so that there are approximately 340 molecules of CO_2 in the solution for each molecule of H_2CO_3.[12] Nevertheless, an increase in the P_{CO_2} increases the $[CO_2]_{dis}$ and, therefore, the H_2CO_3 concentration. Thus, CO_2, which is not an acid, increases the acidity of the solution through the formation of H_2CO_3.

In certain tissues, such as red blood cells and the renal tubular epithelium, the rate of the hydration and dehydration reactions is enhanced by the enzyme carbonic anhydrase. The importance of this enzyme for renal H^+ secretion and HCO_3^- reabsorption will be discussed in Chap. 11.

Dissociation of carbonic acid   The degree to which H_2CO_3 dissociates into $H^+ + HCO_3^-$ [Eq. (10-10)] can be appreciated from the law of mass action for this reaction:

$$K_a = \frac{[H^+] \, [HCO_3^-]}{[H_2CO_3]}$$

Since the K_a is 2.72×10^{-4} and the normal H^+ concentration is $40 \times 10^{-9} \, mol/L$,

---

[*] An additional reaction can occur, as HCO_3^- can dissociate into hydrogen and carbonate ions

$$HCO_3^- \quad \leftrightarrow \quad H^+ + CO_3^{2-}$$

However, the pK_a of this reaction is 9.8, so that only trace elements of carbonate are present in the physiologic pH range.

$$2.72 \times 10^{-4} = \frac{40 \times 10^{-9} \times [HCO_3^-]}{[H_2CO_3]}$$

$$\frac{[HCO_3^-]}{[H_2CO_3]} = 6.8 \times 10^3$$

Thus, there are approximately 6800 molecules of HCO_3^- for each molecule of H_2CO_3.

Law of mass action for bicarbonate/carbon dioxide buffer system Since the concentration of H_2CO_3 is so low in relation to the $[CO_2]_{dis}$ (1 : 340) and the HCO_3^- concentration (1 : 6800), the reactions

$$[CO_2]_{dis} + H_2O \quad \leftrightarrow \quad H_2CO_3 \quad \leftrightarrow \quad H^+ + HCO_3^-$$

can be simplified to

$$[CO_2]_{dis} + H_2O \quad \leftrightarrow \quad H^+ + HCO_3^- \tag{10-12}$$

The law of mass action for this reaction is

$$K_a = \frac{[H^+] [HCO_3^-]}{[CO_2]_{dis} [H_2O]}$$

Since the concentration of water is constant, $(K_a \times [H_2O])$ can be replaced by K_a':

$$K_a' = \frac{[H^+] [HCO_3^-]}{[CO_2]_{dis}} \tag{10-13}$$

If we solve this equation for $[H^+]$,

$$[H^+] = \frac{K_a' \times [CO_2]_{dis}}{[HCO_3^-]}$$

In plasma at 37°C, K_a' is equal to 800 nanomol/L (800×10^{-9} mol/L, pK_a' equals 6.10). Thus,

$$[H^+] = 800 \times \frac{[CO_2]_{dis}}{[HCO_3^-]} \tag{10-14}$$

Substituting $0.03 P_{CO_2}$ for $[CO_2]_{dis}$,

$$[H^+] = 24 \times \frac{P_{CO_2}}{[HCO_3^-]} \tag{10-15}$$

Since the normal H^+ concentration is 40 nanomol/L and the P_{CO_2} is 40 mmHg, the normal HCO_3^- concentration can be calculated from Eq. (10-15):

$$40 = 24 \times \frac{40}{[HCO_3^-]}$$

$$[HCO_3^-] = 24 \, mmol/L^*$$

These relationships also can be expressed by the Henderson-Hasselbalch equation:

$$pH = 6.10 + \log\frac{[HCO_3^-]}{0.03P_{CO_2}} \quad (10\text{-}16)$$

where 6.10 is the pK_a'.

The HCO_3^- concentration usually is measured in the laboratory in one of two ways.[9] The first way is indirect: The arterial pH and P_{CO_2} are measured, and the HCO_3^- concentration is then calculated using the Henderson-Hasselbalch equation. The second method involves adding a strong acid to a venous blood sample and measuring the amount of CO_2 generated by a colorimetric reaction. As the added H^+ combines with plasma HCO_3^-, H_2CO_3 and then CO_2 are formed as Eq. (10-10) is driven to the left. This method, however, measures the *total CO_2 content*, which detects all the forms in which CO_2 is carried in the blood:

$$\text{Total } CO_2 \text{ content} = [HCO_3^-] + [CO_2]_{dis} + [H_2CO_3]$$

Since the H_2CO_3 concentration is very low, it can be omitted. If $0.03P_{CO_2}$ is substituted for $[CO_2]_{dis}$, then

$$[HCO_3^-] = \text{total } CO_2 \text{ content} - 0.03P_{CO_2} \quad (10\text{-}17)$$

At a normal HCO_3^- concentration of 24 mmol/L and a normal P_{CO_2} of 40 mmHg, the total CO_2 content will be $24 + (0.03 \times 40)$ or 25.2 mmol/L. Thus, when the total CO_2 content is measured, Eq. (10-16) must be modified in the following way:

$$pH = \log\frac{\text{total } CO_2 - 0.03P_{CO_2}}{0.03P_{CO_2}} \quad (10\text{-}18)$$

For the sake of simplicity, only the HCO_3^- concentration will be used in this discussion.

Buffering by bicarbonate As noted above, the most efficient buffering occurs within 1.0 pH unit of the pK_a (Fig. 10-2). Although the pK_a' for the HCO_3^-/CO_2 system is 1.30 pH units less than the normal extracellular pH of 7.40, this system is able to *buffer very effectively because the P_{CO_2} can be regulated by changes in alveolar ventilation* (see Chap. 11). An increase in ventilation augments CO_2 excretion and lowers the P_{CO_2}; a reduction in ventilation decreases CO_2 excretion, resulting in an elevation in the P_{CO_2}. Thus, as H_2CO_3 is formed from the buffering of excess H^+ ions by HCO_3^-, a subsequent elevation in the P_{CO_2} [as Eq.

---

* Since HCO_3^- is a univalent anion, this value also represents a concentration of 24 meq/L.

(10-10) is driven to the left] can be prevented by an increase in alveolar ventilation, thereby enhancing the effectiveness of HCO_3^- buffering.

The importance of this ability to regulate ventilation can be illustrated by the following example. Let us assume that 1 liter of plasma, in which HCO_3^- is the only buffer, has the following composition:

$$[H^+] = 40\,\text{nanomol/L} \qquad (pH = 7.40)$$

$$[HCO_3^-] = 24\,\text{mmol/L}$$

$$P_{CO_2} = 40\,\text{mmHg}$$

$$[CO_2]_{\text{dis}} = 1.2\,\text{mmol/L} \qquad (0.03 \times 40 = 1.2)$$

How many millimoles of HCl would have to be added to this solution to raise the H^+ concentration to 80 nanomol/L (pH equals 7.10)? As each millimole of H^+ combines with HCO_3^-, there will be an equimolar *decrease* in the HCO_3^- concentration and *elevation* in the $[CO_2]_{\text{dis}}$ [from Eq. (10-12)]. Thus, the new HCO_3^- concentration will be $24 - x$ and the new $[CO_2]_{\text{dis}}$ will be $1.2 + x$. From Eq. (10-14),

$$[H^+] = 800 \times \frac{[CO_2]_{\text{dis}}}{[HCO_3^-]}$$

$$80 = 800 \times \frac{1.2 + x}{24 - x}$$

$$x = 1.1\,\text{mmol/L}$$

This represents substantial buffering in that the H^+ concentration has increased only from 40 nanomol/L to 80 nanomol/L, even though 1.1 mmol/L (or 1.1 *million* nanomol/L) has been added to the solution. However, this response would be *physiologically inadequate*, since the H^+ concentration has risen to a potentially dangerous level after the addition of only 1.1 mmol of H^+ per liter. The increase in the $[CO_2]_{\text{dis}}$ to 2.3 mmol/L in this setting is equivalent to an elevation in P_{CO_2} to 77 mmHg $(0.03 \times 77 = 2.3)$.

If, however, ventilation could be increased so that the P_{CO_2} remained constant at 40 mmHg (and therefore the $[CO_2]_{\text{dis}}$ remained constant at 1.2 mmol/L), then

$$80 = 800 \times \frac{1.2}{24 - x}$$

$$x = 12\,\text{mmol/L}$$

Thus, the ability to maintain the P_{CO_2} at a constant level *increases the efficiency of HCO_3^- buffering 11-fold*. Furthermore, there will be an additional increase in the buffering capacity of HCO_3^- if ventilation can be sufficiently enhanced to reduce the P_{CO_2} below 40 mmHg. If, for example, the P_{CO_2} were lowered to 20 mmHg $([CO_2]_{\text{dis}} = 0.03 \times 20 = 0.6)$, then *18 mmol of H^+* could be added to each liter of plasma before the H^+ concentration increased to 80 nanomol/L:

$$80 = 800 \times \frac{0.6}{24 - x}$$

$$x = 18 \, \text{mmol/L}$$

These changes in ventilation, which make the HCO_3^-/CO_2 buffering system so effective, occur in humans because the chemoreceptors controlling ventilation are sensitive to alterations in the extracellular H^+ concentration (see Chap. 11). If the H^+ concentration is increased by the addition of HCl to the extracellular fluid, there will be an increase in ventilation, resulting in a reduction in the P_{CO_2}. This is an *appropriate compensatory response*, since the decrease in P_{CO_2} will lower the H^+ concentration toward normal. Conversely, a decrease in the H^+ concentration (or an increase in the pH) will reduce ventilation.

The net effect is that the buffering capacity of the bicarbonate system differs from that of the nonbicarbonate buffers.[13] The latter is determined by the quantity of buffer and the extracellular pH, as depicted in Fig. 10-2. In comparison, the capacity of the bicarbonate system is primarily determined by the plasma HCO_3^- concentration; the ability to vary the P_{CO_2} makes bicarbonate buffering capacity relatively independent of pH.

Isohydric Principle

From the law of mass action [Eq. (10-5)], the acid/base ratio of any weak acid is determined by its K_a and the H^+ concentration of the solution. Since the H^+ concentration affects each buffer, the following relationship is present:

$$[H^+] = K_{a1} \frac{0.03 P_{CO_2}}{[HCO_3^-]} = K_{a2} \frac{[H_2PO_4^-]}{[HPO_4^{2-}]} = K_{a3} \frac{[HA]}{[A^-]} \qquad (10\text{-}19)$$

This is called the *isohydric principle*. If the H^+ concentration is altered, the acid/base ratio of *all* the buffers in the solution is affected. This means that studying the behavior of any one buffer is adequate to predict the behavior of the other buffers in the solution. Clinically, the acid-base status of a patient is expressed in terms of the principal extracellular buffer, the HCO_3^-/CO_2 system:

$$[H^+] = 24 \frac{P_{CO_2}}{[HCO_3^-]}$$

Extracellular Buffers

The body buffers are located in the extracellular and intracellular fluids and in bone. As described above, the ability of a particular buffer to protect the pH is proportional to its concentration and its pK_a in relation to the ambient pH. In the transcellular fluid, HCO_3^- is the most important buffer, as a result of both its relatively high concentration and the ability to vary the P_{CO_2} via changes in alveolar ventilation. If, for example, H_2SO_4 is added to the extracellular fluid from the metabolism of the sulfur-containing amino acids methionine and cysteine,[6] the excess H^+ will be buffered primarily by HCO_3^-:

$$H_2SO_4 + 2NaHCO_3 \quad \rightarrow \quad Na_2SO_4 + 2H_2CO_3 \quad \rightarrow \quad 2CO_2 + 2H_2O \quad (10\text{-}20)$$

The CO_2 produced by this reaction is excreted by the lungs.

Although HCO_3^- is an effective buffer to noncarbonic acids, it *cannot buffer* H_2CO_3, because the combination of H^+ with HCO_3^- results in the regeneration of H_2CO_3:

$$H_2CO_3 + HCO_3^- \rightarrow HCO_3^- + H_2CO_3 \qquad (10\text{-}21)$$

Consequently, H_2CO_3 is buffered primarily by the intracellular buffers (see below).

There are other, quantitatively less important buffers in the extracellular fluid, including inorganic phosphates (plasma phosphate concentration of 1 mmol/L versus 24 mmol/L of HCO_3^-) and the plasma proteins (Pr^-)[5]:

$$H^+ + Pr^- \quad \leftrightarrow \quad HPr \qquad (10\text{-}22)$$

Intracellular and Bone Buffers

The primary intracellular buffers are proteins, organic and inorganic phosphates, and, in the erythrocyte, hemoglobin (Hb^-):

$$H^+ + Hb^- \quad \leftrightarrow \quad HHb \qquad (10\text{-}23)$$

In addition, bone represents an important site of buffering of acid and base loads.[14-17] An acid load, for example, is associated with uptake of some of the excess H^+ ions by bone. This can occur in exchange for surface Na^+ and K^+, and by the *dissolution of bone mineral*, resulting in the release of buffer compounds, such as $NaHCO_3$ and $KHCO_3$ initially and then $CaCO_3$ and $CaHPO_4$, into the extracellular fluid.[14,17,18] This buffering reaction appears to be initiated in part by the fall in the plasma HCO_3^- concentration, since a similar reduction in extracellular pH induced by respiratory acidosis produces much less bone dissolution.[17,18]

The loss of bone mineral with metabolic acidosis is not due simply to the physiochemical release of calcium during the buffering reaction, since a similar response is not seen in dead bone cells. This observation suggests that cell activity must play a role and that both decreased osteoblastic and increased osteoclastic function have been demonstrated.[19] How this occurs is not known.

Although it is difficult to measure the exact contribution of bone buffering, it has been estimated that as much as 40 percent of the buffering of an acute acid load takes place in bone.[20] The role of the bone buffers may be even greater in the presence of a chronic acid retention, as occurs in patients with chronic renal failure.[17,21,22] It has been suggested that parathyroid hormone has a permissive effect on bone buffering,[23] but its physiologic importance remains uncertain.[17]

Bone and intracellular buffers also participate in the pH in the presence of base loads. As an example, increased deposition of carbonate in bone has been demonstrated after the administration of $NaHCO_3$.[20] In addition, the associated reduction in the H^+ concentration drives Eqs. (10-22) and (10-23) to the left, resulting in the release of H^+ from proteins and hemoglobin, and thereby tending to raise the H^+ concentration toward normal.

Clinical Implications   One consequence of bone buffering is that *acid loading directly increases Ca^{2+} release from bone and urinary Ca^{2+} excretion,*[17,24-26] a relationship that may be an important contributing factor in some patients with calcium oxalate stone disease. As described above, a normal diet results in the generation of approximately 50 to 100 meq of H^+ per day, most of which comes from the metabolism of sulfur-containing amino acids. Increasing the acid load by increasing protein intake can promote calcium stone formation via the following effects[25-27]:

- A significant rise in Ca^{2+} excretion.
- A reduction in the excretion of citrate by increasing its reabsorption in the proximal tubule (see page 99). Urinary citrate is normally an important *inhibitor* of stone formation, as it forms a *nondissociable but soluble complex* with Ca^{2+}, thereby decreasing the availability of free Ca^{2+} to precipitate with oxalate.[28]
- A reduction in urine pH. Although calcium oxalate precipitation is not pH-dependent, the more acid urine promotes the conversion of urinary urate to the much less soluble uric acid (urate$^-$ + H^+ → uric acid).[27,29] The possible subsequent precipitation of uric acid can then act as a nidus for calcium stone formation.[29]

Another significant clinical effect of bone buffering is the gradual reduction in bone calcium stores in patients with end-stage renal disease, a disorder associated with progressive acid retention due to impaired urinary acid excretion.[30] Another site of buffering in these patients is skeletal muscle, which can lead to protein breakdown and muscle wasting.[31,32]

Chemical Buffering of Acids and Bases

Acidosis and Alkalosis   The arterial H^+ concentration is abnormal in a variety of clinical conditions (see Chaps. 17 to 21). An increase in the H^+ concentration (or a decrease in the pH) is called *acidemia*; a decrease in the H^+ concentration (or an increase in the pH) is called *alkalemia*. Processes that tend to raise or lower the H^+ concentration are called acidosis and alkalosis, respectively.

In general, acidosis induces acidemia and alkalosis induces alkalemia. However, the difference between these phenomena becomes important in those patients who have mixed acid-base disturbances in which both acidotic and alkalotic processes may coexist. In this setting, the net pH may be acidemic, even though a disorder that induces an alkalosis is also present (see Chap. 17).

From Eq. (10-15), a primary elevation in the P_{CO_2} causes acidemia, whereas a decrease in the P_{CO_2} causes alkalemia. Since the P_{CO_2} is regulated by the rate of alveolar ventilation, these disturbances are referred to as *respiratory acidosis* and *respiratory alkalosis*.

The H^+ concentration also varies inversely with the plasma HCO_3^- concentration. Processes that primarily lower or raise the plasma HCO_3^- concentration are called *metabolic acidosis* and *metabolic alkalosis*, respectively.

Buffer responses to acid and base loads   The importance of the body buffers in protecting the pH can be appreciated from the data in Table 10-2. In these experiments, metabolic acidosis (with acidemia) was induced in dogs by the infusion of HCl. The dogs were nephrectomized to eliminate the effect of changes in renal H^+ excretion. The total extracellular amounts of Na^+, K^+, HCO_3^-, and Cl^- were calculated from the product of the extracellular fluid volume (estimated from the volume of distribution of SO_4^{2-}, which is limited to the extracellular fluid) and the plasma electrolyte concentrations.

An average of 180 mmol of HCl was administered to each dog (the mean weight being 18.9 kg). Let us assume that the total body water was 60 percent of the body weight, or 11.3 liters. If 180 mmol of H^+ were distributed through 11.3 liters of distilled water, the H^+ concentration would be 16 mmol/L (pH of 1.80), a level that is incompatible with life. In the intact animals, however, the arterial pH fell only from 7.40 to 7.07 (H^+ concentration of 86 nanomol/L). This was associated with a reduction in the plasma HCO_3^- concentration from 24 to 7 mmol/L (by the combination of extracellular HCO_3^- with the excess H^+) and with a compensatory increase in alveolar ventilation that lowered the P_{CO_2} from 40

Table 10-2   Summary of data from infusion of HCl into five nephrectomized dogs[a]

Weight, kg	18.9
HCl infused, mmol	180
Final arterial pH	7.07
Change in total extracellular quantity, mmol	
Na^+	+65
K^+	+28
HCO_3^-	−78
Cl^-	+170
Percent neutralized by	
Extracellular HCO_3^-	43
Intracellular buffers	57
Na^+ exchange	36
K^+ exchange	15
Cl^- entry	6

[a] Data adapted from Swan RC, Pitts RF, *J Clin Invest* 34:215, 1955, by copyright permission of the American Society for Clinical Investigation.

to 25 mmHg. Thus, the body buffers were extremely effective in minimizing the degree of acidemia.

The relative contributions of the intracellular and extracellular buffers to this process can be estimated from the changes in the quantities of Na^+, K^+, HCO_3^-, and Cl^- in the extracellular fluid. The administered H^+ ions either remain in the extracellular fluid or enter the cells (Fig. 10-3). The H^+ ions that stay in the extracellular fluid are buffered by HCO_3^- (and, to a much lesser degree, by the plasma proteins), resulting in a decrease in the amount of extra-cellular HCO_3^-. If H^+ ions enter the cells, then, to maintain electroneutrality, either Cl^- will follow H^+ into the cells (a process that primarily occurs in red blood cells, where H^+ is buffered by Hb^-) or Na^+ and K^+ ions will leave the cells (and bone[18]) and enter the extracellular fluid. From Table 10-2, of the 180 mmol of H^+ infused, 78 mmol has been buffered by HCO_3^- and 103 mmol has entered the cells: 65 mmol in exchange for Na^+, 28 mmol in exchange for K^+, and 10 mmol followed by Cl^- (180 mmol of Cl^- was infused, but only 170 mmol remained in the extracellular fluid*). These results are depicted schemically in Fig. 10-4.

Buffering by the extracellular and intracellular buffers follows a characteristic time course that is dependent upon the rapidity with which the administered H^+ ions move into the different fluid compartments. Buffering by plasma HCO_3^- occurs almost immediately, whereas approximately 15 min is required for H^+ to diffuse into the interstitial space to be buffered by interstitial HCO_3^-. H^+ entry into the cells occurs more slowly, as buffering by cell buffers is not complete until 2 to 4 h have elapsed.[33]

A potential serious complication of the transcellular exchange of H^+ for K^+ that follows a H^+ load is an elevation in the plasma K^+ concentration, e.g., from the normal of 4 meq/L to as high as 6 to 7 meq/L in severe metabolic acidemia (see Chap. 12).[34] A similar increase may occur in the plasma Na^+ concentration, because Na^+ also leaves the cells. However, variations of several milliequivalents per liter are not physiologically important, since the normal plasma Na^+ concen-tration is approximately 140 meq/L.

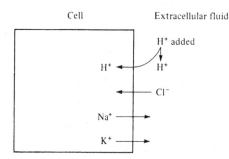

Figure 10-3 Effect of an HCl load on extracellular Cl^-, Na^+, and K^+. As H^+ enters the cells to be buffered, either Cl^- follows H^+ into the cells or intracellular Na^+ and K^+ leave the cells and move into the extracellular fluid. These ion shifts are reversed when H^+ ions are removed from the extracellular fluid.

* An alternative explanation for the intracellular movement of Cl^- is that Cl^- enters the red cell in exchange for intracellular HCO_3^-. This HCO_3^- moves into the extracellular fluid and buffers the excess H^+. The net effect is the same as that of HCl entry into the cell.

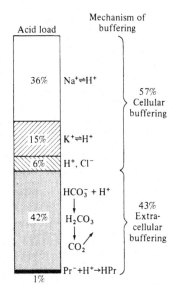

Figure 10-4 Mechanisms of buffering of strong acid infused intravenously in the dog. (*From Pitts RF*, Physiology of the Kidney and Body Fluids, *3d ed. Copyright © 1974 by Year Book Medical Publishers, Inc, Chicago. Used by permission. Adapted from Swan RC, Pitts RF, J Clin Invest 34:205, 1955, by copyright permission of the American Society for Clinical Investigation.*)

The relative contribution of the HCO_3^- and nonbicarbonate buffers in the cells and bone to an acid load varies with the plasma HCO_3^- concentration.[13] In normal subjects, both buffer systems make roughly equivalent contributions. This does not apply, however, in metabolic acidosis or severe chronic respiratory alkalosis, disorders associated with a low plasma HCO_3^- concentration (see below). In these settings, the role of the nonbicarbonate buffers becomes increasingly important, since the cells and bone have a virtually limitless buffering capacity.[13]

Respiratory acidosis   The response to respiratory acidosis (high P_{CO_2}) differs from the response to metabolic acidosis in that there is virtually no extracellular buffering, since HCO_3^- is not an effective buffer for H_2CO_3 [Eq. (10-21)]. As the P_{CO_2} increases, the elevation in H^+ concentration is initially minimized by a buffer-induced rise in the plasma HCO_3^- concentration.* This HCO_3^- is derived from two major sources: (1) Extracellular H_2CO_3 dissociates into HCO_3^- ions and H^+ ions, with the latter moving into the cells (and bone) in exchange for intracellular Na^+ and K^+, and (2) HCO_3^- is released from erythrocytes in exchange for extracellular Cl^- (Fig. 10-5).

The latter process occurs in the following manner. CO_2 diffuses into the erythrocyte, where it combines with H_2O to form H_2CO_3. This reaction is catalyzed by the enzyme carbonic anhydrase. H_2CO_3 is then buffered by Hb:

---

* It is important to remember that the H^+ concentration is determined by the ratio between, not the absolute levels of, P_{CO_2} and HCO_3^-. Thus, the H^+ concentration can be maintained at or near normal when there are parallel changes in the P_{CO_2} and plasma HCO_3^- concentration.

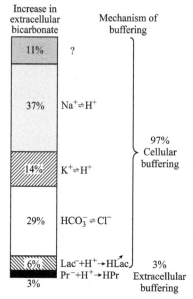

Respiratory acidosis

Figure 10-5 Mechanisms of buffering of CO_2 in respiratory acidosis in the dog. The source of approximately 11 percent of the increase in the extracellular HCO_3^- has not been identified. (*From Pitts RF, Physiology of the Kidney and Body Fluids, 3d ed. Copyright © 1974 by Year Book Medical Publishers, Inc, Chicago. Used by permission. Adapted from Giebisch G, Berger L, Pitts RF, J Clin Invest 34:231, 1955, by copyright permission of the American Society for Clinical Investigation.*)

$$H_2CO_3 + Hb^- \quad \rightarrow \quad HHb + HCO_3^-$$

It is this HCO_3^- that moves into extracellular fluid. Of lesser importance is the uptake of H^+ by the plasma proteins and by extracellular lactate:

$$Na\ lactate + H_2CO_3 \quad \rightarrow \quad lactic\ acid + NaHCO_3$$

The lactic acid produced by this reaction is metabolized within the cells, either into CO_2 and H_2O or via gluconeogenesis into glucose.

In humans, these buffers in the aggregate *increase the plasma HCO_3^- concentration approximately 1 mmol/L for each 10 mmHg elevation in the P_{CO_2}* (see Chap. 20). The degree to which this response protects the H^+ concentration can be appreciated if we calculate the effects of increasing the P_{CO_2} from 40 to 80 mmHg. If there is no buffering and the plasma HCO_3^- concentration remains constant, then the new H^+ concentration will be

$$[H^+] = 24 \times \frac{80}{24}$$

$$= 80\ nanomol/L \qquad (pH = 7.10)$$

However, a 40-mmHg elevation in the P_{CO_2} normally will induce roughly a 4 mmol/L increase in the plasma HCO_3^- concentration. In this setting,

$$[H^+] = 24 \times \frac{80}{28}$$

$$= 69\ nanomol/L \qquad (pH = 7.17)$$

As illustrated by this example, the buffer-induced elevation in the plasma HCO_3^- concentration is not particularly effective in protecting the H^+ concentration in respiratory acidosis. The most effective defense against respiratory acidosis is a further increase in the plasma HCO_3^- concentration, produced by *enhanced renal H^+ excretion* (see Chap. 11). This response, which takes 4 to 5 days to reach completion, results in a *3.5-mmol/L elevation in the plasma HCO_3^- concentration for every 10 mmHg increase in the P_{CO_2}* (see Fig. 20-5). Thus, at a P_{CO_2} of 80 mmHg, the combined buffering and renal responses will raise the plasma HCO_3^- concentration from 24 to about 38 meq/L, resulting in much better protection of the arterial H^+ concentration and pH:

$$[H^+] = 24 \times \frac{80}{38}$$

$$= 50 \,\text{nanomol/L} \qquad (\text{pH} = 7.30)$$

The intracellular and extracellular buffers also protect the pH in metabolic and respiratory alkalosis, as the buffer reactions move in the opposite direction from that observed in the acidemic conditions.[10]* Thus, H^+ ions are released, not taken up, by the buffers. For example,

$$HPr \quad \rightarrow \quad H^+ + Pr^-$$
$$H_2PO_4^- \quad \rightarrow \quad H^+ + HPO_4^{2-}$$

These H^+ ions then react with HCO_3^-, resulting in an *appropriate reduction in the plasma HCO_3^- concentration*, which tends to lower the elevated pH toward normal. To the degree that these H^+ ions are derived from cell buffers, their movement into the extracellular fluid occurs in exchange for extracellular Na^+ and K^+, which enters the cells. Thus, the plasma concentrations of Na^+ and K^+ which tend to rise with acidemia, may fall with alkalemia.[34]

INTRACELLULAR pH

The intracellular pH can be measured using a variety of techniques, including the distribution of a weak acid or base, nuclear magnetic resonance spectroscopy, the insertion of a H^+-sensitive microelectrode, and the use of fluorescent dyes.[35,36] In general, the cytosolic pH has been noted to be lower than that in the extracellular fluid, although it varies from organ to organ. For example, at a normal extracellular pH of 7.40, the mean pH in skeletal or smooth muscle is about 7.06,[35] whereas that in the early proximal convoluted tubule is approximately 7.13.[37]

There is, however, one problem in interpretation of the intracellular pH. In contrast to the value in the extracellular fluid, the *pH within the cell is not uniform* because of the presence of multiple compartments, including the cytosol, mito-

---

*Although similar buffers are involved, the percentage contributions of the individual intracellular and extracellular buffers in alkalemia are somewhat different from those shown in Figs. 10-4 and 10-5 for acidemia.[10]

chondria, endoplasmic reticulum, and nucleus.[2] As depicted in Fig. 10-6, a difference of approximately 0.5 pH unit is obtained when the cell pH of skeletal muscle is measured with both a weak acid, which is preferentially bound to the alkaline regions in the cell, and a weak base, which is preferentially bound to the more acid areas in the cell. At an extracellular pH of 7.40, for example, the respective values for the intracellular pH are 7.17 and 6.69, respectively.

As a result of this heterogeneity, it is difficult to determine which pH reflects the value that regulates the specific cellular function that is being studied. In the proximal tubular cell, for example, extracellular acidemia stimulates NH_4^+ production and secretion, primarily via the breakdown of glutamine (see Chap. 11). It is thought that the initiating signal for this metabolic change is in part the parallel fall that occurs in the intracellular pH.[38] However, studies using both nuclear magnetic resonance and the distribution of a weak acid suggest that although the cytosolic pH declines, the mitochondrial pH may remain relatively stable.[39,40] It may be that this increase in the transmitochondrial pH gradient, rather than the cytosolic pH alone, is the signal to alter the production of NH_4^+.

Several factors contribute to the regulation of intracellular pH, including the rate of metabolic activity, tissue perfusion, and the extracellular pH. As

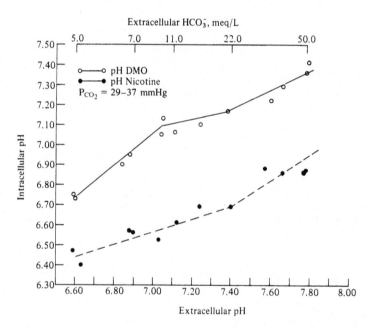

Figure 10-6 Relationship between skeletal muscle cell pH and the extracellular pH in metabolic acidosis and alkalosis, in which the extracellular pH is changed by alterations in the plasma HCO_3^- concentration. A similar relationship is present in respiratory acidosis and alkalosis. The cell pH can be seen to be heterogeneous, as evidenced by the difference between measuring the pH with a weak acid (DMO; 5,5-dimethyl-2,4-oxazolidinedione) or a weak base (nicotine). (*From Adler S, J Clin Invest, 51:256, 1972, by copyright permission of the American Society for Clinical Investigation.*)

illustrated in Fig. 10-6, alterations in the pH of the extracellular fluid produce parallel, although lesser, changes within the cells.[36] The more efficient maintenance of intracellular pH is in part related to the greater buffering capacity within the cells.

This relationship between the pH in the two fluid compartments is extremely important in the clinical setting. The principal physiologic effect of changes in pH is on protein function. Since the cells are the functioning units in the body, it is *the intracellular pH that is of primary importance, yet it is only the extracellular (plasma) pH that can easily be measured in patients.* Fortunately, this still permits an accurate assessment of acid-base status, because of the direct relationship between these two parameters.

The mechanism by which the cells sense alterations in extracellular pH is incompletely understood. Changes in the P_{CO_2} are presumably sensed directly, since CO_2 is lipid-soluble and can freely diffuse across the cell membranes. In comparison, the effect of variations in the plasma HCO_3^- concentration is somewhat indirect. In the proximal convoluted tubule, for example, HCO_3^- leaves the cell across the basolateral membrane via a Na^+-$3HCO_3^-$ carrier (see page 329). This process is stimulated in metabolic acidosis, since the associated reduction in the extracellular HCO_3^- concentration creates a favorable gradient for HCO_3^- exit from the cell.[38] The result is a fall in the intracellular pH, which, as will be described in the next chapter, appears to be an important mediator of the appropriate increase in urinary NH_4^+ excretion that tends to raise the extracellular pH toward normal.

PROBLEMS

10-1 How do buffers minimize change in the H^+ concentration? What factors determine how effective a buffer will be?

10-2 The sequential changes in the plasma HCO_3^- concentration and arterial pH produced by the rapid intravenous administration of 90 meq of HCO_3^- to a 70-kg man are depicted in the following table:

Time, min	HCO_3^-, meq/L	Arterial pH
0	24	7.40
10	32	7.51
20	29	7.48
180	27	7.45

(a) What accounts for the progressive fall in the plasma HCO_3^- concentration between 10 and 180 min?

(b) How will acid-base balance be restored?

10-3 If a patient has a P_{CO_2} that is fixed at 40 mmHg, what factors will determine how much the extracellular pH will fall after an acid load?

APPENDIX: MEASUREMENT OF INTRACELLULAR pH

Newer techniques have largely replaced the indirect measurement of intracellular pH by determining the distribution of a weak acid or base between the extracellular and the intracellular fluids. Fluorescent dyes, for example, permit continuous study of active, functioning cells under conditions in which the pH may be changing.[35] In comparison, the weak acid method is somewhat limited in that continuous measurements cannot be made. Nevertheless, a review of the latter technique is useful at this time, because it demonstrates how the basic principles discussed in this chapter can be applied.

The primary weak acid used has been DMO, which has pK_a of 6.13 at the concentration and temperature of the body fluids.[35,41] Thus, the Henderson-Hasselbalch equation for the reaction

$$HDMO \leftrightarrow H^+ + DMO^-$$

can be written as

$$pH = 6.13 + \log\frac{[DMO^-]}{[HDMO]} \tag{10-24}$$

With DMO, two assumptions are made: (1) that the pK_a in the cell is the same as that in the extracellular fluid; and (2) that the undissociated acid (HDMO), being lipid-soluble, equilibrates across the cell membrane, whereas the polar compound DMO^- crosses the membrane very slowly if at all (Fig. 10-7). Using these assumptions, the intracellular pH can be estimated in the following way:

- The extracellular pH is measured and, from Eq. (10-24), the $[DMO^-]/[HDMO]$ ratio is calculated. At the normal pH of 7.40, this ratio is approximately 20:1.
- The total extracellular DMO concentration, that is, $[DMO^-] + [HDMO]$, is measured and, since the $[DMO^-]/[HDMO]$ ratio is known, the HDMO concentration in the extracellular fluid can be calculated; this value is assumed to be the same as that in the cell.
- The extracellular and the intracellular volumes are measured by using markers limited to these compartments. For example, the distribution of

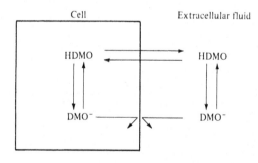

Figure 10-7 Distribution of HDMO and DMO^- between the cell and the extracellular fluid. Since HDMO is lipid-soluble, it is able to equilibrate across the cell membrane, reaching equal concentrations in both compartments. Once in the cell, HDMO dissociates into $H^+ + DMO^-$ (the latter is polar and cannot freely diffuse across the cell membrane). The extent of this reaction is dependent upon the cell pH.

tritiated water (which equilibrates between the extracellular and intracellular compartments) and of sulfate or mannitol (which cannot enter cells) can be used to estimate the total water space and the extracellular fluid volume, respectively. The intracellular fluid volume is equal to the difference between these two measurements.

- The total quantity of DMO in the extracellular fluid is calculated from the product of the extracellular volume and the extracellular DMO concentration.
- The total DMO in the cell is calculated from known amount of DMO administered minus the quantity in the extracellular fluid.
- The cell DMO concentration is then calculated from the total DMO in the cells divided by the intracellular volume.
- Since the DMO$^-$ concentration in the cell equals the total DMO concentration in the cell minus the HDMO concentration in the cell (both of which are known), the intracellular pH can be calculated by inserting these values into Eq. (10-25):

$$pH = 6.13 + \log \frac{[DMO]_{cell} - [HDMO]_{cell}}{[HDMO]_{cell}}$$

REFERENCES

1. Relman AS. Metabolic consequences of acid-base disorders. *Kidney Int* 1:347, 1972.
2. Ganapathy V, Leibach FH. Protons and regulation of biological functions. *Kidney Int* 40(suppl 33):S-4, 1991.
3. Kurtz I, Maher T, Hulter HN. Effect of diet on plasma acid-base composition in normal humans. *Kidney Int* 24:670, 1983.
4. Relman AS. What are "acids" and "bases"? *Am J Med* 17:435, 1954.
5. Madias NE, Cohen JJ. Acid-base chemistry and buffering, in Cohen JJ, Kassirer JP (eds): *Acid/Base*. Boston, Little, Brown, 1982.
6. Lennon EJ, Lemann J Jr, Litzow JR. The effects of diet and stool composition on the net external acid balance of normal subjects. *J Clin Invest* 45:1601, 1966.
7. Hood I, Campbell EJM. Is pK OK? *N Engl J Med* 306;864, 1982.
8. Kruse JA, Hukku P, Carlson RW. Relationship between apparent dissociation constant of blood carbonic acid and disease severity. *J Lab Clin Med* 114:568, 1989.
9. Gennari FG, Cohen JJ, Kassirer JP. Measurement of acid-base status, in Cohen JJ, Kassirer JP (eds): *Acid/Base*. Boston, Little, Brown, 1982.
10. Pitts RF. *Physiology of the Kidney and Body Fluids*. Chicago, Year Book, 1974, chap 11.
11. Hills AG. pH and the Henderson-Hasselbalch equation. *Am J Med* 55:131, 1973.
12. Malnic G, Giebisch G. Mechanism of renal hydrogen ion secretion. *Kidney Int* 1:280, 1972.
13. Fernandez PC, Cohen RM, Feldman GM. The concept of bicarbonate distribution space: The crucial role of body buffers. *Kidney Int* 36:747, 1989.
14. Lemann J Jr, Lennon EJ. Role of diet, gastrointestinal tract and bone in acid-base homeostasis. *Kidney Int* 1:275, 1972.
15. Lemann J Jr, Litzow JR, Lennon EJ. The effects of chronic acid-base loads in normal man: Further evidence for the participation of bone mineral in the defence against chronic metabolic acidosis. *J Clin Invest* 45:1608, 1966.
16. Bettice JA. Skeletal carbon dioxide stores during metabolic acidosis. *Am J Physiol* 247:F326, 1984.

17. Green J, Kleeman CR. Role of bone in regulation of systemic acid-base balance. *Kidney Int* 39:9, 1991.

18. Chabala JM, Levi-Setti R, Bushinsky DA. Alterations in surface ion composition of cultured bone during metabolic, but not respiratory, acidosis. *Am J Physiol* 261:F76, 1991.

19. Kreiger NS, Sessler NE, Bushinsky DA. Acidosis inhibits osteoblastic and stimulates osteoclastic activity in vitro. *Am J Physiol* 262:F442, 1992.

20. Burnell JM. Changes in bone sodium and carbonate in metabolic acidosis and alkalosis in the dog. *J Clin Invest* 50:327, 1971.

21. Litzow JR, Lemann J Jr, Lennon EJ. The effect of treatment of acidosis on calcium balance in patients with chronic azotemic renal disease. *J Clin Invest* 46:280, 1967.

22. Lemann J Jr, Litzow JR, Lennon EJ. Studies on the mechanism by which chronic metabolic acidosis augments urinary calcium excretion in man. *J Clin Invest* 46:1318, 1967.

23. Arruda JAL, Alla V, Rubinstein H, et al. Parathyroid hormone and extrarenal acid buffering. *Am J Physiol* 239:F533, 1980.

24. Lemann J Jr, Adams ND, Gray RW. Urinary calcium excretion in human beings. *N Engl J Med* 301:535, 1979.

25. Lau K, Wolf C, Nussbaum P, et al. Differing effects of acid versus neutral phosphate therapy of hypercalciuria. *Kidney Int* 16:736, 1979.

26. Kok DJ, Iestra JA, Doorenbos CJ, Papapoulos SE. The effects of dietary excesses in animal protein and in sodium on the composition and crystallization kinetics of calcium oxalate monohydrate in urines of healthy men. *J Clin Endocrinol Metab* 71:861, 1990.

27. Breslau NA, Brinkley L, Hill KD, Pak CYC. Relationship of animal protein-rich diet to kidney stone formation and calcium metabolism. *J Clin Endocrinol Metab* 66:140, 1988.

28. Parks JH, Coe FL. A urinary calcium-citrate index for the evaluation of nephrolithiasis. *Kidney Int* 30:85, 1986.

29. Coe FL. Uric acid and calcium oxalate nephrolithiasis. *Kidney Int* 24:392, 1983.

30. Bushinsky DA. The contribution of acidosis to renal osteodystrophy. *Kidney Int* 47:1816, 1995.

31. Bailey JL, Wang X, England BK, et al. The acidosis of chronic renal failure activates muscle proteolysis in rats by augmenting transcription of genes encoding proteins of the ATP-dependent ubiquitin-proteasome pathway. *J Clin Invest* 97:1447, 1996.

32. Graham KA, Reaich D, Channon SM, et al. Correction of acidosis in CAPD decreases whole body protein degradation. *Kidney Int* 49:1396, 1996.

33. Schwartz WB, Orming KJ, Porter R. The internal distribution of hydrogen ions with varying degrees of metabolic acidosis. *J Clin Invest* 36:373, 1957.

34. Adrogué HJ, Madias NE. Changes in plasma potassium concentration during acute acid-base disturbances. *Am J Med* 71:456, 1981.

35. Wray S. Smooth muscle intracellular pH: Measurement, regulation, and function. *Am J Physiol* 254:C213, 1988.

36. Adler S. The simultaneous determination of muscle cell pH using a weak acid and weak base. *J Clin Invest* 51:256, 1972.

37. Pastoriza-Munox E, Harrington RM, Graber ML. Axial heterogeneity of intracellular pH in rat proximal convoluted tubule. *J Clin Invest* 80:207, 1987.

38. Krapf R, Berry CA, Alpern RJ, Rector FC Jr. Regulation of cell pH by ambient bicarbonate, carbon dioxide tension, and pH in rabbit proximal convoluted tubule. *J Clin Invest* 81:381, 1988.

39. Adler S, Shoubridge E, Radda GK. Estimation of cellular pH gradients with ^{31}P-NMR in intact rat renal tubular cells. *Am J Physiol* 247:C188, 1984.

40. Simpson DP, Hager SR. Bicarbonate-carbon dioxide buffer system: A determinant of the mitochondrial pH gradient. *Am J Physiol* 247:F440, 1984.

41. Waddell WJ, Butler TC. Calculation of intracellular pH from the distribution of 5,5-dimethyl-2,4-oxazolidinedione (DMO): Application to skeletal muscle of the dog. *J Clin Invest* 38:720, 1959.

CHAPTER ELEVEN

REGULATION OF
ACID-BASE BALANCE

INTRODUCTION

Acid-base homeostasis can be easily understood if it is viewed in terms of the HCO_3^-/CO_2 buffering system:

$$H^+ + HCO_3^- \quad \leftrightarrow \quad H_2CO_3 \quad \leftrightarrow \quad H_2O + CO_2 \qquad (11\text{-}1)$$

At equilibrium, the relationship between the reactants can be expressed by the law of mass action (see Chap. 10),

$$[H^+] = 24 \times \frac{P_{CO_2}}{[HCO_3^-]} \qquad (11\text{-}2)$$

or by the Henderson-Hasselbalch equation,

$$pH = 6.10 + \log \frac{[HCO_3^-]}{0.03 P_{CO_2}} \qquad (11\text{-}3)$$

This system plays a central role in the maintenance of acid-base balance, because the HCO_3^- concentration and the P_{CO_2} can be *regulated independently*, the former by changes in renal H^+ excretion and the latter by changes in the rate of alveolar ventilation.

These processes are extremely important, because acids and to a lesser degree bases are continually being added to the body through endogenous metabolic processes. The metabolism of carbohydrates and fats (primarily derived from the diet) results in the production of approximately 15,000 mmol of CO_2 per day. Since CO_2 combines with H_2O to form H_2CO_3, severe acidemia would ensue if this CO_2 were not excreted by the lungs.

In addition, the metabolism of proteins and other substances results in the generation of noncarbonic acids and bases.[1-3] The H^+ ions are derived mostly from the oxidation of sulfur-containing (methionine and cysteine) and cationic (arginine and lysine) amino acids, and the hydrolysis of that component of dietary phosphate that exists as $H_2PO_4^-$:

$$\text{Methionine} \quad \rightarrow \quad \text{glucose} + \text{urea} + SO_4^{2-} + 2H^+$$
$$\text{Arginine}^+ \quad \rightarrow \quad \text{glucose (or } CO_2) + \text{urea} + H^+$$
$$\text{R-}H_2PO_4 + H_2O \quad \rightarrow \quad \text{ROH} + 0.8\,HPO_4^{2-}/0.2\,H_2PO_4^- + 1.8\,H^+$$

The major sources of alkali, on the other hand, are the metabolism of anionic amino acids (glutamate and asparatate) and the oxidation or utilization for gluconeogenesis of organic anions (such as citrate and lactate):

$$\text{Glutamate}^- + H^+ \quad \rightarrow \quad \text{glucose} + \text{urea}$$
$$\text{Citrate}^- + 4.5O_2 \quad \rightarrow \quad 5CO_2 + 3H_2O + HCO_3^-$$
$$\text{Lactate}^- + H^+ \quad \rightarrow \quad \text{glucose} + CO_2$$

(The consumption of H^+ ions in the first and third reactions is equivalent to the generation of new HCO_3^- ions in the body.) On a normal western diet, the net effect is the production of *50 to 100 meq of H^+ per day* in adults.[1-3]

The homeostatic response to these acid and base loads occurs in three stages:

- Chemical buffering by the extracellular and intracellular buffers (see Chap. 10).
- Changes in alveolar ventilation to control the P_{CO_2}
- Alterations in renal H^+ excretion to regulate the plasma HCO_3^- concentration

As an example, the H_2SO_4 produced from the oxidation of sulfur-containing amino acids is initially buffered in the extracellular fluid by HCO_3^-:

$$H_2SO_4 + 2NaHCO_3 \quad \rightarrow \quad Na_2SO_4 + 2H_2CO_3 \quad \rightarrow \quad 2H_2O + CO_2 \quad (11\text{-}4)$$

Although this reaction minimizes the increase in the extracellular H^+ concentration, the excess H^+ ions must still be excreted by the kidney to prevent progressive depletion of HCO_3^- and the other body buffers and the development of metabolic acidosis. The CO_2 generated by this reaction is excreted by the lungs.

Under normal conditions, the steady state is preserved, as renal H^+ excretion varies directly with the rate of H^+ production (Fig. 11-1).[1,3] If acid generation is enhanced, for example, some of the excess H^+ is initially retained, resulting in a slight reduction in the plasma HCO_3^- concentration (which may be less than 1 meq/L) and pH.[3] This minimal degree of acidemia, which may be too small to be detected clinically, is at least part of the stimulus to increase net renal acid excretion to a level similar to the new higher rate of acid generation.

The net effect is that the plasma H^+ concentration and pH are maintained within narrow limits. The normal values for these parameters are:

	pH	$[H^+]$, nanoeq/L	P_{CO_2}, mmHg	$[HCO_3^-]$, meq/L
Arterial	7.37–7.43	37–43	36–44	22–26
Venous	7.32–7.38	42–48	42–50	23–27

The decrease in pH (and increase in H^+ concentration) in venous blood is due to the uptake of metabolically produced CO_2 in the capillary circulation.

The remainder of this chapter will mostly discuss the general mechanisms involved in renal H^+ excretion and the factors responsible for the regulation of

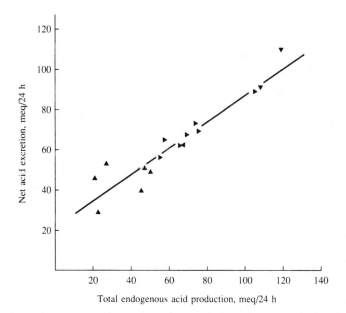

Total endogenous acid production, meq/24 h

Figure 11-1   Relationship between net renal acid excretion and endogenous acid production in the steady state in normal subjects ingesting different diets with varying acid content. (*From Kurtz I, Maher T, Hulter HN, et al*, Kidney Int *24:670, 1983; and Lennon EJ, Lemann J Jr, Litzow JR*, J Clin Invest *45:1601, 1966. Reprinted by permission from* Kidney International *and the American Society for Clinical Investigation.*)

these processes. It is useful to summarize the steps involved in this complex process in advance:

- The kidneys must excrete the 50 to 100 meq of noncarbonic acid generated each day.
- This is achieved by H^+ secretion, although the major mechanisms are different in the proximal tubule and thick ascending limb of the loop of Henle (Na^+-H^+ exchange) and in the collecting tubules (active H^+-ATPase pump).
- The daily acid load cannot be excreted as free H^+ ions, since the free H^+ concentration in the urine is extremely low (< 0.05 meq/L) in the physiologic pH range.
- The daily acid load also cannot be excreted unless *virtually all of the filtered HCO_3^- has been reabsorbed*, because HCO_3^- loss in the urine is equivalent to adding H^+ ions to the body.
- Secreted H^+ ions are excreted by binding either to filtered buffers, such as HPO_4^{2-} and creatinine, or to NH_3 to form NH_4^+. NH_4^+ is generated from the metabolism of glutamine in the proximal tubule; the rate at which this occurs can be varied according to physiologic needs.
- The extracellular pH is the primary physiologic regulator of net acid excretion. In pathophysiologic states, however, the effective circulating volume, aldosterone, and the plasma K^+ concentration all can affect acid excretion, independent of the systemic pH.

RENAL HYDROGEN EXCRETION

The kidneys contribute to acid-base balance by regulating H^+ excretion so that the plasma HCO_3^- concentration remains within appropriate limits. This involves two basic steps: (1) reabsorption of the filtered HCO_3^- and (2) excretion of the 50 to 100 meq of H^+ produced per day.

It is essential to appreciate that loss of filtered HCO_3^- in the urine is equivalent to the addition of H^+ to the body, since both are derived from the dissociation of H_2CO_3. As a result, virtually all of the filtered HCO_3^- must be reabsorbed before the dietary H^+ load can be excreted. The quantitative importance of this process should not be underestimated. A normal subject with a glomerular filtration rate (GFR) of 180 L/day (125 mL/min) and a plasma HCO_3^- concentration of 24 meq/L filters and then must reabsorb approximately *4300 meq* of HCO_3^- each day.

The second step in renal acid-base regulation, excretion of the 50 to 100 meq daily H^+ load, is accomplished by the combination of H^+ ions either with urinary buffers such as HPO_4^{2-} (referred to as titratable acidity) or with ammonia to form amonium—$NH_3 + H^+ \rightarrow NH_4^+$. These processes are important, because the *excretion of free H^+ ions is minimal*. The lowest urine pH that can be achieved in humans is 4.5. Although this is almost 1000 times (3 log units) more acid than the extracellular pH, it still represents an extremely low free H^+ concentration of less than 0.04 meq/L. Remember that the free H^+ concentration at an extracellular pH of 7.40 is only 40 nanomol/L, *one-millionth* the size of the daily acid load.

The reabsorption of HCO_3^- and the formation of titratable acidity and NH_4^+ all involve H^+ secretion from the tubular cell into the lumen (Figs. 11-2 to 11-4).[4,5] Three initial points need to be emphasized:

- The secreted H^+ ions are generated within the tubular cell from the dissociation of H_2O. This process also results in the equimolar production of OH^- ions.
- These OH^- ions bind to the active zinc-containing site of intracellular *carbonic anhydrase*; they then combine with CO_2 to form HCO_3^- ions, which are released into the cytosol and returned to the systemic circulation across the basolateral membrane.[4,6] The net effect is that the *secretion of each H^+ ion is associated with the generation of one HCO_3^- ion in the plasma.* If the secreted H^+ combines with filtered HCO_3^-, the result is HCO_3^- reabsorption (Fig. 11-2). This maintains the plasma HCO_3^- concentration by preventing HCO_3^- loss in the urine. If, however, the secreted H^+ combines with HPO_4^{2-} or NH_3, a *new HCO_3^-* is added to the peritubular capillary (Figs. 11-3 and 11-4). This results in an increase in the plasma HCO_3^- concentration to *replace the HCO_3^- lost in buffering the daily H^+ load* [Eq. (11-4)].
- Different mechanisms are involved in proximal and distal acidification (see below).

Net Acid Excretion

Since the urinary concentration of free H^+ is negligible, the net quantity of H^+ excreted in the urine is equal to the amount of H^+ excreted as titratable acidity and NH_4^+ minus any H^+ added to the body because of urinary HCO_3^- loss:

$$\text{Net acid excretion} = \text{titratable acidity} + NH_4^- - \text{urinary } HCO_3^- \qquad (11\text{-}5)$$

In the steady state, the net amount of H^+ excreted is roughly equal to the normal H^+ load of 50 to 100 meq/day (Fig. 11-1). However, this value can exceed 300 meq/day (primarily through enhanced NH_4^+ excretion) if acid production is increased (see below). Net H^+ excretion also can have a negative value if a large amount of HCO_3^- is lost in the urine. This may appropriately occur after the ingestion of citrate-containing fruit juices, since the metabolism of citrate results in the generation of HCO_3^-. How the kidney is able to make these homeostatic adjustments will be discussed below (see "Regulation of Renal Hydrogen Excretion: Extracellular pH," below).

Proximal Acidification

The primary step in proximal acidification is the secretion of H^+ by the Na^+-H^+ exchanger (or antiporter) in the luminal membrane.[7-10] This transport protein,

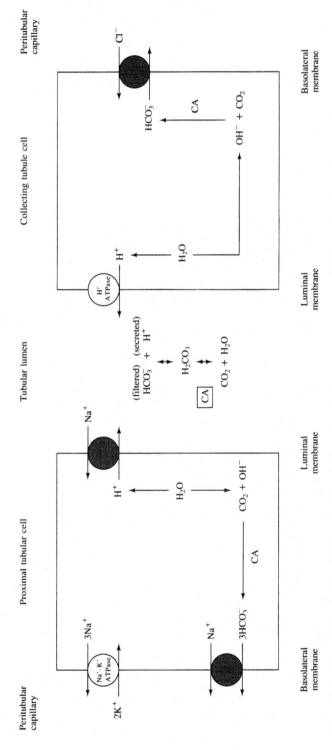

Figure 11-2 Major cellular and luminal events in bicarbonate reabsorption in the proximal tubule and the collecting tubules. Intracellular H_2O breaks down into a H^+ ion and a OH^- ion. The latter combines with CO_2 to form HCO_3^-, via a reaction catalyzed by carbonic anhydrase (CA). In the proximal tubule, the H^+ is secreted into the lumen by the Na^+-H^+ exchanger, whereas the HCO_3^- is returned to the systemic circulation primarily by a Na^+-$3HCO_3^-$ cotransporter. These same processes occur in the collecting tubules, although they are respectively mediated by an active H^+-ATPase pump in the luminal membrane and a Cl^--HCO_3^- exchanger in the basolateral membrane. The secreted H^+ ions combine with filtered HCO_3^- to form carbonic acid (H_2CO_3) and then CO_2 + H_2O, which can be passively reabsorbed. This dissociation of carbonic acid is facilitated when luminal carbonic anhydrase (CA in box) is present, as occurs in the early proximal tubule (see text). The net effect is HCO_3^- reabsorption, even though the HCO_3^- ions returned to the systemic circulation are not the same as those that were filtered. Although not shown, the collecting tubule cells also have H^+-K^+-ATPase pumps in the luminal membrane that are primarily involved in K^+ reabsorption.

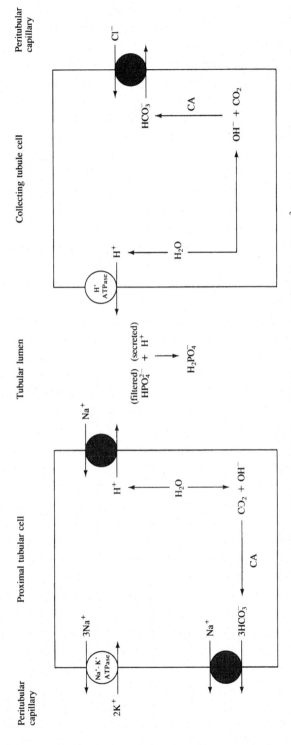

Figure 11-3 Formation of titratable acidity, which is primarily due to buffering of secreted H^+ by filtered HPO_4^{2-} and, to a lesser degree, other buffers such as creatinine. Note that a new HCO_3^- ion is returned to the peritubular capillary for every H^+ ion that is secreted.

331

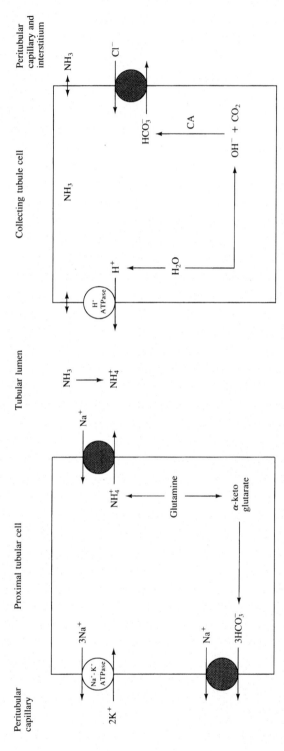

Figure 11-4 Formation of urinary ammonium (NH_4^+). In the proximal tubule, glutamine is taken up by the cells and metabolized into NH_4^+ and α-ketoglutarate. Utilization of the latter results in the generation of HCO_3^-, whereas NH_4^+ substitutes for H^+ on the Na^+-H^+ exchanger and is then secreted directly into the lumen. The mechanism is different in the collecting tubules; nonpolar, lipid-soluble NH_3 diffused from the interstitial fluid into the lumen, where it combines with secreted H^+ to form NH_4^+. Ammonium is lipid-insoluble and is therefore unable to back-diffuse out of the lumen. Note that each NH_4^+ ion that is excreted is associated with the generation of a new HCO_3^- ion that is returned to the peritubular capillary.

which also appears to mediate most of HCO_3^- reabsorption in the thick ascending limb of the loop of Henle,[11,12] preferentially binds filtered Na^+ at its external site and intracellular H^+ at its internal site (Fig. 11-2).[10]

A H^+-ATPase pump, similar to that in the distal nephron, is also present in the proximal tubule.[8,13] Via the use of different experimental methodologies, including genetic deletion, it appears that the Na^+-H^+ exchanger is responsible for approximately two-thirds of proximal H^+ secretion, with the H^+-ATPase pump being responsible for the remainder.[9,14]

The *energy for Na^+-H^+ exchange is indirectly provided by the Na^+-K^+-ATPase pump in the basolateral membrane.* As described in Chap. 3, this pump transports reabsorbed Na^+ into the peritubular capillary and also has two other important effects: It maintains the effective cell Na^+ concentration at a relatively low level (10 to 30 meq/L), and it creates a negative electrical potential in the cell interior. The negative potential is induced by the loss of cation from the cell, because of the $3Na^+ : 2K^+$ stoichiometry of the pump and the back-diffusion of this K^+ out of the cell through K^+ channels in the basolateral membrane. The low cell Na^+ concentration creates a favorable gradient for the passive diffusion of luminal Na^+ into the cell that is large enough to drive H^+ secretion against a concentration gradient via electroneutral Na^+-H^+ exchange.

Proximal acidification also requires that the HCO_3^- formed within the cell be returned to the systemic circulation. As depicted in Fig. 11-2, this is primarily achieved by a Na^+-$3HCO_3^-$ cotransporter* in the basolateral membrane, although a Cl-HCO_3^- exchanger also is present, particularly in the S_3 segment.[11–17] The Na^+-$3HCO_3^-$ transporter (which may actually function as a $Na^+ : CO_3^{2-} : HCO_3^-$ carrier)[17] results in the net movement of negative charge. The energy for this process is provided by the electronegative potential within the cell that is created by the Na^+-K^+-ATPase pump.[18]

Distal Acidification

H^+ secretion in the distal nephron primarily occurs in the *intercalated cells* in the cortical collecting tubule and in the cells in the outer and inner medullary collecting tubules,[19–22] the distal tubule also may contribute but appears to be quantitatively less important.[23] As illustrated in Fig. 11-2, there are three main characteristics of distal acidification:

- H^+ secretion is mediated by active secretory pumps in the luminal membrane.[24–28] Both H^+-ATPase and H^+-K^+-ATPase pumps are present.[24,29,30] The latter is an exchange pump, leading to H^+ secretion and K^+ reabsorption; its main role may be in minimizing K^+ loss during hypokalemia rather than in regulating acid-base balance (see page 393).[24,27,31] Following appro-

---

* The Na^+-$3HCO_3^-$ has an additional function in that it provides the major mechanism by which metabolic acid-base changes are sensed within the cell (see "Regulation of Renal Hydrogen Excretion: Extracellular pH," below).

priate stimuli, such as systemic acidemia (see below), cytoplasmic vesicles containing the H^+-ATPase pumps move to fuse with the luminal membrane, resulting in H^+ secretion.[32] Electroneutrality is maintained in this setting by concurrent secretion of Cl^- via voltage-dependent mechanisms.[19,21]

Note that the Na^+-H^+ antiporter would not be an efficient mechanism of distal acidification, since the *activity of this carrier is limited by the transcellular Na$^+$ gradient* that provides the energy for H^+ secretion. This gradient is diminished in the collecting tubules as a result of the reduction in the tubular fluid Na^+ concentration, which can fall below 30 meq/L in the cortical collecting tubule and, in states of volume depletion, below 5 meq/L in the inner medullary collecting tubule. Furthermore, the gradient against which H^+ must be secreted is markedly increased in these segments. A urine pH of 4.8, for example, represents a H^+ concentration that is 400 times (2.6 log units) greater than that in the extracellular fluid. The net effect is that H^+ secretion by Na^+-H^+ exchange would require a nonphysiologic cell Na^+ concentration well below 1 meq/L. (There is evidence of a basolateral Na^+-H^+ exchanger in the medullary collecting duct; it is likely that this transporter is primarily involved in the regulation of cell pH rather than systemic acid-base balance.[33,34])

- The H^+ secretory cells in the distal nephron do not transport Na^+, since they have few if any of the luminal membrane Na^+ channels or transporters that are required for the entry of luminal Na^+ into the cell.[19,35] However, H^+ secretion by the intercalated cells in the cortical collecting tubule is indirectly influenced by Na^+ reabsorption in the adjacent *principal* cells. The transport of cationic Na^+ through Na^+ channels in the luminal membrane makes the tubular fluid relatively electronegative. This electrical gradient can affect acid handling in two ways: It promotes H^+ accumulation in the lumen by minimizing the degree of back-diffusion,[36,37] and it facilitates the passive reabsorption of HCO_3^-.[23]

- Bicarbonate exit is mediated by a Cl^-/HCO_3^- exchanger in the basolateral membrane, thereby returning HCO_3^- to the systemic circulation.[17,38] This protein is a truncated form of the Cl^-/HCO_3^- exchanger in red cells (which is also called band 3 protein).[39] The energy for Cl^-/HCO_3^- exchange is provided by the inward gradient for Cl^- entry, since the Cl^- concentration in the cells is relatively low.

Regulation of the H^+-ATPase secretory pumps appears to be mediated by a process of membrane insertion and recycling that is similar to the effect of antidiuretic hormone on luminal membrane water channels (see Chap. 6).[32,40] In the medullary collecting tubule and many of the intercalated cells in the cortical collecting tubule, cytoplasmic H^+ pumps are inserted into the luminal membrane with an acid load, thereby facilitating excretion of the excess acid. On the other hand, an alkaline load results in recycling of these transporters from the luminal membrane to cytoplasmic vesicles.[40]

The net effect of H^+ secretion in the collecting tubules is illustrated in Fig. 11-5. The tubular fluid pH falls by about 0.6 units in the proximal tubule; is relatively stable in the loop of Henle and distal tubule, which do not play a major role in urinary acidification; and then falls to its lowest level in the collecting tubules (represented in Fig. 11-5 as the difference between the distal tubule and the final urine).[41]

Impairment of this distal H^+ secretory process results in a reduced net acid excretion, metabolic acidosis, and urine pH that is inappropriately high; this disorder is called type 1 (distal) renal tubular acidosis. A number of different defects can directly or indirectly cause this problem. Patients with Sjögren's syndrome have been described in whom there is complete absence of H^+-ATPase pumps in the intercalated cells.[42,43] How immunologic injury leads to this change is not known. Another mechanism is a mutation in the basolateral Cl^-/HCO_3^- exchanger.[44]

The preceding discussion has emphasized the function of the type A intercalated cells. There is also a second type of intercalated cell (type B) in the cortical collecting tubule that can insert the H^+ pumps into the luminal membrane with an acid load or into the basolateral membrane with an alkaline load.[40] The latter process allows HCO_3^- to be appropriately secreted rather than reabsorbed (see below).

Bicarbonate Reabsorption

Approximately 90 percent of the filtered HCO_3^- is reabsorbed in the proximal tubule, and most of this occurs in the first 1 to 2 mm of this segment.[45,46] The marked reabsorptive capacity of the early proximal tubule appears to be mediated

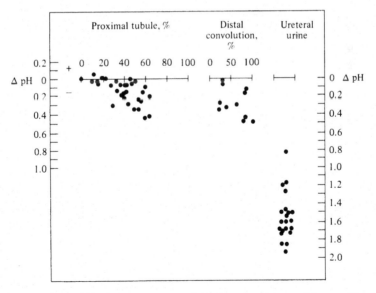

Figure 11-5 Change in pH (ΔpH) of the tubular fluid along the nephron of the rat. (*From Gottschalk CW, Lassiter W, William E, Mylle M, Am J Physiol 198:581, 1960, with permission.*)

by an increased number of Na^+-H^+ exchangers and enhanced permeability to HCO_3^-.[47] The remaining 10 percent of the filtered HCO_3^- is reabsorbed in the more distal segments,[4] and most of this occurs in the thick ascending limb (primarily by Na^+-H^+ exchange)[11,12] and in the outer medullary collecting tubule.[19-21]

Carbonic anhydrase and disequilibrium pH   Carbonic anhydrase within the tubular cells plays a central role in HCO_3^- reabsorption by facilitating the formation of HCO_3^- from the combination of OH^- ions with CO_2 (Fig. 11-2).[6,48-51] The role of *luminal* carbonic anhydrase in the proximal tubule is less well appreciated. As H^+ ions are secreted, two separate reactions occur in the tubular lumen (Fig. 11-2): (1) the combination of H^+ with filtered HCO_3^- to form H_2CO_3 and (2) the dehydration of H_2CO_3 into $CO_2 + H_2O$, which are then reabsorbed:

$$ H^+ + HCO_3^- \overset{1}{\leftrightarrow} H_2CO_3 \overset{2}{\leftrightarrow} CO_2 + H_2O \qquad (11\text{-}6) $$

Step 2, the dehydration of H_2CO_3 into $CO_2 + H_2O$, normally proceeds relatively slowly. However, this reaction is accelerated in the early proximal tubule because the brush border of the tubular cells contains carbonic anhydrase.[48,49] Consequently, there is no accumulation of H_2CO_3 in the proximal tubular fluid. From the law of mass action, the maintenance of a low H_2CO_3 concentration drives reaction 1 in Eq. (11-6) to the right, thereby keeping the free H^+ concentration at a relatively low level. In general, the tubular fluid pH falls only 0.6 pH unit (from 7.40 in the filtrate to about 6.80 by the end of the proximal convoluted tubule), despite the reabsorption of the majority of the filtered HCO_3^- (Fig. 11-5).[41]

This response is extremely important, since, as noted above, the gradient against which H^+ is secreted by the Na^+-H^+ antiporter cannot exceed the favorable inward gradient for Na^+. By minimizing the increase in the tubular fluid H^+ concentration, luminal carbonic anhydrase minimizes the gradient against which H^+ is secreted, thereby allowing continued H^+ secretion and HCO_3^- reabsorption.

The contribution of this system can be appreciated from the response to the administration of a carbonic anhydrase inhibitor that enters the cells to a limited degree and therefore inhibits the luminal but not the intracellular enzyme.[48,49] In this setting, the dehydration of H_2CO_3 in the lumen is slowed, resulting in increases in the H_2CO_3 and H^+ concentrations and thereby *impairing proximal HCO_3^- reabsorption by up to 80 percent*.[49] This ability to induce a HCO_3^- diuresis makes a carbonic anhydrase inhibitor useful in the treatment of some patients with metabolic alkalosis (see Chap. 18).

The role of luminal carbonic anhydrase can also be appreciated by comparing the function of the middle (S_2) and late (S_3) segments of the proximal tubule (see Fig. 3-2). Luminal carbonic anhydrase is present in the former, but absent in the latter.[51,52] As shown in the tubular perfusion experiments in Fig. 11-6, both segments can lower the tubular fluid pH by 0.6 to 0.8 unit. This is associated with a marked reduction in the luminal HCO_3^- concentration in the early proximal tubule, as a result of a relatively high rate of HCO_3^- reabsorption. In

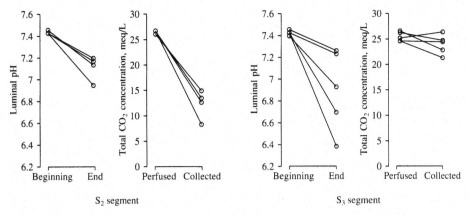

Figure 11-6   Changes in luminal (tubular fluid) pH and total CO_2 concentration as perfusion fluid flows through S_2 (mid) and S_3 (late) segments of the proximal tubule. The total CO_2 concentration is equal to the sum of the concentrations of HCO_3^- and of dissolved CO_2 (equal to $0.03 \times P_{CO_2}$; see page 310). The S_2 segment contains carbonic anhydrase in the lumen; as a result, H^+ secretion results in a fall in luminal pH and in total CO_2 concentration, since a substantial amount of HCO_3^- reabsorption has occurred. In comparison, the S_3 segment lacks luminal carbonic anhydrase. Consequently, the luminal pH falls to a similar degree, even though there has been a relatively small amount of H^+ secretion that is insufficient to lower the total CO_2 concentration. This segment also demonstrates a disequilibrium pH, as the measured value is 6.89, while the calculated value is 7.35 (similar to that in the initial perfusate). The lack of change in the calculated pH from that in the perfusate is a reflection of the stable total CO_2 concentration, whereas the reduction in the measured pH is a reflection of the accumulation of H_2CO_3. There is no disequilibrium pH in the S_2 segment, as the measured and calculated values are the same. (*Adapted from Kurtz I, Star R, Balaban RS, et al. J Clin Invest 78:989, 1986, by copyright permission of the American Society for Clinical Investigation.*)

comparison, there is relatively little HCO_3^- transport in the S_3 segment, since, in the absence of luminal carbonic anhydrase, secreted H^+ ions and H_2CO_3 accumulate in the tubular fluid, producing a rapid fall in luminal pH that limits further H^+ secretion.

It is also possible to demonstrate a *disequilibrium pH* in those segments that lack luminal carbonic anhydrase (the S_3 segment, the cortical collecting tubule, and most of the medullary collecting tubule).[48,52-54] If, for example, the tubular fluid P_{CO_2} and HCO_3^- are measured in the late proximal tubule, the pH can be calculated from the Henderson-Hasselbalch equation [Eq. (11-3)]. However, the *measured pH is almost 0.5 pH unit below the calculated value* (6.89 versus 7.35 in the S_3 segment), a difference that is referred to as a *disequilibrium pH*.[48,52]

The error in the calculated pH results from the fact that the pK_a' of 6.10 can be applied to Eq. (11-6) only when the H_2CO_3 concentration is relatively low in relation to the dissolved CO_2 and HCO_3^- concentrations (see page 308). The 0.5-unit pH difference in this setting is presumably due to the accumulation of excess acid as H_2CO_3. The disequilibrium pH can be dissipated by the addition of carbonic anhydrase to the tubular fluid and is absent in those segments that contain this enzyme.[52,54]

The uneven distribution of luminal carbonic anhydrase may play an important role in urinary acidification. The early proximal tubule has this enzyme and is able to reabsorb about 90 percent of the filtered HCO_3^-. The middle part of the outer medullary collecting tubule also contains luminal carbonic anhydrase[54] and is the most important distal site of HCO_3^- reabsorption.[21] The other distal segments, in comparison, lack luminal carbonic anhydrase and are less able to reabsorb HCO_3^-; however, they play an *essential role in NH_4^+ excretion*, since the exaggerated reduction in tubular fluid pH promotes the diffusion of NH_3 into the lumen, where it combines with the excess H^+ and is trapped as NH_4^+ (see "Ammonium Excretion," below).[5,52-54]

Bicarbonate secretion   Virtually all of the filtered HCO_3^- is reabsorbed in normal subjects, in whom there is a requirement to excrete the daily acid load. However, loss of HCO_3^- in the urine is an appropriate response in patients with metabolic alkalosis (high arterial pH, high plasma HCO_3^- concentration). Although this HCO_3^- diuresis can be achieved by reabsorbing less of the filtered HCO_3^-, it appears that *HCO_3^- secretion by the type B intercalated cells in the cortical collecting tubule* also contributes to this response.[20,40,55,56]

These cells differ from HCO_3^- reabsorbing type A intercalated cells in that the *polarity of the membrane transporters can be reversed*. H^+ and HCO_3^- ions are still produced within the cell; however, the H^+ ions are secreted into the peritubular capillary by the H^+-ATPase pump, which is now inserted in the basolateral, rather than the luminal, membrane (Fig. 11-7).[40,56] The HCO_3^- ions, in comparison, are secreted into the tubular lumen by an anion exchanger in the luminal membrane.[55,56]

Titratable Acidity

Several weak acids are filtered at the glomerulus and may act as buffers in the urine. Their ability to do so is proportional to the quantity of the buffer present and to its pK_a. The latter is important, since maximum buffering occurs at ± 1.0 pH unit from the pK_a (see Fig. 10-2). Because of its favorable pK_a of 6.80 and its relatively high rate of urinary excretion, HPO_4^{2-} is the major urinary buffer (Fig. 11-3), with lesser contributions from other weak acids, such as creatinine ($pK_a = 4.97$) and uric acid ($pK_a = 5.75$).

This process is referred to as *titratable acidity*, since it is measured by the amount of NaOH that must be added to a 24-h urine collection to titrate the urine pH back to the same pH as that in the plasma (approximately 7.40 in normal subjects). Under normal conditions, 10 to 40 meq/day of H^+ is buffered by these weak acids.

The ability of phosphate to buffer H^+ can be illustrated by the following example (Table 11-1). From the Henderson-Hasselbalch equation for the $HPO_4^{2-}/H_2PO_4^-$ system,

Tubular
lumen

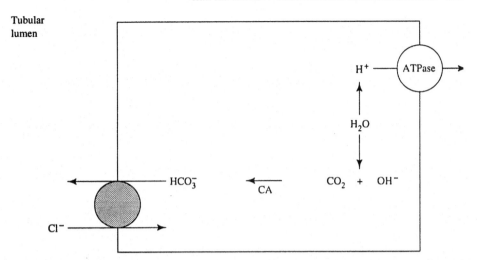

Figure 11-7   Transport mechanisms involved in the secretion of bicarbonate into the tubular lumen in the type B intercalated cells in the cortical collecting tubule. Water within the cell dissociates into hydrogen and hydroxyl anions. The former are secreted into the peritubular capillary by H^+-ATPase pumps in the basolateral membrane. The hydroxyl anions combine with carbon dioxide to form bicarbonate in a reaction catalyzed by carbonic anhydrase (CA). Bicarbonate is then secreted into the tubular lumen via chloride-bicarbonate exchangers in the luminal membrane. The favorable inward concentration gradient for chloride (lumen concentration greater than that in the cell) provides the energy for bicarbonate secretion.

$$pH = 6.80 + \log \frac{[HPO_4^{2-}]}{[H_2PO_4^-]} \tag{11-7}$$

the ratio of HPO_4^{2-} to $H_2PO_4^-$ is $4:1$ at an arterial pH of 7.40. If 50 mmol of phosphate is excreted in the urine (the remainder of the filtered phosphate being reabsorbed), then 40 mmol exists as HPO_4^{2-} and 10 mmol as $H_2PO_4^-$ in the glomerular filtrate. If the tubular fluid pH in the proximal tubule is lowered to 6.8 by H^+ secretion, then, from Eq. (11-7), the ratio of HPO_4^{2-} to $H_2PO_4^-$ will fall to $1:1$.

As a result, there will now be 25 mmol each of HPO_4^{2-} and $H_2PO_4^-$ in the tubule. This represents the buffering of 15 mmol (or 15 million nanomol) of H^+ by

Table 11-1   Effects of a tubular fluid pH on buffering by HPO_4^{2-} if 50 mmol of phosphate is excreted

Segment	pH	Quantity (in mmol) of		Amount buffered by HPO_4^{2-}, mmol
		HPO_4^{2-}	$H_2PO_4^-$	
Filtrate	7.40	40	10	0
Proximal tubule	6.80	25	25	15
Final urine	4.80	0.5	49.5	39.5

HPO_4^{2-}, which an increase in the free H^+ concentration from 40 nanomol/L (pH of 7.40) to only 160 nanomol/L (pH of 6.80). Thus, over 99.99 percent of the secreted H^+ has been buffered. If the tubular fluid pH in the collecting tubules is lowered further to 4.8 (H^+ concentration of 0.016 mmol/L), essentially all the HPO_4^{2-} will be converted to $H_2PO_4^-$, as a total of 39.5 mmol of H^+ will have been buffered by the conversion of HPO_4^{2-} to $H_2PO_4^-$ (Table 11-1).

In summary, the *amount of H^+ buffered by HPO_4^{2-} increases as the tubular fluid pH is reduced.* However, once the urine pH falls below 5.5, virtually all of the urinary phosphate exists as $H_2PO_4^-$ and further buffering cannot occur unless there is an increase in phosphate excretion. To some degree, acid loading decreases proximal phosphate reabsorption[59] by decreasing the activity of the Na^+-phosphate cotransporter that is responsible for the entry of luminal phosphate into the cell.[60,61] This effect may be mediated both by decreased affinity for the interaction with Na^{+}[61] and by conversion of HPO_4^{2-} to $H_2PO_4^-$, which binds less avidly to the cotransporter.[62] In addition, some of the excess H^+ ions may compete for the Na^+ site on the cotransporter, further decreasing phosphate reabsorption.[61]

Nevertheless, the ability to enhance net acid excretion by acidemia-induced phosphaturia is usually limited, and it is *increased NH_4^+ excretion that generally constitutes the major adaptation to an acid load.* An exception occurs in diabetic ketoacidosis, where large amounts of β-hydroxybutyrate ($pK_a = 4.8$) are excreted in the urine (see Chap. 25). These ketoacid anions can act as urinary buffers, augmenting titratable acid excretion by as much as 50 meq/day.[63] This effect is due both to the high concentration of ketoacid anions present and to the proximity of the pK_a of β-hydroxybutyrate to the acid urine pH.

Ammonium Excretion

The ability to excrete H^+ ions as ammonium adds an important degree of flexibility to renal acid-base regulation, because the rate of NH_4^+ production and excretion can be varied according to physiologic needs. The mechanism by which this process occurs has been considered to begin with ammonia (NH_3) production by the tubular cells.[64] Some of the excess NH_3 then freely diffuses into the tubular lumen, where it combines with secreted H^+ ions to form NH_4^+:

$$NH_3 + H^+ \quad \rightarrow \quad NH_4^+ \tag{11-8}$$

These NH_4^+ ions are lipid-insoluble and are therefore "trapped" in the lumen, since back-diffusion cannot occur.

This sequence also explains how NH_3 can act as an effective buffer, even though the pK_a of this system is 9.0, well above that of the plasma or urine. At a urine pH of 6.0, for example, the ratio of NH_3 to NH_4^+ is 1:1000. The combination of this small amount of NH_3 with secreted H^+ ions should rapidly utilize all of the available buffer. This does not occur, however, since the ensuing reduction in the tubular fluid NH_3 concentration results in the diffusion of more NH_3 into the lumen. This ability to replenish the quantity of buffer is not present with titratable acidity; once HPO_4^{2-} has been converted to $H_2PO_4^-$ further buffering by this system cannot occur.

It is now clear that this model represents an oversimplification and that NH_4^+ excretion can be viewed as occurring in three major steps: (1) NH_4^+ is produced, primarily in the early proximal tubular cells; (2) luminal NH_4^+ is partially reabsorbed in the thick ascending limb and the NH_3 is then recycled within the renal medulla; and (3) the medullary interstitial NH_3 reaches high concentrations that allow NH_3 to diffuse into the tubular lumen in the medullary collecting tubule, where it is trapped as NH_4^+ by secreted H^+, as predicted from the classic theory.[64,65]

NH_4^+ production   The initial step in NH_4^+ excretion is the generation of NH_4^+ within the tubular cells from the metabolism of amino acids, particularly but not solely glutamine[2,64,66]:

$$\text{Glutamine} \quad \rightarrow \quad NH_4^+ + \text{glutamate} \quad \rightarrow \quad NH_4^+ + \alpha\text{-ketoglutarate}^{2-}$$

The first of these reactions is catalyzed by phosphate-dependent glutaminase and the second by glutamate dehydrogenase.[67] The subsequent metabolism of α-ketoglutarate results in the generation of two HCO_3^- ions,[2] which are then returned to the systemic circulation by the Na^+-$3HCO_3^-$ cotransporter in the basolateral membrane (Fig. 11-4).

Notice that it is primarily NH_4^+, not NH_3, that is produced by these reactions, which occur mostly in the proximal tubule.[68,69] Lipid-solute NH_3 can freely diffuse out of the cell across both the luminal and basolateral membranes.[70] In comparison, lipid-insoluble NH_4^+ can be secreted only into the tubular lumen, since the required transmembrane transporters are present only in the luminal membrane.[70] This process of NH_4^+ secretion appears to be mediated at least in part by the Na^+-H^+ antiporter, which can also function as a Na^+-NH_4^+ exchanger (Fig. 11-4).[70-72]

Medullary recycling   The NH_4^+ that is produced within the proximal tubule and secreted into the lumen exists in equilibrium with a much smaller quantity of NH_3. This NH_3 is capable of diffusing out of the lumen into the peritubular capillary, thereby reducing net acid excretion. This effect is minimized by the low urine pH, which can lower urinary NH_3 levels well below the level in the plasma. As depicted in Fig. 11-5, however, the urine does not become maximally acidified until the end of the collecting tubules. It is therefore possible that significant quantities of NH_3 could be lost from the lumen, particularly in the medullary collecting tubule, where progressively higher luminal concentrations of NH_4^+ and NH_3 are achieved.

These potential losses of luminal NH_3 are minimized because more than 75 percent of the tubular fluid NH_4^+ is *recycled within the medulla*, thereby maintaining a high interstitial NH_3 concentration (Fig. 11-8).[65,69,73] The primary step in this process is reabsorption in the thick ascending limb by substitution of NH_4^+ for K^+ both on the Na^+-K^+-$2Cl^-$ carrier and, to a much lesser degree, through the K^+ channels in the luminal membrane (see Fig. 4-2).[65,74] The movement of reab-

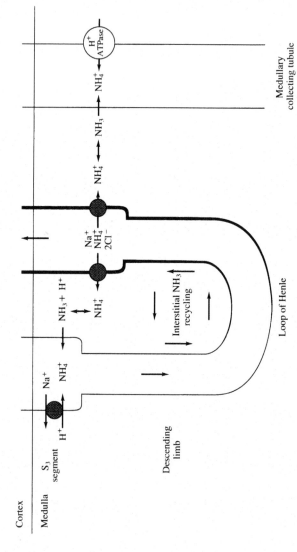

Figure 11-8 Schematic representation of ammonia recycling within the renal medulla. Although NH_4^+ production occurs predominantly in the proximal tubule, most of the NH_4^+ is then reabsorbed in the thick ascending limb, apparently by substitution for K^+ on the $Na^+-K^+-2Cl^-$ carrier in the luminal membrane. Partial dissociation into NH_3 and H^+ then occurs in the less acid tubular cell. The NH_3 diffuses into the medullary interstitium, where it reaches relatively high concentrations; it then diffuses back into those segments that have the lowest pH and therefore have the most favorable gradient: the S_3 segment of the late proximal tubule and, more importantly, the medullary collecting tubule, where the secreted NH_3 is trapped as NH_4^+ and then excreted.

sorbed NH_4^+ into the less acid tubular cell drives Eq. (11-8) to the left, resulting in the formation of NH_3 and H^+. The H^+ ions are then resecreted into the lumen via a Na^+-H^+ exchanger, where they promote HCO_3^- reabsorption by combining with HCO_3^- that is delivered out of the proximal tubule.[75,76]

In comparison, the luminal membrane has the unusual characteristic of being impermeable to NH_3.[76] As a result, the NH_3 formed within the cell will diffuse out across the basolateral membrane into the medullary interstitium, and then into those compartments that have the lowest NH_3 concentration, which in the tubules is a function of both delivery and the tubular fluid pH. As described above, a relatively small amount of H^+ secretion can lead to a large reduction in pH (and the generation of a disequilibrium pH) in those nephron segments that lack luminal carbonic anhydrase (Fig. 11-6). Thus, some of the NH_3 will diffuse into the S_3 segment of the proximal tubule and then be recycled again in the thick ascending limb.[52,74] The net effect is the maintenance of a high medullary interstitial NH_3 concentration, which promotes secretion into the medullary collecting tubule.

Ammonium reabsorption in the thick limb is reduced by hyperkalemia (probably due to competition for the reabsorptive site on the Na^+-K^+-$2Cl^-$ cotransporter, see "Plasma Potassium Concentration," below) and is enhanced by chronic metabolic acidosis due to increased NH_4^- production in and delivery out of the proximal tubule.[73,77] The latter represents an appropriate response, since the ensuing increase in ammonia recycling will facilitate NH_4^- excretion and therefore excretion of the acid load.

NH_3 secretion into the cortical and medullary collecting tubule   The fluid entering the collecting tubules has a relatively low NH_3 concentration because of removal in the loop of Henle. Furthermore, there is no luminal carbonic anhydrase in most of the collecting tubule segments.[28,54] As a result, continued H^+ secretion (by the H^+-ATPase pump) produces a maximally acid urine that further reduces the tubular fluid NH_3 levels. The net effect is that there is a relatively large gradient favoring the free diffusion of interstitial NH_3 into the tubular lumen, where it forms NH_4^+ (Fig. 11-8).[5,69]

For luminal NH_4^+ accumulation to occur with maximum efficiency, the NH_3 and NH_4^+ permeabilities must be different from those in the loop of Henle. In the latter segment, the luminal membrane is permeable to NH_4^+ but not to NH_3; these characteristics permit luminal NH_4^+ to be reabsorbed without NH_3 back-diffusion into the lumen. In contrast, the cell membranes in the collecting tubules are highly permeable to NH_3 but have only a negligible permeability to NH_4^+.[78] As a result, interstitial NH_3 can passively diffuse into the tubular lumen, where it is then trapped as NH_4^+.

The net effect is that NH_3 is secreted into the lumen throughout the collecting tubules.[65] The gradient is greatest in the inner medulla, where the interstitial concentration is highest. However, there is a roughly equivalent degree of NH_3 secretion in the cortex and outer medulla, which have a higher NH_3 permeability, as a result of both an increase in unit permeability and a greater luminal surface area.[65,67]

Response to changes in pH   According to this model, NH_4^+ excretion can be increased in one of two ways: by increasing proximal NH_4^+ production from glutamine and by lowering the urine pH, which will increase NH_3 diffusion into the lumen in the medullary collecting tubule (Fig. 11-9).[65] In humans given an acid load, for example, NH_4^+ excretion begins to increase within 2 h, mostly as a result of the formation of a more acid urine, which increases the efficiency of NH_3 secretion into the medullary collecting tubule.[79] Total NH_4^+ excretion reaches its maximum level at 5 to 6 days, a time at which there is an elevation in both glutamine uptake by the kidney and tubular NH_4^+ production (Fig. 11-10).[5,79-81]

Animal models provide confirmation of this sequence. Phosphate-dependent glutaminase activity increases on the first day and glutamate dehydrogenase activity by day 2 to 3 after an acid load.[82,83] However, NH_4^+ excretion begins to rise on the first day and is much greater than can be explained by the increase in enzyme activity; this response may reflect enhanced efficiency of NH_4^+ trapping or increased glutamine uptake by the cells.[82,83]

The adaptive increase in glutamine metabolism with acidemia begins with increased uptake by the proximal tubular cells.* Under normal conditions, most of the filtered glutamine is reabsorbed by cotransport with Na^+, being driven by the favorable electrochemical gradient for passive Na^+ entry into the cells (see page 75). In the presence of acidemia, however, Na^+-dependent glutamine uptake also occurs from the peritubular capillary across the basolateral membrane.[84,85] The peritubular capillary is a fertile source of glutamine, since only 20 percent of the renal plasma flow and therefore only 20 percent of the glutamine presented to the kidney normally undergoes glomerular filtration.

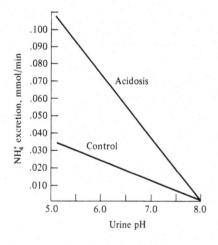

Figure 11-9   Effect of urinary and arterial pH on NH_4^+ excretion. Lowering the arterial pH (that is, acidemia) increases cellular NH_4^+ production from glutamine. Lowering the urine pH enhances the trapping of NH_3 as NH_4^+ in the medullary collecting tubule. (*Redrawn from Pitts RF*, Fed Proc 7:418, 1948, *with permission.*)

* The increment in renal glutamine uptake leads to an initial reduction in circulating glutamine levels.[80] This is then followed by increased glutamine release from skeletal muscle, due in part to activation of glutamine synthetase.

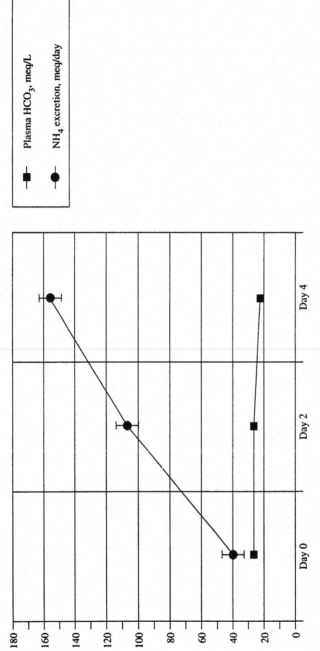

Figure 11-10   Effect of a dietary acid load on the plasma HCO_3^- concentration and urinary NH_4^+ excretion. The latter increases approximately fourfold with a reduction of only a few milliequivalents per liter in the plasma HCO_3^- concentration. (*Data from Welbourne T, Weber M, Bank N, J Clin Invest 51:1852, 1972, with permission.*)

Once glutamine is within the tubular cells, its proximal metabolism is pH-dependent, appropriately increasing with acidemia and decreasing with alkalemia.[68,69] How this occurs is incompletely understood, as several factors may play an important role. With acidemia, for example, the rise in NH_4^+ production may be largely mediated by enhanced activity of the enzymes involved in NH_4^+ production, including phosphate-dependent glutaminase (promoting the metabolism of glutamine to glutamate), glutamate dehydrogenase (promoting the metabolism of glutamate to α-ketoglutarate), and α-ketoglutarate dehydrogenase (promoting the metabolism of α-ketoglutarate).[66,82] These changes in enzyme activity are limited to the proximal tubule,[82] which is consistent with this segment being the site of increased NH_4^+ production in acidemic states.[68]

It is presumed that proximal glutamine metabolism responds to alterations in cell pH that parallel those in the extracellular fluid (see "Extracellular pH," below). In particular, it may be an alteration in the *pH gradient between the cytosol and the mitochondria* that constitutes the signal to change the rate of NH_4^+ production.[66,86] Other, mostly unidentified circulating factors may also contribute, including increased release of glucocorticoids.[87,88]

Regardless of the exact mechanisms involved, the net effect is that NH_4^+ excretion can increase from its normal value of 30 to 40 meq/day to over 300 meq/day with severe metabolic acidosis.[63,89] This response, which is in marked contrast to the limited ability to enhance titratable acid excretion, is appropriate; each NH_4^+ produced results in the equimolar generation of HCO_3^- from the metabolism of α-ketoglutarate.[2] Return of this HCO_3^- to the systemic circulation then raises the plasma HCO_3^- concentration toward normal.

Urine pH

As depicted in Fig. 11-5, the tubular fluid pH falls progressively, reaching its lowest level in the medullary collecting tubule. In humans, the minimum urine pH that can be achieved is 4.5 to 5.0; this represents a maximum plasma-to-tubular fluid H^+ gradient of almost 1:1000 (3 log units). The inability to make the urine more acid may reflect a limit on the strength of the H^+-ATPase pump or on the impermeability of the tubular epithelium, which is required to prevent the passive backflux of secreted H^+ ions out of the lumen.

This ability to lower the urine pH is important, because the formation of both titratable acidity and NH_4^+ is pH-dependent, with both increasing as the urine is made more acid (Table 11-1, Fig. 11-9). If the minimum urine pH were higher, at 5.5 to 6.0 (which is still less than that of the plasma), titratable acid and NH_4^+ excretion would fall, and excretion of the daily H^+ load might be prevented. This appears to be the mechanism responsible for the acidemia in patients with type 1 (distal) renal tubular acidosis (see Chap. 19).

The pH dependence of titratable acidity and NH_4^- formation also means that these processes (as well as HCO_3^- reabsorption) occur throughout the nephron as the urine is made more acid. The sites at which they are most likely to occur can be appreciated from the isohydric principle, which states that all three buffer systems must be in equilibrium:

$$pH = 6.1 + \log\frac{[HCO_3^-]}{0.03P_{CO_2}} = 6.8 + \log\frac{[HPO_4^{2-}]}{[H_2PO_4^-]} = 9.0 + \log\frac{[NH_3]}{[NH_4^+]}$$

Thus, a secreted H^+ ion will preferentially be buffered by that system with the highest concentration and/or the pK_a closest to that of the tubular fluid pH.[69] In the proximal tubule, most secreted H^+ ions are utilized for HCO_3^- reabsorption because of the high concentration of HCO_3^- and the ability to minimize the reduction in pH by the action of luminal carbonic anhydrase. This segment also represents the site in which most NH_4^+ is secreted into the lumen and in which about one-half of the available HPO_4^{2-} is buffered (Table 11-1). In contrast, most H^+ ions secreted in the medullary collecting tubule (where the urine pH is reduced to its lowest value) combine with secreted NH_3, since virtually all the HCO_3^- has been reabsorbed and most of the HPO_4^{2-} has already been buffered (which occurs when the urine pH is below 5.8, that is, more than 1 pH unit from the pK_a of 6.8).

REGULATION OF RENAL HYDROGEN EXCRETION

The preceding section discussed how the kidney excretes H^+ ions. In this section, we will review the factors that determine exactly how much H^+ is excreted. The *extracellular pH* (which is most often measured clinically on a specimen of arterial blood) is the major physiologic regulator of this process, as it allows acid excretion to vary with day-to-day changes in the dietary acid load. In addition, the rate of H^+ secretion also can be influenced by the effective circulating volume, aldosterone, the plasma K^+ concentration, and parathyroid hormone.

Extracellular pH

Net acid excretion tends to vary inversely with the extracellular pH. Acidemia, for example, is characterized by a fall in extracellular pH (or a rise in H^+ concentration) and is associated with an increase in both proximal and distal acidification.[90-93] This is manifested in the proximal tubule by four changes:

- Enhanced luminal Na^+-H^+ exchange,[90,91,94] a response that may be mediated both by binding of excess intracellular H^+ ions to a modifier site on the exchanger[90] and by the synthesis of new exchangers, as evidenced by a rise in mRNA for the Na^+-H^+ antiporter[95]
- Enhanced activity of the luminal H^+-ATPase[13]
- Increased activity of the $Na:3HCO_3^-$ cotransporter in the basolateral membrane, thereby allowing HCO_3^- formed within the cell to be returned to the systemic circulation[91,94,96]
- Increased NH_4^+ production from glutamine[68]

In the collecting tubules, on the other hand, the increase in acidification appears to involve the insertion of preformed cytoplasmic H^+-ATPase pumps into the luminal membrane of the acid-secreting cells,[40,57,97] particularly those in the outer medullary collecting duct.[97] The ensuing reduction in the tubular fluid pH in these segments will promote the diffusion of interstitial NH_3 into the lumen, where it will be trapped as NH_4^+ (Fig. 11-4).[79] The net effect of this increase in acid excretion is enhanced generation of HCO_3^- by the tubules. Return of this HCO_3^- to the systemic circulation will then raise the extracellular pH toward normal.

The extracellular pH is thought to affect net acid excretion in part by *parallel, although lesser, alterations in the renal tubular cell pH*.[98-100] The importance of this local effect, which is independent of other circulating factors, has been demonstrated in experiments with cultured renal proximal tubule cells. Lowering the pH of the bathing medium in this setting leads to a significant increase in the activity of the luminal Na^+-H^+ exchanger.[100] This effect is thought to be mediated by activation of pH-sensitive proteins.[101]

The mechanism by which the intracellular pH changes with the extracellular pH varies with the cause of the acid-base disorder. An elevation in the P_{CO_2}, for example, will lower the pH of the extracellular fluid; this will induce a similar and rapid acidification in the cells, because CO_2 can freely cross cell membranes.

The effect of alterations in the plasma HCO_3^- concentration are less direct, since transcellular diffusion of this anion is limited by the lipid bilayer of the cell membrane. However, the carrier-mediated HCO_3^- exit steps in the basolateral membrane of the proximal tubule (Na^+-$3HCO_3^-$ cotransport)[98,99] and the distal nephron (Cl-HCO_3^-) exchange)[102] are affected by the transmembrane HCO_3^- gradient. Lowering the extracellular pH by reducing the HCO_3^- concentration will make this gradient more favorable, therby promoting HCO_3^- exit from the cell and reducing the cell pH (Fig. 11-11).[98,99] The ensuing increase in acid excretion then raises both the systemic and the intracellular pH toward normal; thus, it may actually be the *intracellular pH* that is primarily being regulated.[102,103]

These adaptive changes in cell pH are determined by the extracellular pH itself, not by the HCO_3^- concentration or P_{CO_2} alone. There is *no alteration in the cell pH* if both the HCO_3^- concentration and the P_{CO_2} are lowered or raised to a similar degree, so that the extracellular pH remains constant.[98] In this setting, there is also no change in net acid excretion.[92]

Metabolic acidosis   Metabolic acidosis is characterized by acidemia that is due to a *reduced* plasma HCO_3^- concentration. Net acid excretion is appropriately and often dramatically increased in this disorder, beginning within a day and reaching its maximum in 5 to 6 days (Fig. 11-10).[5,79,104] This response is mostly due to enhanced NH_4^+ excretion, which is mediated both by increased proximal NH_4^+ secretion[68,79] and by increased distal hydrogen secretion.[40,97]

In comparison, titratable acid excretion is generally limited by the amount of phosphate in the urine, which is modestly increased by an acidemia-induced inhibition of proximal phosphate reabsorption.[59-62] An exception to this rule occurs in

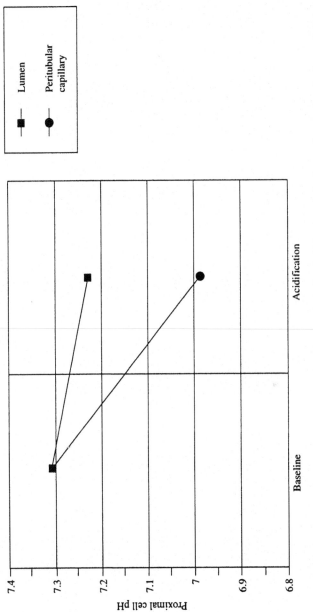

Figure 11-11 Effect of lowering the HCO_3^- concentration and pH in the fluid in the tubular lumen (squares) or in the peritubular capillary (circles) on the proximal tubular cell pH. Only the change in peritubular capillary pH significantly lowers the cell pH, an effect that appears to be mediated by the $Na^+{:}3HCO_3^-$ cotransporter. (*Data from Alpern RJ, Chambers M, J Clin Invest 78:502, 1986, with permission.*)

diabetic ketoacidosis, where urinary ketone anions (particularly β-hydroxybuty-rate) can act as titratable acids. In this setting, net acid excretion can exceed 500 meq/day,[63,89] resulting in the generation of an equivalent quantity of HCO_3^- ions in the extracellular fluid.

The relationship between cell pH and net acid excretion can also be under-stood in terms of the steady state. Suppose a normal subject increases acid gen-eration by going on a high-protein diet. Over a period of days, net acid excretion will rise until it meets the new level of acid production. At this time, the patient is back in a new steady state, but the plasma HCO_3^- concentration must have fallen to provide the signal (lower cell pH) for the higher level of acid excretion. This process is reasonably efficient. As shown in Fig. 11-10, for example, lowering the plasma HCO_3^- concentration by 4 to 5 meq//L leads to a fourfold increase in NH_4^+ excretion.

Metabolic alkalosis   Metabolic alkalosis, on the other hand, is characterized by an alkaline extracellular pH that results from an *elevation* in the plasma HCO_3^- concentration. The normal response to a HCO_3^- load is to excrete the excess HCO_3^- in the urine, both by diminishing its rate of reabsorption and by HCO_3^- secretion in the cortical collecting tubule.[21,55,56] As described above, the latter process occurs in a subpopulation of cortical intercalated cells that are able, in the presence of an elevated pH, to insert H^+-ATPase pumps into the basolateral rather than the luminal membrane (Fig. 11-7).[40]

This protective bicarbonaturic response is extremely efficient. For example, the administration of as much as 1000 meq of $NaHCO_3$ per day to normal subjects induces only a minor elevation in the plasma HCO_3^- concentration, as virtually all of the excess HCO_3^- is excreted in the urine.[105] Thus, maintenance of metabolic alkalosis requires the presence of a defect in HCO_3^- excretion, which is most often due to effective volume and chloride depletion (see below).

Respiratory acidosis and alkalosis   Disturbances in alveolar ventilation induce changes in CO_2 elimination and, consequently, in the P_{CO_2}. Primary hyperventila-tion, for example, enhances CO_2 loss, resulting in a fall in the P_{CO_2} (hypocapnia) and a rise in pH that is called *respiratory alkalosis*. Primary hypoventilation, on the other hand, impairs CO_2 elimination, producing an elevation in the P_{CO_2} (hypercapnia) and a reduction in pH that is called *respiratory acidosis*. Although correction of either of these conditions requires the restoration of nor-mal alveolar ventilation, the kidney can minimize the changes in arterial pH by varying H^+ excretion and HCO_3^- reabsorption.

From Eq. (11-3), the extracellular pH is a function of the HCO_3^-/P_{CO_2} ratio. Thus, the *pH may remain near normal in respiratory acid-base disorders if the P_{CO_2} and HCO_3^- concentration change in the same direction and to a similar degree.* Consequently, an elevation in the plasma HCO_3^- concentration is an appropriate response to hypercapnia, and a reduction in the plasma HCO_3^- concentration is an appropriate response to hypocapnia (see Chaps. 20 and 21).

These changes occur because the P_{CO_2}, via its effect on intracellular pH, is an important determinant of H^+ secretion and HCO_3^- reabsorption (Fig. 11-12).[57,92,93] With chronic respiratory acidosis, for example, there is an increase in net acid excretion (primarily and NH_4^+), resulting in the generation of new HCO_3^- ions in the plasma.[106] The net effect in the steady state (which is achieved within 5 to 6 days) is that the rise is P_{CO_2} is partially offset by an increase in the plasma HCO_3^- concentration that *averages 3.5 meq/L for every 10-mmHg elevation* in the P_{CO_2}.[107]

The renal response is reversed in chronic respiratory alkalosis. In this setting, the concurrent rise in intracellular pH diminishes H^+ secretion, resulting in HCO_3^- loss in the urine and decreased NH_4^+ excretion.[108,109] These changes are manifested by a fall in the plasma HCO_3^- concentration that averages *5 meq/L for every 10-mmHg decline* in the P_{CO_2}.[108]

Chronic metabolic acidosis versus chronic respiratory acidosis   Although chronic metabolic and respiratory acid-base disturbances can produce similar changes in extracellular pH, there are major differences in the renal response that illustrate the role of the intracellular pH in determining the degree of acidification that occurs.[110,111] In chronic metabolic acidosis, for example, the daily acid load must be increased to sustain the acidemia (as with chronic diarrhea). Consequently, net acid and NH_4^+ excretion are persistently above normal (Fig. 11-13).

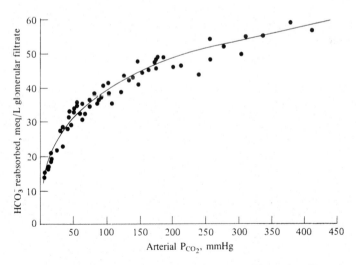

Figure 11-12   Relationship between arterial P_{CO_2} and HCO_3^- reabsorption. Note that the curve is steepest in the physiologic range (P_{CO_2} of 15 to 90 mmHg). (*From Rector FC Jr, Seldin DW, Roberts AD Jr, Smith JS, J Clin Invest 39:1706, 1960, by copyright permission of the American Society for Clinical Investigation.*)

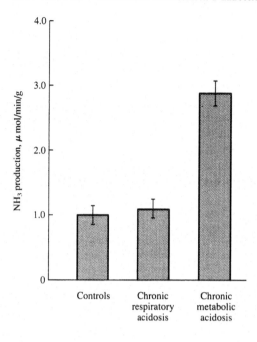

Figure 11-13 Ammonia production by the isolated perfused kidney from control rats and those with chronic respiratory acidosis or chronic metabolic acidosis of 3 days duration. Ammonia production is enhanced only in metabolic acidosis, despite a similar reduction in pH to about 7.30 in both acidotic groups. (*From Rodriguez-Nichols F, Laughrey E, Tannen RL, Am J Physiol 247:F896, 1984, with permission.*)

The same response is seen in respiratory acidosis, as new HCO_3^- ions must be generated to produce the compensatory rise in the plasma HCO_3^- concentration.[92,106] In the new steady state, the pH will be partially corrected, but the daily acid load generated from protein metabolism *will be normal* (assuming that there is no change in dietary intake). As a result, there is *no necessity for increased NH_4^+ excretion* in chronic respiratory acidosis, which returns to a level similar to that in controls (Fig. 11-13).[110]

To summarize, net acid and NH_4^+ excretion are enhanced in chronic metabolic but not respiratory acidosis, despite a similar degree of acidemia in both conditions. This seemingly paradoxical finding may be *explained by differences in proximal tubular cell pH.*[111,112] Both metabolic and respiratory acidosis will produce a similar effect at the basolateral membrane: lowering the cell pH by HCO_3^- exit down a more favorable gradient in metabolic acidosis and by CO_2 entry in respiratory acidosis.[98,99]

The responses are quite different, however, at the luminal membrane. The plasma HCO_3^- concentration and, therefore, the filtered HCO_3^- load are reduced in metabolic acidosis. As a result, less HCO_3^- is reabsorbed in the proximal tubule by Na^+-H^+ exchange. In comparison, the plasma HCO_3^- concentration and filtered HCO_3^- load are elevated in chronic respiratory acidosis. This increase in the tubular HCO_3^- concentration allows more HCO_3^- to be reabsorbed.[113] It is important to remember that proximal acidification is limited by the transcellular Na^+ gradient that provides the energy for the Na^+-H^+ antiporter. When more buffer (as HCO_3^-) is present, more H^+ secretion can occur without an excessive reduction in tubular fluid pH.[113]

The net effect of this increase in H^+ extrusion from the cell is that the *proximal tubular cell pH returns toward normal in chronic respiratory acidosis.*[111,112]* As a result, there is now no stimulus to increase proximal NH_4^+ secretion, incomparison to chronic metabolic acidosis, where the cell pH is persistently reduced.[112] Similar factors may explain why mRNA expression for the Na^+-H^+ exchanger is increased in metabolic acidosis but unchanged in chronic respiratory acidosis.[98]

Effective Circulating Volume

Bicarbonate reabsorption can be influenced by the effective circulating volume, with the most important effect being an increase in HCO_3^- reabsorptive capacity with volume depletion.[113-115] As shown in Fig. 11-14, for example, raising the plasma HCO_3^- concentration by infusing $NaHCO_3$ leads to a plateau in HCO_3^- reabsorption at a level of about 26 meq//L (see page 88). This is a proper response, since it allows virtually all of the filtered HCO_3^- to be reabsorbed as long as the plasma HCO_3^- concentration is within the normal range. Once the latter exceeds 26 meq/L, inappropriate HCO_3^- retention is prevented by excretion of the excess HCO_3^- in the urine.

In contrast, if hypovolemia is induced by the prior administration of a diuretic, then net HCO_3^- reabsorption continues to increase, even at a level above 35 meq/L (Fig. 11-14). This effect can be demonstrated in normals simply by the ingestion of a low-salt diet (10 meq/day), which is sufficient to increase HCO_3^-

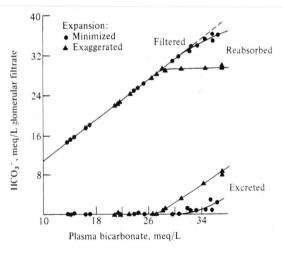

Figure 11-14 Relationship between arterial P_{CO_2} and HCO_3^- reabsorption. Note the curve is steepest in the physiologic range (P_{CO_2} of 15 to 90 mmHG). (*From Rector FC Jr, Seldin DW, Roberts AD Jr, Smith JS, J Clin Invest 39:1706, 1960, by copyright permission of the American Society for Clinical Investigation.*)

---

* It seems likely that distal acidification is similar in metabolic and respiratory acidosis,[93] since the confounding effect of increased HCO_3^- reabsorption is primarily limited to the proximal tubule. However, this preservation of distal function in chronic respiratory acidosis does not lead to a significant increase in net acid excretion, since virtually all of the urinary NH_4^+ is produced proximally.[68,69] Thus, the absence of an elevation in proximal NH_4^+ production in this disorder[110] limits the degree to which distal H^+ secretion can enhance net acid excretion.

reabsorptive capacity by 4 meq/L even though the subject is clinically euvolemic.[116]

The relationship between volume depletion and HCO_3^- transport becomes clinically important in patients with metabolic alkalosis, in whom the inability to excrete the excess HCO_3^- prevents the spontaneous restoration of acid-base balance.[117] In this setting, *the attempt to maintain volume by preventing further Na^+ loss as $NaHCO_3$ occurs at the expense of the systemic pH.*

At least four factors may contribute to this effect on HCO_3^- excretion: (1) a reduction in glomerular filtration rate, (2) activation of the renin-angiotensin-aldosterone system, (3) hypochloremia, and (4) concurrent hypokalemia due to urinary or gastrointestinal losses (see below).[114,127-129] A decline in GFR, for example, may play a permissive role in selected patients. It is not likely to be of primary importance, however, since the rise in the plasma HCO_3^- concentration results in a filtered load of HCO_3^- that is often not diminished. Furthermore, many patients maintain a GFR that is relatively normal; in this setting, increased tubular reabsorption must be responsible for the absence of HCO_3^- excretion.[117,119]

Renin-angiotensin-aldosterone system The hypovolemia-induced increase in renin release can enhance net H^+ secretion and therefore HCO_3^- reabsorption in several ways. Angiotensin II, acting in the early proximal tubule, is a potent stimulator of HCO_3^- transport by increasing the activity of both the luminal Na^+-H^+ antiporter and the basolateral Na^+-$3HCO_3^-$ cotransporter.[120,121]

However, the physiologic significance of this response for acid-base balance is uncertain. Angiotensin II does increase HCO_3^- reabsorption in the early proximal tubule, but the ensuing decrease in delivery out of this segment may result in an equivalent delivery-dependent reduction in HCO_3^- transport in the late proximal tubule.[122,123] Thus, there may be a net neutral effect on HCO_3^- handling, as the major function of the proximal action of angiotensin II is to increase NaCl and water reabsorption, thereby appropriately expanding the extracellular volume.[122]

Aldosterone may play a more important role by stimulating the Na^+-independent H^+-ATPase pump throughout the distal nephron, including the intercalated cells in the critical collecting tubule and the cells in the outer and inner medullary collecting tubule.[124-128]* Aldosterone also increases the activity of the second step in distal acidification, promoting HCO_3^- extrusion from the cell into the peritubular capillary via the basolateral Cl-HCO_3^- exchanger.[102,127]

In addition, aldosterone can indirectly increase net H^+ secretion by the stimulation of Na^+ transport in a different cell population, the principal cells in the cortical collecting tubule (see Chap. 6).[36,37,114] The reabsorption of cationic Na^+ ions creates a lumen-negative potential difference; this electrical gradient then promotes H^+ accumulation in the lumen by minimizing the degree of back-diffusion.

---

*This ability of aldosterone to increase urinary H^+ loss can promote the development of metabolic alkalosis in disorders of primary mineralocorticoid excess, such as primary hyperaldosteronism (see Chap. 18).

Chloride depletion   Hypochloremia is a common concomitant of metabolic alkalosis, since both H^+ and Cl^- ions are lost in most patients, such as those with vomiting or diuretic therapy. This reduction in the filtered Cl^- concentration can enhance H^+ secretion and HCO_3^- reabsorption through both *Na^+-dependent and Na^+-independent* factors. It has been proposed, for example, that the effect of hypochloremia is related to the high level of Na^+ reabsorption seen in volume depletion, often leading to a urine Na^+ concentration below 5 to 10 meq/L. If, as in normal subjects, the filtrate Na^+ concentration is 145 meq/L and the filtrate Cl^- concentration is 115 meq/L, then only 115 meq/L of Na^+ can be reabsorbed with Cl^-. Since Cl^- is the only quantitatively important reabsorbable anion in the filtrate, *further Na^+ reabsorption must be accompanied by H^+ or K^+ secretion to maintain electroneutrality.* These secretory processes, which primarily occur in the collecting tubules, become more important in the presence of hypochloremia, a setting in which less of the filtered Na^+ can be reabsorbed with Cl^-. The net effect is enhanced H^+ secretion, increased HCO_3^- reabsorption, and persistence of the metabolic alkalosis.

The importance of both volume status and the reabsorbability of the anion can be illustrated by the response to an infusion of Na_2SO_4 (SO_4^{2-} being a poorly reabsorbed anion). When given to a euvolemic subject, Na_2SO_4 is rapidly excreted in the urine. In a volume-depleted subject, however, the Na^+ will be retained (in part under the influence of aldosterone), and, since SO_4^{2-} cannot be reabsorbed, H^+ and K^+ secretion must be increased (Fig. 11-15).[129] In contrast, the administration of NaCl in this setting results in both Na^+ and Cl^- reabsorption without affecting H^+ and K^+ secretion.

The reabsorbability of the anion creates a paradoxical situation in patients with hypovolemia and metabolic alkalosis in that the *administration of acid will not necessarily correct the alkalemia.* If, for example, HNO_3 is given (NO_3^- being relatively nonreabsorbable), it will be buffered by extracellular HCO_3^-:

$$HNO_3 + NaHCO_3 \rightarrow NaNO_3 + H_2CO_3 \rightarrow CO_2 + H_2O$$

As the $NaNO_3$ is presented to the cortical collecting tubule, Na^+ will be retained and H^+ excretion enhanced. This is similar to the fate of Na_2SO_4, shown in Fig. 11-15. The net effect is the excretion of the administered HNO_3 as NH_4NO_3.[130] As

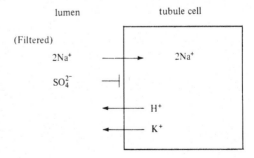

Figure 11-15 Events occurring after Na^+ reabsorption across the luminal membrane of the cortical collecting tubule cell. In a sodium-avid state, the presentation of Na^+ with a nonreabsorbable anion to the cortical collecting tubule enhances H^+ and K^+ secretion. In contrast, if NaCl is presented to this segment, Na^+ will be reabsorbed with Cl^-, with little effect on H^+ and K^+ secretion.

a result, the arterial pH will be unchanged, since an acid urine is excreted despite the presence of systemic alkalemia.

If, in comparison, acid is given as HCl, buffering by $NaHCO_3$ will lead to the generation of NaCl. When this reaches the cortical collecting tubule, the Na^+ will be reabsorbed with Cl^- and not exchanged for H^+. Therefore, the administered H^+ will be retained and the alkalemia will be corrected.

Rather than by giving HCl, the alkalemia can be reversed more easily by promoting HCO_3^- excretion in the urine. This can be achieved by expanding the effective circulating volume with NaCl, eventually allowing the excess HCO_3^- to be excreted as $NaHCO_3$. In comparison, the administration of Na^+ with a different, nonreabsorbable anion, such as SO_4^{2-}, will be ineffective. Thus, the correction of metabolic alkalosis in a volume-depleted (Na^+-avid) subject requires the *administration of the only reabsorbable anion, Cl^-, as either NaCl, HCl, or, if hypokalemia is present, KCl* (see Chap. 18).

The importance of Cl^- may also be related to direct effects on acid-base handling that are *independent of Na^+*.[118,131] In particular, both HCO_3^- secretion by the type B intercalated cells in the cortical collecting tubule and H^+ secretion in the distal nephron can be affected by the local Cl^- concentration.

HCO_3^- secretion into the lumen in the type B intercalated cells appears to be mediated by a Cl-HCO_3^- exchanger in the luminal membrane, the energy for which is provided by the favorable inward gradient for Cl^- (Fig. 11-7).[55,56] Lowering the tubular fluid Cl^- concentration will diminish this gradient, minimizing the ability to secrete HCO_3^-.

With H^+ secretion by the H^+-ATPase pump, Cl^- appears to be passively cosecreted to maintain electroneutrality.[25] The gradient for Cl^- secretion and therefore the ability to secrete H^+ may be enhanced when the tubular fluid Cl^- concentration is reduced.[131]

Both diminished HCO_3^- secretion and enhanced H^+ secretion will contribute to maintenance of the high plasma HCO_3^- concentration and persistence of the alkalemia.

In summary, the effects of hypochloremia on net HCO_3^- reabsorption are most prominent in the collecting tubules. Thus, the appropriate HCO_3^- diuresis induced by fluid and chloride repletion is mostly mediated by decreased net distal HCO_3^- reabsorption (which probably includes a component of HCO_3^- secretion.[132]

Plasma Potassium Concentration

Potassium is another potential influence on renal H^+ secretion, as a reciprocal relationship has been demonstrated between the plasma K^+ concentration and HCO_3^- reabsorption (Fig. 11-16).[133-135] The major proposed mechanism for this relationship is that alterations in K^+ balance lead to *transcellular cation shifts* that affect the intracellular H^+ concentration (Fig. 11-17).

As an example, gastrointestinal or urinary K^+ losses lead to a reduction in the plasma K^+ concentration. As a result, intracellular $K6^+$ moves into the extracellular fluid (through K^+ channels in the cell membrane) down a favorable concen-

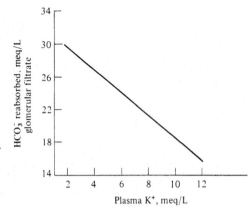

Figure 11-16   Renal tubular reabsorption of HCO_3^- as a function of the plasma K^+ concentration. (*Adapted from Fuller GR, MacLeod MB, Pitts RF, Am J Physiol 182:111, 1956, with permission.*)

tration gradient to replete the extracellular stores. To maintain electroneutrality, H^+ (and Na^+) enter the cell,[136] resulting in an intracellular acidosis.[112,137,138]

This increase in H^+ concentration in the renal tubular cells may account for the enhanced H^+ secretion, HCO_3^- reabsorption, and NH_4^+ excretion observed with K^+ depletion.[133,138,139] In the proximal tubule, for example, hypokalemia is associated with increased activity of both the luminal Na^+-H^+ antiporter and the basolateral Na^+-$3HCO_3^-$ cotransporter, which are required for the elevations in H^+ secretion and HCO_3^- reabsorption.[140]

These changes are reversed with a rise in the plasma K^+ concentration, as K^+ moves into and H^+ out of cells.[141] The ensuing intracellular alkalosis may then account for the associated reductions in HCO_3^- reabsorption and NH_4^+ excretion.[133,138,139]

Factors other than these transcellular shifts also may contribute to the potassium-induced changes in urinary acidification. For example, hyperkalemia reduces NH_4^+ excretion in rats; there is, however, no change in NH_4^+ delivery out of the

Figure 11-17   Reciprocal cation shifts of K^+, H^+, and Na^+ between the cells, including renal tubular cells, and the extracellular fluid. In the presence of hypokalemia, K^+ moves out of the cells down a concentration gradient. Since the cell anions (primarily proteins and organic phosphates) are unable to cross the cell membrane, electroneutrality is maintained by the entry of Na^+ and H^+ into the cell. The increase in cell H^+ concentration may be responsible for the increased H^+ secretion and HCO_3^- reabsorption seen with hypokalemia. On the other hand, hyperkalemia causes H^+ and Na^+ to leave the cells, resulting in a fall in H^+ secretion and HCO_3^- reabsorption.

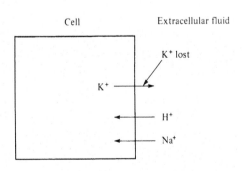

proximal tubule, suggesting that segments distal to the proximal tubule must be involved.[142] There are at least two mechanisms by which distal K^+ and H^+ handling might be related:

- Medullary recycling of NH_4^+ is initiated by substitution of NH_4^+ for K^+ on the Na^+-K^+-$2Cl^-$ carrier in the luminal membrane of the thick ascending limb (Fig. 11-8).[74] Increased luminal K^+ in hyperkalemia could competitively inhibit this process, thereby limiting ammonia accumulation in the medullary interstitium, subsequent secretion into the medullary collecting tubule, and total urinary NH_4^+ excretion.[142,143]
- H^+ secretion in the distal nephron is mediated in part by an electroneutral H^+-K^+-ATPase that also actively reabsorbs K^+.[24,27,29] Active K^+ reabsorption by this pump appears to be stimulated by hypokalemia,[27,144-146] an effect that could in part explain the concurrent increase in H^+ secretion. The net result is that hypokalemia and aldosterone, which stimulate the H^+-K^+-ATPase and H^+-ATPase pumps, respectively, can have a potentiating effect on distal hydrogen secretion and therefore on the development and maintenance of metabolic alkalosis.[147] This synergism has potential clinical importance, since many of the causes of metabolic alkalosis (such as diuretic therapy, vomiting, and primary hyperaldosteronism) are associated with both a reduction in the plasma K^+ concentration and increased aldosterone release (see Chap. 18).

In summary, hypokalemia tends to increase net acid excretion, which promotes the development of metabolic alkalosis. Hyperkalemia, via opposite mechanisms, reduces net acid excretion, which, by causing H^+ retention, favors the development of metabolic acidosis. In some patients with hyperkalemia due to hypoaldosteronism, for example, the associated metabolic acidosis can be corrected solely by lowering the plasma K^+ concentration.[139]

Parathyroid Hormone

Parathyroid hormone (PTH) diminishes proximal HCO_3^- reabsorption by reducing the activity of the Na^+-H^+ exchanger in the luminal membrane[148,149] and the Na^+-$3HCO_3^-$ cotransporter in the basolateral membrane.[150] However, the extra HCO_3^- delivered out of the proximal tubule is mostly picked up in the loop of Henle and more distal segments. Although there may be a slight increase in HCO_3^- excretion, this is generally counteracted by enhanced excretion of phosphate, which can increase net acid excretion by buffering secreted H^+ ions.[151]

This response may be physiologically important, since an acid load stimulates PTH secretion. PTH then minimizes the change in extracellular pH both by promoting bone buffering and by increasing acid and phosphate excretion in the urine.[151,152]

The effect of a chronic excess of PTH on acid-base balance is less clear. Patients with primary hyperparathyroidism, who are also hypercalcemic, tend to have a metabolic acidosis.[153] However, the chronic, continuous administration of PTH to normal humans increases net acid excretion and produces a small eleva- tion, not reduction, in the plasma HCO_3^- concentration.[154]

EFFECT OF ARTERIAL pH ON VENTILATION

Alveolar ventilation provides the oxygen necessary for oxidative metabolism and eliminates the CO_2 produced by these metabolic processes. It is therefore appro- priate that the main physiologic stimuli to respiration are an elevation in the P_{CO_2} and a reduction in the P_{O_2} (hypoxemia).[155,156] The CO_2 stimulus to ventila- tion primarily occurs in chemosensitive areas in the respiratory center in the brain stem, which appear to respond to CO_2-induced changes in the cerebral interstitial pH.[157] This effect is extremely important in the maintenance of the acid-base balance, since roughly 15,000 mmol of CO_2 is produced daily from endogenous metabolism, added to the capillary blood, and then eliminated via the lungs. In contrast, hypoxemia is primarily sensed by peripheral chemorecep- tors in the carotid bodies, which are located near the bifurcation of the carotid arteries.[156,158]

Respiratory Compensation in Metabolic Acidosis and Alkalosis

Alveolar ventilation also is affected by metabolic acid-base disorders.[159-165] In metabolic acidosis, for example, minute ventilation can increase from the normal of approximately 5 L/min to greater than 30 L/min as the arterial pH falls from 7.40 to 7.00 (Fig. 11-18). The initial rise in ventilation is mediated primarily by the peripheral chemoreceptors in the carotid bodies, which immediately sense the reduction in pH. However, the ensuing fall in P_{CO_2} produces an acute *elevation* in cerebrospinal fluid and cerebral interstitial pH, since CO_2 but not HCO_3^- rapidly crosses the blood-brain barrier. As a result, the central chemoreceptors sense alkalemia and act to diminish ventilation, thereby limiting the ventilatory response.[159] If the acidemia persists for hours to days, however, the cerebral pH will fall, as a result of ionic diffusion or the formation of new cerebrospinal fluid that reflects the change in systemic pH.[159,160] This cerebral adaptation allows the full degree of hyperventilation to be seen, usually with 12 to 24 h.[159,161]

The increase in ventilation with metabolic acidosis is an appropriate compen- satory response, since the concomitant reduction in P_{CO_2} will return the extracel- lular pH toward normal.[162,163] Conversely, hypoventilation with a consequent elevation in P_{CO_2} lowers the pH toward normal in metabolic alkalosis, where the plasma HCO_3^- concentration is increased.[164,165]

The potential importance of these respiratory compensations to metabolic acidosis and alkalosis can be appreciated from the following hypothetical example. In diabetic ketoacidosis (see Chap. 25), the increased production of ketoacids is buffered in part in the extracellular fluid, resulting in a decline in the plasma

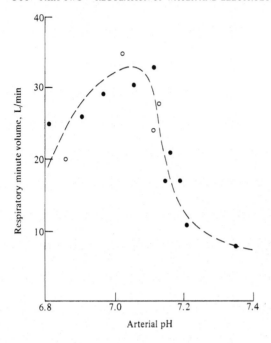

Figure 11-18 Relationship between respiratory minute volume and arterial pH in patients with diabetic ketoacidosis. (*Reproduced from Kety SS, Polis BD, Nadler CS, Schmidt CF, J Clin Invest 27:500, 1948, by copyright permission of the American Society for Clinical Investigation.*)

HCO_3^- concentration. If the latter were reduced to 6 meq/L and the P_{CO_2} remained at the normal 40 mmHg, then

$$pH = 6.1 + \log\frac{6}{0.03 \times 40} = 6.80$$

However, if ventilation were stimulated by the acidemia and the P_{CO_2} fell to 15 mmHg, then

$$pH = 6.1 + \log\frac{6}{0.03 \times 15} = 7.22$$

Thus, the respiratory compensation has turned a life-threatening reduction in pH into one that is much less dangerous.

Limitation of Respiratory Compensation

Despite the effectiveness of the respiratory compensation, the pH is protected for only a few days, since the initially beneficial change in P_{CO_2} then alters renal HCO_3^- reabsorption. In metabolic acidosis, for example, the compensatory fall in P_{CO_2} decreases HCO_3^- reabsorption (Fig. 11-12) and, therefore, the plasma HCO_3^- concentration. The net effect is that, after several days, the *extracellular pH is the same as it would have been if no respiratory compensation had occurred*, since the decline in P_{CO_2} is balanced by a further reduction in the HCO_3^- concentration (Table 11-2).[166] Fortunately, most forms of severe metabolic acidosis

Table 11-2   Arterial pH in chronic metabolic acidosis with and without respiratory compensation

Clinical state	Arterial		
	pH	[HCO$_3^-$], meq/L	P$_{CO_2}$, mmHg
Baseline	7.40	24	40
Metabolic acidosis			
No compensation	7.29	19	40
Compensation			
Acute	7.37	19	34
Chronic	7.29	16	34

are acute (ketoacidosis, lactic acidosis, ingestions), so that the associated hyperventilation does protect the pH.

Similar considerations apply to the compensatory hypoventilation seen with chronic metabolic alkalosis. The rise in P$_{CO_2}$ in this setting leads to increased H$^+$ secretion, a further elevation in the plasma HCO$_3^-$ concentration, and no net improvement in the alkalemia.[167]

It is presumed that alterations in renal tubular cell pH are responsible for these changes in H$^+$ secretion. In metabolic acidosis, for example, the fall in plasma HCO$_3^-$ concentration will produce a parallel reduction in the cell pH that is probably the signal to enhance H$^+$ secretion. Returning the extracellular pH toward normal by increasing ventilation will also raise the cell pH, since reducing the P$_{CO_2}$ will result in CO$_2$ diffusion out of the cell. This will lead to an initially lower level of net acid excretion and therefore a further reduction in the plasma HCO$_3^-$ concentration.

These observations once again illustrate the importance of the steady state. A patient with chronic metabolic acidosis who produces an extra 100 meq of acid per day will enter the steady state only when daily acid excretion increases by 100 meq. The signal to maintain this increment in H$^+$ secretion is probably a reduction in the cell pH; furthermore, the *required level of cellular acidification to enhance acid excretion by 100 meq will be the same whether or not respiratory compensation has occurred.* Thus, the extracellular pH will also be the same in both settings, since it is the primary determinant of changes in the cell pH.[98]

SUMMARY

From the Henderson-Hasselbalch equation, the arterial pH is a function of the [HCO$_3^-$]/0.03P$_{CO_2}$ ratio. Three processes are involved in the maintenance of the arterial pH: (1) The extracellular and intracellular buffers act to minimize changes in pH induced by an acid or base load, (2) the plasma HCO$_3^-$ concentration is held within narrow limits by the regulation of renal H^+ excretion, and (3) the P_{CO_2} is controlled by variations in alveolar ventilation. How these processes interact to protect the pH can be appreciated from the response to a HCl load (Fig. 11-19).

- Extracellular buffering of the excess H^+ by HCO_3^- occurs almost immediately.
- Within several minutes, the respiratory compensation begins, resulting in hyperventilation, a decrease in the P_{CO_2}, and an increase in the pH toward normal.
- Within 2 to 4 h, the intracellular buffers (primarily proteins and organic phosphates) and bone provide further buffering, as H^+ ions enter the cells in exchange for intracellular K^+ and Na^+. These responses act to prevent wide swings in the arterial pH until acid-base homeostasis can be restored by the renal excretion of the H^+ load as NH_4^+ and tritratable acidity.
- The corrective renal response begins on the first day and is complete within 5 to 6 days.[5,79,104]

This sequence tends to be reversed with a $NaHCO_3$ load. The corrective renal response tends to be more rapid than after an acid load, as the excess HCO_3^- is quickly excreted in the urine. Both decreased reabsorption and HCO_3^- secretion in the cortical collecting tubule play a contributory role in this setting.[19-21,55]

Alterations in pH induced by changes in the P_{CO_2} produce a somewhat different response. There is virtually no extracellular buffering, since HCO_3^- cannot effectively buffer H_2CO_3 (see page 313). Similarly, there is no compensatory change in alveolar ventilation, since the primary disturbance is one of abnormal respiration. Thus the intracellular buffers (including hemoglobin) and changes in renal H^+ excretion constitute the only protective mechanisms against respiratory acidosis or alkalosis.

If, for example, the P_{CO_2} is increased, the intracellular buffers will act to increase the plasma HCO_3^- concentration, thereby minimizing the degree of acidemia (Fig. 11-20). This process is complete within 10 to 30 min.[168] The intracellular buffers increase the plasma HCO_3^- concentration by only 1 meq/L for each

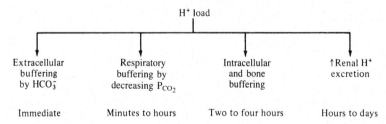

Figure 11-19 Sequential response to a H^+ load, culminating in the restoration of acid-base balance by the renal excretion of the excess H^+.

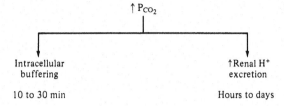

Figure 11-20 Response to an increase in the P_{CO_2}. Although these changes raise the pH toward normal, acid-base homeostasis will not be restored until ventilation is normalized.

10-mmHg rise in the P_{CO_2} and are therefore relatively ineffective in protecting the pH.* If the hypercapnia persists, however, there will be an appropriate increase in renal H^+ excretion, resulting in a further elevation in the plasma HCO_3^- concentration.

It is this renal compensation, which begins within several hours but is not complete for several days,[106] that constitutes the main defense against respiratory acidosis. Even if the P_{CO_2} is chronically elevated at 80 mmHg, the pH usually is not much lower than 7.30 because of the effectiveness of the renal compensation. This sequence is reversed with respiratory alkalosis, as there is an appropriate reduction in the plasma HCO_3^- concentration as a result of intracellular buffering and decreased net acid excretion.[108,109]

The renal responses to alterations in the P_{CO_2} are compensatory but not corrective. Acid-base homeostasis will not be restored unless alveolar ventilation is normalized.

PROBLEMS

11-1 The daily H^+ load is excreted in the urine as titratable acidity and NH_4^+. Would H^+ retention leading to metabolic acidosis occur if there were:

(a) a marked reduction in titratable acid excretion, as a result of a decrease in the plasma phosphate concentration?

(b) a marked reduction in NH_4^+ formation?

11-2 Equal amounts of H^+, as HCl or H_2SO_4, are given over several days to a volume-depleted subject. Which acid will produce the greater degree of acidemia?

11-3 Two patients with a normal GFR of 180 L/day are studied, one with normal acid-base balance and one with metabolic acidosis. The following laboratory data are obtained from the first patient:

$$\text{Plasma } [HCO_3^-] = 24 \, \text{meq/L}$$

$$\text{Titratable acidity} = 30 \, \text{meq/day}$$

$$NH_4^+ \text{ excretion} = 50 \, \text{meq/day}$$

$$\text{Urine pH} = 5.5$$

Similar values in the second patient are

---

* The changes in the plasma HCO_3^- concentration seen with acute and chronic respiratory acidosis and alkalosis are presented in detail in Chaps. 20 and 21.

$$\text{Plasma } [HCO_3^-] = 6\,meq/L$$

$$\text{Titratable acidity} = 75\,meq/day$$

$$NH_4^+ \text{ excretion} = 140\,meq/day$$

$$\text{Urine pH} = 5.0$$

Assuming that all the filtered HCO_3^- is reabsorbed, which is indicated by the low urine pH, calculate:

(a) net acid excretion

(b) total H^+ secretion (which includes that utilized for reabsorption of the filtered HCO_3^-)

11-4 The following values are obtained on a 24-h urine collection:

$$\text{Phosphate} = 60\,mmol$$

$$\text{pH} = 5.8$$

If the arterial pH is 7.40 and the pK_a for phosphate is 6.80, how many millimoles of H^+ are excreted as titratable acidity using HPO_4^{2-} as a buffer? Is NH_4^+ excretion included in the measurement of titratable acidity?

11-5 A patient with persistent vomiting develops metabolic alkalosis as a result of the loss of HCl in gastric juice. Why isn't the condition corrected spontaneously by excretion of the excess HCO_3^- in the urine?

REFERENCES

1. Lennon EJ, Lemann J Jr, Litzow JR. The effects of diet and stool composition on the net external acid balance of normal subjects. *J Clin Invest* 45:1601, 1966.
2. Halperin ML, Jungas RL. The metabolic production and renal disposal of hydrogen ions: An examination of the biochemical processes. *Kidney Int* 24:709, 1983.
3. Kurtz I, Maher T, Hulter HN. Effect of diet on plasma acid-base composition in normal humans. *Kidney Int* 24:670, 1983.
4. DuBose TD Jr, Good DW. Effect of diuretics on renal acid-base transport. *Semin Nephrol* 8:282, 1988.
5. Hamm LL, Simon EE. Roles and mechanisms of urinary buffer excretion. *Am J Physiol* 253:F595, 1987.
6. Soleimani M, Aronson PS. Effects of acetazolamide on Na^+-HCO_3^- contransport in basolateral membrane vesicles in rabbit renal cortex. *J Clin Invest* 83:945, 1989.
7. Malnic G. Hydrogen secretion in renal cortical tubules: Kinetic aspects. *Kidney Int* 32:136, 1987.
8. Kinsella JL, Aronson PS. Properties of the Na^+-H^+ exchanger in renal microvillus membrane vesicles. *Am J Physiol* 238:F461, 1980.
9. Preisig PA, Ives HE, Cragoe EJ Jr, et al. Role of the Na^+/H^+ antiporter in rat proximal tubule bicarbonate absorption. *J Clin Invest* 80:970, 1987.
10. Goldfarb D, Nord EP. Asymmetric affinity of Na^+-H^+ antiporter for Na^+ at the cytoplasmic versus external transport site. *Am J Physiol* 253:F959, 1987.
11. Good DW. Regulation of bicarbonate and ammonium absorption in the thick ascending limb of the rat. *Kidney Int* 40(suppl 33):S-36, 1991.
12. Capasso G, Unwin R, Agulian S, Giebisch G. Bicarbonate transport along the loop of Henle. I. Microperfusion studies of load and inhibitor sensitivity. *J Clin Invest* 88:430, 1991.
13. Maddox DA, Barnes WD, Gennari FJ. Effect of acute increases in filtered HCO_3^- on renal hydrogen transporters: II. $H^{(+)}$-ATPase. *Kidney Int* 52:446, 1997.
14. Schultheis PJ, Clarke LL, Meneton P, et al. Renal and intestinal absorptive defects in mice lacking the NHE3 Na^+/H^+ exchanger. *Nat Genet* 19:282, 1998.
15. Soleimani M, Grassi SM, Aronson PS. Stoichiometry of Na^+-HCO_3^- cotransport in basolateral membrane vesicles isolated from the rabbit renal cortex. *J Clin Invest* 79:1276, 1987.

16. Kurtz I. Basolateral membrane Na^+/H^+ antiport, Na^+/base cotransport, and Na^+- independent Cl^-/base exchange in the rabbit S_3 proximal tubule. *J Clin Invest* 83:616, 1989.

17. Preisig PA, Alpern RJ. Basolateral membrane H/HCO_3 transport in renal tubules. *Kidney Int* 39:1077, 1991.

18. Greger R, Gogelein H. Role of K^+ conductive pathways in the nephron. *Kidney Int* 31:1055, 1987.

19. Levine DZ, Jacobson HR. The regulation of renal acid excretion: New observations from studies of distal nephron segments. *Kidney Int* 29:1099, 1986.

20. Jacobson HR, Furuya H, Breyer MD. Mechanism and regulation of proton transport in the outer medullary collecting duct. *Kidney Int* 40(suppl 33):S-51, 1991.

21. Lombard WE, Kokko JP, Jacobson HR. Bicarbonate transport in cortical and outer medullary collecting tubules. *Am J Physiol* 244:F289, 1983.

22. Tsuruoka S, Schwartz GJ. Metabolic acidosis stimulates H^+ secretion in the rabbit outer medullary collecting duct (inner stripe) of the kidney. *J Clin Invest* 99:1420, 1997.

23. Chan YL, Malnic G, Giebisch G. Renal bicarbonate reabsorption in the rat. III. Distal tubule perfusion study of load dependence and bicarbonate permeability. *J Clin Invest* 84:931, 1989.

24. Garg LC. Respective roles of H-ATPase and H-K-ATPase in ion transport in the kidney. *J Am Soc Nephrol* 2:949, 1991.

25. Stone DK, Xie X-S. Proton translocating ATPases: Issues in structure and function. *Kidney Int* 33:767, 1988.

26. Brown D, Hirsch S, Gluck S. Localization of a proton-pumping ATPase in rat kidney. *J Clin Invest* 82:2114, 1988.

27. Cheval L, Barlet-Bas C, Khadouri C, et al. K^+-ATPase mediated Rb^+ transport in rat collecting tubule: Modulation during K^+ deprivation. *Am J Physiol* 260:F800, 1991.

28. Selvaggio AM, Schwartz JH, Bengele HH, et al. Mechanisms of H^+ secretion by inner medullary collecting duct cells. *Am J Physiol* 254:F391, 1988.

29. Armitage FE, Wingo CS. Luminal acidification in K-replete OMCDi: Contributions of H-K-ATPase and bafilomycin-A1-sensitive H-ATPase. *Am J Physiol* 267:F450, 1994.

30. Wingo CS, Smulka AJ. Function and structure of H-K-ATPase in the kidney. *Am J Physiol* 269:F1, 1995.

31. Kraut JA, Hiura J, Besancon M, et al. Effect of hypokalemia on the abundance of HK alpha 1 and HK alpha 2 protein in the rat kidney. *Am J Physiol* 272:F744, 1997.

32. Brown D. Membrane recycling and epithelial cell function. *Am J Physiol* 256:F1, 1989.

33. Hays SR, Alpern RJ. Apical and basolateral hydrogen extrusion mechanisms in inner stripe of rabbit outer medullary collecting duct. *Am J Physiol* 259:F628, 1990.

34. Hering-Smith KS, Cragoe E Jr, Weiner D, Hamm L. Inner medullary collecting duct Na^+-H^+ exchanger. *Am J Physiol* 260:C1300, 1991.

35. Sauer M, Flemmer A, Thurau K, Beck F X. Sodium entry in principal and intercalated cells of the isolated perfused cortical collecting duct. *Pflugers Arch* 416:88, 1990.

36. Batlle DC. Segmental characterization of defects in collecting tubule acidification. *Kidney Int* 30:546, 1986.

37. Harrington JT, Hulter HN, Cohen JJ, Madias NE. Mineralocorticoid-stimulated renal acidification: The critical role of dietary sodium. *Kidney Int* 30:43, 1986.

38. Star RA. Basolateral membrane sodium-independent Cl^-/HCO_3^- exchange in rat inner medullary collecting duct cell. *J Clin Invest* 85:1959, 1990.

39. Kollert-Jons A, Wagner S, Hubner S, et al. Anion exchanger 1 in human kidney and oncocytoma differs from erythroid AE1 in its NH_2 terminus. *Am J Physiol* 265:F813, 1993.

40. Bastani B, Purcell H, Hemken P, et al. Expression and distribution of renal vacuolar proton-translocating adenosine triphosphatase in response to chronic acid and alkali loads in the rat. *J Clin Invest* 88:126, 1991.

41. DuBose TD Jr, Lucci MS, Hogg RJ, et al. Comparison of acidification parameters in superficial and deep nephrons of the rat. *Am J Physiol* 244:F497, 1983.

42. Cohen EP, Bastani B, Cohen MR, et al. Absence of H^+-ATPase in cortical collecting tubules of a patient with Sjögren's syndrome and distal renal tubular acidosis. *J Am Soc Nephrol* 3:264, 1992.

43. Bastani B, Haragsim L, Gluck S, Siamopoulos KC. Lack of H-ATPase in distal nephron causing hypokalemic distal RTA in a patient with Sjögren's syndrome (letter). *Nephrol Dial Transplant* 10:908, 1995.

44. Karet FE, Gainza FJ, Gyory AZ, et al. Mutations in the chloride-bicarbonate exchanger gene AE1 cause autosomal dominant but not autosomal recessive distal renal tubular acidosis. *Proc Natl Acad Sci U S A* 95:6337, 1998.

45. Liu F-Y, Cogan MG. Axial heterogeneity in the rat proximal convoluted tubule. I. Bicarbonate, chloride, and water transport. *Am J Physiol* 247:F816, 1984.

46. Maddox DA, Gennari JF. The early proximal tubule: A high-capacity delivery-responsive reabsorptive site. *Am J Physiol* 252:F573, 1987.

47. Liu F-Y, Cogan MG. Kinetics of bicarbonate transport in early proximal convoluted tubule. *Am J Physiol* 253:F912, 1987.

48. Lucci MS, Pucacco LR, DuBose TD Jr, et al. Direct evaluation of acidification by rat proximal tubule: Role of carbonic anhydrase. *Am J Physiol* 238:F372, 1980.

49. Lucci MS, Tinker JP, Weiner IM, DuBose TD Jr. Function of proximal tubule carbonic anhydrase defined by selective inhibition. *Am J Physiol* 245:F443, 1983.

50. Sasaki S, Marumo F. Effects of carbonic anhydrase inhibitors on basolateral base transport of rabbit proximal straight tubule. *Am J Physiol* 257:F947, 1989.

51. Lonnerholm G, Wistrand PJ. Carbonic anhydrase in the human kidney: A histochemical and immunocytochemical study. *Kidney Int* 25:886, 1984.

52. Kurtz I, Star R, Balaban RS, et al. Spontaneous disequilibrium pH in S_3 proximal tubules. Role in ammonia and bicarbonate transport. *J Clin Invest* 78:989, 1986.

53. Star RA, Kurtz I, Mejia R, et al. Disequilibrium pH and ammonia transport in isolated perfused cortical collecting tubules. *Am J Physiol* 253:F1232, 1987.

54. Star RA, Burg MB, Knepper MA. Luminal disequilibrium pH and ammonia transport in the outer medullary collecting duct. *Am J Physiol* 252:F1148, 1987.

55. Star RA, Burg MB, Knepper MA. Bicarbonate secretion and chloride absorption by rabbit cortical collecting ducts. Role of chloride/bicarbonate exchange. *J Clin Invest* 76:1123, 1985.

56. Schuster VL. Cortical collecting duct bicarbonate secretion. *Kidney Int* 40(suppl 33):S-47, 1991.

57. Verlander JW, Madsen KM, Tisher CC. Effect of acute respiratory acidosis on two populations of intercalated cells in the rabbit cortical collecting duct. *Am J Physiol* 253:F1142, 1987.

58. Verlander JW, Madsen KM, Low PS, et al. Immunocytochemical localization of band 3 protein in rat collecting duct. *Am J Physiol* 255:F115, 1988.

59. Kempson SA. Effect of metabolic acidosis on renal brush border membrane adaptation to low phosphorus diet. *Kidney Int* 22:225, 1982.

60. Biber J, Custer M, Magagnin S, et al. Renal Na/Pi-cotransporters. *Kidney Int* 49:981, 1996.

61. Busch A, Waldegger S, Herzer T, et al. Electrophysiological analysis of Na^+/Pi cotransport mediated by a transporter cloned from rat kidney and expressed in *Xenopus* oocytes. *Proc Natl Acad Sci U S A* 91:8205, 1994.

62. Quamme GA. Effect of pH on Na^+-dependent phosphate transport in renal outer cortical and outer medullary BBMV. *Am J Physiol* 258:F356, 1990.

63. Owen OE, Licht JH, Sapir DG. Renal function and effects of partial rehydration during diabetic ketoacidosis. *Diabetes* 30:510, 1981.

64. Knepper MA. NH_4^+ transport in the kidney. *Kidney Int* 40(suppl 33):S-95, 1991.

65. DuBose TD Jr, Good DW, Hamm LL, Wall SM. Ammonium transport in the kidney: New physiological concepts and their clinical applications. *J Am Soc Nephrol* 1:1193, 1991.

66. Schoolwerth AC. Regulation of renal ammoniagenesis in metabolic acidosis. *Kidney Int* 40:961, 1991.

67. Wright PA, Knepper MA. Glutamate dehydrogenase activities in microdissected rat nephron segments: Effects of acid-base loading. *Am J Physiol* 259:F53, 1990.

68. Good DW, Burg MB. Ammonia production by individual segments of the rat nephron. *J Clin Invest* 73:602, 1984.
69. Buerkert J, Martin D, Trigg D. Segmental analysis of the renal tubule in buffer production and net acid formation. *Am J Physiol* 244:F442, 1983.
70. Preisig PA, Alpern RJ. Pathways for apical and basolateral membrane NH_3 and NH_4^+ movement in rat proximal tubule. *Am J Physiol* 259:F587, 1990.
71. Simon E, Merli C, Herndon J, et al. Effects of barium and 5-(N-ethyl-N-isopropyl)-amiloride on proximal tubule ammonia transport. *Am J Physiol* 262:F36, 1992.
72. Knepper MA, Packer R, Good DW. Ammonium transport in the kidney. *Physiol Rev* 69:179, 1989.
73. Packer RK, Desai SS, Hornbuckle K, Knepper MA. Role of countercurrent multiplication in renal ammonium handling: Regulation of medullary ammonium accumulation. *J Am Soc Nephrol* 2:77, 1991.
74. Garvin JL, Burg MB, Knepper MA. Active NH_4^+ reabsorption by the medullary thick ascending limb. *Am J Physiol* 255:F57, 1988.
75. Halperin ML. How much "new" bicarbonate is formed in the distal nephron in the process of net acid excretion. *Kidney Int* 35:1277, 1989.
76. Kikeri D, Sun A, Zeidel ML, Hebert SC. Cell membranes impermeable to NH_3. *Nature* 339:478, 1989.
77. Good DW. Adaptation of HCO_3^- and NH_4^+ transport in rat MTAL: Effects of chronic metabolic acidosis and Na^+ intake. *Am J Physiol* 258:F1345, 1990.
78. Flessner MF, Wall SM, Knepper MA. Permeability of rat collecting duct segments to NH_3 and NH_4^+. *Am J Physiol* 260: F264, 1991.
79. Tizianello A, Deferrari G, Garibotto G, et al. Renal ammoniagenesis in early stage of metabolic acidosis in man. *J Clin Invest* 69:240, 1982.
80. Welbourne TC. Interorgan glutamine flow in metabolic acidosis. *Am J Physiol* 253:F1069, 1987.
81. Welbourne T, Weber M, Bank N. The effect of glutamine administration on urinary ammonium excretion in normal subjects and patients with renal disease. *J Clin Invest* 51:1852, 1972.
82. Wright PA, Packer RK, Garcia-Perez A, Knepper MA. Time course of renal glutamate dehydrogenase induction during NH_4Cl loading in rats. *Am J Physiol* 262:F999, 1992.
83. DiGiovanni SR, Madsen KM, Luther AD, Knepper MA. Dissociation of ammoniagenic enzyme adaptation in rat S_1 proximal tubules and ammonium excretion response. *Am J Physiol* 267:F407, 1994.
84. Windus DW, Cohn DE, Klahr S, Hammerman MR. Glutamine transport in renal basolateral vesicles from dogs with metabolic acidosis. *Am J Physiol* 246:F78, 1984.
85. Windus DW, Klahr S, Hammerman MR. Glutamine transport in renal basolateral vesicles from dogs with acute respiratory acidosis. *Am J Physiol* 247:F403, 1984.
86. Simpson DP, Hager SR. Bicarbonate-carbon dioxide buffer system: A determinant of the mitochondrial pH gradient. *Am J Physiol* 247:F440, 1984.
87. Welbourne TC, Givens G, Joshi S. Renal ammoniagenic response to chronic acid loading: Role of glucocorticoids. *Am J Physiol* 254:F134, 1988.
88. Kinsella J, Cujdik T, Sacktor B. Na^+-H^+ exchange activity in renal brush border membrane vesicles in response to metabolic acidosis: The role of glucocorticoids. *Proc Natl Acad Sci U S A* 81:630, 1984.
89. Clarke E, Evans BM, MacIntyre IM. Acidosis in experiment electrolyte depletion. *Clin Sci* 14:421, 1955.
90. Aronson PS, Nee J, Suhm MA. Modifier role of internal H^+ in activation of the Na^+-H^+ exchanger in renal microvillus membrane vesicles. *Nature* 299:161, 1982.
91. Akiba T, Rocco VK, Warnock DG. Parallel adaptation of the rabbit renal cortical sodium/proton antiporter and sodium/bicarbonate cotransporter in metabolic acidosis and alkalosis. *J Clin Invest* 80:308, 1987.
92. Sasaki S, Berry CA, Rector FC Jr. Effect of luminal and peritubular HCO_3^- concentrations and P_{CO_2} on HCO_3^- reabsorption in rabbit proximal convoluted tubules perfused in vitro. *J Clin Invest* 70:639, 1982.

93. Tannen RL, Hamid B. Adaptive changes in renal acidification in response to chronic respiratory acidosis. *Am J Physiol* 248:F492, 1985.
94. Preisig PA, Alpern RJ. Chronic metabolic acidosis causes an adaptation in the apical membrane Na/H antiporter and Na(HCO$_3$)$_3$ symporter in the rat proximal convoluted tubule. *J Clin Invest* 82:1445, 1988.
95. Krapf R, Pearce D, Lynch C, et al. Expression of rat renal Na/H antiporter mRNA levels in response to respiratory and metabolic acidosis. *J Clin Invest* 87:747, 1991.
96. Soleimani M, Lesoine GA, Bergman JA, McKinney T. A pH modifier site regulates activity of the Na$^+$:HCO$_3^-$ cotransporter in basolateral membranes of kidney proximal tubules. *J Clin Invest* 88:1135, 1991.
97. Khadouri C, Marsy S, Barlet-Bas C, et al. Effect of metabolic acidosis and alkalosis on NEM-sensitive ATPase in rat nephron segments. *Am J Physiol* 262:F583, 1992.
98. Krapf R, Berry CA, Alpern RJ, Rector FC Jr. Regulation of cell pH by ambient bicarbonate, carbon dioxide tension, and pH in rabbit proximal convoluted tubule. *J Clin Invest* 81:381, 1988.
99. Alpern RJ, Chambers M. Cell pH in the rat proximal convoluted tubule. Regulation by luminal and peritubular pH and sodium concentration. *J Clin Invest* 78:502, 1986.
100. Horie S, Moe O, Tejedor A, Alpern RJ. Preincubation in acid medium increases Na/H antiporter activity in cultured renal proximal tubule cells. *Proc Natl Acad Sci U S A* 87:4742, 1990.
101. Alpern RJ. Trade-offs in the adaptation to acidosis. *Kidney Int* 47:1205, 1995.
102. Weiner ID, Hamm LL. Regulation of intracellular pH in the rabbit cortical collecting tubule. *J Clin Invest* 85:274, 1989.
103. Kikeri D, Azar S, Sun A, et al. Na$^+$-H$^+$ antiporter and Na$^+$-(HCO$_3^-$)$_n$ symporter regulate intracellular pH in mouse medullary thick limbs of Henle. *Am J Physiol* 258:F445, 1990.
104. Kraut J, Wish J, Sweet S, et al. Failure of increased sodium avidity to facilitate renal acid excretion in dogs fed sulfuric acid. *Kidney Int* 20:50, 1981.
105. Van Goidsenhoven G, Gray OV, Price AV, Sanderson PH. The effect of prolonged administration of large doses of sodium bicarbonate in man. *Clin Sci* 13:383, 1954.
106. Polak A, Haynie GD, Hays RM, Schwartz WB. Effects of chronic hypercapnia on electrolyte and acid-base equilibrium. I. Adaptation. *J Clin Invest* 40:1223, 1961.
107. van Ypersele de Strihou C, Brasseur L, de Coninck J. "Carbon dioxide response curve" for chronic hypercapnia in man. *N Engl J Med* 275:117, 1966.
108. Gennari JF, Goldstein MB, Schwartz WB. The nature of the renal adaptation to chronic hypocapnia. *J Clin Invest* 51:1722, 1972.
109. Gougoux A, Kaehny WD, Cohen JJ. Renal adaptation to chronic hypocapnia: Dietary constraints in achieving H$^+$ retention. *Am J Physiol* 229:1330, 1975.
110. Rodriguez-Nichols F, Laughrey E, Tannen RL. The response of renal NH$_3$ production to chronic respiratory acidosis. *Am J Physiol* 247:F896, 1984.
111. Trivedi B, Tannen RL. Effect of respiratory acidosis on intracellular pH of the proximal tubule. *Am J Physiol* 250:F1039, 1986.
112. Adam WR, Koretsky AP, Weiner MW. ^{31}P-NMR in vivo measurement of renal intracellular pH: Effects of acidosis and potassium depletion in rats. *Am J Physiol* 251:F904, 1986.
113. Cogan MG, Alpern RJ. Regulation of proximal bicarbonate reabsorption. *Am J Physiol* 247:F387, 1984.
114. Sabatini S, Kurtzman NA. The maintenance of metabolic alkalosis: Factors which decrease HCO$_3^-$ excretion. *Kidney Int* 25:357, 1984.
115. Slatopolsky E, Hoffsten P, Purkerson M, Bricker NS. On the influence of extracellular fluid volume expansion and of uremia on bicarbonate reabsorption in man. *J Clin Invest* 49:988, 1970.
116. Cogan MG, Cameiro AV, Tatsuno J, et al. Normal diet NaCl variation can affect the renal set-point for plasma pH-(HCO$_3^-$) maintenance. *J Am Soc Nephrol* 1:193, 1990.
117. Harrington JT. Metabolic alkalosis. *Kidney Int* 26:88, 1984.
118. Galla JH, Gifford JD, Luke RG, Rome L. Adaptations to chloride-depletion alkalosis. *Am J Physiol* 261:R771, 1991.

119. Wesson D. Augmented bicarbonate reabsorption by both the proximal and distal nephron maintained chloride-deplete metabolic alkalosis in rats. *J Clin Invest* 84:1460, 1989.

120. Liu F-Y, Cogan MG. Angiotensin II: A potent regulator of acidification in the rat early proximal convoluted tubule. *J Clin Invest* 80:272, 1987.

121. Geibel J, Giebisch G, Boron WF. Angiotensin II stimulates both Na^+-H^+ exchange and Na^+/HCO_3^- cotransport in rabbit proximal tubule. *Proc Natl Acad Sci U S A* 87:7917, 1990.

122. Cogan MG. Angiotensin II: A potent controller of sodium transport in the early proximal tubule. *Hypertension* 15:451, 1990.

123. Liu F-Y, Cogan MG. Role of angiotensin II in glomerulotubular balance. *Am J Physiol* 259:F72, 1990.

124. Wall SM, Sands JM, Flessner MF, et al. Net acid transport by isolated perfused inner medullary collecting ducts. *Am J Physiol* 258:F75, 1990.

125. Stone DK, Seldin DW, Kokko JP, Jacobson HR. Mineralocorticoid modulation of rabbit kidney medullary collecting duct acidification. A sodium-independent effect. *J Clin Invest* 72:77, 1983.

126. Garg LC, Narang N. Effects of aldosterone on NEM-sensitive ATPases in rabbit nephron segments. *Kidney Int* 34:13, 1988.

127. Hays SR. Mineralocoriticoid modulation of apical and basolateral membrane $H^+/OH^-/HCO_3^-$ transport process in rabbit inner stripe of outer medullary collecting duct. *J Clin Invest* 90:180, 1992.

128. Higashihara E, Carter NW, Pucacco L, Kokko JP. Aldosterone effects on papillary collecting duct pH profile of the rat. *Am J Physiol* 246:F725, 1984.

129. Schwartz WB, Jenson RL, Relman AS. Acidification of the urine and increased ammonium excretion without change in acid-base equilibrium: Sodium reabsorption as a stimulus to the acidifying process. *J Clin Invest* 34:673, 1955.

130. Tannen RL, Bleich HL, Schwartz WB. The renal response to acid loads in metabolic alkalosis: An assessment of the mechanisms regulating acid excretion. *J Clin Invest* 45:562, 1966.

131. Galla JH, Bonduris DN, Luke RG. Effects of chloride and extracellular fluid volume on bicarbonate reabsorption along the nephron in metabolic alkalosis in the rat. Reassessment of the classic hypothesis on the pathogenesis of metabolic alkalosis. *J Clin Invest* 80:41, 1987.

132. Wesson DE. Depressed distal tubule acidification corrects chloride-deplete metabolic alkalosis. *Am J Physiol* 259:F636, 1990.

133. Fuller GR, MacLeod MB, Pitts RF. Influence of administration of potassium salts on the renal tubular reabsorption of bicarbonate. *Am J Physiol* 182:111, 1955.

134. Capasso G, Kinne R, Malnic G, Giebisch G. Renal bicarbonate reabsorption in the rat. I. Effects of hypokalemia and carbonic anhydrase. *J Clin Invest* 78:1558, 1986.

135. Capasso G, Jaeger P, Giebisch G, et al. Renal bicarbonate reabsorption in the rat. II. Distal tubule load dependence and effect of hypokalemia. *J Clin Invest* 80:409, 1987.

136. Cooke RE, Segar W, Cheek DB, et al. The extrarenal correction of alkalosis associated with potassium deficiency. *J Clin Invest* 31:798, 1952.

137. Adler S, Zett B, Anderson B. The effect of acute potassium depletion of muscle cell pH in vitro. *Kidney Int* 2:159, 1972.

138. Jaeger P, Karlmark B, Giebisch G. Ammonia transport in rat cortical tubule: Relationship to potassium metabolism. *Am J Physiol* 245:F593, 1983.

139. Szylman P, Better OS, Chaimowitz C, Rosler A. Role of hyperkalemia in the metabolic acidosis of isolated hypoaldosteronism. *N Engl J Med* 294:361, 1976.

140. Soleimani M, Bergman JA, Hosford MA, McKinney TD. Potassium depletion increases luminal Na^+/H^+ exchange and basolateral $Na^+CO_3^{2-}$:HCO_3^- cotransporter in rat renal cortex. *J Clin Invest* 86:1076, 1990.

141. Altenberg GA, Aristimuno PC, Amorena CE, Taquini AC. Amiloride prevents the metabolic acidosis of a KCl load in nephrectomized rats. *Clin Sci* 76:649, 1989.

142. DuBose TD Jr, Good DW. Effects of chronic hyperkalemia on renal production and proximal tubular transport of ammonium in rats. *Am J Physiol* 260:F680, 1991.

143. DuBose TD Jr, Good DW. Chronic hyperkalemia impairs ammonium transport and accumulation in the inner medulla of the rat. *J Clin Invest* 90:1443, 1992.

144. Wingo C. Active proton secretion and potassium absorption in the rabbit outer medullary collecting duct. Functional evidence for proton-potassium-activated adenosine triphosphatase. *J Clin Invest* 84:361, 1989.

145. Doucet A, Marsy S. Characterization of K-ATPase activity in distal nephron: Stimulation by potassium depletion. *Am J Physiol* 253:F418, 1987.

146. Codina J, Delmas-Mata J, DuBose TD. Expression of HK2 protein is increased selectively in renal medulla by chronic hypokalemia. *Am J Physiol* 275:F433, 1998.

147. Elam-Ong S, Kurtzman NA, Sabatini S. Regulation of collecting tubule adenosine triphosphatases by aldosterone and potassium. *J Clin Invest* 91:2385, 1993.

148. Sasaki S, Marumo F. Mechanisms of inhibition of proximal acidification by PTH. *Am J Physiol* 260:F833, 1991.

149. Fan L, Wiederkehr MR, Collazo R, et al. Dual mechanisms of regulation of Na/H exchanger NHE-3 by parathyroid hormone in rat kidney. *J Biol Chem* 274:11289, 1999.

150. Ruiz OS, Qiu YY, Wang LJ, Arruda JA. Regulation of the renal Na-HCO$_3$ cotransporter: V. Mechanism of the inhibitory effect of parathyroid hormone. *Kidney Int* 49:396, 1996.

151. Bichara M, Mercier O, Borensztein P, Paillard M. Acute metabolic acidosis enhances circulating parathyroid hormone which contributes to the renal response against acidosis in the rat. *J Clin Invest* 86:430, 1990.

152. Arruda JAL, Alla V, Rubinstein H, et al. Parathyroid hormone and extrarenal acid buffering. *Am J Physiol* 239:F533, 1980.

153. Coe FL. Magnitude of metabolic alkalosis in primary hyperparathyroidism. *Arch Intern Med* 134:262, 1974.

154. Hulter HN, Peterson JC. Acid-base homeostasis during chronic PTH excess in humans. *Kidney Int* 28:187, 1985.

155. Lambertsen CJ. Chemical control of respiration at rest, in Mountcastle VB (ed), *Medical Physiology*, 14th ed. St Louis, Mosby, 1980.

156. Berger AJ, Mitchell RA, Severinghaus JW. Regulation of respiration. *N Engl J Med* 297:92, 138,194, 1997.

157. Fencl V, Miller TB, Pappenheimer JR. Studies on the respiratory response to disturbances of acid-base balance, with deductions concerning the ionic composition of cerebral interstitial fluid. *Am J Physiol* 210:459, 1966.

158. Lugliani R, Whipp BJ, Seard C, Wasserman K. Effect of bilateral carotid-body resection on ventilatory control at rest and during exercise in man. *N Engl J Med* 285:1105, 1971.

159. Mitchell RA, Singer MM. Respiration and cerebrospinal fluid pH in metabolic acidosis and alkalosis. *J Appl Physiol* 20:905, 1965.

160. Fencl V, Vale JR, Broch JA. Respiration and cerebral blood flow in metabolic acidosis and alkalosis in humans. *J Appl Physiol* 27:67, 1969.

161. Pierce NF, Fedson DS, Brigham KL, et al. The ventilatory response to acute base deficit in humans. The time course during development and correction of metabolic acidosis. *Ann Intern Med* 72:633, 1970.

162. Albert MS, Dell RB, Winters RW. Quantitative displacement of acid-base equilibrium in metabolic acidosis. *Ann Intern Med* 66:312, 1967.

163. Bushinsky DA, Coe FL, Katzenberg C, et al. Arterial P$_{CO_2}$ in chronic metabolic acidosis. *Kidney Int* 22:311, 1982.

164. Javaheri S, Shore NS, Rose BD, Kazemi H. Compensatory hypoventilation in metabolic alkalosis. *Chest* 81:296, 1982.

165. Javaheri S, Kazemi H. Metabolic alkalosis and hypoventilation in humans. *Am Rev Resp Dis* 136:1011, 1987.

166. Madias N, Schwartz WB, Cohen JJ. The maladaptive renal response to secondary hypocapnia during chronic HCl acidosis in the dog. *J Clin Invest* 60:1393, 1977.

167. Madias NE, Adrogue HH, Cohen JJ. Maladaptive response to secondary hypercapnia in chronic metabolic alkalosis. *Am J Physiol* 238:F283, 1980.

168. Brackett NC Jr, Cohen JJ, Schwartz WB. Carbon dioxide titration curve of normal man. Effect of increasing degrees of a cute hypercapnia on acid-base equilibrium. *N Engl J Med* 272:6, 1965.

TWELVE

POTASSIUM HOMEOSTASIS

INTRODUCTION

The total body K^+ stores in a normal adult are approximately 3000 to 4000 meq (50 to 55 meq/kg body weight). In contrast to Na^+, which is restricted primarily to the extracellular fluid (ECF), K^+ is basically an intracellular cation, with 98 percent of body K^+ being located in the cells. This can be appreciated from the disparity between the K^+ concentrations in the two compartments: cell K^+ concentration of 140 meq/L versus extracellular (and plasma) K^+ concentration of only 4 to 4.5 meq/L. The location of Na^+ and K^+ in the different fluid compartments is maintained by the active Na^+-K^+-ATPase pump in the cell membrane, which pumps Na^+ out of and K^+ into the cell in a $3:2$ ratio (see page 75).[1,2]

Potassium has two major physiologic functions. First, it plays an important role in cell metabolism, participating in the regulation of such processes as protein and glycogen synthesis.[3] As a result, a variety of cell functions may become impaired in conditions of K^+ imbalance. As an example, patients with marked K^+ depletion often complain of polyuria (increased urine output). This is due in part to a reduced ability to concentrate the urine, resulting from decreased responsiveness to antidiuretic hormone (ADH) (see page 172; Fig. 12-1).

Second, the *ratio* of the K^+ concentrations in the cell and the ECF is the major determinant of the resting membrane potential (E_m) across the cell membrane. This relationship can be expressed by the following formula:

$$E_m = -61 \log \frac{r[K^+]_{cell} + 0.01[Na^+]_{cell}}{r[K^+]_{ecf} + 0.01[Na^+]_{ecf}} \qquad (12\text{-}1)$$

where r is the Na^+/K^+ active transport ratio of $3:2$ and 0.01 is the relative membrane permeability of Na^+ to K^+.[4] It is the resting potential that sets the stage for the generation of the action potential that is essential for normal neural and muscular function. Thus, both hypokalemia (low plasma K^+ concentration) and hyperkalemia (high plasma K^+ concentration) can result in potentially fatal muscle paralysis and cardiac arrhythmias, in part by altering conduction in skeletal and cardiac muscle.

The pathophysiologic effects of K^+ imbalance will be discussed in detail in Chaps. 26 to 28. The remainder of this chapter will deal with the two functions responsible for the maintenance of a normal plasma K^+ concentration: (1) the distribution of K^+ between the cells and the extracellular fluid and (2) the urinary excretion of the K^+ added to the extracellular fluid from the diet and endogenous cellular breakdown.

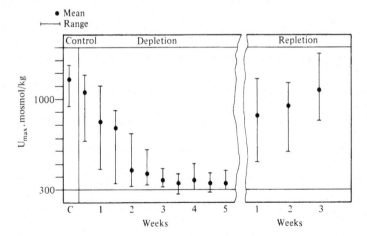

Figure 12-1   Ability to maximally concentrate the urine (U_{max}) in patients with progressive potassium depletion. The average K^+ deficit was 350 meq, or about 10 percent of the total body K^+. (*From Rubini M, J Clin Invest 40:2215, 1961, by copyright permission of the American Society for Clinical Investigation.*)

DISTRIBUTION OF POTASSIUM BETWEEN CELLS AND EXTRACELLULAR FLUID

Regulation of the internal distribution of K^+ must be extremely efficient, since the movement of as little as 1.5 to 2 percent of the cell K^+ into the ECF can result in a potentially fatal increase in the plasma K^+ concentration to as high as 8 meq/L or more. A variety of factors, both physiologic and pathologic, can influence this process (Table 12-1).[5,6] The most important in the day-to-day regulation of K^+ balance are Na^+-K^+-ATPase (the activity of which is increased by catecholamines and insulin) and the plasma K^+ concentration itself.[1]

Sodium-Potassium-ATPase

Normal K^+ distribution is primarily determined by the Na^+-K^+-ATPase pump.[1] The activity of this pump is regulated by several factors, including thyroid hormone and, with regard to K^+ homeostasis, catecholamines, insulin, and the state of K^+ balance.[1]

An example of the importance of this pump in humans can be seen when Na^+-K^+-ATPase is partially inhibited by a massive overdose of digitalis, a drug useful in the treatment of heart disease. In this setting, marked hyperkalemia (plasma K^+ concentration of up to 13.5 meq/L) can occur, because of the relative inability of K^+ to enter the cells.[7]

The result is somewhat different when the pump is impaired chronically.[1] In a variety of chronic diseases such as renal failure and heart failure, Na^+-K^+-ATPase activity is often reduced as a result of an acquired defect in cell function.[8,9] As a result, K^+ leaves and Na^+ enters the cells down passive gradients. The net effect is as much as a 10 to 15 percent reduction in total body K^+ stores in association with

Table 12-1   Factors influencing the distribution of K^+ between the cells and the extracellular fluid

Physiologic
   Na^+-K^+-ATPase
   Catecholamines
   Insulin
   Plasma K^+ concentration
   Exercise
Pathologic
   Chronic diseases
   Extracellular pH
   Hyperosmolality
   Rate of cell breakdown

a high cell Na^+ concentration and a low cell K^+ concentration, but no change in the plasma K^+ concentration because the excess extracellular K^+ has time to be excreted in the urine if renal function is adequate.[8-11] In patients with renal failure, however, the decrease in pump activity can contribute to the development of hyperkalemia.

In addition to the basal distribution of K^+, there is a frequent exchange of K^+ between the ECF and the cells because of variations in dietary intake. For example, three large glasses of orange juice contain approximately 40 meq of K^+. The normal extracellular fluid volume is roughly 17 liters in a 70-kg man. Thus, there would be a potentially dangerous 2.4 meq/L (40 meq $\div$ 17 L) increase in the plasma K^+ concentration if the ingested K^+ remained in the extracellular fluid. This is prevented by the rapid entry of most of the K^+ load into the cells.[6] Within 6 to 8 h, K^+ balance is then restored by the urinary excretion of the excess K^+.[12,13] Although the initial elevation in the plasma K^+ concentration directly promotes the intracellular movement of K^+, both catecholamines and insulin also play an important role in this process.

Catecholamines

Catecholamines can affect internal K^+ distribution, with α-receptors impairing and β_2-receptors promoting the cellular entry of K^+.[14-16] The β_2-receptor-induced stimulation of K^+ uptake is mediated at least in part by activation of the Na^+-K^+-ATPase pump.[1,17] This appears to reflect a *permissive action of basal catecholamine levels*, since there is no evidence that a K^+ load increases the release of epinephrine or norepinephrine.[14]

The physiologic importance of catecholamines in humans can be illustrated by two observations. First, the increment in the plasma K^+ concentration after a K^+ load is greater and more prolonged if the subject has been pretreated with a β-adrenergic blocker, such as propranolol (Fig. 12-2).[14,16,18,19] This difference is due to a substantial reduction in cellular K^+ uptake, most of which normally occurs in skeletal muscle and the liver.[14]

Second, the release of epinephrine during a stress response, such as coronary ischemia, can acutely lower the plasma K^+ concentration by approximately 0.5 to 0.6 meq/L.[20] In this setting, the hypokalemic response also may be mediated by a rise in insulin release. Increased β_2-adrenergic activity enhances insulin secretion both by direct stimulation of the pancreas and by enhancing glycolysis, leading to a rise in the plasma glucose concentration.[21] The net effect can, in patients with preexistent mild diuretic-induced hypokalemia, result in an acute reduction in the plasma K^+ concentration to below 2.8 meq/L (Fig. 12-3).

A similar hypokalemic effect can be induced by the administration of a β_2-adrenergic agonist, such as albuterol, terbutaline, or dobutamine, to treat asthma or heart failure or to prevent premature labor.[22,23] In heart failure, for example, the acute 0.4 meq/L fall in the plasma potassium concentration can enhance the tendency to ventricular arrhythmias.[24]

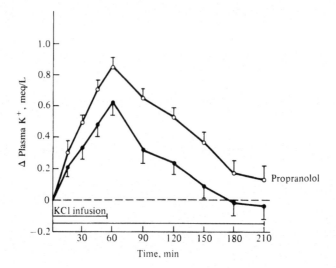

Figure 12-2 Changes in the plasma K^+ concentration after a K^+ load in the absence (solid circles) or presence (open circles) of the β-adrenergic blocker propranol. (*From Rosa RN, Silva P, Young JB, et al, N Engl J Med 302:431, 1980. Reprinted by permission from the* New England Journal of Medicine.)

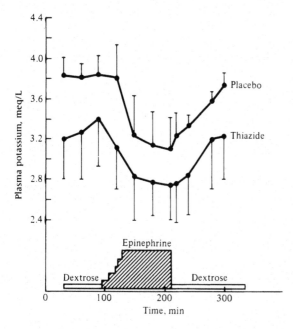

Figure 12-3 Plasma K^+ concentration during an infusion of epinephrine (in physiologic doses) in 6 patients pretreated with a placebo or a thiazide diuretic for 7 days. The plasma K^+ concentration fell in both groups but reached potentially dangerous levels in the diuretic-treated patients, who had mild baseine hypokalemia. (*From Struthers AD, Whitesmith R, Reid JL, Lancet 1:1358, 1983, with permission.*)

Insulin

Insulin promotes the entry of K^+ into skeletal muscle and the liver,[25,26] again by increasing Na^+-K^+-ATPase activity.[1,27] This property, which is independent of any effect on glucose transport,[25] plays a physiologic role in the regulation of the plasma K^+ concentration.[5,6,26,28] For example, the ingestion of glucose (which enhances endogenous insulin release) minimizes the rise in the plasma K^+ concentration induced by concurrent K^+ intake (Fig. 12-4).[19]

On the other hand, the ability to handle a K^+ load is impaired with insulin deficiency (as might be induced by an infusion of somatostatin). In this setting, the baseline plasma K^+ concentration rises (by 0.4 to 0.5 meq/L), and a K^+ load induces a greater than normal degree of hyperkalemia. These changes are reversed by an infusion of insulin.[26] Furthermore, no alteration in K^+ balance is seen when somatostatin is used in type 1 (insulin-dependent) diabetes mellitus, since these patients have little or no endogenous insulin and somatostatin is therefore without effect.[26]

As with catecholamines, it appears that basal *insulin levels permissively allow* K^+ *entry into cells.* The possible presence of a positive feedback loop, in which K^+ stimulates the release of insulin, is uncertain. Initial studies demonstrated a rise in the plasma insulin concentration after an increase in the plasma K^+ concentration of more than 1 meq/L;[28] in comparison, a more physiologic elevation of 0.3 to 0.7 meq/L is without apparent effect.[28,29] It is possible, however, that small elevations in the plasma K^+ concentration can increase insulin release into the portal vein, thereby promoting hepatic K^+ uptake without affecting the peripheral plasma insulin level.[30]

In addition to its physiologic role, the effect of insulin on K^+ distribution is useful in the treatment of *hyperkalemia.* Giving either glucose (to enhance endogenous release) or insulin (with glucose to prevent hypoglycemia) can acutely lower the plasma K^+ concentration by driving K^+ into the cells (see Chap. 28).[31] On the other hand, treating *hypokalemia* by the administration of intravenous K^+ in a dextrose-containing solution can cause an initial further reduction in

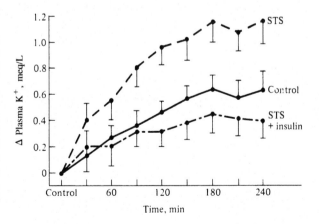

Figure 12-4 Peak increase in the plasma potassium concentration in normal subjects following the ingestion of 0.25 meq/kg of potassium alone (K) or with glucose (K + G), a β-blocker (K + β), or a β blocker and glucose (K + β + G). The degree of hyperkalemia was minimized by glucose (via enhanced release of insulin) and increased by a β-blocker. (*Data from Allon M, Dansby L, Shanklin N,* Am J Med *94:475, 1993, with permission.*)

the plasma K^+ concentration and the possible induction of ventricular arrhythmias.[32] This effect of insulin on K^+ distribution lasts only several hours, since other factors (including the plasma K^+ concentration itself) then cause K^+ to move back into the extracellular fluid.[31]

To summarize, the primary physiologic effect of insulin and catecholamines is to facilitate the disposition of a K^+ load. Although a deficiency of these hormones may initially elevate the baseline plasma K^+ concentration, this is usually transient, since the excess K^+ is readily excreted in the urine. Thus, the *fasting plasma K^+ concentration is typically normal* in patients treated with β-adrenergic blockers and in patients with type 1 diabetes mellitus given enough insulin to prevent marked hyperglycemia.[14,18,26]

Plasma Potassium Concentration

The combination of insulin deficiency and sympathetic blockade impairs but does not prevent the intracellular movement of K^+ after a K^+ load, indicating that other factors must also be involved.[33] One of these is the plasma K^+ concentration itself. After a K^+ load, for example, the initial elevation in the plasma K^+ concentration promotes K^+ entry into the cells, perhaps by passive mechanisms. Conversely, the loss of K^+ from the ECF due to gastrointestinal or renal losses results first in a fall in the plasma K^+ concentration and then in the movement of K^+ from the cells into the ECF to minimize the degree of hypokalemia.

The net effect is that, in most situations, the plasma K^+ concentration varies directly with body K^+ stores, decreasing with K^+ depletion and increasing with K^+ retention.[6] There are, however, some exceptions to this rule, including chronic disease as described above (in which Na^+-K^+-ATPase activity appears to be reduced), exercise, changes in the extracellular pH or rate of cell breakdown, and an increase in the effective plasma osmolality. In these disorders, clinically significant hyperkalemia or hypokalemia may result from redistribution of K^+ between the cells and the ECF without change in body K^+ stores.

Exercise

Potassium is normally released from muscle cells during exercise. This response may in part reflect a delay between K^+ exit during depolarization and subsequent reuptake by the Na^+-K^+-ATPase pump.[1] With moderate to severe exercise, however, an additional factor may become important. Muscle cells have ATP-dependent K^+ channels, in which ATP reduces the number of open channels. Thus, a reduction in ATP levels with marked exercise can open up more channels, thereby promoting K^+ release from the cells.[34]

The release of K^+ during exercise may have a physiologic function. The *local* increase in the plasma K^+ concentration has a vasodilatory effect that contributes to the enhanced blood flow (and therefore energy delivery) to the exercising muscle.[34,35] This response is impaired by K^+ depletion, an abnormality that may contribute to ischemic muscle injury.[35]

The elevation in the systemic plasma K^+ concentration (which is less than that in the local circulation) is related to the degree of exercise: 0.3 to 0.4 meq/L with slow walking,[36] 0.7 to 1.2 meq/L with moderate exercise,[16,37,38] and as much as 2.0 meq/L with severe exercise to exhaustion.[39,40] These changes are reversed after several minutes of rest[37,40] and may be associated with a mild rebound hypokalemia of 0.4 to 0.5 meq/L below the baseline level.[39]

Exercise-induced hyperkalemia is attenuated by physical conditioning.[1,41] Conditioning enhances both the resting cell K^+ concentration and Na^+-K^+-ATPase activity (via an unknown mechanisms); the latter adaptation may be responsible for the lesser degree of K^+ release during exercise.

The hyperkalemia associated with exercise is generally mild and produces no symptoms. However, it can lead to a potentially dangerous elevation in the plasma K^+ concentration in the presence of some other abnormality in K^+ handling. As an example, severe exercise in patients taking a β-adrenergic blocker can acutely raise the plasma K^+ concentration by 1.5 to as much as 4 meq/L.[16,40]

The effect of exercise can also affect the *measurement* of the plasma K^+ concentration. After a tourniquet is applied, the patient is frequently instructed to repeatedly clench and unclench his or her fist in an attempt to increase local blood flow and make the veins more apparent for venipuncture. This can result in as much as a 1 to 2 meq/L elevation in the plasma K^+ concentration, leading to erroneous evaluation of the state of K^+ balance.[42]

Extracellular pH

Changes in acid-base balance may have important effects on the plasma K^+ concentration, particularly in those forms of metabolic acidosis (such as renal failure) that are not due to the accumulation of organic acids.[43] In this setting, 60 percent or more of the excess H^+ ions is buffered in the cells (see Fig. 10-4). Since the major extracellular anion Cl^- enters the cells only to a limited degree, electroneutrality is maintained by the movement of cellular K^+ and Na^+ into the ECF (Fig. 12-5). The result is a *variable increase in the plasma K^+ concentration* of 0.2 to 1.7 meq/L for every 0.1-unit fall in the extracellular pH (the latter is usually measured clinically on an arterial blood specimen).[43,44] (The plasma Na^+ concentration may also rise, but an elevation of a few milliequivalents per liter is not physiologically important, since the normal value is 140 meq/L, not 4 to 4.5 meq/L as with potassium.)

The wide variability in the degree of hyperkalemia is probably related in part to the common presence of other factors that can influence K^+ homeostasis.[43,44] As examples, diarrhea and renal tubular acidosis are associated with increased gastrointestinal and urinary K^+ losses, respectively (see page 623); the negative K^+ balance in these disorders often leads to hypokalemia despite the presence of metabolic acidosis. It should be emphasized, however, that there is still *relative hyperkalemia* in this setting, since correction of the acidemia will lead to a further reduction in the plasma K^+ concentration unless K^+ supplements are administered.

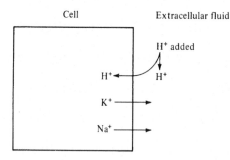

Cell   Extracellular fluid

Figure 12-5 Reciprocal cation shifts of H^+, K^+, and Na^+ between the cells and the extracellular fluid. In the presence of a mineral acid load, H^+ moves into the cells, where it is buffered. To maintain electroneutrality, K^+ and Na^+ leave the cells, resulting in an increase in the plasma K^+ concentration.

The relationship between acidemia and K^+ distribution is also not predictable in the organic acidoses (lactic acidosis and ketoacidosis). In these conditions, the fall in pH appears to be less likely to elevate the plasma K^+ concentration.[43,45-47]* As depicted in Fig. 12-6, for example, the administration of HCl, but not of lactic acid, causes hyperkalemia in dogs. The reason for this difference is not known. One possibility is that the organic anion (such as lactate or β-hydroxybutyrate in ketoacidosis) is able to follow H^+ into the cell, thereby removing the necessity for redistribution of K^+.[43,48] Alternatively, experimental studies suggest that organic anions may act as substrates for the pancreatic β cell, leading to the release of insulin.[49] Insulin then drives K^+ into the cells, counteracting the direct effect of acidemia. However, the applicability of these findings to humans remains to be proven, especially in diabetic ketoacidosis, where insulin deficiency is the primary abnormality.

The change in the plasma K^+ concentration is also much less prominent in metabolic alkalosis.[43] Although H^+ tends to move out of and K^+ into the cells in this disorder, there is generally only a small reduction in the plasma K^+ concentration (unless there are concomitant urinary or gastrointestinal K^+ losses). This relative lack of effect may result in part from less intracellular buffering (and therefore less transcellular H^+ movement) in metabolic alkalosis than in metabolic acidosis (33 percent versus 57 percent).[51] Large changes in the plasma K^+ concentration are also not seen in respiratory acidosis or alkalosis; why this occurs is not well understood.[43]

Hyperosmolality

The plasma K^+ concentration may rise by as much as 0.4 to 0.8 meq/L for every 10 mosmol/kg elevation in the effective plasma osmolality (due to hyperglycemia, hypernatremia, or the administration of hypertonic mannitol).[30,52-55] Hyperosmolality results in the diffusion of water out of cells down an osmotic gradient

---

*Hyperkalemia is a common finding in ketoacidosis and lactic acidosis, but factors other than acidemia are probably of primary importance. In ketoacidosis, for example, both insulin deficiency and hyperosmolality (see below) promote K^+ movement from the cells into the ECF. Thus, the incidence of hyperkalemia is similar in diabetic ketoacidosis and in nonketotic hyperglycemia, where the systemic pH is relatively normal.[50]

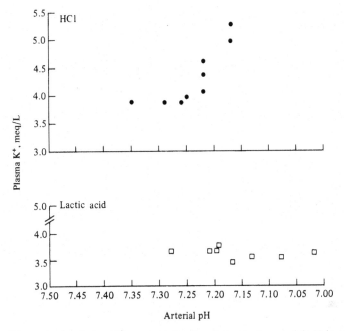

Figure 12-6   Change in the plasma K^+ concentration in relation to the arterial pH in experimentally induced hydrochloric acidosis (HCl is a mineral acid) and lactic acidosis in dogs. (*From Perez GO, Oster JR, Vaamonde CA*, Nephron *27:233, 1981, with permission.*)

(see page 241). In this setting, two factors can contribute to the parallel movement of K^+ into the ECF:

- The loss of water raises the K^+ concentration within the cell, thereby creating a favorable gradient for passive potassium exit through *potassium channels* in the cell membrane.
- The frictional forces between the solvent (water) and solute can result in K^+ being carried along with water through the *water channels* in the cell membrane. This phenomenon, called *solvent drag*, is independent of concentration or electrical gradients for K^+ or other solutes.

A common clinical example of this phenomenon is the increase in the plasma K^+ concentration that commonly accompanies hyperglycemia in uncontrolled diabetes mellitus (Fig. 12-7).[50,52,53] The hyperkalemia partially dissipates with time, as some of the excess extracellular K^+ is excreted in the urine.

Rates of Cell Breakdown and Production

Any condition that enhances cell breakdown (such as severe trauma or the tumor lysis syndrome) results in the release of K^+ (and other intracellular solutes) into

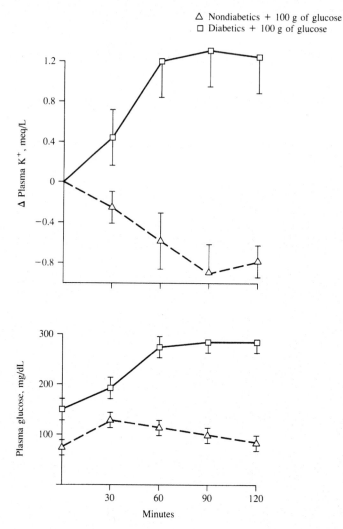

△ Nondiabetics + 100 g of glucose
□ Diabetics + 100 g of glucose

Figure 12-7 Effect of glucose infusion on the plasma K^+ and glucose concentrations in normal subjects (triangles) and in diabetics (squares). The plasma K^+ concentration falls in normals due to the release of insulin, but rises in diabetics because of the development of hyperglycemia and hyperosmolality. (*From Nicholis GL, Kahn T, Sanchez A, Gabrilove JL, Arch Intern Med 141:49, ©1981. Copyright 1981, American Medical Association, with permission.*)

the ECF.[56-58] The degree to which this will elevate the plasma K^+ concentration is related to the ability of other cells to take up the excess K^+ and of the kidney to augment K^+ excretion.

On the other hand, conditions associated with a rapid *increase in cell production* can result in K^+ movement into the cells and hypokalemia. This sequence has been observed after the administration of folic acid or vitamin B_{12} to patients with megaloblastic anemia, who typically respond with an acute and marked increase in the production of red cells and platelets.[59]

Summary

In the basal state, the distribution of K^+ between the cells and the ECF is primarily governed by the Na^+-K^+-ATPase pump in the cell membrane. Although they are not so important in the basal state, catecholamines and insulin play a major role in promoting the cellular uptake of K^+ after a dietary load. This prevents a potentially serious elevation in the plasma K^+ concentration until the kidney can restore K^+ balance by excreting the excess K^+. These hormones appear to act permissively, since their rate of secretion is not enhanced by K^+.

The plasma K^+ concentration may also directly influence K^+ distribution, as K^+ moves into the cells with hyperkalemia and out of the cells with hypokalemia. As a result, the plasma K^+ concentration generally reflects the state of total body K^+ stores. This relationship may be distributed, however, in a variety of conditions (such as exercise, certain forms of metabolic acidosis, or hyperosmolality) in which internal redistribution can alter the plasma K^+ concentration without a similar change in K^+ stores.

RENAL POTASSIUM EXCRETION

Although small amounts of K^+ are lost each day in stool (5 to 10 meq) and sweat (0 to 10 meq), the kidney plays the major role in the maintenance of K^+ balance, appropriately varying K^+ secretion with changes in dietary intake (normal range is 40 to 120 meq/day). The primary event in urinary K^+ excretion is the *secretion of K^+ from the tubular cell into the lumen in the distal nephron*, particularly in the principal cells in the cortical collecting tubule and in the cells in the adjacent connecting segment and outer medullary collecting tubule.[60-62]

Segmental Potassium Handling

The sequential handling of filtered K^+ by the different nephron segments is depicted in the micropuncture experiments in Fig. 12-8.[60,63] The clearance of K^+ is compared to that of inulin, which is filtered and then is neither reabsorbed nor secreted. As a result, a fall in the C_{K^+}/C_{in} ratio indicates that K^+ has been removed from the tubular fluid (or reabsorbed), and an elevation in the ratio indicates that K^+ has been added to the tubular fluid (or secreted). Thus, Fig. 12-8 demonstrates that almost all of the filtered K^+ is reabsorbed in the proximal tubule and the loop of Henle, so that less than 10 percent of the filtered load is delivered to the early distal tubule ($C_{K^+}/C_{in} < 0.1$). Proximal K^+ transport appears to passively follow that of Na^+ and water,[64] whereas reabsorption in the thick ascending limb of the loop of Henle is mediated by the Na^+-K^+-$2Cl^-$ carrier in the luminal membrane (see Fig. 4-2).[62]

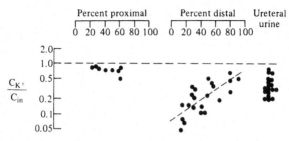

Figure 12-8 Summary of K^+ handling by the rat kidney as a function of the length of the proximal tubule and the cortical distal nephron (which includes the late distal tubule, the connecting segment, and the cortical collecting tubule). Each point in these micropuncture experiments represents a separate sample. A reduction in the C_{K^+}/C_{in} ratio indicates reabsorption, whereas an elevation in the ratio indicates secretion. The function of the loop of Henle and the medullary collecting tubule can be estimated from the difference between late proximal and early distal samples and the difference between late distal and ureteral urine samples, respectively. (*Adapted from Malnic G, Klose RM, Giebisch G, Am J Physiol 211:529, 1966, with permission.*)

In comparison to these reabsorptive processes, K^+ is secreted by the connecting segment, the principal cells in the cortical and outer medullary collecting tubule, and the papillary (or inner medullary) collecting duct (as shown by the rising C_{K^+}/C_{in} ratio in Fig. 12-8).[60,61,65] Secretion in these segments can be varied according to physiologic needs and is generally responsible for most of urinary K^+ excretion.

Distal secretion can be partially counteracted by *K^+ reabsorption* by the intercalated cells in the cortical and outer medullary collecting tubules.[66,67] This process may be mediated by an active H^+-K^+-ATPase pump in the luminal membrane, which results in both H^+ secretion and K^+ reabsorption (see Fig. 5-3).[68-70] The activity of this pump is increased with K^+ depletion[68,70,71] and is reduced with K^+ loading.[72] The former adaptation is probably responsible for the observation that *net K^+ reabsorption, not secretion*, appropriately occurs in the distal nephron with K^+ depletion.[63,66,69] Selective inhibition of the H^+-K^+-ATPase pump in the setting of K^+ depletion abolishes distal K^+ reabsorption.[71]

Medullary recycling The K^+ reabsorbed in the thick ascending limb initially enters the medullary interstitium. Some of this K^+ is then secreted into either the S_3 segment of the late proximal tubule or the thin descending limb of the loop of Henle; this extra K^+ can be reabsorbed again when it enters the outer medulla.[73] Thus, K^+ is *recycled* within the medulla, resulting in the attainment of a relatively high concentration in the interstitium.* The physiologic function of this phenomenon is uncertain. It is possible, for example, that K^+ accumulation in the interstitium promotes K^+ excretion by minimizing the degree of passive backlead out of the collecting tubular lumen (where the highest urine K^+ concentrations are

---

* This process is similar to NH_4^+ recycling between the loop of Henle and the medullary collecting tubule that promotes net NH_4^+ excretion (see page 341).

attained). The high interstitial K^+ concentration also may contribute to K^+ excretion by a second mechanism, by diminishing the gradient for passive K^+ reabsorption via the Na^+-K^+-$2Cl^-$ carrier in the loop of Henle.[74]

Cell Model for Potassium Secretion

Potassium enters the principal cell across the basolateral membrane via the Na^+-K^+-ATPase pump; it is then secreted into the lumen down a favorable electrochemical gradient through K^+ channels in the luminal membrane (Fig. 12-9).[60,75,76] This final step, K^+ movement from the cell into the lumen, appears to be passive[60,63] and therefore is primarily governed by those factors that affect passive transport:

- The *concentration gradient* across the luminal membrane, which is equal to the difference between the cell and tubular fluid K^+ concentrations.

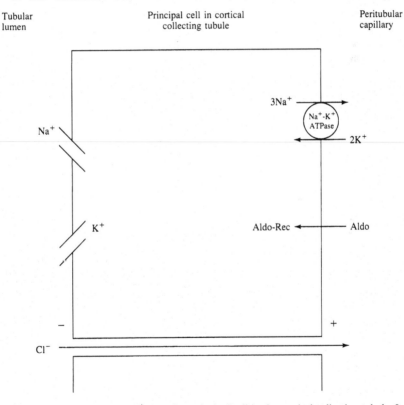

Figure 12-9   Ion transport in the K^+ secreting principal cell in the cortical collecting tubule. Luminal Na^+ enters the cell through Na^+ channels in the luminal membrane, down a concentration gradient created by the Na^+-K^+-ATPase pump. The lumen-negative voltage created by this movement of Na^+ then promotes both the secretion of K^+ (through K^+ channels in the luminal membrane) and the reabsorption of Cl^- (via the paracellular route). These processes are stimulated by aldosterone (Aldo), which enters the cell and combines with its cytosolic receptor (Rec).

Although the total cell K^+ concentration is about 140 to 150 meq/L, ionic interactions with multivalent anions within the cell lower the random movement or activity of cytosolic K^+ to about 80 to 90 meq/L.[77,78] This value is still well above that in the tubular lumen; it is not clear, however, if all or only part of this K^+ represents the transport pool that is available for K^+ secretion.[79] Regardless of its exact composition, the size of this pool is not constant; it appropriately increases after a K^+ load and decreases with K^+ depletion.[79] The plasma K^+ concentration and aldosterone appear to be the prime determinants of this response.

- The *electrical gradient*, which is primarily generated by the reabsorption of Na^+ through Na^+ channels in the luminal membrane.
- The K^+ *permeability* of the luminal membrane, which is a reflection of the number of open K^+ channels.

As will be seen, *aldosterone* and the *plasma K^+ concentration*, acting in concert, are the major physiologic regulators of K^+ secretion.[80] The flow rate to the distal nephron and the potential difference generated by Na^+ reabsorption also are important, but they usually have a permissive rather than a regulatory effect.

Aldosterone

Aldosterone plays a major role in K^+ homeostasis by augmenting K^+ secretion in the principal cells in the cortical collecting tubule and in adjacent cells in the connecting segment and the outer part of the medullary collecting tubule.[81-85] After a K^+ load, for example, aldosterone secretion is directly enhanced, thereby promoting the excretion of the excess K^+ in the urine. This response is very efficient, since a rise in the plasma K^+ concentration of as little as 0.1 to 0.2 meq/L can induce a significant elevation in aldosterone release.[86] Conversely, secretion of this hormone is reduced with K^+ depletion, a response that tends to preserve K^+ balance by minimizing further urinary losses.

Aldosterone appears to result in stimulation of each of the major transport steps depicted in Fig. 12-9: It increases the number of open Na^+ and K^+ channels in the luminal membrane; and it enhances the activity of the Na^+-K^+-ATPase pump in the basolateral membrane (see page 180).[87,88] The *rise in luminal Na^+ permeability is the earliest change*; it promotes Na^+ entry into the cell, and this Na^+ is then returned to the systemic circulation by the Na^+-K^+-ATPase pump. These changes can enhance K^+ secretion by two mechanisms:

- The transport of Na^+ out of the cell by the Na^+-K^+-ATPase pump also results in K^+ movement into the cell, thereby increasing the size of the K^+ transport pool.[1]
- The reabsorption of cationic Na^+ makes the lumen relatively electronegative, thereby increasing the electrical gradient favoring K^+ secretion.

Any persistent increase in K^+ secretion must be accompanied by enhanced Na^+-K^+-ATPase activity; if this did not occur; there would be eventual depletion of cell K^+ stores. It is of interest in this regard that the ratio of Na^+ reabsorption to K^+ secretion in the cortical collecting tubule is $3:2$, similar to the stoichiometry of the Na^+-K^+-ATPase pump.[89] This observation suggests the following sequence: The Na^+-K^+-ATPase pump transports reabsorbed Na^+ out of the cell in exchange for extracellular K^+; most of this K^+ is then secreted into the lumen, rather than leaking back out across the basolateral membrane and being returned to the systemic circulation.[89]

The primacy of the Na^+ reabsorptive effect is also suggested by the response to the diuretic amiloride (see Chap. 15). This agent closes the luminal Na^+ channels and at least transiently prevents the aldosterone-induced increases in K^+ secretion, luminal K^+ permeability, and Na^+-K^+-ATPase activity.[88,90]

Other hormones can also enhance distal K^+ secretion, including ADH, which appears to increase the number of luminal K^+ channels.[91,92] Although ADH is not a primary regulator of K^+ excretion, the elevation in luminal K^+ permeability may be physiologically important. It can counteract the associated reduction in distal flow due to ADH-induced water reabsorption, thereby preventing an undesired decrease in K^+ excretion.[91]

Plasma Potassium Concentration

The plasma K^+ concentration can directly affect K^+ excretion, independent of other factors such as aldosterone.[93] An example of this relationship is illustrated in Fig. 12-10. Dogs were adrenalectomized, given aldosterone replacement at different doses, and then studied at different levels of K^+ intake. As intake was increased, there was a gradual elevation in the plasma K^+ concentration. When aldosterone replacement was at a normal level (50 µg/day, middle curve), urinary K^+ excretion remained at low levels until the plasma K^+ concentration exceeded 4.2 meq/L. At this point, K^+ excretion increased markedly in an attempt to maintain K^+ balance. This presumably reflected a direct effect of the plasma K^+ concentration, since aldosterone levels, Na^+ intake, and the urine output were relatively constant.

In intact animals, however, aldosterone secretion will rise after a K^+ load, resulting in even more rapid excretion of K^+ (left curve, Fig. 12-10). The kidney is normally so efficient in excreting excess K^+ that *chronic hyperkalemia cannot occur unless there is an associated defect in urinary K^+ excretion.*

Studies in adrenalectomized animals have also elucidated the mechanism by which the plasma K^+ concentration affects distal K^+ secretion.[94,95] *Potassium alone replicates all of the changes in the principal cells that are induced by aldosterone*: It increases Na^+ reabsorption and K^+ secretion, luminal membrane permeability to Na^+ and K^+ (by increasing the number of open channels),[75] and the activity of the Na^+-K^+-ATPase pump.[94] How these changes occur is not known. They are, however, less prominent that those seen when a K^+ load is appropriately accompanied by a rise in aldosterone secretion.[96]

The experiments in Fig. 12-10 also demonstrate the effect of chronic changes in aldosterone secretion on the *steady-state plasma K^+ concentration*.[80] If K^+ intake and excretion are normal at 50 meq/day, the plasma K^+ concentration

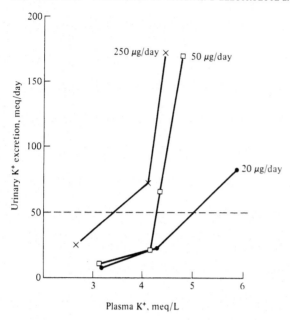

Figure 12-10 Mean values for plasma potassium concentration and steady-state urinary potassium excretion in adrenalectomized dogs given different levels of aldosterone replacement and studied at increasing levels of K^+ intake. The dashed line represents the effects seen when K^+ excretion is 50 meq/day. (*From Young DB, Paulsen AW, Am J Physiol 244:F28, 1983, with permission.*)

will be approximately 4.3 meq/L in dogs receiving physiologic levels of aldosterone (50 µg/day), 3.4 meq/L with hyperaldosteronism (250 µg/day), and 5.0 meq/L with hypoaldosteronism (20 µg/day). When less aldosterone is available, for example, urinary K^+ excretion becomes less efficient; as a result, a higher plasma K^+ concentration is required to establish a new steady state in which intake again equals excretion. Thus, *hypo*aldosteronism is associated with hyperkalemia, whereas primary *hyper*aldosteronism enhances urinary K^+ loss, often leading to a fall in the plasma K^+ concentration (see Chaps. 27 and 28).

Distal Flow Rate

Increasing distal flow rate is another potentially important stimulus of distal K^+ secretion (Fig. 12-11).[97,99] This response is most prominent in the presence of a high-K^+ diet, since the concurrent elevations in aldosterone release and the plasma K^+ concentration produce a high basal level of K^+ secretion. In comparison, K^+ depletion can lead to net reabsorption, not secretion, in the distal nephron.[66] It is not surprising, therefore, that distal flow has little or no effect of K^+ secretion in this setting.[97]

The mechanism by which distal flow affects renal K^+ handling is incompletely understood, but changes in the tubular fluid K^+ concentration appear to play an important role.[98] As described previously, almost all of the filtered K^+ is reab-

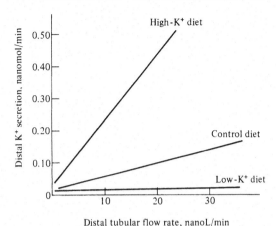

Figure 12-11 Combined effects of dietary intake and distal tubular flow rate on distal K^+ secretion. (*From Khuri RM, Wiederholt M, Strieder N, Giebisch G, Am J Physiol 228:1249, 1975, with permission.*)

sorbed in the proximal tubule and loop of Henle; as a result, the K^+ concentration in the fluid entering the distal nephron may be less than 1 meq/L.

The combination of K^+ secretion and, if ADH is present, water reabsorption in the cortical collecting tubule raises the tubular fluid K^+ concentration.[98] Increasing distal flow washes the secreted K^+ away and replaces it with relatively K^+-free fluid from the more proximal segments. Thus, the K^+ concentration in the lumen is kept at a relatively low level, maintaining a favorable gradient for continued K^+ secretion.[99]

The net effect is that the tubular fluid K^+ concentration remains nearly constant within the physiologic range of flow rate; increasing flow results in more K^+ being secreted without any elevation in the luminal K^+ concentration.[99] There may, however, be a rise in the tubular fluid K^+ concentration when distal flow is substantially diminished due, for example, to volume depletion.[99] In this setting, the high luminal concentration (due to less washout of secreted K^+) and the low urine flow lead to a reduction in the absolute rate of K^+ secretion.

The flow dependence of K^+ secretion may also be related to changes in the delivery of Na^+ to the distal secretory site.[99] Increased distal flow is generally associated with enhanced Na^+ delivery to and reabsorption in the cortical collecting tubule. As noted above, this elevation in Na^+ transport has two effects that favor K^+ secretion: (1) The entry of Na^+ into the cells through its channels in the luminal membrane makes the lumen relatively electronegative, creating an electrical gradient that favors the movement of K^+ from the cells into the lumen (see below), and (2) the subsequent transport of this Na^+ out of the cell by the Na^+-K^+-ATPase pump in the basolateral membrane results in the entry of new K^+ into the cells, thereby providing more K^+ for continued secretion. Thus, the flow dependence of K^+ secretion is probably mediated by the parallel changes in both water[98,100] and Na^+ delivery.[99]

Physiologic role The relationship between K^+ secretion and distal flow rate plays an important role in allowing aldosterone to regulate Na^+ and K^+ balance independently[80] and, as mentioned above, in allowing ADH to regulate H_2O balance without affecting the secretion of K^+ (see page 184).[91,92] As an example, a Na^+ load expands the extracellular volume, resulting in a reduction in the secretion of renin and therefore that of aldosterone. Although the latter change promotes the excretion of the excess Na^+ (by decreasing cortical collecting tubule Na^+ reabsorption), it should also lead to K^+ retention and hyperkalemia. This does not happen, however, since volume expansion tends to increase the glomerular filtration rate (GFR) and to diminish proximal Na^+ reabsorption (see Chap. 8), both of which augment the distal flow rate. The enhanced flow counteracts the fall in aldosterone release, resulting in little or no change in K^+ excretion.[80,101]

The outcome will be different if a Na^+ load is administered in the presence of nonsuppressible aldosterone secretion, as occurs in patients with primary hyperaldosteronism.[102] In this setting, the combination of increased distal flow and normal or elevated aldosterone levels leads to enhanced urinary K^+ excretion and a reduction in the plasma K^+ concentration.[102,103]

These changes are reversed with volume depletion, as the combination of increased aldosterone release and reduced distal flow allows Na^+ to be conserved without substantially affecting K^+ balance.[80,104] These observations explain why untreated patients with heart failure or cirrhosis are *typically normokalemic*, despite the common presence of secondary hyperaldosteronism and high ADH levels. If, however, distal flow is increased, then inappropriate K^+ wasting is likely to ensue. This appears to be the *major mechanism by which the loop and thiazide diuretics induce hypokalemia*.[105] These agents enhance distal delivery by diminishing Na^+ and water reabsorption in the loop of Henle and distal tubule, respectively (see Chap. 15). They also tend to stimulate aldosterone secretion, because of the concomitant reduction in extracellular volume.

Sodium Reabsorption and the Transepithelial Potential Difference

Since K^+ is a charged particle, its secretion is importantly affected by the transepithelial potential difference across the tubular cell. The normal potential difference in the K^+-secreting cells is approximately -15 to -50 mV (lumen negative).[89,106,107] This potential is generated by the transport of Na^+ from the lumen into the peritubular capillary (Fig. 12-12). Since Na^+ is positively charged, its reabsorption makes the lumen relatively electronegative. Cl^- is passively reabsorbed via the paracellular route down this electrical gradient; there is, however, a finite time lag, and it is this delay that is responsible for the observed potential difference.

The importance of Na^+ in the generation of this potential can be illustrated by the response to replacing luminal Na^+ with a nonreabsorbable cation, such as choline$^+$.[106] In this setting, the potential difference falls to zero (Fig. 12-12). On the other hand, replacing luminal Cl^- with a poorly reabsorbed anion, such as SO_4^{2-} increases the anion delay and augments the potential difference.

The central role of the Na^+-generated potential difference on K^+ secretion can be illustrated by the response to the diuretic amiloride.[79,105] This agent impairs the

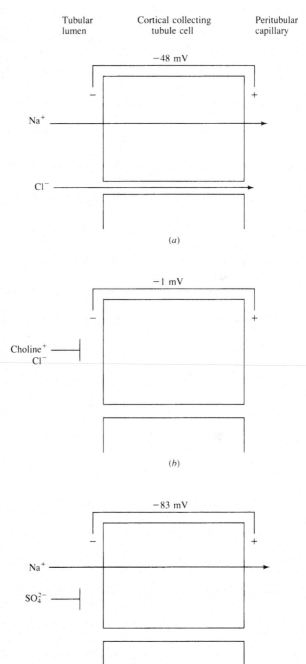

Figure 12-12 Schematic representation of the electrical events in a typical principal cell in the cortical collecting tubule. (*a*) Na^+ is actively transported from the lumen into the capillary. Cl^- follows via the paracellular route after a finite time lag; this delay is responsible for the transepithelial potential difference of −35 to −50 mV, lumen negative. (*b*) Replacing Na^+ in the lumen with the nonreabsorbable cation choline essentially eliminates the potential difference, illustrating the central role of Na^+ transport. (*c*) Replacing Cl^- in the lumen with the non-reabsorbable anion SO_4^{2-} increases the anion delay and enhances the potential difference, thereby favoring the secretion of K^+ into the lumen. (*Data from Giebisch G, Malnic G, Klose RM, Windhager EE, Am J Physiol 211:560, 1966, with permission.*)

entry of luminal Na^+ into the cells of the distal nephron by closing the Na^+ channels in the luminal membrane.[108] The net effect is diminished Na^+ reabsorption and a reduction in the transepithelial potential difference, even in the presence of aldosterone.[79,88,105] There is also a marked fall in K^+ secretion; it is likely that this effect is due to the decrease in potential difference, since amiloride has no known direct influence on K^+ handling.[108]

The stimulatory effect of Na^+ transport on K^+ secretion is more prominent if Na^+ is delivered with an *anion other than Cl^- that is nonreabsorbable*. In this setting, there will be less Cl^- available for reabsorption to dissipate the lumen-negative electrical gradient created by Na^+ entry into the cell. As an example, a volume-depleted subject has a strong stimulus to Na^+ reabsorption in the cortical collecting tubule that is mediated by aldosterone. In this situation, the administration of Na_2SO_4 results in Na^+ reabsorption without SO_4^{2-} and, consequently, increases in the potential difference (Fig. 12-12) and K^+ secretion.[107,109,110] In contrast, if Na^+ balance and therefore both Cl^- delivery and aldosterone secretion are normal, there is no stimulus to retain the excess Na^+, and Na_2SO_4 is excreted with only a small elevation in K^+ secretion.[109,110]

A clinical example of this phenomenon may follow the intravenous administration of the antibiotic carbenicillin, which contains 4.7 meq of Na^+ per gram. Thirty grams of this compound contains approximately 140 meq of the carbenicillin anion; the presence of this nonreabsorbable anion in the tubular fluid can, in some patients, lead to enhanced urinary K^+ loss and hypokalemia.[111,112]

Studies in humans suggest that, in addition to volume status, the nonreabsorbable anion itself may be a determinant of the effect on K^+ secretion.[110] Although the ability of sulfate to enhance K^+ loss is minimized by euvolemia, HCO_3^- is still able to promote K^+ secretion in this setting. How this might occur is not known.

Extracellular pH

As noted above, changes in the extracellular pH produce reciprocal H^+ and K^+ shifts between the cells and the ECF. As a result, K^+ tends to move into cells with alkalemia and out of cells with acidemia. These changes in the cell K^+ concentration will tend to reduce K^+ secretion in acidemia and to increase K^+ secretion in alkalemia.[113-115]

These pH-induced effects, however, are *transient and are frequently overridden by concurrent variations in other factors that affect K^+ handling.*[116,117] In type 2 renal tubular acidosis, for example, proximal HCO_3^- reabsorption is impaired (see Chap. 19). As a result, there is increased delivery of Na^+, the poorly reabsorbable anion HCO_3^-, and water to the distal secretory site. These changes overcome the direct effect of acidosis, and K^+ loss ensues.[118,119] A similar sequence occurs in diabetic ketoacidosis, where Na^+ and water are delivered to the distal nephron with the ketoacid anions, β-hydroxybutyrate and acetoacetate.

Renal Response to Potassium Depletion and Potassium Loading

The regulation of K^+ excretion can be summarized by reviewing the renal responses to changes in K^+ balance.

Potassium depletion K^+ excretion, for example, appropriately falls with K^+ depletion.[63,66,120] This response is initially mediated by diminished release of aldosterone,[120] which represents a direct effect of K^+ on the adrenal zona glomerulosa cells.[121] Within several days, however, a decrease in the cell K^+ concentration in the distal nephron probably assumes primary importance.[120] At this time, neither the administration of aldosterone[120,122] nor increasing distal flow rate (Fig. 12-11) substantially enhances urinary K^+ loss.

The fall in K^+ excretion in this setting is due both to reduced secretion and to active K^+ reabsorption.[61,66] The latter process occurs in the intercalated cells in the cortex and outer medulla[66,67] and appears to be mediated by a luminal H^+-K^+-ATPase pump.[69,71] The activity of this pump, which reabsorbs K^+ and secretes H^+, increases with K^+ depletion.[70,71] This change is associated with an elevation in luminal membrane area in the intercalated cells,[66,67] due at least in part to insertion of new H^+-K^+-ATPase pumps in the luminal membrane.[61]

The net effect is that K^+ excretion can be lowered to 15 to 25 meq/day with a total K^+ deficit of 50 to 150 meq, and to 5 to 15 meq/day with more marked K^+ loss.[123] The inability to conserve K^+ more efficiently may be related to passive leakage down a favorable concentration gradient of cellular K^+ into the tubular lumen through a relatively nonselective cation channel in the terminal nephron segment, the inner medullary collecting duct.[124]

Potassium loading   Urinary K^+ excretion increases after a K^+ load.[60] This response is so efficient that normal subjects can maintain K^+ balance even if K^+ intake is *slowly increased* from the normal level of 60 to 80 meq/day up to 500 meq/day or more.[125,126] This response is mediated both by aldosterone and by a rise in the plasma K^+ concentration.[80,126]

The ability to handle what might be a lethal K^+ load if given acutely is called *K^+ adaptation* and is due primarily to more rapid K^+ excretion in the urine.[127] Early adaptation can be induced by a single normal meal. As an example, rats fed a meal containing K^+ were better able to excrete an intravenous K^+ load several hours later than fasted rats; more rapid urinary excretion meant that there was a smaller elevation in the plasma K^+ concentration.[128]

In addition to increased urinary excretion, two other factors, both of which are promoted by aldosterone, also may contribute to more chronic adaptation: (1) enhanced K^+ entry into extrarenal cells,[129,130] the importance of which is uncertain,[131] and (2) increased gastrointestinal losses due to colonic secretion of K^+.[132,133]

The increase in urinary K^+ excretion during adaptation is due to *enhanced K^+ secretion throughout the late distal nephron*, including the short connecting segment, and the principal cells in the cortical and outer medullary collecting tubules.[66,84,95,96,134] The efficacy of this response is illustrated in Fig. 12-13,

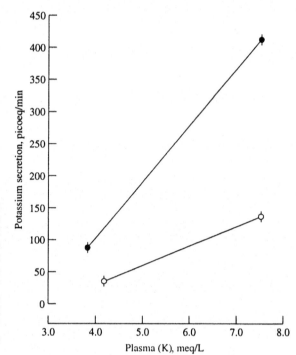

Figure 12-13 Relationship between plasma K^+ concentration (which is elevated by KCl infusion) and distal K^+ secretion in control animals (circles) and adapted animals (squares) given a high-K^+ diet for 4 weeks. At any plasma K^+ concentration, K^+ secretion is two to four times higher in the adapted animals. (*From Stanton BA*, Am J Physiol *257:R989, 1989, with permission.*)

which shows that distal K^+ secretion at a given plasma K^+ concentration is two to four times higher in K^+-adapted rats.[61] In addition to increased secretion, decreased reabsorption in the intercalated cells (mediated by a decrease in activity of the K^+-ATPase pump) also may contribute to the kaliuresis.[72]

Both increased secretion of aldosterone and a small elevation in the plasma K^+ concentration are required for the complete expression of this response.[84,96] They act in part by enhancing Na^+-K^+-ATPase activity in these distal segments,[95,135] either directly or by increasing the entry of luminal Na^+ into the cell.[87,90,94] The morphologic correlate of this increase in Na^+-K^+-ATPase activity is a marked increase in the area of the basolateral membrane, the site at which the Na^+-K^+-ATPase pumps are inserted.[61] This morphologic change begins within the first day of a high K^+ intake and does not reach a plateau until 2 weeks.

The role of these parameters in humans can be illustrated by the response to chronic K^+ loading (400 meq/day) in normal subjects (Fig. 12-14).[126] The plasma K^+ concentration rose from 3.8 to 4.8 meq/L and the plasma aldosterone concentration increased 2.5-fold in the first 2 days. By 20 days, however, both the plasma K^+ concentration (4.2 meq/L) and the plasma aldosterone concentration had partially returned toward baseline levels, even though urinary K^+ excretion remained very high.

The increased efficiency of K^+ secretion at this time was probably related to the hyperkalemia-induced rise in Na^+-K^+-ATPase activity.[126] Indirect evidence in support of this hypothesis was the observation that discontinuing the K^+ load led

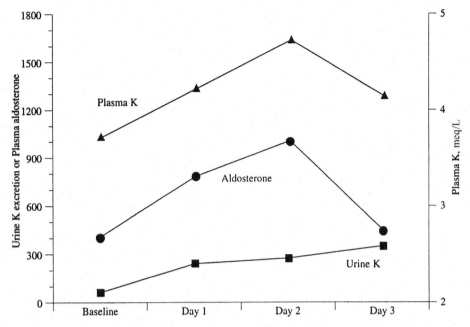

Figure 12-14   Response to increasing K^+ intake to 400 meq/day in normal subjects. Urinary K^+ excretion rises to this level within 2 days and is then maintained. This response is initially driven by elevations in the plasma K^+ and aldosterone concentrations. By day 20, the efficiency of K^+ secretion has increased, resulting in a lesser elevation in the plasma K^+ concentration (to 4.2 meq/L) and normalization of the plasma aldosterone concentration. (*Adapted from Rabelink TJ, Koomans HA, Hené RJ, Dorhout Mees EJ,* Kidney Int *38:942, 1990. Reprinted by permission from* Kidney International.)

to transient Na^+ retention, which could have reflected the time required for distal Na^+-K^+-ATPase activity to fall back to normal.

The major clinical example of K^+ adaptation occurs in chronic renal failure, in which the combination of a constant K^+ intake and fewer functioning nephrons requires an increase in K^+ excretion per nephron.[136,137] This allows K^+ balance to be maintained even in advanced disease as long as intake is not excessive, the urine output and therefore the distal flow rate are adequate, and aldosterone secretion can be appropriately increased.[138,139]

Studies in experimental animals with renal failure have shown that Na^+-K^+-ATPase activity in the distal nephron is elevated, an expected correlate of enhanced K^+ secretion per nephron.[140] However, this elevation in pump activity is seen only when K^+ intake is normal, not when intake is restricted in proportion to the fall in GFR, a setting in which increased K^+ excretion per nephron is not required.[140] This finding suggests that the rise in Na^+-K^+-ATPase activity is *appropriate* and *specific*, not incidentally induced by renal insufficiency.

Enhanced colonic secretion of K^+ also may play an important role in advanced renal disease.[132,141] It has been estimated that increased stool losses may account for the excretion of as much as 30 to 50 percent of dietary K^+ in patients with end-stage renal failure on chronic dialysis.[5,142]

SUMMARY

The maintenance of a normal plasma K^+ concentration is dependent upon the ability of K^+ to enter the cells, where it achieves high concentrations, and upon the urinary excretion of net dietary intake. After a K^+ load, most of the extra K^+ is initially taken up by the cells, a response that is facilitated by basal levels of catecholamines and insulin. This cell uptake minimizes the increase in the plasma K^+ concentration, pending the excretion of the excess K^+ in the urine.

Urinary K^+ excretion is largely a function of secretion in the distal nephron, primarily in the principal cells in the cortical collecting tubule. The main factors modulating this process are aldosterone and the plasma K^+ concentration itself. Distal flow rate and the transepithelial potential difference (which is generated primarily by Na^+ reabsorption) play a more *permissive* role: They do not change directly with K^+ balance, but relatively normal values are required for adequate K^+ secretion.

Understanding these principles can simplify the approach to patients with disorders of K^+ balance. Chronic hyperkalemia, for example, *must be associated with a defect in distal K^+ secretion*, since the adaptation response would normally permit excretion of the excess K^+ (Fig. 12-14). From the preceding discussion, the two major mechanisms by which K^+ secretion might be impaired are *hypoaldosteronism* and *decreased distal flow* (due to a marked volume depletion or advanced renal failure). These conditions therefore constitute most of the differential diagnosis of persistent hyperkalemia (see Chap. 28).

Urinary K^+ wasting and hypokalemia, on the other hand, are due to activation of the distal secretory process. This most often occurs with *hyperaldosteronism* (as long as distal flow is maintained), *increased distal flow* (as long as aldosterone secretion is normal or elevated, as with diuretic therapy), or the delivery of Na^+ to the distal nephron with a *nonreabsorbable anion* (as is seen in ketoacidosis or type 2 renal tubular acidosis).[118,119]

PROBLEMS

12-1   What effect should aldosterone deficiency have on urinary K^+ excretion? What factor ultimately limits the changes that occur?

12-2   In a patient with primary hyperaldosteronism due to an adrenal adenoma, what effect will increased Na^+ intake have on urinary K^+ excretion? How does this differ from the response in normal subjects?

12-3 K^+ depletion is most often due to urinary or gastrointestinal losses of K^+. What test would be helpful in differentiating between these disorders?

12-4   Untreated patients with effective circulating volume depletion due to heart failure or cirrhosis (see Chap. 10) are generally normokalemic even though the activity of the renin-angiotensin-aldosterone system is frequently increased. Why doesn't aldosterone promote excess urinary K^+ loss in this setting? What would happen to K^+ excretion if a diuretic such as furosemide were then given to increase Na^+ and water excretion?

12-5   Which of the following drugs can raise the plasma K^+ concentration?

(a) A converting enzyme inhibitor, which limits the formation of angiotensin II

(b) A thiazide diuretic

(c) A β-adrenergic blocker

(d) An α-adrenergic blocker

(e) An intravenous infusion of glucose

12-6   ADH increases water reabsorption in the collecting tubules. In patients with central diabetes insipidus, the urine output can exceed 10 L/day, because of decreased collecting tubule water reabsorption. What effect will this high-output state have on K^+ excretion?

REFERENCES

1. Clausen T, Everts ME. Regulation of the Na,K-pump in skeletal muscle. *Kidney Int* 35:1, 1989.
2. Doucet A. Function and control of Na-K-ATPase in single nephron segments of the mammalian kidney. *Kidney Int* 34:749, 1988.
3. Knochel JP. Neuromuscular manifestations of electrolyte disorders. *Am J Med* 72:521, 1982.
4. DeVoe RD, Maloney PC. Principles of cell homeostasis, in Mountcastle VB (ed): *Medical Physiology*, 14th ed. St Louis, Mosby, 1980.
5. Brown RS. Extrarenal potassium homeostasis. *Kidney Int* 30:116, 1986.
6. Sterns RH, Cox M, Feig PU, Singer I. Internal potassium balance and the control of the plasma potassium concentration. *Medicine* 60:339, 1981.
7. Reza MJ, Kovick RB, Shine KI, Pearce ML. Massive intravenous digoxin overdose. *N Engl J Med* 291:777, 1974.
8. Kaji D, Kahn T. Na^+-K^+ pump in chronic renal failure. *Am J Physiol* 252:F785, 1987.
9. Edmondson RPS, Thomas RD, Hilton RJ, et al. Leucocyte electrolytes in cardiac and non-cardiac patients receiving diuretics. *Lancet* 1:12, 1974.
10. Casey TH, Summerskill WHJ, Orvis AL. Body and serum potassium in liver disease. I. Relationship to hepatic function and associated factors. *Gastroenterology* 48:198, 1965.
11. Bilbrey GL, Carter NW, White MG, et al. Potassium deficiency in chronic renal failure. *Kidney Int* 4:423, 1973.
12. Winkler AW, Hoff HE, Smith PK. The toxicity of orally administered potassium salts in renal insufficiency. *J Clin Invest* 20:119, 1941.
13. DeFronzo R, Taufield P, Black H, et al. Impaired renal tubular potassium secretion in sickle cell disease. *Ann Intern Med* 90:310, 1979.
14. DeFronzo RA, Bia M, Birkhead G. Epinephrine and potassium homeostasis. *Kidney Int* 20:83, 1981.
15. Brown MJ, Brown DC, Murphy HB. Hypokalemia from β_2-receptor stimulation by circulating epinephrine. *N Engl J Med* 309:1414, 1983.
16. Williams ME, Gervino EV, Rosa RM, et al. Catecholamine modulation of rapid potassium shifts during exercise. *N Engl J Med* 312:823, 1985.
17. Clausen T, Flatman JA. Effect of insulin and epinephrine on Na^+-K^+-ATPase and glucose transport in soleus muscle. *Am J Physiol* 252:E492, 1987.
18. Rosa RM, Silva P, Young JB, et al. Adrenergic modulation of extrarenal potassium disposal. *N Engl J Med* 302:431, 1980.
19. Allon M, Dansby L, Shanklin N. Glucose modulation of the disposal of an acute potassium load in patients with end-stage renal disease. *Am J Med* 94:475, 1993.

20. Struthers AD, Whitesmith R, Reid JL. Prior thiazide treatment increases adrenaline-induced hypokalemia. *Lancet* 1:1358, 1983.
21. Schnack C, Podolsky A, Watzke H, et al. Effect of somatostatin and oral potassium administration on terbutaline-induced hypokalemia. *Am Rev Respir Dis* 139:176, 1989.
22. Lipworth BJ, McDevitt DG, Struthers AD. Prior treatment with diuretic augments the hypokalemic and electrocardiographic effects of inhaled albuterol. *Am J Med* 86:653, 1989.
23. Braden GL, von Oeyen PT, Germain MJ, et al. Ritodrine- and terbutaline-induced hypokalemia in preterm labor: Mechanisms and consequences. *Kidney Int* 51:1867, 1997.
24. Goldenberg IF, Olivari MT, Levine TB, Cohn JN. Effect of dobutamine on plasma potassium in congestive heart failure secondary to idiopathic or ischemic cardiomyopathy. *Am J Cardiol* 63:843, 1989.
25. Zierler KL, Rabinowitz D. Effect of very small concentrations of insulin on forearm metabolism. Persistence of its actions on potassium and free fatty acids without its effects on glucose. *J Clin Invest* 43:950, 1964.
26. DeFronzo RA, Sherwin RS, Dillingham M, et al. Influence of basal insulin and glucagon secretion on potassium and sodium metabolism: Studies with somatostatin in normal dogs and in normal and diabetic human beings. *J Clin Invest* 61:472, 1978.
27. Lytton J, Lin JC, Guidotti G. Identification of two molecular forms of (Na^+, K^+)-ATPase in rat adipocytes. Relation to insulin stimulation of the enzyme. *J Biol Chem* 260:1177, 1985.
28. Dluhy RG, Axelrod L, Williams GH. Serum immunoreactive insulin and growth hormone response to potassium infusion in normal man. *J Appl Physiol* 33:22, 1972.
29. Cox M, Sterns RH, Singer I. The defense against hyperkalemia. The roles of insulin and aldosterone. *N Engl J Med* 299:525, 1978.
30. Kurtzman NA, Gonzalez J, DeFronzo RA, Giebisch G. A patient with hyperkalemia and metabolic acidosis. *Am J Kidney Dis* 15:333, 1990.
31. Blumberg A, Weidmann P, Shaw S, Gnadinger M. Effect of various therapeutic approaches on plasma potassium and major regulating factors in terminal renal failure. *Am J Med* 85:507, 1988.
32. Kunin AS, Surawicz B, Sims EA. Decrease in serum potassium concentration and appearance of cardiac arrhythmias during infusion of potassium with glucose in potassium-depleted patients. *N Engl J Med* 266:228, 1962.
33. DeFronzo RA, Lee R, Jones A, Bia M. Effect of insulinopenia and adrenal hormone deficiency on acute potassium tolerance. *Kidney Int* 17:586, 1980.
34. Daut J, Maier-Rudolph W, von Beckerath N, et al. Hypoxic dilation of coronary arteries is mediated by ATP-sensitive potassium channels. *Science* 247:1341, 1990.
35. Knochel JP, Schlein EM. On the mechanism of rhabdomyolysis in potassium depletion. *J Clin Invest* 51:1750, 1972.
36. Sessard J, Vincent M, Annat G, Bizollon CA. A kinetic study of plasma renin and aldosterone during changes of posture in man. *J Clin Endocrinol Metab* 42:20, 1976.
37. Struthers AD, Quigley C, Brown MJ. Rapid changes in plasma potassium during a game of squash. *Clin Sci* 74:397, 1988.
38. Thomson A, Kelly DT. Exercise stress-induced changes in systemic arterial potassium in angina pectoris. *Am J Cardiol* 63:1435, 1989.
39. Lindinger M, Heigenhauser GJF, McKelvie RS, Jones NL. Blood ion regulation during repeated maximal exercise and recovery in humans. *Am J Physiol* 262:R126, 1992.
40. Lim M, Linton RAF, Wolff CB, Band DM. Propranolol, exercise and arterial plasma potassium. *Lancet* 2:591, 1981.
41. Knochel JP, Blanchley JD, Johnson JH, Carter NW. Muscle cell electrical hyperpolarization and reduced exercise hyperkalemia in physically conditioned dogs. *J Clin Invest* 75:740, 1985.
42. Don BR, Sebastian A, Cheitlin M, et al. Pseudohyperkalemia caused by fist clenching during phlebotomy. *N Engl J Med* 322:1290, 1990.
43. Adrogué HJ, Madias NE. Changes in plasma potassium concentration during acute acid-base disturbances. *Am J Med* 71:456, 1981.

44. Magner PO, Robinson L, Halperin RM, et al. The plasma potassium concentration in metabolic acidosis: A re-evaluation. *Am J Kidney Dis* 11:220, 1988.
45. Fulop M. Serum potassium in lactic acidosis and ketoacidosis. *N Engl J Med* 300:1087, 1979.
46. Orringer CE, Eustace JC, Wunsch CD, Gardner LB. Natural history of lactic acidosis after grand-mal seizures: A model for the study of an anion-gap acidosis not associated with hyperkalemia. *N Engl J Med* 297:796, 1977.
47. Perez GO, Oster JR, Vaamonde CA. Serum potassium concentration in acidemic states. *Nephron* 27:233, 1981.
48. Graber M. A model of the hyperkalemia produced by metabolic acidosis. *Am J Kidney Dis* 22:436, 1993.
49. Adrogué HJ, Chap Z, Ishida T, Field J. Role of endocrine pancreas in the kalemic response to acute metabolic acidosis in conscious dogs. *J Clin Invest* 75:798, 1985.
50. Arieff AI, Carroll HJ, Nonketotic hyperosmolar coma with hyperglycemia: Clinical features, pathophysiology, renal function, acid-base balance, plasma-cerebrospinal fluid equilibria and the effects of therapy in 37 cases. *Medicine* 51:73, 1972.
51. Pitts RF. *Physiology of the Kidney and Body Fluids*. Chicago, Year Book, 1974, chap 11.
52. Nicolis GL, Kahn T, Sanchez A, Gabrilove JL. Glucose-induced hyperkalemia in diabetic subjects. *Arch Intern Med* 41:49, 1981.
53. Viberti GC. Glucose-induced hyperkalaemia: A hazard for diabetics? *Lancet* 1:690, 1978.
54. Conte G, Dal Canton A, Imperatore P, et al. Acute increase in plasma osmolality as a cause of hyperkalemia in patients with renal failure. *Kidney Int* 38:301, 1990.
55. Moreno M, Murphy C, Goldsmith C. Increase in serum potassium resulting from the administration of hypertonic mannitol and other solutions. *J Lab Clin Med* 73:291, 1969.
56. Arseneau JC, Bagley CM, Anderson T, Canellos GP. Hyperkalemia, a sequel to chemo-therapy of Burkitt's lymphoma. *Lancet* 1:10, 1973.
57. Hande KR, Garrow GC. Acute tumor lysis syndrome in patients with high-grade non-Hodgkin's lymphoma. *Am J Med* 94:133, 1993.
58. Drakos P, Bar-Ziv J, Catane R. Tumor lysis syndrome in nonhematologic malignancies. Report of a case and review of the literature. *Am J Clin Oncol* 17:502, 1994.
59. Lawson DH, Murray RM, Parker JLW. Early mortality in the megaloblastic anaemias. *Q J Med* 41:1, 1972.
60. Giebisch G, Wang W. Potassium transport: From clearance to channels and pumps. *Kidney Int* 49:1624, 1996.
61. Stanton BA. Renal potassium transport: Morphological and functional adaptations. *Am J Physiol* 257:R989, 1989.
62. Greger R, Gogelein H. Role of K^+ conductive pathways in the nephron. *Kidney Int* 31:1055, 1987.
63. Malnic G, Klose RM, Giebisch G. Micropuncture study of distal tubular potassium and sodium transport in rat nephron. *Am J Physiol* 211:529, 1966.
64. Kaufman JS, Hamburger RJ. Passive potassium transport in the proximal convoluted tubule. *Am J Physiol* 248:F228, 1985.
65. Diezi J, Michaud P, Aceves J, Giebisch G. Micropuncture study of electrolyte transport across papillary collecting duct of the rat. *Am J Physiol* 224:623, 1973.
66. Stanton BA, Biemesderfer D, Wade JB, Giebisch G. Structural and functional study of the rat distal nephron: Effects of potassium adaptation and depletion. *Kidney Int* 19:36, 1981.
67. Stetson DL, Wade JB, Giebisch G. Morphologic alterations in the rat medullary collecting duct following potassium depletion. *Kidney Int* 17:45, 1980.
68. Garg LC, Narang N. Ouabain-sensitive K-adenosine triphosphatase in distal nephron segments of the rabbit. *J Clin Invest* 81:1204, 1988.
69. Wingo CS, Madsen KM, Smolka A, Tisher CC. H-K-ATPase immunoreactivity in cortical and outer medullary collecting duct. *Kidney Int* 38:985, 1990.
70. Kraut JA, Hiura J, Besancon M, et al. Effect of hypokalemia on the abundance of HK alpha 1 and HK alpha 2 protein in the rat kidney. *Am J Physiol* 272:F744, 1997.

71. Okusa MD, Unwin RJ, Velazquez H, et al. Active potassium absorption by the renal distal tubule. *Am J Physiol* 262:F488, 1992.
72. Garg LC, Narang N. Suppression of ouabain-insensitive K-ATPase activity in rabbit nephron segments during chronic hyperkalemia. *Renal Physiol Biochem* 12:295, 1989.
73. Jamison RL. Potassium recycling. *Kidney Int* 31:695, 1987.
74. Milanes CL, Jamison RL. Effect of acute potassium load on reabsorption in Henle's loop in chronic renal failure in the rat. *Kidney Int* 27:919, 1985.
75. Wong W, Schwab A, Giebisch G. Regulation of small-conductance K$^+$ channel in apical membrane of rat cortical collecting tubule. *Am J Physiol* 259:F494, 1990.
76. Wang WH. View of K$^+$ secretion through the apical K channel of cortical collecting duct. *Kidney Int* 48:1024, 1995.
77. Civan MM. Potassium activities in epithelia. *Fed Proc* 39:2865, 1980.
78. Adam WR, Koretsky AP, Weiner MW. Potassium adaptation: ^{39}K-NMR evidence for intracellular compartmentalization of K$^+$. *Am J Physiol* 254:F401, 1988.
79. Garcia-Filho E, Malnic G, Giebisch G. Effects of changes in electrical potential difference on tubular potassium transport. *Am J Physiol* 238:F235, 1980.
80. Young DB. Quantitative analysis of aldosterone's role in potassium regulation. *Am J Physiol* 255:F811, 1988.
81. Stanton BA. Regulation of Na$^+$ and K$^+$ transport by mineralocorticoids. *Semin Nephrol* 7:82, 1987.
82. Stokes JB, Ingram MJ, Williams AD, Ingram D. Heterogeneity of the rabbit collecting tubule: Localization of mineralocorticoid hormone action to the cortical portion. *Kidney Int* 20:340, 1981.
83. Muto S, Giebisch G, Sansom S. Effect of adrenalectomy on CCD: Evidence for differential response of 2 cell types. *Am J Physiol* 253:F742, 1987.
84. Kashgarian M, Ardito T, Hirsch DJ, Hayslett JP. Response of collecting tubule cells to aldosterone and potassium loading. *Am J Physiol* 253:F8, 1987.
85. Rabinowitz L. Aldosterone and potassium homeostasis. *Kidney Int* 49:1738, 1996.
86. Himathongam T, Dluhy R, Williams GH. Potassium-aldosterone-renin interrelationships. *J Clin Endocrinol Metab* 41:153, 1975.
87. Sansom SC, O'Neil RG. Mineralocorticoid requirement of apical cell membrane Na$^+$ and K$^+$ transport of the cortical collecting duct. *Am J Physiol* 248:F858, 1985.
88. Sansom S, Muto S, Giebisch G. Na-dependent effects of DOCA on cellular transport properties of CCDs from ADX rabbits. *Am J Physiol* 253:F753, 1987.
89. Stokes JB. Sodium and potassium transport by the collecting duct. *Kidney Int* 38:679, 1990.
90. Petty KJ, Kokko JP, Marver D. Secondary effect of aldosterone on Na-K-ATPase activity in the rabbit cortical collecting tubule. *J Clin Invest* 68:1514, 1981.
91. Field MJ, Stanton BA, Giebisch G. Influence of ADH on renal potassium handling: A micropuncture and microperfusion study. *Kidney Int* 25:502, 1984.
92. Cassola AC, Giebisch G, Wong W. Vasopressin increases density of apical low-conductance K$^+$ channels in rat CCD. *Am J Physiol* 264:F502, 1993.
93. Young DB, Paulsen AW. Interrelated effects of aldosterone and plasma potassium on potassium excretion. *Am J Physiol* 244:F28, 1983.
94. Muto S, Sansom S, Giebisch G. Effects of a high potassium diet on electrical properties of cortical collecting ducts from adrenalectomized rabbits. *J Clin Invest* 81:376, 1988.
95. Garg LC, Narang N. Renal adaptation to potassium in the adrenalectomized rabbit. Role of distal tubular sodium-potassium adenosine triphosphatase. *J Clin Invest* 76:1065, 1985.
96. Stanton B, Pan L, Deetjen H, et al. Independent effects of aldosterone and potassium on induction of potassium adaptation in rat kidney. *J Clin Invest* 79:198, 1987.
97. Khuri RM, Wiederholt M, Strieder N, Giebisch G. Effects of flow rate and potassium intake on distal tubular potassium transfer. *Am J Physiol* 228:1249, 1975.
98. Good DW, Wright FS. Luminal influences on potassium secretion: Sodium concentration and fluid flow rate. *Am J Physiol* 236:F192, 1979.

99. Malnic G, Berlioner RW, Giebisch G. Flow dependence of potassium secretion in cortical distal tubules of the rat. *Am J Physiol* 256:F932, 1989.
100. Good DW, Velazquez H, Wright FS. Luminal influences on potassium secretion: Low sodium concentration. *Am J Physiol* 246:F609, 1984.
101. Young DB, McCaa RE. Role of the renin-angiotensin system in potassium control. *Am J Physiol* 238:R359, 1980.
102. George JM, Wright L, Bell NH, Bartter FC. The syndrome of primary aldosteronism. *Am J Med* 48:343, 1970.
103. Young DB, Jackson TE, Tipayamontri U, Scott RC. Effects of sodium intake on steady-state potassium excretion. *Am J Physiol* 246:F772, 1984.
104. Seldin D, Welt L, Cort J. The role of sodium salts and adrenal steroids in the production of hypokalemia alkalosis. *Yale J Biol Med* 29:229, 1956.
105. Duarte CG, Chomety F, Giebisch G. Effect of amiloride, ouabain, and furosemide on distal tubular function in the rat. *Am J Physiol* 221:632, 1971.
106. Giebisch G, Malnic G, Klose RM, Windhager EE. Effect of ionic substitutions on distal potential differences in rat kidney. *Am J Physiol* 211:560, 1966.
107. Velazquez H, Wright FS, Good DW. Luminal influences on potassium secretion: Chloride replacement with sulfate. *Am J Physiol* 242:F46, 1982.
108. Benos DJ. Amiloride: A molecular probe of sodium transport in tissues and cells. *Am J Physiol* 242:C131, 1982.
109. Schwartz WB, Jenson RL, Relman AS. Acidification of the urine and increased ammonium excretion without change in acid-base equilibrium: Sodium reabsorption as a stimulus to the acidifying process. *J Clin Invest* 34:673, 1955.
110. Carlisle EJF, Donnelly SM, Ethier JH, et al. Modulation of the secretion of potassium by accompanying anions in humans. *Kidney Int* 39:1206, 1991.
111. Lipner HT, Ruzany F, Dasgupta M, et al. The behavior of carbenicillin as a nonreabsorbable anion. *J Lab Clin Med* 86:183, 1975.
112. Klastersky J, Vanderkelen B, Daneua D, Mathieu M. Carbenicillin and hypokalemia (letter). *Ann Intern Med* 78:774, 1973.
113. Malnic G, de Mello Aires M, Giebisch G. Potassium transport across renal distal tubules during acid-base disturbances. *Am J Physiol* 221:1192, 1971.
114. Barker ES, Singer RB, Elkinton JR, Clark JK. The renal response in man to acute experimental respiratory alkalosis and acidosis. *J Clin Invest* 36:515, 1957.
115. Stanton BA, Giebisch G. Effects of pH on potassium transport by renal distal tubule. *Am J Physiol* 242:F544, 1982.
116. Gennari FJ, Cohen JJ. Role of the kidney in potassium homeostasis: Lessons from acid-base disturbances. *Kidney Int* 8:1, 1975.
117. Scandling JD, Ornt DB. Mechanism of potassium depletion during chronic metabolic acidosis in the rat. *Am J Physiol* 252:F122, 1987.
118. Sebastian A, McSherry E, Morris RC Jr. Renal potassium wasting in renal tubular acidosis (RTA): It occurrence in types 1 and 2 RTA despite sustained correction of systemic acidosis. *J Clin Invest* 50:667, 1971.
119. Sebastian A, McSherry E, Morris RC Jr. On the mechanism of renal potassium wasting in renal tubular acidosis with the Fanconi syndrome (type 2 RTA). *J Clin Invest* 50:231, 1971.
120. Linas SL, Peterson LN, Anderson RJ, et al. Mechanism of renal potassium conservation in the rat. *Kidney Int* 15:601, 1979.
121. Aguilera G, Catt KJ. Loci of action of regulators of aldosterone biosynthesis in isolated glomerulosa cells. *Endocrinology* 104:1046, 1978.
122. Mujais SK, Chen Y, Nora NA. Discordant aspects of aldosterone resistance in potassium depletion. *Am J Physiol* 262:F972, 1992.
123. Squires RD, Huth EJ. Experimental potassium depletion in normal human subjects. I. Relation of ionic intakes to the renal conservation of potassium. *J Clin Invest* 38:1134, 1959.
124. Light DB, McCann FV, Keller TM, Stanton BA. Amiloride-sensitive cation channel in apical membrane of inner medullary collecting duct. *Am J Physiol* 255:F278, 1988.

125. Talbott JH, Schwab RS. Recent advances in the biochemistry and therapeusis of potassium salts. *N Engl J Med* 222:585, 1940.
126. Rabelink TJ, Koomans HA, Hené RJ, Dorhout Mees EJ. Early and late adjustment to potassium loading in humans. *Kidney Int* 38:942, 1990.
127. Hayslett JP, Binder HJ. Mechanism of potassium adaptation. *Am J Physiol* 243:F103, 1982.
128. Jackson CA. Rapid renal potassium adaptation in rats. *Am J Physiol* 263:F1098, 1992.
129. Alexander EA, Levinsky NG. An extrarenal mechanism of potassium adaptation. *J Clin Invest* 47:740, 1968.
130. Blachley JD, Crider BP, Johnson JH. Extrarenal potassium adaptation: Role of skeletal muscle. *Am J Physiol* 251:F313, 1986.
131. Spital A, Sterns RH. Paradoxical potassium depletion: A renal mechanism for extrarenal potassium adaptation. *Kidney Int* 30:532, 1986.
132. Foster ES, Jones WH, Hayslett JP, Binder HJ. Role of aldosterone and dietary potassium in potassium adaptation in the distal colon of the rat. *Gastroenterology* 88:1985, 1985.
133. Sweiry JH, Binder HJ. Characterization of aldosterone-induced potassium secretion in rat distal colon. *J Clin Invest* 83:844, 1989.
134. Schon DA, Backman KA, Hayslett J. Role of the medullary collecting duct in potassium excretion in potassium-adapted animals. *Kidney Int* 20:655, 1981.
135. Silva P, Hayslett JP, Epstein FH. The role of Na-K-activated adenosine triphosphatase in potassium adaptation. Stimulation of enzymatic activity by potassium loading. *J Clin Invest* 52:2665, 1973.
136. Schultze RG, Taggart DD, Shapiro H, et al. On the adaptation in potassium excretion associated with nephron reduction in the dog. *J Clin Invest* 50:1061, 1971.
137. Bourgoignie JJ, Kaplan M, Pincus J, et al. Renal handling of potassium in dogs with chronic renal insufficiency. *Kidney Int* 20:482, 1981.
138. Gonick HC, Kleeman CR, Rubini ME, Maxwell MH. Functional impairment in chronic renal disease. III. Studies of potassium excretion. *Am J Med Sci* 261:281, 1971.
139. Schambelan M, Sebastian A, Biglieri E. Prevalence, pathogenesis, and functional significance of aldosterone deficiency in hyperkalemic patients with chronic renal insufficiency. *Kidney Int* 17:89, 1980.
140. Schon DA, Silva P, Hayslett JP. Mechanism of potassium excretion in renal insufficiency. *Am J Physiol* 227:1323, 1974.
141. Bastl C, Hayslett JP, Binder HJ. Increased large intestinal secretion of potassium in renal insufficiency. *Kidney Int* 12:9, 1977.
142. Hayes CP Jr, Robinson RR. Fecal potassium excretion in patients on chronic intermittent hemodialysis. *Trans Am Soc Artif Inter Organs* 11:242, 1965.

THREE

PHYSIOLOGIC APPROACH TO ACID-BASE AND ELECTROLYTE DISORDERS

CHAPTER THIRTEEN

MEANING AND APPLICATION OF URINE CHEMISTRIES

As is discussed in the ensuing chapters, measurement of the urinary electrolyte concentrations, osmolality, and pH plays an important role in the diagnosis and management of a variety of disorders. This chapter briefly reviews the meaning of these parameters and the settings in which they may be helpful (Table 13-1). It is important to emphasize that there are *no fixed normal values*, since the kidney varies the rate of excretion to match net dietary intake and endogenous production. Thus, interpretation of a given test requires knowledge of the patient's clinical state. As an example, the urinary excretion of 125 meq of Na^+ per day may be appropriate for a subject on a regular diet, but represents inappropriate renal Na^+ wasting in a patient who is volume-depleted.

In addition to being clinically useful, these tests are simple to perform and widely available. In most circumstances, a random urine specimen is sufficient, although a 24-h collection to determine the daily rate of solute excretion is occasionally indicated. When K^+ depletion is due to extrarenal losses, for example, the urinary K^+ excretion should fall below 25 meq/day. In some patients, however, random measurement may be confusing. If the urine output is only 500 mL/day because of associated volume depletion, then the appropriate excretion of only 20 meq of K^+ per day will be associated with an apparently high urine K^+ concentration of 40 meq/L (20 meq/day $\div$ 0.5 L/day = 40 meq/L).

Table 13-1   Clinical application of urine chemistries

Parameter	Uses
Na^+ excretion	Assessment of volume status Diagnosis of hyponatremia and acute renal failure Dietary compliance in patients with hypertension Evaluation of calcium and uric acid excretion in stone formers
Cl^- excretion	Similar to that for Na^+ excretion Diagnosis of metabolic alkalosis Urine anion gap
K^+ excretion	Diagnosis of hypokalemia
Osmolality or specific gravity	Diagnosis of hyponatremia, hypernatremia, and gravity acute renal failure
pH	Diagnosis of renal tubular acidosis Efficacy of treatment in metabolic alkalosis and uric acid stone disease

SODIUM EXCRETION

The kidney varies the rate of Na^+ excretion to maintain the effective circulating volume, a response that is mediated by a variety of factors, including the renin-angiotensin-aldosterone system and perhaps atrial natriuretic peptide and related peptides (see Chap. 8). As a result, the urine Na^+ concentration can be used as an estimate of the patient's volume status. In particular, a urine Na^+ concentration below 20 meq/L is generally indicative of hypovolemia. This finding is especially useful in the differential diagnosis of both *hyponatremia* and *acute renal failure*. The two major causes of hyponatremia are effective volume depletion and the syndrome of inappropriate antidiuretic hormone secretion (SIADH). The urine Na^+ concentration should be low in the former, but greater than 40 meq/L in the SIADH, which is characterized by water retention but normal Na^+ handling (i.e., output equal to intake; see Chap. 23).

Similar considerations apply to acute renal failure, which is most often due to volume depletion or acute tubular necrosis.[1] The urine Na^+ concentration usually exceeds 40 meq/L in the latter, in part because of the associated tubular damage and a consequent inability to maximally reabsorb Na^+.[1-3] Measuring the fractional excretion of Na^+ and the urine osmolality also can help to differentiate between these conditions (see below).

In normal subjects, urinary Na^+ excretion roughly equals average dietary intake. Thus, measurement of urinary Na^+ excretion (by obtaining a 24-h collection) can be used to check dietary compliance in patients with essential hypertension. Restriction of Na^+ intake is frequently an important component of the therapeutic regimen,[4,5] and adequate adherence should result in the excretion of less than 100 meq/day.

The *concurrent use of diuretics does not interfere with the utility of this test* as long as drug dose and dietary intake are relatively constant. A thiazide diuretic, for example, initially increases Na^+ and water excretion by reducing Na^+ transport in the distal tubule. However, the diuresis is attenuated over a period of days, because the ensuing volume depletion enhances Na^+ reabsorption both in the collecting tubules (via aldosterone) and in the proximal tubule (in part via angiotensin II).[6,7] The net effect is the establishment within 1 week of a new steady state in which the plasma volume is somewhat diminished, but *Na^+ excretion is again equal to intake* (see Fig. 15-2).[8]

Measurement of urinary Na^+ excretion is also important when evaluating patients with recurrent kidney stones. A 24-h urine collection is typically obtained in this setting to determine if calcium or uric acid excretion is increased, both of which can predispose to stone formation.[9,10] However, the tubular reabsorption of both calcium and uric acid is indirectly linked to that of Na^+ (see Chap. 3). Thus, the increased Na^+ reabsorption in hypovolemia can mask the presence of underlying hypercalciuria or hyperuricosuria.[11] In general, Na^+ excretion above 75 to 100 meq/day indicates that volume depletion is not a limiting factor for calcium or uric acid excretion.

Limitations

Despite its usefulness, there are some pitfalls in relying upon the measurement of Na^+ excretion as an index of volume status. A low urine Na^+ concentration, for example, may be seen in normovolemic patients who have *selective renal or glomerular ischemia* due to bilateral renal artery stenosis or acute glomerulonephritis.[2,12] On the other hand, a defect in tubular Na^+ reabsorption can lead to a high rate of Na^+ excretion, despite the presence of volume depletion. This can occur with the use of diuretics,* in aldosterone deficiency, or in advance renal failure.[13]

The urine Na^+ concentration can also be influenced by the rate of water reabsorption. This can be exemplified by central diabetes insipidus, a disorder in which a deficiency of antidiuretic hormone (ADH) can lead to a urine output exceeding 10 L/day. In this setting, the daily excretion of 100 meq of Na^+ will be associated with a urine Na^+ concentration of 10 meq/L or less, incorrectly suggesting the presence of volume depletion. Conversely, a high rate of water reabsorption can raise the urine Na^+ concentration and mask the presence of hypovolemia. To *remove the effect of water reabsorption*, the renal handling of Na^+ can be evaluated directly by calculating the fractional excretion of Na^+ (FE_{Na}).

---

* Although chronic diuretic use does not prevent attainment of a new steady state, urinary Na^+ excretion that is equal to intake is still inappropriately high in a hypovolemic patient.

Fractional Excretion of Sodium

The FE_{Na} can be calculated from a random urine specimen:[2,3,14]

$$FE_{Na}(\%) = \frac{\text{quantity of } Na^+ \text{ excreted}}{\text{quantity of } Na^+ \text{ filtered}} \times 100$$

The quantity of Na^+ excreted is equal to the product of the urine Na^+ concentration (U_{Na}) and the urine flow rate (V); the quantity of Na^+ filtered is equal to the product of the plasma Na^+ concentration (P_{Na}) and the glomerular filtration rate (or creatinine clearance, which is equal to $U_{cr} \times V/P_{cr}$). Thus,

$$FE_{Na} = \frac{U_{Na} \times V}{P_{Na} \times (U_{cr} \times V/P_{cr})} \times 100$$

$$= \frac{U_{Na} \times P_{cr}}{P_{Na} \times U_{cr}} \times 100$$

The primary use of the FE_{Na} is in patients with acute renal failure. As described above, a low urine Na^+ concentration favors the diagnosis of volume depletion, whereas a high value points toward acute tubular necrosis. However, a level between 20 and 40 meq/L may be seen with either disorder.[2,3] This overlap, which is due in part to variations in the rate of water reabsorption, can be minimized by calculating the FE_{Na}.[2,3,14] Na^+ reabsorption is appropriately enhanced in hypovolemic states, and the FE_{Na} is usually less than 1 percent; i.e., more than 99 percent of the filtered Na^+ has been reabsorbed. In contrast, tubular damage leads to a FE_{Na} in excess of 2 to 3 percent in most patients with acute tubular necrosis.

There are, however, exceptions to this general rule, as the FE_{Na} may be less than 1 percent when acute tubular necrosis is superimposed upon chronic effective volume depletion (as occurs in cirrhosis, heart failure, and burns) or when it is induced by radiocontrast media or heme pigment deposition.[1,15-17] The mechanism by which this occurs is uncertain, although tubular function may be better preserved in these disorders.[14]

Limitations   The major limitation in the use of the FE_{Na} is that it is dependent upon the amount of Na^+ filtered, and therefore the *dividing line between volume depletion and normovolemia is not always 1 percent*. This can be best appreciated in patients with normal renal function. If the glomerular filtration rate (GFR) is 180 L/day (125 mL/min) and the plasma Na^+ concentration is 150 meq/L, then 27,000 meq of Na^+ will be filtered each day. As a result, the FE_{Na} will always be under 1 percent as long as daily Na^+ intake is in the usual range of 125 to 250 meq. Since patients with relatively normal renal function should be able to lower daily Na^+ excretion to less than 20 meq/day in the presence of volume depletion, the FE_{Na} should be less than 0.2 percent in this setting. A FE_{Na} of 0.5 percent is indicative of normovolemia, not volume depletion, in such a patient unless there is renal salt wasting. In comparison, a FE_{Na} of 0.5 percent does reflect volume depletion in advanced renal failure, a condition in which the GFR and therefore the filtered Na^+ load are markedly reduced. If, for example, the GFR is only 10 percent of normal, then the filtered Na^+ load is 2700 meq/day; 0.5 percent of this quantity is equal to only 14 meq of Na^+ excreted per day.

The FE_{Na} and the U_{Na} are difficult to interpret with concurrent diuretic therapy, since the ensuing natriuresis will raise these values even in patients who are hypovolemic. Although not widely available, measurement of the fractional clearance of endogenous lithium (which is present in trace amounts) may circumvent this problem. Lithium is primarily reabsorbed in the proximal tubule, which has two important consequences: (1) Proximal reabsorption is increased and therefore lithium excretion is reduced in hypovolemic states, and (2) lithium excretion is not significantly increased by loop diuretics. The fractional excretion of lithium (FE_{Li}) is approximately 20 percent in healthy controls. In one report of patients with acute renal failure, a value below 15 percent (and usually below 10 percent) was highly suggestive of prerenal disease, independent of diuretic therapy.[18] In comparison, the mean FE_{Li} was 26 percent in acute tubular necrosis (ATN).

Given the usual lack of ability to measure trace lithium, other markers for proximal function have been evaluated. Uric acid handling occurs almost entirely in the proximal tubule, and the fractional excretion of uric acid is not affected by loop diuretic therapy. In the study noted above, values below 12 percent were suggestive of prerenal disease (sensitivity 68 percent, specificity 78 percent), while values above 20 percent were suggestive of ATN (sensitivity 96 percent, specificity only 33 percent).[18]

CHLORIDE EXCRETION

Chloride is reabsorbed with sodium throughout the nephron (see Chaps. 3 to 5). As a result, the rate of excretion of these ions is usually similar, and measurement of the urine Cl^- concentration generally adds little to the information obtained from the more routinely measured urine Na^+ concentration.

However, as many as 30 percent of hypovolemic patients have more than a 15-meq/L difference between the urine Na^+ and Cl^- concentrations.[19] This is due to the excretion of Na^+ with another anion (such as HCO_3^- or carbenicillin) or to the excretion of Cl^- with another cation (such as NH_4^+ in metabolic acidosis.[19,20] Thus, it may be helpful to measure the urine Cl^- concentration in a patient who seems to be volume-depleted but has a somewhat elevated urine Na^+ concentration.

This most often occurs in *metabolic alkalosis*, in which acid-base balance can be restored by urinary excretion of the excess HCO_3^- as $NaHCO_3$ (see Chap. 18). Many of these patients, however, are volume-depleted due to vomiting or diuretic use. To the degree that the hypovolemic stimulus to Na^+ retention predominates, there will be low Na^+ and HCO_3^- levels in the urine and persistence of the alkalosis. If, on the other hand, there is a relatively mild volume deficit as compared to the severity of the alkalosis, some $NaHCO_3$ will be excreted, thereby elevating the urine Na^+ concentration (in some cases to over 100 meq/L). In comparison, the urine Cl^- concentration will remain appropriately low (unless some diuretic effect persists), since there is no defect in the reabsorption of NaCl.

Another setting in which measurement of the urine Cl^- concentration may be helpful is in patients with a normal anion gap metabolic acidosis (see Chap. 19).[21,22] In the absence of renal failure, this problem is most often due to diarrhea or to one of the forms of renal tubular acidosis (RTA). The normal response to acidemia is to increase urinary acid excretion, primarily as NH_4^+. When urine NH_4^+ levels are high, the *urine anion gap*,

$$\text{Urine anion gap} = ([Na^+] + [K^+]) - [Cl^-]$$

will have a negative value, since the Cl^- concentration will exceed the concentration of Na^+ and K^+ by the approximate amount of NH_4^+ in the urine. Thus, the urine Cl^- concentration may be inappropriately high in diarrhea-induced hypovolemia because of the need to maintain electroneutrality as NH_4^+ excretion is enhanced.[20]

In comparison, urinary acidification is impaired in RTA, leading to a low level of NH_4^+ excretion and a positive value for the urine anion gap.[21] The urine pH also will be inappropriately high (> 5.3) in this setting.

POTASSIUM EXCRETION

Potassium excretion varies appropriately with intake, a response that is mediated primarily by aldosterone and a direct effect of the plasma K^+ concentration (see Chap. 12). If K^+ depletion occurs, urinary K^+ excretion can fall to a minimum of 5 to 25 meq/day.[23] As a result, measurement of K^+ excretion can aid in the diagnosis of unexplained hypokalemia. An appropriately low value suggests either extrarenal losses (usually from the gastrointestinal tract) or the use of diuretics (if the collection has been obtained after the diuretic effect has worn off). In comparison, the excretion of more than 25 meq of K^+ per day indicates at least a component of renal K^+ wasting.

Measurement of K^+ excretion is less helpful in patients with hyperkalemia. If K^+ intake is increased slowly, normal subjects can take in and excrete more than 40 meq of K^+ per day without a substantial elevation in the plasma K^+ concentration (normal daily intake is 40 to 120 meq).[24,25] Thus, chronic hyperkalemia *must be associated with a defect in urinary K^+ excretion*, since normal renal function would result in the rapid excretion of the excess K^+. As a result, the urine K^+ concentration will be inappropriately low in this setting, most often as a result of renal failure or hypoaldosteronism (see Chap. 28).

URINE OSMOLALITY

Variations in the urine osmolality (U_{osm}) play a central role in the regulation of the plasma osmolality (P_{osm}) and Na^+ concentration. This response is mediated by osmoreceptors in the hypothalamus that influence both thirst and the secretion of ADH (see Chap. 9). After a water load, for example, there is a transient reduction in the P_{osm}, leading to suppression of ADH release. This diminishes water reabsorption in the collecting tubules, resulting in the excretion of the excess water in a dilute urine. Water restriction, on the other hand, sequentially raises the P_{osm}, ADH secretion, and renal water reabsorption, resulting in water retention and the excretion of a concentrated urine.

These relationships allow the U_{osm} to be helpful in the differential diagnosis of both *hyponatremia* and *hypernatremia* (see Chaps. 23 and 24). Hyponatremia with hypoosmolality should virtually abolish ADH release. As a result, a maximally dilute urine should be excreted, with the U_{osm} falling below 100 mosmol/kg. If this is found, then the hyponatremia is probably due to excess water intake at a rate that exceeds normal excretory capacity (a rare disorder called primary polydipsia). Much more commonly, the U_{osm} is inappropriately high and the *hyponatremia results from an inability of the kidneys to excrete water normally*. Lack of suppression of ADH release, due to volume depletion or the syndrome of inappropriate ADH secretion, is the most common cause of this problem.

In contrast, hypernatremia should stimulate ADH secretion, and the U_{osm} should exceed 600 to 800 mosmol/kg. If a concentrated urine is found, then extrarenal water loss (from the respiratory tract or skin) or the administration of Na^+ in excess of water is responsible for the elevation in the plasma Na^+ concentration. On the other hand, a U_{osm} below that of the plasma indicates primary renal water loss due to lack of or resistance to ADH.

The U_{osm} (in addition to the FE_{Na}) also may be helpful in distinguishing volume depletion from postischemic ATN as the cause of the acute renal failure. ADH levels tend to be elevated in both disorders, because hypovolemia is a potent stimulus to the release of ADH (see page 176). However, tubular dysfunction in acute tubular necrosis impairs the response to ADH, leading to the excretion of urine with an osmolality that is generally less than 400 mosmol/kg.[1,3] In comparison, the U_{osm} may exceed 500 mosmol/kg with hypovolemia alone if there is no underlying renal disease. Thus, a high U_{osm} essentially excludes the diagnosis of ATN. The finding of an isosmotic urine, however, is less useful diagnostically. It is consistent with ATN but does not rule out volume depletion, since there may be a concomitant impairment in concentrating ability, a common finding in the elderly or in patients with severe reductions in glomerular filtration rate.[26,27]

Urine Specific Gravity

The solute concentration of the urine (or other solution) also can be estimated by measuring the urine specific gravity, which is defined as the weight of the solution compared with that of an equal volume of distilled water. Plasma is approximately 0.8 to 1.0 percent heavier than water and therefore has a specific gravity of 1.008 to 1.010. Since the specific gravity is proportional to the *weight*, as well as the number, of particles in the solution, its relationship to osmolality is dependent upon the molecular weights of the solutes.

As illustrated in Fig. 13-1, the specific gravity varies with osmolality in a relatively predictable way in normal urine, which contains primarily small solutes such as urea, Na^+, Cl^-, K^+, NH_4^+, and $H_2PO_4^-$. In this setting, each 30 to 35 mosmol/kg raises the specific gravity by approximately 0.001. Thus, a specific gravity of 1.010 usually represents urine osmolality between 300 and 350 mosmol/kg.

However, there will be a disproportionate increase in the specific gravity as compared with the osmolality if larger molecules, such as glucose, are present in high concentrations. Clinical examples of this phenomenon include glucosuria in uncontrolled diabetes mellitus, and the administration of radiocontrast media (mol wt approximately 550) or high doses of the antibiotic carbenicillin. In these settings, the specific gravity can exceed 1.040 to 1.050, even though the urine osmolality may be about 300 mosmol/kg, similar to that of the plasma.[28]

URINE pH

The urine pH generally reflects the degree of acidification of the urine and normally varies with systemic acid-base balance. The major clinical use of the urine pH occurs in patients with metabolic acidosis. The appropriate response to this disorder is to increase urinary acid excretion, so that the urine pH falls below 5.3 and usually below 5.0.[21] Values above 5.3* in adults and 5.6 in children usually indicate abnormal urinary acidification and the presence of renal tubular acidosis;

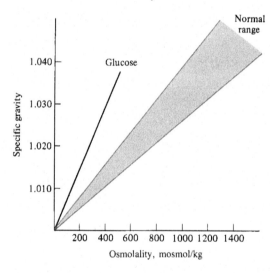

Figure 13-1 Relationship between the specific gravity and osmolality of the urine from normal subjects who have neither glucose nor protein in the urine. For comparison, the relationship between the specific gravity and osmolality for glucose solutions is included. (*Adapted from Miles B, Paton A, deWardener H, Br Med J 2:904, 1954. By permission of the* British Medical Journal.)

---

* The diagnostic use of the urine pH requires that the urine be sterile. Infection with any of the urinary pathogens that produce urease results in the metabolism of urinary urea into ammonia (NH_3). The excess NH_3 directly elevates the urine pH according to the Henderson-Hasselbalch equation (see Chap. 10):

$$pH = 9.3 + \log \frac{NH_3}{NH_4^+}$$

the urine anion gap also tends to have a positive value in this setting, since NH_4^+ excretion is impaired.[21] Distinction between the various types of renal tubular acidosis can then be made by measurement of the urine pH and the fractional excretion of HCO_3^- at different plasma HCO_3^- concentrations (see Chap. 19).

Monitoring the urine pH is also helpful in assessing the efficacy of treatment in metabolic alkalosis and uric acid stone disease. As described above, HCO_3^- reabsorption is often increased in metabolic alkalosis due to concomitant volume depletion. The net effect is that the urine pH is inappropriately acid (< 6.0), since virtually all of the filtered HCO_3^- is reabsorbed. This defect can typically be reversed by NaCl administration; as normovolemia is restored, the excess HCO_3^- can be excreted, resulting in an elevation in the urine pH to above 7.0. A persistently low urine pH usually indicates inadequate volume repletion.

A persistently acid urine is also an important factor in many patients with uric acid stone disease. A high H^+ concentration will drive the reaction

$$H^+ + urate^- \quad \leftrightarrow \quad uric\ acid$$

to the right. The ensuing elevation in the uric acid concentration is physiologically important, since uric acid is much less soluble than urate.[29] Administering alkali, on the other hand, can reverse this problem. The efficacy of therapy can be assessed by monitoring the urine pH, which should be above 6.0 to 6.5.

REFERENCES

1. Rose BD. *Pathophysiology of Renal Disease*, 2d ed. New York, McGraw-Hill, 1987, p. 82.
2. Miller TR, Anderson RJ, Linas SL, et al. Urinary diagnostic indices in acute renal failure: A prospective study. *Ann Intern Med* 89:47, 1978.
3. Espinel CH, Gregory AW. Differential diagnosis of acute renal failure. *Clin Nephrol* 13:73, 1980.
4. Cutler JA, Follmann D, Alexander PS. Randomized trials of sodium reduction: An overview. *Am J Clin Nut* 65(suppl): 643S, 1997.
5. Law MR, Frost CD, Wald NJ. By how much does dietary salt reduction lower blood pressure. I. An analysis of observational data among populations; III. Analysis of data of salt reduction. *Br Med J* 302:811,819, 1991.
6. Wilcox CS, Guzman NJ, Mitch WE, et al. Na^+, K^+ and BP homeostasis in man during furosemide: Effects of prazosin and captopril. *Kidney Int* 131:135, 1987.
7. Bock HA, Stein JH. Diuretics and the control of extracellular fluid volume: Role of counter-regulation. *Semin Nephrol* 8:264, 1988.
8. Maronde R, Milgrom M, Vlachakis ND, Chan L. Response of thiazide-induced hypokalemia to amiloride. *JAMA* 249:237, 1983.
9. Coe FL, Parks JH, Asplin JR. The pathogenesis and treatment of kidney stones. *N Engl J Med* 327:1141, 1992.
10. Parks JH, Coe FL. A urinary calcium-citrate index for the evaluation of nephrolithiasis. *Kidney Int* 30:85, 1986.
11. Muldowney FP, Freaney R, Moloney MF. Importance of dietary sodium in the hypercalciuric syndrome. *Kidney Int* 22:292, 1982.
12. Besarab A, Brown RS, Rubin NT, et al. Reversible renal failure following bilateral renal artery occlusive disease: clinical features, pathology, and the role of surgical revascularization. *JAMA* 235:2838, 1976.

13. Danovitch GM, Bourgoignie JJ, Bricker NS. Reversibility of the "salt-losing" tendency of chronic renal failure. *N Engl J Med* 296:15, 1977.

14. Steiner RW. Interpreting the fractional excretion of sodium. *Am J Med* 77:699, 1984.

15. Planas M, Wachtel T, Frank H, Henderson LW. Characterization of acute renal failure in the burned patient. *Arch Intern Med* 142:2087, 1982.

16. Diamond JR, Yoburn DC. Nonoliguric acute renal failure associated with a low fractional excretion of sodium. *Ann Intern Med* 96:597, 1982.

17. Fang LST, Sirota RA, Ebert TH, Lichtenstein NS. Low fractional excretion of sodium with contrast media–induced acute renal failure. *Arch Intern Med* 140:531, 1980.

18. Steinhaulin F, Burnier M, Magnin JL, et al. Fractional excretion of trace lithium and uric acid in acute renal failure. *J Am Soc Nephrol* 4:1429, 1994.

19. Sherman RA, Eisinger RP. The use (and misuse) of urinary sodium and chloride measurements. *JAMA* 247:3121, 1982.

20. Kamel KS, Ethier JH, Richardson RMA, et al. Urine electrolytes and osmolality: When and how to use them. *Am J Nephrol* 10:89, 1990.

21. Batlle DC, Hizon M, Cohen E, et al. The use of the urine anion gap in the diagnosis of hyperchloremic metabolic acidosis. *N Engl J Med* 318:594, 1988.

22. Goldstein MB, Bear R, Richardson RMA, et al. The urine anion gap: A clinically useful index of ammonium excretion. *Am J Med Sci* 292:198, 1986.

23. Squires RD, Huth EJ. Experimental potassium depletion in normal human subjects. I. Relation on ionic intakes to the renal conservation of potassium. *J Clin Invest* 38:1134, 1959.

24. Talbott JH, Schwab RS. Recent advances in the biochemistry and therapeusis of potassium salts. *N Engl J Med* 222:585, 1940.

25. Rabelink TJ, Koomans HA, Hené RJ, Dorhout Mees EJ. Early and late adjustment to potassium loading in humans. *Kidney Int* 38:942, 1990.

26. Sporn IN, Lancestremere RG, Papper S. Differential diagnosis of oliguria in aged patients. *N Engl J Med* 267:130, 1962.

27. Levinsky NG, Davidson DG, Berliner RW. Effects of reduced glomerular filtration and urine concentration in presence of antidiuretic hormone. *J Clin Invest* 38:730, 1959.

28. Zwelling LA, Balow JE. Hypersthenuria in high-dose carbenicillin therapy. *Ann Intern Med* 89:225, 1978.

29. Coe FL. Uric acid and calcium oxalate nephrolithiasis. *Kidney Int* 24:392, 1983.

HYPOVOLEMIC STATES

In variety of clinical disorders, fluid losses lead to depletion of the extracellular fluid. This problem, if severe, can cause a potentially fatal decrease in tissue perfusion. Fortunately, early diagnosis and treatment can restore normovolemia in almost all cases.

ETIOLOGY

True volume depletion occurs when fluid is lost from the extracellular fluid at a rate exceeding net intake. These losses may occur from the gastrointestinal tract, skin, or lungs; in the urine; or by acute sequestration in the body in a "third space" that is not in equilibrium with the extracellular fluid (Table 14-1).

When these losses occur, two factors tend to protect against the development of hypovolemia. First, dietary Na^+ and water intake are generally far above basal needs. Thus, relatively large losses must occur unless intake is concomitantly reduced (as with anorexia or vomiting). Second, the kidney normally minimizes further urinary losses by enhancing Na^+ and water reabsorption.

The adaptive renal response explains why patients given a diuretic for hypertension do not develop progressive volume depletion. Although a thiazide diuretic

Table 14-1 Etiology of true volume depletion

A. Gastrointestinal losses
   1. Gastric: vomiting or nasogastric suction
   2. Intestinal, pancreatic, or biliary: diarrhea, fistulas, ostomies, or tube drainage
   3. Bleeding
B. Renal losses
   1. Salt and water: diuretics, osmotic diuresis, adrenal insufficiency, or salt-wasting nephropathies
   2. Water: central or nephrogenic diabetes insipidus
C. Skin and respiratory losses
   1. Insensible losses from skin and respiratory tract
   2. Sweat
   3. Burns
   4. Other: skin lesions, drainage and reformation of large pleural effusion, or bronchorrhea
D. Sequestration into a third space
   1. Intestinal obstruction or peritonitis
   2. Crush injury of skeletal fractures
   3. Acute pancreatitis
   4. Bleeding
   5. Obstruction of a major venous system

inhibits NaCl reabsorption in the distal tubule, the initial volume loss stimulates the renin-angiotensin-aldosterone system (and possibly other compensatory mechanisms), resulting in increased proximal and collecting tubule Na^+ reabsorption.[1,2] This balances the diuretic effect, resulting in the attainment *within 1 to 2 weeks* of a *new steady state in which there has been some fluid loss, but, in which Na^+ intake and excretion are again equal* (see Fig. 15-2).[3]

Gastronintestinal Losses

Each day approximately 3 to 6 liters of fluid is secreted by the stomach, pancreas, gallbladder, and intestines into the lumen of the gastrointestinal tract. Almost all this fluid is reabsorbed, with only 100 to 200 mL being lost in the stool. However, volume depletion may ensue if reabsorption is decreased (as with external drainage) or secretion is increased (as with diarrhea).

Acid-base disturbances frequently occur with gastrointestinal losses, depending upon the site from which the fluid is lost. Secretions from the stomach contain high concentrations of H^+ and Cl^-. As a result, vomiting and nasogastric suction are generally associated with metabolic alkalosis. In contrast, intestinal, pancreatic, and biliary secretions are relatively alkaline, with high concentrations of HCO_3^-. Thus, the loss of these fluids due to diarrhea, laxative abuse, fistulas, ostomies, or tube drainage tends to cause metabolic acidosis. Hypokalemia is also commonly associated with these disorders, since K^+ is present in all gastrointestinal secretions.

Acute bleeding from any site in the gastrointestinal tract is another common cause of volume depletion. Electrolyte disturbances usually do not occur in this setting (except for shock-induced lactic acidosis), since it is plasma, not gastrointestinal secretions, that is lost.

Renal Losses

Under normal conditions, renal Na^+ and water excretion is adjusted to match intake. In a normal adult, approximately 130 to 180 liters is filtered across the glomerular capillaries each day. More than 98 to 99 percent of the filtrate is then reabsorbed by the tubules, resulting in a urine output averaging 1 to 2 L/day. Thus, a small (1 to 2 percent) reduction in tubular reabsorption can lead to a 2- to 4-liter increase in Na^+ and water excretion, which, if not replaced, can result in severe volume depletion.

NaCl and water loss A variety of conditions can lead to excessive urinary excretion of NaCl and water (Table 14-1). Diuretics, for example, inhibit active Na^+ transport at different sites in the nephron, resulting in an increased rate of excretion (see Chap. 15). Although they are frequently given to remove fluid in edematous patients, diuretics can produce true hypovolemia if used in excess.

The presence of large amounts of nonreabsorbed solutes in the tubule also can inhibit Na^+ and water reabsorption, resulting in an *osmotic diuresis*. The most common clinical example occurs in uncontrolled diabetes mellitus, in which glucose acts as the osmotic agent. With severe hyperglycemia, urinary losses can contribute to a net fluid deficit of as much as 8 to 10 liters (see Chap. 25).

Variable degrees of Na^+ wasting are also present in many renal diseases. Most patients with renal insufficiency [glomerular filtrate rate (GFR) less than 25 mL/min] are unable to maximally conserve Na^+ if acutely placed on a low-sodium diet. These patients may have an *obligatory* Na^+ loss of 10 to 40 meq/day, in contrast to normal subjects, who can lower Na^+ excretion to less than 5 meq/day.[4,5] This degree of Na^+ wasting is usually not important, since normal Na^+ balance is maintained as long as the patient is on a regular diet.

In rare cases, a more severe degree of Na^+ wasting is present in which obligatory urinary losses may exceed 100 meq of Na^+ and 2 liters of water per day. In this setting, hypovolemia will ensue unless the patient maintains a high Na^+ intake. This picture of a severe *salt-wasting nephropathy* is most often seen in tubular and interstitial diseases, such as medullary cystic kidney disease.[6,7]

Three factors are thought to contribute to this variable salt wasting: the osmotic diuresis produced by increased urea excretion in the remaining functioning nephrons; direct damage to the tubular epithelium, which, in severe cases, can impair the response to aldosterone; and, probably most important in chronic renal disease, an inability to acutely shut off natriuretic forces.[5,6,8] Patients with renal insufficiency tend to have a decreased number of functioning nephrons. If Na^+ intake remains normal, they must be able to augment Na^+ excretion per functioning nephron to maintain Na^+ balance. This requires a fall in tubular Na^+ reabsorption that may be mediated at least in part by a natriuretic hormone, such as atrial natriuretic peptide.

Thus, the salt wasting that occurs when Na^+ intake is abruptly lowered could represent persistent activation of these natriuretic forces. Consistent with this hypothesis is the observation that apparent salt wasters (with acute obligatory losses of as much as 300 meq/day) can maintain Na^+ balance on an intake of only 5 meq/day if intake is gradually reduced over a period of weeks rather than acutely.[5]

Therapy of renal salt wasting must be directed toward establishing the level of Na^+ intake required to maintain Na^+ balance. This can usually be determined empirically, as most patients will tolerate a daily intake above 1.5 to 2 g (60 to 80 meq). It should not be assumed, however, that a patient with salt wasting has a normal ability to excrete a Na^+ load. Some patients with renal insufficiency who become hypovolemic with Na^+ restriction may retain Na^+ and develop edema and hypertension if placed on a high-sodium diet. In these patients, the range of Na^+ intake compatible with the maintenance of Na^+ balance is relatively narrow.

The increase in urine output following relief of bilateral urinary tract obstruction is often considered to represent another example of renal salt wasting. This postobstructive diuresis, however, is in almost all cases *appropriate* in that it represents an attempt to excrete the fluid retained during the period of obstruction.[9,10] Thus, quantitative replacement of the urine output will lead to persistent volume expansion and a urine output that can exceed 10 L/day.

Although the diuresis is largely appropriate, some fluid therapy is required (e.g., 50 to 75 mL/h of half-isotonic saline), since there is often a mild sodium-wasting tendency, the severity of which is limited by the concurrent reduction in glomerular filtration rate and a modest concentrating defect due to downregulation of water channels.[11] Although the risk of volume depletion is minimal with this regimen, the patient should be monitored for signs such as hypotension, decreased skin turgor, or a rise in the blood urea nitrogen (BUN).

Water loss Volume depletion can also result from a selective increase in urinary water excretion. This is due to decreased water reabsorption in the collecting tubules, where antidiuretic hormone (ADH) promotes the reabsorption of water but not Na^+. As a result, an impairment in either ADH secretion (central diabetes insipidus) or the renal response to ADH (nephrogenic diabetes insipidus) may be associated with the excretion of relatively large volumes (over 10 L/day in severe cases) of dilute urine (see Chap. 24). This water loss is usually matched by an equivalent increase in water intake, since the initial elevation in the plasma osmolality and Na^+ concentration stimulates thirst. However, water loss, hypovolemia, and persistent hypernatremia will ensue in infants, comatose patients (neither of whom have ready access to water), or those with a defective thirst mechanism.

Skin and Respiratory Losses

Each day, approximately 700 to 1000 mL of water is lost by evaporation from the skin and respiratory tract (see Chap. 9). Since heat is required for the evaporation of water, these insensible losses play an important role in thermoregulation, allowing the dissipation of some of the heat generated from body metabolism. When external temperatures are high or metabolic heat production is increased (as with fever or exercise), further heat can be lost by the evaporation of sweat (a "sensible" loss) from the skin. Although sweat (Na^+ concentration equals 30 to 50 meq/L) production is low in the basal state, it can exceed 1 to 2 L/h in a subject exercising in a hot, dry climate.[12]*

Negative water balance due to these insensible and sensible losses is usually prevented by the thirst mechanism, similar to that in diabetes insipidus. However, the cumulative sweat Na^+ losses can lead to hypovolemia.

In addition to its role in thermoregulation, the skin acts as a barrier that prevents the loss of interstitial fluid to the external environment. When this barrier is interrupted by burns or exudative skin lesions, a large volume of fluid can be lost. This fluid has an electrolyte composition similar to that of the plasma and contains a variable amount of protein. Thus, the replacement therapy in a burn patient differs from that in a patient with increased insensible or sweat losses.

Although rare, pulmonary losses other than those by evaporation can lead to volume depletion. This most often occurs in patients who have either continuous drainage of an active, usually malignant pleural effusion or an alveolar cell carcinoma with a marked increase in bronchial secretions (Bronchorrhea).

Sequestration into a Third Space

Volume depletion can be produced by the loss of interstitial and intravascular fluid into a third space that is not in equilibrium with the extracellular fluid. For example, a patient with a fractured hip may lose 1500 to 2000 mL of blood into the tissues adjacent to the fracture. Although this fluid will be resorbed back into the extracellular fluid over a period of days to weeks, the acute reduction in blood volume, if not replaced, can lead to severe volume depletion. Other examples of this phenomenon include intestinal obstruction, severe pancreatitis, crush injuries, bleeding (as with trauma or a ruptured abdominal aortic aneurysm), peritonitis, and obstruction of a major venous system.

The main difference between these disorders and, for example, the development of ascites in cirrhosis is the *rate of fluid accumulation*. Cirrhotic ascites develops relatively slowly, allowing time for renal Na^+ and water reten-

---

* These fluid losses represent only a small part of the hemodynamic stress induced by exercise in this setting. The required increases in muscle blood flow (to provide nutrients and remove waste products) and in cutaneous blood flow (to allow heat loss) can exceed 10 L/min in some cases.[12]

tion to replenish the effective circulating volume (see Chap. 16). As a result, cirrhotic patients typically have symptoms of edema rather than those of hypovolemia.

HEMODYNAMIC RESPONSES TO VOLUME DEPLETION

Volume depletion induces a characteristic sequence of compensatory hemodynamic responses. The initial volume deficit results in decreases in the plasma volume and venous return to the heart. The latter is sensed by the cardiopulmonary receptors in the atria and pulmonary veins, leading to sympathetically mediated vasoconstriction in skin and skeletal muscle.[13] This effect, which shunts blood toward the more important cerebral and coronary circulations, is mediated by partial removal of the tonic inhibition of sympathetic tone normally induced by these receptors.

More marked volume depletion leads to a reduction in cardiac output. From the relationship between mean arterial pressure, cardiac output, and systemic vascular resistance,*

Mean arterial pressure = cardiac output × systemic vascular resistance

the fall in cardiac output lowers the systemic blood pressure. This hemodynamic change is sensed by the carotid sinus and aortic arch baroreceptors, which induce a more generalized increase in sympathetic activity that now involves the splanchnic and renal circulations.

The net effect is relative maintenance of cerebral and coronary perfusion and return of the arterial pressure toward normal. The latter is mediated by increases in venous return (mediated in part by active venoconstriction), cardiac contractility, and heart rate (all of which act to elevate the cardiac output) and increases in vascular resistance due both to direct sympathetic effects and to enhanced secretion of renin from the kidney, resulting in the generation of angiotensin II.[13]

If the volume deficit is small (about 10 percent of the blood volume, which is equivalent to donating 500 mL of blood), these sympathetic effects return the cardiac output and blood pressure to normal or near normal, although the heart rate is likely to be increased.[14] In contrast, a marked fall in blood pressure will ensue if the sympathetic response does not occur—for example, because of autonomic insufficiency.[15,16]

With more severe hypovolemia (16 to 25 percent of the blood volume), there is more pronounced sympathetic and angiotensin II–mediated vasoconstriction. Although this may maintain the blood pressure when the patient is recumbent, hypotension can occur when the upright position is assumed, leading to postural dizziness. At this point, the compensatory sympathetic responses are maximal, and

---

* The product of the cardiac output and systemic vascular resistance actually equals the *change in pressure* across the circulation—mean arterial pressure minus mean venous pressure. However, the venous pressure (normal equals 1 to 7 mmHg) is normally much lower than the arterial pressure. As a result, only a slight error results from ignoring the venous pressure.

any further fluid loss will induce marked hypotension, even in recumbency, and eventually shock (see below).[14,17]

SYMPTOMS

Three sets of symptoms can occur in hypovolemic patients: (1) those related to the manner in which fluid loss occurs, such as vomiting, diarrhea, or polyuria; (2) those due to volume depletion; and (3) those due to the electrolyte and acid-base disorders that can accompany volume depletion.

The symptoms induced by hypovolemia are primarily related to the decrease in tissue perfusion. The earliest complaints include lassitude, easy fatigability, thirst, muscle cramps, and postural dizziness. More severe fluid loss can lead to abdominal pain, chest pain, or lethargy and confusion as a result of mesenteric, coronary, or cerebral ischemia. These symptoms usually are reversible, although tissue necrosis may develop if the low-flow state is allowed to persist.

Symptomatic hypovolemia most often occurs in patients with isosmotic Na^+ and water depletion in whom most of the fluid deficit comes from the extracellular fluid. In contrast, in patients with pure water loss due to insensible losses or diabetes insipidus, the elevation in plasma osmolality (and Na^+ concentration) causes water to move down an osmotic gradient from the cells into the extracellular fluid. The net result is that about *two-thirds of the water lost comes from the intracellular fluid.* Consequently, these patients are likely to exhibit the symptoms of hypernatremia (produced by the water deficit) before those of marked extracellular fluid depletion.

A variety of electrolyte and acid-base disorders also may occur, depending upon the composition of the fluid that is lost (see below). The more serious symptoms produced by these disturbances include muscle weakness (hypokalemia and hyperkalemia); polyuria and polydipsia (hypokalemia and hyperglycemia); and lethargy, confusion, seizures, and coma (hyponatremia, hypernatremia, and hyperglycemia).

An additional symptom that appears to occur only in primary adrenal insufficiency is extreme salt craving. Approximately 20 percent of patients with this disorder give a history of heavily salting all foods (including those not usually salted) and even eating salt that they have sprinkled on their hands.[18] The mechanism responsible for this appropriate increase in salt intake is not known.

EVALUATION OF THE HYPOVOLEMIC PATIENT

The evaluation of the patient with suspected hypovolemia includes a careful history for a source of fluid loss, the physical examination, and appropriate laboratory studies. In many patients in whom the history does not provide a clear etiology, a common presumption, particularly in the elderly, is that unreplaced insensible losses are responsible. Evaporative and sweat losses are hypotonic and therefore must produce an elevation in the plasma Na^+ concentration if they are solely responsible for volume depletion. The presence of a normal plasma sodium indicates proportionate salt and water loss if the patient is truly hypovolemic.

These observations also help to avoid the common mistake of assuming that dehydration and volume depletion (or hypovolemia) are synonymous.[19] Volume depletion refers to extracellular volume depletion of any cause, most often due to salt and water loss. In contrast, dehydration refers to the presence of hypernatremia due to pure water loss; such patients are also hypovolemic.

Physical Examination

Although relatively insensitive and nonspecific,[20] certain findings on physical examination may suggest volume depletion. A decrease in the interstitial volume can be detected by examination of the skin and mucous membranes, while a decrease in the plasma volume can lead to reductions in systemic blood pressure and in venous pressure in the jugular veins.

Among patients with hypovolemia due to severe bleeding, the most sensitive and specific findings are severe postural dizziness (preventing measurement of upright vital signs) and/or a postural pulse increment of 30 beats/min or more.[20] Among patients with mild to moderate blood loss or other causes of hypovolemia (vomiting, diarrhea, decreased intake), few findings have proven predictive value, and laboratory confirmation of the presence of volume depletion is typically required.[20]

Skin and mucous membranes   If the skin and subcutaneous tissue on the thigh, calf, or forearm is pinched in normal subjects, it will immediately return to its normally flat state when the pinch is released. This elastic property, called *turgor*, is partially dependent upon the interstitial volume of the skin and subcutaneous tissue. Interstitial fluid loss leads to diminished turgor, and the skin flattens more slowly after the pinch is released. In younger patients, the presence of decreased skin and subcutaneous tissue turgor is a reliable indicator of volume depletion. However, elasticity diminishes with age, so that reduced turgor does not necessarily reflect hypovolemia in older patients (more than 55 to 60 years old). In these patients, skin elasticity is usually best preserved on the inner aspect of the thighs and the skin overlying the sternum. Decreased turgor at these sites is suggestive of volume depletion.

Although reduced skin turgor is an important clinical finding, *normal turgor does not exclude the presence of hypovolemia*. This is particularly true with mild volume deficits, in young patients whose skin is very elastic, and in obese patients, since fat deposits under the skin prevent the changes in subcutaneous turgor from being appreciated.

In addition to having reduced turgor, the skin is usually dry; a dry axilla is particularly suggestive of the presence of hypovolemia.[20] The tongue and oral mucosa may also be dry, since salivary secretions are commonly decreased in this setting.

Examination of the skin also may be helpful in the diagnosis of primary adrenal insufficiency. The impaired release of cortisol in this disorder leads to hypersecretion of adrenocorticotropic hormone (ACTH), which can result in increased pigmentation of the skin, especially in the palmar creases and buccal mucosa.

Arterial blood pressure   As described above, the arterial blood pressure changes from near normal with mild hypovolemia to low in the upright position and then, with progressive volume depletion, to persistently low regardless of posture. Postural hypotension leading to dizziness may be the patient's major complaint and is strongly suggestive of hypovolemia in the absence of an autonomic neuropathy or the use of sympatholytic drugs for hypertension, or in elderly subjects, in whom postural hypotension is common in the absence of hypovolemia.

An important change that can occur with marked fluid loss is that the secondary neurohumoral vasoconstriction leads to decreased intensity of both the Korotkoff sounds (when the blood pressure is being measured with a sphygmomanometer) and the radial pulse.[17,21] As a result, a very low blood pressure suggested by auscultation or palpation may actually be associated with a *near-normal pressure* when measured directly by an intraarterial catheter.

It is important to appreciate that the definition of normal blood pressure in this setting is dependent upon the patient's basal value. Although 120/80 is considered "normal," it is actually low in a hypertensive patient whose usual blood pressure is 180/100.

Venous pressure   The reduction in the vascular volume seen with hypovolemia occurs primarily in the venous circulation (which normally contains 70 percent of the blood volume), leading to a decrease in venous pressure. As a result, measurement of the venous pressure is useful both in the diagnosis of hypovolemia and in assessing the adequacy of volume replacement.[22]

In most patients, the venous pressure can be estimated with sufficient accuracy by examination of the external jugular vein, which runs across the sternocleidomastoid muscle. The patient should initially be recumbent, with the trunk elevated at 15 to 30 degrees and the head turned slightly away from the side to be examined. The external jugular vein can be identified by placing the forefinger just above the clavicle and pressing lightly. This will occlude the vein, which will then distend as blood continues to enter from the cerebral circulation. The external jugular vein usually can be seen more easily by shining a beam of light obliquely across the neck.

At this point, the occlusion at the clavicle should be released and the vein occluded superiorly to prevent distention by continued blood flow. The venous pressure can now be measured, since it will be approximately equal to the *vertical distance* between the upper level of the fluid column within the vein and the level of the right atrium (estimated as being 5 to 6 cm posterior to the sternal angle of Louis). If the vein is distended throughout its length, the patient's trunk should be elevated to 45 or even 90 degrees until an upper level can be seen. In a patient with a markedly increased venous pressure due to right ventricular failure, the external jugular vein may remain distended even when the patient is upright. The normal venous pressure is 1 to 8 cmH_2O or 1 to 6 mmHg (1.36 cmH_2O is equal to 1.00 mmHg).

There are some limitations to the use of this technique. For example, the external jugular vein may not become visible when it is occluded at the clavicle, particularly in those patients with a fat neck. If this occurs, it should not be reported that the venous pressure is very low. Rather, the venous pressure should be measured in some other way, such as by estimation of the *level of pulsations in the internal jugular vein* or directly by insertion of a catheter into the right atrium.

A much less common problem is kinking or obstruction of the external jugular vein at the base of the neck. In this setting, there is an increase in the external jugular venous pressure that does not reflect a similar change in right atrial pressure. This possibility should be suspected if an elevated venous pressure is found in a patient with no evidence or history of cardiac or pulmonary disease.

Relationship between right atrial and left atrial pressures   The filling pressures in the heart are important determinants of cardiac output, since the contractility of cardiac muscle and therefore the stroke volume increases as the filling pressure is increased (Fig. 14-1). If there is no obstruction to flow across the mitral valve, the left atrial pressure will be equal to the left ventricular end-diastolic pressure (LVEDP), that is, to the filling pressure in the left ventricle. The left atrial pressure can be estimated clinically by measurement of the pulmonary capillary wedge pressure with a flow-directed balloon catheter (such as a Swan-Ganz catheter).

In general, there is a predictable relationship between the right and left atrial pressures, with the latter being greater by approximately 5 mmHg (Fig. 14-2).[23] When the right atrial (or central venous) pressure is reduced, the LVEDP also is decreased, and this tends to lower the cardiac output. Conversely, a high central venous pressure is associated with a high left atrial pressure, which predisposes toward the development of pulmonary edema.

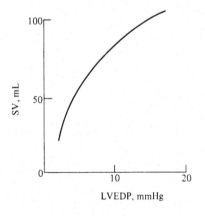

Figure 14-1 Frank-Starling curve relating stroke volume (SV) to left ventricular end-diastolic pressure (LVEDP). (*Adapted from Cohn JN, Am J Med 55:351, 1973, with permission.*)

Although it is the LVEDP (not the right atrial pressure) that is the important determinant of left ventricular output and therefore tissue perfusion, measurement of the central venous pressure is useful because of its direct relationship to the LVEDP. There are, however, two clinical settings in which the central venous or right atrial pressure is not an accurate estimate of the LVEDP (Fig. 14-2). In patients with pure left-sided heart failure (as with an acute myocardial infarction), the wedge pressure is increased but the central venous pressure may remain unchanged if right ventricular function is normal. In this setting, treating a low central venous pressure with volume expanders can precipitate pulmonary edema. On the other hand, the central venous pressure tends to exceed the LVEDP in patients with pure right-sided heart failure (as with cor pulmonale). These patients may have high central venous pressures even in the presence of volume depletion; as a result, the central venous pressure cannot be used as a guide to therapy.

Shock   The symptoms and physical findings that have been described apply to patients with mild to moderate volume depletion who are still able to maintain an adequate level of tissue perfusion. However, as the degree of hypovolemia becomes more severe, due, for example, to the loss of 30 percent of the blood volume from a ruptured aortic aneurysm, there is a marked reduction in tissue perfusion, resulting in a clinical syndrome referred to as hypovolemic shock.[14,17] This syndrome is associated with a marked increase in sympathetic activity and is characterized by tachycardia; cold, clammy extremities; cyanosis; a low urine out-

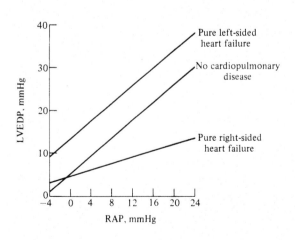

Figure 14-2 Relationship between left ventricular end-diastolic pressure (LVEDP) and mean right atrial pressure (RAP) in three groups of patients. In subjects without cardiopulmonary disease, the LVEDP exceeds the RAP by about 5 mmHg and varies directly with the RAP. In patients with pure right-sided heart failure, e.g., due to chronic pulmonary disease, relatively large changes in the RAP can occur with little change in the LVEDP. In contrast, the LVEDP is much greater than the RAP in patients with pure left-sided heart failure, e.g., due to an acute myocardial infarction. This graph is somewhat simplified, since the standard deviations within each group have been omitted. (*Adapted from Cohn JN, Tristani FE, Khatri IM*, J Clin Invest *48:2008, 1969, by copyright permission of the American Society for Clinical Investigation.*)

put (usually less than 15 mL/h); and agitation and confusion due to reduced cerebral blood flow. Although hypotension is generally present, it is not required for the diagnosis of shock, since some patients vasoconstrict enough to maintain a relatively normal blood pressure. Therapy to restore tissue perfusion must be begun immediately to prevent both ischemic tissue damage and irreversible shock (see below).

Laboratory Data

Hypovolemia can produce a variety of changes in the composition of the urine and blood (Table 14-2). In addition to confirming the presence of volume depletion, these changes can give important clues to the pathogenesis of the fluid loss and to the appropriate replacement therapy.

Urine sodium concentration The response of the kidney to volume depletion is to conserve Na^+ and water in an attempt to expand the extracellular volume. Except in those disorders in which Na^+ reabsorption is impaired, the urine Na^+ concentration in hypovolemic states should be less than 25 meq/L and may be as low as 1 meq/L (Table 14-3). This increase in tubular Na^+ reabsorption is mediated by several factors, including increased activity of the renin-angiotensin-aldosterone system, a fall in systemic blood pressure, and possibly reduced secretion of atrial natriuretic peptide (see Chap. 8).

The urine Cl^- concentration is usually similar to that of Na^+ in hypovolemic states, since Na^+ and Cl^- are generally reabsorbed together. An exception occurs when Na^+ is excreted with another anion.[24] This is most often seen in metabolic alkalosis, where the need to excrete the excess HCO_3^- (as $NaHCO_3$) may raise the urine Na^+ concentration despite the presence of volume depletion. In this setting, the urine Cl^- concentration remains low and is frequently a better index of volume status (see Chap. 18).[25] Thus, the urine Cl^- concentration should be measured when any apparently hypovolemic patient has what seems to be an inappropriately high urine Na^+ concentration.

Even if the physical examination is not diagnostic of hypovolemia, *a low urine Na^+ concentration is virtually pathognomonic of reduced tissue perfusion.* The major exception to this rule occurs with *selective* renal or glomerular hypoperfusion, as with bilateral renal artery stenosis or acute glomerulonephritis.[26,27] In these settings, there is avid renal Na^+ retention independent of systemic fluid balance.

Table 14-2 Laboratory changes in hypovolemic states

Urine N^+ concentration less than 20 meq/L
Urine osmolality greater than 450 mosmol/kg
BUN/plasma creatinine ratio greater than 20:1 with a normal urinalysis
Variable effects on plasma N^+, K^+, and HCO_3^- concentrations
Occasional elevations in the hematocrit and plasma albumin concentration

Table 14-3   Urine Na$^+$ concentration in volume depletion

Less than 20 meq/L	Greater than 40 meq/L
Gastrointestinal losses	Underlying renal disease
Skin losses	Diuretics (while the drug is acting)
Third-space losses	Osmotic diuresis
Diuretics (late)	Hypoaldosteronism
	Some patients with metabolic alkalosis

However, the presence of a low urine Na$^+$ concentration does not necessarily mean that the patient has true volume depletion, since edematous patients with heart failure or hepatic cirrhosis with ascites also avidly conserve Na$^+$. These disorders are characterized by *effective circulating volume depletion* due to a primary reduction in cardiac output (heart failure) or to splanchnic vasodilatation and sequestration of fluid in the peritoneal cavity (cirrhosis) (see Chap. 16). The differentiation between edematous states and true volume depletion usually is made easily from the physical examination.

An alternative to measurement of the urine Na$^+$ concentration is calculation of the fractional excretion of Na$^+$ (FE$_{Na}$). The FE$_{Na}$ is most useful in the differential diagnosis of acute renal failure with a very low glomerular filtration rate; in this setting, the FE$_{Na}$ is usually under 1 percent in hypovolemic patients.[27,28] The FE$_{Na}$ is more difficult to evaluate in patients with a normal glomerular filtration rate, since the filtered Na$^+$ load is so high in this setting that a differential value (FE$_{Na}$ < 0.1 to 0.2 percent) must be used to diagnose volume depletion (see Chap. 13).

Urine osmolality   The renal retention of water in hypovolemic states is mediated in part by ADH, which is secreted in response to the decrease in tissue perfusion (see Chap. 6). As a result, the urine is relatively concentrated, with an osmolality often exceeding 450 mosmol/kg.[27-29] This response may not be seen, however, if concentrating ability is impaired by renal disease, an osmotic diuresis, the administration of diuretics, or central or nephrogenic diabetes insipidus. For example, both severe volume depletion (which impairs urea accumulation in the renal medulla)[28] and hypokalemia (which induces ADH resistance; see Fig. 12-1) can limit the increase in the urine osmolality in some patients. Thus, a high urine osmolality is consistent with hypovolemia, but a relatively isosmotic value does not exclude this disorder.[29]

Urinary concentration can also be assessed by measuring the specific gravity.[30] This test, however, is less accurate than the osmolality, since it is dependent upon the size as well as the number of solute particles in the urine (see Fig. 13-1). As a result, it should be used only if the osmolality cannot be measured; a value above 1.015 is suggestive of a concentrated urine, as is usually seen with hypovolemia.

BUN and plasma creatinine concentration   In most circumstances, the blood urea nitrogen (BUN) and plasma creatinine concentration vary inversely with the GFR, increasing as the GFR falls (see Fig. 2-11). Thus, serial measurements of these parameters can be used to assess the course of renal disease. However, an elevation in the BUN can also be produced by an increase in the rate of urea production or tubular reabsorption. As a result, the plasma creatinine concentration is a more reliable estimate of the GFR, since it is produced at a relatively constant rate by skeletal muscle and is not reabsorbed by the renal tubules.

In normal subjects and those with uncomplicated renal disease, the BUN/plasma creatinine ratio is approximately 10:1. However, this value may be substantially elevated in hypovolemic states, because of the associated increase in tubular reabsorption.[31] In general, approximately 40 to 50 percent of filtered urea is reabsorbed, much of this occurring in the proximal tubule, where it is passively linked to the reabsorption of Na^+ and water (see Chap. 3). Thus, the increase in proximal Na^+ reabsorption in volume depletion produces a parallel rise in urea reabsorption. The net effect is a fall in urea excretion and elevations in the BUN and the BUN/plasma creatinine ratio, often to greater than 20:1. This selective rise in the BUN is called *prerenal azotemia*. The plasma creatinine concentration will increase in this setting only if the degree of hypovolemia is severe enough to lower the GFR.

Although the BUN/plasma creatinine ratio is helpful in the evaluation of hypovolemic patients, it is subject to misinterpretation, since it is also affected by the rate of urea production. A high ratio may be due solely to increased urea production (as with gastrointestinal bleeding), whereas a normal ratio may occur in some patients with hypovolemia if urea production is reduced. This can be illustrated by the following example:

Case History 14-1   A 40-year-old man with a history of peptic ulcer disease is seen after 2 weeks of persistent vomiting. On physical examination, the patient's blood pressure is normal, but his estimated jugular venous pressure is less than $5 \, cmH_2O$ and skin turgor is reduced. The laboratory data include

BUN	=	42 mg/dL
Plasma creatinine	=	3.6 mg/dL
Urine Na^+	=	7 meq/L
Urine osmolality	=	502 mosmol/kg

Comment   The low urine Na^+ concentration, the high urine osmolality, and the physical examination are all suggestive of hypovolemia. This diagnosis was subsequently confirmed by return of the BUN and plasma creatine concentration to normal levels with volume repletion. The failure of the initial BUN to increase out of proportion to the plasma creatinine concentration probably reflected the reduction in protein intake due to vomiting.

Urinalysis Examination of the urine is an important diagnostic tool in patients with elevations in the BUN and plasma creatinine concentration. The urinalysis is generally normal in hypovolemic states, since the kidney is not diseased. This is in contrast to most of the other causes of renal insufficiency, in which the urinalysis reveals protein, cells, and/or casts.[29]

Hypovolemia and renal disease The laboratory diagnosis of hypovolemia may be difficult to establish in patients with underlying renal disease. In this setting, the urine Na^+ concentration may exceed 25 meq/L and the urine osmolality may be less than 350 mosmol/kg, since renal insufficiency impairs the ability to maximally conserve Na^+ and to concentrate the urine.[29,32] In addition, the urinalysis may be abnormal as a result of the primary disease.

Despite these difficulties, making the correct diagnosis is important, since volume depletion is a *reversible* cause of worsening renal function, in contrast to progression of the underlying renal disease. The history and physical examination (possibly vomiting, diarrhea, use of diuretics, or decreased skin turgor) may be helpful in some patients, but these findings are not always present. As a result, a cautious trial of fluid repletion may be warranted in a patient whose renal function has deteriorated without obvious cause.

Plasma sodium concentration A variety of factors can influence the plasma Na^+ concentration in hypovolemic states, and it is the interplay between them that determines the level seen in a given patient (Table 14-4). Volume depletion is a potent stimulus to both ADH release and thirst. The ensuing increases in renal water reabsorption and water intake can lead to water retention and the development of *hyponatremia*. On the other hand, *hypernatremia* can occur when water is lost in excess of solute. This can be seen with unreplaced insensible or sweat losses and with central or nephrogenic diabetes insipidus. Diminished thirst, usually due to impaired mentation, is essential for the plasma Na^+ concentration to rise in these disorders. The ability to increase water intake is normally an effective defense against the development of hypernatremia; patients with diabetes insipidus, for example, typically present with polyuria (that can exceed 10 L/day) and polydipsia, but a relatively normal plasma Na^+ concentration.

The osmotic effect of gastrointestinal losses is variable. Although the fluid lost is generally isosmotic to plasma, it is important to appreciate that the *plasma Na^+ concentration is normally determined by three factors: total exchangeable Na^+, total*

Table 14-4 Plasma Na^+ concentration in volume depletion

May be greater than 150 meq/L	May be less than 135 meq/L
Insensible and sweat losses	All other forms of volume depletion
Central or nephrogenic diabetes insipidus	
Uncontrolled diabetes mellitus	

exchangeable K^+, and total body water (see page 248). Secretory diarrheas, for example, tend to be pure electrolyte solutions, containing Na^+ and K^+ salts in a concentration similar to that in the plasma.[33] As a result, loss of this fluid will lead to volume depletion but no direct change in the plasma Na^+ concentration.

In comparison, osmotic diarrheas (as seen with malabsorption, certain infections, and the administration of lactulose) contain nonreabsorbed solutes and tend to have Na^+ plus K^+ concentrations of 50 to 100 meq/L, well below that in the plasma.[33,34] Thus, water is lost in excess of Na^+ plus K^+, a change that will raise the plasma Na^+ concentration. Hypernatremia may not be seen, however, because of the possible counterbalancing effects of increased water intake and renal water retention. Thus, the *plasma Na^+ concentration may be low, normal, or elevated in patients with diarrhea.*

Similar principles apply to the osmotic diuresis seen with uncontrolled diabetes mellitus. In this setting, the urine is often hyperosmotic to plasma, because of the hypovolemia-induced stimulation of ADH release. Much of the urinary solute, however, is glucose, and the urine Na^+ plus K^+ concentration is typically less than that in the plasma. As a result, the plasma Na^+ concentration will tend to rise. However, this does not usually lead to hypernatremia, since the initial plasma Na^+ concentration is often below normal in these patients. The rise in plasma osmolality induced by hyperglycemia pulls water out of the cells, thereby lowering the plasma Na^+ concentration by dilution (see Chap. 25). Thus, the final plasma Na^+ concentration is variable, being determined by the degree of hyperglycemia, water intake, and the amount of water lost in the urine.

Plasma potassium concentration Either hypokalemia or hyperkalemia can occur in hypovolemic patients. The former is much more common, because there is concurrent K^+ loss from the gastrointestinal tract or in the urine. Hyperkalemia may be seen in several settings. First, the plasma K^+ concentration may be elevated in some forms of metabolic acidosis. As some of the excess H^+ ions enter the cells to be buffered, intracellular K^+ moves into the extracellular fluid to maintain electroneutrality (see Chap. 12). Thus, a patient may have an elevated plasma K^+ concentration even if total body K^+ stores are reduced. Second, there may be an inability to excrete the dietary K^+ load in the urine because of renal failure, hypoaldosteronism, or volume depletion itself, since the delivery of Na^+ and water to the K^+ secretory site in the cortical collecting tubule will be reduced.[35]

Acid-base balance The effect of fluid loss on acid-base balance also is variable. Although many patients maintain a normal extracellular pH, either metabolic alkalosis or metabolic acidosis can occur (Table 14-5). Patients with vomiting or nasogastric suction and those given diuretics tend to develop metabolic alkalosis because of H^+ loss and volume contraction (see Chap. 18). On the other hand, HCO_3^- loss (due to diarrhea or intestinal fistulas) or reduced renal H^+ excretion (due to renal failure or hypoaldosteronism) can lead to metabolic acidosis. In addition, lactic acidosis can occur in shock and ketoacidosis in uncontrolled diabetes mellitus.

Table 14-5 Acid-base disorders that may occur in volume depletion

Metabolic acidosis	Metabolic alkalosis
Diarrhea or loss of other lower intestinal, pancreatic, or biliary secretions	Vomiting or nasogastric suction
Renal failure	Loop or thiazide diuretics
Hypoaldosteronism	
Ketoacidosis in uncontrolled diabetes mellitus	
Lactic acidosis in shock	

Hematocrit and plasma albumin concentration Since the red blood cells and albumin are essentially limited to the vascular space, a reduction in the plasma volume due to volume depletion tends to elevate both the hematocrit and the plasma albumin concentration. These changes, however, are frequently absent because of underlying anemia and/or hypoalbuminemia, due, for example, to bleeding or renal disease.

Summary

An accurate history and physical examination can help to determine both the presence and the etiology of volume depletion. In the patient in whom the diagnosis cannot be made from the history, laboratory data can provide important clues to the correct diagnosis. This can be demonstrated by the following example.

Case History 14-2 A 38-year-old woman is admitted with a 2-day history of weakness and postural dizziness. She denies vomiting, diarrhea, melena, or drugs. On physical examination, the blood pressure is 110/60 recumbent and falls to 80/50 erect. The pulse is 100 and regular. The estimated jugular venous pressure is less than 5 cmH$_2$O, the skin turgor is poor, and the mucous membranes are dry. The laboratory data include

Plasma [Na$^+$]	= 140 meq/L	Arterial pH	=	7.25
[K$^+$]	= 3.2 meq/L	P$_{CO_2}$	=	28 mmHg
[Cl$^-$]	= 116 meq/L	Urine [Na$^+$]	=	9 meq/L
[HCO$_3^-$]	= 12 meq/L	Osmolality	=	584 mosmol/kg
BUN	= 40 mg/dL			
[Creatinine]	= 1.3 mg/dL			

Comment Although the etiology is not apparent from the history, the physical examination is consistent with moderately severe volume depletion. The low urine Na^+ concentration suggests that renal function is normal and that renal salt wasting and adrenal insufficiency are not responsible for the hypovolemia. The presence of metabolic acidosis and hypokalemia suggests that diarrhea is responsible for the fluid loss. Upon closer questioning, a history of laxative abuse with multiple bowel movements each day is obtained.

TREATMENT

Both oral and intravenous replacement fluids can be administered for volume replacement in the hypovolemic patient. The aims of therapy are to restore normovolemia and to correct any associated acid-base or electrolyte disorders that may be present.

Oral Therapy

In patients with mild volume depletion, increasing dietary Na^+ and water intake either by altering the diet or by using NaCl tablets may be sufficient to correct the volume deficit. Oral solutions containing glucose (or cereals that are composed of starch polymers such as rise) and electrolytes can also be used to treat persistent or severe diarrhea, as in cholera.[36-38] The addition of glucose both provides extra calories and promotes small intestinal Na^+ reabsorption, since there is coupled transport of Na^+ and glucose at this site, similar to that in the proximal tubule (see page 90). The rice-based solutions are generally more effective than glucose alone (particularly in cholera), since the digestion of rice provides both more glucose (50 to 80 g/L versus 20 g/L with glucose alone) and amino acids (which can also promote intestinal sodium absorption).[36]

Intravenous Solutions

With more severe hypovolemia or in patients unable to take oral fluids, volume repletion requires the administration of intravenous fluids. A wide variety of intravenous solutions are available. The compositions of the most commonly used solutions are listed in Table 14-6. The content of each solution determines the clinical situation in which it will be most useful.

Dextrose solutions   Since glucose is rapidly metabolized to $CO_2 + H_2O$, the administration of dextrose solutions is physiologically equivalent to administering distilled water.* The main indication for the use of dextrose in water is to provide free water to replace insensible losses or to correct hypernatremia due to a water deficit. More concentrated dextrose solutions (20% and 50%) are available and

---

* Distilled water cannot be given intravenously, because it will produce potentially fatal hemolysis due to water movement into red cells. This problem is prevented by the addition of an osmotically active solute such as dextrose.

are used to provide extra calories (1 g of glucose equals 4 kcal). Hyperglycemia is a potential risk with these solutions, and careful monitoring is warranted.

Saline solutions Most hypovolemic patients are both Na^+- and water-depleted. In this situation, isotonic, hypotonic, or hypertonic saline solutions can be used to correct both deficits. Isotonic saline (0.9%) has a Na^+ concentration of 154 meq/ L, similar to that in the plasma water (see page 000). Half-isotonic saline (0.45%, Na^+ concentration of 77 meq/L) is more dilute than the plasma, and each liter can be viewed as being composed of 550 mL of isotonic saline and 500 mL of free water. On the other hand, hypertonic saline (3%, Na^+ concentration of 513 meq/ L) is more concentrated than the plasma, and each liter can be viewed as containing 1000 mL of isotonic saline plus 359 meq of extra Na^+.

The plasma Na^+ concentration can be used to help determine which solution should be given. For example, half-isotonic saline (or dextrose in quarter-isotonic saline) contains free water and should be administered to patients with hypernatremia, who have a greater deficit of water than of solute. On the other hand, hypovolemic patients with hyponatremia have a greater deficit of solute than of water and should be treated with isotonic or hypertonic saline (see Chap. 23). If the plasma Na^+ concentration is normal, either half-isotonic or isotonic saline can be given. The former has the advantage of containing free water, which can replace continued insensible water losses.

Dextrose in saline solutions The indications for the use of these solutions are the same as those for the saline solutions. The addition of glucose provides a small amount of calories (5% dextrose equals to 50 g/L of glucose or 200 kcal/L).

Alkalinizing solutions The primary uses of $NaHCO_3$ are in the treatment of metabolic acidosis or severe hyperkalemia. $NaHCO_3$ is most commonly administered as a 7.5% solution in 50-mL ampules containing 44 meq of Na^+ and 44 meq of HCO_3^-. This can be given intravenously over 5 min or added to another intravenous solution. However, $NAHCO_3$ should not be added to solutions containing calcium, such as Ringer's lactate, since Ca^{2+} and HCO_3^- can combine to form the insoluble salt $CaCO_3$

Polyionic solutions Ringer's solution contains physiologic concentrations of K^+ and Ca^{2+} in addition to NaCl. Lactated Ringer's solution has a composition even closer to that of the extracellular fluid, containing 28 meq of lactate per liter, which is rapidly metabolized into HCO_3^- in the body. Although they may seem more physiologic, there is no evidence that these solutions offer any advantages when compared with isotonic saline. Furthermore, lactated Ringer's solution should not be used in lactic acidosis, since the ability to convert lactate into HCO_3^- is impaired in this disorder.

Potassium chloride KCl is available in a highly concentrated solution containing 2 meq/mL of K^+. When used to repair a K^+ deficit, 10 to 60 meq of K^+ (5 to

Table 14-6 Composition of commonly used intravenous solutions[a]

Solution	Solute	Concentrations, g/100 mL	Ionic concentration, meq/L					
			[Na$^+$]	[K$^+$]	[Ca^{2+}]	[Cl$^-$]	[HCO$_3^-$]	Total mosmol/L
Dextrose in water								
5.0%	Glucose	5.0	—	—	—	—	—	278
10%	Glucose	10.0	—	—	—	—	—	556
Saline								
Hypotonic (0.45%, half-normal)	NaCl	0.45	77	—	—	77	—	154
Isotonic (0.9%, normal)	NaCl	0.90	154	—	—	154	—	308
Hypertonic	NaCl	3.0	513	—	—	513	—	1026
	NaCl	5.0	855	—	—	855	—	1710
Dextrose in saline								
5% in 0.225%	Glucose	5.0	—	—	—	—	—	—
	NaCl	0.225	38.5	—	—	38.5	—	355
5% in 0.45%	Glucose	5.0	—	—	—	—	—	—
	NaCl	0.45	77	—	—	77	—	432
5% in 0.9%	Glucose	5.0	—	—	—	—	—	—
	NaCl	0.90	154	—	—	154	—	586
Alkalinizing solutions								
Hypertonic sodium bicarbonate (0.6M)	NaHCO$_3$	5.0	595	—	—	—	595	1190
Hypertonic sodium bicarbonate (0.9M)[b]	NaHCO$_3$	7.5	893	—	—	—	893	1786
Polyionic solutions								
Ringer's	NaCl	0.86	147	—	—	156	—	309
	KCl	0.03	—	4	—	—	—	—
	CaCl$_2$	0.03	—	—	5	—	—	—

	Content (g/100 mL)	Na⁺	K⁺	Ca²⁺	Cl⁻	Lactate	mOsm/L
Lactated Ringer's		130	4	3	109	28[c]	274
NaCl	0.60	—	—	—	—	—	—
KCl	0.03	—	—	—	—	—	—
CaCl₂	0.02	—	—	—	—	—	—
Na lactate	0.31	—	—	—	—	—	—
Potassium chloride[d]		—	2	—	2	—	—
KCl	14.85						

[a] Adapted from A. Arieff, *Clinical Disorders of Fluid and Electrolyte Metabolism*, 2d ed, Maxwell MH, Kleeman CR (eds). New York, McGraw-Hill, 1972.

[b] The 0.9M solution of $NaHCO_3$ usually is available in the clinical setting in 50-mL ampuls containing 44 meq of Na^+ and 44 meq of HCO_3^-. This solution can be infused intravenously or added to other solutions.

[c] Lactated Ringer's solution contains 28 meq/L of lactate, which is converted in the body to HCO_3^-.

[d] The KCl solution is available in 20- to 50-mL ampuls, which can be added to other solutions to provide K^+. The K^+ concentration in this solution is 2 meq/mL.

30 mL) can be added to 1 liter of any of the above solutions (see Chap. 27). K^+ should never be given as an intravenous bolus, since it can produce a potentially fatal acute increase in the plasma K^+ concentration.

Plasma volume expanders Since Na^+ salts freely cross the capillary wall, the administration of saline solutions expands both the intravascular and interstitial volumes. When free water is provided, as with dextrose or hypotonic saline solutions, there is also an increase in the intracellular volume, as two-thirds of the free water enters the cells. Thus, dextrose in water expands the extracellular volume only one-third as much as an equivalent volume of isotonic saline, which is limited to the extracellular fluid. In contrast, albumin, polygelatins, and hetastarch are primarily restricted to the vascular space and selectively expand the plasma volume.

Albumin, for example, is available as pooled human albumin that has been treated with heating and filtration to eliminate the risk of infection (such as hepatitis or HIV). When given as a 25% solution (25 g/dL), which is markedly hyperoncotic (normal plasma albumin concentration is 4 to 5 g/dL), albumin increases the plasma oncotic pressure, thereby drawing several times its volume of fluid into the vascular space from the interstitium. Albumin also can be given as a 5% solution in isotonic saline, which is similar to administering plasma.

Blood In patients with anemia, particularly those who are actively bleeding, the administration of blood may be necessary to maintain oxygen transport to the tissues. Blood is usually given as packed red cells, since saline or albumin can be administered in place of the plasma, the components of which (such as platelets and clotting factors) can be used for other purposes.

Which fluid should be used? The composition of the appropriate replacement fluid varies from patient to patient. The type of fluid lost, the plasma K^+ concentration, the plasma osmolality, and acid-base balance all must be taken into account. For example, relatively hypotonic solutions should be used in hyperosmolal patients with hypernatremia or hyperglycemia, and isotonic or hypertonic solutions should be used in hypoosmolal patients with hyponatremia. The one exception to these general rules is that isotonic saline should always be given initially to patients with hypovolemia and hemodynamic compromise (e.g., hypotension or shock).

All the solutes in an intravenous solution must be included when calculating its effective osmolality, since *potassium, the primary intracellular solute, is as osmotically active as sodium.* Thus, 1 liter of isotonic saline is osmotically equivalent to 1 liter of half-isotonic saline (Na^+ concentration of 77 meq/L) to which 77 meq of K^+ has been added. The major exception is glucose, which is rapidly metabolized in the body to CO_2 and H_2O and therefore is only transiently osmotically active.

A patient with diabetes insipidus who develops hypernatremia due to water loss can be treated with dextrose solutions alone. In contrast, a patient who had lost both solutes and water may require more complex replacement therapy. This can be illustrated by the following example.

Case History 14-3   A 37-year-old woman is seen after several days of severe diarrhea and poor oral intake. Findings on the physical examination are consistent with moderately severe volume depletion. The laboratory data include

Plasma [Na^+]	=	142 meq/L	Arterial pH	=	7.22
[K^+]	=	3.7 meq/L	P_{CO_2}	=	20 mmHg
[Cl^-]	=	114 meq/L	Urine [Na^+]	=	4 meq/L
[HCO_3^-]	=	8 meq/L			

Comment   In addition to volume depletion, this patient has metabolic acidosis and probably K^+ depletion, since the plasma K^+ concentration is low-normal in the presence of acidemia. In view of the normal plasma Na^+ concentration and osmolality, the replacement fluid should be mildly hypotonic to provide free water that will replace continuing insensible water losses. An appropriate intravenous solution for this patient would be 1 liter of dextrose in quarter-isotonic saline (Na^+ concentration equal to 38.5 meq/L) to which 44 meq of Na^+ (as $NaHCO_3$) and 40 meq of K^+ (as KCl) have been added. This solution contains HCO_3^- and K^+ to correct the acidemia and K^+ depletion and is slightly hypotonic to plasma, having a Na^+ plus K^+ concentration of 122 meq/L.

The primary indication for the use of albumin- or other colloid-containing solutions is in protein-losing states such as burns or occasionally the nephrotic syndrome.[39] Although these solutions have also been used in the treatment of shock or severe hypovolemia, they appear to offer little or no advantage over the pure electrolyte solutions (see below).

Blood may be required in addition to fluid and electrolytes if the patient is bleeding or has marked anemia. Volume repletion with solutions other than blood expands the plasma volume and lowers the hematocrit by dilution. Thus, the degree of anemia may be masked on admission and become apparent only with volume replacement.

A separate issue in patients with marked hypovolemia due to penetrating torso injuries is whether fluid resuscitation should be delayed until operative intervention to control the bleeding. Animal and some human studies suggest an improved outcome from delayed resuscitation.[40a-42] The presumed mechanism is that aggressive fluid administration might, via augmentation of blood pressure, dilution of clotting factors, and production of hypothermia, disrupt thrombus formation and enhance bleeding. This approach should be considered only if rapid surgical exploration can be performed.[41] In a controlled human trial showing benefit, the mean time from injury to operation was 2 h, results that are not attainable in most circumstances.[40]

Volume Deficit

It is usually difficult to estimate the volume deficit in a hypovolemic patient. Knowledge of the patient's normal weight is helpful, but this information is frequently not obtainable. If hyponatremia or hypernatremia is present, the respective Na^+ and water deficits can be estimated from the following formulas:[*]

$$Na^+ \text{ deficit (in meq)} = 0.6 \times \text{lean body weight (in kg)} \times (140 - \text{plasma } [Na^+])$$

$$\text{Water deficit (in liters)} = 0.5 \times \text{lean body weight (in kg)} \times \left(\frac{\text{plasma } [Na^+]}{140} - 1\right)$$

However, these formulas estimate only the amount of Na^+ in a hyponatremic patient and the volume of water in a hypernatremic patient that would have to be retained to return the plasma Na^+ concentration to the normal value of 140 meq/L. This ignores any isosmotic fluid deficit that may also be present. As an example, the formula for the water deficit is relatively accurate for a patient with diabetes insipidus who has lost only water, but it underestimates the deficit in a hypernatremic patient with diarrhea and increased insensible losses who has lost both Na^+ and water.

The extracellular fluid normally comprises about 20 percent of the lean body weight. Loss of this fluid results in hemoconcentration and an increase in the hematocrit. As a result, the extracellular deficit can be estimated from the change in the hematocrit (Hct) according to a formula similar to that for the water deficit:

$$\text{Extracellular fluid deficit} = 0.2 \times \text{lean body weight} \times \left(\frac{\text{Hct}}{\text{normal Hct}} - 1\right)$$

This formula, however, is useful only if the patient's normal hematocrit is known and if bleeding has not occurred.

In summary, the fluid deficit in a hypovolemic patient usually cannot be calculated precisely. Thus, the adequacy of volume repletion must be evaluated from the findings on physical examination and laboratory data. As volume expansion occurs, the skin turgor should improve and there should be increases in body weight, arterial pressure (if there has been a fall in blood pressure), venous pressure, urine output, and urine Na^+ concentration. For patients who start with a low urine Na^+ concentration, serial measurements of this parameter can be used as an index of the degree to which normovolemia has been restored. If the urine Na^+ concentration remains under 25 meq/L, the kidney is sensing persistent volume depletion, and more fluids should be given.[†]

---

[*] These formulas are derived in Chaps. 23 and 24. The formula for the Na^+ deficit assumes that the patient has true hyponatremia, not pseudohyponatremia due to hyperglycemia or hyperlipidemia (see page 712).

[†] This excludes edematous patients with heart failure or cirrhosis, in whom the low urine Na^+ concentration is an indication of effective circulating volume depletion but not of the need for more fluid.

Rate of Volume Replacement

As with other water and electrolyte disorders, the immediate aim of therapy in hypovolemia is to get the patient out of danger. With the exception of patients with hypotension, shock, or severe associated electrolyte disturbances, *gradual* repletion is preferable, since it will restore normovolemia while minimizing the risk of volume overload and pulmonary edema. The optimal rate of fluid replacement is somewhat arbitrary. A regimen that has been successful is the infusion of the appropriate replacement fluids at the rate of 50 to 100 mL/h *in excess of the sum* of the urine output, estimated insensible losses (approximately 30 to 50 mL/h), and any other losses that may be present (such as diarrhea or tube drainage).

The *aim of therapy is not to administer fluids but to induce positive fluid balance.* Suppose a patient with severe diarrhea has losses averaging 75 mL/h. If fluid is administered at the rate of 75 mL/h plus estimated insensible losses, there will be no positive fluid balance and no correction of the hypovolemic state. A similar problem with continuing losses can occur in central diabetes insipidus, where the urine volume can exceed 500 mL/h. In this setting, the administration of ADH will reduce the urine output and make volume repletion easier to achieve (see Chap. 24).

Hypovolemic Shock

Hypovolemic shock is most often due to bleeding or third-space sequestration, although a similar picture can be produced by any of the causes of true volume depletion. Before discussing the therapy of this disorder, it is important to first review its pathophysiology.[17,43] As described above, progressive volume depletion is associated with increasing degrees of sympathetic and angiotensin II–mediated vasoconstriction. This response initially maintains the blood pressure and cerebral and coronary perfusion. However, the combination of a hypovolemia-induced decrease in cardiac output and intense vasoconstriction results in a marked reduction in splanchnic, renal, and musculocutaneous blood flow that can ultimately lead to ischemic tissue injury and lactic acidosis. The intense ischemia can also result in the release of intracellular contents (such as lysosomal enzymes) into the systemic circulation and to the absorption of endotoxin from the gut.

Early therapy is important to prevent hypovolemic shock from becoming *irreversible.* As depicted in Fig. 14-3a, experimentally induced hemorrhagic shock in a dog can be successfully treated if the blood that has been removed is reinfused within 2 h. However, there is only a transient increase in blood pressure if the return of the shed blood is delayed for 4 h or longer (Fig. 14-3b). A similar phenomenon appears to occur in humans, although substantially more than 4 h may be required before volume repletion becomes ineffective.[44]

Irreversible shock seems to be associated with *pooling of blood in the capillaries and tissues, leading to a further impairment in tissue perfusion.*[44,45] Several factors may contribute to this vasomotor paralysis, including the following:

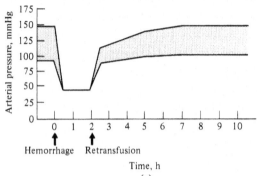

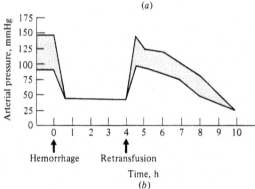

Figure 14-3 Reversibility of experimental hemorrhagic shock in the dog. (*a*) If the mean arterial pressure is reduced to 35 to 40 mmHg for less than 2 h, reinfusion of the shed blood will restore a normal blood pressure. (*b*) If the period of hypotension is extended to 4 h before the shed blood is returned, most of the dogs die within 24 h despite retransfusion. (*From Lillihei RC, Dietzman RH, in Schwartz SI, Lillihei RC, Shires GT, et al. (eds): Principles of Surgery. New York, McGraw-Hill, 1974, with permission.*)

- Hyperpolarization of vascular smooth muscle cells as ATP depletion leads to opening of ATP-dependent K^+ channels, which are normally closed by ATP.[46] Hyperpolarization decreases Ca^{2+} entry through voltage-dependent Ca^{2+} channels, and the ensuing reduction in cell Ca^{2+} concentration can lead to vasodilatation. In experimental models of shock, the administration of the sulfonylura glyburide, an inhibitor of the K^+-ATP channel, led to both vasoconstriction and an elevation in systemic blood pressure.[46] The clinical applicability of this observation remains to be proven.
- Plugging of the capillaries by activated circulating neutrophils.[45]
- A cerebral ischemia–induced impairment in vasomotor regulation, resulting in reversal of the initial increase in peripheral sympathetic tone.[47]
- Increased generation of the vasodilator nitric oxide; in experimental animals, the vascular unresponsiveness in irreversible shock can be overcome by administration of an inhibitor of nitric oxide synthase.[48]
- Generation of iron-dependent, oxygen-derived free radicals.[49] Resuscitation with a free radical–scavenger conjugate of starch and deferoxamine may attenuate derangements in microvascular blood flow.

Regardless of the mechanism, the net effect is that administered fluid is sequestered in the capillary circulation. The ensuing elevation in the capillary hydraulic pressure favors the movement of fluid out of the vascular space into the interstitium.[43-45,47] An increase in capillary permeability also may contribute to this process, as toxic products released from injured tissues or from the local accumulation of neutrophils can damage the capillary wall.[45]

In addition to sequestration in the capillaries, fluid may also be lost into the cells. Tissue ischemia diminishes cellular Na^+-K^+-ATPase activity, thereby reducing the active transport of Na^+ out of the cells. The ensuing rise in cell Na^+ promotes osmotic water entry into the cells.[43] The net effect is more severe plasma volume depletion, hemoconcentration, increased viscosity, and red blood cell aggregation, all of which can further impair the capillary circulation.

With these potential hazards in mind, a rational therapeutic program can be begun. Patients with shock should have careful monitoring of their arterial pressure, central venous pressure (or, preferably, the pulmonary capillary wedge pressure), arterial pH, hematocrit, urine output, and mental status. In addition, therapy must be directed toward the underlying disease—for example, surgery in a patient with a ruptured abdominal aortic aneurysm.

The immediate aim of therapy in hypovolemic shock is to restore tissue perfusion by the administration of fluids. The use of vasopressors such as dopamine or norepinephrine will not correct the underlying volume deficit and may intensify the problem in the capillary circulation, further reducing tissue perfusion and predisposing toward ischemic damage.[50]

Which fluids should be given?   The choice of replacement fluid depends upon the type of fluid lost. Patients who are bleeding may require the administration of large amounts of blood. This can be given most rapidly under pressure through several intravenous catheters. In general, the hematocrit should not be raised over 35 percent. A higher level is not necessary for oxygen transport and may produce an increase in blood viscosity that can lead to stasis in the already impaired capillary circulation. The role of acellular, oxygen-carrying resuscitation fluids when blood is not available is uncertain. In one trial in which patients with traumatic hemorrhagic shock were randomized to receive either a diaspirin cross-linked hemoglobin solution or saline, the patients who received the oxygen-carrying blood substitute had a significantly *higher* mortality at 2 and 28 days (46 versus 17 percent at 28 days).[51]

The optimal form of fluid replacement other than blood is, in most cases, an electrolyte solution, such as isotonic saline or Ringer's lactate.[43] Some physicians have favored the use of a colloid-containing solution (such as albumin, polygelatins, or hetastarch), claiming that it has two advantages: (1) more effective plasma volume expansion, since it remains in the vascular space (in contrast to saline, two-thirds of which enters the interstitium), and (2) a lesser risk of pulmonary edema, since the increase in plasma oncotic pressure favors fluid movement out of the interstitium into the vascular space.[14,52]

However, several controlled studies have *failed to confirm* either of these potential advantages,[53-56] and a review of randomized trails found that resuscitation with colloid solutions was associated with an increased absolute risk of mortality of 4 percent.[57] Albumin and electrolyte solutions are equally effective in producing volume repletion, although 2.5 to 3 times as much saline must be given because of its extravascular distribution.[53] This is not a deleterious effect, however, since saline replaces the interstitial fluid deficit that is induced both by fluid loss and by fluid movement into the cells.

Colloid-containing solutions are also not more effective in preserving pulmonary function.[53,54,58] In general, the *pulmonary circulation is less sensitive than that in the periphery to changes in the plasma albumin concentration.* This difference reflects the normally higher permeability to proteins in the alveolar capillaries, which results in a higher baseline protein concentration and therefore oncotic pressure in the interstitium.[59,60] When the plasma albumin concentration is lowered due, for example, to saline-induced hemodilution, there will initially be a parallel reduction in the interstitial oncotic pressure, since less protein will now cross the capillary wall. The net effect is *maintenance of the balance between Starling's forces and relative resistance to interstitial fluid accumulation* in the absence of severe hypoalbuminemia (see page 485).[58,61]

Thus, the administration of saline to the patient with shock is unlikely to produce pulmonary edema unless there is an excessive elevation in the capillary hydraulic pressure.[61,62] Saline infusion can, however, induce peripheral edema, since the skeletal muscle and subcutaneous capillaries are less permeable to protein. They therefore have a lower baseline interstitial oncotic pressure and a lesser ability to protect against edema by diminishing the accumulation of interstitial proteins.[62] It is important to appreciate that *the development of peripheral edema does not necessarily indicate that fluid repletion should be discontinued,* since it may result from dilutional hypoalbuminemia even though plasma volume depletion persists.[63]

In summary, electrolyte solutions seem to be preferable to colloid in the treatment of severe hypovolemia,[53,55-57] with the possible exception of patients with underlying hypoalbuminemia.[52]

In addition to fluid repletion, military antishock trousers have been used in the treatment of hypovolemic shock. They can rapidly raise the systemic blood pressure both by increasing vascular resistance (by mechanical compression of the legs) and by translocation of fluid from the lower extremities into the cardiopulmonary circulation.[63,64] Prolonged usage should be avoided, since it can lead to an ischemic compartment syndrome or impairment of venous return.[17,64]

Rate of fluid replacement Approximately 1 to 2 liters of fluid should be given in the first hour in an attempt to restore adequate tissue perfusion as quickly as possible. It is impossible to predict what the total fluid deficit in a given patient will be, particularly if bleeding or third-space sequestration continues. Consequently, further fluids should be administered while monitoring the central venous or preferably the pulmonary capillary wedge pressure. Fluids should be given at the initial rapid rate as long as the cardiac filling pressures and the systemic blood pressure remain low.

Lactic acidosis   Marked tissue hypoperfusion in hypovolemic shock is often associated with lactic acidosis. The role of HCO_3^- therapy to raise the extracellular pH in this setting remains controversial. There is evidence that exogenous HCO_3^- can impair net lactate utilization, thereby preventing or minimizing correction of the acidemia.[65] Another potential problem is that measurement of the arterial pH may not give an accurate assessment of the pH at the tissue level in this setting, necessitating evaluation of a mixed-venous blood sample (see page 598).[65]

PROBLEMS

14-1 A 75-year-old woman is admitted to the hospital with the acute onset of severe abdominal pain. When examined, the patient is agitated, her extremities are cold and clammy, and her blood pressure is 60/30. Her abdomen is distended, with diffuse tenderness. The results of the laboratory evaluation include a hematocrit of 53 percent. An arteriogram shows complete occlusion of one of the branches of the superior mesenteric artery.

(a) What is the etiology of the shock state in this patient?

(b) What fluids would you administer?

Prior to surgery, a total of 7 liters of fluid is administered to maintain the blood pressure. Through this period, she is virtually anuric. At surgery, 40 cm of infarcted ileum is removed. Six hours after surgery, the patient is doing well when a marked increased in the urine output to nearly 1000 mL/h is noted. Her urine osmolality is 250 mosmol/kg; her urine Na^+ concentration is 95 meq/L.

(c) What might be responsible for this increase in output?

(d) How would you treat the patient at this time?

14-2 Compare the effects of the loss of water (due to increased insensible losses or diabetes insipidus) and the loss of an equal volume of an isotonic Na^+ solution (due to diuretics or diarrhea) on the extracellular volume and the arterial blood pressure.

14-3 What is the role of pure dextrose solutions in the treatment of hypovolemic shock?

14-4 A 75-year-old woman develops volume depletion as a result of the excessive administration of diuretics. Prior to the administration of diuretics, the patient had a normal BUN and plasma creatinine concentration. After a 6-kg weight loss over 10 days, poor skin turgor is present, and the central venous pressure is 1 cmH_2O. The following laboratory data are obtained:

BUN	=	208 mg/dL
Plasma [creatinine]	=	5.7 mg/dL
Urine [Na^+]	=	5 meq/L
Urine output	=	25 mL/h
Urinalysis	=	normal

After the administration of 5 liters of half-isotonic saline over 18 h, the central venous pressure is 3 cmH_2O, the skin turgor has improved, and the results of repeat laboratory studies are

BUN	=	160 mg/dL
Urine [Na^+]	=	45 meq/L
Urine output	=	80 mL/h

(a) Why have the urine Na^+ concentration and urine output increased?

(b) Does the repeat central venous pressure indicate persistent volume depletion?

(c) Why is the repeat BUN still elevated despite volume repletion?

14-5 A 74-year-old man is admitted from a nursing home with a 3-day history of recurrent vomiting and diarrhea. The results of the physical examination are consistent with volume depletion. The laboratory data reveal

$$\text{Plasma } [Na^+] = 155 \text{ meq/L}$$
$$[K^+] = 3 \text{ meq/L}$$
$$[Cl^-] = 117 \text{ meq/L}$$
$$[HCO_3^-] = 25 \text{ meq/L}$$

(a) What intravenous solution would you use for replacement therapy?

(b) How rapidly should it be administered?

14-6 A 72-year-old woman is found confused on the floor of her apartment. No history is obtainable except that she has a history of hypertension. The physical examination reveals a blood pressure of 110/70, reduced skin turgor, and an estimated jugular venous pressure of less than $5\,\text{cmH}_2\text{O}$. The following laboratory data are obtained:

$$\text{BUN} = 62 \text{ mg/dL}$$
$$\text{Plasma [creatinine]} = 1.8 \text{ mg/dL}$$
$$[Na^+] = 138 \text{ meq/L}$$
$$[K^+] = 3.1 \text{ meq/L}$$
$$[Cl^-] = 100 \text{ meq/L}$$
$$[HCO_3^-] = 29 \text{ meq/L}$$

(a) Is the blood pressure normal?

(b) Could this patient's volume depletion be due to the lack of replacement of insensible losses?

REFERENCES

1. Dirks JH, Cirksena WJ. Micropuncture study of the effect of various diuretics on sodium reabsorption by the proximal tubules of the dog. *J Clin Invest* 45:1875, 1966.
2. Wilcox CS, Guzman NJ, Mitch WE, et al. Na^+, K^+, and BP homeostasis in man during furosemide: Effects of prazosin and captopril. *Kidney Int* 31:135, 1987.
3. Maronde R, Milgrom M, Vlachakis ND, Chan L. Response of thiazide-induced hypokalemia to amiloride. *JAMA* 249:237, 1983.
4. Coleman AJ, Arias M, Carter NW, et al. The mechanism of salt-wasting in chronic renal disease. *J Clin Invest* 45:1116, 1966.
5. Danovitch GM, Bourgoignie JJ, Bricker NS. Reversibility of the "salt-losing" tendency of chronic renal failure. *N Engl J Med* 296:15, 1977.
6. Uribarri J, Oh MS, Carroll HJ. Salt-losing nephropathy. Clinical presentation and mechanisms. *Am J Nephrol* 3:193, 1983.
7. Strauss MB. Clinical and pathological aspects of cystic disease of the renal medulla: An analysis of eighteen cases. *Ann Intern Med* 57:373, 1962.
8. Yeh BPY, Tomko DJ, Stacy WK, et al. Factors influencing sodium and water excretion in uremic man. *Kidney Int* 7:103, 1975.
9. Bishop MC. Diuresis and renal functional recovery in chronic retention. *Br J Urol* 57:1, 1985.
10. Howards SS. Post-obstructive diuresis: A misunderstood phenomenon. *J Urol* 110:537, 1973.
11. Marples FJ, Knepper MA, Nielsen S. Bilateral ureteral obstruction downregulates expression of vasopressin-sensitive AQP-2 water channel in rat kidney. *Am J Physiol* 270:F657, 1996.
12. Better OS. Impaired fluid and electrolyte balance in hot climates. *Kidney Int* 32(suppl 21):S-97, 1987.
13. Daugirdas JT. Dialysis hypotension: A hemodynamic analysis. *Kidney Int* 39:233, 1991.
14. Baskett PJF. ABC of major trauma. Management of hypovolaemic shock. *Br Med J* 300:1453, 1990.
15. Freis ED, Stanton JR, Finnerty FA Jr, et al. The collapse produced by venous congestion of the extremities or by venesection following certain hypotensive agents. *J Clin Invest* 30:435, 1951.

16. Wagner HN Jr. The influence of autonomic vasoregulatory reflexes on the rate of sodium and water excretion in man. *J Clin Invest* 36:1319, 1957.

17. Weil MH, von Planta M, Rackow EC. Acute circulatory failure (shock), in Braunwald E (ed): *Heart Disease. A Textbook of Cardiovascular Medicine*, 3d ed. Philadelphia, Saunders, 1988.

18. Nerup J. Addison's disease. Clinical studies. A report of 108 cases. *Acta Endocrinol (Copenh)* 76:127, 1974.

19. Mange K, Matsuura D, Cizman B, et al. Language guiding therapy: The case of dehydration versus volume depletion. *Ann Intern Med* 127:848, 1997.

20. McGee S, Abernethy WB, Simel DL. Is this patient hypovolemic? *JAMA* 281:1022, 1999.

21. Cohn JN. Blood pressure measurement in shock: Mechanism of inaccuracy in auscultatory and palpatory methods. *JAMA* 199:118, 1967.

22. Franch RH. Examination of the blood, urine, and extravascular fluids, including circulation time and venous pressure, in Hurst JW, Logue RB, Schlant RC, Wenger NK (eds): *The Heart Arteries and Veins*, 3d ed. New York, McGraw-Hill, 1974.

23. Cohn JN, Tristani FE, Khatri IM. Studies in clinical shock and hypotension. VI. Relationship between left and right ventricular function. *J Clin Invest* 48:2008, 1969.

24. Sherman RA, Eisinger RP. The use (and misuse) of urinary sodium and chloride measurements. *JAMA* 247:3121, 1982.

25. Kassirre JP, Schwartz WB. The response of normal man to selective depletion of hydrochloric acid: Factors in the genesis of persistent gastric alkalosis. *Am J Med* 40:10, 1966.

26. Besarab A, Brown RS, Rubin NT, et al. Reversible renal failure following bilateral renal artery occlusive disease: Clinical features, pathology, and the role of surgical revascularization. *JAMA* 235:2838, 1976.

27. Miller TR, Anderson RJ, Linas SL, et al. Urinary diagnostic indices in acute renal failure: A prospective study. *Ann Intern Med* 89:47, 1978.

28. Espinel CH, Gregory AW. Differential diagnosis of acute renal failure. *Clin Nephrol* 13:73, 1980.

29. Rose BD. *Pathophysiology of Renal Disease*, 2d ed. New York, McGraw-Hill, 1987, p. 82.

30. Levinsky NG, Davidson DG, Berliner RW. Effects of reduced glomerular filtration and urine concentration in presence of antidiuretic hormone. *J Clin Invest* 38:730, 1959.

31. Dossetor JB. Creatininemia versus uremia: The relative significance of blood urea nitrogen and serum creatinine concentrations in azotemia. *Ann Intern Med* 65:1287, 1966.

32. Dorhout Mees EJ. Relation between maximal urine concentration, maximal water reabsorption capacity, and mannitol clearance in patients with renal disease. *Br Med J* 1:1159, 1959.

33. Shiau Y-F, Feldman GM, Resnick MA, Coff PM. Stool electrolyte and osmolality measurements in the evaluation of diarrheal disorders. *Ann Intern Med* 102:773, 1985.

34. Nelson DC, McGrew WRG, Hoyumpa AM. Hypernatremia and lactulose therapy. *JAMA* 249:1295, 1983.

35. Popovtzer MM, Katz FH, Pinggera WF, et al. Hyperkalemia in salt-wasting nephropathy: Study of the mechanism. *Arch Intern Med* 132:203, 1973.

36. Gore SM, Fontaine O, Pierce NF. Impact of rice-based oral rehydration solution on stool output and duration of diarrhoea: Meta-analysis of 13 clinical studies. *Br Med J* 304:287, 1992.

37. Carpenter CCJ, Greenough WB, Pierce NF. Oral-rehydration therapy—The role of polymeric substrates. *N Engl J Med* 319:1346, 1988.

38. Alam NJ, Majumder RH, Fuchs GJ, and the CHOICE study group. Efficacy and safety of oral rehydration solution with reduced osmolality in adults with cholera: A randomized double-blind clinical trial. *Lancet* 354:296, 1999.

39. Cureri PW, Luterman A, Burns I, et al, in Schwartz SI, Shires GT, Spencer FC, Storer EH (eds): *Principles of Surgery*, 4th ed. New York, McGraw-Hill, 1984.

40. Bickell WH, Wall MJ Jr, Pepe PE, et al. Immediate versus delayed fluid resuscitation for patients with penetrating torso injuries. *N Engl J Med* 331:1105, 1994.

41. Banerjee A, Jones R. Whither immediate fluid resuscitation? *Lancet* 344:1450, 1994.

42. Solomonov E, Hirsch M, Yahiya A, Krausz MM. The effect of vigorous fluid resuscitation in uncontrolled hemorrhagic shock after massive splenic injury. *Crit Care Med* 28:749, 2000.

43. Holcroft JW, Blaisdell FW. Shock: Causes and management of circulatory collapse, in Sabiston DC Jr (ed): *Textbook of Surgery. The Biological Basis of Modern Surgical Practice.* Philadelphia, Saunders, 1986.
44. Zweifach BW, Fronek A. The interplay of central and peripheral factors in irreversible hemorrhagic shock. *Prog Cardiovasc Dis* 18:147, 1975.
45. Barroso-Aranda J, Schmid-Schonbein GW, Zweifach BW, Engler RL. Granulocytes and noreflow phenomenon in irreversible hemorrhagic shock. *Circ Res* 63:437, 1988.
46. Landry DW, Oliver JA. The ATP-sensitive K^+ channel mediates hypotension in endotoxemia and hypoxic lactic acidosis in dog. *J Clin Invest* 89:2071, 1992.
47. Koyama S, Aibiki M, Kanai K, et al. Role of central nervous system in renal nerve activity during prolonged hemorrhagic shock in dogs. *Am J Physiol* 254:R761, 1988.
48. Thiemermann C, Szabo C, Mitchell JA, Vane JR. Vascular hyporeactivity to vasoconstrictor agents and haemodynamic decompensation in hemorrhagic shock is mediated by nitric oxide. *Proc Natl Acad Sci U S A* 90:267, 1993.
49. Bauer M, Feucht K, Ziegenfuss T, Marzi T. Attenuation of shock-induced hepatic microcirculatory disturbances by the use of a starch-deferoxamine conjugate for resuscitation. *Crit Care Med* 23:316, 1995.
50. Nordin AJ, Makisalo H, Hockerstedt KA. Failure of dobutamine to improve liver oxygenation during resuscitation with a crystalloid solution after experimental haemorrhagic shock. *Eur J Surg* 162:973, 1996.
51. Sloan EP, Koenigsberg M, Gens D, et al. Diaspirin cross-linked hemoglobin (DCLHb) in the treatment of severe traumatic hemorrhagic shock: A randomized controlled efficacy trial. *JAMA* 282:1857, 1999.
52. Rackow EC, Falk JL, Fein IA, et al. Fluid resuscitation in circulatory shock: A comparison of the cardiorespiratory effects of albumin, hetastarch, and saline solutions in patients with hypovolemic and septic shock. *Crit Care Med* 11:839, 1983.
53. Virgilio RW, Rice CL, Smith DE, et al. Crystalloid vs. colloid resuscitation: Is one better? *Surgery* 85:129, 1979.
54. Weaver DM, Ledgerwood AM, Lucas CE, et al. Pulmonary effects of albumin resuscitation for severe hypovolemic shock. *Arch Surg* 113:387, 1978.
55. Moss GS, Lowe RJ, Jilek J, Levine HD. Colloid or crystalloid in the resuscitation of hemorrhagic shock: A controlled clinical trial. *Surgery* 89:434, 1981.
56. Erstad BL, Gales BJ, Rappaport WD. The use of albumin in clinical practice. *Arch Intern Med* 151:901, 1991.
57. Schierhout G, Roberts I. Fluid resuscitation with colloid or crystalloid solutions in critically ill patients: A systematic review of randomised trials. *Br Med J* 316:961, 1998.
58. Holcroft JW, Trunkey DD. Extravascular lung water following hemorrhagic shock in the baboon: Comparison between resuscitation with Ringer's lactate and Plasmanate. *Ann Surg* 180:408, 1974.
59. Taylor AE. Capillary fluid filtration: Starling forces and lymph flow. *Circ Res* 49:557, 1981.
60. Murray JF. The lung and heart failure. *Hosp Pract* 20(4):55, 1985.
61. Gallagher TJ, Banner MJ, Barnes PA. Large volume crystalloid resuscitation does not increase extravascular lung water. *Anesth Analg* 64:623, 1985.
62. Zarins CK, Rice CL, Peters RM, Virgilio RW. Lymph and pulmonary response to isobaric reduction in plasma oncotic pressure in baboons. *Circ Res* 43:925, 1978.
63. Shine KI, Kuhn M, Young LS, Tillisch JH. Aspects of the management of shock. *Ann Intern Med* 93:723, 1980.
64. Kaback KR, Sanders AB, Meslin HW. MAST suit update. *JAMA* 252:2598, 1984.
65. Adrogué HJ, Rashad MN, Gorin AD, et al. Assessing acid-base status in circulatory failure: Differences between arterial and central venous blood. *N Engl J Med* 320:1312, 1989.

CLINICAL USE OF DIURETICS

Diuretics are among the most commonly used drugs. They primarily act by diminishing NaCl reabsorption at different sites in the nephron, thereby increasing urinary sodium and H_2O losses. This ability to induce negative fluid balance has made diuretics useful in the treatment of a variety of conditions, particularly edematous states and hypertension. This chapter will review the mechanism of action of diuretics, the time course of their action, the fluid and electrolyte complications that can occur, and an approach to the patient with refractory edema, with particular emphasis on the problems that can occur in the patient with cirrhosis. A more complete discussion of the different edematous states will then be presented in the following chapter.

MECHANISM OF ACTION

The diuretics are generally divided into three major classes, which are distinguished by the site at which they impair Na^+ reabsorption: loop diuretics in the thick ascending limb of the loop of Henle; thiazide-type diuretics in the distal tubule and connecting segment (and perhaps the early cortical collecting tubule); and potassium-sparing diuretics in the aldosterone-sensitive principal cells in the cortical collecting tubule (Table 15-1).[1,2,3]

To appreciate how this occurs, it is first necessary to review the general mechanism by which Na^+ is reabsorbed. As was described in Chaps. 3 to 5, each of the Na^+-transporting cells contains Na^+-K^+-ATPase pumps in the basolateral membrane.[4] These pumps perform two major functions: They return reabsorbed Na^+ to the systemic circulation, and they maintain the cell Na^+ concentration at relatively low levels. The latter effect is particularly important, since it allows filtered Na^+ to passively enter the cells down a favorable concentration gradient. This process must be mediated by a transmembrane carrier or a Na^+ channel, since charged particles cannot freely cross the lipid bilayer of the cell membrane. Each of the major nephron segments has a *unique Na^+ entry mechanism*, and the ability to specifically inhibit this step explains the nephron segment at which each of the different classes of diuretics acts.[3]

- The thick ascending limb of the loop of Henle has a Na^+-K^+-$2Cl^-$ cotransporter in the luminal membrane that is inhibited by loop diuretics.
- The distal tubule has a Na^+-Cl^- cotransporter in the luminal membrane that is inhibited by thiazide-type diuretics.
- The principal cells in the collecting tubules have Na^+ channels in the luminal membrane that are directly inhibited by amiloride or triamterene and indirectly inhibited by the aldosterone antagonist spironolactone.

Table 15-1 Physiologic characteristics of commonly used diuretics

Site of action	Carrier or channel inhibited	Percent filtered Na^+ excreted

Loop of Henle
  Furosemide
  Bumetanide
  Ethacrynic acid
	Na^+-K^+-$2Cl^-$ carrier	Up to 25

Distal tubule and connecting segment
  Thiazides
  Chlorthalidone
  Metolazone
	Na^+-Cl^- carrier	Up to 3 to 5

Cortical collecting tubule
  Spironolactone
  Amiloride
  Triamterene
	Na^+ channel	Up to 1 to 2

The site of action within the nephron is a major determinant of diuretic potency. Most of the filtered Na^+ is reabsorbed in the proximal tubule (about 55 to 60 percent) and the loop of Henle (25 to 35 percent; see Table 8-3). It might be expected, therefore, that a proximally acting diuretic, such as the carbonic anhydrase inhibitor acetazolamide, could induce relatively large losses of Na^+ and H_2O. This does not occur, however, because most of the excess fluid delivered out of the proximal tubule can be reabsorbed more distally, particularly in the loop of Henle. Transport in the latter segment is primarily flow-dependent, varying directly with the delivery of Cl^- (see Fig. 4-3).[5,6]

A similar process of distal compensation occurs with the loop diuretics. The distal tubule is able to increase its rate of reabsorption, as evidenced by tubular hypertrophy and a rise in Na^+-K^+-ATPase activity with chronic loop diuretic administration.[7-10] However, the reabsorptive capacity of the distal and collecting tubules is relatively limited, and in most circumstances the natriuretic response to a loop diuretic is not seriously impaired.[2]

Loop Diuretics

The loop diuretics—furosemide, bumetanide, torsemide, and ethacrynic acid—can lead to the excretion of up to 20 to 25 percent of the filtered Na^+ when given in maximum dosage.[1,11] They act in the medullary and cortical aspects of the thick ascending limb, including the macula densa cells in the early distal tubule. At each of these sites, Na^+ entry is primarily mediated by a Na^+-K^+-$2Cl^-$ carrier in the luminal membrane that is activated when all four sites are occupied (see Chap. 4).[1,3,6,12,13] The loop diuretics appear to compete for the Cl^- site on this carrier, thereby diminishing net reabsorption.[13,14]

The loop diuretics also have important effects on renal Ca^{2+} handling. The reabsorption of Ca^{2+} in the loop of Henle is primarily passive, being driven by the gradient created by NaCl transport (see page 92).[15,16] As a result, inhibiting the reabsorption of NaCl leads to a parallel reduction in the reabsorption of Ca^{2+} thereby increasing Ca^{2+} excretion. This effect is clinically important, because enhancing urinary Ca^{2+} losses with saline and a loop diuretic is a mainstay of therapy in patients with hypercalcemia.[17]

One potential concern is that the calciuric response can lead to kidney stones and/or nephrocalcinosis. These complications have been primarily reported in premature infants, in whom a loop diuretic can induce more than a 10-fold rise in Ca^{2+} excretion.[18,19]

Thiazide-Type Diuretics

The thiazide-type diuretics primarily inhibit NaCl transport in the distal tubule,[1,2,3,20,21] the connecting segment at the end of the distal tubule,[22] and possibly the early cortical collecting tubule (although this finding is controversial).[23,24] These segments normally reabsorb less of the filtered load than does the loop of Henle; as a result, the thiazide-type diuretics are less potent and, when given in maximum dosage, inhibit the reabsorption of at most 3 to 5 percent of the filtered Na^+.[1,2] Furthermore, the net diuresis may be partially limited by increased reabsorption in the cortical collecting tubule.[8,25] These responses make the thiazides less useful in the treatment of edematous states but are not a problem in uncomplicated hypertension, where marked fluid loss is neither necessary nor desirable.

Thiazide-sensitive Na^+ entry in the distal nephron is mediated by neutral *Na^+-Cl^- cotransport*.[3,26] Both a Na^+-Cl^- cotransporter[27-29] and, to a lesser degree, parallel Na^+-H^+ and Cl^--HCO_3^- exchangers are responsible for NaCl reabsorption at these sites (see page 145).[22,26]

The thiazides inhibit NaCl reabsorption in these segments by competing for the Cl^- site on the Na^+-Cl^- cotransporter.[30]* Some of these drugs (chlorothiazide but not bendroflumethazide, for example) also modestly impair Na^+ transport in the proximal tubule, due in part to partial inhibition of carbonic anhydrase.[21,31] This does not normally contribute to the net diuresis, however, since the excess fluid delivered out of the proximal tubule is reclaimed in the loop of Henle.[21]

Like the loop diuretics, the thiazides also can importantly affect Ca^{2+} handling.[32] The distal tubule is the major site of active Ca^{2+} reabsorption in the nephron, an effect that is independent of Na^+ transport.[15] Although the thiazides inhibit the reabsorption of Na^+ in this segment, they are able at the same time to *increase the reabsorption of Ca^{2+}*.[33] A similar response appears to occur in the cortical collecting tubule, as the K^+-sparing diuretic amiloride also can promote Ca^{2+} reabsorption.[33] The fall in Ca^{2+} excretion can be useful in the treatment of recurrent kidney stones due to hypercalciuria;[34] this response is mediated by diuretic-induced alterations in intracellular composition and electrical potential (see page 92).[35]

Potassium-Sparing Diuretics

The three major K^+ sparing diuretics—amiloride, spironolactone, and triamterene—act in the principal cells in the cortical collecting tubule (and possibly in the papillary or inner medullary collecting duct).[1,3,36,37] Na^+ entry in these segments occurs through aldosterone-sensitive *Na^+ channels*, rather than being carrier-mediated.[38,39] The reabsorption of cationic Na^+ without an anion creates a lumen-negative electrical gradient that then favors the secretion of K^+ (through selective K^+ channels) and H^+. Thus, inhibition of Na^+ reabsorption at this site can lead to hyperkalemia and metabolic acidosis as a result of the concurrent reductions in K^+ and H^+ excretion.[1,2]

---

*The loop diuretics are generally ineffective in this segment, although furosemide may have a small inhibitory effect.[20]

These drugs act by decreasing the number of open Na^+ channels, amiloride and triamterene directly and spironolactone by competitively inhibiting the effect of aldosterone.[36,37] Another cation, the antibiotic trimethoprim, also can act as a K^+-sparing diuretic when given in very high doses in patients with AIDS[40] and occasionally when given in conventional doses.[41]

The K^+-sparing diuretics have relatively weak natriuretic activity, leading to the maximum excretion of only 1 to 2 percent of the filtered Na^+.[1] Thus, they are primarily used in combination with a loop or thiazide diuretic, either to diminish the degree of K^+ loss or to increase the net diuresis in patients with refractory edema.[1,2] In addition, spironolactone may have the surprising effect of being particularly potent in patients with cirrhosis and ascites (see "Refractory Edema," below).

An additional use of amiloride has been demonstrated in patients with polyuria and polydipsia due to lithium-induced nephrogenic diabetes insipidus (see Chap. 24). The resistance to antidiuretic hormone (ADH) in this disorder appears to result from lithium accumulation in the collecting tubule cells by movement through the Na^+ channels in the luminal membrane. Blocking these channels with amiloride has been shown to partially reverse and may even prevent the concentrating defect, presumably by diminishing lithium entry into the tubular cells.[42]

Amiloride is generally the best tolerated of this diuretic class. It can be given once a day and is associated with few side effects other than hyperkalemia. Triamterene, in comparison, is a potential nephrotoxin,[43] possibly leading to crystalluria and cast formation (in up to one-half of patients)[44] and rarely to triamterene stones[45] or to acute renal failure due to either intratubular crystal deposition or the concurrent use of a nonsteroidal anti-inflammatory drug.[46,47]

It is estimated, for example, that triamterene accounts for 1 in every 200 to 250 stones.[45] These stones, which are more likely to occur in patients with a prior history of stone disease, are faintly radiopaque; their formation is pH-independent, and they usually contain some calcium oxalate (although pure triamterene stones can occur).[45,48]

Acetazolamide

Acetazolamide inhibits the activity of carbonic anhydrase, which plays an important role in proximal HCO_3^-, Na^+, and Cl^- reabsorption (see page 335). As a result, this agent produces both NaCl and $NaHCO_3$ loss.[49,50] The net diuresis, however, is relatively modest for two reasons: (1) Most of the excess fluid delivered out of the proximal tubule is reclaimed in the more distal segments, particularly the loop of Henle; and (2) the diuretic action is progressively attenuated by the metabolic acidosis that results from the loss of HCO_3^- in the urine. The major indication for the use of acetazolamide as a diuretic is in edematous patients with metabolic alkalosis, in whom loss of the excess HCO_3^- in the urine will tend to restore acid-base balance.[50]

Mannitol

Mannitol is a nonreabsorbable polysaccharide that acts as an osmotic diuretic, inhibiting Na^+ and water reabsorption in the proximal tubule and more importantly the loop of Henle.[51,52] In contrast to other diuretics, mannitol produces a relative water diuresis in which water is lost in excess of Na^+ and K^+.[57]

The major clinical use of mannitol as a diuretic has been in the early stages of oliguric, postischemic acute renal failure in an attempt to prevent progression to acute tubular necrosis.[53,54] The benefit of this approach is uncertain. Mannitol is not generally used in edematous states, since initial retention of the hypertonic mannitol can induce further volume expansion, which, in heart failure, can precipitate pulmonary edema.

Mannitol can also produce a clinically important increase in the plasma osmolality by two different mechanisms. First, the preferential water diuresis induced by the repeated administration of mannitol can, if the losses are not replaced, lead to a water deficit and hypernatremia.[55] Second, hypertonic mannitol may be retained in patients with renal failure, directly increasing the plasma osmolality. In this setting, water movement out of the cells down an osmotic gradient will lower the plasma Na^+ concentration by dilution.[56,57] This is an important condition to recognize, since treatment must be aimed at the hyperosmolality, not the hyponatremia (see page 668).

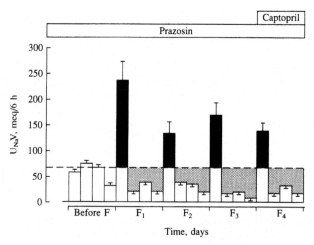

Figure 15-1   Values for 6-hourly rates of Na^+ excretion in normal subjects ingesting 270 meq of Na^+ per day after being given 40 mg of furosemide. The dashed horizontal line represents the level of Na^+ intake, which in the control period is roughly equal to the rate of Na^+ excretion. The latter rose markedly after the diuretic but fell below control levels (shaded areas) once the diuretic effect dissipated. The end result is no net diuresis at the end of the day. Blocking the renin-angiotensin-aldosterone system with captopril and the effect of norepinephrine with the α_1-adrenergic blocker prazosin did not alter this response. (*From Wilcox CS, Guzman NJ, Mitch WE, et al*, Kidney Int *31:135, 1987. Reprinted by permission from* Kidney International.)

TIME COURSE OF DIURESIS

The efficacy of a diuretic is related to a number of factors, including its site of action, its duration of action, and dietary Na^+ intake. The importance of the last two factors is illustrated in Fig. 15-1, which depicts the effect of a short-acting loop diuretic (furosemide) on the pattern of daily Na^+ excretion.[58,59] As expected, a significant natriuresis is noted during the 6-h period that the diuretic is acting. However, Na^+ excretion falls to very low levels during the remaining 18 h of the day, because the associated volume depletion leads to the activation of Na^+-retaining mechanisms.

The net result in these patients on a high Na^+ intake (270 meq/day) is that there is *no net Na^+ loss*. In this setting, one or more of the following changes must be present to induce negative Na^+ balance.

- The patient can be placed on a low-Na^+ diet, thereby minimizing the degree of Na^+ retention once the diuretic has worn off.[59] This is the preferred method, since it can also limit concurrent K^+ losses (see below).[60]
- The diuretic can be given twice a day.
- The dose of the diuretic can be increased, although the larger initial diuresis may induce symptomatic hypovolemia.

Several factors contribute to the compensatory antinatriuresis following the institution of diuretic therapy.[61] The initial fluid loss leads to activation of the renin-angiotensin-aldosterone and sympathetic nervous systems; angiotensin II, aldosterone, and norepinephrine can all promote tubular Na^+ reabsorption (see Chaps. 2 and 6).[62-64] However, blocking both of these pathways with prazosin (an α_1-adrenergic blocker) and captopril (an angiotensin converting enzyme inhibitor) does not prevent the secondary renal Na^+ retention (Fig. 15-1). In this setting, in which both vasoconstrictor hormones are inhibited, there is a mean *13-mmHg fall in the systemic blood pressure.*[58] Hypotension, in the absence of neurohumoral activation, directly promotes Na^+ retention via the pressure natriuresis phenomenon (see page 272).[64]

These observations permit a more complete understanding of the volume regulatory actions of angiotensin II and norepinephrine. In the presence of volume depletion, the combined vasoconstrictor and Na^+-retaining effects of these hormones result in both maintenance of the systemic blood pressure and an appropriate fall in Na^+ excretion. If, on the other hand, there were no stimulation of Na^+ reabsorption, then the persistent normotensin would, by pressure natriuresis, promote further Na^+ loss and exacerbation of the hypovolemic state.

Reestablishment of the Steady State

Even if a net diuresis is induced, the response is short-lived, as a *new steady state is rapidly established, in which Na^+ intake and output are again equal* but the extracellular volume has fallen due to the initial period of negative Na^+ balance. In this setting, the diuretic-induced Na^+ losses are counterbalanced, as in Fig. 15-1, by several factors:[65]

- Neurohumorally mediated increases in tubular reabsorption at non-diuretic-sensitive sites, such as the proximal tubule (angiotensin II and to a lesser degree norepinephrine) and the collecting tubules (aldosterone).[61,62]
- Flow-mediated increases in tubular reabsorption distal to the site of action of the diuretic as distal Na^+ delivery is enhanced.[2,10] As mentioned above, administration of a loop diuretic leads to hypertrophy and increased Na^+-K^+-ATPase activity in both the distal and collecting tubules.[7-9] A thiazide diuretic, on the other hand, acts in the distal tubule and the more distal adaptations are limited to the Na^+-reabsorbing cells in the collecting tubules.[8,25]
- Diminished diuretic entry into the urine also may contribute at a later stage if renal perfusion becomes impaired.[67]

The attainment and maintenance of the new steady state requires that both *diuretic dose and Na^+ intake be relatively constant*. This limitation on the net diuresis is physiologically appropriate, since progressive volume depletion and shock would eventually ensue if urinary Na^+ excretion were persistently greater than intake. What is generally underappreciated, however, is how rapidly the steady state is reestablished. Figure 15-2 illustrates the response of three normal subjects on a constant Na^+ and K^+ intake to the administration of 100 mg of hydrochlorothiazide per day, a relatively high initial dose.[68] As can be seen, *Na^+ is lost for only 3 days and K^+ for 6 to 9 days*; after this period, intake and output of these ions are again equal. A similar course in which there is a limited net diuresis also occurs in edematous states such as heart failure and cirrhosis. In heart failure, for example, the diuretic-induced reduction in cardiac filling pressures leads to a decline in cardiac output and activation of the renin-angiotensin system.[69]

These findings are very important clinically. As long as dose and dietary intake are stable, *all of the fluid and electrolyte complications associated with diuretic therapy occur within the first 2 to 3 weeks of drug administration*. Suppose, for example, that 25 mg of hydrochlorothiazide is given each day to a patient with essential hypertension. At 3 weeks, the blood pressure has fallen to the goal level, and the blood urea nitrogen (BUN) and plasma creatinine, Na^+, and K^+ concentrations remain within the normal range. In this setting, late hypokalemia or hyponatremia is not likely to occur, and *repeat blood tests at every visit are not necessary* unless some new problem, such as vomiting or diarrhea, is superimposed.

As an example, sequential evaluation of patients with hypertension has revealed that all of the fall in the plasma K^+ concentration following therapy with a thiazide diuretic occurs within the first 2 to 4 weeks, with subsequent stabilization at the new level.[70] Similar considerations apply to the use of a K^+-

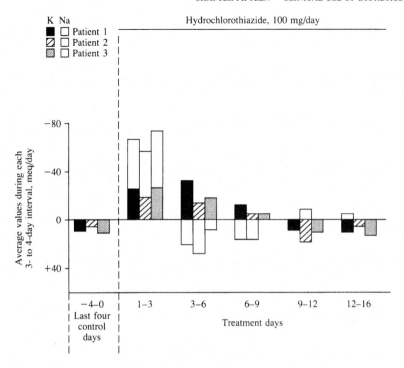

Figure 15-2   Sodium and potassium balance in three nonedematous patients treated with 100 mg of hydrochlorothiazide per day. Data for each patient reflect the average balance for each 3- or 4-day period. Net loss of Na⁺ is seen for only 3 days and of K⁺ for 6 to 9 days before a new steady state is reestablished. (*Adapted from Maronde RF, Milgrom M, Vlachakis ND, Chan L, JAMA 249:237, 1983. Copyright 1983, American Medical Association.*)

sparing diuretic to correct thiazide-induced hypokalemia; the plasma K^+ concentration rises during the first 2 to 3 weeks and then remains relatively constant.[71]

There is one other clinical correlate of these counterregulatory responses. Assuming no limitation in drug absorption and constant drug dosage, the *maximum diuresis will occur with the first dose of the diuretic.* As soon as fluid loss occurs, activation of Na^+-retaining mechanisms limit the response to the second dose. This concept is illustrated by the findings in Fig. 15-3; patients with stable chronic renal failure were treated with either intravenous boluses or a constant infusion of bumetanide.[72] The response to the second bolus was approximately one-third less than that to the first dose, whereas there is a gradually falling natriuresis with a constant infusion.

The sequence is somewhat different in patients who are markedly volume-expanded as a result of renal sodium retention. In this setting, the renin-angiotensin system is suppressed and will not be activated by initial Na^+ loss, since hypervolemia persists. Thus, the second and subsequent doses may produce as large a natriuresis as the original dose until most of the excess fluid has been removed. Even in this setting, however, the first dose still represents the maximum response that will be seen.

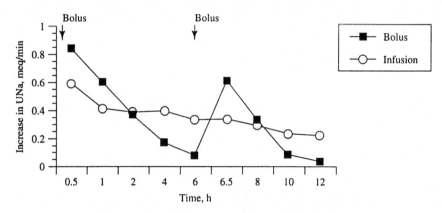

Figure 15-3 Maximum first-dose increase in urinary sodium excretion (UNa) after intravenous bolus or infusion of bumetanide in patients with stable chronic renal failure. With an intravenous bolus (dark squares), the peak natriuretic response to the second dose is 25 percent less than that to the first. With a continuous intravenous infusion (open circles), the natriuresis gradually declines over the 12-h period. The infusion produced a greater overall natriuresis, since an optimal rate of diuretic excretion was maintained. (*Adapted from Rudy DW, Voelker JR, Greene PK, et al, Ann Intern Med 115:360, 1991, with permission.*)

FLUID AND ELECTROLYTE COMPLICATIONS

A review of the toxic and idiosyncratic side effects that can be induced by the different diuretics is beyond the scope of this discussion. It is important, however, to understand the pathogenesis and frequency of the major fluid and electrolyte disturbances that can occur (Table 15-2).

Volume Depletion

Although the duration of Na^+ loss is limited, some patients have a relatively large initial diuretic response and develop true volume depletion. This problem can be seen in patients with hypertension and also in those with mild edema who are

Table 15-2 Fluid and electrolyte complications of diuretic therapy

Volume depletion
Azotemia
Hypokalemia
Metabolic alkalosis
Hyperkalemia and metabolic acidosis with K^+-sparing diuretics
Hyponatremia, especially with the thiazides
Hyperuricemia
Hypomagnesemia

started on daily diuretic therapy, which is then continued even after the edema has disappeared. Symptoms that can develop in this setting include weakness, malaise, muscle cramps, and postural dizziness.

Effective circulating volume depletion also can develop in patients who remain edematous. Although fluid overload persists, there may be a sufficient reduction in intracardiac filling pressures and cardiac output to produce a clinically important reduction in tissue perfusion (see the sections on treatment of heart failure and cirrhosis in the following chapter).

Azotemia

A reduction in the effective circulating volume with diuretic therapy also can diminish renal perfusion and secondarily the glomerular filtration rate. This problem, which is manifested by elevations in the BUN and plasma creatinine concentration, is called *prerenal azotemia*, since the defect is in renal perfusion, not in renal function, and there is a greater rise in the BUN than in the plasma creatinine concentration (see page 92).[73]

Increased passive reabsorption of urea, which follows the hypovolemia-induced increments in Na^+ and water reabsorption, plays a major role in the more pronounced elevation in BUN. In addition, as much as one-third of the rise in the BUN may reflect increased urea production; it is possible, for example, that reduced perfusion to skeletal muscle leads to enhanced local proteolysis.[74] The amino acids that are released are then converted into urea in the liver.

Hypokalemia and Use of Diuretics in Hypertension

The loop and thiazide diuretics tend to increase urinary K^+ losses[1,2,75] and often lead to the development of hypokalemia. For example, the administration of 50 mg of hydrochlorothiazide per day to treat hypertension is associated with a mean reduction in the plasma K^+ concentration of about 0.4 to 0.6 meq/L, with roughly 15 percent of patients falling to or below 3.5 meq/L.[70,76] The degree of potassium wasting is even greater with 50 mg of the longer-acting chlorthalidone; in this setting, the mean fall in the plasma K^+ concentration is 0.8 to 0.9 meq/L.[76]

Two factors appear to be responsible for the kaliuresis in this setting: increased delivery of Na^+ and H_2O to the distal secretory site, as a result of inhibition of reabsorption in the more proximal segments, and enhanced secretion of aldosterone, as a result of both the underlying disease (heart failure or cirrhosis) and the induction of volume depletion.[2,75]

The clinical significance of mild hypokalemia (plasma K^+ concentration between 3.0 and 3.5 meq/L) remains controversial, particularly in the treatment of patients with essential hypertension.[77] Some physicians have argued that mild K^+ depletion is usually a benign condition and that corrective therapy is not required in the absence of symptoms. Although this may be generally true, some patients appear to be at risk. As an example, results from the Multiple Risk Factor Intervention Trial (MRFIT) and other studies suggest that antihypertensive therapy in selected patients might be associated with an *increase in the incidence of sudden death* (Fig. 15-4).[78-80]

The mechanism by which diuretics might increase coronary risk is uncertain. These agents produce a variety of metabolic abnormalities that could contribute to this problem, including hypokalemia, hypomagnesemia (see below), hyperlipidemia, and hyperglycemia.[81-83] The possible role of any of these factors is, of course, difficult to prove. Hypokalemia has been shown in some studies to be associated with an increased incidence of ventricular arrhythmias.[84] In a report from the Framingham Heart Study, an association was noted between complex or frequent ($\geq 30/h$) ventricular premature beats and hypokalemia.[85] It was estimated that the risk of these arrhythmias increased by 27 percent with each 0.5 meq/L reduction in the plasma potassium concentration.

In the basal state, the development of ventricular arrhythmias may not be seen until the plasma K^+ concentration falls to or below 3.0 meq/L.[76] However, mild hypokalemia can become severe hypokalemia during a stress response, with the plasma K^+ concentration falling, for example, from 3.3 meq/L to below 2.8 meq/L in some patients (see Fig. 12-3). This response appears to be mediated by epinephrine, which derives K^+ into the cells via activation of the β_2-adrenergic receptors.[86]

These observations suggest the following scenario: Coronary ischemia leads to the release of epinephrine, which exacerbates preexistent diuretic-induced hypokalemia. The combination of coronary ischemia and a marked reduction in the plasma K^+ concentration then facilitates the development of potentially fatal ventricular arrhythmias, particularly in patients with underlying left ventricular

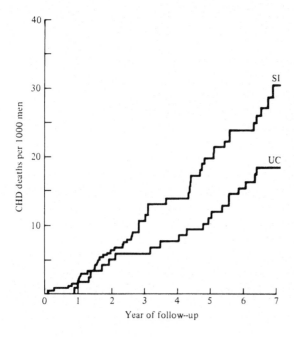

Figure 15-4 Cumulative coronary heart disease (CHD) mortality rates for hypertensive men with an abnormal resting electrocardiogram in the special intervention (SI) and usual care (UC) groups at 7 years in the MRFIT trial. The mortality rate was 68 percent higher in the treated (SI) group. (*Adapted from Multiple Risk Factor Intervention Trial Research Group,* Am J Cardiol *55:1, 1985, with permission.*)

hypertrophy. There is some evidence in support of this hypothesis, as the incidence of ventricular fibrillation following an acute myocardial infarction is increased more than twofold in patients who are initially hypokalemic.[87]

The thiazide diuretic dose may be an important determinant of risk. Many patients in the studies in which diuretics were associated with an increased risk of sudden death were treated with more than 50 mg/day of hydrochlorothiazide or chlorthalidone.[78-80] However, *lower and probably safer* doses can be used in many patients. As little as 12.5 mg of hydrochlorothiazide or 15 mg of chlorthalidone generally produce as large an antihypertensive effect as higher doses, with little or no change in the plasma concentrations of K^+, glucose, or uric acid (Fig. 15-5).[88-92] No increase in ventricular ectopic activity is observed with these lower doses,[93] and low-dose thiazide therapy is one of the recommended first-line modalities for the treatment of hypertension.[99] The greater degree of volume depletion induced by higher diuretic doses may not lead to a more prominent fall in blood pressure because of increased activity of the renin-angiotensin system.

Metabolic Alkalosis

Loop or thiazide diuretic–induced hypokalemia is often accompanied by metabolic alkalosis. Two factors contribute to this problem: increased urinary H^+ loss, due in part to secondary hyperaldosteronism, and, to a lesser degree, contraction of the extracellular volume around a constant amount of extracellular HCO_3^- (called a contraction alkalosis; see Chap. 18).[95,96] Aldosterone contributes to H^+-loss in this setting both by stimulating the distal H^+ ATPase pump and by

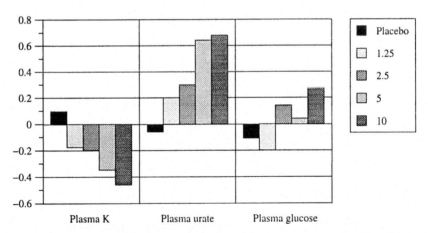

Figure 15-5 Metabolic complications induced by bendrofluazide in relation to dose (multiply by 10 to get equivalent doses of hydrochlorothiazide). Increasing the dose led to progressive hypokalemia and hyperuricemia and a greater likelihood of a mild elevation in the plasma glucose concentration, all without a further reduction in the systemic blood pressure. Each treatment group contained approximately 52 patients. (*Data from Carlsen JE, Kober L, Torp-Pedersen C, Johannsen P,* Br Med J *300:975, 1990, with permission.*)

promoting the reabsorption of cationic Na^+. The latter effect creates a lumen-negative electrical potential that promotes H^+ accumulation in the lumen by minimizing the degree of back-diffusion (see page 354).

The loop diuretics can also increase net H^+ loss by increased H^+ secretion in the cortical aspect of the thick ascending limb.[97] This segment has two luminal mechanisms for Na^+ entry: via Na^+-K^+-$2Cl^-$ transport and Na^+-H^+ exchange. Inhibition of the former with a loop diuretic will tend to increase Na^+ reabsorption in exchange for H^+

Although NaCl will reverse the alkalemia, this is not desirable in patients with edema. In this setting, acetazolamide may restore acid-base balance by promoting HCO_3^- loss in the urine.

Hyperkalemia and Metabolic Acidosis

The K^+-sparing diuretics reduce both K^+ and H^+ secretion in the collecting tubules. As a result, their use can result in both hyperkalemia and metabolic acidosis.[98,99] Prevention is the best therapy, as these drugs should be used with great caution, if at all, in patients with renal failure or those being treated with either an angiotensin converting enzyme inhibitor (which diminishes the release of aldosterone) or a K^+ supplement.

Hyponatremia

Hyponatremia is a relatively common abnormality in edematous patients with heart failure or cirrhosis. This problem can be exacerbated or produced de novo in hypertensives by diuretic therapy. The mechanism by which hyponatremia is induced is related both to effective volume depletion, leading to enhanced secretion of ADH, and to an increase in water intake.[100,101] The net effect is that ingested water is retained, lowering the plasma Na^+ concentration by dilution.

Almost all cases are due to therapy with a thiazide-type diuretic.[57,100,101] Although loop diuretics also induce volume depletion, they do so by impairing NaCl reabsorption in the thick ascending limb, thereby decreasing the generation of the medullary osmolal gradient (see Chap. 4). As a result, the ability of ADH to increase water reabsorption and promote the development of hyponatremia is limited.* The thiazides, in comparison, act in the cortex and do not interfere with concentrating ability.[102]

Hyperuricemia

Hyperuricemia is a relatively common finding in patients on diuretic therapy.[103,104] In general, this problem reflects increased urate reabsorption in the proximal

---

* The reduction in the urine osmolality induced by a loop diuretic actually increases free water excretion, making these agents *useful in the treatment of hyponatremia* in the syndrome of inappropriate ADH secretion (see page 729).

tubule, a process that appears to be mediated by parallel Na^+-H^+ and $urate^-$-OH^- exchangers in the luminal membrane (see Fig. 3-13a).[103,105] Net urate reabsorption varies directly with proximal Na^+ transport, and in patients with diuretic-induced volume depletion, both Na^+ and urate excretion are reduced.[106] If, on the other hand, the fluid losses are replaced, there is no stimulus to compensatory Na^+ retention and no hyperuricemia.[107]

The mechanism by which urate reabsorption is increased in this setting is incompletely understood. Angiotensin II, released in response to hypovolemia, may play a role by enhancing the activity of the Na^+-H^+ exchanger, which can then lead to a parallel increase in $urate^-$-OH^- exchange. In addition, enhanced proximal water reabsorption will elevate the tubular fluid urate concentration, thereby promoting passive urate reabsorption.

Treatment of diuretic-induced hyperuricemia is *not necessary in asymptomatic patients*, even though the plasma urate concentration may exceed 12 mg/dL.[104,108] Goutly arthritis is uncommon in this setting, occurring primarily in patients with a personal or family history of gout. Renal damage due to the intratubular precipitation of uric acid is also not a problem, since the hyperuricemia is due to an initial decrease in the distal delivery and subsequent excretion or uric acid.

Hypomagnesemia

Magnesium depletion, which is generally mild, can be induced by diuretic therapy.[109-111] Most of the filtered magnesium is reabsorbed in the loop of Henle, a process that can be inhibited directly with loop diuretics.[112] The thiazides, in comparison, have little acute effect on magnesium handling but may be associated with chronic magnesium depletion, perhaps because of the effects of hypokalemia or secondary hyperaldosteronism. Hypokalemia may directly inhibit distal tubular cell magnesium uptake, thereby increasing magnesium excretion.[112]

How aldosterone enhances urinary magnesium excretion is not clear, but the following mechanisms may contribute. The extrusion of reabsorbed magnesium across the basolateral membrane in the cortical collecting tubule may be mediated by a Na^+-Mg^{2+} exchanger that relies on the favorable inward gradient for Na^+ to enter the cell. Increasing Na^+ reabsorption with aldosterone raises the cell Na^+ concentration, thereby diminishing the gradient for Na^+ entry across the basolateral membrane and therefore the degree of Mg^{2+} extrusion.[113] The observation that decreasing the aldosterone effect with a K^+-sparing diuretic tends to diminish urinary magnesium losses is compatible with this hypothesis.[111,114]

DETERMINANTS OF DIURETIC RESPONSE

Before discussing the problem of resistant edema, it is important to first review the factors that influence the natriuretic response to a given diuretic. As described above, two important determinants are the site of action of the diuretic and the possible presence of counterbalancing antinatriuretic forces, such as angiotensin II, aldosterone, and a fall in the systemic blood pressure. In addition, the *rate of drug excretion* also plays a major role, particularly with the loop diuretics.[115-117]

Almost all of the commonly used diuretics, particularly the loop diuretics, are highly protein-bound.[118] As a result, they are not well filtered and enter the urine primarily via the organic anion or organic cation secretory pump in the proximal tubule (see Fig. 3-13*b*).[116,119] Their subsequent ability to inhibit Na^+ reabsorption is in part dose-dependent, being influenced by the rate at which the diuretic is delivered to its tubular site of action (Fig. 15-6). Thus, higher doses of a loop diuretic will in general produce a greater rate of both diuretic and Na^+ excretion. On the other hand, impaired diuretic entry into the lumen is one of the causes of diuretic resistance (see below).

It should be noted, however, that the natriuretic response tends to plateau at higher rates of diuretic excretion, presumably because of complete inhibition of the diuretic-sensitive carrier or channel. In normal subjects, for example, the *maximum diuresis is seen with 40 mg of furosemide or 1 mg of bumetanide given intravenously*. The oral dose equivalent is similar for bumetanide, which is almost completely absorbed, but is increased to 80 mg for furosemide, only about one-half of which undergoes intestinal absorption. These doses often must be adjusted upward in edematous patients as a result of decreased net drug entry into the lumen.

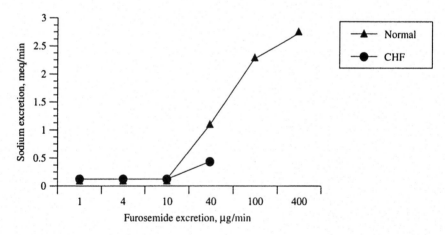

Figure 15-6 Relation between the rate of furosemide excretion and the increase in sodium excretion in normals and in patients with congestive heart failure (CHF). A diuresis is not seen until a threshold rate of furosemide excretion is reached; at this point, sodium excretion increases in a dose-dependent manner until a maximum effect is seen. Patients with CHF show relative resistance at a given rate of diuretic excretion as a result of increased sodium reabsorption in other nephron segments. (*Data from Brater DC, Day B, Burdette A, Anderson S, et al*, Kidney Int 26:183, 1984, with permission.)

REFRACTORY EDEMA

Although the treatment of the different edematous states will be discussed in the following chapter, the same principles apply to all patients who are resistant to conventional diuretic therapy. The causes of this problem and possible corrective measures are depicted in Table 15-3.[1,3,120] In general, therapy is begun with a loop diuretic, since these agents are the most potent and give the most predictable response. The initial aim is to find the *effective single dose*. In patients with advanced renal insufficiency or congestive heart failure, for example, 40 mg of intravenous furosemide may not induce a diuresis because of a reduction in drug entry into the tubular lumen. In this setting, giving 40 mg twice a day will also be ineffective, since adequate urinary levels are never achieved.[115] A more appropriate regimen is to *double the individual dose* until a diuresis is obtained or a maximum dose of 160 to 200 mg (or 320 to 400 mg of oral furosemide due to incomplete intestinal absorption) is reached.[115,116]

Excess Sodium Intake

Assuming that the patient is taking the diuretic, maintenance of a high-Na^+ diet can, as shown in Fig. 15-1, prevent net fluid loss even though an adequate diuresis is achieved. This possibility can be confirmed by a 24-h urine collection. A value above 100 to 150 meq/day indicates the necessity for either better dietary compliance or the use of higher doses or more frequent drug administration.

This problem with diet is often seen after patients are discharged from the hospital, when Na^+ intake may be less carefully regulated. As a result, a previously

Table 15-3   Pathogenesis and treatment of refractory edema

Problem	Treatment
Excess sodium intake	Measure urine sodium excretion; attempt more rigorous dietary restriction if greater than 100 meq/day
Decreased or delayed intestinal drug absorption	Bowel wall edema can reversibly impair oral drug absorption; switch to intravenous loop diuretic if high-dose oral therapy is ineffective
Decreased drug entry into the tubular lumen	Increase to maximum effective dose of a loop diuretic (160 to 200 mg of intravenous furosemide or 4 to 5 mg of bumetanide); use of spironolactone in cirrhosis; mixture of albumin and loop diuretic if marked hypoalbuminemia
Increased distal reabsorption	Multiple daily doses if partial diuretic response; add thiazide-type and/or K^+-sparing diuretic
Decreased loop sodium delivery due to low GFR and/or enhanced proximal reabsorption	Attempt to increase delivery out of proximal tubule with acetazolamide or corticosteroids; diuretic administration in supine posture or head-down tilt; dialysis or hemofiltration if severe renal or heart failure

well-controlled patient may develop recurrent edema in the absence of any exacerbation of his or her underlying disease. Enhanced activity in the outpatient setting also may play a role. With congestive heart failure, for example, the cardiac output may be relatively normal at rest but unable to increase appropriately with exertion (see "Decreased Loop Sodium Delivery," below). This low-output state will exacerbate the tendency to Na^+ retention.

Decreased or Delayed Intestinal Drug Absorption

Some edematous patients who are resistant to as much as 240 mg of oral furosemide respond to as little as 40 mg given intravenously.[121] This problem, which has been described in advanced heart failure and cirrhosis, reflects a delay in intestinal absorption, leading to urinary excretion of the drug at suboptimal levels.[121-123] Decreased intestinal perfusion, reduced intestinal motility, and perhaps mucosal edema all may contribute to the delay in absorption.[122,123] Both removal of edema with intravenous diuretic therapy and, in heart failure, stabilization of cardiac function may at least partially correct this absorptive defect, thereby restoring the efficacy of oral therapy.

Decreased Drug Entry into the Tubular Lumen

Decreased drug excretion can limit the diuretic response in patients with advanced heart failure, renal failure, cirrhosis, or hypoalbuminemia.[120,124] For example, thiazide-type diuretics generally produce little effect once the glomerular filtration rate is below 20 mL/min[125] unless either a loop diuretic is given concurrently[126] or very high doses of the thiazide are used.[127] The loop diuretics, on the other hand, may be effective even in advanced renal failure (Fig. 15-3).[72,119,128] As will be described below, there may be advantages to the use of intravenous infusions rather than bolus injections of loop diuretics in some patients.

Renal failure   Diuretic excretion is often limited in renal failure, in part because of the retention of organic anions such as hippurate that compete for secretion by the proximal secretory pump.[116,119] In this setting, a higher than normal dose is often required to produce the desired diuretic effect.

Studies with furosemide indicate that the peak response can usually be achieved by increasing the single intravenous dose from 40 mg up to a maximum of 160 to 200 mg.[107,128] This dose can be given two or even three times a day if necessary, since there is a relatively short-lived diuretic response. Similar considerations apply to bumetanide, which is usually 40 times more potent than furosemide on a weight basis and is therefore given in one-fortieth the dose. In renal failure, however, there is a relative increase in the extrarenal clearance of bumetanide; as a result, the dose must be increased to one-twentieth that of furosemide, or a maximum of 8 to 10 mg.[116]

Some studies have advocated the use of extremely high doses of furosemide (up to 2400 mg per day) in resistant patients. Although this may increase the urine output in selected cases, it is also associated with an enhanced risk of ototoxicity and possible permanent deafness, particularly if given as an intravenous bolus (with the attendant very high peak plasma levels) rather than being infused slowly over 20 to 60 min.[129,130] Observations in animals suggest that this complication may be due to inhibition of a Na^+-K^+-$2Cl^-$ carrier (similar to that in the thick ascending limb) in the endolymph-producing cells.[131] Ethacrynic acid appears to have the highest ototoxic potential; its use is generally limited to patients allergic to one of the other agents, since it is the *only loop or thiazide diuretic that is not a sulfonamide derivative.*

Cirrhosis   Spironolactone is the diuretic of choice for the initial treatment of fluid overload in the setting of cirrhosis. It may be more effective than loop diuretics alone[132,133] and does not induce hypokalemia, which may precipitate hepatic encephalopathy.

One possible explanation for the surprising efficacy of spironolactone compared to loop diuretics is that patients with cirrhotic ascites have marked hyperaldosteronism and therefore reclaim the excess fluid delivered out of the loop of Henle in the cortical collecting tubule. As depicted in Fig. 15-7, however, the slope of the relationship between the rate of furosemide excretion and the diuretic response in cirrhotic patients may be similar to that in normals, suggesting that there is only minor intraluminal resistance to furosemide.

As mentioned above, most loop diuretics are highly protein-bound; as a result, they enter the tubular lumen by secretion in the proximal tubule, not by glomerular filtration. In many cases, the resistance to loop diuretics in cirrhosis results from a decreased rate of drug secretion into the lumen ($< 20\,mg/h$), perhaps as a result of competition from other organic anions such as bile salts for the organic anion secretory pump.[117] Spironolactone may be uniquely effective in this setting because it is the only *diuretic that does not require access to the tubular lumen.*[37] It enters the tubular cell from the plasma across the basolateral membrane and then competes with aldosterone for its cytosolic receptor.

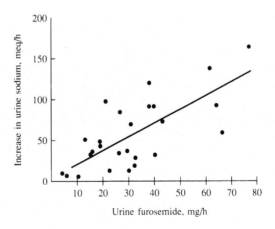

Figure 15-7 Relationship between the rate of furosemide excretion and the increase in the rate of Na^+ excretion in patients with alcoholic liver disease. The slope of this line is similar to that in normal subjects, with the natriuresis being limited in those patients with a low rate of furosemide excretion. (*From Pinzani M, Daskalopoulos G, Laffi G, et al*, Gastroenterology, *92:294, 1987. Copyright 1987 by The American Gastroenterological Association. Used with permission.*)

For patients who do not respond to dietary Na^+ restriction and spironolactone alone, the most successful therapeutic regimen is the combination of single morning oral doses of spironolactone and furosemide, beginning with 100 mg and 40 mg, respectively.[133,134] This combination in this ratio usually maintains normokalemia. The doses can be doubled if a clinical response is not evident. The maximum recommended doses are spironolactone 400 mg/day and furosemide 160 mg/day.

Hypoalbuminemia Marked hypoalbuminemia (plasmin albumin concentration usually under 2 g/dL) is another condition that may be associated with decreased diuretic entry into the lumen.[135] The protein-binding of drugs and toxins largely restricts the volume of distribution to the vascular space. This has two potentially protective effects: It limits access to the cells, and it maximizes the rate of delivery to the kidney, where rapid excretion can occur. When binding of a loop diuretic is diminished because of a reduction in the plasma albumin concentration, however, there is increased entry into the interstitial space and a slower rate of drug excretion.

A second mechanism may be operative when hypoalbuminemia is due to heavy proteinuria in the nephrotic syndrome. In this setting, free drug that is secreted into the tubular lumen may be bound to filtered albumin, thereby becoming inactive.[136,137] In experimental animals, for example, nephrotic-range albuminuria can diminish the response to intraluminal furosemide by about 50 percent.[137] Filtered IgG, in comparison, does not bind furosemide or interfere with its effect.[137]

Some patients with the nephrotic syndrome and severe hypoalbuminemia are resistant to conventional diuretic therapy. Some of these patients have been treated with 40 to 80 mg of furosemide added to 6.25 to 12.5 g of salt-poor albumin. Infusion of the furosemide-albumin complex is thought to act by increasing diuretic delivery to the kidney and can, in some cases, lead to a modest increase in sodium excretion.[138]

Intravenous infusion of loop diuretics A possibly safer and more effective alternative to bolus injections in patients requiring high-dose therapy is to administer the loop diuretic as a continuous intravenous infusion. Studies in patients with stable chronic renal failure suggest that a constant infusion of bumetanide (1 mg bolus followed by 1 mg per hour) can produce as much as a 33 percent greater increment in sodium excretion compared to standard bolus therapy (6 mg every 6 to 12 h) (Fig. 15-3).[72] This difference is probably related to differences in the rate of drug excretion. Bolus therapy may be transiently associated with periods of both supramaximal and submaximal excretion, resulting in some of the drug being excreted ineffectively. In comparison, a constant infusion maintains an optimal rate of drug excretion on the ascending portion of the curve in Fig. 15-6. (Similar findings have been demonstrated in normal subjects, as 4 mg of intravenous furosemide per hour produces a greater diuresis than a 40-mg bolus.[139]

The main utility of continuous intravenous loop diuretics is in hospitalized patients in the intensive care unit with marked edema who show a response to a standard intravenous bolus that is not sustained. Patients who show no response to a large bolus (such as 240 to 320 mg of furosemide) are *unlikely to respond to an infusion*, since bolus therapy results in higher initial plasma and urinary diuretic levels.

After the initial bolus, we generally begin with furosemide at a dose of 20 mg/h. If the diuresis is not sustained, a second bolus is given followed by a higher infusion rate of 40 mg/h. The risk associated with still higher infusion rates of 80 to 160 mg/h must be weighed against those of alternative strategies such as the addition of a thiazide-type diuretic or fluid removal via hemofiltration (see below). Equivalent doses are 1 mg/h increasing to 2 mg/h for bumetanide and 10 mg/h increasing to 20 mg/h for torsemide.

Increased Distal Reabsorption

The effect of a loop or thiazide diuretic is in part blunted by increased Na^+ reabsorption in the more distal segments, because of both the direct effect of the increase in Na^+ delivery and the action of aldosterone in the collecting tubules.[3,8,10,25] As an example, patients with moderate to advanced heart failure typically have a lower maximal diuretic response even if there is adequate drug entry into the lumen (Fig. 15-6).[115] In this setting, the *single response may be insufficient and drug administration two or even three times a day may be required.* In comparison, there is little to be gained from increasing the single dose above 120 to 160 mg of intravenous furosemide (or 3 to 4 mg of bumetanide), since there is already maximal inhibition of the Na^+-K^+-$2Cl^-$ carrier.[115]

In some patients, however, the increase in distal reabsorption results in resistance to loop diuretic therapy. This problem can often be overcome by the addition of a thiazide with or without a K^+-sparing diuretic to block Na^+ transport at multiple sites in the nephron.[120,126,140-142] The K^+-sparing diuretic is usually given to minimize K^+ loss, since it induces only a minor increment in Na^+ excretion.[120]

The efficacy of the addition of a thiazide may be related to both the *proximal and distal* actions of the drug. The former normally plays a minor role, because the excess fluid delivered out of the proximal tubule is reabsorbed in the loop of Henle;[21] concurrent use of a loop diuretic, however, blocks this compensatory response and can unmask the proximal effect. Furthermore, there is a compensatory rise in distal tubule Na^+ reabsorption induced by the increase in delivery out of the loop of Henle; as a result, blocking this response with a thiazide will now produce a larger than normal increment in Na^+ excretion.[2,10] In one study of patients pretreated with furosemide or placebo, for example, the natriuretic response to the addition of a thiazide was approximately 20 percent greater in the furosemide group, suggesting increased reabsorption at a thiazide-sensitive site (Fig. 15-8).[10]

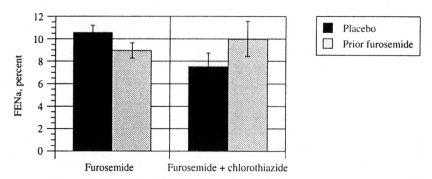

Figure 15-8   Diuretic responsiveness in patients previously treated for 1 month with placebo or the loop diuretic furosemide. The subjects who had been treated with furosemide had a lesser increase in the fractional excretion of sodium (FENa) after the administration of furosemide (left panel) but a greater natriuretic response to the addition of chlorothiazide (right panel). These findings are compatible with increased tubular sodium reabsorption at the thiazide-sensitive site in the distal tubule when distal sodium delivery is chronically increased by furosemide. (*Data from Loon NR, Wilcox CS, Unwin RJ,* Kidney Int *36:682, 1989, with permission.*)

The beneficial effect of adding a thiazide can be demonstrated even in patients with advanced renal failure. One study, for example, evaluated patients with a mean creatinine clearance of 13 mL/min.[142] The addition of the equivalent of 30 mg of hydrochlorothiazide almost doubled the increase in Na^+ excretion induced by the equivalent of 150 to 200 mg of furosemide alone.

It had been proposed that metolazone is more effective than other thiazides in this setting.[127] However, this study used very large doses; at equivalent doses, there is little evidence of a response different from that to other thiazide-type diuretics.[3,126,142]

Careful monitoring is required when combination therapy is initiated, because an excessive diuretic response may be seen. Some previously refractory patients, for example, can lose as much as 5 liters of fluid and 200 meq of K^+ per day.[140] It is prudent, therefore, to begin with low doses of a thiazide (such as 250 mg of chlorothiazide, 25 mg of hydrochlorothiazide, or 1.25 to 5 mg of metolazone) and probably to add a K^+-sparing diuretic unless the patient has baseline hyperkalemia. As described above, monitoring is most important on the first day, when the diuretic response is likely to be greatest (Fig. 15-3).

Decreased Loop Sodium Delivery

In some patients with severe heart failure or cirrhosis, the combination of a reduction in glomerular filtration rate (as a result of the decline in renal perfusion) and an increase in proximal reabsorption (mediated in part by angiotensin II) markedly reduces the delivery of fluid to the diuretic-sensitive sites in the more distal nephron segments.[124,143] In this setting, the addition of acetazolamide may substantially enhance the diuretic response by diminishing proximal reabsorption.[144]

Improving renal perfusion by changes in *posture* is an additional modality that may be successful in selected cases. Patients with heart failure and cirrhosis tend to have effective volume depletion and renal vasoconstriction, mediated in part by the associated increases in angiotensin II and norepinephrine. These changes are most prominent in the upright position, because of the effects of gravity and an inability in heart failure to appropriately increase cardiac output with exertion.[145] On the other hand, assumption of the supine position or a 10-degree head-down tilt maximizes cardiac output in relation to needs and may enhance venous return to the heart; the net effect is a rise in creatinine clearance of as much as 40 percent and a possible doubling of Na^+ excretion both in the basal state and after the administration of a loop diuretic.[146,147]

Some patients with advanced heart failure or renal failure will not respond to any of the above modalities. In this setting, either dialysis or hemofiltration can be used to remove the excess fluid.[148-150] With continuous arteriovenous hemofiltration, for example, catheters are inserted into an artery and a vein. Arterial pressure is used to perfuse a hemofilter (similar to a dialysis cartridge); the blood leaving the filter then returns to the patient through the venous catheter. Careful monitoring is essential, since the rate of filtration can exceed 500 to 1000 mL/h with this procedure.[148,150]

OTHER USES OF DIURETICS

The preceding discussion has reviewed the use of diuretics in edematous states, hypertension, hypercalcemia, and hypercalciuria. These agents are also useful in the treatment of a variety of other conditions, including metabolic alkalosis, renal tubular acidosis, diabetes insipidus, hyponatremia due to the syndrome of inappropriate ADH secretion, and hypokalemia due to primary hyperaldosteronism (see the relevant chapters elsewhere in the book).

DIURETICS AND PROSTAGLANDINS

The loop diuretics and to a lesser degree the thiazides increase the renal production of prostaglandins.[151-153] The local release of vasodilator prostaglandins may have important hemodynamic actions, leading to an acute increase in renal blood flow,[151,152] venodilation, and a rise in venous capacitance.[154,155] The last effect is helpful in the treatment of acute pulmonary edema, since the associated pooling of blood in the venous system will diminish fluid delivery to the heart, thereby lowering the cardiac filling pressures prior to the onset of the diuresis.[156]

Nonsteroidal anti-inflammatory drugs, which impair prostaglandin synthesis, minimize the diuresis induced by furosemide in humans.[157,158] It is not clear, however, whether this reflects reversal of a natriuretic effect of the prostaglandins (which may inhibit Na^+ reabsorption in the thick ascending limb and cortical collecting tubule) or renal ischemia due to the unopposed vasoconstrictor actions of angiotensin II and norepinephrine.[159]

Inhibition of vasodilator prostaglandin synthesis by nonsteroidal anti-inflammatory drugs may have two additional deleterious effects in patients treated with diuretics: (1) an elevation in blood pressure in hypertensives[160,161] and (2) a further reduction in cardiac output in severe heart failure due to the rise in vascular resistance.[162]

Vasoconstrictor Response to Loop Diuretics

Loop diuretics are one of the initial mainstays of therapy in severe heart failure, because of the combination of venodilation (in acute pulmonary edema) and enhanced urine output. However, there may be an acute deleterious effect in some patients with chronic heart failure. This maladaptive response, which lasts for up to 1 h, is characterized by arteriolar vasoconstriction and a rise in systemic blood pressure; the ensuing increase in afterload then induces an elevation in pulmonary capillary wedge pressure and a reduction in cardiac output.[163] The plasma renin activity and plasma norepinephrine levels are increased in this setting and are presumably responsible for the rise in vascular resistance. By 4 h, in comparison, there is an improvement in cardiac function as the vasoconstrictor hormones return to the basal levels and the diuretic effect lowers the cardiac filling pressures.

Early vasoconstriction also occurs in some patients with cirrhosis, in whom furosemide can acutely lower both renal plasma flow and the glomerular filtration rate by 30 to 40 percent.[164]

PROBLEMS

15-1 Match the clinical setting with the preferred form of diuretic therapy.

   (a) Acetazolamide
   (b) Loop diuretic
   (c) Thiazide-type diuretic
   (d) Spironolactone

   (1) Recurrent nephrolithiasis due to hypercalciuria
   (2) Cirrhosis with ascites
   (3) Metabolic alkalosis following diuretic therapy for heart failure
   (4) Hypercalcemia
   (5) Hyponatremia due to the syndrome of inappropriate ADH secretion

15-2 What are the mechanisms by which the following can limit the response to a diuretic?

   (a) Hypoalbuminemia
   (b) Activation of the renin-angiotensin system
   (c) Hypotension

REFERENCES

1. Rose BD. Diuretics. *Kidney Int* 39:336, 1991.
2. Hropot M, Fowler N, Karlmark B, Giebisch G. Tubular action of diuretics: Distal effects on electrolyte transport and acidification. *Kidney Int* 28:477, 1985.
3. Ellison DH. Diuretic drugs and the treatment of edema: From clinic to bench and back again. *Am J Kidney Dis* 23:623, 1994.
4. Katz AI. Distribution and function of classes of ATPases along the nephron. *Kidney Int* 29:21, 1986.
5. Wright FS. Flow-dependent transport processes: Filtration, absorption, secretion. *Am J Physiol* 243:F1, 1982.
6. Greger R, Velazquez H. The cortical thick ascending limb and early distal convoluted tubule in the urine concentrating mechanism. *Kidney Int* 31:590, 1987.
7. Ellison DH, Velasquez H, Wright FS. Adaptation of the distal convoluted tubule of the rat. Structural and functional effects of dietary salt intake and chronic diuretic infusion. *J Clin Invest* 83:113, 1989.
8. Stanton BA, Kaissling B. Regulation of renal ion transport and cell growth by sodium. *Am J Physiol* 257:F1, 1989.
9. Scherzer P, Wald H, Popovtzer MM. Enhanced glomerular filtration and Na^+-K^+-ATPase with furosemide administration. *Am J Physiol* 252:F910, 1987.
10. Loon NR, Wilcox CS, Unwin RJ. Mechanism of impaired natriuretic response to furosemide during prolonged therapy. *Kidney Int* 36:682, 1989.
11. Stanton BA, Kaissling B. Adaptation of distal tubule and collecting duct to increased Na delivery. II. Na^+ and K^+ transport. *Am J Physiol* 255:F1269, 1988.
12. Hebert SC, Reeves WB, Molony RA, Andreoli TE. The medullary thick limb: Function and modulation of the single effect multiplier. *Kidney Int* 31:580, 1987.
13. O'Grady SM, Palfrey HC, Field M. Characteristics and functions of Na-K-2Cl cotransport in epithelial tissues. *Am J Physiol* 253:C177, 1987.
14. Amsler K, Kinne R. Photoinactivation of S-P-Cl cotransport in $LLC\text{-}PK_1/Cl$ 4 cells by bumetanide. *Am J Physiol* 250:C799, 1986.
15. Bronner F. Renal calcium transport: Mechanisms and regulation—An overview. *Am J Physiol* 257:F707, 1989.
16. Friedman PA. Basal and hormone-activated calcium absorption in mouse renal thick ascending limbs. *Am J Physiol* 254:F62, 1988.
17. Bilezikian JP. Drug therapy: Management of acute hypercalcemia. *N Engl J Med* 326:1196, 1992.
18. Hufnagel KG, Khan SN, Penn D, et al. Renal calcifications: A complication of long-term furosemide therapy in pre-term infants. *Pediatrics* 70:360, 1982.
19. Short A, Cooke RWI. The incidence of renal calcification in preterm infants. *Arch Dis Child* 66:412, 1991.
20. Velazquez H, Wright FS. Effect of diuretic drugs on Na, Cl, and K transport in the rat renal distal tubule. *Am J Physiol* 250:F1013, 1986.
21. Kunau RT Jr, Weller DR, Webb HL. Clarification of the site of action of chlorothiazide in the rat nephron. *J Clin Invest* 56:401, 1975.
22. Shimizu T, Yoshitomi K, Nakamura M, Imai M. Site and mechanism of action of trichlormethazide in rabbit distal nephron segments perfused in vitro. *J Clin Invest* 82:721, 1988.
23. Terada Y, Knepper MA. Thiazide-sensitive NaCl absorption in rat cortical collecting duct. *Am J Physiol* 259:F519, 1990.
24. Rouch AJ, Chen L, Troutman SL, Schafer JA. Na^+ transport in isolated CCD: Effects of bradykinin, ANP, clonidine, and hydrochlorothiazide. *Am J Physiol* 260:F86, 1991.
25. Garg LC, Narang N. Effects of hydrochlorothiazide on Na^+-K^+-ATPase activity along the rat nephron. *Kidney Int* 31:918, 1985.
26. Stanton BA. Cellular actions of thiazide diuretics in the distal tubule. *J Am Soc Nephrol* 1:836, 1990.

27. Plotkin MD, Kaplan MR, Verlander JW, et al. Localization of the thiazide-sensitive Na-Cl cotransporter, rTSC1, in the rat kidney. *Kidney Int* 49:174, 1996.
28. Gamba G, Saltzberg SN, Lombardi M, et al. Primary structure and functional expression of a cDNA encoding the thiazide-sensitive electroneutral sodium-chloride cotransporter. *Proc Natl Acad Sci U S A* 90:2749, 1993.
29. Gamba G. Molecular biology of distal nephron sodium transport mechanisms. *Kidney Int* 56:1606, 1999.
30. Tran JM, Farrell MA, Fanestil DD. Effect of ions on binding of the thiazide-type diuretic metolazone to the kidney membrane. *Am J Physiol* 258:F908, 1990.
31. Boer WH, Koomans HA, Dorhout Mees EJ. Acute effects of the thiazides, with and without carbonic anhydrase inhibiting activity, on lithium and free water clearance in man. *Clin Sci* 76:539, 1989.
32. Sutton RAL. Disorders of renal calcium excretion. *Kidney Int* 23:665, 1983.
33. Costanzo LS. Localization of diuretic action in microperfused rat distal tubules: Ca and Na transport. *Am J Physiol* 248:F527, 1985.
34. Coe FL, Parks JH, Asplin JR. The pathogenesis and treatment of kidney stones. *N Engl J Med* 327:1141, 1992.
35. Gesek FA, Friedman PA. Mechanism of calcium transport stimulation by chlorothiazide in mouse distal collecting tubule cells. *J Clin Invest* 90:429, 1992.
36. Kleyman TR, Cragoe EJ Jr. The mechanism of action of amiloride. *Semin Nephrol* 8:242, 1988.
37. Horisberger J-D, Giebisch G. Potassium-sparing diuretics. *Renal Physiol* 10:198, 1987.
38. Frindt G, Sackin H, Palmer LG. Whole-cell currents in rat cortical collecting tubule: Low-Na diet increases amiloride-sensitive conductance. *Am J Physiol* 258:F502, 1990.
39. Sansom S, Muto S, Giebisch G. Na-dependent effects of DOCA on cellular transport properties of CCDs from ADX rabbits. *Am J Physiol* 253:F753, 1987.
40. Gamba G. Molecular biology of distal nephron sodium transport mechanisms. *Kidney Int* 56:1606, 1999.
41. Alappan R, Perazella MA, Buller GK. Hyperkalemia in hospitalized patients treated with trimethoprim-sulfamethoxazle. *Ann Intern Med* 124:316, 1996.
42. Batlle DC, von Riotte AB, Gaviria M, Grupp M. Amelioration of polyuria by amiloride in patients receiving long-term lithium therapy. *N Engl J Med* 312:408, 1985.
43. Sica DA, Gehr TWB. Triamterene and the kidney. *Nephron* 51:454, 1989.
44. Fairley KF, Woo KT, Birch BF, et al. Triamterene-induced crystalluria and cylinduria: Clinical and experimental studies. *Clin Nephrol* 26:169, 1986.
45. Carr MC, Prien EL Jr, Babayan RK. Triamterene nephrolithiasis: Renewed attention is warranted. *J Urol* 144:1339, 1990.
46. Farge D, Turner MW, Roy DR, Jothy S. Dyazide-induced reversible acute renal failure associated with intratubular crystal deposition. *Am J Kid Dis* 8:445, 1986.
47. Weinberg MS, Quigg RJ, Salant DJ, Bernard DB. Anuric renal failure precipitated by indomethacin and triamterene. *Nephron* 40:216, 1985.
48. Woolfson RG, Mansell MA. Does triamterene cause renal calculi? *Br Med J* 303:1217, 1991.
49. Leaf A, Schwartz WB, Relman AS. Oral administration of a potent carbonic anhydrase inhibitor ("Diamox"): I. Changes in electrolyte and acid-base balance. *N Engl J Med* 250:759, 1954.
50. Preisig PA, Toto RD, Alpern RJ. Carbonic anhydrase inhibitors. *Renal Physiol* 10:136, 1987.
51. Seely JF, Dirks JH. Micropuncture study of hypertonic mannitol diuresis in the proximal and distal tubule of the dog kidney. *J Clin Invest* 48:2330, 1969.
52. Mathisen O, Raeder M, Kiil F. Mechanism of osmotic diuresis. *Kidney Int* 19:431, 1981.
53. Lieberthal W, Levinsky NG. Treatment of acute tubular necrosis. *Semin Nephrol* 10:571, 1990.
54. Lieberthal W, Sheridan AM, Valeri CR. Protective effect of atrial natriuretic factor and mannitol following renal ischemia. *Am J Physiol* 258:F1266, 1990.
55. Gipstein RM, Boyle JD. Hypernatremia complicating prolonged mannitol diuresis. *N Engl J Med* 272:1116, 1965.

56. Aviram A, Pfau A, Czackes JW, Ullman TD. Hyperosmolality with hyponatremia caused by inappropriate administration of mannitol. *Am J Med* 42:648, 1967.
57. Singer I, Oster JR. Hyponatremia, hyposmolality, and hypotonicity. *Arch Intern Med* 159:333, 1999.
58. Wilcox CS, Guzman NJ, Mitch WE, et al. Na$^+$, K$^+$, and BP homeostasis in man during furosemide: Effects of prazosin and captopril. *Kidney Int* 31:135, 1987.
59. Wilcox CS, Mitch WE, Kelly RA, et al. Response of the kidney to furosemide: I. Effects of salt intake and renal compensation. *J Lab Clin Med* 102:450, 1983.
60. Ram CVS, Garrett BN, Kaplan NM. Moderate sodium restriction and various diuretics in the treatment of hypertension. Effects on potassium wastage and blood pressure control. *Arch Intern Med* 141:1015, 1981.
61. Bock HA, Stein JH. Diuretics and the control of extracellular fluid volume: Role of counterregulation. *Semin Nephrol* 8:264, 1988.
62. Cogan MG. Angiotensin II: A potent controller of sodium transport in the early proximal tubule. *Hypertension* 15:451, 1990.
63. Stanton BA. Regulation of Na$^+$ and K$^+$ transport by mineralocorticoids. *Semin Nephrol* 7:82, 1987.
64. Osborn JL, Holdaas H, Thames MD, DiBona GF. Renal adrenoreceptor mediation of antinatriuretic and renin secretion responses to low frequency renal nerve stimulation in the dog. *Circ Res* 53:298, 1983.
65. Guyton AC. Blood pressure control—Special role of the kidneys and body fluids. *Science* 252:1813, 1991.
66. Dirks JH, Cirksena WJ. Micropuncture study of the effect of various diuretics on sodium reabsorption by the proximal tubules of the dog. *J Clin Invest* 45:1875, 1966.
67. Nomua A, Yasuda H, Minami M, et al. Effect of furosemide in congestive heart failure. *Clin Pharmacol Ther* 30:177, 1981.
68. Maronde R, Milgrom M, Vlachakis ND, Chan L. Response of thiazide-induced hypokalemia to amiloride. *JAMA* 249:237, 1983.
69. Ikram H, Chan W, Espiner EA, Nicholls MG. Hemodynamic and hormone responses to acute and chronic frusemide therapy in congestive heart failure. *Clin Sci* 59:443, 1980.
70. Morgan DB, Davidson C. Hypokalemia and diuretics: An analysis of publications. *Br Med J* 280:905, 1980.
71. Ridgeway NA, Ginn DR, Alley K. Outpatient conversion of treatment to potassium-sparing diuretics. *Am J Med* 80:785, 1986.
72. Rudy DW, Voelker JR, Greene PK, et al. Loop diuretics for chronic renal failure: A continuous infusion is more efficacious than bolus therapy. *Ann Intern Med* 115:360, 1991.
73. Dossetor JB. Creatininemia versus uremia: The relative significance of blood urea nitrogen and serum creatinine concentrations in azotemia. *Ann Intern Med* 65:1287, 1966.
74. Kamm DE, Wu L, Kuchmy BL. Contribution of the urea appearance rate to diuretic-induced azotemia in the rat. *Kidney Int* 32:47, 1987.
75. Duarte CG, Chomety F, Giebisch G. Effect of amiloride, ouabain, and furosemide on distal tubular function in the rat. *Am J Physiol* 221:632, 1971.
76. Siegel D, Hully SB, Black DM, et al. Diuretics, serum and intracellular electrolyte levels, and arrhythmias in hypertensive men. *JAMA* 267:1083, 1992.
77. Tannen RL. Diuretic-induced hypokalemia. *Kidney Int* 28:988, 1985.
78. Multiple Risk Factor Intervention Trial Research Group. Baseline resting electrocardiographic abnormalities, antihypertensive treatment, and mortality in the Multiple Risk Factor Intervention Trial. *Am J Cardiol* 55:1, 1985.
79. Kuller LH, Hulley SB, Cohen JD, Neaton J. Unexpected effects of treating hypertension in men with electrocardiographic abnormalities: A critical analysis. *Circulation* 73:114, 1986.
80. Siscovick DS, Raghunathan TE, Psaty BM, et al. Diuretic therapy for hypertension and the risk of primary cardiac arrest. *N Engl J Med* 330:1852, 1994.
81. Kasiske BL, Ma JZ, Kalil RS, Louis TA. Effects of antihypertensive therapy on serum lipids. *Ann Intern Med* 122:133, 1995.

82. Houston MC. The effects of antihypertensive drugs on glucose intolerance in hypertensive non-diabetics and diabetics. *Am Heart J* 115:640, 1988.

83. Hoes AW, Grobbee DE, Lubsen JL, et al. Diuretics, beta blockers, and the risk for sudden cardiac death in hypertensive patients. *Ann Intern Med* 123:481, 1995.

84. Cohen JD, Neaton JD, Prineas RJ, et al. Diuretics, serum potassium and ventricular arrhythmias in the Multiple Risk Factor Intervention Trial. *Am J Cardiol* 60:548, 1987.

85. Tsuji H, Venditti FJ Jr, Evans JC, et al. The associations of levels of serum potassium and magnesium with ventricular premature complexes (the Framingham Heart Study). *Am J Cardiol* 74:237, 1994.

86. Brown MJ, Brown DC, Murphy MB. Hypokalemia from beta$_2$-receptor stimulation by circulating epinephrine. *N Engl J Med* 309:1414, 1983.

87. Nordrehaug JE, von der Lippe G. Hypokalemia and ventricular fibrillation in acute myocardial infarction. *Br Heart J* 50:525, 1983.

88. Carlsen JE, Kober L, Torp-Pedersen C, Johannsen P. Relation between dose of bendrofluazide, antihypertensive effect, and adverse biochemical effects. *Br Med J* 300:975, 1990.

89. Johnston GD, Wilson R, McDermott BJ, et al. Low-dose cyclopenthiazide in the treatment of hypertension: A one-year community-based study. *Q J Med* 78:135, 1991.

90. Vardan S, Mehotra KG, Mookherjee S, et al. Efficacy and reduced metabolic side effects of a 15 mg chlorthalidone formulation in the treatment of mild hypertension. A multicenter study. *JAMA* 258:484, 1987.

91. McVeigh G, Galloway DG, Johnston D. The case for low dose diuretics in hypertension: Comparison of low and conventional doses of cyclopenthiazide. *Br Med J* 297:95, 1988.

92. Dahlof B, Hansson L, Acousta JH, et al. Controlled trial of enalapril and hydrochlorothiazide in 200 hypertensive patients. *Am J Hypertens* 1:38, 1988.

93. Kostis JB, Lacy CR, Hall WD, et al. The effect of chlorthalidone on ventricular ectopic activity in patients with isolated systolic hypertension. *Am J Cardiol* 74:464, 1994.

94. Joint National Committee. The sixth report of the Joint National Committee on Detection, Evaluation, and Treatment of High Blood Pressure. *Arch Intern Med* 157:2413, 1997.

95. Cannon PJ, Heinemann HO, Albert MS, et al. "Contraction" alkalosis after diuresis of edematous patients with ethacrynic acid. *Ann Intern Med* 62:979, 1965.

96. Garella S, Chang BS, Kahn SI. Dilution acidosis and contraction alkalosis: Review of a concept. *Kidney Int* 8:279, 1975.

97. DuBose TD Jr, Good DW. Effect of diuretics on renal acid-base transport. *Semin Nephrol* 8:282, 1988.

98. Greenblatt DJ, Koch-Weser J. Adverse reactions to spironolactone. *JAMA* 225:40, 1973.

99. Gabow PA, Moore S, Schrier RW. Spironolactone-induced hyperchloremic acidosis in cirrhosis. *Ann Intern Med* 90:338, 1979.

100. Ashraf N, Locksley R, Arieff AI. Thiazide-induced hyponatremia associated with death or neurologic damage in outpatients. *Am J Med* 70:1163, 1981.

101. Friedman E, Shadel M, Halkin H, Farfel Z. Thiazide-induced hyponatremia. Reproducibility by single-dose challenge and an analysis of pathogenesis. *Ann Intern Med* 110:24, 1989.

102. Szatalowicz VL, Miller PD, Lacher JW, et al. Comparative effects of diuretics on renal water excretion in hyponatremic oedematous disorders. *Clin Sci* 62:345, 1982.

103. Kahn AM. Effect of diuretics on the renal handling of urate. *Semin Nephrol* 8:305, 1988.

104. Langford HG, Blaufox MD, Borhani NO, et al. Is thiazide-produced uric acid elevation harmful? Analysis of data from the Hypertension Detection and Follow-up Program. *Arch Intern Med* 147:645, 1987.

105. Kahn AM. Indirect coupling between sodium and urate transport in the proximal tubule. *Kidney Int* 36:378, 1989.

106. Weinman EJ, Eknoyan G, Suki WN. The influence of the extracellular fluid volume on the tubular reabsorption of uric acid. *J Clin Invest* 55:283, 1975.

107. Steele TH, Oppenheimer S. Factors affecting urate excretion following diuretic administration in man. *Am J Med* 47:564, 1969.

108. Liang MH, Fries JF. Asymptomatic hyperuricemia: The case for conservative management. *Ann Intern Med* 88:666, 1978.
109. Swales JD. Magnesium deficiency and diuretics. *Br Med J* 285:1377, 1982.
110. Dorup I, Skajaa K, Clausen T, Kjeldsen K. Reduced concentrations of potassium, magnesium, and sodium-potassium pumps in human skeletal muscle during treatment with diuretics. *Br Med J* 296:455, 1988.
111. Ryan MP. Diuretics and potassium/magnesium depletion. Directions for treatment. *Am J Med* 82(suppl 3A):38, 1987.
112. Quamme GA. Renal magnesium handling: New insights in understanding old problems. *Kidney Int* 52:1180, 1997.
113. Dai L-J, Friedman PA, Quamme GA. Cellular mechanisms of chlorothiazide and potassium depletion on Mg^{2+} uptake in mouse distal convoluted tubule cells. *Kidney Int* 51:1008, 1997.
114. Dyckner T, Wester P-O, Widman L. Amiloride prevents thiazide-induced intracellular potassium and magnesium losses. *Acta Med Scand* 224:25, 1988.
115. Brater D, Voelker JR. Use of diuretics in patients with renal disease, in Bennett WM, McCarron DA (eds): *Contemporary Issues in Nephrology. Pharmacotherapy of Renal Disease and Hypertension.* New York, Churchill Livingstone, 1987.
116. Voelker JR, Cartwright-Brown D, Anderson S, et al. Comparison of loop diuretics in patients with chronic renal insufficiency. *Kidney Int* 32:572, 1987.
117. Pinzani M, Daskalopoulos G, Laffi G, et al. Altered furosemide pharmacokinetics in chronic alcoholic liver disease with ascites contributes to diuretic resistance. *Gastroenterology* 92:294, 1987.
118. Friedman PA. Biochemistry and pharmacology of diuretics. *Semin Nephrol* 8:198, 1988.
119. Rane A, Villeneuve JP, Stone WJ, et al. Plasma binding and disposition of furosemide in the nephrotic syndrome and in uremia. *Clin Pharmacol Ther* 24:199, 1978.
120. Ellison DH. The physiologic basis of diuretic synergism: Its role in treating diuretic resistance. *Ann Intern Med* 114:886, 1991.
121. Odlund BOG, Freeman B. Diuretic resistance: Reduced bioavailability and effect of oral frusemide. *Br Med J* 280:1577, 1980.
122. Vasko MR, Brown-Cartwright D, Knochel JP, et al. Furosemide absorption altered in decompensated congestive heart failure. *Ann Intern Med* 102:314, 1985.
123. Fredrick MJ, Pound DC, Hall SD, Brater DC. Furosemide absorption in patients with cirrhosis. *Clin Pharmacol Ther* 49:241, 1991.
124. Kramer BK, Schweda F, Rieger GA. Diuretic treatment and diuretic resistance in heart failure. *Am J Med* 106:90, 1999.
125. Reubi FC, Cottier PT. Effect of reduced glomerular filtration rate on responsiveness to chlorothiazide and mercurial diuretics. *Circulation* 23:200, 1961.
126. Wollam GL, Tarazi RC, Bravo EL, Dustan HP. Diuretic potency of combined hydrochlorothiazide and furosemide therapy in patients with azotemia. *Am J Med* 72:929, 1982.
127. Dargie HJ, Allison MEM, Kennedy AC, Gray MJB. High dosage metolazone in chronic renal failure. *Br Med J* 4:196, 1972.
128. Brater DC, Anderson S, Brown-Cartwright D. Response to furosemide in chronic renal insufficiency: Rationale for limited doses. *Clin Pharmacol Ther* 40:134, 1986.
129. Brown CB, Ogg CS, Cameron JS. High dose frusemide in acute renal failure: A controlled trial. *Clin Nephrol* 15:90, 1981.
130. Gallagher KL, Jones JK. Furosemide-induced ototoxocity. *Ann Intern Med* 91:744, 1979.
131. Ferrary E, Bernard C, Oudar O, et al. Sodium transfer from endolymph through a luminal amiloride-sensitive channel. *Am J Physiol* 257:F182, 1989.
132. Perez-Ayuso RM, Arroyo V, Planas R, et al. Random comparative study of efficacy of furosemide vs spironolactone in nonazotemic cirrhosis with ascites: Relationship between the diuretic response and the activity of the renin-aldosterone system. *Gastroenterology* 84:961, 1983.
133. Fogel MR, Sawhney VK, Neal EA, et al. Diuresis in the ascitic patient: A randomized controlled trial of three regimens. *J Clin Gastroenterol* 3(suppl 1):73, 1981.

134. Runyon BA. Management of adult patients with ascites caused by cirrhosis. *Hepatology* 27:264, 1998.
135. Inoue M, Okajima K, Itoh K, et al. Mechanism of furosemide resistance in analbuminemic rats and hypoalbuminemic patients. *Kidney Int* 32:198, 1987.
136. Kirchner KA, Voelker JR, Brater DC. Binding inhibitors restore furosemide potency in tubule fluid containing albumin. *Kidney Int* 40:418, 1991.
137. Kirchner KA, Voelker JR, Brater DC. Intratubular albumin blunts the response to furosemide—A mechanism for diuretic resistance in the nephrotic syndrome. *J Pharmacol Exp Ther* 252:1097, 1990.
138. Fliser D, Zurbruggen I, Mutschler E, et al. Coadministration of albumin and furosemide in patients with the nephrotic syndrome. *Kidney Int* 55:629, 1999.
139. van Meyel JJM, Smits P, Russel FGM, et al. Diuretic efficiency of furosemide during continuous administration versus bolus injection in healthy volunteers. *Clin Pharmacol Ther* 51:440, 1992.
140. Oster JR, Epstein M, Smoller S. Combination therapy with thiazide-type and loop diuretic agents for resistant sodium retention. *Ann Intern Med* 99:405, 1983.
141. Kiyingi A, Field MJ, Pawsey CC, et al. Metolazone in treatment of severe refractory congestive cardiac failure. *Lancet* 335:29, 1990.
142. Fliser D, Schroter M, Neubeck M, Ritz E. Coadministration of thiazide diuretics increases the efficacy of loop diuretics even in patients with advanced renal failure. *Kidney Int* 46:482, 1994.
143. Wald H, Scherzer P, Popovtzer MM. Na,K-ATPase in isolated nephron segments in rats with experimental heart failure. *Circ Res* 68:1051, 1991.
144. Brest AN, Seller R, Onesti G, et al. Clinical selection of diuretic drugs in the management of cardiac edema. *Am J Cardiol* 22:168, 1968.
145. Millard RW, Higgins CB, Franklin D, Vatner SF. Regulation of the renal circulation during severe exercise in normal dogs and dogs with experimental heart failure. *Circ Res* 31:881, 1972.
146. Ring-Larsen H, Hendriksen JH, Wilken C, et al. Diuretic treatment in decompensated cirrhosis and congestive heart failure: Effect of posture. *Br Med J* 292:1351, 1986.
147. Karnad DR, Tembulkar P, Abraham P, Desai NK. Head-down tilt as a physiologic diuretic in normal controls and in patients with fluid retaining states. *Lancet* 2:525, 1987.
148. Health and Public Policy Committee, American College of Physicians. Clinical competence in continuous arteriovenous hemofiltration. *Ann Intern Med* 108:900, 1988.
149. Marenzi G, Grazi S, Giraldi F, et al. Interrelation of humoral factors, hemodynamics, and fluid and salt metabolism in congestive heart failure: Effects of extracorporeal ultrafiltration. *Am J Med* 94:49, 1993.
150. Agostoni P, Marenzi G, Lauri G, et al. Sustained improvement in functional capacity after removal of body fluid with isolated ultrafiltration in chronic cardiac insufficiency: Failure of furosemide to provide the same result. *Am J Med* 96:191, 1994.
151. Patak RV, Fadem SZ, Rosenblatt SG, et al. Diuretic-induced changes in renal blood flow and prostaglandin E excretion in the dog. *Am J Physiol* 236:F494, 1979.
152. Wilson TW, Loadholt CB, Privitera PJ, Halushka PV. Furosemide increases 6-keto-prostaglandin F_1 alpha. Relation to natriuresis, vasodilation, and renin release. *Hypertension* 4:634, 1982.
153. Kirchner KA, Brandon S, Mueller RA, et al. Mechanism of attenuated hydrochlorthiazide response during indomethacin administration. *Kidney Int* 31:1097, 1987.
154. Bourland WA, Day DK, Williams HE. The role of the kidney in the early nondiuretic action of furosemide to reduce elevated left atrial pressure in the hypervolemic dog. *J Pharmacol Exp Ther* 202:221, 1977.
155. Johnston GD, Hiatt WR, Nies AS, et al. Factors modulating the early nondiuretic vascular effects of furosemide in man. The possible role of renal prostaglandins. *Circ Res* 53:630, 1983.
156. Dikshit K, Vyden JK, Forrester JS, et al. Renal and extrarenal hemodynamic effects of furosemide in congestive heart failure after acute myocardial infarction. *N Engl J Med* 288:1087, 1973.
157. Brater DC. Analysis of the effect of indomethacin on the response to furosemide in man: Effect of dose of furosemide. *J Pharmacol Exp Ther* 210:386, 1979.

158. Laiwah ACY, Mactier RA. Antagonist effect of non-steroidal anti-inflammatory drugs on fru-semide-induced diuresis in cardiac failure. *Br Med J* 283:714, 1981.
159. Patrono C, Dunn MJ. The clinical significance of inhibition of renal prostaglandin synthesis. *Kidney Int* 32:1, 1987.
160. Puddey IE, Beilin EJ, Vandongen R, et al. Differential effects of sulindac and indomethacin on blood pressure in treated essential hypertensive subjects. *Clin Sci* 69:327, 1985.
161. Wong DG, Spence JD, Lamki L, et al. Effect of non-steroidal anti-inflammatory drugs on con-trol of hypertension by β-blockers and diuretics. *Lancet* 1:997, 1986.
162. Dzau VJ, Packer M, Lilly LS, et al. Prostaglandins in severe congestive heart failure. Relation to activation of the renin-angiotensin system and hyponatremia. *N Engl J Med* 310:347, 1984.
163. Francis GS, Siegel RM, Goldsmith SR, et al. Acute vasoconstrictor response to intravenous furosemide in chronic congestive heart failure. Activation of the neurohumoral axis. *Ann Intern Med* 103:1, 1985.
164. Daskalopoulos G, Laffi G, Morgan T, et al. Immediate effects of furosemide on renal hemody-namics in chronic liver disease with ascites. *Gastroenterology* 92:1859, 1987.

CHAPTER
SIXTEEN

EDEMATOUS STATES

Edema is defined as a palpable swelling produced by expansion of the interstitial fluid volume. A variety of clinical conditions are associated with the development of edema, including heart failure, cirrhosis, and the nephrotic syndrome. This chapter will review the basic principles governing the pathophysiology of edema formation and the treatment of the different edematous states. The review of the clinical use of diuretics presented in Chap. 15 should be read before proceeding with this discussion, since these agents constitute the mainstay of therapy for most generalized edematous states.

PATHOPHYSIOLOGY OF EDEMA FORMATION

There are two basic steps involved in edema formation:

- There is an *alteration in capillary hemodynamics* that favors the movement of fluid from the vascular space into the interstitium.
- *Dietary Na$^+$ and water are retained by the kidney.*

The importance of the kidneys in the development of edema should not be underestimated. Edema does not become clinically apparent until the interstitial volume has increased by at least 2.5 to 3 liters. Since the normal plasma volume is only about 3 liters, edematous patients would develop marked hemoconcentration and shock if the edema fluid were derived only from the plasma.

These complications do not occur because of the sequence depicted in Fig. 16-1. The initial movement of fluid from the vascular space into the interstitium reduces the plasma volume and consequently tissue perfusion. In response to these changes, the kidney retains Na^+ and water (see Chap. 8). Some of this fluid stays in the vascular space, returning the plasma volume toward normal. However, the alteration in capillary hemodynamics results in most of the retained fluid entering the interstitium and eventually becoming apparent as edema. The net effect is a marked expansion of the total extracellular volume (as edema) with maintenance of the plasma volume at close to normal levels.

This example illustrates an important point to which we will return in the sections on therapy: In most edematous states, renal Na^+ and water retention is an *appropriate* compensation in that it restores tissue perfusion, even though it also augments the degree of edema. On the other hand, removing the edema fluid with diuretic therapy will improve symptoms but may diminish tissue perfusion, occasionally to clinically significant levels.

The hemodynamic effects are somewhat different when the primary abnormality is *inappropriate* renal fluid retention. In this setting, both the plasma and

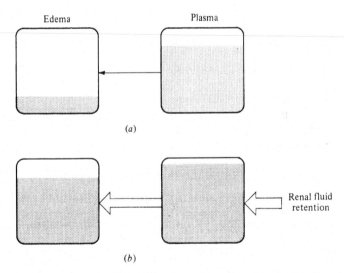

Figure 16-1 Pathophysiology of edema formation when there is an alteration in capillary hemodynamics, such as an elevated capillary hydraulic pressure, that favors the movement of fluid out of the vascular space into the interstitium. The normal plasma volume is depicted as the full size of the plasma square. The shaded area in the edema square refers to the increase in the interstitial fluid volume as edema. The initial reduction in the plasma volume produced by the loss of fluid into the interstitium (*a*) stimulates renal Na^+ and water retention (*b*). This appropriately restores the plasma volume toward normal, but, because of the altered capillary hemodynamics, much of the retained fluid enters the interstitium and becomes apparent as edema.

interstitial volumes are expanded and there are no deleterious hemodynamic effects from removal of the excess fluid. This is an example of *overfilling* of the vascular tree, in contrast to the *underfilling* described above. It occurs most often with primary renal disease but may also be seen in early cirrhosis and with the use of certain drugs.

Capillary Hemodynamics

The exchange of fluid between the plasma and the interstitium is determined by the hydraulic and oncotic pressures in each compartment. The relationship between these parameters can be expressed by Starling's law (see Chap. 7).[1-3]

$$\text{Net filtration} = \text{LpS } (\Delta \text{ hydraulic pressure} - \Delta \text{ oncotic pressure})$$

$$= \text{LpS } \left[\left(P_{cap} - P_{if} \right) - \sigma \left(\pi_{cap} - \pi_{if} \right) \right] \qquad (16\text{-}1)$$

where Lp is the unit permeability or porosity of the capillary wall, S is the surface area available for filtration, P_{cap} and P_{if} are the capillary and interstitial fluid hydraulic pressures, π_{cap} and π_{if} are the capillary and interstitial fluid oncotic pressures, and σ represents the reflection coefficient of proteins across the capillary wall (with values ranging from 0 if completely permeable to 1 if completely impermeable).

The normal values for Starling's forces in experimental animals and humans are uncertain, largely because of difficulties in the measurement of these parameters (with the exception of the capillary oncotic pressure). Furthermore, capillary hemodynamics are not necessarily uniform within an organ (as both open and closed capillaries may be present), and capillaries in different organs have unique hemodynamic and permeability characteristics.

Despite these difficulties, important differences in the magnitude of Starling's forces have been identified in skeletal muscle and subcutaneous tissue (the sites of peripheral edema), the liver, and the lung (Table 16-1).[2,4,5] Approximate normal values in a skeletal muscle capillary are shown in Fig. 16-2. As can be seen, the mean capillary hydraulic pressure (17 mmHg), which pushes fluid out of the capillary, and the plasma oncotic pressure (28 mmHg), which pulls fluid into the vascular space, are quantitatively the most important. There is normally a small mean gradient of about 0.3 mmHg favoring filtration out of the vascular space;* the fluid that is filtered is then returned to the systemic circulation by the lymphatics so that fluid accumulation in the interstitium is prevented.

Starling's forces are substantially different in the liver. The hepatic sinusoids are highly permeable to proteins; as a result, the capillary and interstitial oncotic pressures are roughly equal, and there is little transcapillary oncotic pressure

---

* This gradient is not uniform within the capillary circulation. The hydraulic pressure within most of the capillary is relatively high at 25 to 30 mmHg, resulting in filtration throughout the capillary.[1,3,6] Most of this excess fluid is then returned to the vascular space in the highly permeable postcapillary venules, where the hydraulic pressure falls to 10 mmHg, a level below the oncotic pressure gradient.[3]

Table 16-1   Approximate normal values for Starling's forces in skeletal muscle and lung[a]

	Skeletal muscle	Alveoli
Hydraulic pressure		
Capillary (mean)	17.3	8
Interstitium	−3.0	−2
Mean gradient	20.3	10
Oncotic pressure		
Capillary (mean)	28	26
Interstitium	8	18
Mean gradient	20	8
Net gradient favoring filtration ($\Delta P - \Delta \pi$)	0.3	2

[a] Units are millimeters of mercury. Values are from Refs. 1, 2, and 4.

gradient.[2] The net effect is that the *hydraulic pressure gradient favoring filtration is essentially unopposed.* To some degree, filtration is minimized by a lower capillary hydraulic pressure than in skeletal muscle, since approximately two-thirds of hepatic blood flow is derived from the portal vein, a low-pressure system. Nevertheless, there is still a larger gradient favoring filtration; however, edema does not normally occur, because the filtered fluid is again removed by the lymphatics.

The alveolar capillaries are somewhat similar to the hepatic sinusoids. They have a relatively low capillary hydraulic pressure (due to perfusion from the low-pressure system in the right ventricle), but they are also more permeable to proteins than skeletal muscle, resulting in a lesser transcapillary oncotic pressure gradient (Table 16-1).[4,5] The clinical significance of this difference will be discussed below.

Edema formation   The development of edema requires an alteration in one or more of Starling's forces in a direction that favors an increase in net filtration.

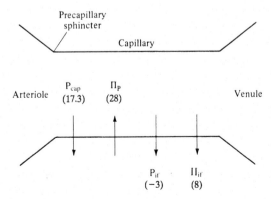

Figure 16-2   Schematic representation of the hemodynamic factors controlling fluid movement across the capillary wall in subcutaneous tissue. The numbers in parentheses represent the approximate normal values, in millimeters of mercury, for each of the factors. The negative value for P_{if} is probably generated by the removal of interstitial fluid by the lymphatic vessels. The net effect is a small gradient favoring filtration of 0.3 mmHg.

This can be produced by an elevation in capillary hydraulic pressure, capillary permeability, or interstitial oncotic pressure, or by a reduction in the plasma oncotic pressure (Table 16-2). Edema can also be induced by lymphatic obstruction, since the fluid that is normally filtered is not returned to the systemic circulation.

Table 16-2 Major causes of edematous states

Increased capillary hydraulic pressure
  A. Increased plasma volume due to renal Na^+ retention
    1. Heart failure, including cor pulmonale
    2. Primary renal Na^+ retention
      a. Renal disease, including the nephrotic syndrome
      b. Drugs: minoxidil, diazoxide, calcium channel blockers (?), nonsteroidal anti-inflammatory drugs, fludrocortisone, estrogens
      c. Refeeding edema
      d. Early hepatic cirrhosis
    3. Pregnancy and premenstrual edema
    4. Idiopathic edema, when diuretic-induced
  B. Venous obstruction
    1. Hepatic cirrhosis or hepatic venous obstruction
    2. Acute pulmonary edema
    3. Local venous obstruction
  C. Decreased arteriolar resistance
    1. Calcium channel blockers (?)
    2. Idiopathic edema (?)
Decreased plasma oncotic pressure (primarily when plasma albumin concentration < 1.5 to 2 g/dL)
  A. Protein loss
    1. Nephrotic syndrome
    2. Protein-losing enteropathy
  B. Reduced albumin synthesis
    1. Liver disease
    2. Malnutrition
Increased capillary permeability
  A. Idiopathic edema (?)
  B. Burns
  C. Trauma
  D. Inflammation or sepsis
  E. Allergic reactions, including certain forms of angioedema
  F. Adult respiratory distress syndrome
  G. Diabetes mellitus
  H. Interleukin 2 therapy
  I. Malignant ascites
Lymphatic obstruction or increased interstitial oncotic pressure
  A. Nodal enlargement due to malignancy
  B. Hypothyroidism
  C. Malignant ascites

Increased capillary hydraulic pressure Capillary hydraulic pressure, although generated by cardiac contraction, is relatively insensitive to alterations in arterial pressure. This stability is due to autoregulatory changes in resistance at the precapillary sphincter (Fig. 16-2), which determine the extent to which the arterial pressure is transmitted to the capillary (see page 250). If the arterial pressure is increased, for example, the sphincter constricts, minimizing the elevation in capillary hydraulic pressure. This explains why patients with hypertension do not develop edema. Conversely, the sphincter dilates when the arterial pressure is reduced. This decreases the pressure drop across the sphincter, allowing the capillary pressure (as well as blood flow) to be maintained.

In contrast, the resistance at the venous end of the capillary is not well regulated. Consequently, changes in venous pressure result in parallel alterations in capillary hydraulic pressure. The venous pressure is increased in two settings: (1) when the blood volume is expanded, augmenting the volume in the venous system, and (2) when there is venous obstruction. Examples of edema due to volume expansion include heart failure and renal disease; edema due to venous obstruction, on the other hand, is commonly seen with cirrhosis, in which there is a marked increase in hepatic sinusoidal pressure, and with deep venous thrombosis in the lower extremities.

Decreased plasma oncotic pressure Hypoalbuminemia due to albumin loss in the urine in the nephrotic syndrome or to decreased hepatic albumin synthesis is another potential cause of edema. However, hypoalbuminemia alone may be a less common cause of edema than was previously suspected (see "Safety Factors," below).

Increased capillary permeability An increase in capillary permeability due to vascular injury promotes the development of edema both directly and by permitting albumin to move into the interstitium, thereby diminishing the oncotic pressure gradient. This problem may be operative in the following clinical settings:

- Burns, in which both histamine and oxygen free radicals can induce microvascular injury.[7]
- Therapy with interleukin-2, which appears to directly increase capillary permeability.[8,9]
- Episodic idiopathic capillary leak syndromes, which may be mediated by increased expression of interleukin-2 receptors on circulating mononuclear cells or by increased generation of kinins.[10-13] Affected patients often have an associated monoclonal gammopathy and, during episodes, have a massive leak of proteins and fluids out of the vascular space, with the hematocrit rising acutely to as high as 70 to 80 percent.[12] The mortality rate is high in this disorder. Preliminary evidence suggests that the combination of aminophylline (an inhibitor of phosphodiesterase) and terbutaline (a relatively selective β_2-adrenergic agonist) may prevent episodes.[12] It is not clear, however, why these drugs are effective.

- Any of the conditions associated with the adult respiratory distress syndrome (Table 16-2). In this disorder, ischemia- or sepsis-induced release of cytokines, such as interleukin 1, interleukin 8, or tumor necrosis factor, may play an important role in the increase in pulmonary capillary permeability, at least in part via the recruitment of neutrophils.[14-16]

Capillary permeability is also moderately increased in patients with diabetes mellitus.[17,18] This abnormality may be mediated in part by hyperglycemia-induced accumulation of both diacylglycerol (with subsequent activation of protein kinase C; see Fig. 6-3) and advanced glycosylation end products derived from the combination of glucose with circulating proteins.[19,20] The net effect is to enhance the severity of edema, which, in these patients, is usually due to heart failure or the nephrotic syndrome.

Lymphatic obstruction or increased interstitial oncotic pressure Lymphatic obstruction is an unusual cause of edema that is most often seen with nodal enlargement due to malignancy. This process is called lymphedema.[21] With hypothyroidism (myxedema), on the other hand, there is a marked increase in the interstitial accumulation of albumin and other proteins.[22] Although this may be due in part to an elevation in capillary permeability, the excess interstitial protein and fluid would normally be returned to the systemic circulation by the lymphatics. However, lymphatic flow is low or normal in myxedema,[22] not increased as in other edematous states.[23] This may be due to binding of the filtered proteins to excess interstitial mucopolysaccharides, thereby preventing their removal by the lymphatics.[22]

Establishing the diagnosis of these forms of edema is important, since they should not be treated with diuretics. When diuretics are given to treat the usual forms of peripheral edema, the initial fluid loss comes from the intravascular space. The ensuing reduction in venous and therefore intracapillary pressure allows the edema fluid to be mobilized and the plasma volume to be maintained. However, this sequence does not occur with lymphatic obstruction or myxedema, since edema fluid cannot be easily mobilized into the vascular space. Similar considerations apply to peripheral edema due to localized venous disease of the lower extremities.

Safety factors Since there is normally a small gradient favoring filtration, it might be expected that even a minor change in these hemodynamic forces would lead to edema. However, experimental and clinical observations indicate that there must be at least a *15-mmHg increase in the gradient favoring filtration before edema can be detected.*[1,2,5] Three factors contribute to this protective response:

- Increased lymphatic flow can initially remove the excess filtrate.
- Fluid entry into the interstitium lowers the interstitial oncotic pressure, both by dilution and by lymphatic-mediated removal of interstitial proteins. For

example, interstitial oncotic pressure falls to very low levels in congestive heart failure, while the plasma oncotic pressure is relatively normal.[24] The associated increase in the transcapillary oncotic pressure gradient ($\pi_{cap} - \pi_{if}$) counterbalances the rise in capillary hydraulic pressure, thereby minimizing the degree of edema formation.

- The increase in interstitial fluid volume will raise the hydraulic pressure; edema cannot occur until the normally negative value (generated by lymphatic fluid removal) becomes positive.[1]

As an example, two safety factors limit the degree of ascites formation in patients with cirrhosis. Increased lymph flow (which can rise more than 10-fold as intrasinusoidal hypertension augments the rate of filtration) provides the initial protection. However, once the rate of fluid movement out of the sinusoids is sufficient to overcome the ability of the lymphatics to remove the excess fluid, the ensuing elevation in intraperitoneal pressure eventually limits continued fluid accumulation in the peritoneum.[25,26]

Hypoalbuminemia and edema   The magnitude of the reduction that can occur in interstitial oncotic pressure is related to the baseline level. If, as listed in Table 16-1, the normal value in skeletal muscle and subcutaneous tissue is only 8 mmHg, then loss of interstitial proteins could account for a maximum safety factor of only 8 mmHg. However, more recent studies suggest that the normal level in humans may be as high as 12 to 15 mmHg.[27-29]

The potential clinical relevance of this observation can be illustrated by studies in patients with heavy proteinuria due to the nephrotic syndrome. The fall in the plasma albumin concentration in this disorder leads to a parallel decline in the interstitial oncotic pressure as a result of less entry of albumin into the interstitium (Fig. 16-3). As a result, the *transcapillary oncotic pressure gradient is initially maintained*, with a protective factor that is increased up to twofold if the interstitial oncotic pressure is 12 to 15 mmHg rather than 8 mmHg.

The relative roles of hypoalbuminemia and primary renal sodium retention (induced by the underlying disease) in individual patients with the nephrotic syndrome appear to be variable.[30] Some findings in both animals and humans with the nephrotic syndrome are compatible with the hypothesis that Na^+ retention, not hypoalbuminemia, is primarily responsible for edema formation:[29-35]

- Minimal change disease is a common cause of the nephrotic syndrome. When a remission is induced by corticosteroids, there is an increase in glomerular filtration rate and a substantial rise in sodium excretion (with partial resolution of the edema) *before any significant elevation in the plasma albumin concentration* (Fig. 16-4).[35] This finding suggests that the renal disease, rather than hypoalbuminemia, is responsible for the initial Na^+ retention.

- If underfilling due to hypoalbuminemia were the primary initiating factor in edema formation, then removal of the edema with diuretics should lead to

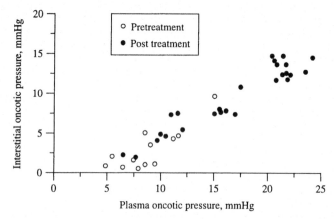

Figure 16-3 Relationship between plasma and interstitial oncotic pressures in nephrotic patients with minimal change disease before (open circles) and after (closed circles) corticosteroid-induced remission of the proteinuria. These values are reduced in parallel during active disease with little change in the transcapillary oncotic pressure gradient. (*Adapted from Koomans HA, Kortlandt W, Geers AB, Dorhout Mees EJ*, Nephron *40:391, 1985, with permission.*)

plasma volume depletion and azotemia. However, the plasma volume appears to remain relatively constant in this setting unless there is excessive fluid removal.[31]

Experimental models of glomerular disease show a primary increase in Na^+ reabsorption that appears to occur in the collecting tubules.[33,36] How this might occur

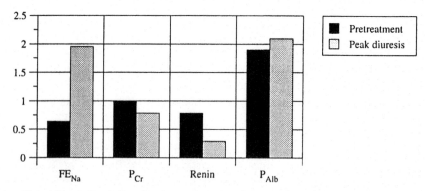

Figure 16-4 Changes in the fractional excretion of Na^+ (percent), plasma creatinine concentration (mg/dL), plasma renin activity (ng/mL/h), and plasma albumin concentration (g/dL) before corticosteroid therapy, during the peak diuresis, and after remission has been induced. The peak diuresis is associated with a fall in the plasma creatinine concentration and plasma renin activity toward normal, but occurs before there has been any significant rise in the plasma albumin concentration. (*From Koomans HA, Boer WH, Dorhout Mees EJ*, Nephron *47:173, 1987, with permission.*)

is not well understood.[34,37] Other studies, however, suggest an important role for hypoalbuminemia in at least some patients:[38]

- The administration of albumin to raise the plasma oncotic pressure can increase sodium excretion and lead to resolution of edema in some patients.[39,40]
- Some patients have very low rates of sodium excretion, elevated plasma renin activity, and symptoms of hypovolemia.[41,42]

Severe and acute hypoalbuminemia are settings in which underfilling edema can occur. In patients with severe hypoalbuminemia (plasma albumin less than 1.5 g/dL), washout of the interstitial oncotic pressure would eventually be complete, leading to a reduction in the transcapillary oncotic pressure gradient and a tendency to underfilling.[42] On the other hand, the rapid administration of large volumes of saline to patients with marked hypovolemia leads to acute hypoalbuminemia, with no time for the interstitial albumin concentration to fall.[43] As a result, the transcapillary oncotic pressure gradient is reduced and peripheral edema can occur before the restoration of normal intracardiac filling pressures.

In summary, the relative roles of primary renal sodium retention and hypoalbuminemia in individual patients with the nephrotic syndrome appear to be variable.[38,41,42] A study in children with minimal change disease sheds some light on the often conflicting findings.[41] Thirty children with minimal change disease in remission were monitored carefully and studied within a few days of the onset of relapse as indicated by persistent 3^+ findings on the urine dipstick for protein. When the children were first evaluated, three different groups were noted:

- Nine children were relatively normoalbuminemic [mean plasma albumin concentration 3.7 g/dL (37 g/L)]. They had a reduced fractional excretion of sodium and signs of modest volume expansion (weight gain, increased blood volume) but no overt edema. These findings appear to represent primary renal sodium retention.
- Eight children had edema, overt nephrotic syndrome, and a mean plasma albumin concentration of 1.8 g/dL (18 g/L), but no signs of hypovolemia.
- Thirteen children had edema, overt nephrotic syndrome, a mean plasma albumin concentration of 1.6 g/dL (16 g/L), and clear evidence of hypovolemia, provided by one or more symptoms suggestive of volume depletion (tachycardia, peripheral vasoconstriction, oliguria) and marked elevation in the plasma renin activity and concentrations of aldosterone and norepinephrine. These children also had a low glomerular filtration rate. In one child, the symptoms and neurohumoral activation were transiently improved by albumin infusion.

Pulmonary edema   As mentioned above, the pulmonary circulation has a greater baseline permeability to albumin and therefore a higher interstitial oncotic pressure of about 18 mmHg (Table 16-1).[2,4,5] As a result, there is a larger safety factor against edema due to hypoalbuminemia than that seen in skeletal muscle, since there can be a greater parallel decline in the interstitial oncotic pressure. Thus, in the absence of a concurrent rise in left atrial and pulmonary capillary pressures, pulmonary edema is not usually seen with hypoalbuminemia, even at a plasma albumin concentration acutely low enough to induce peripheral edema.[43]

Kwashiorkor   Edema is common in the malnutrition syndrome kwashiorkor. This complication has been ascribed to hypoalbuminemia, but the preceding discussion casts doubt on this hypothesis. As an alternative, it has been suggested that increased generation of cysteinyl leukotrienes may be of primary importance in the edema of kwashiorkor by increasing capillary permeability.[44]

Renal Sodium Retention

The retention of fluid by the kidney in edematous states results from one of two basic mechanisms. In some patients, the primary problem is an inability to excrete the Na^+ and water that have been ingested. This most often occurs in patients with renal disease, such as the nephrotic syndrome or glomerulonephritis, as noted above.[33,36,37] More commonly, renal fluid retention is an *appropriate compensatory response* to effective arterial or circulating volume depletion, with the urine Na^+ concentration often being less than 25 meq/L (Fig. 16-1).[45,46] As reviewed in detail in Chap. 8, the effective circulating volume is an unmeasurable entity that refers to the pressure that is perfusing the arterial baroreceptors, such as those in the carotid sinus and glomerular afferent arteriole.[46] In most instances, the effective circulating volume is directly proportional to the cardiac output. Thus, when the cardiac output is reduced because of underlying cardiac disease, the kidney attempts to restore the effective circulating volume by retaining Na^+ and water.

However, effective tissue perfusion and the cardiac output are not always related, since the former can also be reduced by a decrease in peripheral vascular resistance.[46] For example, creation of an arteriovenous fistula is associated with no initial change in cardiac output, yet tissue perfusion is reduced since the blood flowing through the fistula is bypassing the capillary circulation. In response to this hemodynamic change, the kidney retains Na^+ and water, thereby increasing the blood volume and cardiac output.[47] The new steady state is characterized by a cardiac output that exceeds the baseline level by an amount equal to the flow rate through the fistula.

A common clinical correlate of this experiment occurs in patients with cirrhosis and ascites, who frequently have an elevated cardiac output.[48] Despite this, they behave as if they were volume-depleted, as evidenced by avid renal Na^+ retention[49] and a progressive rise in secretion of the three *hypovolemic hormones*—renin, norepinephrine, and antidiuretic hormone (ADH).[46,50-52]

The disparity between the high cardiac output and the renal and neurohumoral responses in cirrhosis is due both to splanchnic vasodilatation and to the presence of multiple arteriovenous fistulas throughout the body, such as spider angiomata in the skin; the net effect is a marked fall in systemic vascular resistance and a reduction in systemic blood pressure.[46,53] Much of the cardiac output is circulating ineffectively, as there is a progressive reduction in renal and eventually musculocutaneous perfusion.[53] (See "Cirrhosis," below, for a discussion of the possible pathogenesis of these hemodynamic changes.)

The renal Na^+ and water retention seen in heart failure or advanced cirrhosis results from both a hypovolemia-induced fall in glomerular filtration rate (GFR) and, much more importantly, an increase in tubular reabsorption. The latter may occur throughout the nephron, as enhanced proximal, loop, and collecting tubular reabsorption all may occur with effective volume depletion.[54-60] The initial decline in effective circulating volume primarily affects the distal nephron as collecting tubular Na^+ reabsorption is enhanced, a response that is largely mediated by an increase in the secretion of aldosterone (and perhaps a reduction in the release of natriuretic peptides).[54,61] As the disease progresses, proximal reabsorption is also stimulated,[54] probably as a result of increased levels of angiotensin II and renal sympathetic neural tone.[61,62]

The compensated state   Although the renin-angiotensin-aldosterone system undoubtedly contributes to Na^+ retention in disorders such as heart failure and cirrhosis, the plasma renin activity is normal in some patients with these disorders.[63,64] A partial explanation for this seemingly paradoxical finding is that the patient has entered a *compensated state* in which the initial fluid retention has increased venous return to the heart, thereby allowing systemic hemodynamics to be stabilized (at least in the resting state) and removing the stimulus for continued renin release.[61,63]

This sequence is depicted in Fig. 16-5, which shows the changes that occur with chronic thoracic inferior vena cava constriction, an experimental model that simulates the changes seen in heart failure in humans.[61] The new steady state seen after 6 to 7 days is characterized by plasma volume expansion but normalization of the systemic blood pressure, urinary Na^+ excretion, and renin and aldosterone release.

In many patients, however, stable heart failure is associated with a persistent reduction in cardiac output, and it is not clear why the plasma renin activity should be normal.[63] One possible explanation is that circulating renin may not reflect the degree of activation of tissue renin angiotensin systems (see page 30). Studies in animals with congestive heart failure, for example, have shown that there is persistent, hypoperfusion-induced activation of the *intrarenal* renin-angiotensin system even though the plasma concentrations of renin and angiotensin II are not elevated.[65]

Summary

The development of edema requires both an alteration in capillary hemodynamics (favoring fluid movement into the interstitium) and renal Na^+ and water retention. When the former predominates (as with major venous obstruction), there is an initial fall in the plasma volume. Edema then occurs because the compensatory retention of Na^+ and water by the kidney permits the plasma volume to be

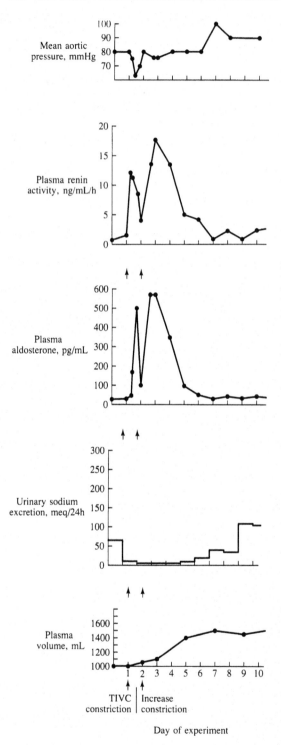

Figure 16-5 Sequential changes in mean aortic pressure, plasma renin activity, plasma aldosterone concentration, urinary sodium excretion, and plasma volume in a dog with moderate thoracic inferior vena cava constriction. There is initial hypotension, activation of the renin-angiotensin-aldosterone system, and a marked reduction in urinary Na$^+$ excretion. By day 7, however, a new steady state is achieved in which renin and aldosterone levels and Na$^+$ excretion have returned to baseline levels. The associated plasma volume expansion is responsible for restoring venous return to the heart, thereby allowing systemic hemodynamics to be normalized. (*From Watkins L Jr, Burton JA, Haber E, et al, J Clin Invest 57:1606, 1976, by copyright permission of the American Society for Clinical Investigation.*)

maintained at near normal levels, while much of the excess fluid accumulates in the interstitium (Fig. 16-1).

However, *generalized edema will not develop if* Na^+ *retention is prevented by eliminating* Na^+ *from the diet.* In this setting, the initial movement of fluid into the interstitium will significantly reduce the plasma volume. This will decrease both the arterial and venous pressures and consequently the capillary hydraulic pressure, thereby diminishing further fluid entry into the interstitium.

Similar considerations apply to heart failure and cirrhosis, which also represent conditions of effective circulating volume depletion. In these disorders, however, there is plasma volume expansion, because fluid retention is stimulated not by a fall in plasma volume but by a primary reduction in either cardiac output or systemic vascular resistance (due primarily to splanchnic vasodilatation), respectively.

SYMPTOMS AND DIAGNOSIS

A complete discussion of the many diseases that can produce heart failure, cirrhosis, or the nephrotic syndrome and the methods used in their diagnosis is beyond the scope of this chapter. The mechanism of edema formation and treatment of the individual disorders will be discussed in the next section. It is useful, however, to first review the general findings of physical examination that can aid in establishing the proper diagnosis. Three factors are of particular importance (Table 16-3):

- The *pattern of distribution of edema*, which reflects those capillaries with altered hemodynamic forces
- The *central venous pressure*
- The presence or absence of *pulmonary edema*

Pulmonary Edema

Patients with pulmonary edema complain primarily of shortness of breath and orthopnea. Chest pain also may be a prominent symptom when pulmonary edema

Table 16-3 Physical findings in major edematous states

Disorder	Pulmonary edema	Central venous pressure	Ascites and/or pedal edema
Left-sided heart failure	+	Variable	—
Right-sided heart failure	—	↑	+
Hepatic cirrhosis	—	↓ −Nl	+
Renal disease	Variable	↑	+
Nephrotic syndrome	—	Variable	+
Idiopathic edema	—	↓ −Nl	+

is due to an acute myocardial infarction. Physical examination usually reveals a tachypneic, diaphoretic patient with wet rales on auscultation of the chest and possibly gallop rhythms and heart murmurs. The diagnosis should be confirmed by a chest x-ray, since other disorders that require different therapy may produce similar findings.

Although cardiac disease is the most common cause of pulmonary edema, it can also be produced by those disorders associated with primary renal Na^+ retention or the acute respiratory distress syndrome (ARDS). If the correct diagnosis cannot be established from the history, physical examination, and laboratory data, measurement of the pulmonary capillary wedge pressure can be extremely helpful. The wedge pressure exceeds 18 to 20 mmHG when pulmonary edema is due to heart disease or primary renal Na^+ retention,[66] but is relatively normal in the setting of increased capillary permeability in the acute respiratory distress syndrome.[67]

In contrast to cardiac and renal disease, uncomplicated cirrhosis is not associated with pulmonary edema. The postsinusoidal obstruction in this disorder leads to selective increases in venous and capillary pressures *below the hepatic vein*[68] and to a normal or reduced blood volume in the cardiopulmonary circulation.[51]

Peripheral Edema and Ascites

In comparison to the potentially life-threatening nature of pulmonary edema, peripheral edema and ascites are cosmetically undesirable but produce less serious symptoms. These include swollen legs, difficulty in walking, increased abdominal girth, and shortness of breath due to pressure on the diaphragm in patients with tense ascites.

Peripheral edema can be detected by the presence of pitting after pressure is applied to the edematous area. Since peripheral edema locates preferentially in the dependent areas, it is primarily found in the lower extremities in ambulatory patients and over the sacrum in patients at bed rest. Ascites, on the other hand, is associated with abdominal distention and shifting dullness and a fluid wave on percussion of the abdomen. Patients with the nephrotic syndrome may also have prominent periorbital edema due to the low tissue pressure in this area.

The distribution of edema and estimation of the central venous pressure can aid in the differential diagnosis of heart failure, cirrhosis, primary renal Na^+ retention, and the nephrotic syndrome (Table 16-3). This is particularly important in some patients with chronic right-sided heart failure, in whom the cardiac disease can lead to both cirrhosis (due to chronic passive congestion of the liver) and hemodynamically mediated proteinuria, which on rare occasions can approach the nephrotic range.[69]

Heart failure   Patients with right-sided heart failure have peripheral edema and, in severe cases, ascites and edema of the abdominal wall. Shortness of breath is commonly present and may be due to underlying pulmonary disease or coexistent left ventricular failure. The edema in these disorders is due to an increase in venous pressure behind the right side of the heart. Thus, the pressures in the right atrium and subclavian vein are elevated, changes that can be detected by estimation of the jugular venous pressure or by direct measurement with a central venous pressure catheter.*

Cirrhosis   Cirrhotic patients can develop ascites and then edema in the lower extremities because of an increase in venous pressure below the diseased liver. As a result, the venous pressure above the hepatic vein—i.e., in the vena cava, jugular veins, and right atrium—usually is reduced or normal,[51,68] not elevated as in right-sided heart failure. One exception to this general rule can occur in patients with tense ascites, in whom upward pressure on the diaphragm can increase the intrathoracic pressure. Although elevated initially in this setting, the central venous pressure rapidly falls to normal following the removal of a small amount of ascitic fluid, which substantially reduces the intraperitoneal pressure.[68]

A portal pressure > 12 mmHg appears to be required for fluid retention in patients with cirrhosis; neither ascites nor edema is seen in patients without portal hypertension.[70,71] The presence of other signs of portal hypertension, such as distended abdominal wall veins and splenomegaly, also is suggestive of primary hepatic disease. However, these findings are not necessarily specific, since chronic right-sided heart failure can produce hepatic injury.

The potential difficulties in distinguishing between primary hepatic and cardiac disease can be illustrated by the following example.

Case History 16-1   A 56-year-old man has a 3-year history of ascites, which now requires removal of 3 to 4 liters of ascitic fluid by paracentesis every 3 weeks. The patient has been told that he has cirrhosis, although a liver biopsy has not been performed. He has no history of hepatic disease and is only a social drinker. The physical examination reveals no acute distress, a soft abdomen with marked ascites, and moderate pedal edema. The heartbeat is irregularly irregular. The heart sounds are distant, and no murmurs are heard. Several spider angiomata are present. The estimated jugular venous pressure is greater than $15\,\mathrm{cmH_2O}$.

The electrocardiogram shows arterial fibrillation and low voltage. There is 3^+ proteinuria by dipstick; the plasma albumin concentration is $2.9\,\mathrm{g/dL}$; and the liver function tests are mildly abnormal.

Comment   Despite the features suggestive of cirrhosis, the elevated jugular venous pressure in the absence of tense ascites pointed toward right-sided heart failure. The central venous pressure was measured directly and found to be $21\,\mathrm{cmH_2O}$ (normal is 1 to $7\,\mathrm{cmH_2O}$). Further evaluation confirmed the diagnosis of constrictive pericarditis. After pericardiectomy, the patient had a

---

* The technique for evaluating jugular venous pressure is discussed on page 423.

complete recovery, including reversal of the liver function abnormalities and the proteinuria.

Primary renal sodium retention   The physical findings associated with primary renal Na^+ retention are similar to those seen with biventricular failure: Both pulmonary and peripheral edema may be present and the jugular venous pressure should be elevated, since these patients are truly *volume-expanded*. An abnormal urinalysis (particularly if there are signs of active renal disease, such as red cell casts) will usually distinguish underlying renal disease from heart failure. However, this differentiation may be difficult in some patients, since cardiac disease can produce both renal insufficiency (due to diminished renal perfusion) and proteinuria.[69] In this setting, the diagnosis may be established by the presence of normal cardiac function by echocardiography.

Nephrotic syndrome   Patients with the nephrotic syndrome typically present with periorbital and peripheral edema and occasionally ascites. The central venous pressure is usually normal to high-normal in the nephrotic syndrome, a reflection of the primary role of renal Na^+ retention in most patients. However, as described above, some patients have underfilling, which should be associated with a low central venous pressure.[38,41,42]

The diagnosis of the nephrotic syndrome can be confirmed by documenting the presence of both heavy proteinuria (usually greater than 3 g/day) and hypoalbuminemia. Lipiduria and hyperlipidemia are also seen in many patients; the former reflects the abnormal glomerular filtration of large lipoprotein molecules, and the latter reflects both increased hepatic lipoprotein synthesis (induced by the fall in plasma oncotic pressure) and decreased clearance of triglycerides.[72]

Other   Patients with idiopathic edema behave as if they were volume-depleted because of the exaggerated fall in the plasma volume in the erect position and the concomitant use of diuretics (see "Idiopathic Edema," below). As a result, they have peripheral edema, but the central venous pressure is normal or low-normal and pulmonary edema does not occur.

In addition to the above disorders, edema may result from local changes in capillary hemodynamics. For example, a patient with a postphlebitic syndrome after an episode of thrombophlebitis may develop *unilateral* pedal edema due to an increase in venous pressure that is limited to that extremely. This is different from the generalized edematous states, in which bilateral edema should be present.

ETIOLOGY AND TREATMENT

General Principles of Treatment

Before discussing the therapy of the specific edematous disorders, it is important to consider the following questions that apply to all edematous states:

- When must edema be treated?
- What are the consequences of the removal of edema fluid?
- How rapidly should edema fluid be removed?

When must edema be treated?   Pulmonary edema is the only form of generalized edema that is life-threatening and demands immediate treatment.* In all other edematous states, the removal of the excess fluid can proceed more slowly, since it is of no danger to the patient. This is particularly true in cirrhosis, where hypokalemia, metabolic alkalosis, and rapid fluid shifts induced by diuretics can precipitate hepatic coma or the hepatorenal syndrome (see "Cirrhosis and Ascites," below).

What are the consequences of the removal of edema fluid?   As described above, the retention of Na^+ and water by the kidney in heart failure, cirrhosis, and capillary leak syndromes is *compensatory* in that it acts to raise the effective circulating volume toward normal (see Fig. 16-1). In comparison, fluid accumulation is *inappropriate* with primary renal Na^+ retention, where the effective circulating volume as well as the total extracellular volume is expanded.

If the retention of edema fluid is compensatory, then *removal of the fluid with diuretics should diminish the effective circulating volume*. To the degree that the fluid lost by diuresis comes from the plasma volume, there will be a decrease in venous return to the heart and therefore in the cardiac filling pressures. From the Frank-Starling relationship (Fig. 16-6), this reduction in the left ventricular end-diastolic filling pressure (LVEDP) should lower the stroke volume in both normal and failing hearts, possibly resulting in a fall in cardiac output and consequently in tissue perfusion.

There is a great deal of evidence that this sequence occurs commonly in edematous states. First, the administration of diuretics to patients with either acute or chronic heart failure frequently leads to a reduction in cardiac output.[73-75] A similar sequence can occur in cirrhosis, particularly in patients who are rapidly diuresed.[76,77] Second, diuretic-induced fluid removal leads to *increased secretion of the three 'hypovolemic" hormones*—renin, norepinephrine, and ADH—in many patients with heart failure or cirrhosis.[49,77,78]

Despite the reduction that may occur in the effective circulating volume, *most patients benefit from the appropriate use of diuretics*. As an example, the diminished exercise tolerance and symptoms of pulmonary congestion in patients with heart failure are often improved by diuretic therapy, even though the cardiac output may fall by an average of 20 percent.[74] This observation suggests that small reductions in the cardiac output can be well tolerated. Similarly, relief of symptoms of fatigue and bloating are common in patients with noncardiac causes of edema.

---

*Laryngeal edema, due to an allergic reaction, and angioedema also are potentially fatal. However, these conditions are special forms of localized edema requiring epinephrine, corticosteroids, and, if needed, tracheostomy, not fluid removal.

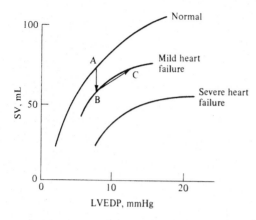

Figure 16-6 Frank-Starling curves relating stroke volume (SV) to left ventricular end-diastolic pressure (LVEDP) in normal subjects and patients with heart failure. The onset of mild heart failure results in an initial reduction in cardiac function (middle curve, point B), a change that can initially be normalized by raising the LVEDP via renal fluid retention (point C). In comparison, normalization of stroke volume is not attainable with severe heart failure. (*Adapted from Cohn JN, Am J Med 55:131, 1973, with permission.*)

However, the decrease in the effective circulating volume is sufficient to significantly impair tissue perfusion in selected cases. This occurs most commonly in two settings:

- When there is a low baseline effective circulating volume, as in severe cardiac failure
- After the excessive or overly rapidly use of diuretics[76]

The adequacy of tissue perfusion can be estimated simply by monitoring the blood urea nitrogen (BUN) and plasma creatinine concentration. *As long as these parameters remain constant, it can be assumed that diuretic therapy has not led to a significant impairment in perfusion to the kidney or, therefore, to other organs.*

Otherwise unexplained significant elevations in the BUN and plasma creatinine concentration after diuretic therapy indicate that *further fluid removal should be avoided* and that other therapeutic measures aimed at improving the underlying disease should be attempted. The decline in tissue perfusion in this setting also can lead to weakness, fatigue, postural dizziness, and lethargy and confusion due to decreased cerebral blood flow. These problems can be illustrated by the following example.

Case History 16-2   A previously well 46-year-old man is admitted to the hospital with pulmonary edema due to an acute myocardial infarction. As part of his initial therapy, he is given intravenous furosemide and then continued on an oral furosemide dose of 40 mg/day. The pulmonary edema rapidly clears, and the patient is having an uneventful recovery when it is noted on the tenth hospital day that his BUN has risen from 10 mg/dL on admission to 110 mg/dL and his plasma creatinine concentration has increased from 1 to 4.5 mg/dL. There has been a 6-kg weight loss since admission.

The physical examination reveals that the patient is in no acute distress. The vital signs show a small reduction in blood pressure since admission. The chest is clear to percussion and auscultation, and there are no murmurs or gallops on cardiac examination. Estimated jugular venous pressure is less than 5 cmH$_2$O, there is no peripheral edema, and the skin turgor is diminished.

Examination of the urine reveals a normal sediment, no proteinuria, a urine Na$^+$ concentration of 2 meq/L, and a urine osmolality of 550 mosmol/kg.

Comment   There are many signs in this patient pointing toward volume depletion secondary to *excessive diuresis* as the cause of the acute renal failure. These include weight loss, decreased skin turgor, low central venous pressure, a low urine Na$^+$ concentration and high urine osmolality, and an increase in BUN out of proportion to the elevation in the plasma creatinine concentration. This previously well patient presented with a normal extracellular volume, a small quantity of which had been translocated into the alveoli. Thus, continued fluid removal in this setting must lead to extracellular volume depletion.

Diuretic therapy was discontinued and the patient was given a high-sodium diet while being carefully observed for the recurrence of heart failure. After 6 days of this regimen, his skin turgor, BUN, and plasma creatinine concentration had returned to normal.

However, a reduction in the effective circulating volume in response to diuretic therapy is not always due to overdiuresis. This can be illustrated by the following case history.

Case History 16-3   A 64-year-old woman with chronic congestive heart failure due to atherosclerotic heart disease is admitted to the hospital. In addition to pulmonary edema, she also has signs of right-sided heart failure, including distended neck veins and pedal edema. After 3 days of diuretic therapy, there has been a 5-kg weight loss with marked clinical improvement, although a mild degree of pulmonary congestion persists. During this period, the BUN has risen from 20 to 60 mg/dL, with an increase in the plasma creatinine concentration from 1.2 to 2.3 mg/dL. The urinary findings are similar to those in Case History 16-2.

Comment   This case represents another example of reduced tissue perfusion due to diuretic therapy. However, edema persists. Thus, this patient has such severe heart disease that she cannot both be edema-free and have a stable plasma creatinine concentration on diuretic therapy alone. As shown in Fig. 16-6, the stroke volume can vary directly with the LVEDP even in severe heart failure. In this patient, the cardiac output was better maintained only at filling pressures so high that they caused both pulmonary and peripheral edema. When the filling pressures were reduced to a degree sufficient to diminish the edema, the cardiac output and tissue perfusion were sacrificed.

In contrast to the adverse hemodynamic changes that may be seen in heart failure, cirrhosis, or some cases of the nephrotic syndrome, impaired renal perfusion should not occur after the appropriate use of diuretics in patients with primary renal Na^+ retention (Table 16-2). In these conditions, the effective circulating volume is increased by fluid retention. Although diuretics reduce the effective circulating volume, it will be from an initially high level back toward normal.

As noted above, localized edema due to lymphatic obstruction, deep vein thrombosis, or hypothyroidism should *not* be treated with diuretics. Edema in these settings cannot be mobilized by a diuresis-induced reduction in venous pressure. As a result, diuretic therapy will predictably lead to volume depletion. Similar considerations apply to malignant ascites due to peritoneal carcinomatosis.[79]

How rapidly should edema fluid be removed?   When diuretics are administered, the fluid that is lost initially comes from the plasma. This results in a reduction in the venous pressure and consequently in capillary hydraulic pressure, thereby promoting restoration of the plasma volume by the mobilization of edema fluid into the vascular space. The rapidity with which this occurs is variable. In patients with generalized edema due to heart failure, the nephrotic syndrome, or primary Na^+ retention, the edema fluid can be mobilized rapidly, since most capillary beds are involved. Thus, removal of 2 to 3 liters of edema fluid or more in 24 h can often be accomplished in such patients with marked edema without much reduction in the plasma volume.

One important exception occurs in patients with cirrhosis and ascites but *no peripheral edema.*[76,77] In this setting, the excess ascitic fluid can be mobilized only via the peritoneal capillaries. Direct measurements have indicated that 500 to 750 mL/day is the maximum level that can be safely achieved by most patients.[76,77,80] If diuresis proceeds more rapidly, the ascitic fluid will be unable to completely replenish the plasma volume, resulting in azotemia and the possible precipitation of the hepatorenal syndrome (Fig. 16-7). This limitation does not apply to patients who also have peripheral edema, since the rate of fluid mobilization is again relatively unlimited in this setting.

Heart Failure

Heart failure can be produced by a variety of disorders, including coronary artery disease, hypertension, the cardiomyopathies, valvular disease, and cor pulmonale. The edema in the different causes of heart failure is due to an increase in venous pressure that produces a parallel rise in capillary hydraulic pressure. Despite the similarity in pathogenesis, the *site of edema accumulation* is variable and is dependent upon the nature of the cardiac disease.

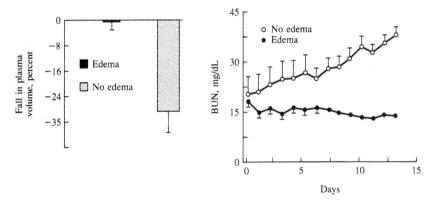

Figure 16-7   Change in plasma volume (left panel) and BUN (right panel) following diuretic-induced fluid loss of over 1 L/day in patients with cirrhosis with or without peripheral edema. A limited rate of ascites mobilization in the latter patients resulted in plasma volume depletion and progressive azotemia. These problems did not occur when peripheral edema was present. (*From Pockros PJ, Reynolds TJ,* Gastroenterology *90:1827, 1986. Copyright 1986 by The American Gastroenterological Association.*)

- Coronary or hypertensive heart disease tends to preferentially impair left ventricular function. As a result, patients with one of these disorders typically present with pulmonary but not peripheral edema.
- Cor pulmonale, in comparison, is initially associated with pure right ventricular failure, resulting in prominent edema in the lower extremities and perhaps ascites.
- Cardiomyopathies tend to produce equivalent involvement of both the right and left ventricles, often leading to the *simultaneous onset* of pulmonary and peripheral edema.

In acute pulmonary edema due to a myocardial infarction or ischemia, the left ventricular disease results in elevation in left ventricular end-diastolic and left atrial pressures, which are transmitted *back* through the pulmonary veins to the pulmonary capillaries. In general, the pulmonary capillary pressure must exceed 18 to 20 mmHg (normal equals 5 to 12 mmHg) before pulmonary edema occurs.[66,81]

The pathogenesis of edema formation is somewhat different in chronic heart failure. In this setting, the increase in capillary pressure is a result of plasma volume expansion, not solely the obstructive effect of a diseased heart. This is called the *forward hypothesis* of heart failure, in which the primary event is a reduction in cardiac output (Fig. 16-8).[46,82,83] This decrease in tissue perfusion leads to activation of the sympathetic and renin-angiotensin systems, which have a variety of cardiovascular and renal effects (see Chaps. 2 and 8).[84,85] Catecholamines, for example, stimulate both heart rate and cardiac contractility, changes that can initially return the cardiac output to normal, at least at rest. Norepinephrine and angiotensin II also cause both arteriolar constriction, which

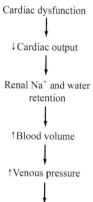

Cardiac dysfunction

↓ Cardiac output

Renal Na⁺ and water
retention

↑ Blood volume

↑ Venous pressure

Edema

Figure 16-8 Forward hypothesis of heart failure in which a primary reduction in cardiac output leads to fluid retention and edema.

can normalize the systemic blood pressure, and enhanced renal Na^+ reabsorption (which is in part due to angiotensin II–induced secretion of aldosterone).

The net effect in patients with relatively well-preserved cardiac function is an initially mild impairment in Na^+-excretory ability. Edema is often absent at this time, unless there is a high level of Na^+ intake.[88]* With more advanced disease, however, forward output can be restored only by plasma volume expansion and intracardiac filling pressures that are high enough to promote edema formation.

The effect of fluid retention on cardiac function is illustrated in Fig. 16-6. The upper curve represents the normal Frank-Starling relationship between stroke volume and LVEDP, in which *increasing cardiac stretch enhances cardiac contractility*.[73,89,90] The development of mild cardiac failure (middle curve) will, if the sympathetic stimulation of cardiac function is insufficient, lower both stroke volume and cardiac output (line AB). The ensuing renal Na^+ and water retention can reverse these abnormalities, since the increments in plasma volume and LVEDP will augment cardiac contractility (line BC).

At this point, the patient is in a new steady state of *compensated heart failure* in which the stroke volume and cardiac output are normal, Na^+ excretion matches Na^+ intake, and the activity of the renin-angiotensin-aldosterone system has returned to normal (Fig. 16-5).[61,63] The restoration of tissue perfusion in this setting has occurred only after there has been an elevation in the LVEDP, perhaps to a level sufficient to produce pulmonary edema.

There are several points that deserve emphasis in this simple example of mild to moderate heart failure:

---

* This hypothesis is also applicable to high-output heart failure due, for example, to hyperthyroidism (where the hypermetabolic state leads to an increase in energy requirements) or to arteriovenous fistulas (where blood flowing through the fistulas is bypassing the capillary circulation). In these conditions, the patients still behave as if they are effectively volume-depleted, since the cardiac output is inappropriately low in relation to tissue needs.[47,86,87]

- It demonstrates again the dual effects of fluid retention in edematous states: a beneficial increment in cardiac output and a potentially harmful elevation in venous pressure. The major increase in cardiac output occurs as the LVEDP rises to 12 to 15 mmHg. There is little further effect on cardiac function about this level, but pulmonary edema becomes more likely.[81] These relationships have important implications for therapy (see "Treatment," below).

- It illustrates that vascular congestion (that is, an elevated LVEDP) and a low cardiac output do not have to occur together in patients with heart disease. At point B, the patient is in a low-output state, but there is no congestion; at point C, the patient is congested but has a normal cardiac output.

- The Frank-Starling relationship in Fig. 16-6 varies with exercise. Patients with moderate heart disease may have a normal cardiac output at rest but may be unable to increase the output adequately with even mild exertion.[91] This relative decrease in tissue perfusion can lead sequentially to further neurohumoral activation, renal vasoconstriction and ischemia, Na^+ retention, and ultimately edema.[92,93] In this setting, limiting physical activity may produce substantial improvement. Simply assuming the supine position for 1 to 2 h, for example, maximizes the cardiac output in relation to tissue needs. This can induce as much as a 40 percent rise in glomerular filtration rate and a doubling of the natriuretic response to a diuretic.[94]

- Patients with mild to moderate heart disease may have no edema with dietary Na^+ restriction but may retain Na^+ and possibly become edematous if given a Na^+ load.[88] Suppose points A and C in Fig. 16-6 reflect the hemodynamic state on a low-Na^+ diet. An increase in Na^+ intake will initially expand the intravascular volume and raise the LVEDP. In the normal subject (point A), who is still on the ascending limb of the Frank-Starling curve, the increase in filling pressure will enhance stroke volume and cardiac output, which will then promote the excretion of the excess Na^+. In contrast, a similar elevation in the LVEDP in the patient with heart failure (point C), who is on a flatter part of the curve, will produce less of an increment both in cardiac output and consequently in Na^+ excretion. Limiting dietary Na^+ intake in this setting may be sufficient to alleviate the edema.

The situation is somewhat different with severe heart failure (lower curve, Fig. 16-6). In this case, the plateau in stroke volume occurs earlier and at a lower level than in mild heart failure, and increasing the LVEDP cannot normalize the stroke volume. Two factors appear to account for this plateau. First, the heart may simply have reached its maximum capacity to increase contractility in response to increasing stretch.[95] Second, the Frank-Starling relationship actually applies to left ventricular end-diastolic *volume*, since it is the stretching of cardiac muscle that is responsible for the enhanced contractility.[90] The more easily measured LVEDP is used clinically since, in relatively normal hearts, pressure and volume vary in parallel. However, cardiac compliance may be greatly reduced with severe heart disease.[96] As a result, a *small increase in volume produces a large elevation in LVEDP* but no substantial stretching of the cardiac muscle and therefore little change in cardiac output.[97]

Systolic versus diastolic dysfunction   The decrease in cardiac output that is initially seen in heart failure can occur by one of two mechanisms: *systolic dysfunction*, in which impaired cardiac contractility is the primary abnormality; and *diastolic dysfunction*, in which there is a limitation in diastolic filling and therefore in forward output due to increased ventricular stiffness. Two factors may contribute to the latter problem: delayed postsystolic relaxation, which may reflect impaired calcium efflux from the myocardial cells, and decreased ventricular compliance, which impairs ventricular filling during late diastole.[93,94] Diastolic dysfunction is most often seen with hypertensive and less commonly with ischemic heart disease.[98,100].

The distinction between these two, not mutually exclusive types of heart failure can be made by measurement of the ejection fraction with ultrasonography or radionuclide scanning. The ejection fraction will be normal (55 to 70 percent) with isolated diastolic dysfunction, since contractility is not impaired.[98-100] Establishing the correct diagnosis is important clinically, because each mechanism requires a different approach to therapy (see below).

Decreased diastolic compliance can also explain the development of "flash" pulmonary edema during an episode of ischemia. In this setting, lack of cardiac distensibility during diastolic filling can result in a marked elevation in left heart pressures and subsequent fluid movement into the alveoli. Some of these patients do not require chronic therapy for heart failure, since spontaneous or anatomic correction of the ischemic lesion can lead to restoration of normal cardiac function.[101-103] Recovery, however, may not be complete for several days to as long as 2 weeks, due to the phenomenon of the "stunned" postischemic myocardium.[101,103,104]

Neurohumoral adaptation: initial benefit but long-term adverse effects   The reduction in tissue perfusion associated with progressive cardiac dysfunction leads to increasing release of norepinephrine, renin, and ADH, all of which are systemic and renal vasoconstrictors.[84,85,105-107] These neurohumoral changes, which begin before the onset of clinically evident congestion,[106] are initially beneficial, since they raise the cardiac output and systemic blood pressure toward normal. *Excessive* vasoconstriction is prevented in this setting by increased secretion of both renal vasodilator prostaglandins and atrial natriuretic peptide (ANP);[85,107-110] renal ischemia and the elevation in atrial and ventricular pressures are the respective stimuli for the release of these hormones (see Chap. 6).

The physiologic significance of prostaglandins in heart failure can be illustrated by the response to a nonsteroidal anti-inflammatory drug, which blocks prostaglandin synthesis. Removal of prostaglandin-induced vasodilation can lead to two deleterious effects in these patients: a decline in glomerular filtration rate, since the vasoconstrictor actions of angiotensin II and norepinephrine are now unopposed; and a fall in cardiac output, due to the association rise in systemic vascular resistance and therefore in cardiac afterload.[107]

An adverse response to a nonsteroidal anti-inflammatory drug is most likely to occur when prostaglandin synthesis is enhanced—namely, in those patients with advanced heart failure in whom circulating angiotensin II and norepinephrine levels are most likely to be elevated. The presence of *otherwise unexplained hyponatremia* is a good marker for patients at risk, since the combination of decreased renal perfusion and the associated rise in ADH release impairs the ability to excrete ingested water.[107]

The function of ANP in heart failure is less well defined. The chronic increase in cardiac filling pressures leads to the release of ANP and brain natriuretic peptide (BNP) from the atria and, to a lesser degree, the ventricles (see Chap. 6).[111-114] Both the cardiac and circulating levels of these hormones rise in parallel with the severity of the heart disease, even though the patients remain Na^+-avid and vasoconstricted.[112-114] It is possible that ANP and BNP play a modulating role in this setting, minimizing but not preventing the systemic and renal effects, such as the degree of sodium retention and vasoconstriction.[109]

In addition to these peptides' possible physiologic role, measurement of plasma levels of ANP and BNP may be useful as a noninvasive marker of the presence of mild left ventricular dysfunction, which is usually estimated by echocardiography or radionuclide scanning.[112-116]

Long-term effects   Although neurohumoral vasoconstriction initially maintains circulatory hemodynamics, this response is clearly *maladaptive in the long term,* because the failing heart has to pump against a higher resistance. The slowing of disease progression and improvement in patient survival observed with use of angiotensin converting enzyme (ACE) inhibitors in patients with systolic dysfunction suggest that there is, over time, a net negative effect of the neurohumoral adaptations of ventricular function (see below).

Treatment: acute pulmonary edema   An extensive discussion of the treatment of acute pulmonary edema and chronic heart failure is beyond the scope of this chapter. It is useful, however, to review those therapeutic modalities directed toward preventing edema accumulation and preserving normal renal function.

Acute pulmonary edema is a medical emergency requiring immediate therapy to restore tissue oxygenation and perfusion.[117] The initial regimen generally includes the administration of humidified oxygen via a face mask; intravenous morphine, which allays anxiety and induces venodilation, thereby diminishing venous return and lowering cardiac filling pressures; and an intravenous loop diuretic (such as 40 mg of furosemide) for fluid removal and for possible venodilation.[118] If these modalities are ineffective, intravenous nitroglycerin or intravenous nitroprusside can be added to further reduce venous return.[119] The initial aim of therapy is to lower the pulmonary capillary wedge pressure (if it is being measured) to 15 to 18 mmHg, a level that is low enough to alleviate pulmonary edema but not so low as to further reduce the cardiac output.[81,120]

Patients with systolic dysfunction who remain in pulmonary edema despite the above modalities may benefit from intravenous inotropic support to improve cardiac performance and systemic perfusion. This is usually achieved by beta-agonist therapy (e.g., dobutamine), a phosphodiesterase inhibitor (e.g., milrinone), or both.[121,122]

Patients with acute pulmonary edema may also have severe acid-base disturbances, such as respiratory and metabolic acidosis (primarily lactic acidosis).[123,124] Specific therapy may not be necessary, since reversal of the pulmonary edema is usually sufficient to restore acid-base balance by improving gas exchange and by allowing metabolism of the excess lactate into bicarbonate.[123,124]

Treatment: chronic heart failure   There are now five drugs that are often used in the treatment of chronic heart failure due to systolic dysfunction. Two improve symptoms (digoxin and loop diuretics), and three improve survival (ACE inhibitors, beta blockers, if tolerated, and, in advanced heart failure, spironolactone). Important adjunctive measures include dietary Na^+ restriction (1 to 2 g/day of sodium) and periods of rest. Some patients have a cardiac output that is relatively normal at rest but does not increase adequately with exertion.[91] It is during this latter period that renal Na^+ retention is most intense.[92,93] Thus, limiting physical activity may produce substantial clinical improvement, since maximizing tissue perfusion in relation to needs will maximize Na^+ excretion.[94]

Loop diuretics   Diuretics (loop diuretics are usually used) have the advantage of directly removing the excess fluid, thereby controlling the congestive symptoms (e.g., pulmonary and peripheral edema.[125-127] However, they do not reverse the impairment in cardiac function.

Other potential difficulties with diuretic therapy in heart failure are reviewed in Chap. 15.[128] In some patients with marked edema, for example, impaired gastrointestinal function (due to decreased perfusion or mucosal edema) can delay the absorption and thereby minimize the efficacy of an oral loop diuretic; this defect can often be reversed after a period of intravenous diuretic therapy. Even if drug delivery to the kidney is adequate, the associated increases in angiotensin II and aldosterone enhance Na^+ reabsorption, thus diminishing the maximum diuretic response. In this setting, the effective single dose [up to a maximum oral dose of 160 to 240 mg of furosemide (only about one-half of which is absorbed) or 2 to 3 mg of oral or intravenous bumetanide] may have to be given twice a day to induce an adequate net diuresis.[128]

Loop diuretic therapy alone can also induce hypokalemia and hypomagnesemia, which can predispose to serious arrhythmias. There is evidence that loop diuretics may increase arrhythmic mortality, an effect that can be prevented by the concurrent administration of a potassium-sparing diuretic.[129]

Spironolactone Administration of the potassium-sparing diuretic spironolactone, which competes with aldosterone for the mineralocorticoid receptor, significantly reduces mortality in patients with advanced heart failure (Fig. 16-9).[130] Two possible explanations for this benefit are that aldosterone has a deleterious effect on the failing heart or that maintaining a higher plasma potassium concentration is beneficial. The observation that non-potassium-sparing diuretics increase arrhythmic mortality in patients with mild to moderate heart failure, an effect that can be prevented by a potassium-sparing diuretic, suggests that hypokalemia plays at least a contributory role.[129] Based upon these findings, it has been suggested that spironolactone (25 to 50 mg/day) may have a role in any stage of heart failure requiring diuretic therapy.

Digoxin Digoxin can improve cardiac performance, especially in patients with rapid atrial fibrillation, in whom slowing of the ventricular rate allows better ventricular filling.[131] Its long-term efficacy in patients with normal sinus rhythm is less predictable. Initial studies showed that stable patients treated with digoxin are much more likely to deteriorate if they are switched to placebo than if they are maintained on digoxin.[132,133] This symptomatic benefit (5 versus 27 percent worsening with placebo in one study) occurs even in patients already receiving an ACE inhibitor.[132]

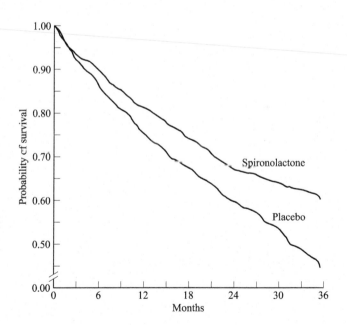

Figure 16-9 Spironolactone reduces mortality in heart failure. Kaplan-Meier analysis of survival among 1663 patients with advanced heart failure in the RALES trial shows that spironolactone reduces mortality by 30 percent (35 versus 46 percent for placebo, p < 0.001). (*Redrawn from Pitt B, Zannad F, Remme WJ, et al, N Engl J Med 341:709, 1999, with permission.*)

The DIG (Digoxin Investigation Group) trial of almost 6800 patients is the definitive study of the effectiveness of digoxin.[134] Digoxin therapy was associated with symptomatic improvement, as shown by a reduction in the combined endpoints of hospitalization for worsening chronic heart failure and mortality due to chronic heart failure. However, there was no improvement in total survival with digoxin therapy (Fig. 16-10); the small improvement in death from worsening heart failure was counterbalanced by an apparent increase in arrhythmic death.

Digoxin is generally ineffective in those patients with heart failure who have normal ventricular contractility. This problem may be seen with isolated diastolic dysfunction or with obstruction to flow in severe mitral stenosis.[100,135,136]

Vasodilators   Vasodilator therapy with an ACE inhibitor or the combination of hydralazine and isosorbide dinitrate (HI) was the first pharmacologic approach shown to improve survival in patients with heart failure due to systolic dysfunction. Both can improve patient survival by decreasing progressive cardiac dysfunction and, in mild disease, by diminishing the incidence of sudden death,[137,138] although a comparative study suggests that the benefit is more pronounced with the ACE inhibitors.[138]

The benefit of ACE inhibition has been demonstrated in the entire spectrum of patients with heart failure, ranging from asymptomatic left ventricular dysfunction[139] to mild to moderate heart failure[137,138,140] to severe disease.[141] The selective angiotensin II–receptor antagonists appear to have an efficacy similar to that of the ACE inhibitors.[142]

Since ACE inhibitors produce more benefit than the direct vasodilators hydralazine and isosorbide dinitrate and since other oral vasodilators are less effective,[143] the mechanism of action of ACE inhibition probably involves more

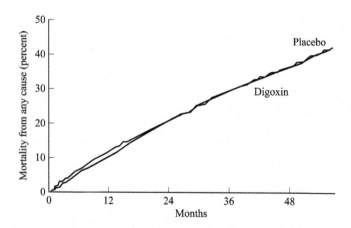

Figure 16-10   Digoxin has no effect on survival in heart failure. No difference in mortality was observed in patients with symptomatic congestive heart failure and a low left ventricular ejection fraction (≤ 45 percent) who were randomized to either digoxin or placebo. (*Redrawn from the Digitalis Investigation Group, N Engl J Med 336:525, 1997, with permission.*)

than simply reducing afterload. One possibility is inhibition of the local intra-cardiac renin-angiotensin system.[144] Such an effect may more efficiently reverse deleterious actions of angiotensin II on cardiac function. In addition, vasodilation-induced increases in the release of the vasoconstrictors angiotensin II and norepi-nephrine are seen with HI but not with the ACE inhibitors.[145]

Since ACE inhibitors increase cardiac output and renal blood flow, it might be assumed that they would improve the glomerular filtration rate as well. However, this occurs in less than 10 percent of cases, while the plasma creatinine concentration actually rises in about 30 percent of patients.[146-148] The latter complication is generally seen in the first week of therapy as angiotensin II levels are acutely reduced.[146] It is most likely to occur in those settings in which maintenance of the glomerular filtration rate is dependent upon high ambient angiotensin II levels:[146,147,149] (1) when there has been an excessive diuretic response, with the LVEDP falling below 15 mmHg; (2) when the mean arterial pressure falls below 65 mmHg, and (3) when the pretreatment plasma Na^+ concentration is below 137 meq/L, which is a marker for marked neurohumoral activation.[107]

Thus, the mechanism of reversible renal insufficiency in this setting is similar to that seen in some patients with bilateral renal artery stenosis (see page 42). Restoration of baseline renal function can often be achieved by lowering the diuretic dose or, if a long-acting agent is used, possibly switching to captopril.[147,150] If this is unsuccessful, HI should be used, since these agents do not interfere with angiotensin II production and therefore are less likely to impair glomerular filtration.[47]

Beta blockers   Since beta blockers have negative inotropic activity, the presence of heart failure has been considered a contraindication to their use. However, an increasing number of studies have demonstrated that at least some beta blockers (e.g., carvedilol, metoprolol, and bisoprolol) can lead to symptomatic improve-ment and improved survival in patients with heart failure (Fig. 16-11).[151-154] Compared to those treated with placebo, patients treated with a beta blocker had an approximate 30 percent reduction in mortality during an average follow-up of 13 months.[154] Most patients in these trials were treated with ACE inhibitors, suggesting that beta blockers provide an additive survival benefit.[151-153]

How beta blockers might act in this setting is not well understood. Among the proposed mechanisms are prevention of a toxic effect of the increased concentra-tions of circulating norepinephrine on the heart, a reduction in the plasma con-centration of vasoconstrictors, and upregulation of β_1-adrenergic receptors.

It has been recommended that the beta blockers used in the above studies (carvedilol, metoprolol, and bisoprolol) be considered in patients with New York Heart Association class II and III congestive heart failure (CHF) who have been stabilized on an ACE inhibitor, digoxin, and diuretics. An important concern is that many patients have a substantial period of worsening heart failure, often lasting 3 to 4 months, after the initiation of beta-blocker therapy.[155] This is more likely to occur in patients with advanced disease.

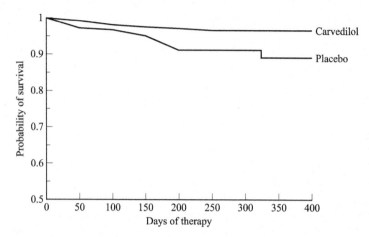

Figure 16-11 Carvedilol improves survival in heart failure. Among patients with CHF who were treated with digoxin, diuretics, and an angiotensin converting enzyme inhibitor, those randomized to carvedilol had significantly improved survival compared to individuals given placebo. (*Redrawn from Packer M, Bristow MR, Cohn JN, et al for the US Carvedilol Heart Failure Study Group, N Engl J Med 334:1349, 1996, with permission.*)

Guidelines have been published for the safe initiation of therapy.[156] It is particularly important that therapy be begun in *very low doses* and the dose doubled at weekly intervals until the target dose is reached or symptoms become limiting. Initial and target doses are 3.125 mg bid and 25 to 50 mg bid (the higher doses being used in subjects over 85 kg) for carvedilol, 6.25 mg bid and 50 to 75 mg bid for metoprolol or 12.5 or 25 mg daily and titrated up to 200 mg/day for therapy with extended-release metoprolol, and 1.25 mg qd and 5 to 10 mg qd for bisoprolol. Dose increases are generally made at 2-week intervals. Even lower starting doses should be given to patients with recent decompensation of a systolic pressure below 85 mmHg. Every effort should be made to achieve the target dose, since the improvement appears to be dose-dependent. It is recommended that such therapy be initiated under the consultative guidance of a heart failure center that has experience with this regimen.

Cor Pulmonale

The pathogenesis of edema in cor pulmonale due to chronic obstructive pulmonary disease is different from that in other forms of heart failure. In this disorder, the cardiac output and GFR are usually normal or near normal both in the resting state and with exercise.[157-159]

Edema seems to occur almost exclusively in patients with hypercapnia, suggesting that the high P_{CO_2} rather than cardiac dysfunction may be responsible for Na^+ retention in this disorder.[159] Hypercapnia is associated with an appropriate increase in proximal HCO_3^- reabsorption, which serves to minimize the fall in arterial pH (see Chap. 21). This increase in proximal HCO_3^- transport, which occurs via Na^+-H^+ exchange, may be responsible for edema formation in cor pulmonale, since it also promotes the reabsorption of NaCl and H_2O (see page 78).

Another contributing factor to sodium retention may be hypoxemia. Hypoxemia can cause renal vasoconstriction, leading to a reduction in urinary sodium excretion.[160]

Therapy of edema in cor pulmonale consists of improving pulmonary function (if possible) and the use of diuretics. Correction of hypoxemia, with continuous low-flow oxygen if necessary, also may be helpful. As in other edematous states, the BUN and plasma creatinine concentration should be monitored during diuretic therapy, with further fluid removal being deferred if renal function deteriorates. In addition, diuretic-induced metabolic alkalosis should be avoided, since the rise in extracellular pH can further depress net alveolar ventilation.[161] The carbonic anhydrase inhibitor acetazolamide may be particularly effective in this setting; it tends to produce a $NaHCO_3$ diuresis, thereby correcting both the fluid overload and the alkalosis (see Chap. 15).

Cirrhosis and Ascites

Ascites refers to the accumulation of fluid in the peritoneal cavity. It can be seen in a variety of conditions, including severe acute or chronic hepatic disease (particularly cirrhosis), heart failure, the nephrotic syndrome, and with tumor implants on the peritoneum. In the last condition, both lymphatic obstruction and increased capillary permeability contribute to ascites formation.[79]

In patients with liver disease, the ascitic fluid is derived from the hepatic sinusoids and enters the peritoneum by moving across the hepatic capsule. The principal factor in the development of hepatic ascites is *sinusoidal obstruction* (due to fibrosis or hepatic venous occlusion), leading to an increase in the hydraulic pressure in the sinusoids.[70,162] A portal pressure > 12 mmHg appears to be required for fluid retention in patients with cirrhosis; neither ascites nor edema is seen in patients without portal hypertension[70,71] or in those without sinusoidal hypertension (e.g., portal vein thrombosis).

Hypoalbuminemia due to increased hepatic synthesis may also be present; it does not, however, play an important role in hepatic ascites, since the sinusoids are normally freely permeable to albumin. Thus, the transcapillary oncotic pressure gradient is normally very low and does not act to hold fluid in the vascular space.[2,25]

Mechanisms of ascites formation   The possible mechanisms responsible for fluid retention and ascites formation in cirrhosis are illustrated in Fig. 16-12. Impaired Na^+ excretion can be demonstrated early in the course of the disease, prior to the presence of clinically evident edema and despite normal renal function and appropriate suppression of renin secretion.[163,164] Similar findings can be demonstrated in experimental models of hepatic disease in which Na^+ retention precedes the development of ascites.[165]

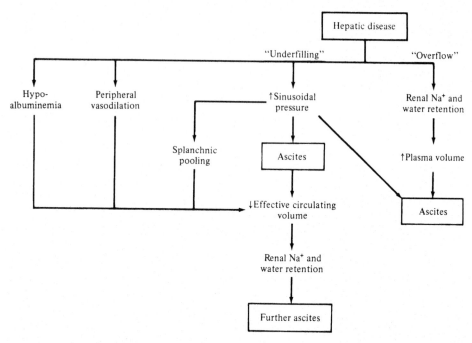

Figure 16-12 Underfilling and overflow theories of the pathogenesis of fluid retention and ascites formation in hepatic disease. In some patients, both mechanisms may be operative. In addition, the combination of increased femoral venous pressure (resulting from an ascites-induced elevation in intraperitoneal pressure) and perhaps marked hypoalbuminemia can lead to peripheral edema.

These observations have suggested that there might be an initial *overflow* phenomenon in which hepatic disease directly stimulates renal Na^+ reabsorption independent of any change in systemic hemodynamics.[166,167] How this might occur is incompletely understood. Studies in experimental animals indicate that increased intrasinusoidal pressure, rather than portal venous pressure, is required.[167] This hemodynamic change may then activate a hepatorenal reflex, resulting in an elevation in renal sympathetic nerve activity.[168,169] The ensuing combination of a diminished renal perfusion and enhanced Na^+ reabsorption can then promote fluid retention.[168] The elevation in intrasinusoidal pressure promotes the accumulation of most of this excess fluid in the peritoneum.

It is likely, however, that effective circulating volume depletion or *underfilling* of the arterial circulation (rather than overflow) is primarily responsible for the sodium retention in cirrhosis.[46,170] The earliest change appears to be a decrease in systemic vascular resistance due primarily to splanchnic vasodilatation.[46,170] In some experimental models, vasodilatation clearly precedes the onset of renal sodium retention.[171]

A similar finding may occur in humans. When patients with cirrhosis and no ascites or edema are volume-expanded with a high-salt diet plus a mineralocorticoid, some patients become progressively edematous and do not undergo aldosterone escape (see page 185).[169] These patients, when compared to those who excreted sodium normally, where already vasodilated, as evidenced by a much lower systemic vascular resistance and a higher cardiac output.

The role of increasing splanchnic vasodilation in humans with progressive cirrhosis can be illustrated by the sequential changes in systemic and renal hemodynamics that are seen in this disorder. Early in the course of the disease—stable cirrhosis, no ascites—the vasodilatory substances that affect the portal circulation also involve the kidney, and the glomerular filtration rate may be as high as 50 percent above normal.[172] In addition to nitric oxide, vasodilator prostaglandins also may contribute to the glomerular hyperfiltration.[173]

As the hepatic disease and splanchnic vasodilation become more severe, a progressive fall in systemic vascular resistance and blood pressure ensues; these alterations lead to increased renal and femoral vascular resistance (and reduced flow to these sites) that results in part from the hypotension-induced activation of the renin-angiotensin system.[53] The observation that the central blood volume (that volume present in the cardiopulmonary circulation and the arterial tree) is progressively reduced in cirrhosis is also consistent with a reduction in extra-splanchnic perfusion.[57]

The mechanism responsible for vasodilatation and the hyperdynamic circulation in cirrhosis are not well understood. Research has focused upon *nitric oxide (NO)* and its role in splanchnic vasodilation in cirrhosis.[174] In cirrhotic rats, for example, inhibition of the synthesis of NO significantly increases the arterial pressure and systemic vascular resistance, decreases the cardiac index,[175,176] and reverses the impaired response to vasopressors.[177,178] Although human studies are limited, the observation that serum levels of nitrite and nitrate, an index of in vivo NO synthesis, are significantly higher in cirrhotic patients than in controls is also compatible with the NO hypothesis.[179]

The reason for enhanced NO production in cirrhosis is unclear. One mechanism may be that endotoxin absorbed from the gut is not normally inactivated in the liver because of portal-systemic shunting. The ensuing endotoxinemia is a known stimulus to nitric oxide synthesis; increased release of cytokines also may play a contributory role.[174,180,181] Among patients with cirrhosis, support for this hypothesis is provided by the following observations:[180]

- Blood in the portal veins contains higher NO concentrations than blood from the peripheral veins.
- The oral administration of an antibiotic significantly reduces plasma levels of endotoxin, nitrite, and nitrate.

The importance of splanchnic vasodilatation–induced underfilling for the impairment in renal function in cirrhosis can also be demonstrated by the response to ornipressin, an analog of ADH. This vasoconstrictor acutely raises splanchnic resistance, leading sequentially to an elevation in mean arterial pressure; reductions in the plasma renin activity and norepinephrine concentration; a decrease in renal vascular resistance; and elevations in renal blood flow, glomerular filtration rate (from 18 to 29 mL/min in this study), and Na^+ excretion.[182] The therapeutic significance of this observation remains to be determined.

Indirect evidence of underfilling in cirrhosis has also come from studies of patients who are acutely volume-expanded by immersion to the neck in warm water (in which the hydrostatic pressure of the water on the lower extremities results in the translocation of fluid to the central cardiopulmonary circulation; see page 264) or by the insertion of a peritoneovenous shunt (in which ascitic fluid is reinfused into the internal jugular vein) or a transjugular intrahepatic porto-systemic shunt (in which a low-resistance channel is created between the hepatic vein and the intrahepatic portion of the portal vein).[183–186] These modalities are often able to induce a marked natriuresis and a reduction in the plasma renin activity and norepinephrine concentration, all of which suggest improved tissue perfusion.

The net effect, as described earlier, is that patients with advanced cirrhosis have very low rates of Na^+ excretion (< 10 meq/day in some cases),[49]* a systemic blood pressure that is often below normal,[187] increased secretion of the three hypovolemic hormones (renin, norepinephrine, and ADH),[50,51,183] and a progressive decline in the glomerular filtration rate.[50,188]

Hepatorenal syndrome The progressive hemodynamically mediated fall in GFR is, when clinically apparent, called the hepatorenal syndrome.[190-192] This disorder is induced by intense renal vasoconstriction that is thought to reflect an imbalance between the high level of vasoconstrictors and a relatively low level of protective renal vasodilators (such as prostaglandins and perhaps kinins). Studies in nonazotemic cirrhotics with ascites suggest that the approximate incidence of the hepatorenal syndrome is 18 percent at 1 year and 39 percent at 5 years.[193] An episode of gastrointestinal bleeding or infection may be a precipitating event, and patients at highest risk are those with hyponatremia and a high plasma renin activity, signs of marked neurohumoral activation that reflect more severe effective circulating volume depletion.[193] Progression to renal failure is typically associated with a fall in mean arterial pressure, another indicator of increasing systemic vasodilatation.

The decline in GFR in patients with cirrhosis is initially *masked* because both urea and creatinine production are often markedly reduced due to the liver disease and to decreased muscle mass, respectively. As a result, some cirrhotic patients with a plasma creatinine concentration within the "normal" range (1.0 to 1.3 mg/dL) have a glomerular filtration rate as low as 20 to 60 mL/min.[194,195] Calculation of the creatinine clearance will partially overcome this problem, since the reduction in creatinine production will be accounted for by a decline in creatinine excretion. However, the clearance value obtained will, because of

---

* Sodium retention and ascites formation are not prominent in all liver diseases, being relatively late events in primary biliary cirrhosis.[190] The renal vasodilator and natriuretic effects of retained bile salts may be responsible for the relative preservation of renal function in this disorder.

increased creatinine secretion, tend to overestimate the true GFR by as much as 40 percent or more in patients with renal insufficiency.[195]

These renal manifestations of underfilling progress in parallel to the severity of the hepatic disease and may be prognostically important. For example, patients with Na^+ excretion below 10 meq/day or a plasma Na^+ concentration below 125 to 130 meq/L (indicative of impaired water excretion due in part to higher levels of ADH) have a mean survival time as low as 5 to 6 months, in comparison to over 2 years in patients with ascites but without these findings.[49,183] Mean survival in the hepatorenal syndrome is only a few weeks, with 90 percent of patients dying within 3 months.[193]

In summary, underfilling appears to be of primary importance in the sodium retention seen in cirrhosis in humans.[46,170] Splanchnic vasodilatation, lowering both systemic vascular resistance and the systemic blood pressure, may be the primary change, with increased hepatic sinusoidal pressure resulting in the preferential accumulation of the excess fluid in the peritoneum.

Vasodilator hormones   As in heart failure, the degree of renal vasoconstriction induced by angiotensin II and norepinephrine is initially minimized in cirrhosis by increased renal secretion of vasodilator prostaglandins and kinins.[50,196,197] These hormones also may limit the degree of Na^+ retention, since prostaglandin E_2 and perhaps bradykinin appear to decrease tubular Na^+ reabsorption (see Chap. 6).

Treatment   The treatment of edema in cirrhosis varies with the severity of the disease.[162] Patients with mild to moderate disease usually have a *baseline rate of Na^+ excretion of at least 40 meq/day and a relatively normal plasma Na^+ concentration.*[49,50,183] These findings are a reflection of the less severe state of underfilling and therefore lower levels of renin and ADH. In this setting, the first step is restriction of sodium intake. An 88 meq (2000 mg) per day sodium diet is the most practical yet successful level of sodium restriction.[198,199] It can be followed in an outpatient setting without the purchase of special food.

Water intake also may need to be restricted to about 1000 mL/day. As noted above, a reduction in the plasma Na^+ concentration is a common problem in advanced disease, since the combination of progressive renal ischemia and increasing ADH levels markedly limits the ability to excrete water.[50,183,200] These changes parallel the severity of the hepatic disease, and, as in congestive heart failure,[149] hyponatremia is a marker for decreased patient survival.[200]

However, this diet alone will be effective only in the small subset of patients whose urinary sodium excretion is more than 78 meq/day (88 meq intake minus 10 meq of nonurinary losses). Thus, most patients with cirrhosis and ascites will require diuretic therapy. However, the use of diuretics in patients with cirrhosis is associated with several relatively unusual concerns, including the rate of fluid removal and a potential risk from the development of diuretic-induced hypokalemia and metabolic alkalosis.

Rate of fluid loss   As described previously, the presence or absence of peripheral edema is an important determinant of the rate at which fluid can be safely removed in cirrhosis. After induction of fluid loss with a diuretic, peripheral edema can be mobilized to protect the plasma volume in a relatively rate-unlimited fashion; in comparison, most patients can safely mobilize only about 300 to 500 mL of ascitic fluid per day.[76,77,80] As a result, more rapid fluid loss should be avoided in those patients who have *only ascites*, since it can lead to plasma volume depletion and azotemia (Fig. 16-7). Furthermore, rapid diuresis is not necessary in this setting because, in the absence of very tense ascites, the excess fluid is of no immediate danger to the patient.

The issue of fluid mobilization is even more important in patients with malignant ascites due to peritoneal carcinomatosis or chylous malignant ascites. The tumor-induced lymphatic obstruction in this setting largely prevents mobilization of the ascitic fluid.[79] Thus, even slow diuresis is likely to produce plasma volume depletion and azotemia unless the patient also has peripheral edema. Patients with massive hepatic metastases appear to represent an exception to this general rule. The ascites in this condition is due to intrahepatic hypertension and can be treated in a similar fashion to cirrhotic ascites.[79]

Avoidance of hypokalemic alkalosis   Therapy with loop diuretics alone should be avoided in cirrhosis because some patients have *developed hepatic coma coincident with the onset of hypokalemic alkalosis* and then awakened following no therapy other than KCl replacement.[201,202] Hypokalemia may promote the development of hepatic coma by increasing ammonia (NH_3) production by the renal tubular cells,[203,204] thereby adding to the already high blood ammonia levels that are often present in severe liver disease. This renal effect of hypokalemia appears to be mediated by a *transcellular cation exchange* in which K^+ leaves the cell (to replete the extracellular stores) and electroneutrality is maintained in part by the movement of extracellular H^+ ions into the cell; the ensuing intracellular acidosis is a potent stimulus to ammonia production (see page 344).

Concomitant metabolic alkalosis may also contribute to this problem. From the Henderson-Hasselbalch equation for the ammonia/ammonium buffer system,

$$pH = 9.0 + \log\frac{[NH_3]}{[NH_4^+]}$$

an elevation in extracellular pH will tend to convert NH_4^+ into NH_3. The latter is lipid-soluble and can therefore diffuse down its concentration gradient into the brain cells, thereby increasing the degree of cerebral dysfunction.

Diuretic regimen   Spironolactone, an aldosterone antagonist, is the diuretic of choice for the initial treatment of fluid overload in the setting of cirrhosis. It is more effective than furosemide alone in patients with more severe disease,[205,206] and it does not induce hypokalemia; to the contrary, this potassium-sparing diuretic may induce hyperkalemia. Spironolactone, which can cause painful gynecomastia, is often more effective than amiloride, another potassium-sparing diuretic that directly closes the aldosterone-sensitive luminal sodium channels in the collecting tubules but produces a lesser diuresis in patients with marked hyperaldosteronism.[207]

The surprising finding that the normally weak diuretic spironolactone may be more effective than a loop diuretic in cirrhotic ascites seems to be related to a slower rate of drug excretion in the urine.[208] Most diuretics are highly protein-bound in the plasma and therefore enter the tubular lumen by secretion in the proximal tubule, not by glomerular filtration. This process appears to be impaired in cirrhosis as a result of the retention of substances such as bile salts, which may have a competitive or toxic effect on tubular secretion.[208] Spironolactone, in comparison, is the only commonly used diuretic that does not require access to the tubular lumen. It passively diffuses from the plasma into the cell across the basolateral membrane; it then competitively inhibits the aldosterone receptor.[209]

The most successful therapeutic regimen is the combination of single morning oral doses of spironolactone and furosemide, beginning with 100 mg and 40 mg, respectively.[199,206] This combination in this ratio usually maintains normokalemia. The doses can be doubled if a clinical response is not evident.

Massive ascites Patients with ascites that is massive or symptomatic (such as shortness of breath or impending rupture of an umbilical hernia) cannot easily be treated with diuretic therapy, given the recommendation of a maximum 300 to 500 mL/day net fluid loss in the absence of peripheral edema. Such patients are often treated with total paracentesis.

Paracentesis differs from diuretic therapy in three important ways: Fluid removal is easier to achieve, fluid is removed more quickly, and the risk of plasma volume depletion is related to the *rate of ascites reaccumulation* rather than the rate of fluid loss. It may also reduce intravariceal pressure and variceal wall tension, possibly reducing the risk of variceal bleeding.[210]

Total (or large-volume) paracentesis can be safely performed in patients with massive or tense ascites, resulting in *a shorter period of hospitalization and a lesser incidence of azotemia and electrolyte disturbances* when compared to therapy with diuretics alone.[211-214]

The need for colloid replacement after total paracentesis in an attempt to slow ascites reaccumulation and therefore minimize effective circulating volume depletion remains a controversial issue.[211,212,215] In a randomized trial, patients with tense ascites undergoing total paracentesis who received albumin (10 g/L of ascites removed) were less likely to show signs of hemodynamic deterioration such as an increase in the plasma renin activity, worsening renal function, and/or severe hyponatremia.[212]

However, improved survival has not been proven, and it has not been possible to identify patients in advance who may benefit.[215,216] In addition, the groups that use plasma expanders administer one-half of the expander at the end of the paracentesis and the remainder 6 h later; this converts an otherwise simple outpatient procedure into an all-day visit or an overnight stay in the hospital. These factors, as well as the cost and current shortage of albumin, make its routine use currently difficult to justify.

Resistant ascites A patient is not considered to be diuretic-resistant unless the individual is excreting less than 78 meq of sodium (88 meq dietary intake minus 10 meq nonurinary excretion) per day while being administered diuretics at the doses recommended above.[216] Patients excreting more than 78 meq of sodium per day should be losing weight. If they are not, they are noncompliant with the diet and should visit the dietitian again. Patients may also be considered diuretic-resistant if they develop significant diuretic-related complications, such as progressive azotemia, hepatic encephalopathy, or progressive electrolyte imbalance.

Diuretic-resistant ascites commonly occurs in association with advanced cirrhosis, enhanced neurohumoral activation, and extremely low sodium excretion.[217,218] Neurohumoral activation causes renal vasoconstriction and enhanced sodium reabsorption (in the proximal tubule and collecting tubules). Even in those not resistant to diuretics, a greater degree of neurohumoral activation occurs in patients with diminished diuretic responsiveness.[205]

Progressive liver disease is the most common cause of the development of true diuretic resistance in a patient previously sensitive to diuretics.[191,219] Two other complications of cirrhosis, hepatocellular carcinoma and portal vein thrombosis, may also underlie this development.

Three options exist for fluid control in diuretic-resistant patients: paracentesis, insertion of a transjugular intrahepatic portosystemic shunt, and liver transplantation.[198,199,220] If there are no contraindications, the development of ascites in a previously compensated cirrhotic patient is an accepted indication for listing for liver transplantation. Patients who are first listed only after the development of diuretic resistance may not live long enough to receive a new liver because of the organ shortage and long waiting times in the United States.

The role of serial total paracenteses in the treatment of recurrent tense ascites is less clear than that of paracentesis used as initial therapy. Most of these patients are noncompliant with their sodium-restricted diet and/or medications and are masquerading as diuretic-resistant, preferring to have their ascites removed rather than follow the diet and take their medications. The problem with this approach is that repeated paracentesis can cause protein and complement depletion compared to diet/diuretic therapy and may indirectly predispose to ascitic fluid infection.[216]

Intrahepatic and portal pressures can be lowered by insertion of a transjugular intrahepatic portosystemic shunt (TIPS). In approximately 75 percent of patients with refractory ascites, uncontrolled observations suggest that this modality leads to an increase in urine output, a marked or complete reduction in ascites, and cessation of diuretic therapy or the use of much lower diuretic doses.[221,222] However, a randomized controlled trial that compared TIPS to paracentesis found a higher mortality in the TIPS group (33 percent versus 17 percent).[223]

TIPS placement is also associated with a variety of complications, including hepatic encephalopathy (approximately 30 percent of patients).[224,225] Another significant problem is early thrombosis or delayed shunt stenosis. Thus, enthusiasm for this technique has waned.

A peritoneovenous shunt, which drains into the internal jugular vein, reinfuses ascites into the vascular space and was popularized as a "physiologic" treatment of resistant ascites (and of the hepatorenal syndrome). However, because of an excessive rate of complications and no survival advantage compared with medical therapy, this procedure has been virtually abandoned.[226,227] Probably the only indication for this technique is the rare patient with diuretic-resistant cirrhotic ascites who is not a candidate for transplantation and who has too many abdominal surgical scars to permit safe, successful paracentesis.[216]

Primary Renal Sodium Retention

Patients with normal cardiac and hepatic function may develop edema if there is a primary renal abnormality preventing the excretion of Na^+ and water (Fig. 16-13). This is most frequently seen with acute or chronic renal failure in which the low GFR favors Na^+ retention. Patients with acute glomerulonephritis or the nephrotic syndrome, for example, are particularly prone to develop edema. In these disorders, the glomeruli are diseased and the filtration rate is reduced, but tubular function is initially normal. Thus, the kidney behaves as if it is underperfused and avidly reabsorbs Na^+,[228,229] particularly in the collecting tubules.[33,36,37] The net effect is edema formation, suppression of renin release, high ANP levels, and frequently hypertension that is directly induced by volume expansion.[230,231] At a similar degree of weight gain, patients with nephrotic syndrome have less suppression of renin release and less stimulation of ANP secretion than patients with acute glomerulonephritis.[231] These observations suggest a smaller increase in plasma volume in the nephrotic syndrome, perhaps due to the low oncotic pressure (see "Nephrotic Syndrome," below).

Renal Na^+ handling may be somewhat different with chronic disease, as the glomerular injury is associated with secondary tubular dysfunction. As a result, the tendency to edema formation is reduced in some patients, because of an impairment in tubular Na^+ reabsorption.[228] Similar considerations apply to

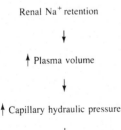

Renal Na^+ retention

↓

↑ Plasma volume

↓

↑ Capillary hydraulic pressure

↓

Edema

Figure 16-13   Pathogenesis of edema in primary renal Na^+ retention, which is most often due to glomerular disease, advanced renal failure, or the use of potent vasodilators in the treatment of hypertension.

primary tubulointerstitial diseases such as chronic pyelonephritis, in which early Na^+ retention is unusual due to the predominant tubular damage.

With advanced renal failure, however, the glomerular filtration rate falls to very low levels and Na^+ retention again becomes a problem. In this setting, there may be a very *narrow range in which Na^+ balance can be maintained*, since the ability to acutely conserve Na^+ on a low-Na^+ diet is also impaired.[232] Thus, the optimal Na^+ intake to prevent both volume depletion and volume expansion must be empirically determined.

Drugs   Certain drugs can enhance renal Na^+ reabsorption (Table 16-2). This is most likely to occur in patients with hypertension who are treated with *direct vasodilators*, such as minoxidil and diazoxide.[233,234] Patients treated with minoxidil, for example, often require therapy with high doses of a loop diuretic (such as 160 to 240 mg of furosemide) to prevent edema formation. Edema can also be induced by calcium-channel blockers, particularly the dihydropyridines. It is unclear, however, whether leakage out of the capillary due to dilatation of the precapillary sphincter or primary renal Na^+ retention is responsible for the edema.[235]

The mechanism by which these agents stimulate Na^+ retention is uncertain. The fall in blood pressure itself probably plays an important role via the pressure natriuresis phenomenon (see page 272). In addition, direct vasodilators also activate the renin-angiotensin-aldosterone and sympathetic nervous systems, both of which stimulate Na^+ retention.[233,236] The ability of sympathetic agents to directly diminish renin release and of ACE inhibitors to diminish angiotensin II production may therefore explain why these drugs do not produce edema even though they lead to an equivalent reduction in blood pressure.

It has also been suggested that vasodilators may directly enhance Na^+ reabsorption.[233] However, two observations make this unlikely. First, the tendency to edema formation is directly related to vasodilator potency, with the effect of minoxidil being greater than that of hydralazine and the effect of nifedipine being greater than that of other calcium channel blockers.[234] Second, diazoxide produces Na^+ retention only if it is given systemically and lowers the blood pressure, not if it is infused directly into the renal artery.[237]

Nonsteroidal anti-inflammatory drugs are widely used in the treatment of rheumatologic disorders and primarily act by inhibiting renal prostaglandin synthesis. Since protaglandins maintain renal perfusion and may promote Na^+ excretion (see Chap. 6), decreasing their production can lead to Na^+ retention and edema.[238] Fluid retention is particularly likely to occur in patients with underling heart failure or cirrhosis—conditions of effective hypovolemia in which the effect of prostaglandins is enhanced because high angiotensin II levels stimulate prostaglandin synthesis.

Fludrocortisone is a synthetic mineralocorticoid used in the treatment of hypoaldosteronism. Although this drug initially causes fluid retention, edema is unusual because of the phenomenon of mineralocorticoid escape (see page 185). Estrogens (alone or in oral contraceptives) also may promote Na^+ retention, primarily in patients with impaired estrogen metabolism due to hepatic disease.[239,240]

Pregnancy   Normal pregnancy is associated with the retention of 900 to 1000 meq of Na^+ and 6 to 8 L of water.[241] This is commonly associated with mild peripheral edema, particularly in the third trimester, a time at which partial obstruction of the inferior vena cava by the enlarged uterus also may play a contributory role.

The degree of fluid retention in pregnancy is generally independent of alterations in Na^+ intake, suggesting that Na^+ balance is being strictly regulated. It is possible, for example, that Na^+ retention reflects an *appropriate* response to systemic vasodilatation (which increases vascular capacity) and relative hypotension rather than a defect in renal function.[46,242]

Refeeding edema   Another example of primary renal Na^+ retention occurs in refeeding edema. Patients who have fasted for as little as 3 days display marked Na^+ retention and possibly edema after refeeding with carbohydrates.[243] A similar phenomenon may be seen during the treatment of diabetic ketoacidosis[244] and in some women with idiopathic edema (see "Idiopathic Edema," below).[245]

The mechanism by which these changes in Na^+ handling are mediated is incompletely understood, but increased availability of insulin is thought to play a major role. Insulin indirectly stimulates Na^+ reabsorption in the proximal tubule and perhaps in the loop of Henle and distal tubule as well.[246-248] In addition, fluid losses occur during fasting, driven in part by the excretion of ketoacid anions with Na^+ to maintain electroneutrality. This leads to the activation of the renin-angiotensin system, which, when combined with increased Na^+ intake during refeeding, can lead to rebound fluid overload.[245]

Treatment   Nonpregnant patients with primary renal sodium retention can be safely treated with diuretics. Unless an excessive diuresis is induced, there is no risk of effective volume depletion, since these patients are truly volume-expanded. However, high doses of a loop diuretic (such as a maximum of 160 to 200 mg of intravenous furosemide, or twice this amount orally due to incomplete absorption)[128] with or without a thiazide are often required with advanced renal failure or with minoxidil or diazoxide therapy for severe hypertension.[234,249] Either dialysis or hemofiltration is an effective alternative for refractory edema in patients with renal failure.

In comparison, edema during pregnancy is considered to be a physiologic rather than a pathologic event. As a result, diuretic therapy is not required and may actually have a deleterious effect by diminishing uterine perfusion.

Refeeding or insulin-induced edema is usually a transient phenomenon. In some cases, however, the edema persists, and patients may be treated as if they had idiopathic edema (see below).

Nephrotic Syndrome

The nephrotic syndrome can be produced by a variety of renal disorders and is characterized by an increase in the permeability of the glomerular capillary wall to proteins, leading to an increase in protein excretion. As described previously, primary renal Na^+ retention (and consequent volume expansion) appears to be a major factor in nephrotic edema.[29-36,35] This has important implications for treatment, since appropriate removal of the edema fluid with diuretics usually does not lead to either plasma volume depletion or azotemia.[31]

The second, not mutually exclusive mechanism of nephrotic edema is underfilling due to hypoalbuminemia.[38,41,42] This is most likely to occur with the acute onset of nephrosis or in patients with severe hypoalbuminemia (plasma albumin concentration below 1.5 g/dL).[41,42] To the degree that underfilling is present, diuretic therapy may lead to signs of volume depletion.

Treatment   The main aim of therapy in the nephrotic syndrome is, if possible, to reverse the glomerular disease, as with corticosteroids in minimal change disease.[29,250] Pending this potential response, a loop diuretic and dietary Na^+ restriction can be used to control the edema.[30] Diuretic resistance can occur, particularly in patients with marked hypoalbuminemia (plasma albumin concentration below 2 g/dL) or advanced renal insufficiency. This problem is in part due to binding of free drug in the tubular lumen by filtered albumin, thereby rendering the diuretic inactive.[251,252]

In addition, marked hypoalbuminemia can lead sequentially to diminished plasma binding of the diuretic, increased diffusion of unbound drug out of the vascular space, and a decreased rate of drug delivery to and subsequent excretion in the urine.[252] In this setting, mixing the loop diuretic with albumin prior to infusion can partially overcome the diuretic resistance, leading to an increase in Na^+ excretion.[253,254]

Other therapeutic options include higher doses of the loop diuretic (to a maximum similar to that in primary renal Na^+ retention above) and combination therapy with a loop and a thiazide diuretic.[249] Tight wrapping of the legs and periodic elevation of the lower extremities also may be helpful by maximizing venous return to the heart.[255]

Idiopathic Edema

Idiopathic edema refers to a disorder occurring in young, menstruating women in the absence of cardiac, hepatic, or renal disease.[245,256-258] Fluid retention may initial occur premenstrually but often becomes persistent. Emotional problems (including depression and neurotic symptoms) and obesity are commonly part of this syndrome.[259]

Role of capillary leak   The etiology of idiopathic edema is uncertain. Many women with this disorder have an *abnormal response to assumption of the upright posture*. Normal subjects develop a mild degree of plasma volume depletion in this setting because of pooling of fluid in the lower extremities. As a result, there is a fall in urinary Na^+ excretion[240] and a daytime weight gain that averages 0.5 to 1.5 kg.[256,257] In comparison, women with idiopathic edema lose much more fluid from the vascular space with standing,[257,261] leading to often marked elevations in the release of renin, norepinephrine, and ADH and to a larger morning-to evening weight gain that can exceed 5 kg in severe cases.[256-258]

These observations suggest that idiopathic edema may represent a *capillary leak* syndrome, in which increased capillary permeability favors the movement of fluid out of the vascular space, particularly when standing.[256,261] This primary tendency to plasma volume depletion also explains why the jugular venous pressure is in the low-normal range and pulmonary edema does not occur, even in the presence of marked peripheral edema.

The factors responsible for fluid leakage out of the capillaries are not well understood: Either primary capillary injury[262] or altered capillary hemodynamics could be responsible. It is possible, for example, that dilatation of the precapillary sphincter plays a central role by permitting more of the systemic pressure to be transmitted to the capillary, thereby increasing the capillary hydraulic pressure. Women with idiopathic edema often have impaired hypothalamic function, resulting in abnormal release of prolactin, luteinizing hormone, and perhaps other hormones.[263] These changes might then affect control of the capillary circulation.

Refeeding Women with idiopathic edema are typically very conscious of their weight and may drastically cut down on food intake for days at a time in an effort to lose weight. The subsequent end of this fast can lead to rapid weight gain via the phenomenon of refeeding edema (see above).[245]

Diuretic-induced edema Another theory postulates that idiopathic edema may be paradoxically *induced by the chronic administration of diuretics.*[245,264] According to this hypothesis, patients are initially begun on a diuretic for a minor degree of fluid retention. As therapy is continued, persistent diuretic-induced hypovolemia results in the activation of Na^+-retaining mechanisms, particularly the renin-angiotensin-aldosterone system. If the diuretic is then stopped, the patient may be unable to *acutely* shut of these Na^+-retaining mechanisms, resulting in rapid edema formation and the *mistaken* assumption that chronic diuretic therapy is indicated. If, however, the patient is maintained without diuretics for 1 to 3 weeks, a spontaneous diuresis will frequently ensue, with resolution of the edema (Fig. 16-14).

The frequency with which diuretics are responsible for idiopathic edema is uncertain. Some investigators have proposed that most cases are diuretic-induced,[245,264] while others have found that most patients have no history or signs (volume depletion, hypokalemia, positive urine assay) of diuretic use.)[265]

Diagnosis The diagnosis of idiopathic edema is one of exclusion and should be considered only in menstruating women who have a normal plasma albumin concentration, normal jugular venous pressure, and no evidence of cardiac, hepatic, or renal disease. Idiopathic edema should also be differentiated from pre-

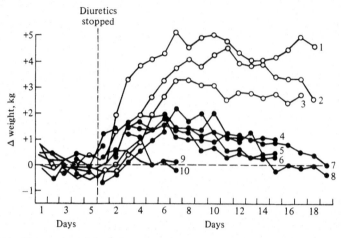

Figure 16-14 Changes in weight before and after stopping diuretics in 10 patients with idiopathic edema. Patients 4 to 10 returned to their baseline weight within 20 days. Patients 1 to 3 maintained their weight gain but eventually lost the extra weight after the institution of a low-sodium diet. (*From MacGregor GA, Roulston JE, Markandu ND, Jones JC, deWardener HE*, Lancet *1:397, 1979, with permission.*)

menstrual edema. The latter disorder occurs in many women; it is mild and self-limited, with a diuresis beginning with or shortly after the onset of menses. The fluid retention in this setting is thought to be humorally mediated, as estrogens or possibly prolactin may be responsible for the fluid retention.

Some women are already receiving diuretic therapy at the initial evaluation by a new physician, sometimes in massive doses that can exceed 600 mg of furosemide per day.[266] As a result, hypokalemia is a common problem, with the plasma K^+ concentration in severe cases being persistently below 3 meq/L. This uncontrolled therapy can lead to two potential complications: rhabdomyolysis (which may be due in part to K^+ depletion; see page 859) and chronic renal insufficiency that, on renal biopsy, is characterized by prominent tubulointerstitial scarring and atrophy and by intimal thickening of the interlobular arteries.[266,267] Both chronic hypokalemia and, rarely, an interstitial nephritis secondary to the diuretic may contribute to the renal injury. Discontinuation of diuretic therapy generally leads to at least partial recovery of renal function.[266]

Treatment Since diuretic-induced edema appears to be operative in at least some patients, initial therapy should consist of a low-Na^+ diet and *cessation of diuretic therapy* for 3 to 4 weeks (Fig. 16-14). The patient should be advised that this will initially lead to weight gain and reassured that diuretics can be always be reinstituted if a spontaneous diuresis does not ensue. If it becomes evident that a diuretic is required, the lowest effective dose should be used and it should be given in the early evening, since the edema primarily accumulates during the daytime, when the patient is erect.[257]

In patients who are not taking diuretics and those who fail to respond to diuretic withdrawal, it has been suggested that a diet restricted in sodium and carbohydrate (approximately 90 g/day) leads to resolution of edema in many cases.[265] It is presumed that this effect is the reverse of the sodium retention seen with refeeding.

Patients who are resistant to this conservative regimen are often difficult to treat effectively. High-dose loop diuretic therapy can be used with careful monitoring of the plasma K^+ and creatinine concentrations.[266] An alternative that has been effective in some cases is blockade of the renin-angiotensin system with an ACE inhibitor.[261,268] Minimizing the degree of secondary hyperaldosteronism may diminish the quantity of fluid retained during the day. It does not, however, prevent the capillary leak or plasma volume depletion. As a result, these agents often lower the systemic blood pressure by 5 to 10 mmHg, producing symptoms of hypotension in some patients.[261]

Two additional modalities have been tried in refractory idiopathic edema. Selected patients have responded to therapy aimed at reversing a possible dopamine deficiency by the administration of the dopamine agonist bromocriptine or a levodopa-carbidopa combination.[256,269,270] The efficacy of these agents, however, remains unproven, and their use may be associated with unacceptable side effects.

Increasing sympathetic activity with low-dose amphetamines or the sympathetic agonist ephedrine (15 to 60 mg TID) also has had some success.[257,271,272] These drugs may act by constricting the precapillary sphincter, thereby lowering the capillary hydraulic pressure and retarding fluid movement out of the capillary. Ephedrine has been given successfully with an ACE inhibitor.[272] Side effects can be minimized by using lower ephedrine doses.

PROBLEMS

16-1 The appropriate use of diuretics may induce or exacerbate effective circulating volume depletion in which of the following edematous states?

(a) Congestive heart failure
(b) Nephrotic syndrome with a plasma albumin concentration of 2.8 g/dL
(c) Renal failure
(d) Cirrhosis and ascites

What is the simplest way to detect this change?

(a) Measurement of the urine Na^+ concentration
(b) Measurement of the BUN
(c) Estimation of the jugular venous pressure
(d) Measurement of the systemic blood pressure

16-2 A previously well 45-year-old man is admitted with the acute onset of crushing chest pain and dyspnea. Medical evaluation confirms the diagnosis of acute myocardial infarction with pulmonary edema. After treatment with oxygen, intermittent positive-pressure breathing, and diuretics, he becomes edema-free. Because of the diuresis, his weight has fallen by 3 kg within 24 h after admission and his estimated jugular venous pressure is less than 5 cmH$_2$O. At this time, he is noted to be oliguric with a urine Na^+ concentration of 4 meq/L. His BUN has increased from 10 to 28 mg/dL.

(a) What are two most likely causes of the oliguria and increase in BUN?
(b) Would a normal ejection reaction necessarily distinguish between these possibilities?
(c) Does the low jugular venous pressure exclude the presence of cardiac dysfunction?
(d) Is his total extracellular volume greater than, equal to, or less than normal?
(e) What modes of therapy might return his BUN and urine output to normal?

REFERENCES

1. Guyton AC. *Textbook of Medical Physiology*, 8th ed. Philadelphia, Saunders, 1991, chap. 16.
2. Taylor AE. Capillary fluid filtration: Starling forces and lymph flow. *Circ Res* 49:557, 1981.
3. Renkin EM. Regulation of the microcirculation. *Microvasc Res* 30:251, 1985.
4. Murray JF. The lung and heart failure. *Hosp Prac* 20(4):55, 1985.
5. Crandall ED, Staub NC, Goldberg HS, Effros RM. Recent developments in pulmonary edema. *Ann Intern Med* 99:808, 1983.
6. Davis MJ. Control of bat wing capillary pressure and blood flow during reduced renal perfusion pressure. *Am J Physiol* 255:H1114, 1988.
7. Deitch EA. Current concepts: The management of burns. *N Engl J Med* 323:1249, 1990.
8. Belldegrun A, Webb D, Austin HA III, et al. Effects of interleukin-2 on renal function in patients receiving immunotherapy for advanced cancer. *Ann Intern Med* 106:817, 1987.
9. Gold PJ, Thompson JA, Markowitz DR, et al. Metastatic renal cell carcinoma: Long-term survival after therapy with high-dose continuous-infusion interleukin-2. *Cancer J Sci Am* 3(suppl):S85, 1997.
10. Teelucksingh S, Padfield PL, Edwards CRW. Systemic capillary leak syndrome. *Q J Med* 75:515, 1990.
11. Cicardi M, Gardinali M, Bisiani G, et al. The systemic capillary leak syndrome: Appearance of interleukin-2-receptor-positive cells during attacks. *Ann Intern Med* 113:475, 1990.
12. Droder RM, Kyle RA, Griepp PR. Control of systemic capillary leak syndrome with aminophylline and terbutaline. *Am J Med* 92:523, 1992.
13. Amoura Z, Papo T, Ninet J, et al. Systemic capillary leak syndrome: Report on 13 patients with special focus on course and treatment. *Am J Med* 103:514, 1997.
14. Ohlsson K, Björk P, Bergenfeldt M, et al. Interleukin-1 receptor antagonist reduces mortality from septic shock. *Nature* 348:550, 1990.
15. Colletti LM, Remick DG, Burtch GD, et al. Role of tumor necrossis factor-*a* in the pathophysiologic alterations after hepatic ischemia/reperfusion injury in the rat. *J Clin Invest* 85:1936, 1990.
16. Miller EJ, Cohen AB, Matthay MA. Increased interleukin-8 concentrations in the pulmonary edema fluid of patients with acute respiratory distress syndrome from sepsis. *Crit Care Med* 24:1448, 1996.
17. Bollinger A, Frey J, Jäger K, et al. Patterns of diffusion through skin capillaries in patients with long-term diabetes. *N Engl J Med* 307:1305, 1982.
18. Hommel E, Mathiesen ER, Aukland K, Parving H-H. Pathophysiological aspects of edema formation in diabetic nephropathy. *Kidney Int* 38:1187, 1990.
19. Wolf BA, Williams JR, Easom RA, et al. Diacyglycerol accumulation and microvascular abnormalities induced by elevated glucose levels. *J Clin Invest* 87:31, 1991.
20. Brownlee M. Glycation products and the pathogenesis of diabetic complications. *Diabetes Care* 15:1835, 1992.
21. Szuba A, Rockson SG. Lymphedema: Classification, diagnosis and therapy. *Vasc Med* 3:145, 1998.
22. Parving HH, Hansen JM, Nielsen SL, et al. Mechanisms of edema formation in myxedema: Increased protein extravasation and relatively slow lymphatic drainage. *N Engl J Med* 301:460, 1979.

23. Hollander W, Reilly P, Burrows BA. Lymphatic flow in human subjects as indicated by the disappearance of I^{131}-labeled albumin for the subcutaneous tissue. *J Clin Invest* 40:222, 1961.

24. Kwan T, Pintea M, Garcia Morino F, et al. Transcapillary oncotic pressure in the edema of congestive heart failure. *Nephron* 54:21, 1990.

25. Zink J, Greenway CV. Intraperitoneal pressure in formation and reabsorption of ascites in cats. *Am J Physiol* 233:H185, 1977.

26. Henriksen JH, Stage JG, Schlichting P, Winkler K. Intraperitoneal pressure: Ascitic fluid and splanchnic vascular pressures, and their role in prevention and formation of ascites. *Scand J Clin Lab Invest* 40:493, 1980.

27. Fauchald PF. Transcapillary colloid osmotic pressure gradient and body fluid volumes in renal failure. *Kidney Int* 29:895, 1986.

28. Koomans HA, Kortlandt W, Geers AB, Dorhout Mees EJ. Lowered protein content of tissue fluid in patients with the nephrotic syndrome: Observations during disease and recovery. *Nephron* 40:391, 1985.

29. Humphreys MH. Mechanisms and management of nephrotic edema. *Kidney Int* 45:266, 1994.

30. Rose BD. Mechanism and treatment of edema in nephrotic syndrome, in Rose BD (ed): *UpToDate in Medicine*. Wellesley, MA, UpToDate, 2000.

31. Geers AB, Koomans HA, Roos JC, Dorhout Mees EJ. Preservation of blood volume during edema removal in nephrotic subjects. *Kidney Int* 28:562, 1985.

32. Kaysen GA, Paukert TT, Menke DJ, et al. Plasma volume expansion is necessary for edema formation in the rat with Heymann nephritis. *Am J Physiol* 248:F247, 1985.

33. Ichikawa I, Rennke HG, Hoyer JR, et al. Role for intrarenal mechanisms in the impaired salt excretion of experimental nephrotic syndrome. *J Clin Invest* 71:91, 1983.

34. Perico N, Delaini F, Lupini C, et al. Blunted excretory response to atrial natriuretic peptide in experimental nephrosis. *Kidney Int* 36:57, 1989.

35. Koomans HA, Boer WH, Dorhout Mees EJ. Renal function during recovery from minimal lesions nephrotic syndrome. *Nephron* 47:173, 1987.

36. Buerkert J, Martin DR, Trigg D, Simon EE. Sodium handling by deep nephrons and the terminal collecting duct in glomerulonephritis. *Kidney Int* 39:850, 1991.

37. Valentin J-P, Qiu C, Muldowney WP, et al. Cellular basis for blunted volume expansion natriuresis in experimental nephrotic syndrome. *J Clin Invest* 90:1302, 1992.

38. Schrier RW, Fassett RG. A critique of the overfill hypothesis of sodium and water retention in the nephrotic syndrome. *Kidney Int* 53:1111, 1998.

39. Eder HA, Lauson HD, Chinard FP, et al. A study of the mechanisms of edema formation in patients with the nephrotic syndrome. *J Clin Invest* 33:636, 1954.

40. Luetscher JA Jr, Hall AD, Kremer VL. Treatment of nephrosis with concentrated human serum albumin. II. Effects of renal function and on excretion of water and some electrolytes. *J Clin Invest* 29:896, 1950.

41. Vande Walle JG, Donckerwolcke RA, van Isselt JW, et al. Volume regulation in children with early relapse of minimal-change nephrosis with or without hypovolaemic symptoms. *Lancet* 346:148, 1995.

42. Vande Walle JG, Donckerwolcke RA, Koomans HA. Pathophysiology of edema formation in children with nephrotic syndrome not due to minimal change disease. *J Am Soc Nephrol* 10:323, 1999.

43. Zarins CK, Rice CL, Peters RM, Virgilio RW. Lymph and pulmonary response to isobaric reduction in plasma oncotic pressure in baboons. *Circ Res* 43:925, 1978.

44. Mayatepek E, Becker K, Gana L, et al. Leukotrienes in the pathophysiology of kwashiorkor. *Lancet* 342:958, 1993.

45. Schrier RW. Body fluid volume regulation in health and disease: A unifying hypothesis. *Ann Intern Med* 113:155, 1990.

46. Schrier RW. An odyssey into the milieu intérieur: Pondering the enigmas. *J Am Soc Nephrol* 1:1549, 1992.

47. Epstein FH, Ferguson TB. The effect of the formation of an arteriovenous fistula upon blood volume. *J Clin Invest* 34:434, 1955.
48. Kowalski HJ, Abelmann WH. The cardiac output at rest in Laennec's cirrhosis. *J Clin Invest* 32:1025, 1953.
49. Aroyo V, Bosch J, Gaya-Beltran J, et al. Plasma renin activity and urinary sodium excretion as prognostic indicators in nonazotemic cirrhosis with ascites. *Ann Intern Med* 94:198, 1981.
50. Perez-Ayuso RM, Arroyo V, Campos J, et al. Evidence that renal prostaglandins are involved in renal water metabolism in cirrhosis. *Kidney Int* 26:72, 1984.
51. Henriksen JH, Bendtsen F, Gerbes AL, et al. Estimated central blood volume in cirrhosis: Relationship to sympathetic nervous activity, β-adrenergic blockade and atrial natriuretic factor. *Hepatology* 16:1163, 1992.
52. Gines P, Arroyo V. Hepatorenal syndrome. *J Am Soc Nephrol* 10:1833, 1999.
53. Fernandez-Seara J, Prieto J, Quiroga J, et al. Systemic and renal hemodynamics in patients with liver cirrhosis and ascites with and without functional renal failure. *Gastroenterology* 97:1304, 1989.
54. Stein JH, Osgood RW, Boonjarern S, et al. Segmental sodium reabsorption in rats with mild and severe volume depletion. *Am J Physiol* 227:351, 1974.
55. Bell NJ, Schedl HP, Bartter FC. An explanation for abnormal water retention and hypoosmolality in congestive heart failure. *Am J Med* 36:C, 1964.
56. Schedl HP, Bartter FC. An explanation for and experimental correction of the abnormal water diuresis in cirrhosis. *J Clin Invest* 39:248, 1960.
57. Chou S-Y, Porush JG, Faubert PF. Renal medullary circulation: Hormonal control. *Kidney Int* 37:1, 1990.
58. Faubert PF, Chou S-Y, Porush JG, et al. Papillary plasma flow and tissue osmolality in chronic caval dogs. *Am J Physiol* 242:F370, 1982.
59. Chou S-Y, Reiser I, Porush JG. Reversal of Na$^+$ retention in chronic caval dogs by verapamil: Contribution of medullary circulation. *Am J Physiol* 263:F642, 1992.
60. Grausz H, Lieberman R, Earley LE. Effect of plasma albumin on sodium reabsorption in patients with nephrotic syndrome. *Kidney Int* 1:47, 1972.
61. Watkins L Jr, Burton JA, Haber E, et al. The renin-angiotensin-aldosterone system in congestive failure in conscious dogs. *J Clin Invest* 57:1606, 1976.
62. DiBona GF, Herman PJ, Sawin LL. Neutral control of renal function in edema-forming states. *Am J Physiol* 254:R1017, 1988.
63. Dzau VJ, Colucci WS, Hollenberg NK, Williams GH. Relation of the renin angiotensin-aldosterone system to clinical state in congestive heart failure. *Circulation* 63:645, 1981.
64. Chonko AM, Bay WH, Stein JH, Ferris TF. The role of renin and aldosterone in the salt retention of edema. *Am J Med* 63:881, 1977.
65. Schunkert H, Ingelfinger JR, Hirsch AT, et al. Evidence for tissue specific activation of renal angiotensinogen mRNA expression in chronic stable experimental heart failure. *J Clin Invest* 90:1523, 1992.
66. McHugh TJ, Forrester J, Adler L, et al. Pulmonary vascular congestion in acute myocardial infarction: Hemodynamic and radiologic correlations. *Ann Intern Med* 76:29, 1972.
67. Kollef MH, Schuster DP. The acute respiratory distress syndrome. *N Engl J Med* 332:27, 1995.
68. Guazzi M, Polese A, Margrini F, et al. Negative influences of ascites on the cardiac function of cirrhotic patients. *Am J Med* 59:175, 1975.
69. Carrie BJ, Hilberman M, Schroeder JS, Myers BD. Albuminuria and the permselective properties of the glomerulus in heart failure. *Kidney Int* 17:507, 1980.
70. Gines P, Fernandez-Esparrach G, Arroyo V, et al. Pathogenesis of ascites in cirrhosis. *Semin Liver Dis* 17:175, 1997.
71. Morali GA, Sniderman KW, Deitel KM, et al. Is sinusoidal portal hypertension a necessary factor for the development of hepatic ascites? *J Hepatol* 16:249, 1992.
72. Wheeler DC, Bernard DB. Lipid abnormalities in the nephrotic syndrome: Causes, consequences, and treatment. *Am J Kidney Dis* 23:331, 1994.

73. Cohn JN. Blood pressure and cardiac performance. *Am J Med* 55:351, 1973.
74. Stampfer M, Epstein SE, Beiser GD, Braunwald E. Hemodynamic effects of diuresis at rest and during intense exercise in patients with impaired cardiac function. *Circulation* 37:900, 1968.
75. Lal S, Murtagh JG, Pollock AM, et al. Acute hemodynamic effects of furosemide in patients with normal and raised left atrial pressures. *Br Heart J* 31:711, 1969.
76. Pockros PJ, Reynolds TB. Rapid diuresis in patients with ascites from chronic liver disease: The importance of peripheral edema. *Gastroenterology* 90:1827, 1986.
77. Shear L, Ching S, Gabuzda GJ. Compartmentalization of ascites and edema in patients with hepatic cirrhosis. *N Engl J Med* 282:1391, 1970.
78. Duncan LE Jr, Bartter FC. The effect of changes in body sodium on extracellular fluid volume and aldosterone and sodium excretion by normal and edematous men. *J Clin Invest* 35:1299, 1956.
79. Pockros PJ, Esrason KT, Nguyen C, et al. Mobilization of malignant ascites with diuretics is dependent on ascitic fluid characteristics. *Gastroenterology* 103:1302, 1992.
80. Boyer TD. Removal of ascites: What's the rush. *Gastroenterology* 90:2022, 1986.
81. Forrester JS, Diamond G, Chatterjee K, Swan HJC. Medical therapy of acute myocardial infarction by application of hemodynamic subsets. *N Engl J Med* 295:1356, 1976.
82. Starr I Jr. The role of "static blood pressure" in abnormal increments of venous pressure, especially in heart failure: Clinical and experimental studies. *Am J Med Sci* 199:40, 1940.
83. Warren JV, Stead EA. Fluid dynamics in chronic congestive heart failure: An interpretation of the mechanisms producing the edema, increased plasma volume, and elevated venous pressure in certain patients with prolonged congestive failure. *Arch Intern Med* 73:138, 1944.
84. Dzau VJ. Renal and circulatory mechanisms in congestive heart failure. *Kidney Int* 31:1402, 1987.
85. Packer M. Neurohumoral interactions and adaptations in congestive heart failure. *Circulation* 77:721, 1988.
86. Schrier RW. Pathogenesis of sodium and water retention in high-output and low-output cardiac failure, nephrotic syndrome, cirrhosis, and pregnancy. *N Engl J Med* 319:1065,1127, 1988.
87. Winaver J, Hoffman A, Burnett JC Jr, Haramati A. Hormonal determinants of sodium excretion in rats with high-output heart failure. *Am J Physiol* 254:R776, 1988.
88. Braunwald E, Plauth WH, Morrow AG. A method for the detection and quantification of impaired sodium excretion. *Circulation* 32:223, 1965.
89. Noble MIM. The Frank-Starling curve. *Clin Sci* 54:1, 1978.
90. Lakatta EG. Starling's law of the heart is explained by an intimate interaction of muscle length and myofilament calcium activation. *J Am Coll Cardiol* 10:1157, 1987.
91. Reddy HK, Weber KT, Janicki JS, McElroy PA. Hemodynamic, ventilatory and metabolic effects of light isometric exercise in patients with chronic heart failure. *J Am Coll Cardiol* 12:353, 1988.
92. Higgins CB, Vatner SF, Franklin D, Braunwald E. Effects of experimentally produced heart failure on the peripheral vascular response to severe exercise in conscious dogs. *Circ Res* 31:186, 1972.
93. Millard RW, Higgins CB, Franklin D, Vatner SF. Regulation of the renal circulation during severe exercise in normal dogs and dogs with experimental heart failure. *Circ Res* 31:881, 1972.
94. Ring-Larsen H, Hendriksen JH, Wilken C, et al. Diuretic treatment in decompensated cirrhosis and congestive heart failure: Effect of posture. *Br Med J* 292:1351, 1986.
95. Schwinger RH, Bohm M, Koch A, et al. The failing human heart is unable to use the Frank-Starling mechanism. *Circ Res* 74:959, 1994.
96. Gault JH, Covell JW, Braunwald E, Ross J Jr. Left ventricular performance following correction of free aortic regurgitation. *Circulation* 42:773, 1970.
97. Komamura K, Shannon RP, Ihara T, et al. Exhaustion of Frank-Starling mechanism in conscious dogs with heart failure. *Am J Physiol* 265:H1119, 1993.
98. Bonow RO, Udelson JE. Left ventricular diastolic dysfunction as a cause of congestive heart failure. Mechanisms and management. *Ann Intern Med* 117:502, 1992.

99. Grossman W. Diastolic dysfunction in congestive heart failure. *N Engl J Med* 325:1557, 1991.

100. Soufer R, Wohlgelertner D, Vita NA, et al. Intact left ventricular function in clinical congestive heart failure. *Am J Cardiol* 55:1032, 1985.

101. Kloner RA, Przyklenk K. Hibernation and stunning of the myocardium. *N Engl J Med* 325:1877, 1991.

102. Braunwald E, Rutherford JD. Reversible ischemic left ventricular dysfunction: Evidence of the "hibernating myocardium." *J Am Coll Cardiol* 8:1467, 1986.

103. Gerber BL, Wijns W, Vanoverschelde JL, et al. Myocardial perfusion and oxygen consumption is reperfused noninfarcted dysfunctional myocardium after unstable angina: Direct evidence for myocardial stunning in humans. *J Am Coll Cardiol* 34:1939, 1999.

104. Marban E. Myocardial stunning and hibernation. The physiology behind the colloquialisms. *Circulation* 83:681, 1991.

105. Mettauer B, Rouleau J-L, Bichet D, et al. Sodium and water excretion abnormalities in congestive heart failure. *Ann Intern Med* 105:161, 1986.

106. Francis GC, Benedict C, Johnstone DE, et al. Comparison of neuroendocrine activation in patients with left ventricular dysfunction with and without congestive heart failure. A substudy of the Studies of Left Ventricular Dysfunction (SOLVD). *Circulation* 82:1724, 1990.

107. Dzau VJ, Packer M, Lilly LS, et al. Prostaglandins in severe congestive heart failure. Relation to activation of the renin-angiotensin system and hyponatremia. *N Engl J Med* 310:347, 1984.

108. Raine AEG, Erne P, Burgisser E, et al. Atrial natriuretic peptide and atrial pressure in patients with congestive heart failure. *N Engl J Med* 315:533, 1986.

109. Awazu M, Imada T, Kon V, et al. Role of endogenous atrial natriuretic peptide in congestive heart failure. *Am J Physiol* 257:R641, 1989.

110. Creager MA, Hirsch AT, Navel EG, et al. Responsiveness of atrial natriuretic factor to reduction in right atrial pressure in patients with chronic congestive heart failure. *J Am Coll Cardiol* 6:1191, 1988.

111. Yasue H, Obata K, Okamura K, et al. Increased secretion of atrial natriuretic polypeptide from the left ventricle in patients with dilated cardiomyopathy. *J Clin Invest* 83:46, 1989.

112. Lerman A, Gibbons RJ, Rodenheffer RJ, et al. Circulating N-terminal atrial natriuretic peptide as a marker for symptomless left-ventricular dysfunction. *Lancet* 341:1105, 1993.

113. Motwani JG, McAlpine H, Kennedy N, Struthers AD. Plasma brain natriuretic peptide as an indicator for angiotensin-converting-enzyme inhibition after myocardial infarction. *Lancet* 341:1109, 1993.

114. Richards AM, Nicholls MG, Yandle TG, et al. Plasma N-terminal pro-brain natriuretic peptide and adrenomedullin: New neurohormonal predictors of left ventricular function and prognosis after myocardial infarction. *Circulation* 97:1921, 1998.

115. Davidson NC, Naas AA, Hanson JK, et al. Comparison of atrial natriuretic peptide, B-type natriuretic peptide, and N-terminal proatrial natriuretic peptide as indicators of left ventricular systolic dysfunction. *Am J Cardiol* 77:828, 1996.

116. McDonagh TA, Robb SD, Murdoch DR, et al. Biochemical detection of left-ventricular systolic dysfunction. *Lancet* 351:9, 1998.

117. Gropper MA, Wiener-Kronish J, Hashimoto S. Acute cardiogenic pulmonary edema. *Clin Chest Med* 15:501, 1994.

118. Dikshit K, Vyden JK, Forrester JS, et al. Renal and extrarenal hemodynamic effects of furosemide in congestive heart failure after acute myocardial infarction. *N Engl J Med* 288:1087, 1973.

119. Cotter G, Metzkor E, Faigenberg Z, et al. Randomized trial of high-dose isosorbide dinitrate plus low-dose isosorbide dinitrate in severe pulmonary edema. *Lancet* 351:389, 1998.

120. Crexells C, Chatterjee K, Forrester JS, et al. Optimal level of filling pressure in the left side of the heart in acute myocardial infarction. *N Engl J Med* 289:1263, 1973.

121. Gage J, Rutman H, Lucido D, et al. Additive effects of dobutamine and amrinone on myocardial contractility and ventricular performance in patients with severe heart failure. *Circulation* 74:367, 1986.

122. Mager G, Klocke RK, Kux A, et al. Phosphodiesterase III inhibition or adrenoreceptor stimulation: Milrinone as an alternative to dobutamine in the treatment of severe heart failure. *Am Heart J* 121:1974, 1991.

123. Aberman A, Fulop M. The metabolic and respiratory acidosis of acute pulmonary edema. *Ann Intern Med* 76:173, 1972.

124. Fulop M, Horowitz M, Aberman A, Jaffee E. Lactic acidosis in pulmonary edema due to left ventricular failure. *Ann Intern Med* 79:180, 1973.

125. ACC/AHA Task Force Report. Guidelines for the evaluation and management of heart failure. *J Am Coll Cardiol* 26:1376, 1995.

126. Richardson A, Bayliss J, Scriven AJ, et al. Double blind-comparison of captopril alone versus fusemide plus amiloride in mild heart failure. *Lancet* 2:709, 1987.

127. Cowley AJ, Stainer K, Wynne RD, et al. Symptomatic assessment of patients with heart failure: Double-blind comparison of increasing doses of diuretics and captopril in moderate heart failure. *Lancet* 2:770, 1986.

128. Brater D, Voelker JR. Use of diuretics in patients with renal disease, in Bennett WM, McCarron DA (eds): *Contemporary Issues in Nephrology. Pharmacotherapy of Renal Disease and Hypertension.* New York, Churchill Livingstone, 1987.

129. Cooper HA, Dries DL, Davis CE, et al. Diuretics and risk of arrhythmic death in patients with left ventricular dysfunction. *Circulation* 100:1311, 1999.

130. Pitt B, Zannad F, Femme WJ, et al. The effect of spironolactone on morbidity and mortality in patients with severe heart failure. *N Engl J Med* 341:709, 1999.

131. Smith TW. Digitalis: Mechanisms of action and clinical use. *N Engl J Med* 318:358, 1988.

132. Packer M, Gheorghiade M, Young JB, et al. Withdrawal of digoxin from patients with chronic heart failure treated with angiotensin-converting-enzyme inhibitors. *N Engl J Med* 329:1, 1993.

133. Uretsky BF, Young JB, Shahidi FE, et al. Randomized study assessing the effect of digoxin withdrawal in patients with mild to moderate chronic congestive heart failure: Results for the PROVED trial. *J Am Coll Cardiol* 22:955, 1993.

134. The Digitalis Investigation Group. The effect of digoxin on mortality and morbidity in patients with heart failure. *N Engl J Med* 336:525, 1997.

135. Topol EJ, Traill TA, Fortuin NJ. Hypertensive hypertrophic cardiomyopathy of the elderly. *N Engl J Med* 312:277, 1985.

136. Beiser GD, Epstein SE, Stampfer M, et al. Studies on digitalis. XVII. Effects of ouabain on the hemodynamic response to exercise in patients with mitral stenosis in normal sinus rhythm. *N Engl J Med* 278:131, 1968.

137. The SOLVD Investigators. Effect of enalapril on survival in patients with reduced left ventricular ejection fractions and congestive heart failure. *N Engl J Med* 325:293, 1991.

138. Cohn J, Johnson G, Ziesche S, et al. A comparison of enalapril with hydralazine-isosorbide dinitrate in the treatment of chronic congestive heart failure. *N Engl J Med* 325:303, 1991.

139. The SOLVD Investigators. Effect of enalapril on mortality and the development of heart failure in asymptomatic patients with reduced left ventricular ejection fractions. *N Engl J Med* 327:685, 1992.

140. Pfeffer MA, Baunwald E, Moyé LA, et al. Effect of captopril on mortality in patients with left ventricular dysfunction after myocardial infarction. Results from the Survival and Ventricular Enlargement trial. *N Engl J Med* 327:669, 1992.

141. The CONSENSUS Trial Study Group. Effects of enalapril on mortality in severe congestive heart failure: Results of the Cooperative North Scandinavia Enalapril Survival Study (CONSENSUS). *N Engl J Med* 316:1429, 1987.

142. Sharmna D, Buyse M, Pitt B, et al. Meta-analysis of observed mortality data from all-controlled, double-blind, multiple-dose studies of losartan in heart failure. *Am J Cardiol* 85:187, 2000.

143. Cohn JN, Archibald DG, Ziesche S, et al. Effect of vasodilator therapy on mortality in chronic congestive heart failure: Results of a Veterans Administration Cooperative Study. *N Engl J Med* 314:1547, 1986.

144. Dzau VJ. Tissue renin-angiotensin system in myocardial hypertrophy and failure. *Arch Intern Med* 153:937, 1993.

145. Braunwald E. ACE inhibitors—A cornerstone of the treatment of heart failure. *N Engl J Med* 325:351, 1991.

146. Ljungman S, Kjekshus J, Swedberg K. Renal function in severe congestive heart failure during treatment with enalapril (the Cooperative North Scandinavian Enalapril Survival Study [CONSENSUS] trial). *Am J Cardiol* 70:492, 1992.

147. Packer M, Lee WH, Medina N, et al. Functional renal insufficiency during long-term therapy with captopril and enalapril in severe chronic heart failure. *Ann Intern Med* 106:346, 1987.

148. Packer M, Lee WH, Medina N, Yushak M. Influence of renal function on the hemodynamic and clinical responses to long-term captopril therapy in severe chronic heart failure. *Ann Intern Med* 104:147, 1986.

149. Packer M, Lee WH, Kessler PD, et al. Identification of hyponatremia as a risk factor for the development of functional renal insufficiency during converting enzyme inhibition in severe chronic heart failure. *J Am Coll Cardiol* 10:837, 1987.

150. Packer M, Lee WH, Yushak M, Medina N. Comparison of captopril and enalapril in patients with severe chronic heart failure. *N Engl J Med* 315:847, 1986.

151. Packer M, Bristow MR, Cohn JN, et al for the US Carvedilol Heart Failure Study Group. The effect of carvedilol on morbidity and mortality in patients with chronic heart failure. *N Engl J Med* 334:1349, 1996.

152. MERIT-HF Study Group. Effect of metoprolol CR/XL in chronic heart failure: Metoprolol CR/XL Randomised Intervention Trial in Congestive Heart Failure (MERIT-HF). *Lancet* 353:2001, 1999.

153. CIBIS-II Investigators and Committees. The Cardiac Insufficiency Bisoprolol Study II (CIBIS-II): A randomised trial. *Lancet* 353:9, 1999.

154. Lechat P, Packer M, Chalon S, et al. Clinical effects of β-adrenergic blockade in chronic heart failure: A meta-analysis of double-blind, placebo-controlled, randomized trials. *Circulation* 98:1184, 1998.

155. Macdonald PS, Keogh AM, Aboyoun CL, et al. Tolerability and efficacy of carvedilol in patients with New York Heart Association class IV heart failure. *J Am Coll Cardiol* 33:924, 1999.

156. Eichhorn EJ, Bristow MR. Practical guidelines for initiation of beta-adrenergic blockade in patients with chronic heart failure. *Am J Cardiol* 79:794, 1997.

157. Campbell EJM, Short DS. The cause of oedema in cor pulmonale. *Lancet* 1:1184, 1960.

158. Richens JM, Howard P. Oedema in cor pulmonale. *Clin Sci* 62:255, 1982.

159. Farber MO, Roberts LR, Weinberger MH, et al. Abnormalities of sodium and H_2O handling in chronic obstructive lung disease. *Arch Intern Med* 142:1326, 1982.

160. Reihman DH, Farber MO, Weinberger MH, et al. Effect of hypoxemia on sodium and water excretion in chronic obstructive lung disease. *Am J Med* 78:87, 1985.

161. Bear R, Goldstein M, Philipson M, et al. Effect of metabolic alkalosis on respiratory function in patients with chronic obstructive lung disease. *Can Med Assoc J* 117:900, 1977.

162. Runyon BA. Ascites and spontaneous bacterial peritonitis, in Feldman M, Scharschmidt BF, Sleisenger MH (eds): *Sleisenger and Fordtran's Gastronintestinal and Liver Disease. Pathophysiology/Diagnosis/Treatment.* Philadelphia, Sanders, 1998, p. 1310.

163. Naccarato R, Messa P, D'Angelo A, et al. Renal handling of sodium and water in early chronic liver disease. *Gastroenterology* 81:205, 1981.

164. La Villa G, Salmeron JM, Arroyo V, et al. Mineralocorticoid escape in patients with compensated cirrhosis and portal hypertension. *Gastroenterology* 102:2114, 1992.

165. Levy M. Sodium retention and ascites formation in dogs with experimental portal cirrhosis. *Am J Physiol* 233:F572, 1977.

166. Better OS, Schrier RW. Disturbed volume homeostasis in patients with cirrhosis of the liver. *Kidney Int* 23:303, 1983.

167. Unilowsky B, Wexler MJ, Levy M. Dogs with experimental cirrhosis of the liver but without intrahepatic hypertension do not retain sodium or form ascites. *J Clin Invest* 72:1594, 1983.

168. DiBona GF. Renal neural activity in hepatorenal syndrome. *Kidney Int* 25:841, 1984.

169. Levy M, Wexler MJ. Hepatic denervation alters first-phase urinary sodium excretion in dogs with cirrhosis. *Am J Physiol* 253:F664, 1987.
170. Schrier RW, Arroyo V, Bernardi M, et al. Peripheral arterial vasodilation hypothesis: A proposal for the initiation of renal sodium and water retention in cirrhosis. *Hepatology* 8:1151, 1988.
171. Albilos A, Colombato LA, Groszmann RJ. Vasodilation and sodium retention in prehepatic portal hypertension. *Gastroenterology* 102:931, 1992.
172. Wong F, Massie D, Colman J, Dudley F. Glomerular hyperfiltration in patients with well compensated hepatic cirrhosis. *Gastroenterology* 104:884, 1993.
173. Wong F, Massie D, Hsu P, Dudley F. Indomethacin-induced renal dysfunction in patients with well-compensated hepatic cirrhosis. *Gastroenterology* 104:869, 1993.
174. Vallance P, Moncada S. Hyperdynamic circulation in cirrhosis: A role for nitric oxide? *Lancet* 337:776, 1991.
175. Pizcueta P, Pique JM, Fernandez M, et al. Modulation of the hyperdynamic circulation of cirrhotic rats by nitric oxide inhibition. *Gastroenterology* 103:1909, 1992.
176. Claria J, Jimenez W, Ros J, et al. Pathogenesis of arterial hypotension in cirrhotic rats with ascites: Role of endogenous nitric oxide. *Hepatology* 15:343, 1992.
177. Sieber CC, Lopez Talavera JC, Groszmann RJ. Role of nitric oxide in the in vitro splanchnic vascular hyperactivity in ascitic cirrhotic rats. *Gastroenterology* 104:1750, 1993.
178. Sieber CC, Groszmann RJ. Nitric oxide mediates hyporeactivity to vasopressors in mesenteric vessels of portal hypertensive rats. *Gastroenterology* 103:235, 1992.
179. Guarner C, Soriano G, Tomas A, et al. Increased serum nitrite and nitrate levels in patients with cirrhosis: Relationship to endotoxemia. *Hepatology* 18:1139, 1993.
180. Battista S, Bar F, Mengozzi G, et al. Systemic and portal nitric oxide and endothelin-1 levels in cirrhotic patients. *J Hepatol* suppl 1:73(a), 1995.
181. Sherlock S. The kidneys in hepatic cirrhosis: Victims of portal-systemic venous shunting (portal-systemic nephropathy). *Gastroenterology* 104:931, 1993.
182. Lenz K, Hortnagl H, Druml W, et al. Ornipressin in the treatment of functional renal failure in decompensated liver cirrhosis. Effects on renal hemodynamics and atrial natriuretic factor. *Gastroenterology* 101:1060, 1991.
183. Nicholls KM, Shapiro MD, Groves BS, Schrier RW. Factors determining response to water immersion in non-excretor cirrhotic patients. *Kidney* 30:417, 1986.
184. Shapiro MD, Nicolls KM, Groves BM, et al. Interrelationship between cardiac output and vascular resistance as determinants of effective arterial blood volume in cirrhotic patients. *Kidney Int* 28:206, 1985.
185. Shaw-Stiffel T, Campbell PJ, Sole MJ, et al. Renal prostaglandin E$_2$ and other vasoactive modulators in refractory hepatic ascites: Response to peritoneovenous shunting. *Gastroenterology* 95:1332, 1988.
186. Guevara M, Gines P, Bandi JC, et al. Transjugular intrahepatic portosystemic shunt in hepatorenal syndrome: Effects on renal function and vasoactive systems. *Hepatology* 28:416, 1998.
187. Tristani RE, Cohn JN. Systemic and renal hemodynamics in oliguric hepatic failure: Effect of volume expansion. *J Clin Invest* 46:1894, 1967.
188. Epstein M, Berk DP, Hollenberg NK, et al. Renal failure in patients with cirrhosis. *Am J Med* 49:175, 1970.
189. Better OS. Renal and cardiovascular dysfunction in liver disease. *Kidney Int* 29:598, 1986.
190. Epstein M. Hepatorenal syndrome: Emerging perspectives of pathophysiology and therapy. *J Am Soc Nephrol* 4:1735, 1994.
191. Gines P, Arroyo V. Hepatorenal syndrome. *J Am Soc Nephrol* 10:1833, 1999.
192. Badalamenti S, Graziani G, Salerno F, Ponticelli C. Hepatorenal syndrome: New perspectives in pathogenesis and treatment. *Arch Intern Med* 153:1957, 1993.
193. Gines A, Escorsell A, Gines P, et al. Incidence, predictive factors, and treatment of the hepatorenal syndrome with ascites. *Gastroenterology* 105:229, 1993.
194. Papadakis MA, Arieff AI. Unpredictability of clinical evaluation of renal function in cirrhosis. Prospective study. *Am J Med* 82:945, 1987.

195. Caregaro L, Menon F, Angeli P, et al. Limitation of serum creatinine level and creatinine clearance as filtration markers in cirrhosis. *Arch Intern Med* 154:201, 1994.

196. Laffi G, La Villa G, Pinzani M, et al. Altered renal and platelet arachidonic acid metabolism in cirrhosis. *Gastroenterology* 90:274, 1986.

197. Wong PY, Talamo RC, Williams GH. Kallikrein-kinin and renin-angiotensin systems in cirrhosis of the liver. *Gastroenterology* 73:1114, 1977.

198. Runyon BA. Care of patients with ascites. *N Engl J Med* 330:337, 1994.

199. Runyon BA. Management of adult patients with ascites caused by cirrhosis. *Hepatology* 27:264, 1998.

200. Papadakis MA, Fraser CL, Arieff AI. Hyponatraemia in patients with cirrhosis. *Q J Med* 76:675, 1990.

201. Gabuzda GJ, Hall PW III. Relation of potassium depletion to renal ammonium metabolism and hepatic coma. *Medicine* 45:481, 1966.

202. Artz SA, Paes IC, Faloon WW. Hypokalemia-induced hepatic coma in cirrhosis: Occurrence despite neomycin therapy. *Gastroenterology* 51:1046, 1966.

203. Baertl JM, Sancelta SM, Gabuzda GJ. Relation of acute potassium depletion to renal ammonium metabolism in patients with cirrhosis. *J Clin Invest* 42:696, 1963.

204. Jaeger P, Karlmark B, Giebisch G. Ammonia transport in rat cortical tubule: Relationship to potassium metabolism. *Am J Physiol* 245:F593, 1983.

205. Perez-Ayuso RM, Arroyo V, Planas R, et al. Random comparative study of efficacy of furosemide vs spironolactone in nonazotemic cirrhosis with ascites: Relationship between the diuretic response and the activity of the renin-aldosterone system. *Gastroenterology* 84:961, 1983.

206. Fogel MR, Sawhney VK, Neal EA, et al. Diuresis in the ascitic patient: A randomized controlled trial of three regimens. *J Clin Gastroenterol* 3(suppl 1):73, 1981.

207. Angeli P, Dalla Pria M, De Bei E, et al. Randomized clinical study of the efficacy of amiloride and potassium canrenoate in nonazotemic cirrhotic patients with ascites. *Hepatology* 19:72, 1994.

208. Pinzani M, Daskalopoulos G, Laffi G, et al. Altered furosemide pharamacokinetics in chronic alcoholic liver disease with ascites contributes to diuretic resistance. *Gastroenterology* 92:294, 1987.

209. Horisberger J-D, Giebisch G. Potassium-sparing diuretics. *Renal Physiol* 10:198, 1987.

210. Kravetz D, Romero G, Argonz J, et al. Total volume paracentesis decreases variceal pressure, size, and variceal wall tension in cirrhotic patients. *Hepatology* 25:59, 1997.

211. Gines P, Arroyo V, Quintero E, et al. Comparison of paracentesis and diuretics in the treatment of cirrhotics with tense ascites. Results of a randomized study. *Gastroenterology* 93:234, 1987.

212. Gines P, Tito L, Arroyo V, et al. Randomized comparative study of therapeutic paracentesis with and without intravenous albumin in cirrhosis. *Gastroenterology* 94:1493, 1988.

213. Garcia-Tsao G. Treatment of ascites with a single total paracentesis. *Hepatology* 13:1005, 1991.

214. Gines A, Fernandez Esparrach G, Monescillo A, et al. Randomized trial comparing albumin, dextran 70, and polygeline in cirrhotic patients with ascites treated with paracentesis. *Gastroenterology* 111:1002, 1996.

215. Runyon BA. Patient selection is important in studying the impact of large-volume paracentesis on intravascular volume. *Am J Gastroenterol* 92:371, 1997.

216. Runyon BA. Treatment of diuretic-resistant ascites in patients with cirrhosis, in Rose BD (ed): *UpToDate in Medicine*. Wellesley, MA, UpToDate, 2000.

217. Arroyo V, Epstein M, Gallu G, et al. Refractory ascites in cirrhosis: Mechanism and treatment. *Gastroenterol Int* 2:195, 1989.

218. Runyon BA. Refractory ascites. *Semin Liver Dis* 13:343, 1993.

219. Gines P, Quintero E, Arroyo V, et al. Compensated cirrhosis: Natural history and prognostic factors. *Hepatology* 7:122, 1987.

220. Epstein M. Treatment of refractory ascites. *N Engl J Med* 321:1675, 1989.

221. Ochs A, Rössle M, Haag K, et al. The transjugular intrahepatic portosystemic stent-shunt procedure for refractory ascites. *N Engl J Med* 332:1192, 1995.
222. Somberg KA, Lake JR, Tomlanovich SJ, et al. Transjugular intrahepatic portosystemic shunts for refractory ascites: Assessment of clinical and hormonal response and renal function. *Hepatology* 21:709, 1995.
223. Lebrec D, Giuily N, Hadengue A, et al. Transjugular intrahepatic portosystemic shunts: Comparison with paracentesis in patients with cirrhosis and refractory ascites: A randomized trial. French Group of Clinicians and a Group of Biologists. *J Hepatol* 25:135, 1996.
224. Martinet JP, Fenyves D, Legault L, et al. Treatment of refractory ascites using transjugular intrahepatic portosystemic shunt (TIPS): A caution. *Dig Dis Sci* 42:161, 1997.
225. Sanyal AJ, Freedman AM, Shiffman ML, et al. Portosystemic encephalopathy after transjugular intrahepatic portosystemic shunt: Results of a prospective controlled study. *Hepatology* 20:46, 1994.
226. Stanley MM, Ochi S, Lee KK, et al. Peritoneovenous shunting as compared with medical treatment in patients with alcoholic cirrhosis and massive ascites. *N Engl J Med* 321:1632, 1989.
227. Gines P, Arroyo V, Vargas V, et al. Paracentesis with intravenous infusion of albumin as compared with peritoneovenous shunting in cirrhosis with refractory ascites. *N Engl J Med* 325:829, 1991.
228. Wagnild JP, Gutman FD. Functional adaptation of nephrons in dogs with acute progressing to chronic experimental glomerulonephritis. *J Clin Invest* 57:1575, 1976.
229. Miller TR, Anderson RJ, Linas SL, et al. Urinary diagnostic indices in acute renal failure: A prospective study. *Ann Intern Med* 89:47, 1978.
230. Rodriguez-Iturbe B, Baggio B, Colina-Chourio J, et al. Studies of the renin-aldosterone system in the acute nephritic syndrome. *Kidney Int* 19:445, 1981.
231. Rodriguez-Iturbe B, Colic D, Parra G, Gutkowska J. Atrial natriuretic factor in the acute nephritis and nephrotic syndromes. *Kidney Int* 38:512, 1990.
232. Danovitch GM, Bourgoignie JJ, Bricker NS. Reversibility of the "salt-losing" tendency of chronic renal failure. *N Engl J Med* 296:15, 1977.
233. Markham RV Jr, Gilmore A, Pettinger WA, et al. Central and regional hemodynamic effects and neurohumoral consequences of minoxidil in severe congestive heart failure and comparison to hydralazine and nitroprusside. *Am J Cardiol* 52:774, 1983.
234. Mroczek WJ, Lee WR. Diazoxide therapy: Use and risks. *Ann Intern Med* 85:529, 1976.
235. Russell RP. Side effects of calcium channel blockers. *Hypertension* 11(suppl II):II-42, 1988.
236. Pettinger WA, Keeton K. Altered renin release and propranolol potentiation of vasodilator drug hypotension. *J Clin Invest* 55:236, 1975.
237. Greene JA Jr. Effects of diazoxide on renal function in the dog. *Proc Soc Exp Biol Med* 125:275, 1976.
238. Clive DM, Stoff JS. Renal syndromes associated with nonsteroidal antiinflammatory drugs. *N Engl J Med* 310:563, 1984.
239. Christy NP, Shaver JC. Estrogens and the kidney. *Kidney Int* 6:366, 1974.
240. Preedy JRK, Aitken EH. The effect of estrogen on water and electrolyte metabolism. II. Hepatic disease. *J Clin Invest* 35:430, 1956.
241. Lindheimer MD, Katz AI. Sodium and diuretics in pregnancy. *N Engl J Med* 288:891, 1973.
242. Nadel AS, Ballerman BJ, Anderson S, Brenner BM. Interrelationships between atrial peptides, renin, and blood volume in pregnant rats. *Am J Physiol* 254:R793, 1988.
243. Veverbrants E, Arky RA. Effects of fasting and refeeding. I. Studies on sodium, potassium and water excretion on a constant electrolyte and fluid intake. *J Clin Endocrinol Metab* 29:55, 1969.
244. Saudek CD, Boulter PR, Knopp RH, Arky RA. Sodium retention accompanying insulin treatment of diabetes mellitus. *Diabetes* 23:240, 1974.
245. de Wardener HE. Idiopathic edema: Role of diuretic abuse. *Kidney Int* 19:881, 1981.
246. DeFronzo RA, Cooke CR, Andres R, et al. The effect of insulin on renal handling of sodium, potassium, calcium, and phosphate in man. *J Clin Invest* 55:845, 1975.

247. Baum M. Insulin stimulates volume absorption in rabbit proximal convoluted tubule. *J Clin Invest* 79:1104, 1987.

248. Nakamura R, Emmanouel DS, Katz AI. Insulin binding sites in various segments of the rabbit nephron. *J Clin Invest* 72:388, 1983.

249. Wollam GL, Tarazi RC, Bravo EL, Dustan HP. Diuretic potency of combined hydrochlorothiazide and furosemide therapy in patients with azotemia. *Am J Med* 72:929, 1982.

250. Rose BD, Appel GB. Treatment of minimal change disease, in Rose BD (eds): *UpToDate in Medicine*. Wellesley, MA, UpToDate, 2000.

251. Kirchner KA, Voelker JR, Brater DC. Binding inhibitors restore furosemide potency in tubule fluid containing albumin. *Kidney Int* 40:418, 1991.

252. Smith DE, Hyneck ML, Berardi RR, Port FK. Urinary protein binding, kinetics and dynamics of furosemide in nephrotic patients. *J Pharm Sci* 74:603, 1985.

253. Inoue M, Okajima K, Itoh K, et al. Mechanism of furosemide resistance in analbuminemic rats and hypoalbuminemic patients. *Kidney Int* 32:198, 1987.

254. Fliser D, Zurbruggen I, Mutschler E, et al. Coadministration of albumin and furosemide in patients with nephrotic syndrome. *Kidney Int* 55:629, 1999.

255. Bank N. External compression for treatment of resistant edema (letter). *N Engl J Med* 302:969, 1980.

256. Badr K. Idiopathic edema, in Brenner BM, Stein JH (eds): *Contemporary Issues in Nephrology: Body Fluid Homeostasis*. New York, Churchill Livingstone, 1987.

257. Streeten DHP. Idiopathic edema: Pathogenesis, clinical features, and treatment. *Metabolism* 25:353, 1978.

258. Edwards OM, Bayliss RIS. Idiopathic oedema of women. *Q J Med* 45:125, 1976.

259. Pelosi AJ, Sykes RA, Lough JRM, et al. A psychiatric study of idiopathic edema. *Lancet* 2:999, 1986.

260. Epstein FH, Goodyer AN, Laurason FD, Relman AS. Studies of the antidiuresis of quiet standing: The importance of changes in plasma volume and glomerular filtration rate. *J Clin Invest* 30:62, 1951.

261. Suzuki H, Fujimaki M, Nakane H, et al. Effect of angiotensin converting enzyme inhibitor, captopril (SQ 14,225), on orthostatic sodium and water retention in patients with idiopathic edema. *Nephron* 39:244, 1985.

262. Coleman M, Horwith M, Brown JL. Idiopathic edema: Studies demonstrating protein-leaking angiopathy. *Am J Med* 49:106, 1970.

263. Young B, Brownjohn AM, Chapman C, Lee MR. Evidence for a hypothalamic disturbance in cyclical oedema. *Br Med J* 286:1691, 1983.

264. MacGregor GA, Markandu ND, Roulston JE, et al. Is "idiopathic" oedema idiopathic? *Lancet* 1:397, 1979.

265. Peloski AJ, Czapla K, Duncan A, et al. The role of diuretics in the aetiology of idiopathic oedema. *Q J Med* 88:49, 1995.

266. Schichiri M, Shiigai T, Takeuchi J. Long-term furosemide treatment in idiopathic edema. *Arch Intern Med* 144:2161, 1984.

267. Riemenschneider T, Bohle A. Morphologic aspects of low-potassium and low-sodium nephropathy. *Clin Nephrol* 19:271, 1983.

268. Docci D, Turci F. Captopril in idiopathic edema (letter). *N Engl J Med* 308:1102, 1983.

269. Sowers J, Catamia R, Paris J, Tuck M. Effects of bromocriptine on renin, aldosterone, and prolactin responses to posture and metoclopramide in idiopathic edema. *J Clin Endocrinol Metab* 54:510, 1982.

270. Edwards OM, Dent RG. Idiopathic edema. *Lancet* 1:1188, 1979.

271. Speller PJ, Streeten DHP. Mechanism of the diuretic action of D-amphetamine. *Metabolism* 13:453, 1964.

272. Edwards BD, Hudson WA. A novel treatment for idiopathetic oedema of women. *Nephron* 58:369, 1991.

SEVENTEEN

INTRODUCTION TO SIMPLE AND MIXED ACID-BASE DISORDERS

Disturbances of acid-base homeostasis are common clinical problems that will be discussed in detail in Chaps. 18 to 21. This chapter will first review the basic principles of acid-base physiology, the general mechanisms by which abnormalities can occur, and an approach to evaluating patients with simple and mixed acid-base disorders.

ACID-BASE PHYSIOLOGY

Free H^+ ions are present in the body fluids in extremely low concentrations. The normal H^+ concentration in the extracellular fluid is roughly 40 nanoeq/L, approximately *one-millionth* the milliequivalent-per-liter concentrations of Na^+, K^+, Cl^-, and HCO_3^-* However, H^+ ions are small and highly reactive, allowing them to bind more strongly to negatively charged portions of molecules than Na^+ or K^+. As a result, maintenance of a stable H^+ ion level is required for normal cellular function, since small fluctuations in the H^+ concentration have important

---

* These concentrations can also be expressed in terms of molarity. Since the valence of H^+ is 1^+, 40 nanoeq/L equals 40 nanomol/L.

effects on the activity of cellular enzymes (see Fig. 10-1). There is a relatively narrow range of extracellular H^+ concentration that is compatible with life, from 16 to 160 nanoeq/L (pH equals 7.80 to 6.80).

Under normal conditions, the H^+ concentration varies little from the normal value of 40 nanoeq/L. The body buffers play an important role in this regulatory process, as they are able to take up or release H^+ ions to prevent large changes in the H^+ concentration. There are a variety of buffers in the extracellular and intracellular fluids, most of which are weak acids (which can release H^+ ions) and their ionized salts (which can take up H^+ ions) (see Chap. 10). The most important extracellular buffer is HCO_3^-, which combines with H^+ according to the following reaction:

$$H^+ + \underset{\text{salt}}{HCO_3^-} \quad \leftrightarrow \quad \underset{\text{weak acid}}{H_2CO_3} \quad \leftrightarrow \quad H_2O + CO_2 \qquad (17\text{-}1)$$

In most circumstances, the concentration of H_2CO_3 is very low in relation to that of HCO_3^- and CO_2. As a result, the law of mass action for Eq. (17-1) can be expressed solely in terms of the concentrations of H^+, HCO_3^-, and CO_2 (see page 308):

$$[H^+] = \frac{K_a' \times 0.03 P_{CO_2}}{[HCO_3^-]} \qquad (17\text{-}2)$$

where K_a' is the dissociation constant for this reaction and $0.03 P_{CO_2}$ represents the solubility of CO_2 in the plasma. If the H^+ concentration is measured in nanomoles per liter (nanomol/L), the value of K_a' is approximately 800 nanomol/L. If this is substituted in Eq. (17-2), then

$$[H^+] = 24 \times \frac{P_{CO_2}}{[HCO_3^-]} \qquad (17\text{-}3)$$

Equation (17-2) can also be expressed in logarithmic terms as the Henderson-Hasselbalch equation:

$$pH = 6.10 + \log \frac{[HCO_3^-]}{0.03 P_{CO_2}} \qquad (17\text{-}4)$$

where pH equals $-\log [H^+]$ (the H^+ concentration being measured in moles per liter) and 6.10 equals $-\log pK_a'$ (or $-\log 800 \times 10^{-9}$ mol/L). At the normal H^+ concentration of 40 nanomol/L (or 40×10^{-9} mol/L),

$$pH = -\log (40 \times 10^{-9})$$

$$= -(\log 40 + \log 10^{-9})$$

Since $\log 40$ equals 1.6 and $\log 10^{-9}$ equals -9,

$$pH = -(1.6 - 9)$$

$$= 7.40$$

Although the acidity of the extracellular fluid is measured as the pH, it is frequently easier to think in terms of the H^+ concentration and Eq. (17-3). As a result, the following chapters will use both the pH and H^+ concentration to permit the reader to become familiar with these concepts. It is important to recognize the inverse relationship between the pH and the H^+ concentration. An increase in the H^+ concentration reduces the pH, and a decrease in the H^+ concentration raises the pH (Table 17-1).

Measurement of pH

The pH and P_{CO_2} are determined on blood drawn anaerobically (to prevent the loss of CO_2 from the blood into the air) into a heparinized syringe.[1,2] The pH is measured by an electrode permeable only to H^+ ions (see page 302) and the P_{CO_2} by a CO_2 electrode. The HCO_3^- concentration can then be calculated from the Henderson-Hasselbalch equation or measured directly. The latter procedure involves the addition of a strong acid to the plasma sample and measurement by a colorimetric reaction of the amount of CO_2 generated.[1] The added H^+ ions will combine with plasma HCO_3, leading to the formation of H_2CO_3 and then CO_2 as Eq. (17-1) is driven to the right. Thus, this method measures the *total* CO_2 *content*, since it also includes the dissolved CO_2 (equals to $0.03P_{CO_2}$, which in the physiologic range adds 1 to 2 meq/L to the HCO_3^- concentration). For the sake of simplicity, the following discussion will refer only to the HCO_3^- concentration, since it is this parameter that is directly affected by changes in renal H^+ secretion and by the addition of acid or alkaline loads to the extracellular fluid.

Although the calculated and measured values for the plasma HCO_3^- concentration are generally similar, they may occasionally differ by as much as 7 to 8 meq/L. Some observers have suggested that the measured value is likely to be

Table 17-1 Relationship between the arterial pH and H^+ concentration in the physiologic range

pH	$[H^+]$, nanomol/L
7.80	16
7.70	20
7.60	26
7.50	32
7.40	40
7.30	50
7.20	63
7.10	80
7.00	100
6.90	125
6.80	160

more accurate in this setting, since calculation of the HCO_3^- level assumes, perhaps incorrectly, that the pK_a of 6.10 and the solubility constant for CO_2 of 0.03 are unchanged in acute acid-base disturbances.[3] On the other hand, other investigators claim that the calculated value is usually a better estimate, since there may be errors in the automated test used to directly measure the total CO_2 content[4] and since the pK_a seems to vary little in most clinical conditions.[5] This issue is at present unresolved. Fortunately, the difference is usually small, and the only clinical problem may occur with calculation of the anion gap, where accurate determination of the plasma bicarbonate concentration is important (see Chap. 19).[4]

The normal values for the major acid-base variables in arterial and venous blood are

	pH	$[H^+]$, nanoeq/L	P_{CO_2}, mmHg	$[HCO_3^-]$, meq/L
Arterial	7.37–7.43	37–43	36–44	22–26
Venous	7.32–7.38	42–48	42–50	23–27

The decrease in pH (and increase in H^+ concentration) in venous blood is due to the uptake of metabolically produced CO_2 in the capillary circulation.

In general, arterial rather than venous blood is used to measure the extracellular pH. Arterial blood allows concurrent measurement of arterial oxygenation and is not as influenced by local changes in tissue perfusion. However, venous blood is easier to obtain and just as accurate for pH determination if drawn without a tourniquet from a well-perfused area.

Pitfalls   There are several pitfalls that can lead to inaccurate results when the extracellular pH is measured. In addition to preventing CO_2 loss into the air by drawing the blood sample anaerobically,[2] rapid measurement or cooling to 4°C is required. At room temperature, continued anaerobic glycolysis by red cells and white cells leads to the production of organic acids that can induce small reductions in the pH and the plasma HCO_3^- concentration.[1]

If air bubbles occupy more than 1 to 2 percent of the blood volume in the syringe, an artifactually high arterial P_{O_2} and an underestimation of the true arterial P_{CO_2} may result from equilibration of these gases between air bubbles and the specimen.[6] The magnitude of this error is greatest when the difference in gas tensions between blood and air are high, when the surface area of bubbles is maximized by agitation, and when the time between specimen collection and analysis is prolonged.[7,8]

Dilution of the blood specimen with heparin is another potential problem. For example, patients in an intensive care unit often have their pH measured using arterial blood drawn from an indwelling intraarterial catheter that is routinely flushed with heparin. To minimize contamination of the blood sample, the first 8 to 10 mL should be discarded. Use of the first 2 mL (which mostly contains heparin) can lead to erroneous values for pH and P_{CO_2} as low as 6.50 and 3.5 mmHg, respectively.[9]

A similar error can occur with the use of a heparinized syringe.[10] There should be enough heparin to coat the sides of the syringe, but the volume of anticoagulant solution should be less than 5 percent of the volume of the blood sample.

Lastly, it is not always correct to assume that the arterial pH reflects the pH at the tissue level. This is a particular problem in patients with severe circulatory failure or cardiac arrest, in whom pulmonary blood flow is often substantially reduced. In this setting, blood that is delivered to the lungs may be adequately cleared of CO_2, resulting in a relatively normal or even diminished arterial P_{CO_2}. However, the low cardiac output slows the return of CO_2-containing blood from the periphery. As a result, the *mixed venous* P_{CO_2}, which represents blood that has not yet entered the pulmonary circulation, may be markedly higher than the P_{CO_2} in arterial blood.[11,12] In one study, for example, patients with a mean arterial pH of 7.42 and P_{CO_2} of 32 mmHg during cardiopulmonary resuscitation had respective mixed venous values of 7.14 and 74 mmHg.[11] If the latter results more closely reflect the pH at the cellular level, then arterial measurements can lead to the misleading assumption that acid-base balance is being maintained.

In addition to testing of mixed venous blood samples, the presence of diminished pulmonary blood flow may be suggested from measurement of the *end-tidal* CO_2 *concentration*.[13] A value above 1.5 percent suggests adequate pulmonary perfusion and the likelihood that arterial and mixed venous blood have a similar pH and P_{CO_2}. A value below 1 percent, however, is often indicative of a significant impairment in venous return.

Regulation of Hydrogen Concentration

The HCO_3^-/CO_2 system is the principal buffer in the extracellular fluid, because of both the high concentration of HCO_3^- and the ability to control the plasma HCO_3^- concentration and the P_{CO_2} independently (see Chap. 11). The former is regulated by *changes in the rate of H^+ secretion from the renal tubular cell into the tubular lumen*. Most of the secreted H^+ ions combine with filtered HCO_3^-, so that the final urine is virtually HCO_3^- free. Reabsorption of the filtered HCO_3^- is essential if acid-base balance is to be maintained, since loss of HCO_3^- in the urine is equivalent to the retention of H^+ (both H^+ and HCO_3^- being derived from the dissociation of H_2CO_3).

In addition, some secreted H^+ ions combine either with HPO_4^{2-} (to form $H_2PO_4^-$) or with NH_3 (to form NH_4^+). These processes play a central regulatory role, since they result in the generation of *new HCO_3^- ions* in the extracellular fluid (see Figs. 11-3 and 11-4). Thus, an increase in net H^+ secretion (as $H_2PO_4^-$ and NH_4^+) leads to a rise in the plasma HCO_3^- concentration, whereas a reduction in net H^+ secretion results in H^+ retention and a fall in the plasma HCO_3^- concentration.

CO_2, on the other hand, is eliminated by the lungs. Thus, the P_{CO_2} is regulated by the *rate of alveolar ventilation*. Hyperventilation enhances CO_2 excretion and lowers the P_{CO_2}; hypoventilation reduces CO_2 excretion and raises the P_{CO_2}. Although CO_2 is not an acid, since it contains no H^+ ions, it acts as an acid in the body by combining with water to form H_2CO_3 [Eq. (17-1)].

The kidneys and lungs play a central role in the maintenance of acid-base balance, because they can adjust the rate of acid excretion to meet homeostatic needs. Each day, approximately 15,000 mmol of CO_2 is produced by endogenous metabolism and then excreted by the lungs. Similarly, a normal diet generates 50 to 100 meq of H^+ per day, derived mostly from the metabolism of sulfur-containing amino acids and the subsequent generation of H_2SO_4.[14,15] These H^+ ions are initially buffered by HCO_3^- and the cellular and bone buffers to minimize the fall in extracellular pH (see page 315). Acid-base balance is then restored by urinary H^+ excretion, which regenerates the HCO_3^- lost in the original buffering reaction.

When acid-base disturbances do occur, renal and respiratory function change in an attempt to normalize the pH. From the law of mass action,

$$[H^+] = 24 \times \frac{P_{CO_2}}{[HCO_3^-]}$$

it can be seen that the H^+ concentration is related to the $P_{CO_2}/[HCO_3^-]$ ratio, not to the absolute value of either compound. If the H^+ concentration is increased, regardless of cause, it can be reduced toward normal by a decrease in the P_{CO_2} and/or an elevation in the plasma HCO_3^- concentration. Both of these changes occur, as both alveolar ventilation and urinary H^+ excretion are enhanced in this setting. At least part of the signal for these adaptations appears to be a parallel increase in H^+ concentration (or reduction in pH) in the cerebral interstitium surrounding the central respiratory centers and in the renal tubular cells.[16-18]

Conversely, alveolar ventilation and H^+ secretion are diminished when the H^+ concentration is reduced. The resultant increase in the P_{CO_2} and decline in the plasma HCO_3^- concentration raise the H^+ concentration toward normal.

ACID-BASE DISORDERS

Definitions

A change in the extracellular pH may be seen when renal or respiratory function is abnormal or when an acid or base load overwhelms excretory capacity. *Acidemia* is defined as a decrease in the blood pH (or an increase in the H^+ concentration), and *alkalemia* as an elevation in the blood pH (or a reduction in the H^+ concentration).

On the other hand, *acidosis* and *alkalosis* refer to processes that tend to lower and raise the pH, respectively. In most conditions, an acidotic process leads to acidemia and an alkalotic process to alkalemia. However, this may not be true in patients with mixed acid-base disturbances, in whom the final pH depends upon the balance between the different disorders that are present (see below).

Changes in the plasma H^+ concentration and pH can be induced by alterations in the P_{CO_2} or plasma HCO_3^- concentration [Eqs. (17-3) and (17-4)]. Since the P_{CO_2} is regulated by respiration, primary abnormalities in the P_{CO_2} are called *respiratory acidosis* (high P_{CO_2}) and *respiratory alkalosis* (low P_{CO_2}). In contrast, primary changes in the plasma HCO_3^- concentration are referred to as *metabolic acidosis* (low HCO_3^-) and *metabolic alkalosis* (high HCO_3^-).

In each of these disorders, compensatory renal or respiratory responses act to minimize the change in H^+ concentration by minimizing the alteration in the $P_{CO_2}/[HCO_3^-]$ ratio (Table 17-2). To achieve this, the compensatory response always *changes in the same direction* as the primary disturbance. Thus, a high P_{CO_2} in respiratory acidosis results in enhanced renal H^+ excretion and an appropriate elevation in the plasma HCO_3^- concentration.

Table 17-2 also demonstrates that the diagnosis of an acid-base disorder requires *measurement of the extracellular pH*. Simply looking at the plasma HCO_3^- concentration (which is routinely measured with the plasma Na^+, K^+, and Cl^- concentrations) is not sufficient. A high value, for example, can be seen both in metabolic alkalosis (where it is the primary problem) and in respiratory acidosis (where it represents the appropriate renal compensation). These disorders can be differentiated by measurement of the pH.

Metabolic Acidosis

Metabolic acidosis is characterized by a fall in the plasma HCO_3^- concentration and a low pH (or high H^+ concentration). It can be induced either by HCO_3^- loss (as with diarrhea) or by the buffering of a noncarbonic acid, such as lactic acid or retained diet-generated sulfuric acid (as occurs in renal failure):

$$H_2SO_4 + 2NaHCO_3 \quad \rightarrow \quad Na_2SO_4 + 2H_2CO_3 \quad \rightarrow \quad 2CO_2 + 2H_2O$$

The reduction in pH stimulates ventilation, resulting in a compensatory decrease in the P_{CO_2}.[19,20] Ultimate restoration of the pH usually depends upon renal excretion of the excess acid, a process that takes several days.

Table 17-2   Characteristics of the primary acid-base disturbances

Disorder	pH	[H^+]	Primary disturbance	Compensatory response
Metabolic acidosis	↓	↑	↓ [HCO_3^-]	↓ P_{CO_2}
Metabolic alkalosis	↑	↓	↑ [HCO_3^-]	↑ P_{CO_2}
Respiratory acidosis	↓	↑	↑ P_{CO_2}	↑ [HCO_3^-]
Respiratory alkalosis	↑	↓	↓ P_{CO_2}	↓ [HCO_3^-]

Metabolic Alkalosis

Metabolic alkalosis results from an elevation in the plasma HCO_3^- concentration and is associated with a high pH (or low H^+ concentration). This disorder can be produced by HCO_3^- administration or, more commonly, by H^+ loss, as with vomiting or the use of diuretics. The respiratory compensation consists of hypoventilation and an elevation in the P_{CO_2}.[21,22]

Renal excretion of the excess HCO_3^- (as $NaHCO_3$) should rapidly correct the pH. However, this does not occur in patients with metabolic alkalosis because HCO_3^- reabsorptive capacity is enhanced, usually because of concomitant volume depletion and chloride (see Chap. 18).

Respiratory Acidosis

Respiratory acidosis is due to decreased effective alveolar ventilation, resulting in reduced pulmonary excretion of CO_2 and an increase in the extracellular P_{CO_2} (hypercapnia). The renal compensation consists of enhanced H^+ excretion, which raises the plasma HCO_3^- concentration.[23,24] This response takes 3 to 5 days to reach completion.[23] As a result, two different acid-base disorders may occur: *acute* respiratory acidosis, in which there may be a dramatic fall in pH, and *chronic* respiratory acidosis, in which the pH is relatively well protected as a result of the renal compensation (see Chap. 20). Similar considerations apply to respiratory alkalosis but not to metabolic acidosis or alkalosis, since the respiratory compensation in these disorders is rapid, beginning within minutes and being complete within 12 to 24 h.[20]

Respiratory Alkalosis

The primary disturbance in respiratory alkalosis is hyperventilation, resulting in a fall in the extracellular P_{CO_2} (hypocapnia) and an increase in pH (or reduction in H^+ concentration). The compensatory response consists of diminished renal H^+ secretion, producing HCO_3^- loss in the urine and an appropriate decrease in the plasma HCO_3^- concentration. As with respiratory acidosis, the renal compensation is time-dependent, so that both acute and chronic respiratory alkalosis can occur.[25-27]

Mixed Acid-Base Disorders

It is not uncommon for more than one of the above primary disorders to be present. Suppose a patient has a low arterial pH and is therefore acidemic. In this setting, a low plasma HCO_3^- concentration indicates metabolic acidosis and a high P_{CO_2} indicates respiratory acidosis. If both are present, then the patient has a *combined* metabolic and respiratory acidosis. Similar reasoning can lead to the diagnosis of a combined metabolic and respiratory alkalosis in a patient with an elevated pH, a high plasma HCO_3^- concentration, and a low P_{CO_2}.

Knowledge of the extent of the renal and respiratory compensations allows more complex disturbances to be diagnosed.* The responses listed in Table 17-3 have been empirically derived from observations in humans with different acid-base disorders.[19-26] A simple example can illustrate how this information can be utilized. A patient with a salicylate overdose is found to have the following arterial blood values:

$$pH = 7.45$$

$$P_{CO_2} = 20 \text{ mmHg}$$

$$[HCO_3^-] = 13 \text{ meq/L}$$

Evaluation of acid-base status begins with the pH. The slightly high pH indicates that the patient is alkalemic. This can be due to a high HCO_3^- concentration or a low P_{CO_2}. Since only the latter is present, the primary diagnosis is respiratory alkalosis, most likely acute given the history. In this disorder, the body buffers will reduce the plasma HCO_3^- concentration by 2 meq/L for every 10 mmHg decrease in the P_{CO_2} (Table 17-3).[25,26] Thus, the $[HCO_3^-]$ should fall from 24 to 20 meq/L as the P_{CO_2} drops acutely from 40 to 20 mmHg. The actual $[HCO_3^-]$ of 13 meq/L is lower than expected, suggesting that the patient has a combined respiratory alkalosis and metabolic acidosis, a common finding with salicylate intoxication.[27]

Table 17-3   Renal and respiratory compensation to primary acid-base disturbances in humans

Disorder	Primary change	Compensatory response
Metabolic acidosis	↓ $[HCO_3^-]$	1.2 mmHg decrease in P_{CO_2} for every 1 meq/L fall in $[HCO_3^-]$
Metabolic alkalosis	↑ $[HCO_3^-]$	0.7 mmHg elevation in P_{CO_2} for every 1 meq/L rise in $[HCO_3^-]$
Respiratory acidosis	↑ P_{CO_2}	
Acute		1 meq/L increases in $[HCO_3^-]$ for every 10 mmHg rise in P_{CO_2}
Chronic		3.5 meq/L elevation in $[HCO_3^-]$ for every 10 mmHg rise in P_{CO_2}
Respiratory alkalosis	↓ P_{CO_2}	
Acute		2 meq/L reduction in $[HCO_3^-]$ for every 10 mmHg fall in P_{CO_2}
Chronic		4 meq/L decrease in $[HCO_3^-]$ for every 10 mmHg reduction in P_{CO_2}

* Calculation of the anion gap and the ratio of the rise in the anion gap to the fall in the plasma HCO_3^- concentration also may be diagnostically important in patients with metabolic acidosis (see Chap. 19).

The renal and respiratory compensations return the pH *toward* but rarely *to* normal. Thus, a normal pH in the presence of changes in the P_{CO_2} and plasma HCO_3^- concentration immediately suggests a mixed disorder. For example, the following arterial blood values:

$$pH = 7.40$$

$$P_{CO_2} = 60 \, mmHg$$

$$[HCO_3^-] = 36 \, meq/L$$

are due to a combination of respiratory acidosis (elevated P_{CO_2}) and metabolic alkalosis (high plasma HCO_3^- concentration). This disorder is most often due to diuretic therapy in a patient with severe chronic lung disease.

Finally, an arterial P_{CO_2} of 40 mmHg or a plasma HCO_3^- concentration of 24 meq/L is not always normal. A patient with metabolic acidosis should hyperventilate to minimize the reduction in pH. On the average, the P_{CO_2} falls 1.2 mmHg for every 1 meq/L fall in the plasma HCO_3^- concentration.[19] Thus, a 16-meq/L reduction in the plasma HCO_3^- concentration from 24 to 8 meq/L should lower the P_{CO_2} by about 19 mmHg (16 × 1.2), from 40 to 21 mmHg. In this setting, the new pH will be 7.20. If, however, the P_{CO_2} remains at 40 mmHg, then the degree of acidemia will be more severe,

$$pH = 6.10 + \frac{8}{0.03 \times 40}$$

$$= 6.92$$

Since the P_{CO_2} of 40 mmHg is *inappropriately high* by 19 mmHg, this patient has a combined metabolic and respiratory acidosis.

Acid-Base Map

If the relationship between the arterial pH (or H^+ concentration), P_{CO_2}, and HCO_3^- concentration in the different acid-base disorders is plotted, the result is the *acid-base map* in Fig. 17-1. The stippled areas represent the responses of otherwise normal subjects to metabolic and respiratory acidosis and alkalosis, including the appropriate compensations that should be present. Thus, a given increase in the P_{CO_2} is associated with a greater reduction in pH in acute, as compared to chronic, respiratory acidosis. This difference is due to the compensatory elevation in the plasma HCO_3^- concentration seen with chronic hypercapnia.

Values between the stippled areas, on the other hand, represent mixed acid-base disturbances. This can be appreciated by plotting the three mixed disorders described above: Point A lies between respiratory alkalosis and metabolic acidosis, point B between respiratory acidosis and metabolic alkalosis (even though the pH is normal), and point C between metabolic and respiratory acidosis.

As mentioned above, the diagnostic approach used in this and the following four chapters is based upon the observed in vivo compensatory responses of

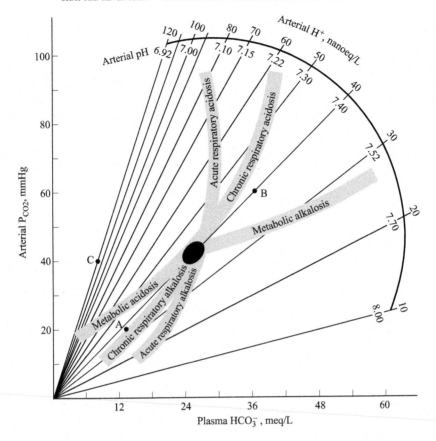

Figure 17-1   Acid-base map describing the relationships between the arterial pH, H^+ concentration, P_{CO_2}, and HCO_3^- concentration. The dark area in the center represents the range of normal values for these parameters; the stippled areas represent the different simple acid-base disturbances. Points A, B, and C indicate the three mixed acid-base disorders discussed in the text. (*From Harrington JT, Cohen JJ, Kassirer JP, Mixed acid-base disturbances, in Cohen JJ, Kassirer JP (eds):* Acid/Base. *Little, Brown, Boston, 1982, with permission.*)

patients with the different acid-base disorders.[19-26] In vitro measurements such as the base deficit, whole blood buffer base, and standard bicarbonate offer no advantages and frequently are confusing.[28] Consequently, they will not be used in this text.

CLINICAL USE OF HYDROGEN CONCENTRATION

Although the acidity of the blood is measured in terms of pH, it is somewhat difficult to use logarithms at the bedside. In contrast, the calculation of the H^+ concentration is much easier. As stated in Eq. (17-3),

$$[H^+] = 24 \times \frac{P_{CO_2}}{[HCO_3^-]}$$

If the normal arterial P_{CO_2} is 40 mmHg and the HCO_3^- concentration is 24 meq/L, then the normal H^+ concentration is 40 nanoeq/L. To use this formula, one only has to know how to convert the measured pH into H^+ concentration, a process involving a few simple calculations (Table 17-1).[29] If one begins at a pH of 7.40 and a H^+ concentration of 40 nanoeq/L, then for every 0.10 increase in pH, the H^+ concentration must be multiplied by 0.8; for every 0.10 decrease in pH, the H^+ concentration must be multiplied by 1.25. For example,

$$pH = 7.30 \quad [H^+] = 40 \times 1.25 = 50\,\text{nanoeq/L}$$

$$pH = 7.20 \quad [H^+] = 40 \times 1.25 \times 1.25 = 63\,\text{nanoeq/L}$$

$$pH = 7.50 \quad [H^+] = 40 \times 0.8 = 32\,\text{nanoeq/L}$$

Values at less than 0.10-unit steps can be estimated from interpolation. A pH of 7.27 is three-tenths of the way between 7.30 and 7.20. Since the H^+ concentration increases by 13 nanoeq/L (from 50 to 63 nanoeq/L) as the pH falls from 7.30 to 7.20, the H^+ concentration at a pH of 7.27 can be calculated from

$$[H^+] = 50 + (0.3 \times 13) = 54\,\text{nanoeq/L}$$

The following example illustrates how this equation can be used in the clinical setting. Suppose a patient with salicylate intoxication is found to have the following arterial values, which are consistent with a mild metabolic acidosis:

$$pH = 7.32$$

$$P_{CO_2} = 30\,\text{mmHg}$$

$$[HCO_3^-] = 15\,\text{meq/L}$$

An important facet of therapy in this disorder is to alkalinize the blood, which will decrease the concentration of salicylate in the tissues (see Chap. 19). Thus, the initial aim of therapy is to raise the arterial pH to 7.45 (H^+ concentration equal to 36 nanoeq/L). Assuming that the P_{CO_2} remains constant, the level to which the plasma HCO_3^- concentration has to be raised to achieve this goal can be estimated from

$$[H^+] = 24 \times \frac{P_{CO_2}}{[HCO_3^-]}$$

$$36 = 24 \times \frac{30}{[HCO_3^-]}$$

$$[HCO_3^-] = 20\,\text{meq/L}$$

POTASSIUM BALANCE IN ACID-BASE DISORDERS

There are important interactions between potassium and acid-base balance that involve both transcellular cation exchanges and alterations in renal function.

Metabolic Acid-Base Disorders

In metabolic acidosis, more than one-half of the excess hydrogen ions are buffered in the cells. In this setting, electroneutrality is maintained in part by the movement of intracellular potassium into the extracellular fluid. Thus, metabolic acidosis results in a plasma potassium concentration that is elevated in relation to total body stores. The net effect in some cases is overt hyperkalemia; in other patients, who are potassium-depleted due to urinary or gastrointestinal losses, the plasma potassium concentration is normal or even reduced.[30] There is still relative hyperkalemia, however, as evidenced by a further fall in the plasma potassium concentration if the acidemia is corrected.

On average, the plasma potassium concentration will rise by 0.6 meq/L (the range is 0.2 to 1.7 meq/L) for every 0.1-unit reduction in extracellular pH.[31] The wide range, however, means that the degree to which the plasma potassium concentration will fall with treatment of the acidemia cannot be accurately predicted. Thus, careful monitoring is required.

A fall in pH is much less likely to raise the plasma potassium concentration in patients with lactic acidosis or ketoacidosis.[31,32] The hyperkalemia that is commonly seen in diabetic ketoacidosis, for example, is more closely related to insulin deficiency and hyperosmolality than to the degree of acidemia.[31,32] Why this occurs is not well understood.

Just as metabolic acidosis can cause hyperkalemia, a rise in the plasma potassium concentration can induce a mild metabolic acidosis. Two factors contribute to this phenomenon. First, a transcellular exchange occurs, as the entry of most of the excess potassium into the cells is balanced in part by intracellular hydrogen ions moving into the extracellular fluid.[33] The net effect is an extracellular acidosis and an intracellular alkalosis. Second, the rise in cell pH within the renal tubular cells reduces ammonium and therefore net acid excretion. In patients with hypoaldosteronism, for example, the mild metabolic acidosis is primarily due to the associated hyperkalemia.

The net effect of these changes in cation distribution and renal function is that metabolic acidosis and relative hyperkalemia are often seen together. For similar reasons, when the above ionic changes are reversed, hypokalemia and metabolic alkalosis are also a common combination.[12,13]

Respiratory Acid-Base Disorders

Respiratory acidosis and alkalosis induce relatively small changes in potassium balance. The reason for this minor effect is not well understood.

Concurrent Disorders of Potassium Balance

The preceding discussion has emphasized the effect of pH on potassium distribution between the cells and extracellular fluid. However, some patients have concurrent disorders of potassium balance that can affect this relationship. In particular, although metabolic acidosis typically produces relative hyperkalemia, patients may be hypokalemic at presentation if there is a source of potassium loss. Examples include diarrhea and renal tubular acidosis. On the other hand, true hyperkalemia (i.e., associated with increased body potassium stores) is present in patients with hypoaldosteronism (type 4 renal tubular acidosis) as a result of impaired urinary potassium excretion.

The situation may be more complicated in patients with diabetic ketoacidosis. These patients are often markedly potassium-depleted because of urinary and gastrointestinal losses; however, hyperkalemia is found in approximately one-third of patients at presentation because of the hyperosmolality and insulin deficiency, not, as noted above, the metabolic acidosis. The administration of insulin typically leads to hypokalemia, unmasking the true state of potassium balance (see Chap. 25).

PROBLEMS

17-1 Convert the following values for arterial pH to H^+ concentration:

(a) 7.60

(b) 7.15

(c) 7.24

17-2 What acid-base disorders are represented by the following sets of arterial blood tests:

	pH	P_{CO_2}, mmHg	$[HCO_3^-]$, meq/L
(a)	7.32	28	14
(b)	7.47	20	14
(c)	7.08	49	14
(d)	7.51	49	38

17-3 A patient with severe diarrhea has the following laboratory tests:

$$\text{Arterial pH} = 6.98$$

$$P_{CO_2} = 13 \text{ mmHg}$$

$$[HCO_3^-] = 3 \text{ meq/L}$$

(a) What is the acid-base disorder?

To get the patient out of danger, the initial aim of therapy is to increase the pH to 7.20 by the administration of $NaHCO_3$. Assuming that the P_{CO_2} remains constant:

(b) To what level must the plasma HCO_3^- concentration be raised to reach a pH of 7.20?

If the P_{CO_2} increased to 18 mmHg with therapy, due to partial removal of the acidemic stimulus to hyperventilation:

(c) To what level must the plasma HCO_3^- concentration now be increased to achieve a pH of 7.20?

REFERENCES

1. Gennari FG, Cohen JJ, Kassirer JP. Measurement of acid-base status, in Cohen JJ, Kassirer JP (eds): *Acid/Base*. Boston, Little Brown, 1982.
2. Biswas CK, Ramos JM, Agroyannis B, Kerr DNS. Blood gas analysis: Effect of air bubbles in syringe and delay in estimation. *Br Med J* 1:923, 1982.
3. Hood I, Campbell EJM. Is pK OK? *N Engl J Med* 306:864, 1982.
4. Mohler JG, Mohler PA, Pallivatchuval RG. Failure of the serum CO_2 determined by automation to estimate the plasma bicarbonate. *Scand J Clin Lab Invest* 47(suppl 188):61, 1987.
5. Kruse JA, Hukku P, Carlson RW. Relationship between apparent dissociation constant of blood carbonic acid and disease severity. *J Lab Clin Med* 114:568, 1989.
6. Williams AJ. ABC of oxygen—Assessing and interpreting arterial blood gases and acid-base balance. *Br Med J* 317:1213, 1998.
7. Harsten A, Berg B, Inerot S, Muth L. Importance of correct handling of samples for the results of blood gas analysis. *Acta Anaesthesiol Scand* 32:365, 1988.
8. Mueller RG, Lang GE, Beam JM. Bubbles in samples for blood gas determinations: A potential source of error. *Am J Clin Pathol* 65:242, 1976.
9. Ng RH, Dennis RC, Yeston N, et al. Factitious cause of unexpected arterial blood-gas results (letter). *N Engl J Med* 310:1189, 1984.
10. Hutchison AD, Ralston SH, Dryburgh FJ, et al. Too much heparin: Possible source of error on blood gas analysis. *Br Med J* 287:1131, 1983.
11. Weil MH, Rackow EC, Trevino R, et al. Difference in acid-base state between venous and arterial blood during cardiopulmonary resuscitation. *N Engl J Med* 315:153, 1986.
12. Adrogué HJ, Rashad MN, Gorin AD, et al. Assessing acid-base status in circulatory failure: Differences between arterial and central venous blood. *N Engl J Med* 320:1312, 1989.
13. Falk JL, Rackow EC, Weil MH. End-tidal carbon dioxide concentration during cardiopulmonary resuscitation. *N Engl J Med* 318:607, 1988.
14. Lennon EJ, Lemann J Jr, Litzow JR. The effects of diet and stool composition on the net external acid balance of normal subjects. *J Clin Invest* 45:1601, 1966.
15. Breslau NA, Brinkley L, Hill KD, Pak CYC. Relationship of animal protein-rich diet to kidney stone formation and calcium metabolism. *J Clin Endocrinol Metab* 66:140, 1988.
16. Berger AJ, Mitchell RA, Severinghaus JW. Regulation of respiration. *N Engl J Med* 297:92,138,194, 1977.
17. Coates EL, Li A, Nattie E. Widespread sites of brain stem ventilatory chemoreceptors. *J Appl Physiol* 75:5, 1993.
18. Krapf R, Berry CA, Alpern RJ, Rector FC Jr. Regulation of cell pH by ambient bicarbonate, carbon dioxide tension, and pH in rabbit proximal convoluted tubule. *J Clin Invest* 81:381, 1988.
19. Bushinsky DA, Coe FL, Katzenberg C, et al. Arterial P_{CO_2} in chronic metabolic acidosis. *Kidney Int* 22:311, 1982.
20. Pierce NF, Fedson DS, Brigham KL, et al. The ventilatory response to acute base deficit in humans. The time course during development and correction of metabolic acidosis. *Ann Intern Med* 72:633, 1970.
21. Javaheri S, Kazemi H. Metabolic alkalosis and hypoventilation in humans. *Am Rev Respir Dis* 136:1011, 1987.
22. Javaheri S, Shore NS, Rose BD, Kazemi H. Compensatory hyperventilation in metabolic alkalosis. *Chest* 81:296, 1982.
23. Polak A, Haynie GD, Hays RM, Schwartz WB. Effects of chronic hypercapnia on electrolyte and acid-base equilibrium. I. Adaptation. *J Clin Invest* 40:1223, 1961.
24. van Ypersele de Strihou C, Brasseur L, de Coninck J. "Carbon dioxide response curve" for chronic hypercapnia in man. *N Engl J Med* 275:117, 1966.
25. Arbus GS, Herbert LA, Levesque PR, et al. Characterization and clinical application of the "significance band" for acute respiratory alkalosis. *N Engl J Med* 280:117, 1969.

26. Gennari JF, Goldstein MB, Schwartz WB. The nature of the renal adaptation to chronic hypocapnia. *J Clin Invest* 51:1722, 1972.
27. Gabow PA, Anderson R, Potts DE, Schrier RW. Acid-base disturbances in the salicylate-intoxicated adult. *Arch Intern Med* 138:1481, 1978.
28. Schwartz WB, Relman AS. A critique of the parameters used in the evaluation of acid-base disorders: "Whole blood buffer base" and "standard bicarbonate" compared with blood pH and plasma bicarbonate concentration. *N Engl J Med* 268:1382, 1963.
29. Fagan TJ. Estimation of hydrogen ion concentration (letter). *N Engl J Med* 288:915, 1973.
30. Magner PO, Robinson L, Halperin RM, et al. The plasma potassium concentration in metabolic acidosis: A re-evaluation. *Am J Kidney Dis* 11:220, 1988.
31. Adrogué HJ, Madias NE. Changes in plasma potassium concentration during acute acid-base disturbances. *Am J Med* 71:456, 1981.
32. Adrogué HJ, Chap Z, Ishida T, Field J. Role of endocrine pancreas in the kalemic response to acute metabolic acidosis in conscious dogs. *J Clin Invest* 75:798, 1985.
33. Altenberg GA, Aristimuno PC, Amorena CE, Taquini AC. Amiloride prevents the metabolic acidosis of a KCl load in nephrectomized rats. *Clin Sci* 76:649, 1989.

METABOLIC ALKALOSIS

The introduction to acid-base disorders presented in Chap. 17 should be read before proceeding with this discussion. Primary metabolic alkalosis is characterized by an elevation in the arterial pH (or a reduction in the H^+ concentration), an increase in the plasma HCO_3^- concentration, and compensatory hypoventilation, resulting in a rise in the P_{CO_2}. A high HCO_3^- concentration, however, is not diagnostic of metabolic alkalosis, since it can also represent the renal compensation to chronic respiratory acidosis. These disorders can be differentiated by measurement of the extracellular pH, which is reduced in chronic respiratory acidosis. In addition, a plasma HCO_3^- concentration of 40 meq/L or more indicates at least some degree of metabolic alkalosis, since this level is greater than that generally achieved by the renal compensation to severe chronic hypercapnia.

PATHOPHYSIOLOGY

The pathophysiology of metabolic alkalosis is most easily understood by asking two separate questions:

- How do patients become alkalotic?
- Why do they remain alkalotic, since renal excretion of the excess HCO_3^- should rapidly restore normal acid-base balance?

Generation of Metabolic Alkalosis

A primary elevation in the plasma HCO_3^- concentration is usually induced by H^+ loss from the gastrointestinal tract (as with vomiting or nasogastric suction) or in the urine (as with the diuretic therapy) (Table 18-1). These H^+ ions are derived from the intracellular dissociation of H_2CO_3:

$$CO_2 + H_2O \leftrightarrow H_2CO_3 \leftrightarrow H^+ + HCO_3^-$$

Thus, there will be an *equimolar generation of HCO_3^- for each milliequivalent of H^+ that is lost.*

Metabolic alkalosis can also be produced by the administration of HCO_3^-, by H^+ movement into the cells, and by certain forms of volume contraction. A transcellular H^+ shift typically occurs with hypokalemia. As the plasma K^+ concentration falls, K^+ moves out of the cells down a favorable concentration gradient to partially replete the extracellular stores. Electroneutrality is main-

Table 18-1   Causes of metabolic alkalosis

Loss of hydrogen
  A. Gastrointestinal loss
      1. Removal of gastric secretions—vomiting or nasogastric suction[a]
      2. Antacid therapy, particularly with cation-exchange resin
      3. Chloride-losing diarrhea
  B. Renal loss
      1. Loop or thiazide-type diuretics[a]
      2. Mineralocorticoid excess[a]
      3. Postchronic hypercapnia
      4. Low chloride intake
      5. High-dose carbenicillin or other penicillin derivative
      6. Hypercalcemia, including the milk-alkali syndrome
  C. H^+ movement into cells
      1. Hypokalemia[a]
      2. Refeeding (?)
Retention of bicarbonate
  A. Massive blood transfusion
  B. Administration of $NaHCO_3$
  C. Milk-alkali syndrome
Contraction alkalosis
  A. Loop or thiazide-type diuretics
  B. Gastric losses in patients with achlorhydria
  C. Sweat losses in cystic fibrosis

[a] Most common causes.

tained in this setting by a reciprocal shift of H^+ (and Na^+) into the cells.[1,2] The net effect is an *extracellular alkalosis with a paradoxical intracellular acidosis*.[3,4] K^+ repletion can reverse the H^+ shift and lower the extracellular pH toward normal.[1,2]

A *contraction alkalosis* occurs when the fluid that is lost contains Cl^- but little or no HCO_3^-. In this setting, which is most commonly due to diuretics, the extracellular volume contracts around a relatively constant quantity of extracellular HCO_3^-. As a result, the plasma HCO_3^- concentration rises (Fig. 18-1).[5] The severity of this process is generally limited by buffering of the excess extracellular HCO_3^- by cell and bone buffers.[6]

Patients with metabolic alkalosis are almost always *hypochloremic*, usually because of chloride loss with H^+ with gastrointestinal or renal losses. As described in the next section, hypochloremia is thought to play a major role in the maintenance of metabolic alkalosis by limiting HCO_3^- excretion.

Maintenance of Metabolic Alkalosis

The kidney possesses the ability to correct a metabolic alkalosis by excreting the excess HCO_3^- in the urine. For example, normal subjects given 1000 meq of $NaHCO_3$ per day for 2 weeks excrete virtually all of the excess HCO_3^- and develop only a minor increase in the plasma HCO_3^- concentration.[7] Since the disorders that cause metabolic alkalosis are associated with a much smaller HCO_3^- load, the *perpetuation of metabolic alkalosis requires an impairment in renal HCO_3^- excretion*

Extracellular fluid

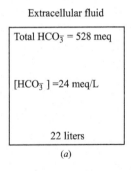

Total HCO_3^- = 528 meq

$[HCO_3^-]$ =24 meq/L

22 liters

(a)

Figure 18-1 Mechanism of contraction alkalosis. (*a*) The volume and HCO_3^- concentration of the extracellular fluid in an as yet untreated 70-kg man whose extracellular volume has increased from 17 to 22 liters because of congestive heart failure. (*b*) If the excess NaCl is lost isotonically after the administration of diuretic, there will be a reduction in the extracellular volume. Since the quantity of extracellular HCO_3^- is initially unchanged, the HCO_3^- concentration in the extracellular fluid will increase from 24 to 31 meq/L.

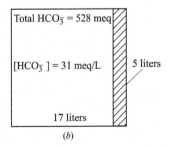

Total HCO_3^- = 528 meq

$[HCO_3^-]$ = 31 meq/L

5 liters

17 liters

(b)

(Table 18-2).* Both a reduction in glomerular filtration rate (and therefore in the filtered HCO_3^- load) and an elevation in tubular reabsorption contribute to this process.[8-11] It is likely that the latter is more important, since a low filtration rate alone, as in chronic renal insufficiency, does not appear to predispose to metabolic alkalosis.

As was reviewed in Chap. 11, HCO_3^- reabsorption occurs by H^+ secretion from the tubular cell into the lumen. The proximal tubule plays the major role in this process, reabsorbing approximately 90 percent of the filtered HCO_3^-, mostly via Na^+-H^+ exchange. The remaining HCO_3^- is primarily reabsorbed in the loop of Henle via Na^+-H^+ exchange and in the collecting tubules via an active H^+-ATPase pump in the luminal membrane.

A variety of factors may contribute to the increase in HCO_3^- reabsorption that is seen in metabolic alkalosis, including volume and chloride depletion, hyper-aldosteronism, and hypokalemia.

Effective circulating volume depletion The increase in net HCO_3^- reabsorption in effective volume depletion (which includes edematous states such as heart failure and cirrhosis; see page 259) can be viewed as an appropriate response from the viewpoint of volume regulation. If the excess HCO_3^- were excreted in the urine, it would obligate concurrent Na^+ loss to maintain electroneutrality, further dimin-ishing tissue perfusion.

The effect of volume status on HCO_3^- reabsorption is dependent upon the degree of volume depletion. As an example, a 4-meq/L increase in HCO_3^- reab-sorptive capacity (from 25 to 29 meq/L of glomerular filtration rate) can be seen with the ingestion of a very low Na^+ diet (10 meq/day), even though the patient is clinically euvolemic.[12] On the other hand, HCO_3^- reabsorptive capacity can exceed 35 meq/L with marked reductions in tissue perfusion, thereby allowing a relatively severe metabolic alkalosis to persist.[9,10]

Table 18-2 Causes of impaired HCO_3^- excretion that allow metabolic alkalosis to persist

---

Decreased glomerular filtration rate
  A. Effective circulating volume depletion
  B. Renal failure (usually associated with metabolic acidosis)
Increased tubular reabsorption
  A. Effective circulating volume depletion
  B. Chloride depletion (also decreases bicarbonate secretion)
  C. Hypokalemia
  D. Hyperaldosteronism

---

* In this regard, metabolic alkalosis is similar to other "excess" disorders, such as hyponatremia (too much water), hyperkalemia (too much K^+), and edema (too much Na^+). In each of these condi-tions, renal excretory capacity for the retained solute or water is normally so high that a defect in renal excretion must be present for the disorder to persist.

Despite the clear relationship between hypovolemia and increased HCO_3^- reabsorption, the mechanism by which this occurs is incompletely understood. Micropuncture studies in experimental animals suggest that increased proximal reabsorption, if it occurs, cannot quantitatively explain the reduction in HCO_3^- excretion.[13-15] It is probable that this relative lack of change reflects the interaction of several counterbalancing factors.[16] Both angiotensin II, released in response to hypovolemia, and the elevated tubular fluid HCO_3^- concentration increase proximal HCO_3^- reabsorption—the former by enhancing the activity of the Na^+-H^+-exchanger,[17] and the latter by allowing more H^+ ions to be secreted before approaching the minimum pH that the proximal tubule can achieve.[15,16] On the other hand, metabolic alkalosis itself decreases the activity of the Na^+-H^+ antiporter, an effect that is probably mediated in part by a parallel rise in renal tubular cell pH.[18]

The net effect is that the decrease in HCO_3^- excretion in metabolic alkalosis associated with volume depletion is primarily due to enhanced net HCO_3^- reabsorption in the distal nephron.[14,15] Secondary hyperaldosteronism may contribute to this response. Aldosterone directly stimulates the H^+-ATPase pump in the cortical and medullary collecting tubules.[19,20] In addition, aldosterone can indirectly increase net H^+ secretion (and therefore HCO_3^- reabsorption) by promoting Na^+ transport in the cortical collecting tubule.[21,22] The reabsorption of cationic Na^+ creates a lumen-negative potential difference; this electrical gradient then promotes H^+ accumulation in the lumen by minimizing the rate of passive back-diffusion.

Concurrent Cl^- depletion (induced by vomiting or diuretics) and hypokalemia also appear to play an important role in the increase in distal HCO_3^- reabsorption. To the degree that *Na^+ is reabsorbed but Cl^- cannot follow to dissipate the electrical gradient*, there will be a greater increase in luminal negativity and therefore a greater stimulus to H^+ secretion.[23] The net effect of the almost complete reabsorption of filtered HCO_3^- is the paradoxical finding of *an acid urine despite the presence of extracellular alkalemia.*[23]

These changes are reversed with correction of the fluid and chloride deficits. In this setting, reversal of the metabolic alkalosis requires increased HCO_3^- excretion, a change that is primarily mediated by decreased net HCO_3^- reabsorption in the distal nephron.[24]

Chloride depletion   The above discussion has suggested a central role for volume depletion in the maintenance of metabolic alkalosis. It has been suggested, however, that it is *Cl^- depletion*, rather than decreased tissue perfusion, that is actually of primary importance.[13,14,25] Consistent with this hypothesis is the observation that repair of the volume deficit by the administration of albumin does not reverse the increase in distal HCO_3^- reabsorption and does not correct the alkalosis.[14] On the other hand, the administration of non-Na^+-containing Cl^- salts (such as potassium or choline chloride) does not restore normovolemia but does result in decreased net acid excretion and a reduction in the plasma HCO_3^- to normal.[13,14,25]

There are three mechanisms by which Cl^- depletion could perpetuate a metabolic alkalosis, independent of Na^+ balance[13]:

- The activity of the Na^+-K^+-$2Cl^-$ carrier in the luminal membrane of the macula densa cell is primarily determined by the availability of Cl^- (see Fig. 4-3). Thus, hypochloremia will decrease Cl^- delivery to the macula densa, resulting in less NaCl reabsorption. The latter change will promote the release of renin, leading to secondary hyperaldosteronism[26] and increased distal H^+ secretion.
- The luminal H^+-ATPase pump in the intercalated cells in the collecting tubules is probably associated with passive cosecretion of Cl^- to maintain electroneutrality.[27] A decline in the tubular fluid Cl^- concentration will facilitate this process by maximizing the transtubular gradient for Cl^- secretion.
- It has been assumed that the appropriate HCO_3^- loss in metabolic alkalosis results from diminished reabsorption of filtered HCO_3^-. It now appears, however, that at least some of the urinary HCO_3^- is derived from *HCO_3^- secretion* by a subpopulation of intercalated cells in the cortical collecting tubule in which the H^+-ATPase pump is located on the basolateral rather than the luminal membrane (see page 338) (Fig. 18-2).[28,29] The final step in this process seems to involve Cl^-/HCO_3^- exchange across the luminal mem-

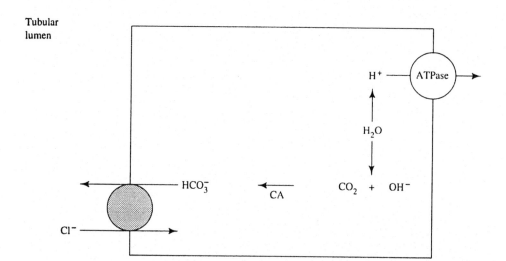

Figure 18-2   Transport mechanisms involved in the secretion of bicarbonate into the tubular lumen in the type B intercalated cells in the cortical collecting tubule. Water within the cell dissociates into hydrogen and hydroxyl anions. The former are secreted into the peritubular capillary by H-ATPase pumps in the basolateral membrane. The hydroxyl anions combine with carbon dioxide to form bicarbonate in a reaction catalyzed by carbonic anhydrase (CA). Bicarbonate is then secreted into the tubular lumen via chloride-bicarbonate exchangers in the luminal membrane. The favorable inward concentration gradient for chloride (lumen concentration greater than that in the cell) provides the energy for bicarbonate secretion.

brane. The energy for this transport is supplied by the highly favorable inward gradient for Cl^-, since the cell Cl^- concentration is very low. Lowering the tubular fluid Cl^- concentration in metabolic alkalosis will diminish this gradient, thereby minimizing the ability to secrete HCO_3^-.

In summary, the relative roles of volume and Cl^- depletion are unresolved. This issue is not of great clinical importance, however, since the administration of NaCl will simultaneously correct both problems and allow the excess HCO_3^- to be excreted in the urine (see "Treatment," below).[9,29,30] This HCO_3^- diuresis is primarily due to diminished distal HCO_3^- reabsorption and/or enhanced distal HCO_3^- secretion.[13,24,28,29]

It is important to emphasize that hypovolemia has *two separate and independent effects* in metabolic alkalosis. To the degree that renal HCO_3^- reabsorption is enhanced, volume and chloride depletion from any cause will tend to perpetuate an alkalosis. However, hypovolemia will *produce* an alkalosis only when the fluid lost contains an excess of H^+ ions or an excess of Cl^- in relation to HCO_3^-, thereby raising the plasma HCO_3^- concentration by contraction (Fig. 18-1). Thus, the vomiting or diuretic therapy often induce a metabolic alkalosis, but bleeding, which is associated with the loss of Cl^- and HCO_3^- in concentrations similar to those in the plasma, does not.

Hypokalemia   Hypokalemia is a potent stimulus to H^+ secretion and HCO_3^- reabsorption (see Fig. 11-16).[31,32] At least three factors may contribute to this relationship:

- The concurrent intracellular acidosis, induced by transcellular K^+/H^+ exchange,[1,2] will tend to increase H^+ secretion.
- There is a second proton pump in the distal nephron, a H^+-K^+-ATPase that actively reabsorbs K^+ as well as secreting H^+.[33-35] Electroneutrality is maintained by H^+ and K^+ movement in opposite directions across the luminal membrane. Active K^+ reabsorption by this pump appears to be appropriately stimulated by hypokalemia, an effect that could also enhance H^+ secretion.[33,35-37] Thus, hypokalemia and aldosterone, which stimulate the H^+-K^+-ATPase and H^+-ATPase pumps, respectively, appear to have a potentiating effect on distal hydrogen secretion and therefore on the development and maintenance of metabolic alkalosis.[38] It is of interest in this regard that many of the causes of metabolic alkalosis (such as diuretic therapy, vomiting, and primary hyperaldosteronism) are associated with both a reduction in the plasma K^+ concentration and increased aldosterone release.
- Severe hypokalemia may cause, by an unknown mechanism, a reduction in chloride reabsorption in the distal nephron.[39,40] As a result, Na^+ reabsorption at this site is associated with a greater luminal electronegativity and therefore a greater tendency for H^+ secretion.[40]

The effect of hypokalemia is relatively small when HCO_3^- reabsorption is already stimulated by volume depletion (Fig. 18-3).[41] It appears to be of primary importance, however, in states of primary mineralocorticoid excess, as with an aldosterone-producing adrenal adenoma.[40-42] In this setting, aldosterone-induced Na^+ retention is transient, with marked volume expansion and edema being prevented by the phenomenon of aldosterone escape (see page 185). As a result, Na^+ intake and excretion are roughly equal, and it is hypokalemia, not volume depletion, that is now responsible for perpetuation of the alkalosis. Correction of the K^+ deficit returns the plasma HCO_3^- concentration toward normal in this setting, both by decreasing net acid excretion in the urine[9,40-42] and, as most of the exogenous K^+ enters the cells to replete cellular stores, by movement of H^+ ions back into the extracellular fluids.[1,2]

Respiratory Compensation

The development of alkalemia is sensed by the respiratory chemoreceptors, resulting in a decline in ventilation and an *appropriate* elevation in the P_{CO_2}. On average, the P_{CO_2} rises 0.7 mmHg for every 1.0-meq/L increment in the plasma HCO_3^- concentration.[43,49] Thus, if the plasma HCO_3^- concentration is 34 meq/L (or 10 meq/L greater than normal), there should be a 7 mmHg increase in the P_{CO_2} to approximately 47 mmHg.

Values significantly different from this predicted value represent superimposed respiratory acidosis or alkalosis.

The respiratory compensation may be partially or completely impaired in the presence of underlying respiratory alkalosis or hypoxemia. As an example, patients with heart failure or cirrhosis frequently develop metabolic alkalosis as a result of diuretic therapy. However, both of these disorders are often associated with a primary respiratory alkalosis (see Chap. 21), which can prevent the appropriate compensatory hypoventilation.

Hypoxemia, on the other hand, is generally less likely to affect the ventilatory response. Hypoventilation will lower the P_{O_2} at the same time as it raises the P_{CO_2}.[45] However, the hypoxemic stimulation to respiration in alkalemic patients does not become prominent until the P_{O_2} is below 50 mmHg (see page 649). Thus,

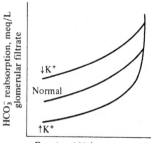

Fractional Na⁺ reabsorption

Figure 18-3 HCO_3^- reabsorption as a function of the fraction of the filtered Na^+ that is reabsorbed and the state of K^+ balance. HCO_3^- reabsorption is enhanced by both volume depletion (high fractional Na^+ reabsorption) and hypokalemia, conditions that therefore can perpetuate metabolic alkalosis. (*Redrawn form Kurtzman NA, White MG, Rogers PW, Arch Intern Med 131:702, 1973. By permission of the American Medical Association, copyright 1973.*)

in the absence of underlying lung disease, the fall in P_{O_2} in metabolic alkalosis will not usually be sufficient to impair the compensatory response. As a result, the P_{CO_2} in a previously normal subject can exceed 60 mmHg in severe metabolic alkalosis.[36]

What is less clear is the degree to which the change in respiration actually protects the extracellular pH. Studies in experimental animals indicate that the rise in P_{CO_2} in metabolic alkalosis increases net H^+ excretion and therefore *further elevates the plasma HCO_3^- concentration.*[47] These changes probably result from a reduction in renal tubular cell pH induced by the increment in P_{CO_2}; the relative intracellular acidosis will stimulate H^+ secretion, thereby raising the plasma HCO_3^- concentration. The net effect is that, after several days, the *arterial pH is the same as it would have been if no respiratory compensation had occurred,* because of equivalent elevations in the extracellular P_{CO_2} and HCO_3^- concentration (see page 580).[47]

ETIOLOGY

Metabolic alkalosis can be produced by a variety of disorders, most of which are characterized by enhanced HCO_3^- reabsorption due to volume, Cl^-, and/or K^+ depletion (Table 18-1).[11]

Gastrointestinal Hydrogen Loss

Removal of gastric secretions   Gastric juice contains high concentrations of HCl and lesser concentrations of KCl. Each milliequivalent of H^+ secreted generates 1 meq of HCO_3^-. Under normal conditions, the increase in the plasma HCO_3^- concentration is only transient, since the entry of the acid into the duodenum stimulates an equal amount of pancreatic HCO_3^- secretion.[48] However, there is no stimulus to HCO_3^- secretion if the gastric juice is removed, either by vomiting or by nasogastric suction. The net result is an increase in the plasma HCO_3^- concentration and metabolic alkalosis.[23,49,50] The tendency toward alkalosis is enhanced by the concomitant volume and K^+ depletion.

Metabolic alkalosis also can occur after removal of gastric acid secretions in patients with achlorhydria (little or no gastric acid secretion). In this setting, contraction (due to the loss of a high Cl^- low HCO_3^- fluid) rather than H^+ loss is responsible for the elevation in the plasma HCO_3^- concentration.

A somewhat similar sequence can be induced by chronic therapy with an antacid, such as magnesium hydroxide. The hydroxide component buffers gastric H^+, while the magnesium combines with pancreatic HCO_3^- to form insoluble magnesium carbonate. If only these reactions occurred, there would be equivalent H^+ and HCO_3^- loss and no change in acid-base balance. However, some of the magnesium combines with other constituents in the intestinal lumen, such as fats and phosphates. As a result, some of the secreted HCO_3^- remains soluble and is absorbed, leading to a mild alkaline load that produces no problems as long as renal function is normal.[51]

The outcome may be different in patients with advanced renal failure who are also treated with a cation-exchange resin (Kayexalate) for hyperkalemia.[49,52] In this setting, some of the magnesium binds to the resin, leaving more HCO_3^- in a soluble form in the intestinal lumen and able to be absorbed. The renal failure is important in perpetuating the alkalosis, since it prevents excretion of the excess HCO_3^-.

Congenital chloridorrhea   Since the enteric fluids below the stomach are alkaline, diarrhea usually leads to metabolic acidosis. However, a rare condition, *congenital chloridorrhea*, is associated with a specific intestinal defect in Cl^- reabsorption and HCO_3^- secretion, resulting in a high fecal Cl^- concentration that can reach 140 meq/L and a low fecal pH.[49,53] Loss of this fluid tends to produce metabolic alkalosis; a similar problem can occur in some patients with a villous adenoma.[49]

Congenital chloridorrhea is induced by mutations in the down-regulated adenoma gene, which is presumably an intestinal anion transporter or a regulator of such a transporter.[54] Treatment generally consists of a high chloride intake to prevent volume depletion. However, such an approach also increases the severity of the diarrhea because of the chloride malabsorption. Decreasing gastric chloride secretion with a proton pump inhibitor such as omeprazole may produce 15 to 20 percent reductions in stool volume and Cl^- excretion.[55]

Factitious diarrhea   Factitious diarrhea due to laxative abuse is often associated with metabolic acidosis resulting from loss of HCO_3^--containing fluid.[49,56] However, many patients develop metabolic alkalosis.[49,56,57] How this occurs is not well understood, but hypokalemia may play an important role.

Renal Hydrogen Loss

Mineralocorticoid excess and hypokalemia   The conditions associated with primary mineralocorticoid excess, such as primary hyperaldosteronism, are discussed in Chap. 27, since hypokalemia is typically the most prominent abnormality in these patients. As described above, aldosterone can promote H^+ secretion and the development of metabolic alkalosis by directly stimulating the distal H^+-ATPase pump and by making the lumen more electronegative via enhanced Na^+ reabsorption.[19-22] These transport processes involve different cells in the cortical and medullary collecting tubule, with Na^+ reabsorption occurring in the principal cells and H^+ secretion occurring in the intercalated cells (see Chap. 5).

Hypokalemia due to concomitant urinary K^+ loss plays an essential role in the maintenance of the metabolic alkalosis in this setting.[9,40-42] If K^+ depletion is prevented, there is a lesser increment in net H^+ excretion and only a minor elevation in the plasma HCO_3^- concentration.[42]

For these effects on H^+ and K^+ secretion to occur, there must be *adequate delivery of Na^+ and water to the distal secretory site* (see page 184). This is not a problem in primary hyperaldosteronism, in which the patient tends to be mildly volume-expanded due to the stimulus to distal Na^+ retention. However, distal delivery is reduced in patients with effective circulating volume depletion. As a result, the associated secondary hyperaldosteronism does not lead to excessive H^+ and K^+ loss.[22,58] Thus, uncomplicated patients with heart failure or cirrhosis typically have a normal K^+ concentration and are not alkalemic. However, hypokalemia and metabolic alkalosis may rapidly ensue if distal delivery is enhanced by the administration of diuretics.

Diuretics   The loop and thiazide-type diuretics are commonly associated with metabolic alkalosis, the severity of which varies directly with the degree of diuresis. Both volume contraction and, more importantly, increased urinary H^+ loss contribute to this problem.[5,6,59] The latter is primarily due to enhanced distal H^+ secretion, which results from the interplay of three factors: hypersecretion of aldosterone due to the associated hypovolemia; increased distal flow, since these agents inhibit NaCl and water reabsorption proximal to the H^+ secretory sites in the collecting tubules; and the concomitant development of hypokalemia.

Posthypercapnic alkalosis   Chronic respiratory acidosis is associated with a compensatory increase in H^+ secretion and therefore in renal HCO_3^- reabsorption (see Chap. 20).[60] This represents an appropriate response, since the rise in the plasma HCO_3^- concentration returns the extracellular pH toward normal. The net effect is that acidemia is not a major problem in uncomplicated patients.

Treatment with mechanical ventilation in this disorder can lead to a rapid reduction in the P_{CO_2}. The plasma HCO_3^- concentration, however, will remain elevated, resulting in the development of metabolic alkalosis and, because of the fall in P_{CO_2}, an acute rise in cerebral pH that can produce serious neurologic abnormalities and death.[61] As a result, the P_{CO_2} should be lowered slowly and carefully in patients with chronic hypercapnia; there is no need for rapid lowering, since the extracellular pH is generally well protected.[60]

Several factors may contribute to maintenance of the alkalosis in this setting. Initially, there may be a "memory" effect, as the hypercapnia-induced stimulation of HCO_3^- reabsorption persists even though the P_{CO_2} has been returned toward normal.[62] How this occurs is not clear; however, the original increment in H^+ secretion takes 3 to 5 days to reach its maximum level,[60] and reversal of this process may be equally slow. Chronic respiratory acidosis is also associated with both hypoxemia (which can lead to renal vasoconstriction)[63] and Cl^- loss in the urine, resulting in hypochloremia and volume depletion.[64] Increased cosecretion of Cl^- with the distal H^+-ATPase pump may be in part responsible for the chloruresis.[27] As a result, a posthypercapnic alkalosis will tend to persist until Cl^- balance is restored.[64]

Low chloride intake   Metabolic alkalosis may be induced in infants by the inadvertent administration of formula containing Na^+ but almost no Cl^-.[65] The ensuing Cl^- depletion diminishes the amount of Cl^- in the tubular lumen, which can promote the development of metabolic alkalosis by two mechanisms: Tubular Na^+ reabsorption must occur in exchange for H^+ (or K^+), since less Cl^- is available,[22,23] and there is a more favorable gradient for Cl^- to be cosecreted into the lumen with H^+ by the H^+-ATPase pump.[27] Once the alkalosis has developed, the decrease in Cl^- delivery will, as noted above, contribute to perpetuation of the high plasma HCO_3^- concentration by impairing HCO_3^- secretion.[28,29]

High-dose carbenicillin or penicillin A similar problem can occur with the intravenous administration of high doses of Na^+ carbenicillin or some other penicillin derivatives.[66,67] Intravenous carbenicillin, for example, contains 4.7 meq/g of Na^+, or 141 meq if 30 g is given. As the Na^+ carbenicillin is filtered, carbenicillin acts as a nonreabsorbable anion. Consequently, some distal Na^+ reabsorption must occur in exchange for K^+ and H^+, resulting in hypokalemia and metabolic alkalosis.[68] The relatively low tubular fluid Cl^- concentration in this setting also may play a contributory role.

Hypercalcemia Renal H^+ secretion and HCO_3^- reabsorption are increased by hypercalcemia,[69,70] possibly leading to a mild metabolic alkalosis.[71] Both the mechanism by which this might occur and the role of concurrent changes in parathyroid hormone (PTH) secretion are unclear. Patients with primary hyperparathyroidism tend to have a mild metabolic acidosis, a change that has been thought to result from a decrease in proximal HCO_3^- reabsorption.[72] However, some other factor may be important in this setting, since the chronic continuous administration of PTH to normal humans *increases* net acid excretion and produces a small elevation, not a reduction, in the plasma HCO_3^- concentration.[73]

Regardless of the mechanism, similar factors probably contribute in the *milk-alkali syndrome*, in which the chronic ingestion of milk and/or calcium carbonate–containing antacids leads to hypercalcemia and metabolic alkalosis.[74-76] The carbonate load raises the plasma HCO_3^- concentration, while the combination of hypercalcemia and renal insufficiency (which is mostly due to the hypercalcemia) prevents the urinary excretion of the excess HCO_3^-.[75] The most common cause at present is the administration of calcium carbonate as a phosphate binder to patients with chronic renal failure.[76]

Intracellular Shift of Hydrogen

Hypokalemia Hypokalemia is a frequent finding in patients with metabolic alkalosis. This association is due to several factors: (1) The common causes of metabolic alkalosis (vomiting, diuretics, mineralocorticoid excess) directly induce both H^+ and K^+ loss, (2) hypokalemia causes a transcellular shift in which K^+ leaves and H^+ enters the cells, thereby raising the extracellular pH,[1,2] and (3) hypokalemia increases net acid excretion and HCO_3^- reabsorption,[31,32,40-42] an effect that is probably due in part to the associated intracellular acidosis.

Refeeding   Patients who are refed carbohydrate after a prolonged fast can acutely develop metabolic alkalosis.[77] Since there is neither volume contraction nor a demonstrable increase in urinary acid excretion, it has been proposed that an intracellular shift of H^+ may be responsible. The mechanism by which this might occur is unknown.

Refeeding is also associated with Na^+ retention, which may be responsible for perpetuation of the alkalosis.[77] Increased secretion of insulin, resulting from the carbohydrate ingestion, may contribute to this response.

Retention of Bicarbonate

Because of the ability of the kidney to excrete HCO_3^-, it is difficult to produce more than a small increment in the plasma HCO_3^- concentration by the chronic administration of as much as 1000 meq of HCO_3^- per day.[7] However, a significant alkalemia can be produced by the acute infusion of base or by the chronic administration of alkali in a patient in whom renal HCO_3^- excretion is impaired (as in the milk-alkali syndrome).

Administration of organic anions   Organic anions, such as lactate, are rapidly metabolized in the body to HCO_3^-.[78] For example,

$$CH_3CHOHCOO^- \text{(lactate)} + 3O_2 \quad \rightarrow \quad 2CO_2 + 2H_2O + HCO_3^-$$

The same is true for acetate, citrate, and, in the presence of insulin, the anions of the ketoacids.[79]

As a result, the administration of organic anions can lead to the development of metabolic alkalosis. Most bank blood, for example, is anticoagulated with acid-citrate-dextran. Each unit (500 mL) of blood contains 16.8 meq of citrate, which generates HCO_3^- as it is metabolized. Although citric acid also is present, it has only a transient effect on the systemic pH, since it is rapidly converted into CO_2 and H_2O. In general, more than eight units of blood must be given acutely to produce a significant elevation in the plasma HCO_3^- concentration.[80]

Citrate-induced alkalosis also may occur when citrate is used in place of heparin as an anticoagulant in hemodialysis patients who are at high risk for bleeding.[81] In this setting, the rise in the plasma HCO_3^- concentration may persist for several days because of the absence of renal function.

A similar problem may occur after the administration of some human plasma protein fractions (Protenate, Plasmatein), which are used as volume expanders.[82] The solutions contain acetate (as a source of HCO_3^-) and citrate (as a preservative) in a total concentration of 40 to 50 meq/L. The metabolism of these anions can lead to a significant elevation in the plasma HCO_3^- concentration.

Administration of sodium bicarbonate   The most common indication for $NaHCO_3$ therapy is in the treatment of metabolic acidosis. However, HCO_3^- therapy can result in metabolic alkalosis if given in excessive amounts. This is particularly true in lactic acidosis[83] and ketoacidosis,[79] in which endogenous HCO_3^- is replaced during the initial buffering reaction by lactate or β-hydroxybutyrate. As a result, there is *no loss of potential* HCO_3^- (excluding those anions excreted in the urine), since the organic anion can be metabolized back to HCO_3^- once the underlying abnormality is corrected.

The net effect is that the administration of HCO_3^- in these disorders* creates an excess of potential HCO_3^-, leading to a post-correction metabolic alkalosis. In extreme cases, the systemic pH has reached 7.90, with the plasma HCO_3^- concentration exceeding 60 to 70 meq/L, after the indiscriminate use of $NaHCO_3$ during cardiopulmonary resuscitation.[83] A similar problem can occur with massive $NaHCO_3$ ingestion as long as there is an underlying defect in HCO_3^- excretion, such as renal insufficiency.[84]

Contraction Alkalosis

The mechanism of a contraction alkalosis, in which NaCl and water are lost without HCO_3^-, is illustrated in Fig. 18-1. This problem is most commonly seen with loop or thiazide-type diuretics;[5] it can, however also occur with vomiting (even in patients with achlorhydria, in whom NaCl replaces HCl in the gastric secretions) or with cystic fibrosis (where the sweat Cl^- concentration can exceed 70 to 100 meq/L, while the HCO_3^- concentration is well below that of the plasma).[85]

In the absence of massive fluid losses, the direct effect of contraction is largely minimized by the release of H^+ from cell buffers, thereby lowering the plasma HCO_3^- concentration toward normal:[6]

$$HCO_3^- + HBuf \quad \rightarrow \quad Buf^- + H_2CO_3 \quad \rightarrow \quad CO_2 + H_2O$$

Thus, with diuretic therapy or vomiting, it is the urinary or gastrointestinal losses of H^+ that are primarily responsible for the metabolic alkalosis.[6] The major contribution of volume contraction is in maintenance of the alkalosis by preventing excretion of the excess HCO_3^- in the urine.

SYMPTOMS

Patients with metabolic alkalosis may be asymptomatic or complain of symptoms related either to volume depletion (weakness, muscle cramps, postural dizziness) or to hypokalemia (polyuria, polydipsia, muscle weakness). Complaints directly related to alkalemia, however, are uncommon. Paresthesias, carpopedal spasm, and light-headedness occur in acute respiratory alkalosis but are seen much less frequently in metabolic alkalosis. This difference is probably related to the degree of alkalosis in the central nervous system: HCO_3^-, a polar compound, crosses the blood-brain barrier much more slowly than the lipid-soluble CO_2, producing a

---

* The indications for the use of HCO_3^- in lactic acidosis and ketoacidosis are discussed in Chaps. 19 and 25.

lesser increase in the cerebrospinal fluid pH.[86] Thus, the potentially severe neuro-logic abnormalities that may be seen in posthypercapnic alkalosis[61] are probably due to the sudden fall in P_{CO_2}, not the persistent elevation in the plasma HCO_3^- concentration.

The physical examination is not usually helpful, revealing only signs of volume depletion, such as reduced skin turgor, low estimated jugular venous pressure, and postural hypotension, in selected cases. There may, however, be relatively specific findings in patients with self-induced vomiting. These include ulcers, calluses, and scarring on the dorsum of the hand; dental erosions due to chronic exposure to the acid gastric secretions; and puffy cheeks resulting from hypertrophy of the salivary glands.[50]

DIAGNOSIS

The etiology of metabolic alkalosis almost always is obtainable from the history. If there is no pertinent history, then the most likely diagnoses are *surreptitious vomiting or diuretic ingestion or one of the causes of mineralocorticoid excess*. The urine Cl^- concentration can be helpful in differentiating between these conditions (Table 18-3).

Urine Chloride Concentration

The combination of hypovolemia and hypochloremia in patients with vomiting or cystic fibrosis or those taking diuretics should induce maximum renal Cl^- conservation, usually lowering the urine Cl^- concentration to less than 25 meq/L. (This excludes the period during which the diuretic is acting, when Cl^- excretion is elevated.) These patients may also show the physical findings of volume depletion or of self-induced vomiting described above. In contrast, the signs of hypovolemia are absent and the urine Cl^- concentration exceeds 40 meq/L in patients with mineralocorticoid excess or alkali loading, who are generally volume-expanded and in whom Cl^- excretion is equal to intake.

Metabolic alkalosis is the major clinical setting in which the *urine Cl^- concentration may be a more accurate estimate of volume status than is the urine Na^+*

Table 18-3   Urine Cl^- concentration in patients with metabolic alkalosis

Less than 25 meq/L	Greater than 40 meq/L
Vomiting or nasogastric suction	Primary mineralocorticoid excess
Diuretics (late)	Diuretics (early)
Factitious diarrhea	Alkali load (bicarbonate or other organic anion)
Posthypercapnia	Bartter's or Gitelman's syndrome
Cystic fibrosis	Severe hypokalemia (plasma $[K^+] < 2.0$ meq/L)
Low chloride intake	

concentration.[87] Although hypovolemia leads to Na^+ retention, this may be counteracted by the necessity for Na^+ to be excreted with the excess HCO_3^-. As depicted in Fig. 18-3, the maximum reabsorptive capacity for HCO_3^- may be markedly increased by volume depletion and the associated Na^+ retention. This response, however, takes 3 to 4 days to reach completion, leading to variability in the urinary findings (Table 18-4).[23,49]

In the first few days of vomiting, there is a high filtered HCO_3^- concentration and hyperaldosteronism but an inability to maximally conserve HCO_3^-. As a result, some of the excess HCO_3^- is delivered out of the proximal tubule as $NaHCO_3$, and some of this Na^+ is then exchanged for K^+ in the cortical collecting tubule under the influence of aldosterone. The net effect is relatively high rates of Na^+, K^+, and HCO_3^- excretion, the latter leading to an alkaline urine pH. The urinary loss of potentially large amounts of K^+ during this early period is primarily responsible for the K^+ depletion that commonly occurs with persistent or massive vomiting; gastric losses play a lesser role, since K^+ concentration in gastric secretions is only 5 to 10 meq/L. The urine Cl^- concentration is appropriately reduced at this time, the only urinary sign pointing toward hypovolemia.

The urinary chemistries change dramatically once HCO_3^- reabsorptive capacity increases sufficiently to reabsorb all of the filtered HCO_3^-.[23] At this time, excretion of Na^+, K^+, HCO_3^-, and Cl^- are all reduced, and there is a paradoxically acid urine pH (Table 18-4). This late phase is dependent upon volume and Cl^- depletion being severe enough to allow all of the filtered HCO_3^- to be reabsorbed. Some patients ingest enough NaCl so that the filtered HCO_3^- concentration remains above reabsorptive capacity, leading to persistent urinary changes similar to those in the early phase. Again, it is the low urine Cl^- concentration that will point toward the correct diagnosis.

The urine Cl^- concentration may not be useful in patients who are unable to maximally conserve Cl^- because of a defect in tubular reabsorption. This abnormality may occur with renal insufficiency or with severe hypokalemia (plasma K^+ concentration below 2.0 meq/L), in which distal Cl^- reabsorption appears to be impaired.[39,40,88] In these settings, the urine Cl^- concentration may be elevated despite the presence of volume depletion.

Metabolic Alkalosis versus Respiratory Acidosis

An elevated plasma HCO_3^- concentration, hypercapnia, and hypoxemia all may be found in chronic respiratory acidosis as well as in metabolic alkalosis (see Chap.

Table 18-4 Variation in urine electrolytes with vomiting

Time	$[Na^+]$	$[K^+]$	$[Cl^-]$	$[HCO_3^-]$	pH
Days 1–3	↑	↑	↓	↑	> 6.5
Late	↓	↓	↓	↓	< 5.5

20). If uncomplicated, these disorders can be easily differentiated by measuring the arterial pH. However, this distinction becomes more difficult when the patient with underlying chronic lung disease develops a superimposed metabolic alkalosis. As an example, consider the following case history:

Case History 18-1   A 45-year-old man with a long smoking history reports 1 week of recurrent vomiting and has the following arterial blood values on room air:

$$pH = 7.49$$

$$P_{CO_2} = 55 \text{ mmHg}$$

$$[HCO_3^-] = 40 \text{ meq/L}$$

$$P_{CO_2} = 68 \text{ mmHg}$$

Comment   The high P_{CO_2} is compatible with either an appropriate respiratory compensation to metabolic alkalosis or underlying lung disease in this chronic smoker. The simplest way to establish the correct diagnosis is to treat the metabolic alkalosis and follow the P_{CO_2}, which should return to normal if there is no impairment in pulmonary function.

It also may be helpful in selected cases to calculate the alveolar-arterial (A-a) oxygen gradient (see page 663):[89]

$$(\text{A-a}) \text{ O}_2 \text{ gradient} = P_{I_{O_2}} - 1.25 P_{CO_2} - P_{a_{O_2}}$$

$$= 150 - (1.25 \times 55) - 68$$

$$= 13 \text{ mmHg}$$

where $P_{I_{O_2}}$ refers to the partial pressure of oxygen in the inspired air (150 mmHg at sea level) and $P_{a_{O_2}}$ is the partial pressure of oxygen in arterial blood. A normal (A-a) O_2 gradient suggests that pulmonary function is normal and that this patient has a pure metabolic alkalosis. However, the converse is not necessarily true. An increased gradient is not diagnostic of chronic respiratory acidosis, since it can be seen in many acute and chronic pulmonary diseases not associated with CO_2 retention.

TREATMENT

Metabolic alkalosis can be corrected most easily be the urinary excretion of the excess HCO_3^-. This does not occur spontaneously because, in the patient with relatively normal renal function, volume, Cl^-, and/or K^+ depletion leads to enhanced net HCO_3^- reabsorption.[9-11] Therefore, the aim of therapy is to repair these deficits, which will have two beneficial effects: a decrease in HCO_3^- reabsorption, thereby allowing the excess HCO_3^- to be excreted, and, with K^+ repletion, a direct reduction in the plasma HCO_3^- concentration because of the reciprocal shift of K^+ into and H^+ out of the cells.[1,2] As will be seen, this requires the *administration of Cl^-, as NaCl, KCl, or HCl.*[30,90,91]

Treatment should also be directed at the underlying disease and at diminishing further H^+ loss. In patients with continued vomiting or nasogastric suction, for example, the administration of an H_2-blocker or proton pump inhibitor can markedly reduce the rate of gastric H^+ secretion.[92]

Saline-Responsive Alkalosis

The most common causes of metabolic alkalosis are vomiting, nasogastric suction, and diuretic therapy. In these disorders (and with posthypercapnia and a low chloride intake), the increase in HCO_3^- reabsorption that maintains the alkalosis can be reversed by the oral or intravenous administration of NaCl and water, e.g., as half-isotonic or isotonic saline (Table 18-5).[30,90,91] This regimen can lower the plasma HCO_3^- concentration in three ways:

- By reversal of the contraction component.
- By removing the stimulus to renal Na^+ retention, thereby permitting $NaHCO_3$ excretion in the urine.
- By increasing distal Cl^- delivery, which will promote HCO_3^- secretion in the cortical collecting tubule. Studies in experimental animals suggest that increased HCO_3^- secretion is the primary factor responsible for the corrective bicarbonaturia following NaCl administration.[29]

The therapeutic effectiveness of this regimen can be followed at the bedside by measuring the *urine pH*. The urine pH is often below 5.5 prior to therapy as a result of enhanced H^+ secretion. However, when volume and Cl^- replacement are sufficient to allow the excess HCO_3^- to be excreted, the urine pH will exceed 7.0 and occasionally 8.0. The urine Cl^- concentration will remain below 25 meq/L until the Cl^- is corrected.

The efficacy of fluid repletion is dependent upon the administration of Na^+ with the only *reabsorbable* anion, Cl^-.[90,93] As this Na^+ enters the glomerular filtrate, it is reabsorbed with Cl^-, resulting in volume expansion. The outcome

Table 18-5 Causes of metabolic alkalosis according to saline responsiveness

Saline-responsive	Saline-resistant
Vomiting or nasogastric suction	Edematous states
Diuretics	Mineralocorticoid excess
Posthypercapnia	Severe hypokalemia
Low chloride intake	Renal failure

is different if Na^+ is given with an impermeant anion, such as SO_4^{2-}. Reabsorption of this Na^+ in the distal nephron must now be accompanied by H^+ (or K^+) secretion to maintain electroneutrality.[93] The resulting increase in H^+ secretion will generate more HCO_3^- in the plasma, leading to exacerbation of the alkalosis.

Although adequate NaCl repletion will usually normalize the plasma HCO_3^- concentration, it will not reverse any K^+ depletion that might be present. As with Na^+, the administration of K^+ with any anion other than Cl^- results in an increase in H^+ secretion, preventing correction of the alkalosis.[90,94] This is important clinically, since many of the commercial K^+ supplements contain HCO_3^-, acetate, or citrate. Only KCl will be effective.

The requirement for Cl^- replacement also applies to those patients who are treated with an acid infusion (see below). HCl will be effective, because the initial buffering of the excess acid will generate NaCl:

$$HCl + NaHCO_3 \quad \rightarrow \quad NaCl + H_2CO_3 \quad \rightarrow \quad CO_2 + H_2O \qquad (18\text{-}1)$$

In comparison, the administration of nitric acid will generate $NaNO_3$:

$$HNO_3 + NaHCO_3 \quad \rightarrow \quad NaNO_3 + H_2CO_3 \quad \rightarrow \quad CO_2 + H_2O$$

The delivery of this Na^+ to the distal nephron with impermeant NO_3^- will again increase distal H^+ secretion.[95] The net effect is excretion of the administered acid and persistence of the alkalosis.

With the exception of patients with hypotension, shock, or severe associated electrolyte disturbances, *gradual* saline or half-isotonic saline repletion is preferable, since it will restore normovolemia while minimizing the risk of volume overload and pulmonary edema. The optimal rate of fluid replacement is somewhat arbitrary. A regimen that has been successful is the infusion of the appropriate replacement fluid at the rate of 50 to 100 mL/h *in excess of the sum* of the urine output, estimated insensible losses (approximately 30 to 50 mL/h), and any other losses that may be present (such as diarrhea or tube drainage).

Saline-Resistant Alkalosis

The administration of saline is occasionally ineffective in correcting the alkalosis. This typically occurs in edematous states and in those disorders in which K^+ depletion, not hypovolemia, is responsible for perpetuation of the alkalosis (Table 18-5).

Edematous states Patients with heart failure, cirrhosis, or the nephrotic syndrome often develop metabolic alkalosis following diuretic therapy. Both a reduction in the effective circulating volume, leading to Na^+-avidity, and renal insufficiency can contribute to the inability to excrete the excess HCO_3^- in these disorders. However, the administration of saline is not indicated, since it will increase the degree of edema, perhaps precipitating pulmonary edema in the presence of heart failure. Corrective therapy consists of withholding diuretics if possible, acetazolamide, HCl, or dialysis.

Acetazolamide (250 to 375 mg, once or twice a day, given orally or intravenously) is a carbonic anhydrase inhibitor that increases the renal excretion of $NaHCO_3$ (see Chap. 15).[96,97] This serves the dual purpose of treating both the edema and the alkalosis. As with the use of saline in saline-responsive states, the efficacy of acetazolamide can be assessed by monitoring the urine pH, which should exceed 7.0 if HCO_3^- excretion is substantially enhanced. K^+ balance must be carefully followed, since acetazolamide increases urinary K^+ excretion.[96,97]

Acetazolamide can also be used in edematous patients with cor pulmonale and chronic hypercapnia.[98,99] Correction of the alkalemia may be particularly important in this setting, since the rise in pH can further depress ventilation.[98] There are, however, some potential problems, as acetazolamide can induce both a transient, further elevation in the P_{CO_2} (usually 3 to 7 mmHg) and marked acidemia if there is an excessive reduction in the plasma HCO_3^- concentration.[100,101] The exacerbation of the hypercapnia, which is generally not clinically important, is due to partial inhibition of carbonic anhydrase in red cells. This enzyme catalyzes the hydration of CO_2 to H_2CO_3, a reaction that is essential for CO_2 transport by the red cells and therefore for the elimination of CO_2 by the lungs.

If acetazolamide is ineffective and the alkalemia is moderately severe, HCl can be used to lower the plasma HCO_3^- concentration.[102,103] The amount of HCl required to normalize the plasma HCO_3^- concentration is equal to the HCO_3^- excess, which can be estimated from

$$HCO_3^- \text{ excess} = HCO_3^- \text{ space} \times HCO_3^- \text{ excess per liter}$$

In metabolic alkalosis, the HCO_3^- space is approximately 50 percent of the lean body weight.[104] If the normal plasma HCO_3^- concentration is 24 meq/L, then

$$HCO_3^- \text{ excess} = 0.5 \times \text{lean body weight (kg)} \times (\text{plasma } [HCO_3^-] - 24)$$

Thus, in a 60-kg patient with a plasma HCO_3^- concentration of 40 meq/L,

$$HCO_3^- \text{ excess} = 0.5 \times 60 \times (40 - 24)$$

$$= 480 \text{ meq}$$

It should be noted that this formula *underestimates* the acid requirement of a patient in a nonsteady state. As an example, continued losses from nasogastric suction must be added on to the initial estimate of the HCO_3^- excess.

HCl is usually given as an isotonic solution (150 meq each of H^+ and Cl^- in 1 liter of distilled water) over 8 to 24 h.[11,102] Since HCl is very corrosive, it should be infused into a major vein, such as the subclavian or femoral vein. However, a peripheral vein can be safely used if the HCl is buffered in an amino acid solution and infused with a fat emulsion.[103]

Ammonium chloride and arginine hydrochloride, which result in the formation of HCl, should not be given, since they may lead to appreciable toxicity. Ammonium chloride is converted into HCl and ammonia in the liver; the ensuing accumulation of ammonia makes this drug contraindicated in patients with advanced liver disease. Furthermore, an ammonia-related metabolic encephalo-pathy, characterized by lethargy and coma, may occur even in patients with nor-mal hepatic and renal function.[105] Arginine hydrochloride, on the other hand, can induce potentially life-threatening hyperkalemia.[106,107] This effect is thought to result from the movement of cellular potassium into the extracellular fluid as the cationic arginine enters the cells.

Mineralocorticoid excess   States of primary mineralocorticoid excess are charac-terized by mild volume expansion and a rate of urinary Na^+ excretion that is equal to intake (due to aldosterone escape; see page 185). The alkalosis in this setting is resistant to saline, since neither renal Na^+ avidity nor Cl^- depletion is the limiting factor in HCO_3^- excretion.[41] In contrast, it is the combination of hypo-kalemia and hypersecretion of aldosterone that is responsible for perpetuation of the alkalosis.[9,10,41,42] Correction of the hypokalemia tends to lower the plasma HCO_3^- concentration in two ways:[41] by allowing increased HCO_3^- excretion and by causing H^+ ions to move out of the cells into the extracellular fluid.[1,2]

Successful treatment requires the restoration of normal mineralocorticoid activity (see Chap. 27). This can be achieved by surgical removal of an adrenal adenoma or by the use of a K^+-sparing diuretic, such as amiloride or the aldo-sterone antagonist spironolactone.[108]

Severe hypokalemia   Patients with metabolic alkalosis and hypovolemia may be resistant to saline therapy in the presence of severe K^+ depletion.[88] In this setting, the total K^+ deficit usually is greater than 800 to 1000 meq, the plasma K^+ concentration generally is less than 2.0 meq/L, and the urine Cl^- concentration exceeds 15 meq/L despite the presence of volume depletion. This defect in Cl^- conservation, which appears to be due to diminished distal Cl^- reabsorption,[39,40] may explain the negative response to saline. If Cl^- reabsorption is impaired and the availability of K^+ for exchange with Na^+ is limited, then Na^+ reabsorption must be accompanied by increased H^+ secretion and HCO_3^- reabsorption,[40] thereby preventing a HCO_3^- diuresis. Diminished Cl^- reabsorption could also impair corrective HCO_3^- secretion in the cortical collecting tubule, a process that appears to be mediated by Cl^-/HCO_3^- exchange.

These effects of severe hypokalemia are readily reversible. The replacement of only one-half of the K^+ deficit will normalize Cl^- reabsorption and restore saline responsiveness, as the administration of saline will now correct the alkalosis.[88]

Renal failure   Rarely, a patient with renal failure develops metabolic alkalosis, usually as a result of marked gastric losses by nasogastric suction. In this setting, either HCl or dialysis can be used if the alkalemia is severe.[109] However, a special, low-buffer dialysis solution must be used, since normal solutions contain 35 to 40 meq/L of bicarbonate or an organic anion (such as acetate), which generates HCO_3^- when metabolized.[109]

PROBLEMS

18-1 A patient with cirrhosis and ascites is admitted to the hospital with acute gastrointestinal bleeding due to ruptured esophageal varices. He is taken to surgery, where a portacaval shunt is performed. He is given a total of 19 units of blood before and during the surgery. Although the ascites was removed during the surgery, it begins to reaccumulate postoperatively. His laboratory tests were normal preoperatively, but the following values are obtained 12 h after surgery:

$$\text{arterial pH} = 7.53$$

$$P_{CO_2} = 50 \text{ mmHg}$$

$$[HCO_3^-] = 40 \text{ meq/L}$$

(a) What is responsible for the development of the metabolic alkalosis?
(b) What would you expect the urine pH and Na^+ concentration to be?
(c) How would you correct the alkalosis?

18-2 A 45-year-old woman with peptic ulcer disease reports 6 days of persistent vomiting. On physical examination, the blood pressure is found to be 100/60 without postural change, the skin turgor is decreased, and the jugular neck veins are flat. The initial laboratory data are

Plasma [Na$^+$]	=	140 meq/L	BUN	=	80 mg/dL
[K$^+$]	=	2.2 meq/L	[Creatinine]	=	1.9 mg/dL
[Cl$^-$]	=	86 meq/L	Urine pH	=	5.0
[HCO$_3^-$]	=	42 meq/L	[Na$^+$]	=	2 meq/L
Arterial pH	=	7.53	[K$^+$]	=	21 meq/L
P$_{CO_2}$	=	53 mmHg	[Cl$^-$]	=	3 meq/L

(a) How would you treat this patient?

Twenty-four hours after appropriate therapy has been started, the plasma HCO$_3^-$ concentration is 30 meq/L. The following urinary values are obtained:

$$\text{Urine } [Na^+] = 100 \text{ meq/L}$$

$$[K^+] = 20 \text{ meq/L}$$

$$[Cl^-] = 3 \text{ meq/L}$$

(b) How do you account for the discrepancy between the high urine Na$^+$ concentration and the low urine Cl$^-$ concentration?

18-3 A 22-year-old woman complains of easy fatigability and weakness for 1 year. She has no other symptoms. The physical examination is unremarkable, including a normal blood pressure. The following laboratory tests have been repeatedly present during this time:

$$\text{Plasma } [Na^+] = 141 \text{ meq/L}$$

$$[K^+] = 2.1 \text{ meq/L}$$

$$[Cl^-] = 85 \text{ meq/L}$$

$$[HCO_3^-] = 45 \text{ meq/L}$$

$$\text{Urine } [Na^+] = 80 \text{ meq/day}$$

$$[K^+] = 170 \text{ meq/day}$$

(a) What is the differential diagnosis?
(b) What test would you order next?

REFERENCES

1. Cooke RE, Segar W, Cheek DB, et al. The extrarenal correction of alkalosis associated with potassium deficiency. *J Clin Invest* 31:798, 1952.
2. Orloff J, Kennedy T Jr, Berliner RW. The effect of potassium in nephrectomized rats with hypokalemic alkalosis. *J Clin Invest* 32:538, 1953.
3. Adler S, Zett B, Anderson B. The effect of acute potassium depletion on muscle cell pH in vitro. *Kidney Int* 2:159, 1972.
4. Adam WR, Koretsky AP, Weiner MW. ^{31}P-NMR in vivo measurement of renal intracellular pH: Effects of acidosis and potassium depletion in rats. *Am J Physiol* 251:F904, 1986.
5. Cannon PJ, Heinemann HO, Albert MS, et al. "Contraction" alkalosis after diuresis of edematous patients with ethacrynic acid. *Ann Intern Med* 62:979, 1965.
6. Garella S, Chang BS, Kahn SI. Dilution acidosis and contraction alkalosis: Review of a concept. *Kidney Int* 8:279, 1975.
7. Van Goidsenhoven G, Gray OV, Price AV, Sanderson PH. The effect of prolonged administration of large doses of sodium bicarbonate in man. *Clin Sci* 13:383, 1954.
8. Berger BE, Cogan MG, Sebastian A. Reduced glomerular filtration rate and enhanced bicarbonate reabsorption maintain metabolic alkalosis in humans. *Kidney Int* 26:205, 1984.
9. Jacobson HR, Seldin DW. On the generation, maintenance, and correction of metabolic alkalosis. *Am J Physiol* 245:F425, 1983.
10. Sabatini S, Kurtzman NA. The maintenance of metabolic alkalosis: Factors which decrease HCO$_3^-$ excretion. *Kidney Int* 25:357, 1984.
11. Palmer BF, Alpern RJ. Metabolic alkalosis. *J Am Soc Nephrol* 8:1462, 1997.
12. Cogan MG, Cameiro AV, Tatsuno J, et al. Normal diet NaCl variation can affect the renal set-point for plasma pH-(HCO$_3^-$) maintenance. *J Am Soc Nephrol* 1:193, 1990.
13. Galla JH, Gifford JD, Luke RG, Rome L. Adaptations to chloride-depletion alkalosis. *Am J Physiol* 261:R771, 1991.
14. Galla JH, Bonduris DN, Luke RG. Effects of chloride and extracellular fluid volume on bicarbonate reabsorption along the nephron in metabolic alkalosis in the rat. Reassessment of the classic hypothesis on the pathogenesis of metabolic alkalosis. *J Clin Invest* 80:41, 1987.
15. Wesson D. Augmented bicarbonate reabsorption by both the proximal and distal nephron maintains chloride-deplete metabolic alkalosis in rats. *J Clin Invest* 84:1460, 1989.
16. Cogan MG, Alpern RJ. Regulation of proximal bicarbonate reabsorption. *Am J Physiol* 247:F387, 1984.
17. Liu F-Y, Cogan MG. Angiotensin II stimulates early proximal bicarbonate absorption in the rat by decreasing cyclic adenosine monophosphate. *J Clin Invest* 84:83, 1989.
18. Akiba T, Rocco VK, Warnock DG. Parallel adaptation of the rabbit renal cortical sodium/proton antiporter and sodium/bicarbonate cotransporter in metabolic acidosis and alkalosis. *J Clin Invest* 80.308, 1987.
19. Stone DK, Seldin DW, Kokko JP, Jacobson HR. Mineralocorticoid modulation of rabbit kidney medullary collecting duct acidification. A sodium-independent effect. *J Clin Invest* 72:77, 1983.
20. Garg LC, Narang N. Effects of aldosterone on NEM-sensitive ATPases in rabbit nephron segments. *Kidney Int* 34:13, 1988.
21. Batlle DC. Segmental characterization of defects in collecting tubule acidification. *Kidney Int* 30:546, 1986.
22. Harrington JT, Hulter HN, Cohen JJ, Madias NE. Mineralocorticoid-stimulated renal acidification: The critical role of dietary sodium. *Kidney Int* 30:43, 1986.
23. Kassirer JP, Schwartz WB. The response of normal man to selective depletion of hydrochloric acid: Factors in the genesis of persistent gastric alkalosis. *Am J Med* 40:10, 1966.
24. Wesson DE. Depressed distal tubule acidification corrects chloride-deplete metabolic alkalosis. *Am J Physiol* 259:F636, 1990.
25. Rosen RA, Julian BA, Dubovsky EV, et al. On the mechanism by which chloride corrects metabolic alkalosis in man. *Am J Med* 84:449, 1988.

26. Kotchen TA, Luke RG, Ott CE, et al. Effect of chloride on renal and blood pressure responses to sodium chloride. *Ann Intern Med* 98(part 2):817, 1983.

27. Stone DK, Xie X-S. Proton translocating ATPases: Issues in structure and function. *Kidney Int* 33:767, 1988.

28. Bastani B, Purcell H, Hemken P, et al. Expression and distribution of renal vacuolar proton-translocating adenosine triphosphatase in response to chronic acid and alkali loads in the rat. *J Clin Invest* 88:126, 1991.

29. Wesson DE, Dolson GM. Enhanced HCO_3 secretion by distal tubule contributes to NaCl-induced correction of chronic alkalosis. *Am J Physiol* 264:F899, 1993.

30. Kassirer JP, Schwartz WB. Correction of metabolic alkalosis in man without repair of potassium deficiency. *Am J Med* 40:19, 1966.

31. Capasso G, Jaeger P, Giebisch G, et al. Renal bicarbonate reabsorption in the rat. II. Distal tubule load dependence and effect of hypokalemia. *J Clin Invest* 80:409, 1987.

32. Capasso G, Kinne R, Malnic G, Giebisch G. Renal bicarbonate reabsorption in the rat: I. Effects of hypokalemia and carbonic anhydrase. *J Clin Invest* 78:1558, 1986.

33. Garg LC. Respective roles of H-ATPase and H-K-ATPase in ion transport in the kidney. *J Am Soc Nephrol* 2:949, 1991.

34. Wingo C. Active proton secretion and potassium absorption in the rabbit outer medullary collecting duct. Functional evidence for proton-potassium-activated adenosine triphosphatase. *J Clin Invest* 84:361, 1989.

35. Wingo CS, Smulka AJ. Function and structure of H-K-ATPase in the kidney. *Am J Physiol* 269:F1, 1995.

36. Doucet A, Marsy S. Characterization of K-ATPase activity in distal nephron: Stimulation by potassium depletion. *Am J Physiol* 253:F418, 1987.

37. Codina J, Delmas-Mata J, DuBose TD. Expression of HK2 protein is increased selectively in renal medulla by chronic hypokalemia. *Am J Physiol* 275:F433, 1998.

38. Elam-Ong S, Kurtzman NA, Sabatini S. Regulation of collecting tubule adenosine triphosphatases by aldosterone and potassium. *J Clin Invest* 91:2385, 1993.

39. Luke RG, Wright FS, Fowler N, et al. Effects of potassium depletion on renal tubular chloride transport in the rat. *Kidney Int* 14:414, 1978.

40. Hulter HN, Sigala JF, Sebastian A. K^+ deprivation potentiates the renal alkalosis-producing effect of mineralocorticoid. *Am J Physiol* 235:F298, 1978.

41. Kurtzman NA, White MG, Rogers PW. Pathophysiology of metabolic alkalosis. *Arch Intern Med* 131:702, 1973.

42. Kassirer JP, London AM, Goldman DM, Schwartz WB. On the pathogenesis of metabolic alkalosis in hyperaldosteronism. *Am J Med* 49:306, 1970.

43. Javaheri S, Shore NS, Rose BD, Kazemi H. Compensatory hypoventilation in metabolic alkalosis. *Chest* 81:296, 1982.

44. Javaheri S, Kazemi H. Metabolic alkalosis and hypoventilation in humans. *Am Rev Respir Dis* 136:1011, 1987.

45. Berger AJ, Mitchell RA, Severinghaus JW. Regulation of respiration. *N Engl J Med* 297:92, 138, 194, 1977.

46. Javaheri S, Nardell EA. Severe metabolic alkalosis: A case report. *Br Med J* 2:1016, 1981.

47. Madias NE, Adrogue HH, Cohen JJ. Maladaptive response to secondary hypercapnia in chronic metabolic alkalosis. *Am J Physiol* 238:F283, 1980.

48. Wilkes JM, Garner A, Peters TJ. Mechanisms of acid disposal and acid-stimulated alkaline secretion by gastroduodenal mucosa. *Dig Dis Sci* 33:361, 1988.

49. Perez GO, Oster JR, Rogers A. Acid-base disturbances in gastrointestinal disease. *Dig Dis Sci* 32:1033, 1987.

50. Mitchell JE, Seim HC, Colon E, Pomeroy C. Medical complications and medical management of bulimia. *Ann Intern Med* 107:71, 1987.

51. Stemmer CL, Oster JR, Vaamonde CA, et al. Effect of routine doses of antacid on renal acidification. *Lancet* 2:3, 1986.

52. Madias NE, Levey AS. Metabolic alkalosis due to absorption of "nonabsorbable" antacids. *Am J Med* 74:155, 1983.

53. Gorden P, Levitin H. Congenital alkalosis with diarrhea: A sequel to Darrow's original description. *Ann Intern Med* 78:876, 1973.
54. Hoglund P, Haila S, Socha J, et al. Mutations of the Down-regulated adenoma (DRA) gene cause congenital chloride diarrhoea. *Nat Genet* 14:316, 1996.
55. Aichbichler BW, Zerr CH, Santa Ana CA, et al. Proton-pump inhibition of gastric chloride secretion in congenital chloridorrhea. *N Engl J Med* 336:106, 1997.
56. Labowitz J, Wald A. Factitious diarrhea and Munchausen's syndrome, in Rose BD (ed): *UpToDate in Medicine*, Wellesley, MA, UpToDate, 2000.
57. Oster JR, Materson BJ, Rogers AI. Laxative abuse syndrome. *Am J Gastroenterol* 74:451, 1980.
58. Seldin D, Welt L, Cort J. The role of sodium salts and adrenal steroids in the production of hypokalemic alkalosis. *Yale J Biol Med* 29:229, 1956.
59. Hropot M, Fowler N, Karlmark B, Giesbisch G. Tubular action of diuretics: Distal effects on electrolyte transport and acidification. *Kidney Int* 28:477, 1985.
60. Polak A, Haynie GD, Hays RM, Schwartz WB. Effects of chronic hypercapnia on electrolyte and acid-base equilibrium: I. Adaptation. *J Clin Invest* 40:1223, 1961.
61. Rotheram EB Jr, Safar P, Robin ED. CNS disorder during mechanical ventilation in chronic pulmonary disease. *JAMA* 189:993, 1964.
62. Cogan MG. Chronic hypercapnia stimulates proximal bicarbonate reabsorption in the rat. *J Clin Invest* 74:1942, 1984.
63. Reihman DH, Farber MO, Weinberger MH, et al. Effect of hypoxemia on sodium and water excretion in chronic obstructive lung disease. *Am J Med* 78:87, 1985.
64. Schwartz WB, Hays RM, Polak A, Haynie G. Effects of chronic hypercapnia on electrolyte and acid-base equilibrium: II. Recovery with special reference to the influence of chloride intake. *J Clin Invest* 40:1238, 1961.
65. Linshaw MA, Harrison HL, Gruskin AB, et al. Hypochloremic alkalosis in infants associated with soy protein formula. *J Pediatr* 96:635, 1980.
66. Klastersky J, Vanderkelen B, Daneua D, Mathieu M. Carbenicillin and hypokalemia (letter). *Ann Intern Med* 78:744, 1973.
67. Brunner FP, Frick PG. Hypokalemia, metabolic alkalosis, and hypernatremia due to "massive" sodium penicillin therapy. *Br Med J* 4:550, 1968.
68. Lipner HT, Ruzany F, Dasgupta M, et al. The behavior of carbenicillin as a nonreabsorbable anion. *J Lab Clin Med* 86:183, 1975.
69. Crumb CK, Martinez-Maldonado M, Eknoyan G, Suki W. Effects of volume expansion, purified parathyroid extract, and calcium on renal bicarbonate absorption in the dog. *J Clin Invest* 54:1287, 1974.
70. Hulter HN, Sebastian A, Toto RD, et al. Renal and systemic acid-based effects of the chronic administration of hypercalcemia-producing agents: Calcitriol, PTH, and intravenous calcium. *Kidney Int* 21:445, 1982.
71. Heinemann HO. Metabolic alkalosis in patients with hypercalcemia. *Metabolism* 14:1131, 1965.
72. Coe FL. Magnitude of metabolic acidosis in primary hyperparathyroidism. *Arch Intern Med* 134:262, 1974.
73. Hulter HN, Peterson JC. Acid-base homeostasis during chronic PTH excess in humans. *Kidney Int* 28:187, 1985.
74. McMillan DE, Freeman RB. The milk-alkali syndrome: A study of the acute disorder with comments on the development of the chronic condition. *Medicine* 44:485, 1965.
75. Kapsner P, Langsdorf L, Marcus R, et al. Milk-alkali syndrome in patients treated with calcium carbonate after cardiac transplantation. *Arch Intern Med* 146:1965, 1986.
76. Beall DP, Scofield RH. Milk-alkali syndrome associated with calcium carbonate consumption. *Medicine* 74:89, 1995.
77. Stinebaugh BJ, Schloeder FX. Glucose-induced alkalosis in fasting subjects: Relationship to renal bicarbonate reabsorption during fasting and refeeding. *J Clin Invest* 51:1326, 1972.

78. Fulop M, Horowitz M, Aberman A, Jaffee E. Lactic acidosis in pulmonary edema due to left ventricular failure. *Ann Intern Med* 79:180, 1973.
79. Seldin DW, Tarail R. The metabolism of glucose and electrolytes in diabetic acidosis. *J Clin Invest* 29:552, 1950.
80. Litwin M, Smith L, Moore FD. Metabolic alkalosis following massive transfusion. *Surgery* 45:805, 1959.
81. Kelleher SP, Schulman G. Severe metabolic alkalosis complicating regional citrate hemodialysis. *Am J Kidney Dis* 9:235, 1987.
82. Rahilly GT, Berl T. Severe metabolic alkalosis caused by administration of plasma protein fraction in end-stage renal failure. *N Engl J Med* 301:824, 1979.
83. Mattar JA, Weil MH, Shubin H, Stein L. Cardiac arrest in the critically ill: II. Hyperosmolal states following cardiac arrest. *Am J Med* 56:162, 1974.
84. Levin T. What this patient didn't need: A dose of salts. *Hosp Pract* 18(7):95, 1983.
85. Kennedy JD, Dinwiddie R, Daman-Willems C, et al. Pseudo-Bartter's syndrome in cystic fibrosis. *Arch Dis Child* 65:786, 1990.
86. Mitchell RA, Carman CT, Severinghaus JW, et al. Stability of cerebrospinal fluid pH in chronic acid-base disturbances in blood. *J Appl Physiol* 20:443, 1965.
87. Sherman RA, Eisinger RP. The use (and misuse) of urinary sodium and chloride measurements. *JAMA* 247:3121, 1982.
88. Garella S, Chazan JA, Cohen JJ. Saline-resistant metabolic alkalosis or "chloride-wasting nephropathy." *Ann Intern Med* 73:31, 1970.
89. Snider GL. Interpretation of the arterial oxygen and carbon dioxide partial pressure. *Chest* 63:801, 1973.
90. Schwartz WB, van Ypersele de Strihou CE, Kassirer JP. Role of anions in metabolic alkalosis and potassium deficiency. *N Engl J Med* 279:630, 1968.
91. Cohen JJ. Correction of metabolic alkalosis by the kidney after isometric expansion of extracellular fluid. *J Clin Invest* 47:1181, 1968.
92. Barton CH, Vaziri ND, Ness RI, et al. Cimetidine in the management of metabolic alkalosis induced by nasogastric drainage. *Arch Surg* 114:70, 1979.
93. Schwartz WB, Jenson RL, Relman AS. Acidification of the urine and increased ammonium excretion without change in acid-base equilibrium: Sodium reabsorption as a stimulus to the acidifying process. *J Clin Invest* 34:673, 1955.
94. Bleich HL, Tannen RL, Schwartz WB. The induction of metabolic alkalosis by correction of potassium deficiency. *J Clin Invest* 45:573, 1966.
95. Tannen RL, Bleich HL, Schwartz WB. The renal response to acid loads in metabolic alkalosis: An assessment of the mechanisms regulating acid excretion. *J Clin Invest* 45:562, 1966.
96. Leaf A, Schwartz WB, Relman AS. Oral administration of a potent carbonic anhydrase inhibitor ("Diamox"): I. Changes in electrolyte and acid-base balance. *N Engl J Med* 250:759, 1954.
97. Preisig PA, Toto RD, Alpern RJ. Carbonic anhydrase inhibitors. *Renal Physiol* 10:136, 1987.
98. Bear R, Goldstein M, Philipson M, et al. Effect of metabolic alkalosis on respiratory function in patients with chronic obstructive lung disease. *Can Med Assoc J* 117:900, 1977.
99. Miller PD, Berns AS. Acute metabolic alkalosis perpetuating hypercapnia: A role for acetazolamide in chronic obstructive pulmonary disease. *JAMA* 238:2400, 1977.
100. Bell ALL, Smith CN, Andreae E. Effects of the carbonic anhydrase inhibitor "6063" (Diamox) on respiration and electrolyte metabolism of patients with respiratory acidosis. *Am J Med* 18:536, 1955.
101. Dorris R, Olivia JV, Rodman T. Dichlorphenamide, a potent carbonic anhydrase inhibitor: Effect on alveolar ventilation, ventilation-perfusion relationships and diffusion in patients with chronic lung disease. *Am J Med* 36:79, 1964.
102. Abouna G, Veazey P, Terry D Jr. Intravenous infusion of hydrochloric acid for treatment of severe metabolic alkalosis. *Surgery* 75:194, 1974.
103. Knutsen OH. New method for administration of hydrochloric acid in metabolic alkalosis. *Lancet* 1:953, 1983.

104. Androgué JH, Brensilver J, Cohen JJ, Madias NE. Influence of steady-state alterations in acid-base equilibrium on the fate of administered bicarbonate in the dog. *J Clin Invest* 71:867, 1983.
105. Warren SE, Swerdlin ARH, Steinberg SM. Treatment of alkalosis with ammonium chloride: A case report. *Clin Pharmacol Ther* 25:624, 1979.
106. Bushinsky DA, Gennari FJ. Life-threatening hyperkalemia induced by arginine. *Ann Intern Med* 89:632, 1978.
107. Hertz P, Richardson JA. Arginine-induced hyperkalemia in renal failure patients. *Arch Intern Med* 130:778, 1972.
108. Griffing GT, Cole AG, Aurecchia SA, et al. Amiloride in primary hyperaldosteronism. *Clin Pharmacol Ther* 31:56, 1982.
109. Swartz RD, Rubin JE, Brown RS, et al. Correction of postoperative metabolic alkalosis and renal failure by hemodialysis. *Ann Intern Med* 86:52, 1977.

NINETEEN

METABOLIC ACIDOSIS

The introduction to acid-base disorders in Chap. 17 should be read before proceeding with this discussion. Metabolic acidosis is a clinical disturbance characterized by a low arterial pH (or an increased H^+ concentration), a reduced plasma HCO_3^- concentration, and compensatory hyperventilation, resulting in a decrease in the P_{CO_2}. A low plasma HCO_3^- concentration, however, is not diagnostic of metabolic acidosis, since it also results from the renal compensation to chronic respiratory alkalosis. These disorders can be easily differentiated by measurement of the arterial pH. In addition, a plasma HCO_3^- concentration of 10 meq/L or less is indicative of metabolic acidosis, as the renal compensation to chronic hypocapnia does not produce this degree of hypobicarbonatremia (see Chap. 21).

PATHOPHYSIOLOGY

From the reaction of H^+ with the primary extracellular buffer, HCO_3^-.

$$H^+ + HCO_3^- \leftrightarrow H_2CO_3 \leftrightarrow CO_2 + H_2O \qquad (19\text{-}1)$$

it can be appreciated that metabolic acidosis can be produced in two ways: by the addition of H^+ ions or by the loss of HCO_3^- ions. The latter increases the extracellular H^+ concentration by driving the buffering reaction to the left.

Response to an Acid Load

The response of the body to an increase in the arterial H^+ concentration involves four processes (see Chaps. 10 and 11): extracellular buffering, intracellular and bone buffering, respiratory compensation, and the renal excretion of the H^+ load. The first three act to minimize the increase in H^+ concentration until the kidneys restore acid-base balance by eliminating the excess H^+ in the urine. Since each of these processes has important clinical implications, they will be considered separately.

Extracellular buffering Because of its high concentration, HCO_3^- is the most important buffer in the extracellular fluid. The ability of HCO_3^- to prevent large changes in the arterial pH (or H^+ concentration) can be appreciated if we use the law of mass action to express the relationship between H^+, HCO_3^-, and P_{CO_2} (see page 308):

$$[H^+] = 24 \times \frac{P_{CO_2}}{[HCO_3^-]} \qquad (19\text{-}2)$$

If the normal P_{CO_2} is 40 mmHg and the plasma HCO_3^- concentration is 24 meq/L (equal to 24 mmol/L), then

$$[H^+] = 24 \times \frac{40}{24}$$

$$= 40 \, \text{nanoeq/L} \qquad (pH = 7.40)$$

Let us assume that 12 meq of H^+ is added to each liter of the extracellular fluid. As this H^+ is buffered by HCO_3^-, the plasma HCO_3^- concentration will fall from 24 to 12 meq/L. If the P_{CO_2} remains constant,

$$[H^+] = 24 \times \frac{40}{12}$$

$$= 80 \, \text{nanoeq/L} \qquad (pH = 7.10)$$

Even though 12 meq (or 12 million nanoeq) of H^+ has been added to each liter, the free H^+ concentration has increased by only 40 nanoeq/L or 40×10^{-6} meq/L. Thus, more than 99.99 percent of the extra H^+ ions has been taken up by HCO_3^-, thereby preventing the H^+ concentration from exceeding 160 nanoeq/L (pH equals 6.80), the highest level that is generally compatible with life.

Intracellular buffering and the plasma potassium concentration H^+ ions also are able to enter the cells and be taken up by the cell and bone buffers, including proteins, phosphates, and bone carbonate:

$$H^+ + Pr^- \quad \leftrightarrow \quad HPr$$

On the average, 55 to 60 percent of an acid load will eventually be buffered by the cells and bone, although higher values may occur with severe acidemia when extracellular HCO_3^- stores are markedly reduced.[1-3] As a result, the addition of 12 meq of H^+ to each liter of extracellular fluid will lower the plasma HCO_3^- concentration by 5 meq/L or less, not by 12 meq/L. If the new plasma HCO_3^- concentration is 19 meq/L and the P_{CO_2} remains at 40 mmHg, then

$$[H^+] = 24 \times \frac{40}{19}$$

$$= 51 \, \text{nanoeq/L} \qquad (\text{pH} = 7.29)$$

Thus, the contribution of cellular and bone buffers results in better maintenance of the extracellular H^+ concentration than was seen above when only extracellular HCO_3^- buffering was available (pH = 7.10).

The intracellular entry of H^+ ions in metabolic acidosis is associated in part with the movement of K^+ out of the cells to maintain electroneutrality.[4-6] This response leads to a variable rise in the plasma K^+ concentration that is most prominent in those forms of metabolic acidosis that are due to an excess of non-organic acid, as occurs with renal failure or diarrhea.[5] In the latter setting, the plasma K^+ concentration may be below normal as a result of concurrent intestinal losses, but it is still higher than it would have been in the absence of acidemia.[6]

For reasons that are incompletely understood, the fall in pH in the organic acidosis (such as ketoacidosis, lactic acidosis, or that following certain ingestions) seems to have little effect on K^+ distribution (see page 379).[5,7,8] Hyperkalemia is often present in these disorders, but is primarily due to other factors. In diabetic ketoacidosis and nonketotic hyperglycemia, for example, the combination of insulin deficiency (which retards K^+ entry into cells) and hyperglycemia (which pulls water and, by solvent drag, K^+ out of the cells) frequently leads to hyperkalemia, despite usually marked K^+ depletion due to urinary and gastrointestinal losses.[7,9] Correction of these problems with insulin therapy results in a rapid fall in the plasma K^+ concentration, thereby unmasking the true state of K^+ balance. Hyperkalemia can also occur in lactic acidosis, but it is due to hypoperfusion-induced tissue breakdown and renal failure, not to acidemia.

Respiratory compensation   Metabolic acidosis stimulates both the central and peripheral chemoreceptors controlling respiration, resulting in an increase in alveolar ventilation. The ensuing fall in P_{CO_2} will then raise the extracellular pH toward normal. This increase in ventilation begins within 1 to 2 h and reaches its maximum level at 12 to 24 h.[10] It is characterized more by an increase in tidal volume than by an increase in respiratory rate, and may, if the acidemia is severe, reach a maximum of as much as 30 L/min (normal equals 5 to 6 L/min).[11] This degree of hyperventilation (called Kussmaul's respiration) is usually apparent on physical examination and should alert the physician to a possible underlying metabolic acidosis.

Studies in otherwise normal patients with metabolic acidosis have revealed that, on the average, the P_{CO_2} *will fall 1.2 mmHg for every 1.0-meq/L reduction in the plasma* HCO_3^- *concentration* down to a minimum P_{CO_2} of 10 to 15 mmHg.[12] Suppose, for example, that an acid load lowers the plasma HCO_3^- concentration to 9 meq/L. This decrease of 15 meq/L should be associated with an 18 mmHg (15 × 1.2) fall in the P_{CO_2} to approximately 22 mmHg (pH equals 7.23). Thus, in pure metabolic acidosis with a plasma HCO_3^- concentration of 9 meq/L, the *normal* P_{CO_2} *is roughly 22 mmHg, not 40 mmHg.*

Values substantially different from the predicted P_{CO_2} represent mixed acid-base disorders (Table 19-1). Thus, a "normal" P_{CO_2} of 40 mmHg (pH equals 6.98) in this setting is indicative of a combined metabolic and respiratory acidosis, as might occur in a patient with chronic lung disease. On the other hand, a lower than expected P_{CO_2} of 15 mmHg (pH equals 7.40) suggests a combined metabolic acidosis and respiratory alkalosis, as might be seen with salicylate intoxication (see below).

Although compensatory hyperventilation minimizes the degree of acidemia, this *protective effect appears to last for only a few days.* This limitation occurs because the fall in P_{CO_2} directly lowers renal HCO_3^- reabsorption, resulting in HCO_3^- loss in the urine and a further reduction in the plasma HCO_3^- concentration.[13] It is thought that these changes reflect a hypocapnia-induced rise in renal tubular cell pH, which diminishes H^+ secretion and HCO_3^- reabsorption (see page 360).

The net effect is that the *arterial pH in chronic metabolic acidosis is the same whether or not the respiratory compensation has occurred.*[13] As shown in the example in Table 19-2, for example, the arterial pH is 7.29 in uncompensated metabolic acidosis. The compensatory 6 mmHg decrease in the P_{CO_2} then lowers the plasma HCO_3^- concentration from 19 to 16 meq/L, returning the arterial pH to 7.29. Fortunately, severe metabolic acidosis is usually acute (lactic acidosis, ketoacidosis, ingestions), and the hypocapnia is protective in this setting.

Renal hydrogen excretion   The metabolism of a normal adult diet results in the generation of 50 to 100 meq of H^+ per day, which must then be excreted in the urine if acid-base balance is to be maintained.[14] This process involves two basic steps: reabsorption of the filtered HCO_3^- and secretion of the dietary acid load.

Table 19-1   Arterial measurements in hypothetical acid-base disorders

Acid-base status	Plasma [HCO_3^-], meq/L	P_{CO_2}, mmHg	Arterial pH
Normal	24	40	7.40
Pure metabolic acidosis	9	22	7.23
Combined metabolic and respiratory acidosis	9	40	6.98
Combined metabolic acidosis and respiratory alkalosis	9	15	7.40

Table 19-2 Arterial pH in chronic metabolic acidosis with and without respiratory compensation

Clinical state	Arterial		
	pH	$[HCO_3^-]$, meq/L	P_{CO_2}, mmHg
Baseline	7.40	24	40
Metabolic acidosis			
No compensation	7.29	19	40
Compensation			
Acute	7.37	19	34
Chronic	7.29	16	34

The filtered HCO_3^- must be reabsorbed, since urinary HCO_3^- loss will increase the net acid load and lower the plasma HCO_3^- concentration. Ninety percent of HCO_3^- reabsorption occurs in the proximal tubule and the remainder in the thick ascending limb and the distal nephron (see Chap. 11).

The dietary acid load is excreted by the secretion of H^+ ions from the tubular cell into the lumen. These H^+ ions then combine either with the urinary buffers (particularly HPO_4^{2-} in a process called titratable acidity) or with NH_3:[15]

$$H^+ + HPO_4^{2-} \quad \rightarrow \quad H_2PO_4^- \tag{19-3}$$

$$H^+ + NH_3 \quad \rightarrow \quad NH_4^+ \tag{19-4}$$

In general, 10 to 40 meq of H^+ is excreted each day as titratable acidity and 30 to 60 meq as NH_4^+. These processes are essential for the maintenance of acid-base balance, because the rate of excretion of *free* H^+ ions is extremely low. At the minimum urine pH of 4.50, for example, the free H^+ concentration is less than 0.05 meq/L.

In the absence of therapy with $NaHCO_3$, the correction of metabolic acidosis usually requires the urinary excretion of the excess H^+. The kidney responds to this increased H^+ load by augmenting cellular NH_4^+ production and subsequent excretion,[15,16] changes that may be mediated by the extracellular acidemia producing a parallel reduction in the renal tubular cell pH (see page 347).[17,18] The net effect is that NH_4^+ excretion can exceed 250 meq/day with severe acidemia.[19,20]

In contrast, there generally is only a limited ability to enhance titratable acidity, since phosphate excretion remains relatively constant.[15] One exception occurs in diabetic ketoacidosis, where excreted ketone anions (particularly β-hydroxybutyrate) can act as urinary buffers, increasing titratable acid excretion by up to 50 meq/day.[19] The net effect is that total acid excretion can reach a maximum rate of 500 meq/day (more than five times normal) in patients with severe metabolic acidosis.[19,20]

Generation of Metabolic Acidosis

From this discussion, it can be seen that metabolic acidosis can be induced by two basic mechanisms: an inability of the kidney to excrete the dietary H^+ load or an increase in the generation of H^+ as a result of either the addition of H^+ or the loss of HCO_3^- (Table 19-3). Decreased H^+ excretion produces a *slowly developing acidemia*, since only that fraction of the 50- to 100-meq daily H^+ load that is not excreted will be retained. In comparison, an acute increase in the H^+ load (as with lactic acidosis) can overwhelm renal excretory capacity, leading to the *rapid onset* of severe metabolic acidosis.

Anion Gap

Calculation of the anion gap is often helpful in the differential diagnosis of metabolic acidosis (Table 19-4).[21-23] The anion gap is equal to the difference between the plasma concentrations of the major cation (Na^+) and the major measured anions ($Cl^- + HCO_3$):

Table 19-3   Causes of metabolic acidosis

Inability to excrete the dietary H^+ load
- A. Diminished NH_4^+ production
  1. Renal failure[a]
  2. Hypoaldosteronism (type 4 renal tubular acidosis)[a]
- B. Diminished H^+ secretion
  1. Type 1 (distal) renal tubular acidosis

Increased H^+ load or HCO_3^- loss
- A. Lactic acidosis[a]
- B. Ketoacidosis[a]
- C. Ingestions
  1. Salicylates
  2. Methanol or formaldehyde
  3. Ethylene glycol
  4. Paraldehyde
  5. Sulfur
  6. Toluene
  7. Ammonium chloride
  8. Hyperalimentation fluids
- D. Massive rhabdomyolysis
- E. Gastrointestinal HCO_3^- loss
  1. Diarrhea[a]
  2. Pancreatic, biliary, or intestinal fistulas
  3. Ureterosigmoidostomy
  4. Cholestyramine
- F. Renal HCO_3^- loss
  1. Type 2 (proximal) renal tubular acidosis

[a] Most common causes.

Table 19-4 Anion gap in major causes of metabolic acidosis

High anion gap[a]
- A. Lactic acidosis: lactate, D-lactate
- B. Ketoacidosis: β-hydroxybutyrate
- C. Renal failure: sulfate, phosphate, urate, hippurate
- D. Ingestions
  - 1. Salicylate: ketones, lactate, salicylate
  - 2. Methanol or formaldehyde: formate
  - 3. Ethylene glycol: glycolate, oxalate
  - 4. Paraldehyde: organic anions
  - 5. Toluene: hippurate (usually presents with normal anion gap)
  - 6. Sulfur: SO_4^{2-}
- E. Massive rhabdomyolysis

Normal anion gap (hyperchloremic acidosis)
- A. Gastrointestinal loss of HCO_3^-
  - 1. Diarrhea
- B. Renal HCO_3^- loss
  - 1. Type 2 (proximal) renal tubular acidosis
- C. Renal dysfunction
  - 1. Some cases of renal failure
  - 2. Hypoaldosteronism (type 4 renal tubular acidosis)
  - 3.. Type 1 (distal) renal tubular acidosis
- D. Ingestions
  - 1. Ammonium chloride
  - 2. Hyperalimentation fluids
- E. Some cases of ketoacidosis, particularly during treatment with insulin

---

[a] The substances after the colon represent the major retained anions in the high anion gap acidoses.

$$\text{Anion gap} = [Na^+] - ([Cl^-] + [HCO_3^-]) \qquad (19\text{-}5)$$

The approximate normal values for these ions are 140, 108, and 24 meq/L, respectively, leading to an anion gap of 5 to 11 meq/L. (This is lower than previously measured values, since a higher plasma Cl^- concentration is measured with the newer autoanalyzers.[24] As a result, knowing the normal range in a particular laboratory is often essential if the anion gap is to be interpreted properly.

The negative charges on the plasma proteins account for most of the missing anions, as the charges on the other cations (K^+, Ca^{2+}, and Mg^{2+}) and anions (phosphate, sulfate, and organic anions) tend to balance out. Thus, the normal value for the anion gap must be adjusted downward in patients with hypoalbuminemia; the approximate correction is a reduction in the anion gap of 2.5 meq/L for every 1 g/dL decline in the plasma albumin concentration.[22]

The factors that can affect the anion gap can be more easily appreciated if Eq. (19-5) is rewritten in the following way. In addition to being equal to the difference between measured cations and anions, the anion gap is also equal to the difference between *unmeasured* anions and cations:

$$\text{Anion gap} = \text{unmeasured anions} - \text{unmeasured cations} \qquad (19\text{-}6)$$

Thus, an increase in anion gap can be produced by a fall in unmeasured cations (hypocalcemia, hypokalemia, or hypomagnesemia, where the change is only 1 to 3 meq/L) or, more importantly, by an elevation in the amount of unmeasured anions. This can be induced by a high plasma albumin concentration (as with hypovolemia-induced hemoconcentration) or by the accumulation of a variety of different anions.

These relationships can be applied to the different causes of metabolic acidosis, in which there is rapid extracellular buffering of the excess acid by HCO_3. If the acid is HCl, then

$$HCl + NaHCO_3 \rightarrow NaCl + H_2CO_3 \rightarrow CO_2 + H_2O \qquad (19\text{-}7)$$

In this setting, there is a milliequivalent-for-milliequivalent replacement of extracellular HCO_3^- by Cl^-; thus, there is no change in the anion gap, since the sum of ($[Cl^-] + [HCO_3^-]$) remains constant. This disorder is called a *hyperchloremic acidosis*, because of the associated increase in the plasma Cl^- concentration.

Gastrointestinal or renal loss of $NaHCO_3$ indirectly produces the same result. The kidney retains NaCl in this setting in an effort to preserve the extracellular volume, leading to a net exchange of HCO_3^- for Cl^-.

Conversely, if H^+ accumulates with any anion other than Cl^-, extracellular HCO_3^- will be replaced by an unmeasured anion (A^-):

$$HA + NaHCO_3 \quad \rightarrow \quad NaA + H_2CO_3 \quad \rightarrow \quad CO_2 + H_2O \qquad (19\text{-}8)$$

The ensuing accumulation of A^- leads to an elevation in the anion gap. In this setting, identification of the specific disease process usually can be obtained by measuring the plasma concentrations of creatinine, glucose, and lactate and by checking the plasma for the presence of ketones and intoxicants (particularly salicylates, methanol, and ethylene glycol) (Table 19-4).

A simple example of how this approach can be used is illustrated by the following case history:

Case History 19-1   A 27-year-old man with insulin-dependent diabetes mellitus has not been taking his insulin and is admitted to the hospital in a semicomatose condition. The following laboratory data are obtained:

Plasma $[Na^+]$	=	140 meq/L	Arterial pH	=	7.10
$[K^+]$	=	7.0 meq/L	P_{CO_2}	=	20 mmHg
$[Cl^-]$	=	105 meq/L	[Glucose]	=	800 mg/dL
$[HCO_3^-]$	=	6 meq/L	Plasma ketones	=	4+
Anion gap	=	29 meq/L			

Comment The high anion gap, hyperglycemia, and ketonemia all point to the diagnosis of diabetic ketoacidosis. Note that the increase in the anion gap of approximately 18 meq/L (from 11 to 29) is the same as the fall in the plasma HCO_3^- concentration (from 24 to 6 meq/L).

Although a high anion gap is helpful in the differential diagnosis of metabolic acidosis, it is not always possible to identify the extra unmeasured anions.[22-25] This is particularly true when there is only a minor elevation in the anion gap (to less than 20 meq/L); in this setting, the correct diagnosis may not be evident, since ketones, lactate, renal failure, and ingestions all may be missing. In comparison, one of these disorders is generally present when the anion gap exceeds 25 meq/L.

Another potential problem is that the distinction between a high and a normal anion gap acidosis is not always absolute. Patients with diarrhea, for example, tend to develop a normal anion gap acidosis because of HCO_3^- loss in the stool. If the fluid losses are severe, however, hemoconcentration (leading to hyperalbuminemia), lactic acidosis (due to hypoperfusion), and hyperphosphatemia (resulting from acidemia-induced release of phosphate from the cells) all may combine to raise the anion gap.[26] This combination of normal and high anion gap acidosis can be detected by comparing the change (Δ) in anion gap to the change (Δ) in plasma HCO_3^- concentration.

Δ Anion gap/Δ plasma HCO_3^- concentration In addition to the level of the anion gap, the relationship between the increase in the anion gap and the fall in the plasma HCO_3^- concentration may be helpful diagnostically. Use of this parameter is dependent upon an accurate assumption of the change in anion gap, which requires an estimate of the normal anion gap if no prior measurements are available. As described above, the normal value of approximately 8 meq/L[24] must be adjusted downward in patients with hypoalbuminemia, with the approximate correction being a 2.5-meq/L fall in the anion gap for every 1-g/dL reduction in the plasma albumin concentration.[22]

Failure to make this correction will underestimate the change in anion gap. Suppose, for example, the anion gap is 15 meq/L in a patient with a plasma albumin concentration of 2 g/dL. The Δ anion gap is 7 meq/L using 8 meq/L as the baseline value; however, accounting for the hypoalbuminemia leads to a baseline anion gap of roughly 3 meq/L [8 − (2.5 × 2)], resulting in a higher Δ anion gap of 12 meq/L.

Although Eq. (19-8) seems to imply that there should be a 1:1 relationship between the elevation in anion gap and the fall in plasma HCO_3^- concentration, this is usually not the case. As described above, more than 50 percent of the excess H^+ is buffered by the cells, *not by HCO_3^-*. In contrast, *most of the excess anions remain in the extracellular fluid*, since their distribution is pH-dependent. The extracellular fluid has a slightly higher pH (and lower H^+ concentration) than the cells; as a result, the following reaction is driven to the left:

$$H^+ + BHB^- \quad \leftrightarrow \quad HBHB$$

where BHB^- refers to the β-hydroxybutyrate$^-$ anion and HBHB refers to the undissociated β-hydroxybutryric acid. The net effect is that the extracellular fluid has, in relation to the cells, a relatively high concentration of β-hydroxy-butyrate$^-$, which is less able to enter the cells because anions cannot easily cross the lipid bilayer of the cell membrane.

As a result, the *elevation in the anion gap usually exceeds the fall in the plasma HCO_3^- concentration*; in lactic acidosis, for example, the Δ/Δ ratio averages about $1.6 : 1$.[27] It should be appreciated, however, that hydrogen buffering in cells and bone takes several hours to reach completion. Thus, the ratio may be close to $1 : 1$ with very acute lactic acidosis (as with seizures or exercise to exhaustion), since there has not been time for nonextracellular buffering to occur.

Although the same principles apply to ketoacidosis, the ratio is often close to $1 : 1$ in this disorder because the *loss of ketoacid anions in the urine* (which lowers the anion gap) tends to balance the effect of intracellular buffering of H^+.[27-30] The adequacy of renal function appears to be an important determinant of the rise in anion gap in ketoacidosis. Patients in whom the glomerular filtration rate is relatively normal have an elevation in filtered ketoacid load that exceeds tubular reabsorptive capacity.[31] As a result, they can excrete a large quantity of ketoacid anions in the urine,* thereby minimizing the rise in the anion gap and therefore in the Δ/Δ ratio.[28,30] In comparison, the anion gap will be higher when renal function is impaired, usually because of underlying renal disease or volume depletion induced by the glucose osmotic diuresis (see Chap. 25).[28,30] Anion loss in the urine is much less prominent in lactic acidosis, because the associated state of marked tissue hypoperfusion usually results in little or no urine output.

The loss of ketoacid anions in the urine also accounts for the observation that a *normal anion gap acidosis typically occurs during the treatment phase of ketoacidosis*.[28,30] In the above case history, there is a 20-meq/L elevation in the anion gap and a roughly equivalent decline in the plasma HCO_3^- concentration. After the administration of insulin, these ketoacid anions will be metabolized to HCO_3^- (see below). Thus, the anion gap will return to normal, but the plasma HCO_3^- concentration will increase by about 8 meq/L, not 20 meq/L, since *most of the generated HCO_3^- will effectively enter the cells to replenish the cell buffers*. At this time, the plasma HCO_3^- concentration will be 14 meq/L and the pH will still be acid, but here will be no excess unmeasured anions (i.e., the patient will have a normal anion gap acidosis). The acidemia in this setting is due to two factors: the previous production of ketoacids and the excretion of the ketoacid anions, which, if retained, could have been converted back into HCO_3^- after the administration of insulin; thus, loss of these anions is physiologically equivalent to the loss of HCO_3^-.

---

* Only those ketones that are excreted as the Na^+ or K^+ salt will lower the Δ/Δ ratio. Both β-hydroxybutyrate and acetoacetate also may be excreted as the intact acid or as the NH_4^+ salt. In these settings, H^+ is effectively lost with the anion, thereby correcting both the high anion gap and the fall in the plasma HCO_3^- concentration.

In addition to this sequence during treatment, some patients with ketoacidosis excrete ketones in the urine so efficiently that the anion gap is relatively normal *before* any therapy has been instituted.[29,30] A similar sequence, in which patients who overproduce organic acids can present with a normal anion gap, may occur in two other settings: D-lactic acidosis and toluene exposure (glue-sniffing). Filtered L-lactate, the normal isomer produced in humans, is reabsorbed in the proximal tubule via a Na^+-L-lactate cotransporter in the luminal membrane. This transporter is stereospecific and does not bind D-lactate, which may be overproduced in patients with a short bowel syndrome (see below). As a result, D-lactate is rapidly excreted in the urine, lowering the anion gap toward normal. However, the acidosis persists, since the H^+ ion is still retained.

Anion loss is even more rapid with toluene ingestion, which is associated with overproduction of hippuric acid.[32] Hippurate is both *filtered and secreted*; as a result, almost all of the hippurate delivered to the kidney enters the tubular lumen and is then excreted, since there is little hippurate reabsorption. The net effect is that many patients present with a normal anion gap and are mistakenly thought to have renal tubular acidosis.[32]

Summary In summary, the Δ/Δ ratio is normally between 1 and 2 in patients with an uncomplicated high anion gap metabolic acidosis. A value below $1:1$ suggests a *combined high and normal anion gap acidosis*, as might occur when hemoconcentration and lactic acidosis are superimposed on severe diarrhea.[26] On the other hand, a value above $2:1$ suggests that the fall in the plasma HCO_3^- concentration is less than expected because of a concurrent metabolic alkalosis. Consider the following case history:

Case History 19-2 A previously well 55-year-old woman is admitted with a complaint of severe vomiting for 5 days. Physical examination reveals postural hypotension, tachycardia, and diminished skin turgor. The laboratory findings include the following:

Plasma [Na^+]	= 140 meq/L	Arterial pH	=	7.23
[K^+]	= 3.4 meq/L	P_{CO_2}	=	22 mmHg
[Cl^-]	= 77 meq/L	Plasma ketones	=	trace
HCO_3^-	= 9 meq/L	[Creatinine]	=	2.1 mg/dL
Anion gap	= 54 meq/L			

Comment This patient has a high anion gap metabolic acidosis. Lactic acidosis is most likely in view of the physical findings and lack of significant ketonemia, renal failure, or history of an ingestion. However, the anion gap of 54 meq/L is markedly increased (45 meq/L above normal) while the reduction in the plasma HCO_3^- concentration is much smaller (15 meq/L, giving 9 meq/L), leading to a Δ/Δ ratio of $3:1$. This disparity can be explained by a concomitant metabolic alkalosis due to vomiting, which raised the plasma HCO_3^-

concentration without affecting the anion gap. Proof of this diagnosis came from evaluating the response to fluid repletion. As tissue perfusion was restored and metabolism of the excess lactate generated HCO_3^- (see below), the plasma HCO_3^- concentration rose from 9 to 37 meq/L and the pH became alkalemic. Thus, the 45-meq/L elevation in the anion gap was actually associated with a 28-meq/L fall in the plasma HCO_3^- concentration, a 1.7:1 ratio that is typical of lactic acidosis.[27]

Anion gap in renal failure   To understand the changes in the anion gap that can occur in renal failure, it is first necessary to review the normal handling of acids. The dietary acid load is primarily due to the generation of H_2SO_4 from the metabolism of sulfur-containing amino acids.[14,33,34] This acid is rapidly buffered by HCO_3^- and other buffers, leading to the formation of Na_2SO_4:

$$H_2SO_4 + 2NaHCO_3 \rightarrow Na_2SO_4 + 2H_2CO_3 \rightarrow 2CO_2 + 2H_2O$$

To maintain the steady state, both the $2H^+$ and the SO_4^{2-} must be excreted in the urine. As described above, the excretion of H^+, primarily as NH_4^+, is a tubular function. In comparison, the excretion of SO_4^{2-} is determined by the difference between filtration and some degree of tubular reabsorption. In general, progressive renal diseases lead to parallel impairments in glomerular filtration rate and tubular function; as a result, both the H^+ and SO_4^{2-} are retained, producing a high anion gap metabolic acidosis.[35,36] (Other retained anions in renal failure include phosphate, urate, and hippurate.[37]

These findings are different, however, if there is more prominent impairment in tubular function. In this setting, both H^+ secretion and SO_4^{2-} reabsorption will be diminished, with the latter maintaining the rate of SO_4^{2-} excretion (as Na_2SO_4) at near normal levels. Na^+ depletion is prevented by an equivalent increase in NaCl reabsorption. The net effect is H^+ and Cl^- retention, maintenance of SO_4^{2-} balance, and a normal anion gap metabolic acidosis.[35,36]

Anion gap in other conditions   Small changes in the anion gap can occur in a variety of disorders other than metabolic acidosis.[21-23] A high anion gap, for example, can occur in nonketotic hyperglycemia with no or only mild metabolic acidosis as a result of the release of phosphate and perhaps other anions from the cells.[9]

An elevation in unmeasured plasma anions is also a common finding in metabolic alkalosis.[22,38] Three factors may contribute to this finding: (1) a rise in the plasma albumin concentration as a result of extracellular volume depletion; (2) an increase in the number of negative charges per albumin molecule, since the pH is further away from the isoelectric point for albumin of approximately 5.4; and (3) an appropriate alkalemia-induced increase in lactate production in an attempt to lower the pH toward normal. A high anion gap can also result from a reduction in unmeasured cations; this effect, however, is generally of minor importance, since hypokalemia, hypocalcemia, or hypomagnesemia will raise the anion gap by only a few milliequivalents per liter.

There are also settings in which a low anion gap (less than 5 meq/L) may be found. From Eq. (19-6), this phenomenon can be induced by a fall in unmeasured anions (primarily hypoalbuminemia) or by a rise in unmeasured cations.[39] The latter can occur with hyperkalemia, hypercalcemia, hypermagnesemia, severe lithium intoxication, or some cases of multiple myeloma in which a cationic IgG paraprotein is produced.[22,40,41]

In rare cases, the anion gap has a negative value.[42] This is most often due to a laboratory artifact in severe hypernatremia (at levels above 170 meq/L, the true concentration of sodium is underestimated), marked hyperlipidemia (where light scattering in the colorimetric assay can result in marked overestimation of the plasma chloride concentration, occasionally to above 200 meq/L), or bromide intoxication.[20,42,43] The last problem may be seen in patients taking pyridostigmine bromide for myasthenia gravis; it does not occur with Bromo-Seltzer, which no longer contains bromide.[42] In several of the commonly used laboratory assays for chloride, there is a greater affinity for bromide; as a result, each milliequivalent of bromide may be measured as 2 meq of chloride, leading to overestimation of the plasma chloride concentration and a low or even negative anion gap.

Urine anion gap Calculation of the urine anion gap may be helpful diagnostically in some cases with a normal anion gap metabolic acidosis.[44,45] The major measured cations and anions in the urine are Na^+, K^+, and Cl^-; thus, the urine anion gap is equal to

$$\text{Urine anion gap} = ([Na^+] + [K^+]) - [Cl^-] \tag{19-9}$$

$$\text{Urine anion gap} = \text{unmeasured anions} - \text{unmeasured cations} \tag{19-10}$$

In normal subjects excreting between 20 and 40 meq of NH_4^+ per liter (NH_4^+ being the major unmeasured urinary cation), the urine anion gap generally has a positive value or is near zero.[44,46] In metabolic acidosis, however, the excretion of NH_4^+ (and of Cl^- to maintain electroneutrality) should increase markedly if renal acidification is intact, resulting in a value that varies from -20 to more than -50 meq/L; the negative value in this setting occurs because the Cl^- concentration now exceeds that of Na^+ plus K^+. In comparison, the acidemia in renal failure and types 1 and 4 renal tubular acidosis is primarily due to impaired H^+ and NH_4^+ excretion, and the urine anion gap typically retains its normal positive value (Fig. 19-1).[44] Thus, use of the urine anion gap in conjunction with the urine pH and plasma K^+ concentration can help in arriving at the correct diagnosis (see "Renal Tubular Acidosis," below).

One simple example can illustrate the potential utility of the urine anion gap. Hypokalemia is a stimulus to renal NH_3 production, an effect that may be related to an intracellular acidosis induced by the transcellular shift of K^+ out of and H^+ into the cells (see page 356).[47] Diffusion of some of this excess NH_3 into the urine will drive Eq. (19-4) to the right, thereby lowering the H^+ concentration and raising the urine pH. Thus, a patient with diarrhea and hypokalemia may have metabolic acidosis and, because of the effect of NH_3, an increase in urine pH similar to that in type 1 renal tubular acidosis. The correct diagnosis in this setting

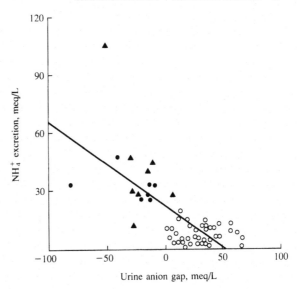

Figure 19-1 The relationship between the urine anion gap and the rate of NH_4^+ excretion in normal subjects receiving ammonium chloride (closed circles), in patients with metabolic acidosis due to diarrhea (closed triangles), and in patients with impaired urinary acidification due to type 1 or 4 renal tubular acidosis (open circles). The urine anion gap has a positive value in the last group, indicative of the defect in NH_4^+ excretion. (*From Batlle DC, Hizon M, Cohen E, et al.* N Engl J Med *318:594, 1988. By permission from the* New England Journal of Medicine.)

can be established by calculation of the urine anion gap, which will have a positive value in renal tubular acidosis but will be appropriately negative with diarrhea, since renal NH_4^+ excretion is not impaired in this disorder.[44]

There are, however, two conditions in which the urine anion gap cannot be used. The first is a high anion gap acidosis, such as ketoacidosis, where the excretion of unmeasured ketoacid anions in the urine will counteract the effect of NH_4^+.[44,45] As a result, the urine anion gap may be positive even though there is an appropriate increase in the rate of NH_4^+ excretion. The second is volume depletion with avid Na^+ retention (urine Na^+ concentration $< 25\,meq/L$).[44] The associated decrease in distal Na^+ delivery impairs distal acidification, resulting in a reversible form of type 1 renal tubular acidosis, even though diarrhea may be the primary abnormality. Viewed in terms of the urine anion gap, the concurrent increase in Cl^- reabsorption prevents the excretion of NH_4Cl and the development of a negative anion gap.

The decreased acid excretion with volume depletion may play an important role in the genesis of the metabolic acidosis that may be seen with severe or persistent diarrhea.[45] Diarrheal fluid may contain as much as 50 meq/L of base. If renal function were normal, however, the fall in the plasma bicarbonate concentration would be limited by increased ammonium excretion, which can reach 150 to 200 meq/day. Concurrent volume depletion will limit this adaptive response, thereby increasing the severity of the acidosis.

Urine osmolal gap When the urine anion gap is positive and it is unclear whether increased excretion of unmeasured anions is responsible, the urine ammonium concentration can be estimated from calculation of the urine osmolal gap.[32,45] This calculation requires measurement of the urine osmolality and the urine sodium, potassium, urea nitrogen, and, if the dipstick is positive, glucose concentrations. The calculated urine osmolality can then be estimated from

$$\text{Calculated urine osmolality} = 2 \times ([\text{Na}^+ + \text{K}]) + \frac{[\text{urea nitrogen}]}{2.8} + \frac{[\text{glucose}]}{18}$$

The multiple of 2 accounts for the anions accompanying sodium and potassium, while the divisors 2.8 and 18 reflect adjustments required to convert from the routinely used units of mg/dL to mmol/L or mosmol/kg.

The gap between the measured and calculated urine osmolality should largely represent ammonium salts. This calculation is not affected by unmeasured anions (such as β-hydroxybutyrate), since these anions will be accounted for by the cations sodium, potassium, and ammonium. Suppose, for example, that there is a 100-mosmol/kg difference between the measured and calculated urine osmolality; ammonium excretion in this setting should be approximately one-half this value (because of accompanying anions) or 50 meq/L, a level that is appropriate with metabolic acidosis.[48]

One circumstance in which the urine gap will be inaccurate is when large quantities of an intact (undissociated) acid are excreted, as most often occurs with β-hydroxybutyric acid in ketoacidosis. In this setting, the osmolal gap may be due primarily to β-hydroxybutyric acid rather than to ammonium salts. This error is likely to be small, however, since β-hydroxybutyric acid is excreted primarily as the ketoacid anion as a result of the relatively low pKa (4.7) of this acid. In one careful study of patients with diabetic ketoacidosis, the concentration of undissociated β-hydroxybutyric acid was less than 4 meq/L, while the concentration of ketoacid anions was more than six times higher.[19] Furthermore, the diagnosis of ketoacidosis is usually easily established from the history and routine laboratory data and does not require calculation of the urine anion or osmolal gaps.

ETIOLOGY AND DIAGNOSIS

This section will review the pathogenesis, etiology, and diagnosis of the different disorders that can cause metabolic acidosis. It will also include some specific aspects of therapy, although the general principles involved in the treatment of metabolic acidosis will be discussed separately later in the chapter.

Lactic Acidosis

Lactic acid is derived from the metabolism of pyruvic acid; this reaction is catalyzed by lactate dehydrogenase and involves the conversion of NADH into NAD$^+$ (reduced and oxidized nicotine adenine dinucleotide, respectively) (Fig. 19-2). Normal subjects produce 15 to 20 mmol/kg of lactic acid per day, most of which is generated from glucose via the glycolytic pathway or from the deamination of alanine.[49,50]

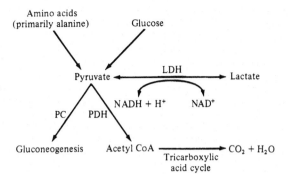

Figure 19-2 Major pathways of pyruvate and lactate metabolism. LDH is lactate dehydrogenase, PDH is pyruvate dehydrogenase, PC is pyruvate carboxylase, and NADH and NAD^+ are reduced and oxidized nicotine adenine dinucleotide, respectively.

Lactic acid is rapidly buffered, in part by extracellular HCO_3^-, resulting in the generation of lactate:

$$CH_3-CHOH-COOH + NaHCO_3 \quad \rightarrow \quad Na^+lactate^-$$
$$+ H_2CO_3 \quad \rightarrow \quad CO_2 + H_2O \tag{19-11}$$

In the liver and, to a lesser degree, the kidney, lactate is metabolized back to pyruvate, which is then converted into either CO_2 and H_2O (80 percent, catalyzed in part by pyruvate dehydrogenase) or glucose (20 percent, catalyzed in part by pyruvate carboxylase; Fig. 19-2). Either of these processes results in the *regeneration of the HCO_3^-* lost in the initial buffering of lactic acid:

$$\text{Lactate} + 3O_2 \quad \rightarrow \quad HCO_3^- + 2CO_2 + 2H_2O \tag{19-12}$$

$$2\,\text{Lactate} + 2H_2O + 2CO_2 \quad \rightarrow \quad 2HCO_3^- + \text{glucose} \tag{19-13}$$

These reactions require both the entry of pyruvate into the mitochondria and normal oxidative metabolism. In comparison, pyruvate will be preferentially converted into lactate in the cytosol in the presence of mitochondrial dysfunction or a marked reduction in tissue perfusion.

The normal plasma lactate concentration is 0.5 to 1.5 meq/L. Lactic acidosis is considered to be present if the plasma lactate level exceeds 4 to 5 meq/L in an acidemic patient.

Pathogenesis and etiology   Excess lactate can accumulate when there is increased lactate production and/or diminished lactate utilization.[49-52] The former can occur by three mechanisms: enhanced pyruvate production, reduced pyruvate utilization, or, most commonly, an altered redox state within the cell in which pyruvate is preferentially converted into lactate (Table 19-5).[49,50] During glycolysis, NADH is generated and then reoxidized to NAD^+ in the mitochondria. If oxidation is impaired, however, NADH will accumulate, further promoting the conversion of pyruvate to lactate (Fig. 19-2). In this setting, the associated adenosine triphosphate (ATP) depletion may lead to vasodilatation and a further decline in systemic blood pressure. ATP normally closes ATP-dependent K^+ channels. Thus, ATP depletion in lactic acidosis leads to opening of these channels, resulting

Table 19-5 Etiology of lactic acidosis

Increased lactate production
- A. Increased pyruvate production
  1. Enzymatic defects in glycogenolysis of gluconeogenesis (as with type 1 glycogen storage disease)[53]
  2. Respiratory alkalosis, including salicylate intoxication[49,54]
  3. Pheochromocytoma[55,56]
- B. Impaired pyruvate utilization
  1. Decreased activity of pyruvate dehydrogenase or pyruvate carboxylase
      a. Congential[57]
      b. Possibly a role in diabetes mellitus, Reye's syndrome[58,59]
- C. Altered redox state favoring pyruvate conversion to lactate
  1. Enhanced metabolic rate
      a. Grand mal seizure[60]
      b. Severe exercise[61,62]
      c. Hypothermic shivering[63]
      d. Severe asthma[64]
  2. Decreased oxygen delivery
      a. Shock[45]
      b. Cardiac arrest
      c. Acute pulmonary edema[58]
      d. Carbon monoxide poisoning ($\downarrow O_2$ uptake by hemoglobin)[65]
      e. Severe hypoxemia ($P_{O_2} < 25$ to 30 mmHg)[66]
      f. Pheochromocytoma[55,56]
  3. Reduced oxygen utilization
      a. Cyanide intoxication ($\downarrow$ oxidative metabolism), which may result from cyanide poisoning[67] or, during a fire, from smoke inhalation of vapors derived from the thermal decomposition of nitrogen-containing materials such as wool, silk, and polyurethane[68]
      b. Drug-induced mitochondrial dysfunction due to zidovudine or stavudine[69-72]
- D. D-Lactic acidosis[73-76]

Primary decrease in lactate utilization
- A. Hypoperfusion and marked acidemia[51,52,77]
- B. Alcoholism[78]
- C. Liver disease[49]

Mechanism uncertain
- A. Malignancy[79-82]
- B. Diabetes mellitus,[49] including metformin[83,84] in the absence of tissue hypoxia
- C. Acquired immune deficiency syndrome[85]
- D. Hypoglycemia[49]
- E. Idiopathic

sequentially in K^+ movement out of the cells, hyperpolarization of vascular smooth muscle cells, and decreased Ca^{2+} entry into these cells through voltage-dependent Ca^{2+} channels.[86] The fall in cell Ca^{2+} concentration produces smooth muscle relaxation and a reduction in systemic vascular resistance.

In certain disorders, the primary role of lactate overproduction is clear. As an example, plasma lactate levels may transiently be as high as 15 meq/L during a grand mal seizure[60] and 20 to 25 meq/L with maximal exercise, with the systemic pH falling to as low as 6.80.[61,87] Studies in these patients have demonstrated rapid recovery of acid-base balance, with a maximum rate of lactate utilization that can reach 320 meq/h.[49]

This high rate of lactate metabolism suggests that there must be some component of *decreased utilization* in those disorders in which lactate overproduction occurs more slowly. In shock, for example, the reduction in perfusion to the liver and an associated intracellular acidosis may combine to substantially diminish hepatic lactate metabolism.[51,52,88] The importance of these events has been demonstrated experimentally by the observation that infusing lactic acid to otherwise normal animals is associated with increased hepatic utilization and relative difficulty in lowering the extracellular pH.[51,52]

Most cases of lactic acidosis are due to marked tissue hypoperfusion in shock or during a cariodpulmonary arrest.[49,50,89] The prognosis is generally poor unless tissue perfusion can be rapidly restored.

The association of lactic acidosis with *diabetes mellitus* is less certain, since many cases in the past were associated with the use of phenformin and some of those today with metformin.[83,84] Nevertheless, a moderate degree of lactic acidosis may be seen in some patients with diabetic ketoacidosis.[49,90] How this occurs is not clear, although marked hypovolemia is likely to play an important role. Documentation of concurrent lactic acidosis may be clinically important, since the altered redox state in this setting also converts acetoacetate into β-hydroxybutyrate. Only the former is recognized by the nitroprusside tablet or dipstick used to detect the presence of ketones; as a result, a falsely negative result may be obtained and the diagnosis of ketoacidosis obscured when there is preferential production of β-hydroxybutyrate.[90]

The pathogenesis of the lactic acidosis found with *malignancies* is also unclear.[79-82] Anaerobic metabolism due to dense clusters of tumor cells and/or metastatic replacement of the hepatic parenchyma have been proposed, but lactic acidosis has occurred in patients with relatively small tumor burdens.[79,81] Direct lactate production by the neoplastic cells has also been suggested, but this would not explain the rarity of tumor-induced lactic acidosis. Regardless of the mechanism, removal of the tumor (or by chemotherapy, irradiation, or surgery) leads to correction of the acidosis.[79,81,82]

A mild degree of lactic acidosis also may be seen with *alcoholism*.[78] In this condition, lactate production is usually normal, but lactate utilization is diminished because of impaired hepatic gluconeogenesis. Although lactate levels generally do not exceed 3 meq/L in this setting, alcohol ingestion can potentiate the severity of other disorders that are associated with the overproduction of lactate.

There are rare patients with the acquired immune deficiency syndrome (AIDS) in whom lactic acidosis is associated with drug-induced mitochondrial dysfunction in the absence of sepsis or hypotension. Such an association has been described in patients with zidovudine-induced myopathy, characterized by elevated plasma creatine kinase concentrations and proximal muscle weakness,[91] and zidovudine- or stavudine-induced hepatic steatosis and hepatic failure.[69,70] The latter complication may, in some cases, be due to a concurrent deficiency of riboflavin, a precursor to a number of cofactors necessary for mitochondrial energy production. In several patients, nucleoside-induced lactic acidosis has been reversed by riboflavin therapy.[71,72] In addition, a seemingly idiopathic form of lactic acidosis can occur in the absence of zidovudine.[85]

D-lactic acidosis A unique form of lactic acidosis can occur in patients with jejunoileal bypass or, less commonly, small bowel resection or other cause of the short bowel syndrome. In these settings, glucose and starch are metabolized in the colon into D-lactic acid, which is then absorbed into the systemic circulation.[73-76] The ensuing acidemia tends to persist, since D-lactate is not recognized by L-lactate dehydrogenase, the enzyme that catalyzes the conversion of the physiologically occurring L-lactate into pyruvate.

Two factors tend to contribute to the overproduction of D-lactic acid in this disorder.[74] First, there is overgrowth of gram-positive anaerobes, such as lactobacilli, which are most able to produce D-lactate. Second, there is usually relatively little glucose and starch delivered to the colon because of extensive small-intestinal absorption. However, delivery of these substrates is markedly enhanced when the small bowel is bypassed, removed, or diseased.

Patients with this disorder present with episodic metabolic acidosis (usually occurring after high-carbohydrate meals) and characteristic neurologic abnormalities, including confusion, cerebellar ataxia, slurred speech, and loss of memory.[73-75] They may complain of feeling or appearing to be drunk in the absence of ethanol intake. It is not clear whether these symptoms are due to D-lactate itself or to some other toxin produced in the colon and then absorbed in parallel with D-lactate.

The classic neurologic findings plus the metabolic acidosis and the history of intestinal disease should strongly suggest the presence of D-lactic acidosis. Confirmation of the diagnosis requires a special enzymatic assay that uses D-lactate dehydrogenase and measures the generation of NADH as lactate is converted to pyruvate.[73-75] In contrast, the standard assay for lactate uses L-lactate dehydrogenase, which will not detect D-lactate.

An additional source of confusion may occur in D-lactic acidosis. Filtered D-lactate is *rapidly excreted* in the urine, being unable to bind to the Na^+-L-lactate cotransporter in the luminal membrane of the proximal tubule that normally promotes L-lactate reabsorption. As a result, patients with this disorder may have an anion gap that is normal or less than expected from the degree of reduction in the plasma HCO_3^- concentration.

Therapy in D-lactic acidosis consists of acute sodium bicarbonate administration to correct the acidemia and oral antimicrobial agents (such as metronidazole, neomycin, or vancomycin) to decrease the number of D-lactate producing organisms.[74-76] A low-carbohydrate diet (or the use of starch polymers rather than simple sugars) also is helpful, by diminishing carboyhydrate delivery to the colon.

Diagnosis Although the diagnosis of lactate acidosis can be made definitively only by the demonstration of an elevated plasma lactate concentration, there are often many suggestive clues in the history, physical examination, laboratory data, and response to therapy. These include a high anion gap; the presence of one of the disorders that can cause lactic acidosis; cool, clammy extremities and hypotension if shock is present; and continuing production of acid, as evidenced by an inability of exogenous HCO_3^- to raise the plasma HCO_3^- concentration.

The presence of an organic acidosis (primarily lactic acidosis or ketoacidosis) should also be suspected if effective treatment of the underlying problem (such as fluid repletion in hypovolemic shock) leads to a *spontaneous elevation in the plasma HCO_3^- concentration*. This occurs because metabolism of the organic anion, in this case lactate, results in the regeneration of HCO_3^- [Eqs. (19-12) and (19-13)].

Treatment Correction of the underlying disorder is the primary therapy in lactic acidosis. Reversal of circulatory failure, for example, will reduce further lactate production and allow metabolism of the excess lactate to HCO_3^-. (This spontaneous regeneration of HCO_3^- does not occur in D-lactic acidosis, since D-lactate cannot be metabolized.)

The role of $NaHCO_3$ administration in lactic acidosis has been a source of great controversy.[92] Proponents argue that raising the arterial pH may improve tissue perfusion, by reversing acidemia-induced vasodilatation and impaired cardiac contractility, and may diminish the risk of serious arrhythmias (see "Symptoms," below).[50,93] These potential benefits, however, must be weighed against the possible risks, which include volume overload, hypernatremia (a 5 percent $NaHCO_3$ solution contains almost 900 meq of Na^+ per liter), and overshoot metabolic alkalosis after normal hemodynamics has been restored.[94] In addition, metabolic acidosis may be in part protective during ischemia by minimizing hypoperfusion-induced tissue injury.[95]

In addition, both experimental[88,96,97] and human studies[80,97,98] have suggested that HCO_3^- therapy may be relatively ineffective, *producing only a transient elevation in the plasma HCO_3^- concentration* and possibly *worsening the intracellular acidosis*.[88,99,100] The seeming lack of efficacy of alkali therapy appears to be due in part to an associated *increase in net lactic acid production* (which also leads to a further rise in the anion gap).[88,96]

This unexpected change in lactate metabolism may be induced by the continued generation of CO_2, as a result of both cellular metabolic activity (including fibrillating myocardial cells during cardiac arrest)[99] and buffering of the excess H^+ ions by exogenous HCO_3^- [Eq. (19-1)].[88,101] This CO_2 then accumulates in the tissues, since pulmonary blood flow is reduced as part of the shock state.[102-104] The ensuing local hypercapnia can exacerbate the intracellular acidosis, leading to decreased lactate utilization in hepatic cells and a decline in contractility in cardiac cells.[82,96,99,101] The latter effect can reduce the cardiac output, a change that will promote further lactic acid production.*

It must also be emphasized that this problem of CO_2 accumulation may *not be detectable in arterial blood.*[103,104] Blood entering the pulmonary circulation may be adequately cleared of CO_2, resulting in a relatively normal arterial P_{CO_2}. However, total CO_2 elimination is diminished because of the reduction in pulmonary blood flow with severe circulatory failure or cardiac arrest. As a result, the P_{CO_2} at the tissue level may be markedly elevated, a change that can be detected by measurement of *mixed venous blood.* In one study of patients undergoing cardiopulmonary resuscitation, the mean arterial pH and P_{CO_2} were 7.42 and 32 mmHg, respectively, whereas the mixed venous values were 7.14 and 74 mmHg.[103] This problem may be exacerbated by $NaHCO_3$ therapy, in part because buffering of H^+ ions in the blood by HCO_3^- increases the generation of CO_2.[103,104]

In summary, these findings make the optimal therapy of lactic acidosis uncertain at the present time. Some physicians have concluded that there is little indication for $NaHCO_3$ administration,[97] particularly during cardiac arrest.[100] However, most physicians give small amounts of $NaHCO_3$ to maintain the arterial pH above 7.10, since more severe acidemia can result in a deterioration in cardiovascular function. Careful monitoring, including measurement of mixed or central venous pH, is required to minimize side effects related to HCO_3^- administration.

There are three possible experimental alternatives to HCO_3^- therapy. One is the administration of Na_2CO_3 as a source of alkali: Buffering of excess H^+ ions by this compound will generate HCO_3^-, not CO_2, thereby minimizing the tendency to exacerbate the intracellular acidosis.[88,101] However, this agent has not been effective during cardiac arrest in experimental animals.[99,100] Although the extracellular pH may be increased, there is no improvement in the progressive decline in myocardial cell pH that results from continued CO_2 production by the fibrillating cells.

The second alternative is the administration of dichloroacetate (DCA). This compound stimulates pyruvate dehydrogenase activity, thereby minimizing lactate production by allowing pyruvate to be oxidized to CO_2 and H_2O (Fig. 19-2). Although there is evidence of benefit in experimental models of lactic acidosis, a controlled trial in humans showed that DCA produced a minor increase in the plasma bicarbonate concentration and arterial pH but no improvement in systemic hemodynamics or mortality.[106]

The third option is tromethamine (THAM). THAM is an inert amino alcohol that buffers acids and CO_2 by virtue of its amine ($-NH^2$) moiety via the following reactions:[107]

---

* Increased lactate accumulation following HCO_3^- administration may also diminish cardiac function by a second mechanism. Patients who undergo prolonged cardiopulmonary resuscitation often have up to a 50 percent reduction in the ionized Ca^{2+} concentration in the plasma, a change that can directly impair cardiac contractility.[105] The total plasma Ca^{2+} concentration, however, remains normal, indicating that increased binding of Ca^{2+} must be present. This effect is directly related to the severity of the acidemia and could represent Ca^{2+} binding to lactate.

$$THAM-NH_2 + H^+ = THAM-NH_3^+$$

$$THAM-NH_2 + H_2O + CO_2 = THAM-NH_3^+ + HCO_3^-$$

Protonated THAM is excreted in the urine at a slightly higher rate than creatinine clearance in conjunction with either chloride or bicarbonate. Thus, THAM supplements the buffering capacity of blood without generating carbon dioxide but is less effective in patients with renal failure. Reported toxicities include hyperkalemia, hypoglycemia, and respiratory depression; the last complication probably results from the ability of THAM to rapidly increase the pH and decrease the P_{CO_2} in the central nervous system.

Published clinical experience with THAM is limited, but the drug has been used to treat severe acidemia due to sepsis, hypercapnia, diabetic ketoacidosis, renal tubular acidosis, gastroenteritis, and drug intoxication.[107] Its clinical efficacy compared to that of sodium bicarbonate in the treatment of metabolic acidosis remains unproven, and THAM is of uncertain safety.

These findings are consistent with the primary importance of reversing the underlying disorder. Patients generally die from tissue ischemia rather than from acidemia itself.

Ketoacidosis

The biochemistry of ketoacidosis is discussed in detail in Chap. 25. Stated briefly, free fatty acids are converted in the liver into triglycerides, CO_2, and H_2O or into the ketoacids, acetoacetic acid and β-hydroxybutyric acid. Overproduction of ketoacids resulting in metabolic acidosis requires two factors: (1) an increase in free fatty acid delivery to the liver due to enhanced lipolysis, and (2) a resetting of hepatocyte function such that the free fatty acids are converted preferentially into ketoacids and not triglycerides.[108-110] *Both diminished activity of insulin and enhanced secretion of glucagon* (due in part to the insulin deficiency) contribute to these changes: the lack of insulin by increasing lipolysis, and the excess of glucagon by indirectly increasing fatty acyl CoA entry into the hepatic mitochondria, where it can be converted into ketones.[108-110]

Etiology Uncontrolled diabetes mellitus is the most common cause of ketoacidosis. Hyperglycemia is invariably present in this setting, with the plasma glucose concentration usually exceeding 400 mg/dL.

Fasting Fasting can also result in ketosis, as the appropriate hormonal milieu (low insulin, high glucagon) is established by the lack of carbohydrate intake. In comparison to the potentially severe ketoacidosis that can occur in uncontrolled diabetes, ketoacid levels do not exceed 10 meq/L with fasting. This limitation in the degree of ketone formation may reflect the ability of ketonemia to promote insulin secretion, eventually limiting the availability of free fatty acids.[111,112]

Alcoholic ketoacidosis The combination of alcohol ingestion and poor dietary intake is another cause of ketoacidosis.[113-115] The decrease in carbohydrate intake plus the inhibition of gluconeogenesis by alcohol[49] result in the necessary changes in insulin and glucagon secretion. In addition, ethanol directly enhances lipolysis, further increasing the supply of free fatty acids.[116]

The net effect may be a relatively severe acidosis that is often due to factors other than ketoacidosis alone.[115,117] Concurrent hypovolemia can lead to enhanced lactic acid production, and some of the ethanol will be metabolized into acetic acid.

These patients also frequently present with a mixed-base disturbance:[115]

- Metabolic alkalosis may result from vomiting, which is a common complicating problem. In some cases, the arterial pH may be relatively normal, and only the elevated anion gap points toward the presence of ketoacidosis.
- Patients with underlying chronic hepatic disease may have a chronic respiratory alkalosis (see Chap. 21).
- Urinary loss of the ketoacid anions can lead to a relatively normal anion gap in comparison to the fall in the plasma bicarbonate concentration (see "Anion Gap," above).

Other Increased ketoacid production can also occur in a variety of congenital organic acidemias (such as methylmalonic or isovaleric acidemia)[118,119] and may contribute to the acidemia associated with salicylate intoxication.[22] The mechanisms responsible for the increased ketone synthesis in these disorders are not completely understood.

Diagnosis The presence of alcoholic ketoacidosis should be suspected in a patient with a history of alcohol abuse who is found to have an otherwise unexplained high anion gap metabolic acidosis with a normal or only slightly elevated plasma glucose concentration. The osmolal gap—the difference between the measured and calculated plasma osmolality (see page 607)—also tends to be increased as a result of the accumulation of glycerol (derived from fat breakdown) and acetone and the possible presence of ethanol.[120] This finding, however, is of limited diagnostic utility, since the osmolal gap is also increased in other high anion gap acidoses, such as that due to methanol or ethylene glycol intoxication (see below).[121]

Confirmation of the presence of ketoacidosis requires the demonstration of ketonemia. This is generally done with nitroprusside (Acetest) tablets or reagent sticks. A 4+ reaction with serum diluted 1:1 is strongly suggestive of ketoacidosis. However, nitroprusside reacts with acetoacetate and acetone (produced by the decarboxylation of acetoacetic acid), but not with β-hydroxybutyrate.[90] The latter ketoacid is formed from the reduction of the β-aldehyde group of acetoacetate in a reaction utilizing NADH. β-Hydroxybutyrate makes up about 75 percent of the circulating ketones in diabetic ketoacidosis, but this value can reach 90 percent when NADH levels are elevated with concurrent lactic acidosis[90] or in alcoholic ketoacidosis (where NADH is generated from the oxidation of ethanol to acetic acid).[113]

In these settings, the nitroprusside test may underestimate the degree of ketonemia and ketonuria. Clinical awareness of the possibility of ketoacidosis is essential, since an assay for β-hydroxybutyrate is not available in most hospitals. An indirect method to circumvent this problem is to add a few drops of hydrogen peroxide to a urine specimen. This will nonenzymatically convert β-hydroxybutyrate into acetoacetate, which will then be detectable by nitroprusside.[122] An alternative, if available, is to directly measure β-hydroxybutyrate in the blood.

A different problem in diagnosis arises with sulfhydryl drugs, particularly captopril, which is widely used in the treatment of diabetic nephropathy and hypertension in diabetics. These drugs can interact with the nitroprusside reagent to produce a false-positive ketone test.[123] Thus, a positive nitroprusside test for ketonuria or ketonemia cannot be reliably interpreted in patients treated with captopril. In this setting, the diagnosis of diabetic ketoacidosis must be made on clinical grounds (otherwise unexplained high anion gap metabolic acidosis in a patient with uncontrolled diabetes) or by direct measurement of β-hydroxybutyrate.

Treatment Although insulin is the keystone to therapy in diabetic ketoacidosis, it may be dangerous in alcoholism or fasting, where the baseline plasma glucose concentration may be low. In these conditions, the administration of glucose and saline will augment endogenous insulin secretion, diminish that of glucagon, normalize fatty acid metabolism, and correct any fluid deficit that may be present.[114,115]

The role of HCO_3^- therapy is uncertain in ketoacidosis, as it is in lactic acidosis. Most patients with ketoacidosis will derive no benefit from exogenous alkali, since insulin-induced metabolism of the ketoacid anions will result in the rapid regeneration of HCO_3^- and at least partial correction of the acidemia.[30,124,125] There are, however, two settings in which HCO_3^- therapy may be beneficial: with marked acidemia (arterial pH < 7.00 to 7.10), and with a relatively normal anion gap, due to excretion of ketoacid anions in the urine.[30,93] In the latter condition, the quantity of HCO_3^- that can be generated from organic anion metabolism is minimized, and, in the absence of alkali therapy, restoration of acid-base balance will be a slow process, requiring renal excretion of the excess acid as NH_4^+.[30]

Hypophosphatemia is also a frequent complication of the treatment of ketoacidosis, since the rise in insulin levels promotes phosphate movement from the extracellular fluid into the cells. However, phosphate administration is generally not required unless marked hypophosphatemia occurs. When present, severe hypophosphatemia may be associated with marked and possibly life-threatening complications in these patients, including myocardial dysfunction.[126]

Renal Failure

Metabolic acidosis is a common complication of advanced renal disease and results from an inability of the diseased kidney to excrete the daily dietary acid load.[35,36,127] The acidemia is generally not severe, although alkali therapy may still have a variety of beneficial effects.

Pathogenesis   Renal insufficiency can affect all of the parameters involved in net acid excretion. With the initial reduction in glomerular filtration rate (GFR), hydrogen balance is maintained by increased ammonium excretion per functioning nephron.[127-130] However, total ammonium excretion begins to fall when the GFR is less than 40 to 50 mL/min (Fig. 19-3).[130,131] The net effect is the development of metabolic acidosis, resulting from an *inability to excrete all of the daily H^+ load*.[35,36,130]

Both decreased titratable acidity (primarily as phosphate) and reduced HCO_3^- reabsorption also may contribute to the decline in net acid excretion. Phosphate excretion is initially maintained in renal failure, in part by the associated secondary hyperparathyroidism (see page 202). However, net phosphorus absorption and therefore urinary excretion are diminished in patients with advanced disease, because of both dietary restriction and the use of oral phosphate binders, such as calcium carbonate, to prevent hyperphosphatemia.[130]

The role of impaired HCO_3^- reabsorption is uncertain;[127] the need to increase Na^+ excretion per functioning nephron to maintain Na^+ balance may lead to a modest increase in HCO_3^- excretion.[130,132,133] This defect, however, does not appear to play an important role in most cases.[133,134]

The fall in total ammonium excretion in renal failure usually does not represent tubular dysfunction per se. Ammonium excretion per total GFR (to account for the reduction in functioning renal mass) is three to four times normal, a level similar to the maximum achieved in normal subjects following an acid load.[127,129] This suggests that the reduction in total ammonium excretion reflects the *limited number of functioning nephrons*, since ammonium production is already proceeding at a maximal rate.[129]

As the patient approaches end-stage renal failure, the plasma HCO_3^- concentration usually, but not always, falls and then stabilizes at 12 to 20 meq/L.[35,36,130,135] Although H^+ ions continue to be retained, a further reduction in the plasma HCO_3^- concentration is prevented by buffering of the excess acid, primarily by bone buffers.[135,136] This process is manifested in part by the release of calcium from bone and its subsequent excretion in the urine. This negative calcium balance can be reversed with alkali therapy;[135] if it is untreated, however, the calcium loss can, over a prolonged period, lead to osteopenia.[136]

A plasma HCO_3^- concentration below 10 to 12 meq/L is usually due to a superimposed abnormality, such as hypoaldosteronism (in which hyperkalemia is a prominent finding; see Chap. 28), or another cause of metabolic acidosis, as with diarrhea. The latter problem can lead to a severe reduction in pH, since patients with renal failure cannot compensate for the increased H^+ load by increasing renal acid excretion.

Treatment   Exogenous alkali therapy has not in the past been used to correct asymptomatic metabolic acidosis in adults with renal failure. The limited fall in the

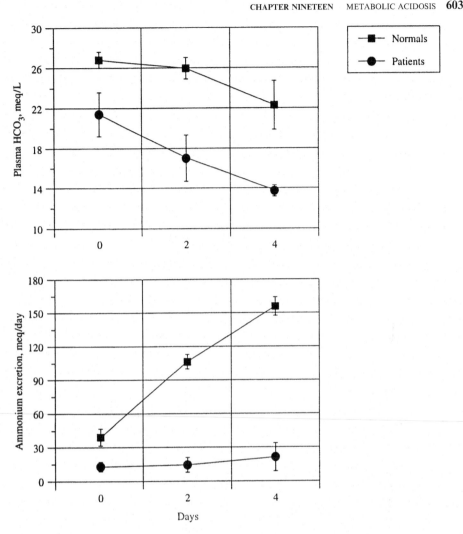

Figure 19-3   Effect of a dietary acid load on the plasma HCO_3^- concentration and urinary NH_4^+ excretion in normals (squares) and patients with chronic renal failure (circles). Normal subjects increase NH_4^+ excretion approximately fourfold with only a few meq/L reduction in the plasma HCO_3^- concentration. The patients with chronic renal disease had a low rate of NH_4^+ excretion at baseline (despite already having a mild metabolic acidosis) and showed no increment following the acid load. (*Data from Welbourne T, Weber M, Bank N, J Clin Invest 51:1852, 1972, with permission.*)

plasma HCO_3^- concentration plus the respiratory compensation usually maintain the arterial pH near 7.30, a level that poses no danger to the patient. Furthermore, raising the pH in the presence of hypocalcemia can precipitate tetany, and the associated Na^+ load can increase the tendency toward volume expansion. As a result, the major indications for $NaHCO_3$ therapy have included a fall in the plasma HCO_3^- concentration below 12 meq/L; symptoms such as dyspnea, and persistent hyperkalemia, since raising the pH will drive K^+ into the cells; and acidemia in children, which can impair growth.[137]

In adults, in whom growth is not an issue, there are least three potential reasons why even mild metabolic acidosis should be treated in the patient with renal failure:[138]

- Minimizing bone buffering of excess H^+ ions may minimize the loss of bone calcium and possibly prevent or delay the development of osteopenia.[135,136] Correction of the acidosis also can prevent progression of hyperparathyroid bone disease,[139] an effect that may be related to a diminished stimulus to secondary hyperparathyroidism.[138]
- Metabolic acidosis can lead to increased skeletal muscle breakdown and decreased albumin synthesis,[141-145] an effect that can be reversed by correction of the acidemia.[146,147] The catabolic state, which appears to be mediated in part by increased release of cortisol and diminished release of insulin-like growth factor-I (IGF-I), may contribute to loss of lean body mass and muscle weakness.[143,144] These problems may be exacerbated by the low-protein diet that may be prescribed in an attempt to slow the rate of progression of the renal failure (see page 48).[142]
- The adaptive increase in NH_3 production per nephron can lead to local complement activation and tubulointerstitial damage.[148] Preventing this response with alkali therapy may protect the kidney and slow the rate of progression of the underlying disease.[148]

Definitive studies on the treatment of metabolic acidosis in chronic renal failure in humans have not yet been performed. Nevertheless, some physicians have advocated the earlier use of alkali therapy in this setting, particularly in view of the observation that $NaHCO_3$ is better excreted (perhaps reflecting the impairment in HCO_3^- reabsorption) and therefore less likely to produce fluid overload than an equivalent quantity of NaCl.[149]

If alkali therapy is given, $NaHCO_3$ is the treatment of choice, while sodium citrate (citrate is rapidly metabolized to HCO_3^-) should be *avoided*. Citrate can markedly increase passive aluminum absorption, possibly predisposing to aluminum intoxication in patients with renal failure who are taking aluminum hydroxide to control hyperphosphatemia (see page 205).[150,151] Two factors are thought to contribute to this effect: (1) Citrate combines with aluminum to form a nondissociable but soluble and absorbable complex, and (2) citrate combines with Ca^{2+} in the intestinal lumen, leading to a reduction in the free Ca^{2+} concentration that increases the permeability of tight junctions.[150]

Ingestions

Salicylates   Aspirin (acetylsalicylic acid) is rapidly converted into salicylic acid in the body. Although there is no absolute correlation between the plasma salicylate concentration and symptoms, most patients show signs of intoxication when the plasma level exceeds 40 to 50 mg/dL (therapeutic range is 20 to 35 mg/dL).[156] Early symptoms include tinnitus, vertigo, nausea, vomiting, and diarrhea; more severe intoxication can cause altered mental status, coma, noncardiac pulmonary edema, and death. Fatal overdosage can occur after the ingestion of 10 to 30 g by adults and as little as 3 g by children. The diagnosis can be made with certainty only by measurement of the plasma salicylate concentration.

Increasing doses of aspirin cause a progressively greater risk of toxicity because of *saturation of protective mechanisms.*[157] At therapeutic levels, 90 percent of salicylate is protein bound and therefore limited to the vascular space; the drug is then partially glycinated in the liver to salicyluric acid, which is both less toxic and more rapidly excreted by the kidney than salicylate. With salicylate toxicity, however, the degree of protein binding falls to 50 percent and salicyluric acid formation becomes saturated. Thus, more drug is now able to reach the tissues, and, because of the decline in renal excretion, toxic levels persist for a longer period of time.

A variety of acid-base disturbances can occur with salicylate intoxication.[158] Salicylates stimulate the respiratory center directly,[159] resulting in a fall in the P_{CO_2} and respiratory alkalosis as the earliest abnormality.[156,158,160] Metabolic acidosis may then ensue, primarily because of the accumulation of organic acids, including lactate and ketoacids.[22,49,161] The respiratory alkalosis, which normally promotes lactic acid production in an attempt to minimize the rise in pH,[54] appears to play a contributory role in this process. In experimental animals, lactate accumulation is not seen if the initial fall in P_{CO_2} is prevented but gradually becomes more prominent if hypocapnia is allowed to occur.[161] Salicylic acid itself (mol wt 180) has only a minor effect, since a plasma level of 50 mg/dL represents a concentration that is less than 3 meq/L.

The net effect of these changes is that most adults have either a respiratory alkalosis or a mixed respiratory alkalosis–metabolic acidosis; pure metabolic acidosis is unusual.[158] In addition, approximately one-third of adults will also ingest one or more other medications, many of which are respiratory depressants and can lead to concurrent respiratory acidosis.[158]

Treatment   The serious neurologic toxicity of salicylates, including death, is related to the cerebral tissue salicylate concentration; thus, a reduction in this level must be the first goal of therapy. This can in part be achieved by *alkalinization of the plasma* to an arterial pH between 7.45 and 7.50. To appreciate how this works, it is important to note that salicylic acid (HS) is a weak acid with a pK_a of 3.0. Thus, the Henderson-Hasselbalch equation for the reaction

$$H^+ + S^- \quad \leftrightarrow \quad HS \qquad (19\text{-}14)$$

can be expressed as

$$pH = 3.0 + \log\frac{[S^-]}{[HS]} \qquad (19\text{-}15)$$

where S^- represents the salicylate anion.

At the normal pH of 7.40, the ratio of HS to S$^-$ is about 1:25,000; that is, only 0.004 percent of the total extracellular salicylate exists as HS. HS is nonpolar, lipid-soluble, and able to cross cell membranes; S$^-$ is polar and crosses membranes poorly. As a result, the plasma and central nervous system (CNS) HS concentrations are in diffusion equilibrium, but not the S$^-$ concentrations (Fig. 19-4).

If the systemic pH is increased, Eq. (19-14) will move to the left. As the plasma HS concentration falls, HS will leave the CNS (and other tissues) down a concentration gradient, where it will be trapped in the plasma as S$^-$. The fall in the CNS HS concentration then causes Eq. (19-14) to move to the right in the brain cell. This maintains the cellular HS concentration, thereby promoting further drug movement out of the CNS. For example, increasing the arterial pH from 7.20 to 7.50 will decrease the fractional concentration of HS from 0.006 to 0.003 percent. Although this change appears small, it will promote a significant reduction in tissue salicylate concentration. Note that alkalinization leads to an initial increment in the plasma salicylate concentration, but it is the tissue levels that are dangerous to the patient.

A second goal of treatment is rapid elimination of the drug from the body. Since salicylate is highly protein bound, it enters the urine primarily via secretion by the organic anion secretory pathway in the proximal tubule (see Chap. 3) rather than by glomerular filtration. The rate of salicylate excretion can be markedly enhanced by alkalinization of the urine, which, by the same process of nonionic diffusion, converts urinary HS to S$^-$, thereby minimizing the back-diffusion of secreted HS out of the tubular lumen.[162] As an example, raising the urine pH from 6.5 to 8.1 by the administration of NaHCO$_3$ can increase total salicylate excretion more than fivefold.[163]

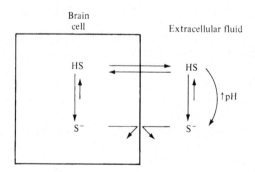

Figure 19-4 Schematic representation of the equilibrium distribution of salicylate (S$^-$) and salicylic acid (HS) between the extracellular fluid and the brain cell. HS is lipid-soluble and is in diffusion equilibrium; S$^-$ is not in equilibrium, since it is charged and cannot readily cross the cell membrane. Alkalinization of the extracellular fluid causes the reaction, H$^+$ + S$^-$ ↔ HS, to move to the left, reducing the extracellular HS concentration. This allows cellular HS to diffuse into the extracellular fluid down a concentration gradient. The decrease in the cellular HS concentration then causes some cellular S$^-$ to be converted to HS, thereby promoting continued HS diffusion out of the brain. Similar considerations explain the increased movement of salicylate from the tubular cell into the lumen when the urine is alkalinized.

The efficiency of salicylate removal can also be enhanced by hemodialysis.[156,157,164] This procedure should be considered when the plasma salicylate concentration exceeds 80 mg/dL or the patient is comatose or has impaired renal function or fluid overload.

Another frequent problem of uncertain etiology is a low cerebrospinal fluid glucose concentration, which may contribute to the neurologic abnormalities.[156] Thus, the administration of glucose should be part of the initial therapy in all patients with salicylate intoxication.

In summary, the administration of alkali is an important component of therapy in the patient with salicylate intoxication and metabolic acidosis. If, however, respiratory alkalosis is the primary disturbance, further alkalinization is not necessary.

Methanol   Methanol (wood alcohol, CH_3OH) is a component of shellac, varnish, deicing solutions, sterno, and other commercial preparations. It is metabolized to formaldehyde (in a reaction catalyzed by alcohol dehydrogenase) and then formic acid (Fig. 19-5). Symptoms and the high anion gap metabolic acidosis are usually delayed for 12 to 36 h after ingestion, since they are due to accumulation of these metabolites, particularly formic acid.[157,165,166] Early complaints include weakness, nausea, headache, and decreased vision, which can then progress to blindness, coma, and death. Funduscopic examination may reveal a retinal sheen due to retinal edema.

The minimum lethal dose is 50 to 100 mL, although smaller amounts can lead to permanent blindness. Similar clinical and acid-base disturbances may result from the ingestion of formaldehyde.[167]

Osmolal gap   The diagnosis of methanol ingestion is made by a specific serum assay for methanol. In addition, the presence of methanol intoxication may be suspected indirectly by the demonstration of an *osmolal gap* between the measured and calculated plasma osmolality:[168,169]

$$\text{Calculated } P_{osm} - 2 \times \text{plasma } [Na^+] + \frac{[\text{glucose}]}{18} + \frac{BUN}{2.8} \qquad (19\text{-}16)$$

Methanol is a small molecule (mol wt 32) that can achieve high osmolal concentration in the plasma. A level of 80 mg/dL, for example, is equivalent to 25 mosmol/kg. Thus, the measured plasma osmolality will exceed the calculated value in Eq. (19-16) by this amount. A similar but less prominent effect can be induced by ethylene glycol, which is a larger molecule (mol wt 62) that is present in lower molar concentrations than methanol. Salicylates, on the other hand, have only a minor effect, since their plasma level is almost always less than 5 mosmol/kg.[168]

Thus, a high osmolal gap in a patient with an *otherwise unexplained* high anion gap metabolic acidosis has been thought to be suggestive of the presence of either methanol or ethylene glycol intoxication. However, an elevated osmolal gap is a relatively nonspecific finding, since it is also seen in other high anion gap acidosis,

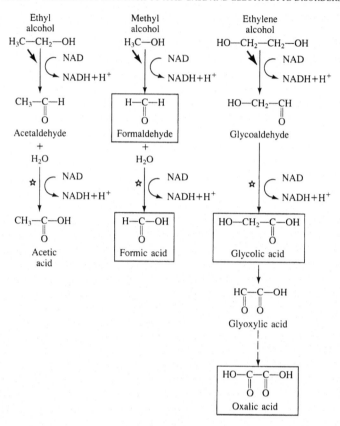

Figure 19-5 Pathways of metabolism of ethyl alcohol (ethanol), methyl alcohol (methanol), and ethylene glycol. Alcohol dehydrogenase (bold arrow) is a cytosolic enzyme that catalyzes the first oxidative step for each alcohol. Aldehyde dehydrogenase (star) is a mitochondrial enzyme that then catalyzes the second oxidative step. The products in boxes are those responsible for the major reactions associated with methanol or ethylene glycol intoxication. (*Adapted from Garella S*, Kidney Int *33:735, 1988. Reprinted by permission from* Kidney International.)

such as diabetic or alcoholic ketoacidosis, lactic acidosis, and in chronic, but not acute, renal failure (due to the retention of unidentified small solutes).[120,121,170,171] Furthermore, the osmolal gap must be correlated with concomitant measurement of the plasma ethanol concentration, since patients ingesting methanol or ethylene glycol often abuse alcohol as well.[121]*

The factors responsible for the osmolal gap in ketoacidosis and lactic acidosis have not been defined. In one study of alcoholic ketoacidosis and lactic acidosis, for example, the osmolal gap in these disorders averaged 27 and 17

---

* Detection of an osmolal group with an alcohol intoxication can be achieved only if the plasma osmolality is measured by freezing-point depression. In comparison, the osmotic contribution of volatile alcohols is not detected when a vapor pressure osmometer is used, since this technique assumes that only water is in the vapor phase.[172,173]

mosmol/kg, respectively.[121] Although ethanol contributed in many of these patients, the gap remained at 10 to 11 mosmol/kg after the effect of ethanol was subtracted. Several possibilities can explain at least part of the persistent osmolal gap in this setting:

- The release from the cells of smaller products of glycogen breakdown (other than lactate) into the circulation
- The accumulation of acetone in ketoacidosis

The net effect of these observations is that an elevated osmolal gap alone is not diagnostic of a particular disorder in the patient with a high anion gap metabolic acidosis. If, however, the history is not suggestive of either lactic acidosis or ketoacidosis, then a high osmolal gap (particularly if $\geq$ 25 mosmol/kg) strongly points toward methanol or ethylene glycol intoxication.[121] In this setting, prophylactic ethanol infusion can be initiated to prevent the formation of toxic metabolites, pending results of the assays for these toxins (see below).

An osmolal gap can also be found in a number of other conditions that are *not associated with metabolic acidosis*, including ethanol or isopropyl alcohol ingestions or after the administration of intravenous glycine (during transurethral resection of the bladder or prostate; see page 713) or mannitol.[170]

Treatment Prompt treatment is required to prevent death or permanent residue such as blindness after a methanol overdose. In addition to correcting the acidemia with $NaHCO_3$ and administering oral charcoal to minimize further drug absorption,[174] there are two basic aspects of therapy in the presence of severe poisoning: (1) administration of ethanol or fomepizole to prevent the formation of toxic metabolites and (2) hemodialysis to remove both the parent compound and metabolites.[175-177]

Intravenous or oral ethanol is an effective therapy because alcohol dehydrogenase, the enzyme that is necessary for the metabolism of methanol and ethylene glycol into their toxic metabolites (Fig. 19-5), has more than a 10-fold greater affinity for ethanol than for other alcohols.[157,176,178] This effect is most prominent when the plasma ethanol concentration is about 100 to 200 mg/dL, a level that can generally be achieved by the following regimen: a loading dose of 0.6 g/kg plus an hourly maintenance dose of 66 mg/kg in nondrinkers, 154 mg/kg in drinkers, and 240 mg/kg once hemodialysis is started.[176,179] If oral ethanol is given, the dose may have to be doubled if charcoal has been administered.[179] Regardless of the mode of administration, the plasma ethanol concentration should be monitored, since adjustments in dosage will be required in some patients.

The effect of ethanol has also been demonstrated in selected patients who become intoxicated with both methanol and ethanol.[180] In this setting, there may be very high plasma methanol levels, but no symptoms and no metabolic acidosis, since formaldehyde and formate production are minimized.

An alternative to ethanol is the administration of fomepizole (Antizol), which rapidly and competitively inhibits alcohol dehydrogenase more potently than ethanol.[181-183] Small studies or case series have documented dramatic improvements in acidemia and prevention of renal injury when fomepizole is used to treat ethylene glycol intoxication.[184,185] Fomepizole also prolongs the half-life of ethanol; thus, the simultaneous use of both agents is *not* recommended. Fomepizole is usually well tolerated but occasionally produces headache, nausea, bradycardia, dizziness, eosinophilia, or mild, transient elevation in liver enzymes.

Hemodialysis is used to remove both the parent compound and metabolites.[157] Sorbent-based hemodialysis systems should be avoided, since drug clearance may be impaired because of rapid saturation of the cartridges.[186] Drug removal is also much slower with peritoneal dialysis,[177] which should not be used unless hemodialysis is not available.

In general, ethanol is begun at the time of diagnosis and continued until the plasma methanol concentration is below 20 mg/dL.[175] Hemodialysis should also be instituted if the plasma level is greater than 50 mg/dL, more than 30 mL have been ingested, acidemia is present, or visual acuity is decreased.[175]

Ethylene glycol Ethylene glycol is a component of antifreeze and solvents that is metabolized via alcohol dehydrogenase into a variety of toxic metabolites (Fig. 19-5). The most important appear to be glycolic acid and oxalic acid, which are responsible for both the clinical symptoms and the metabolic acidosis.[157,187,188] After ingestion, there are three clinical stages of varying severity.[189,190] During the first 12 h, neurologic symptoms predominate, ranging from drunkenness to coma. This is followed by the onset of cardiopulmonary abnormalities, such as tachypnea and pulmonary edema, and then flank pain and renal failure. The latter is primarily due to glycolate-induced damage to the tubules, although plugging of the tubular lumen by precipitated oxalate crystals may also contribute.[188,191] The lethal dose of ethylene glycol is approximately 100 mL.

The diagnosis, suspected from the history and the possible presence of envelope- and needle-shaped oxalate crystals in the urine,[191] can be confirmed by the demonstration of ethylene glycol in the serum. The standard assay using sodium periodate and Schiff's aldehyde reagent is generally accurate but can give a false-positive result if mannitol has been given to induce a diuresis.[192] The diagnosis may also be suspected indirectly by the presence of an osmolal gap in the plasma, although this is generally less prominent than with methanol, which is a smaller molecule (see "Methanol," above).

Treatment The specific treatment of ethylene glycol intoxication is identical to that for methanol: ethanol or fomepizole and hemodialysis.[157,178,179,182,184,185,189] Other modalities that may be helpful include a forced diuresis to minimize tubular blockade by oxalate crystals and the administration of pyridoxine and thiamine, which respectively promote the conversion of glyoxylate into glycine and α-hydroxy-β-ketoadipate, rather than the more toxic oxalate.[169]

Other toxins A variety of other toxins can rarely lead to metabolic acidosis. Sniffing of *toluene*, a component of paint thinners, model glues, and transmission fluid, can produce a metabolic acidosis, primarily via metabolism to hippuric acid.[32] However, the hippurate anion is both filtered and secreted and is therefore rapidly excreted in the urine. As a result, the patient may present with a minimally elevated or even normal anion gap, incorrectly suggesting the possible presence of renal tubular acidosis.[32] The ingestion of *elemental sulfur*, used as a folk remedy, is associated with the generation of sulfuric acid.[193] The anion gap remains normal in this disorder, since the excess sulfate is rapidly excreted in the urine. Inhalation of chlorine gas leads to the production of hydrochloric acid, producing a normal anion gap acidosis.[199]

Hyperalimentation fluids   The administration of hyperalimentation fluids can produce a metabolic acidosis by two mechanisms. First, some of these solutions contain an excess of cationic amino acids, such as arginine and lysine. When these amino acids are utilized, H^+ ions are formed:[195]

$$R-NH_3^+ + O_2 \quad \rightarrow \quad urea + CO_2 + H_2O + H^+$$

This is in addition to the H^+ ions generated by the sulfur-containing amino acids in the solution. Second, starved patients may become hypophosphatemic when fed, resulting in a fall in phosphate and therefore titratable acid excretion. In this setting, the H^+ load associated with the metabolism of the administered protein is not as efficiently excreted, and metabolic acidosis is more likely to ensue.[196]

Gastrointestinal Loss of Bicarbonate

Diarrhea and fistulas   The intestinal fluids below the stomach, including pancreatic and biliary secretions, are relatively alkaline. The net base in these fluids, which may have a total concentration of 50 to 70 meq/L,[197] consists of HCO_3^- as well as organic anions, which, if absorbed, would be metabolized to HCO_3^-.[198] As a result, diarrhea, a villous adenoma, or the removal of pancreatic, biliary, or intestinal secretions (by tube drainage, fistulas, or vomiting if there is intestinal obstruction) can lead to metabolic acidosis,[26,197] particularly if volume depletion or underlying renal disease limits the ability of the kidneys to adapt by increasing NH_4^+ excretion.[45]

The same sequence can occur in occult laxative abuse, which should be considered in any patient with a hyperchloremic metabolic acidosis and/or chronic diarrhea of unknown etiology.[199,200] As many as 15 percent of patients referred to tertiary care centers for evaluation of chronic diarrhea are found to have laxative abuse as the cause of their diarrhea.[201] However, for reasons that are not well understood, many patients with laxative abuse present with metabolic alkalosis rather than acidosis.[197,202]

The increase in stool output in diarrheal states can result from either increased intestinal secretion or decreased absorption of fluids that have been secreted.[203] Secretion, for example, may be increased with cholera, toxigenic *Escherichia coli*, or humoral substances released from tumors, such as vasoactive intestinal peptide.

Ureterosigmoidostomy and other forms of urinary division Implantation of the ureters into the sigmoid colon or, more recently, a short loop of ileum that opens at the abdominal wall (ureteroileostomy) has been used to treat patients with obstructive uropathy due to locally invasive tumor, surgical removal of the bladder for carcinoma, or less often neurologic bladder dysfunction. A hyperchloremic metabolic acidosis is a relatively common complication of ureterosigmoidostomy (occurring in up to 80 percent of cases) and is due to two factors:[197,204-207]

- The colon has an anion exchange pump, with luminal Cl^- being reabsorbed as HCO_3^- is secreted. Thus, when urinary Cl^- enters the colon, it will exchange for HCO_3^-, which will then be lost in the stool.[208]
- The colon can directly absorb NH_4^+, which is derived both from the urine and from urea-splitting bacteria in the colon.[197,204] In the liver, the NH_4^+ is metabolized into NH_3 and H^+. Hyperammonemic encephalopathy can occur in patients with underlying liver disease or a marked ammonia load due to a urinary tract infection with a urea-splitting organism.[209]

Metabolic acidosis is much less likely with a ureteroileostomy, since rapid drainage of urine into an ileostomy bag means that contact time between the urine and the intestine is normally too short for significant changes in urinary composition to occur. However, metabolic acidosis can be seen if contact time is increased because of malfunction of the loop (most often due to stomal stenosis).[204-207] Thus, a loopogram should be performed when an otherwise unexplained metabolic acidosis develops in a patient with a ureteroileostomy. Reabsorption of urinary ammonium appears to be more important to the fall in the plasma bicarbonate concentration in this setting than is secretion of bicarbonate in the ileum.[204,205]

Cholestyramine Cholestyramine chloride is an orally administered resin used in the treatment of hypercholesterolemia. It is nonreabsorbable and can act as an anion-exchange resin, exchanging its Cl^- for endogenous HCO_3^- and producing a metabolic acidosis.[210] This problem is most likely to occur if there is underlying renal disease, which can minimize renal excretion of the excess acid.

Renal Tubular Acidosis

Renal tubular acidosis (RTA) refers to those conditions in which metabolic acidosis results from diminished net tubular H^+ secretion.[211,212] There are three major types of RTA, the characteristics of which are summarized in Table 19-6. Although these disorders are relatively unusual in adults (with the exception of type 4 RTA), they provide interesting examples of the different ways in which the renal regulation of acid-base balance can be impaired.

The acidosis associated with renal failure could also be included in this group. However, NH_4^+ excretion per total GFR in this disorder is equal to that achieved in acidemic patients with normal renal function.[129] Thus, as mentioned above, the

Table 19-6   Characteristics of different types of renal tubular acidosis[a]

	Type 1 (distal)	Type 2 (proximal)	Type 4
Basic defect	Decreased distal acidification	Diminished proximal HCO_3^- reabsorption	Aldosterone deficiency or resistance
Urine pH during acidemia	> 5.3	Variable: > 5.3 if above reabsorptive threshold; < 5.3 if below	Usually < 5.3
Plasma [HCO_3^-], untreated	May be below 10 meq/L	Usually 14 to 20 meq/L	Usually above 15 meq/L
Fractional excretion of HCO_3^- at normal plasma [HCO_3^-]	< 3% in adults, may reach 5%–10% in young children	> 15%–20%	< 3%
Diagnosis	Response to $NaHCO_3$ or NH_4Cl	Response to $NaHCO_3$	Measure plasma aldosterone concentration
Plasma [K^+]	Usually reduced or normal; elevated with voltage defect	Normal or reduced	Elevated
Dose of HCO_3^- to normalize plasma [HCO_3^-], meq/kg per day	1–2 in adults, 4–14 in children	10–15	1–3; may require no alkali if hyperkalemia corrected
Nonelectrolyte complications	Nephrocalcinosis and renal stones	Rickets or osteomalacia	None

[a] What had been called type 3 RTA is actually a variant of type 1 RTA (see below).

major problem in renal failure is too few functioning nephrons, not diminished tubular function. In addition, the ability to maximally acidify the urine (urine pH ≤ 5.3) is usually maintained in renal failure, in contrast to type 1 and, in some circumstances, type 2 RTA.[127,130,131]

Type 1 (distal) RTA   Type 1 RTA is characterized by a decrease in net H^+ secretion in the collecting tubules such that the urine pH, which can normally be lowered to a minimum of 4.5 to 5.0 in these segments, remains above 5.3. This defect in acidification diminishes NH_4^+ and titratable acid excretion, thereby preventing complete excretion of the dietary acid load. As a result, there is continued H^+ retention, leading to a progressive reduction in the plasma HCO_3^- concentration, which may fall below 10 meq/L.

Pathogenesis   Acidification in the collecting tubules is primarily achieved via H^+ secretion by a luminal H^+-ATPase pump (see Fig. 5-3). This pump is located both in the cortex (where it is present only in the *intercalated* cells) and in the medulla.[213,214] Although the H^+ secretory cells in the distal nephron do not transport Na^+,[213,215] net H^+ secretion in the cortical collecting tubule is indirectly influenced by Na^+ reabsorption in the adjacent *principal* cells (see Fig. 5-2). The removal of cationic Na^+ from the tubular fluid makes the lumen more electronegative, thereby promoting the accumulation of H^+ ions in the lumen by minimizing the degree of passive back-diffusion.[213,216,217] In comparison, H^+ secretion in the medulla largely occurs in the absence of Na^+ reabsorption by adjacent cells and therefore is essentially *Na^+-independent*.[213,218]

This brief review of distal acidification suggests that there are three mechanisms by which type 1 RTA can occur.[211,212,217]

- The most common problem is thought to be a defect in the H^+-ATPase pump, which may be present in the cortex and/or the medulla. It is likely that a number of different defects can directly or indirectly cause this problem: Three patients with Sjögren's syndrome have been described in whom immunocytochemical analysis of tissue obtained by renal biopsy showed complete absence of H^+-ATPase pumps in the intercalated cells.[219,220] How immunologic injury leads to this change is not known.

  There are also genetic forms of type 1 RTA. In patients with autosomal dominant disease, mutations in the gene for the chloride-bicarbonate exchanger (AE1 or band 3) have often been described.[221-223] This exchanger is responsible for returning bicarbonate generated within the cell during hydrogen secretion to the systemic circulation. Mutations have also been described in the gene encoding the B subunit of the H^+-ATPase pump; this disorder is associated with sensorineural deafness, suggesting that the pump is also required for normal function of the inner ear.[224]

- There can be a reduction in cortical Na^+ reabsorption, thereby diminishing the degree of luminal negativity and producing a *voltage-dependent defect*. This abnormality will lead to a concurrent impairment in K^+ secretion, which is also driven in part by the favorable electrical gradient (see Chap. 12).[225] Thus, hyperkalemia will accompany the metabolic acidosis; this problem has most often been described in patients with urinary tract obstruction and sickle cell disease.[217,226-228] In the former disorder, for example, a reduction in Na^+-K^+-ATPase activity may be responsible for the reduction in Na^+ reabsorption; there may also be a concomitant decrease in H^+-ATPase activity in the outer medulla, further decreasing the ability to secrete hydrogen ions.[229] Impaired distal hydrogen and potassium secretion may also occur with any cause of marked volume depletion, where the diminished distal delivery of Na^+ can induce a readily reversible form of type 1 RTA.[44,230]

  An alternative mechanism may explain the development of hyperkalemic type 1 RTA in some cases.[231] These patients may have two different defects:

(1) an impairment in the H^+-ATPase pump, which is responsible for the RTA, and (2) hypoaldosteronism or aldosterone resistance induced by tubular injury, which is responsible for the hyperkalemia.

- There can be an increase in membrane permeability, which allows the back-diffusion of H^+ ions (or possibly H_2CO_3). A urine pH of 5.0, for example, is associated with a H^+ concentration that is *250 times greater* than that in the extracellular fluid. This gradient can be maintained only if the luminal membrane and tight junction are relatively impermeable to H^+. A *gradient defect* has been documented only in patients treated with amphotericin B, which is a potent tubular toxin.[211,232]

The possible site and mechanism of the acidification defect in type 1 RTA have been partially elucidated by the responses to furosemide and Na_2SO_4.[217] Both agents enhance luminal electronegativity by increasing Na^+ delivery to and reabsorption in the cortical collecting tubule; in addition, the presence of the impermeant anion SO_4^{2-} will tend to make the lumen more electronegative, since the gradient created by Na^+ transport cannot be dissipated by SO_4^{2-} reabsorption.

The changes that these agents induce in H^+ and K^+ excretion in normal subjects and those with type 1 RTA are shown in Table 19-7:[217,228]

- Normal subjects with metabolic acidosis will have an acid urine pH (< 5.3) that can be further lowered with furosemide or Na_2SO_4; the increase in electronegativity will also enhance K^+ excretion in this setting.
- Patients with diffuse impairment in the H^+-ATPase pump (due to decreased function or number) will have a persistently alkaline urine pH but a normal rise in K^+ excretion, since principal cell function is intact. A similar result will be seen if the pump dysfunction is limited to the cortical collecting tubule.

Table 19-7   Response to furosemide in normals and different types of type 1 renal tubular acidosis[a]

Type of defect	Site	Urine		K^+ excretion	
		Acidosis	Furosemide	Baseline	Furosemide
Normal		< 5.3	Further decline	Normal	Increased
H^+-ATPase pump	Diffuse or CCT alone	> 5.5	> 5.5	Normal	Increased
H^+-ATPase pump	MCT	> 5.5	< 5.5	Normal	Increased
Voltage or Na^+ reabsorptive	CCT	> 5.5	> 5.5	Decreased	No response

[a] Similar responses will occur to Na_2SO_4. CCT equals cortical collecting tubule; MCT equals medullary collecting tubule.

- Patients with a pump defect that is *limited to the medulla* will have a relatively normal increase in both H^+ and K^+ excretion because cortical function is appropriately stimulated by the rise in luminal electronegativity.
- Patients with a primary impairment in cortical Na^+ reabsorption (a *voltage defect*) will have baseline hyperkalemia and no posttherapy increase in H^+ or K^+ excretion, since there is no enhancement in luminal electronegativity.[228,233] It is not possible to exclude the possibility that there is also a defect in pump function in this setting.

Although proximal HCO_3^- reabsorption is intact in this disorder, variable degrees of *fixed* bicarbonaturia are obligated by the high urine pH. If, for example, the urine P_{CO_2} is 46 mmHg (similar to that in venous blood), then, from the Henderson-Hasselbalch equation, the urinary HCO_3^- concentration will vary with the urine pH*:

$$\text{Urine pH} = pK_a' + \log\frac{[HCO_3^-]}{0.03 P_{CO_2}} \qquad (19\text{-}17)$$

At a urine pH below 6.0, the urinary HCO_3^- concentration is negligible. In adults with type 1 RTA, the urine pH is usually less than 6.5, resulting in a relatively mild degree of urinary HCO_3^- loss with less than 3 percent of the filtered HCO_3^- being excreted (Fig. 19-6). The latter can be calculated from a formula similar to that for the fractional excretion of Na^+ (see page 407), using a random urine specimen collected under oil to minimize the evaporative loss of CO_2:

$$FE_{HCO_3^-}(\%) = \frac{\text{urine } [HCO_3^-] \times \text{plasma [creatinine]}}{\text{plasma } [HCO_3^-] \times \text{urine [creatinine]}} \times 100 \qquad (19\text{-}18)$$

In children, however, the minimum urine pH is generally higher and fixed HCO_3^- losses, which can be calculated from Eq. (19-17), are greater. When the urine pH exceeds 7.0, for example, the fractional excretion of HCO_3^- can reach 5 to 10 percent, thereby making an important contribution to the acidemia. This syndrome, which has been called *type 3 RTA*, occurs in infants, who within a few years have a lower urine pH and follow a course more typical of type 1 RTA.[235]

Plasma K^+ concentration The different types of acidification defects produce different changes in K^+ balance. Those patients who have an impairment in the H^+-ATPase pump or increased permeability to H^+ back-diffusion tend to have *urinary K^+ wasting and hypokalemia prior to therapy.*[236,237] Three factors may contribute to this problem:

- Single net distal H^+ secretion is diminished, more Na^+ reabsorption must now occur in exchange for K^+.

---

* The urine pK_a' varies with total electrolyte concentration and may be somewhat different from the plasma value of 6.10.[234]

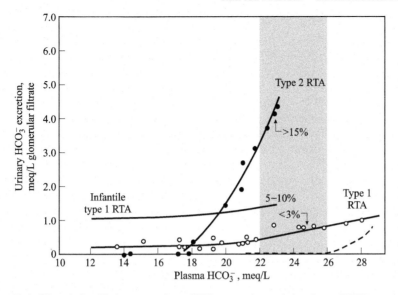

Figure 19-6   The relationship between urinary HCO_3^- excretion and the plasma HCO_3^- concentration in normal subjects (dashed line) and in patients with type 1 and type 2 RTA as $NaHCO_3$ is administered to raise the plasma HCO_3^- concentration toward normal. In the last condition, there is little urinary HCO_3^- and an acid urine pH when the plasma HCO_3^- concentration is below the maximal reabsorptive capacity. Above this level, however, there is a rapid increase in HCO_3^- excretion such that more than 10 to 15 percent of the filtered HCO_3^- is excreted at a normal plasma HCO_3^- concentration (shaded area). Patients with type 1 RTA, on the other hand, are similar to normal subjects except that there is a fixed degree of bicarbonaturia obligated by the high urine pH. In adults, this is generally less than 3 percent of the filtered load, but it can reach 5 to 10 percent in infantile type 1 RTA, in which there is a higher minimal urine pH. (*Adapted from Sebastian A, McSherry E, Morris RC Jr, in Brenner BM, Rector FC Jr (eds): The Kidney. Philadelphia, Saunders, 1976, chap 16, with permission.*)

- There may be a concurrent decrease in the activity of the second proton pump in the luminal membrane of the cortical and outer medullary collecting tubules, the H^+-K^+-ATPase pump that reabsorbs K^+ as well as secreting H^+ (see Chap. 11).[214,238] The main function of this pump may be to reabsorb K^+ in states of K^+ depletion, rather than to maintain acid-base balance. As a result, its inhibition may promote urinary K^+ wasting and hypokalemia as well as metabolic acidosis.[239]
- Metabolic acidosis leads to increased NaCl and water delivery out of the proximal tubule; the ensuing Na^+-wasting results in secondary hyperaldosteronism and increased K^+ losses. The latter defect in proximal function is a probable reflection of the low plasma HCO_3^- concentration and therefore the less quantity of HCO_3^- reabsorption by Na^+-H^+ exchange in the proximal tubule. The Na^+-H^+ exchanger plays an important role in proximal NaCl reabsorption, both by creating a gradient for passive Cl^- transport and by promoting active Cl^- transport by operating in parallel with a Cl^- formate$^-$ exchanger (see page 79).

Thus, any cause of metabolic acidosis will tend to diminish net proximal fluid reabsorption.[240] Acidemia can also directly impair Cl^- transport (via an unknown mechanism) in the cortical aspect of the thick ascending limb.[241]

These abnormalities and most of the urinary K^+ wasting can be reversed by correction of the acidemia.[236,237] Some defect may persist, however, in those patients with impaired pump activity, since there will still be a requirement to secrete more than normal amounts of K^+ in exchange for Na^+ in the cortical collecting tubule.[236,242]

In comparison, those patients with a voltage defect due to diminished distal Na^+ transport will have a lesser degree of luminal electronegativity and therefore will excrete less H^+ and K^+, resulting in *hyperkalemia* as well as metabolic acidosis.[211,217,226-228,243] These patients appear to have normal amounts of H^+-ATPase in the intercalated cells.[243] Although hyperkalemic acidosis is also found in type 4 RTA, this disorder is associated with low aldosterone levels and usually intact ability to reduce the urine pH below 5.3.[44,226]

Nephrocalcinosis   Hypercalciuria, hyperphosphaturia, nephrolithiasis (with calcium phosphate or struvite stones), and nephrocalcinosis are frequently associated with untreated type 1 RTA.[244-248] In some families, hypercalciuria precedes the metabolic acidosis, suggesting that calcium-induced tubular damage is then responsible for the RTA.[244,245] In most cases, however, acidemia is directly responsible, both by increasing calcium phosphate release from bone during buffering of the excess H^+[135,249,250] and by directly reducing (via an uncertain mechanism) the tubular reabsorption of these ions.[251-253] The degree of hypercalciuria is generally proportional to the fall in the plasma HCO_3^- concentration.[254]

In addition to hypercalciuria and hyperphosphaturia, two other factors increase the tendency to stone formation in type 1 RTA: the persistently high urine pH, which promotes the precipitation of calcium phosphate, and low levels of citrate excretion. Citrate normally inhibits crystallization by forming a non-dissociable but soluble complex with calcium, thereby decreasing the amount of free calcium available for stone formation[245-248,255] Both metabolic acidosis and hypokalemia may contribute to the hypocitraturia by lowering the tubular cell pH in the proximal tubule, the former directly and the latter by transcellular K^+/H^+ exchange (see page 356).[256,257] Intracellular acidosis promotes citrate utilization, leading sequentially to low citrate levels in the cell, a more favorable gradient for citrate reabsorption from the tubular lumen, and a decline in citrate excretion.[256] The acidemia-induced fall in luminal pH in the proximal tubule also may contribute to this response by converting filtered $citrate^{3-}$ into the more reabsorbable $citrate^{2-}$.[258]

Stone disease is less common in incomplete type 1 RTA.[248,260] In this setting, low urinary citrate levels may be of primary importance (see below).

All of the above changes in complete type 1 RTA typically respond to early and complete correction of the acidemia: less calcium phosphate release from bone, enhanced tubular reabsorption of these ions, an increase in urinary citrate excretion (although not necessarily to normal,[246,248,255] and prevention of nephrocalcinosis and nephrolithiasis,[246-248,261] even in the incomplete form.[248]

In general, *potassium citrate* (citrate is rapidly metabolized in HCO_3^-) is the preferred therapy.[248] It is better tolerated than HCO_3^- solutions, correction of hypokalemia will further increase citrate excretion, and the natriuresis associated with *sodium* citrate leads to an undesirable increase in calcium excretion, since Na^+ and calcium handling are indirectly linked in the proximal tubule and loop of Henle (see Chap. 3).[262,263]

In contrast, alkali therapy alone is less likely to prevent nephrocalcinosis in those patients with hereditary RTA in whom hypercalciuria is the primary defect.[244,245] In this setting, conventional therapy for calcium stones, such as a thiazide diuretic to diminish calcium excretion and neutral phosphate to increase the excretion of the crystallization inhibitor pyrophosphate, may be effective.[264-266]

Incomplete type 1 RTA   Some patients with defective urinary acidification do not become acidemic, a syndrome that is referred to as *incomplete* type 1 RTA.[131,267,268] Patients with the incomplete form have a normal rate of ammonium excretion despite a high urine pH. Why this occurs is not clear, but the observation that they also have a low rate of citrate excretion (similar to the complete form) suggests that there may be a primarily abnormality in the proximal tubule, such as an intracellular acidosis.[268] This will promote proximal ammonium and H^+ secretion; by the mechanisms described above, both the intracellular and intraluminal acidosis can then enhance net citrate reabsorption.

The proposed increase in proximal ammonia production in combination with hypocitraturia can then explain the other findings in incomplete type 1 RTA:[268]

- The increase in ammonia production will drive the reaction, $NH_3 + H_4^+ \leftrightarrow NH_4^+$, to the right, thereby lowering the free hydrogen concentration and raising the urine pH, even though total ammonium excretion is normal.
- The combination of a high urine pH and low citrate excretion can promote the precipitation of calcium phosphate in the tubules and the interstitium, possibly leading to kidney stones or nephrocalcinosis.
- The direct toxic effect of NH_3 (which is freely diffusible and can accumulate in the medulla) and perhaps calcium phosphate precipitation may explain the occasional progression of incomplete to complete type 1 RTA with metabolic acidosis. According to this hypothesis, the impairment in collecting tubule function is a secondary process induced by the primary abnormality in the proximal tubule.

Etiology   Many different conditions have been associated with type 1 RTA (Table 19-8).[212] The most common identifiable causes in adults are autoimmune disorders, such as Sjögren's syndrome and rheumatoid arthritis, hypercalciuria which is the primary defect in some families), toluene sniffing in

Table 19-8 Major causes of type 1 renal tubular acidosis

Primary
  A. Idiopathic or sporadic
Hereditary
  A. Familial, including hypercalciuria as the primary abnormality
  B. Marfan's syndrome
  C. Wilson's disease
  D. Ehlers-Danlos syndrome
Disorders of calcium metabolism and nephrocalcinosis
  A. Idiopathic or familial hypercalciuria
  B. Primary hyperparathyroidism
  C. Hypervitaminosis D
  D. Medullary sponge kidney
Autoimmune diseases
  A. Sjögren's syndrome
  B. Rheumatoid arthritis
  C. Systemic lupus erythematosus
  D. Chronic active hepatitis
  E. Primary biliary cirrhosis
  F. Hypergammaglobulinemia in cirrhosis
  G. Thyroiditis
Drugs and toxins
  A. Amphotericin B
  B. Ifosfamide
  C. Lithium carbonate
  D. Analgesic abuse
  E. Light chains in multiple myeloma
  F. Toluene
Associated with hyperkalemia
  A. Urinary tract obstruction
  B. Sickle cell anemia
  C. Renal transplant rejection
  D. Systemic lupus erythematosus
Marked volume depletion of any cause

recreational drug users (although, as noted above, overproduction of hippuric acid is the probable mechanism in this setting),[32] and marked volume depletion;[219,220,230,244,245,269,270] in comparison, hereditary RTA is most common in children.[261] In selected patients with Sjögren's syndrome, the correct diagnosis is delayed because the renal tubular acidosis can precede the characteristic extrarenal manifestations by 5 years or more.[269,271]

Clinical manifestations Patients with type 1 RTA are often asymptomatic, although they may have complaints related to stone disease, to severe acidemia itself (see "Symptoms," below), or to hypokalemia (weakness, fatigue, polyuria, polydipsia). The situation is potentially more serious in children, in whom failure to thrive (in infants) and decreased linear growth are common and reversible findings.[137,261]

Diagnosis The presence of type 1 RTA should be suspected in any patient with a normal anion gap metabolic acidosis and a urine pH greater than 5.3 in adults[44,131,132] or 5.6 in children.[242] In the absence of a high urine pH due to infection with a urea-splitting organism, the only other conditions that can produce this combination are type 2 RTA, volume depletion,[44,230] and hypokalemia (which increases urinary NH_3 production).[47] Measurement of the urine Na^+ concentration and the urine anion gap should be helpful in evaluating the contribution of the last two conditions: (1) a low urine Na^+ concentration (< 25 meq/L) can raise the urine pH by limiting distal Na^+ delivery and reabsorption,[44,230] and (2) the urine anion gap should be appropriately negative with hypokalemia alone, since there is no defect in NH_4^+ excretion in this setting.[44,272]

Types 1 and 2 RTA can be differentiated by the response to raising the plasma HCO_3^- concentration with $NaHCO_3$ (infused at a rate of 0.5 to 1.0 meq/kg/h). The urine pH and fractional excretion of HCO_3^- will remain constant in type 1 disease but will rise markedly in type 2 RTA, since the reabsorptive threshold for HCO_3^- is excreted in this setting (Fig. 19-6).

A different approach is required in patients with incomplete type 1 RTA, in whom the plasma HCO_3^- is normal. This disorder is usually suspected because the urine pH is persistently above 5.5 in a patient with a positive family history of RTA or calcium stone disease.[131,248,260,267] The diagnosis can be established by giving an acid load as NH_4Cl in a dose of 0.1 g/kg.[131,267] This should induce a 4- to 5-meq/L fall in the plasma HCO_3^- concentration within 4 to 6 h. The urine pH will remain above 5.3 in type 1 RTA but will be less than this value and usually below 5.0 in normal subjects, in whom acidemia stimulates maximal urinary acidification.

Treatment Correction of the acidosis is generally indicated in type 1 RTA to allow normal growth to occur in children;[137,273] to minimize stone formation, nephrocalcinosis, and possible osteopenia due to calcium loss from bone;[246-248,254] and to diminish inappropriate urinary K^+ losses.[236,237] The alkali requirement in this setting is variable, being equal to the fraction of the dietary H^+ load that is not excreted *plus* the fixed HCO_3^- losses obligated by the high urine pH (Fig. 19-6). In adults, the latter are relatively small, and only 1 to 2 meq/kg per day of alkali is usually necessary. In children, however, the urine pH and HCO_3^- losses are higher, and as much as 4 to 14 meq/kg per day in divided doses may be required.[137]

Many patients can be treated only with $NaHCO_3$ or sodium citrate* (Bicitra), since K^+ wasting is markedly diminished when the acidemia is corrected.[236,237]

---

* As described earlier, citrate should be avoided in patients who have developed renal failure, since it increases intestinal permeability and can lead to excessive aluminum absorption and tissue accumulation.[150] This is most likely to occur in patients with renal failure who are taking aluminum-containing antacids to control hyperphosphatemia (see page 206).

However, potassium citrate, alone or with sodium citrate (Polycitra), is indicated for hypokalemia or for calcium stone disease or nephrocalcinosis.[248,262,263]

Type 2 (proximal) RTA   A different problem is present in type 2 RTA: decreased proximal HCO_3^- reabsorption (Table 19-6).[212,261] Normal subjects who are euvolemic reabsorb essentially all the filtered HCO_3^- until the HCO_3^- concentration in the plasma and, therefore, in the glomerular filtrate exceeds 26 to 28 meq/L (see Chap. 3). Above this level, the excess HCO_3^- is appropriately excreted in the urine. Approximately 90 percent of this HCO_3^- reabsorption occurs in the proximal tubule.

In type 2 RTA, proximal HCO_3^- reabsorption is reduced, as is total HCO_3^- reabsorptive capacity. If, for example, only 17 meq/L of glomerular filtrate can be reabsorbed, then HCO_3^- will be lost in the urine until the plasma HCO_3^- concentration reaches 17 meq/L. At this point, all the filtered HCO_3^- can again be reclaimed and a new steady state is achieved. Thus, type 2 RTA is a *self-limiting disorder* in which the plasma HCO_3^- concentration is usually between 14 and 20 meq/L.[261]

The absence of more severe acidemia in this condition is a probable reflection of the *intact reabsorptive capacity of the distal nephron*, particularly the outer medullary collecting tubule.[218] In experimental animals, for example, the administration of a carbonic anhydrase inhibitor can block up to 80 percent of proximal HCO_3^- reabsorption, but only 30 percent of the filtered HCO_3^- appears in the urine as a result of enhanced distal reabsorption.[274] A similar effect probably occurs in humans, as the *total absence* of proximal reabsorption lowers the plasma HCO_3^- concentration to only 11 to 12 meq/L.[275]

The clinical difference between types 1 and 2 RTA can be appreciated by examining the relationship between urinary HCO_3^- excretion and the plasma HCO_3^- concentration (Fig. 19-6). In normal subjects, HCO_3^- does not significantly appear in the urine until the plasma HCO_3^- concentration exceeds 26 meq/L. This relationship is shifted to a lower level in type 2 RTA. If maximal reabsorptive capacity is 17 meq/L, then administering alkali to raise the plasma HCO_3^- concentration above this level will lead to the excretion of increasing amounts of HCO_3^-. By the time the plasma HCO_3^- concentration reaches the normal range, more than 15 percent of the filtered HCO_3^- will appear in the urine, and the urine pH will exceed 7.5. In contrast, the urine can be made maximally acid (pH < 5.3) if the plasma HCO_3^- concentration is below 17 meq/L, since all the filtered HCO_3^- can now be absorbed and distal acidification is normal.

In comparison, the curve relating urinary HCO_3^- excretion and the plasma HCO_3^- concentration in type 1 RTA is similar to that in normal subjects except that the elevated urine pH obligates a fixed degree of bicarbonaturia. However, the distal defect prevents the excretion of all of the dietary acid load, and progressive and severe acidemia can occur.

The defect in HCO_3^- reabsorption in type 2 RTA may occur alone or as part of the Fanconi syndrome, in which a variety of other proximal functions are impaired, including the reabsorption of phosphate, glucose, amino acids, and urate.[265,266] In this setting, metabolic acidosis may be accompanied by hypophosphatemia, hypouricemia, aminoaciduria, and/or glucosuria at a normal plasma glucose concentration.

Pathogenesis   The factors responsible for the defects in proximal transport in type 2 RTA are incompletely understood.[276] As described in Chap. 11, three factors are of primary importance in proximal HCO_3^- reabsorption: (1) the Na^+-H^+ exchanger in the luminal membrane, (2) the Na^+-K^+-ATPase pump in the basolateral membrane that provides the energy of Na^+-H^+ exchange by maintaining a low cell Na^+ concentration and therefore a favorable gradient for passive Na^+ entry into the cell, and (3) the enzyme carbonic anhydrase, which is located both in the cells, where it results in the generation of H^+ and HCO_3^-, and in the lumen, where it facilitates HCO_3^- reabsorption by catalyzing the dehydration of the H_2CO_3 that is formed by the combination of filtered HCO_3^- with secreted H^+.

It is likely that one or more of these factors must be impaired to account for the HCO_3^- reabsorptive defect in type 2 RTA.[276] As examples, defective carbonic anhydrase activity and, in cystinosis, ATP depletion have been described in selected patients.[277-279] In addition, the administration of a carbonic anhydrase inhibitor, such as acetazolamide in glaucoma or a topical sulfonamide antibiotic in extensive burns, often results in a mild metabolic acidosis.[280,281]

Proximal tubular dysfunction can also be seen in multiple myeloma, which may be the most common cause of type 2 RTA in adults.[282,283] It is likely that toxic light chains are reabsorbed by and then accumulate in the proximal tubular cells, leading via an uncertain mechanism to impaired tubular function.[284]

Another cause of type 2 RTA is the anticancer drug ifosfamide;[285,286] it is unclear whether the tubular toxicity is mediated by the parent drug or by the metabolite chloracetaldehyde.[287] In addition to HCO_3^- loss, other findings that may occur include phosphate wasting and hypophosphatemia (possibly leading to rickets in children), renal glucosuria, and aminoaciduria. Signs of distal damage also may be seen, including type 1 RTA and polyuria due to nephrogenic diabetes insipidus.[285]

K$^+$ *balance*   Urinary K^+ wasting and hypokalemia are common in type 2 RTA, although the degree to which this occurs is variable.[236,288] Prior to treatment, the patient is in a steady state in which virtually all of the filtered HCO_3^- can be reabsorbed. In this setting, however, there is often persistent hyperaldosteronism and mild hypokalemia.[288] As described above, these changes are probably related to the decrease in proximal transport of HCO_3^-, which leads to diminished active and passive proximal NaCl reabsorption and a tendency to Na^+ wasting.[240] An additional problem is added with alkali therapy, as the elevation in the filtered HCO_3^- concentration above the reabsorptive threshold results in a marked increase in HCO_3^- and water delivery to the cortical collecting tubule (Fig. 19-6). This elevation in distal flow with the relatively nonreabsorbable anion HCO_3^- plus persistent hyperaldosteronism combine to further enhance urinary K^+ losses (Fig. 19-7).[288]

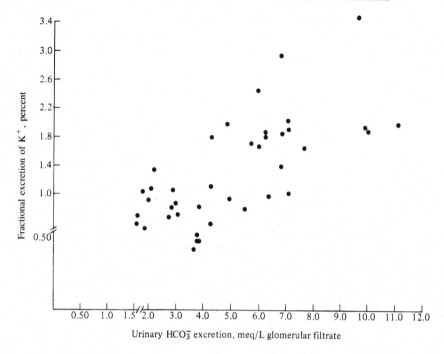

Figure 19-7   Relationship between the fractional excretion of filtered K^+ and urinary HCO_3^- excretion in patients with type 2 RTA in whom the plasma HCO_3^- concentration is maintained at normal levels (22 to 26 meq/L). (*Adapted from Sebastian A, McSherry E, Morris RC Jr, J Clin Invest 50:231, 1971, by copyright permission of The American Society for Clinical Investigation.*)

Bone disease   Rickets in children and osteomalacia or osteopenia in adults are relatively common in type 2 RTA, occurring in up to 20 percent of cases.[247] Although these skeletal abnormalities may also be present in other acidemic states, their frequency in type 2 RTA may be due in part to phosphate wasting and subsequent hypophosphatemia and to acquired vitamin D deficiency, since the proximal tubule is a major site of formation of calcitriol, the most active form of vitamin D (see Chap. 6). In addition, acidemia can directly impair growth in children.[261,273]

Nephrocalcinosis and nephrolithiasis do not occur in this disorder, in contrast to their frequency in type 1 RTA.[247] Two factors may combine to protect against this complication: the ability to lower the urine pH, which increases the solubility of calcium phosphate, and the presence of nonreabsorbed amino acids and organic anions (including citrate), which can form soluble complexes with calcium, thereby limiting the amount of free calcium available to precipitate with phosphate or oxalate.[247]

Etiology   A variety of congenital and acquired disorders can cause type 2 RTA (Table 19-9). Idiopathic RTA and cystinosis are most common in children;

Table 19-9   Major causes of type 2 renal tubular acidosis

Primary
    A. Idiopathic or sporadic, may be transient in children
Hereditary
    A. Cystinosis
    B. Hereditary fructose intolerance (during fructose administration)
    C. Familial osteopetrosis (where there may be diminished carbonic anhydrase activity)
    D. Tyrosinemia
    E. Glycogen storage disease, type 1
    F. Wilson's disease
    G. Pyruvate carboxylase deficiency
    H. Lowe's syndrome
    I. Galactosemia
Acquired disorders
    A. Multiple myeloma, latent or fully expressed
    B. Hypocalcemia and vitamin D deficiency
    C. Drugs and toxins
        1. Ifosfamide
        2. Acetazolamide or other carbonic anhydrase inhibitor
        3. Streptozotocin
        4. Outdated tetracycline
        5. Lead
        6. Cadmium
        7. Mercury
    D. Amyloidosis
    E. Renal transplant rejection
    F. Sjögren's syndrome

carbonic anhydrase inhibitors and multiple myeloma (which may be latent) are most often responsible in adults.[238,282]

Diagnosis   The presence of type 2 RTA should be suspected in any patient with an unexplained normal anion gap metabolic acidosis, even if the urine pH is below 5.3. Other findings suggestive of proximal tubule dysfunction may be very helpful in this setting, including hypophosphatemia, hypouricemia, and renal glucosuria.

    The diagnosis of type 2 RTA can be established by raising the plasma HCO_3^- concentration toward normal with an infusion of $NaHCO_3$ (at a rate of 0.5 to 1.0 meq/kg/h). The urine pH, even if initially acid, will increase rapidly once the reabsorptive threshold for HCO_3^- is exceeded. As a result, the urine pH will be greater than 7.5 and the fractional excretion of HCO_3^- greater than 15 to 20 percent as the plasma HCO_3^- concentration approaches normal (Fig. 19-6).

Treatment   Correction of the acidemia will allow normal growth to occur in children[261,273] and will promote healing of the bone disease (with phosphate and vitamin D supplementation if hypophosphatemia is also present).[247] The adequately treated patient should be asymptomatic (unless there is a complicating systemic disease) and able to lead a normal life. Furthermore, idiopathic type 2 RTA in children may be transient, disappearing spontaneously after several years.[273]

Reversal of the acidemia is often difficult, however, because the exogenous alkali is rapidly excreted in the urine. As a result, 10 to 15 meq/kg/day of alkali is typically required to stay ahead of urinary excretion. In addition, an empirically determined fraction must be given as the K^+ salt, since the associated bicarbonaturia leads to increased urinary K^+ losses (Fig. 19-7).[288] Serial monitoring is also required in children, since growth can lead to substantial changes in alkali requirement.

Either HCO_3^- or citrate can be used as the source of alkali. In general, the latter is better tolerated and, when given in such high doses, may actually be slightly safer. The buffering of gastric H^+ ions by administered HCO_3^- can lead to the rapid formation of up to several hundred milliliters of CO_2 in the stomach. There are isolated case reports in which patients taking more than 20 meq of $NaHCO_3$ after eating a large meal developed gastric rupture due to the sudden increase in gastric volume.[289]

When large doses of alkali are ineffective or not well tolerated, the addition of a thiazide diuretic may be helpful.[290] The ensuing mild volume depletion will increase the proximal reabsorption of Na^+ and secondarily that of HCO_3^- (see Chap. 3).

Type 4 RTA   Type 4 RTA refers to metabolic acidosis resulting from aldosterone deficiency or resistance. Aldosterone normally promotes distal K^+ and H^+ secretion as well as Na^+ reabsorption (see Chap. 6). The effect on H^+ secretion results both from direct stimulation of the H^+-ATPase pump[291] and from increased luminal electronegativity created by Na^+ reabsorption.[216] As a result, hypoaldosteronism impairs these processes, leading to hyperkalemia (which is generally more prominent) and metabolic acidosis (see Chap. 28).

In addition to the direct effect of aldosterone deficiency, hyperkalemia plays an important role in the metabolic acidosis by impairing NH_4^+ production and excretion.[292-294] This effect may result in part from an increase in the tubular fluid K^+ concentration competitively inhibiting the binding of NH_4^+ to the K^+ site on the Na^+-K^+-$2Cl^-$ carrier in the loop of Henle. As a result, there will be sequential reductions in NH_4^+ recycling within the medulla and in NH_3 secretion into the medullary collecting tubule (see page 341).[295] Reversing this process by correcting the hyperkalemia often leads to increased NH_4^+ excretion and correction of the metabolic acidosis.[294]

The metabolic acidosis seen with hypoaldosteronism is generally mild, with the plasma HCO_3^- concentration usually remaining above 15 meq/L. The urine pH in this disorder is generally but not always below 5.3,[44,296] distinguishing this disorder from the hyperkalemic form of type 1 RTA.[233] The low urine pH is also compatible with diminished NH_4^+ production as the primary abnormality, since total acid excretion is reduced because of the lack of available buffers, not impaired acidification.

The clinical characteristics of type 4 RTA are discussed in detail in Chap. 28 because of the general prominence of hyperkalemia in this disorder. Although mineralocorticoid replacement may be effective in treating the hyperkalemia and metabolic acidosis,[296,297] most patients have underlying renal insufficiency, and the associated Na^+ retention can exacerbate edema or hypertension. As a result, the combination of a low K^+ diet and a loop diuretic is often used.[298] The latter, by increasing distal Na^+ delivery, results in greater luminal electronegativity and an increase in K^+ and H^+ secretion.[228]

Massive Rhabdomyolysis

A rare cause of a high anion gap metabolic acidosis is massive rhabdomyolysis.[299] The presumed mechanism is the release of H^+ and organic anions from the damaged cells. This diagnosis should be suspected if there is a marked elevation in the plasma level of creatine kinase (as well as that of other muscle enzymes) and no other apparent cause for the acidemia.

SYMPTOMS

Metabolic acidosis can result in changes in pulmonary cardiovascular, neurologic, and musculoskeletal function. Since the respiratory compensation results in as much as a four- to eightfold increase in minute ventilation (see Fig. 11-16),[11,12] the patient may complain of dyspnea on exertion and, with severe acidemia, even at rest. Furthermore, the observation of hyperpnea (affecting the depth more than the rate of ventilation) on physical examination may be the only clue suggesting the presence of an underlying acidemic state.

A fall in the arterial pH to less than 7.00 to 7.10 can predispose toward potentially fatal ventricular arrhythmias and can reduce both cardiac contractility and the inotropic response to catecholamines.[93,300,301] The last effect may be mediated in part by decreased delivery of calcium to myofilaments and by decreased responsiveness of the myofilaments to calcium; how these changes might occur is not known.[301] This decrease in ventricular function may play an important role in the perpetuation of shock-induced lactic acidosis, and partial correction of the acidemia may be required before tissue perfusion can be restored.[93] As noted above, however, alkali therapy may actually worsen the intracellular acidosis in patients with circulatory failure.[99,100]

Neurologic symptoms ranging from lethargy to coma have been described in metabolic acidosis. These symptoms appear to be more closely related to the fall in pH in the cerebrospinal fluid (CSF) than to that in the plasma.[302] In general, neurologic abnormalities are much less prominent in metabolic acidosis than in respiratory acidosis. This may be due to the ability of lipid-soluble CO_2 to cross the blood-brain barrier much more rapidly than water-soluble HCO_3^-, thereby producing a greater fall in CSF pH.[303,304] When neurologic symptoms do occur in metabolic acidosis, a concurrent problem is more likely to be responsible, such as the toxic effects of ingestions, diminished cerebral perfusion in shock, and hyperosmolality due to hyperglycemia in diabetic ketoacidosis.[305]

Chronic acidemia, as with renal failure or renal tubular acidosis, can lead to a variety of skeletal problems that are probably due in part to release of Ca^{2+} and phosphate during bone buffering of the excess H^+ ions.[135,249,250,264,306] Of particular importance is impaired growth in children.[137,271,307] Other abnormalities that may occur include osteitis fibrosa (from secondary hyperparathyroidism), rickets in children, and osteomalacia or osteopenia in adults.[247,308]

Correction of the acidemia may reverse these changes in patients without renal failure.[308] Therapy is generally less successful with advanced renal disease, since other factors also contribute to the bone abnormalities, such as hyperparathyroidism, vitamin D deficiency, and poor nutrition due to anorexia.[307,309,310] (The pathophysiology of renal osteodystrophy is reviewed in Chap. 6.)

In infants and young children, acidemia may also be associated with a variety of nonspecific symptoms, such as anorexia, nausea, weight loss, muscle weakness, and listlessness.[261] The last two symptoms may result in part from loss of lean body mass as a result of alterations in muscle protein metabolism.[141,145,146] These changes are reversible with the restoration of acid-base balance.

TREATMENT

The specific aspects of therapy for individual disorders have been discussed in the appropriate sections above. It is important, however, to review the general principles, particularly the type, quantity, and rate of alkali replacement.

General Principles

In most clinical situations, correction of the acidemia can be achieved by the administration of $NaHCO_3$. There are, however, some exceptions to this recommendation, since no alkali therapy may be required in lactic or ketoacidosis (where metabolism of the organic anions will regenerate HCO_3^-), and sodium and/or potassium citrate may be preferable for chronic treatment in renal tubular acidosis. THAM and sodium lactate have also been used but offer no particular advantage over $NaHCO_3$.[311,312]

The initial therapeutic goal in patients with severe acidemia is to raise the systemic pH to about 7.20, a level at which arrhythmias become less likely and cardiac contractility and responsiveness to catecholamines will be restored. Attainment of this pH usually requires only a small increment in the plasma HCO_3^- concentration. As an example, the following arterial blood values are obtained from a patient with chronic diarrhea:

$$\text{Arterial pH} = 7.10$$

$$P_{CO_2} = 20 \text{ mmHg}$$

$$[HCO_3^-] = 6 \text{ meq/L}$$

The level to which the plasma HCO_3^- concentration must be raised for the pH to reach 7.20 can be calculated from the Henderson-Hasselbalch equation:

$$pH = 6.10 + \frac{[HCO_3^-]}{0.03 P_{CO_2}}$$

If we assume that the P_{CO_2} will remain constant, then

$$7.20 = 6.10 + \frac{[HCO_3^-]}{0.03 \times 20}$$

Since this equation is difficult to solve at the bedside, it is easier to express the relationship between these parameters in nonlogarithmic terms [Eq. (19-2)]:

$$[H^+] = 24 \times \frac{P_{CO_2}}{[HCO_3^-]}$$

Since the H^+ concentration is 63 nanoeq/L at a pH of 7.20 (see Table 19-1),

$$63 = 24 \times \frac{20}{[HCO_3^-]}$$

$$[HCO_3^-] = 8 \text{ meq/L}$$

This calculation slightly underestimates the initial HCO_3^- requirement, since the drive to compensatory hyperventilation will diminish as the acidemia is corrected, resulting in an elevation in the P_{CO_2}. If we assume that the P_{CO_2} will rise from 20 to 25 mmHg, then

$$63 = 24 \times \frac{25}{[HCO_3^-]}$$

$$[HCO_3^-] = 10 \text{ meq/L}$$

Thus, *only a small increase in the plasma HCO_3^- concentration is necessary to get the patient out of danger if there is a normal respiratory compensation.*

Rapid administration of HCO_3^- is important only in patients with severe metabolic acidosis. In this setting, even a minimal additional reduction in the plasma HCO_3^- concentration can result in a large percentage change and therefore can induce an immediately life-threatening degree of acidemia. For example, lowering the plasma HCO_3^- concentration from 24 to 22 meq/L in a patient with an initial pH of 7.40 and P_{CO_2} of 40 mmHg will have only a minor effect on the pH and H^+ concentration:

$$[H^+] = 24 \times \frac{40}{22}$$

$$= 44 \text{ nanoeq/L} \qquad (pH = 7.36)$$

However, a similar 2-meq/L reduction in a patient with an initial pH of 7.11, a plasma HCO_3^- concentration of 4 meq/L, and a P_{CO_2} of 13 mmHg will now decrease the pH to 6.81:

$$[H^+] = 24 \times \frac{13}{2}$$

$$= 156 \text{ nanoeq/L} \qquad (pH = 6.81)$$

Regardless of the initial severity, rapid correction of the pH to above 7.20 to 7.25 not only is unnecessary but can induce potentially important reductions in the CSF pH and in tissue oxygen delivery. The administration of $NaHCO_3$ will tend to lower minute ventilation and raise the P_{CO_2}. Since CO_2 crosses the blood-brain barrier much more rapidly than HCO_3^-, the brain will acutely sense only the elevation in the P_{CO_2}. Thus, the CSF pH will become more acid, with possible aggravation of the neurologic symptoms.[302] The increase in the arterial pH will also shift the hemoglobin dissociation curve to the left, increasing the affinity of hemoglobin for oxygen and possibly reducing tissue oxygen delivery.

Bicarbonate Deficit

The amount of HCO_3^- required to correct the acidemia can be estimated from the following formula:

$$HCO_3^- \text{ deficit} = HCO_3^- \text{ space} \times HCO_3^- \text{ deficit per liter} \qquad (19\text{-}19)$$

The apparent bicarbonate space is a reflection of total body buffering capacity. It is therefore determined both by the quantity of extracellular HCO_3^- and by the intracellular (proteins and phosphates) and bone (carbonate) buffers.[3] It has been measured empirically by administering HCO_3^- and then observing the ensuing elevation in the plasma HCO_3^- concentration.[2] If, for example, 100 meq raises the plasma HCO_3^- concentration by 5 meq/L, then the apparent bicarbonate space is 20 L.

At a normal plasma HCO_3^- concentration of 24 meq/L, excess H^+ ions are buffered proportionately through the total body water, and the apparent HCO_3^- space is about 50 percent of lean body weight (Fig. 19-8). However, the HCO_3^- space rises in metabolic acidosis, since the fall in the plasma HCO_3^- concentration means that there is an ever-increasing contribution from the nonbicarbonate buffers. Thus, the bicarbonate space is approximately 60 percent of lean body weight in mild to moderate metabolic acidosis, but can reach 70 percent or more as the plasma HCO_3^- concentration falls below 8 to 10 meq/L (Fig. 19-8).[2,3]

The bicarbonate space can be estimated from:[3]

$$\text{Bicarbonate space} = \left[0.4 + \left(2.6/P_{HCO_3^-}\right)\right] \times \text{lean body weight} \qquad (19\text{-}20)$$

It can exceed total body water or even lean body weight in severe metabolic acidosis, because almost all of the buffering is occurring within the cells and bone, where there is a virtually inexhaustible supply of buffer.

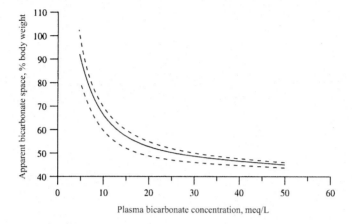

Figure 19-8 Variation in the apparent bicarbonate space according to the plasma bicarbonate concentration. At values below 10 meq/L, most of the buffering is performed by the intracellular and bone buffers, leading to a marked rise in the space of distribution that can exceed 70 percent of lean body weight in severe metabolic acidosis. (*From Fernandez PC, Cohen RM, Feldman GM*, Kidney Int *36:747, 1989. Reprinted by permission from* Kidney International.)

In the above patient with diarrhea, for example, the initial aim of therapy is to raise the plasma HCO_3^- concentration from 6 to 10 meq/L. If this patient weighed 70 kg, then

$$HCO_3^- \text{ deficit} = 0.7 \times 70 \times (10 - 6)$$

$$= 196 \text{ meq}$$

Thus, 196 meq of HCO_3^- can be given intravenously over the first several hours. If this is effective in raising the pH to a safe level, further HCO_3^- may be unnecessary, since increased renal H^+ excretion will slowly regenerate the lost HCO_3^-. Similarly, *exogenous alkali may not be required* if the initial arterial pH is greater than 7.20, the patient is asymptomatic, and the underlying process, such as diarrhea, can be controlled.

Needless to say, these are only rough guidelines and cannot replace serial measurements of the extracellular pH. In particular, the formula assumes a reasonably accurate estimate of lean body weight and assumes that the patient is in a steady state. If, for example, there is continuing acid production, as with severe diarrhea, then the HCO_3^- requirements will increase with time.

The degree to which exogenous HCO_3^- will raise the plasma HCO_3^- concentration and pH is also dependent upon when the measurements are made. As described above, excess H^+ ions are buffered first in the extracellular fluid and then in the cells. A similar sequence occurs when HCO_3^- is given to correct a metabolic acidosis. Acutely, the added HCO_3^- is limited to the vascular space, producing a large increase in the plasma HCO_3^- concentration. However, this change is attenuated as the exogenous HCO_3^- equilibrates through the total extracellular fluid, which occurs within 15 min, and then equilibrates with the intracellular and bone buffers, which occurs in 2 to 4 h.

If, for example, we assume that the extracellular volume is 15 liters and the total HCO_3^- space is 49 liters in the above 70-kg patient with diarrhea, then the rapid infusion of 100 meq of HCO_3^- will produce a 7-meq/L increase in the plasma HCO_3^- concentration at 15 min, but only a 2-meq/L increase at 2 to 4 h. Thus, the extracellular pH will be greater if it is measured at 15 min, before equilibration with the intracellular buffers has occurred. As a result, it should be recognized that measurement of the pH shortly after HCO_3^- has been given may overestimate the final effect of therapy.

Plasma Potassium Concentration

K^+ depletion is common in patients with metabolic acidosis associated with gastrointestinal and/or renal losses of K^+. Despite this, the initial plasma K^+ concentration may be relatively normal, since metabolic acidemia (except for the organic acidoses) causes K^+ to move out of the cells into the extracellular fluid (see page 379).[5,8]

A similar effect frequently occurs in diabetic ketoacidosis, in which the combination of insulin deficiency and hyperglycemia (rather than acidemia) promotes K^+ movement into the extracellular fluid. Thus, patients with this disorder are commonly hyperkalemic at presentation, despite moderate to marked K^+ depletion (see Chap. 25).[9] The administration of insulin will reverse this sequence, redistributing K^+ into the cells and unmasking the true state of K^+ balance. As a result, careful monitoring of the plasma K^+ concentration is essential during the initial phases of therapy.

The potential risks of treatment are more immediate in the acidemic patient who is already hypokalemic at presentation. In this setting, there is a very large K^+ deficit, and the restoration of normal pH (or treatment with insulin in diabetic ketoacidosis) will further reduce the plasma K^+ concentration. Thus, initial therapy should consist of KCl alone (if the acidemia is not severe) or KCl with $NaHCO_3$ with careful monitoring of the pH, the plasma K^+ concentration, muscle strength, and the electrocardiogram. As much as 40 meq/h of KCl may be required to prevent life-threatening hypokalemia in some patients (see Chap. 27).

Metabolic Acidosis and Heart Failure

Sodium bicarbonate therapy is potentially dangerous in patients with left ventricular failure, since it can lead to increasing pulmonary congestion. Fortunately, alkali therapy is usually unnecessary when the underlying disorder is lactic acidosis due to acute pulmonary edema. In this setting, improvement in pulmonary function leads to spontaneous resolution of the acidemia as a result of HCO_3^- generation from the metabolism of lactate.[58]

However, specific therapy may be required in patients with severe acidemia (arterial pH < 7.10 to 7.15), particularly if the patient does not have a self-correcting organic acidosis, such as lactic or ketoacidosis. Acutely, small doses of NaHCO$_3$ (45 to 90 meq) can be cautiously administered. The risk of this regimen is relatively small, since more than one-half of the HCO$_3^-$ will enter the cells to replenish the intracellular buffers.[1,2] Thus, there will be much less volume expansion than with an equivalent quantity of NaCl, which is restricted to the extracellular fluid.

Alternatively, peritoneal dialysis or hemodialysis can be used to correct both the fluid overload and the acidemia. The former is generally preferred in patients with severe heart disease, since it avoids the hemodynamic instability often associated with hemodialysis. The dialysate should preferably contain HCO$_3^-$ as a source of alkali rather than lactate or acetate, which may not be normally metabolized in severe heart failure.[313]

PROBLEMS

19-1 The following laboratory tests are obtained from two patients. Would you administer NaHCO$_3$ to either one?

(a)   Plasma [Na$^+$] $= 140$ meq/L

[K$^+$] $= 4.2$ meq/L

[Cl$^-$] $= 114$ meq/L

[HCO$_3^-$] $= 16$ meq/L

(b)   Plasma [Na$^+$] $= 140$ meq/L

[K$^+$] $= 4.7$ meq/L

[Cl$^-$] $= 122$ meq/L

[HCO$_3^-$] $= 7$ meq/L

Arterial pH $= 7.32$

P$_{CO_2}$ $= 14$ mmHg

19-2 A 31-year-old man with a history of epilepsy has a grand mal seizure. Laboratory tests taken immediately after the seizure has stopped reveal

Arterial pH $= 7.14$

P$_{CO_2}$ $= 45$ mmHg

Plasma [Na$^+$] $= 140$ meq/L

[K$^+$] $= 4.0$ meq/L

[Cl$^-$] $= 98$ meq/L

[HCO$_3^-$] $= 17$ meq/L

(a) What is the acid-base disturbance?

(b) Does the patient need NaHCO$_3$?

(c) What will happen to his plasma K$^+$ concentration as the acidemia is corrected?

19-3 If HCO$_3^-$ therapy sufficient to normalize the plasma HCO$_3^-$ concentration is suddenly stopped, match the subsequent course with the type of RTA:

(a) Type 1 RTA in adults (minimum urine pH $= 6.5$)

(b) Type 1 RTA in infants (minimum urine pH = 7.2)
(c) Type 2 RTA

1. Rapid fall in plasma HCO_3^- concentration, which stabilizes at 16 meq/L
2. Rapid decrease in plasma HCO_3^- concentration, which falls below 10 meq/L
3. Slowly progressive decrease in plasma HCO_3^- concentration to less than 10 meq/L

If the plasma HCO_3^- concentration is raised to 22 meq/L with exogenous $NaHCO_3$, how would you distinguish among these three disorders?

19-4 Match the laboratory findings with the appropriate cause of a normal anion gap metabolic acidosis. The units in the table are meq/L.

	$[Na^+]$	$[K^+]$	$[Cl^-]$	$[HCO_3^-]$	Urine pH	Urine anion gap
1.	140	2.9	115	14	6.4	−45
2.	137	5.3	113	17	5.2	+18
3.	139	3.1	120	11	6.1	+23

(a) Hypoaldosteronism (type 4 RTA)
(b) Diarrhea due to laxative abuse
(c) Type 1 RTA

19-5 A 58-year-old man with a history of chronic bronchitis develops severe diarrhea caused by pseudomembranous colitis. It is noted that the volume of diarrheal fluid is approximately 1 L/h. Results of the initial laboratory tests are

$$Plasma\ [Na^+] = 138\ meq/L$$
$$[K^+] = 3.8\ meq/L$$
$$[Cl^-] = 115\ meq/L$$
$$[HCO_3^-] = 9\ meq/L$$
$$Arterial\ pH = 6.97$$
$$P_{CO_2} = 40\ mmHg$$

(a) What is the acid-base disorder?
(b) Assuming that the P_{CO_2} remains at 40 mmHg, to what level does the plasma HCO_3^- concentration have to be raised to increase the pH to 7.20?
(c) How much HCO_3^- would be required to raise the plasma HCO_3^- concentration to the desired level, assuming that the patient has a lean body weight of 80 kg?
(d) After the administration of this amount of HCO_3^- over 4 h, the plasma HCO_3^- concentration is still 9 meq/L. What is responsible for this inability to correct the acidemia?
(e) What would you estimate the total body K^+ stores in this patient to be?

19-6 A 50-year-old woman has severe chronic renal failure. The following laboratory data are obtained:

$$Plasma\ [Na^+] = 137\ meq/L$$
$$[K^+] = 5.4\ meq/L$$
$$[Cl^-] = 102\ meq/L$$
$$[HCO_3^-] = 10\ meq/L$$
$$Arterial\ pH = 7.22$$
$$P_{CO_2} = 25\ mmHg$$

(a) Why does metabolic acidosis develop in renal failure?
Thirty minutes after the administration of 88 meq of HCO_3^-, repeat blood tests reveal the following:

Arterial pH = 7.38

$$P_{CO_2} = 28 \text{ mmHg}$$

$$[HCO_3^-] = 16 \text{ meq/L}$$

In view of the improvement in the pH, no further HCO_3^- is given. However, on the next day, blood tests showed:

Arterial pH = 7.28

$$P_{CO_2} = 26 \text{ mmHg}$$

$$[HCO_3^-] = 12 \text{ meq/L}$$

(b) What factors might have been responsible for this reduction in the arterial pH?

REFERENCES

1. Schwartz WB, Orming KJ, Porter R. The internal distribution of hydrogen ions with varying degrees of metabolic acidosis. *J Clin Invest* 36:373, 1957.
2. Adrogué JH, Brensilver J, Cohen JJ, Madias NE. Influence of steady-state alterations in acid-base equilibrium on the fate of administered bicarbonate in the dog. *J Clin Invest* 71:867, 1983.
3. Fernandez PC, Cohen RM, Feldman GM. The concept of bicarbonate distribution space: The crucial role of body buffers. *Kidney Int* 36:747, 1989.
4. Burnell JM, Villamil MF, Uyeno BT, Scribner BH. The effect in humans of extracellular pH change on the relationship between serum potassium concentration and intracellular potassium. *J Clin Invest* 35:935, 1956.
5. Adrogué HJ, Madias NE. Changes in plasma potassium concentration during acute acid-base disturbances. *Am J Med* 71:456, 1981.
6. Magner PO, Robinson L, Halperin RM, et al. The plasma potassium concentration in metabolic acidosis: A re-evaluation. *Am J Kidney Dis* 11:220, 1988.
7. Fulop M. Serum potassium in lactic acidosis and ketoacidosis. *N Engl J Med* 300:1087, 1979.
8. Adrogué HJ, Chap Z, Ishida T, Field J. Role of endocrine pancreas in the kalemic response to acute metabolic acidosis in conscious dogs. *J Clin Invest* 75:798, 1985.
9. Arieff AI, Carroll HJ. Nonketotic hyperosmolar coma with hyperglycemia: Clinical features, pathophysiology, renal function, acid-base balance, plasma-cerebrospinal fluid equilibria and the effects of therapy in 37 cases. *Medicine* 51:73, 1972.
10. Pierce NF, Fedson DS, Brigham KL, et al. The ventilatory response to acute base deficit in humans: The time course during development and correction of metabolic acidosis. *Ann Intern Med* 72:633, 1970.
11. Kety SS, Polis BD, Nadler CS, Schmidt CF. The blood flow and oxygen consumption of the human brain in diabetic acidosis and coma. *J Clin Invest* 27:500, 1948.
12. Bushinsky DA, Coe FL, Katzenberg C, et al. Arterial P_{CO_2} in chronic metabolic acidosis. *Kidney Int* 22:311, 1982.
13. Madias N, Schwartz WB, Cohen JJ. The maladaptive renal response to secondary hypocapnia during chronic HCl acidosis in the dog. *J Clin Invest* 60:1393, 1977.
14. Kurtz I, Maher T, Hulter HN. Effect of diet on plasma acid-base composition in normal humans. *Kidney Int* 24:670, 1983.
15. Hamm LL, Simon EE. Roles and mechanisms of urinary buffer excretion. *Am J Physiol* 253:F595, 1987.
16. Tizianello A, Deferrari G, Garibotto G, et al. Renal ammoniagenesis in an early stage of metabolic acidosis in man. *J Clin Invest* 69:240, 1982.
17. Krapf R, Berry CA, Alpern RJ, Rector FC Jr. Regulation of cell pH by ambient bicarbonate, carbon dioxide tension, and pH in rabbit proximal convoluted tubule. *J Clin Invest* 81:381, 1988.

18. Horie S, Moe O, Tejedor A, Alpern RJ. Preincubation in acid medium increases Na/H antiporter activity in cultured renal proximal tubule cells. *Proc Natl Acad Sci U S A* 87:4742, 1990.
19. Owen OE, Licht JH, Sapir DG. Renal function and effects of partial rehydration during diabetic ketoacidosis. *Diabetes* 30:510, 1981.
20. Clarke E, Evans BM, MacIntyre IM. Acidosis in experimental electrolyte depletion. *Clin Soc* 14:421, 1955.
21. Emmett M, Narins RG. Clinical use of the anion gap. *Medicine* 56:38, 1977.
22. Gabow PA. Disorders associated with an altered anion gap. *Kidney Int* 27:472, 1985.
23. Gabow PA, Kaehny WD, Fennessey PV, et al. Diagnostic importance of an increased anion gap. *N Engl J Med* 303:854, 1980.
24. Winter SD, Pearson R, Gabow PA, et al. The fall of the serum anion gap. *Arch Intern Med* 150:311, 1990.
25. Rackow EC, Mecher C, Astiz ME, et al. Unmeasured anion during severe sepsis with metabolic acidosis. *Circ Shock* 30:107, 1990.
26. Wang F, Butler T, Rabbani GH, Jones PK. The acidosis of cholera: Contributions of hyperproteinemia, lactic acidemia, and hyperphosphatemia to an increased anion gap. *N Engl J Med* 315:1591, 1986.
27. Oh MS, Carroll HJ, Goldstein DA, Fein IA. Hyperchloremic acidosis during the recovery phase of diabetic ketosis. *Ann Intern Med* 89:925, 1978.
28. Oh MS, Carroll HJ, Uribarri J. Mechanism of normochloremic and hyperchloremic acidemia in diabetic ketoacidosis. *Nephron* 54:1, 1990.
29. Androgué HJ, Wilson H, Boyd AE, et al. Plasma acid-base patterns in diabetic ketoacidosis. *N Engl J Med* 307:1603, 1982.
30. Androgué HJ, Eknoyan G, Suki WK. Diabetic ketoacidosis: Role of the kidney in the acid-base homeostasis re-evaluated. *Kidney Int* 25:591, 1984.
31. Ferrier B, Martin M, Janbon B, Baverel G. Transport of β-hydroxybutyrate and acetoacetate along rat nephron: A micropuncture study. *Am J Physiol* 262:F762, 1992.
32. Carlisle EJF, Donnelly SM, Vasuvattakul S, et al. Glue-sniffing and distal renal tubular acidosis: Sticking to the facts. *J Am Soc Nephrol* 1:1019, 1991.
33. Lennon EJ, Lemann J Jr, Litzow JR. The effects of diet and stool composition on the net external acid balance of normal subjects. *J Clin Invest* 45:1601, 1966.
34. Halperin ML, Jungas RL. The metabolic production and renal disposal of hydrogen ions: An examination of the biochemical processes. *Kidney Int* 24:709, 1983.
35. Wallia R, Greenberg A, Piraino B, et al. Serum electrolyte patterns in end-stage renal disease. *Am J Kidney Dis* 8:98, 1986.
36. Widmer B, Gerhardt RE, Harrington JT, Cohen JJ. Serum electrolyte and acid-base composition: The influence of graded degrees of chronic renal failure. *Arch Intern Med* 139:1099, 1979.
37. Seligson D, Bluemle LW Jr, Webster GD Jr, et al. Organic acids in body fluids of the uremic patient. *J Clin Invest* 38:1042, 1959.
38. Madias NE, Ayus JC, Adrogué HJ. Increased anion gap in metabolic alkalosis: The role of plasma-protein equivalency. *N Engl J Med* 300:1421, 1979.
39. Figge J, Jabor A, Kazda A, Fenci V. Anion gap and hypoalbuminemia. *Crit Care Med* 26:1807, 1998.
40. Kelleher SP, Raciti A, Arbeit LA. Reduced or absent serum anion gap as a marker for severe lithium carbonate intoxication. *Arch Intern Med* 146:1839, 1986.
41. DeTroyer A, Stolarczyk A, Zegers de Beyl D, Stryckmans P. Value of anion-gap determination in multiple myeloma. *N Engl J Med* 296:858, 1977.
42. Wacks I, Oster JR, Perez GO, Kett DH. Spurious hyperchloremia and hyperbicarbonatemia in a patient receiving pyridostigmine bromide therapy for myasthenia gravis. *Am J Kidney Dis* 16:76, 1990.
43. Graber ML, Quigg RJ, Stempsey WE, Weis S. Spurious hyperchloremia and decreased anion gap in hyperlipidemia. *Ann Intern Med* 98:607, 1983.

44. Batlle DC, Hizon M, Cohen E, et al. The use of the urine anion gap in the diagnosis of hyperchloremic metabolic acidosis. *N Engl J Med* 318:594, 1988.
45. Halperin ML, Vasuvattakul S, Bayoumi A. A modified classification of metabolic acidosis. A pathophysiologic approach. *Nephron* 60:129, 1992.
46. Inase N, Ozawa K, Sasaki S, Marumo F. Is the urine anion gap a reliable index of ammonium excretion in most situations? *Nephron* 54:180, 1990.
47. Tannen RL. The effect of uncomplicated potassium depletion on urinary acidification. *J Clin Invest* 49:813, 1970.
48. Halperin ML. Modified urine osmolal gap: An accurate method for estimating the urinary ammonium concentration (letter). *Nephron* 69:100, 1995.
49. Kreisberg RA. Lactate homeostasis and lactic acidosis. *Ann Intern Med* 92:227, 1980.
50. Madias NE. Lactic acidosis. *Kidney Int* 29:752, 1986.
51. Arieff AI, Park R, Leach WJ, Lazarowitz VC. Pathophysiology of experimental lactic acidosis in dogs. *Am J Physiol* 239:F135, 1980.
52. Arieff AI, Graf H. Pathophysiology of type A hypoxic lactic acidosis in dogs. *Am J Physiol* 253:E271, 1987.
53. Israels S, Haworth JC, Dunn HG, Applegarth DA. Lactic acidosis in childhood. *Adv Pediatr* 22:267, 1976.
54. Huckabee WE. Relationships of pyruvate and lactate during anaerobic metabolism: I. Effects of infusion of pyruvate or glucose and of hyperventilation. *J Clin Invest* 37:244, 1958.
55. Bornemann M, Hill SC, Kidd GS II. Lactic acidosis in pheochromocytoma. *Ann Intern Med* 105:880, 1986.
56. Madias NE, Goorno WE, Herson S. Severe lactic acidosis as a presenting feature of pheochromocytoma. *Am J Kidney Dis* 10:250, 1987.
57. Robinson BH, MacKay N, Petrova-Benedict R, et al. Defects in the E_2 lipoyl transacetylase and the x-lipoyl containing component of the pyruvate dehydrogenase complex in patients with lactic acidemia. *J Clin Invest* 85:1821, 1990.
58. Fulop M, Horowitz M, Aberman A, Jaffee E. Lactic acidosis in pulmonary edema due to left ventricular failure. *Ann Intern Med* 79:180, 1973.
59. Tonsgard JH, Huttenlocher PR, Thisted RA. Lactic acidemia in Reye's syndrome. *Pediatrics* 69:64, 1982.
60. Orringer CE, Eustace JC, Wunsch CD, Gardner LB. Natural history of lactic acidosis after grand-mal seizures: A model for the study of an anion-gap acidosis not associated with hyperkalemia. *N Engl J Med* 297:796, 1977.
61. Osnes JB, Hermansen L. Acid-base balance after maximal exercise of short duration. *J Appl Physiol* 32:59, 1972.
62. McKelvie RS, Lindinger MI, Heigenhauser GJF, et al. Renal responses to exercise-induced lactic acidosis. *Am J Physiol* 257:R102, 1989.
63. Reuler JB. Hypothermia: Pathophysiology, clinical settings, and management. *Ann Intern Med* 89:519, 1978.
64. Appel D, Rubenstein R, Schrager K, Williams MH Jr. Lactic acidosis in severe asthma. *Am J Med* 75:580, 1983.
65. Buehler JH, Berns AS, Webster JR, et al. Lactic acidosis from carboxyhemoglobinemia after smoke inhalation. *Ann Intern Med* 82:803, 1975.
66. Eldridge F. Blood lactate and pyruvate in pulmonary insufficiency. *N Engl J Med* 274:878, 1966.
67. Graham DL, Laman D, Theodore J, Robin ED. Acute cyanide poisoning complicated by lactic acidosis and pulmonary edema. *Arch Intern Med* 137:1051, 1977.
68. Baud FJ, Barriot P, Toffis V, et al. Elevated blood cyanide concentrations in victims of smoke inhalation. *N Engl J Med* 325:1761, 1991.
69. Sundar K, Suarez M, Banogon PE, Shapiro JM. Zidovudine-induced fatal lactic acidosis and hepatic failure in patients with acquired immunodeficiency syndrome: Report of two patients and review of the literature. *Crit Care Med* 25:1425, 1997.
70. Lenzo NP, Garas BA, French MA. Hepatic steatosis and lactic acidosis associated with stavudine treatment in an HIV patient: A case report. *AIDS* 11:1294, 1997.

71. Fouty B, Frerman F, Reves R. Riboflavin to treat nucleoside analogue-induced lactic acidosis. *Lancet* 32:291, 1998.
72. Luzzati R, Del Bravo P, Di Perri G, et al. Riboflavine and severe lactic acidosis. *Lancet* 353:901, 1999.
73. Stolberg L, Rolfe R, Gitlin N, et al. D-lactic acidosis due to abnormal gut flora. *N Engl J Med* 306:1344, 1982.
74. Halperin ML, Kamel KS. D-lactic acidosis: Turning sugars into acids in the gastrointestinal tract. *Kidney Int* 49:1, 1996.
75. Uribarri J, Oh MS, Carroll HJ. D-lactic acidosis. *Medicine* 77:73, 1998.
76. Mayne AJ, Dandy DJ, Preece MA, et al. Dietary management of D-lactic acidosis in short bowel syndrome. *Arch Dis Child* 65:229, 1990.
77. Cohen RD, Iles RA. Lactic acidosis: Some physiological and clinical considerations. *Clin Sci Mol Med* 53:405, 1977.
78. Kreisberg RA, Owen WC, Siegal AM. Ethanol-induced hyperlacticacidemia: Inhibition of lactate utilization. *J Clin Invest* 50:166, 1971.
79. Field M, Block JB, Levin R, Rall DP. Significance of blood lactate elevations among patients with acute leukemia and other neoplastic proliferative disorders. *Am J Med* 40:528, 1966.
80. Fraley DS, Adler S, Bruns FJ, Zett B. Stimulation of lactate production by administration of bicarbonate in a patient with a solid neoplasma and lactic acidosis. *N Engl J Med* 303:1100, 1980.
81. Nadiminti Y, Wang JC, Chou S-Y, et al. Lactic acidosis associated with Hodgkin's disease. *N Engl J Med* 303:15, 1980.
82. Rice K, Schwartz SH. Lactic acidosis with small cell carcinoma: Rapid response to chemotherapy. *Am J Med* 79:501, 1985.
83. Gan SC, Barr J, Arieff AI, Pearl RG. Biguanide-associated lactic acidosis: Case report and review of the literature. *Arch Intern Med* 152:2333, 1992.
84. Stang M, Wysowski DK, Butler Jones D. Incidence of lactic acidosis in metformin users. *Diabetes Care* 22:925, 1999.
85. Chattha G, Arieff AI, Cummings C, Tierney LM Jr. Lactic acidosis complicating the acquired immunodeficiency syndrome. *Ann Intern Med* 118:37, 1993.
86. Landry DW, Oliver JA. The ATP-sensitive K$^+$ channel mediates hypotension in endotoxemia and hypoxic lactic acidosis in dog. *J Clin Invest* 89:2071, 1992.
87. Lindinger M, Heigenhauser GJF, McKelvie RS, Jones NL. Blood ion regulation during repeated maximal exercise and recovery in humans. *Am J Physiol* 262:R126, 1992.
88. Bersin RM, Arieff AI. Improved hemodynamic function during hypoxia with carbicarb, a new agent for the management of acidosis. *Circulation* 77:227, 1988.
89. Weil MH, Afifi AA. Experimental and clinical studies on lactate and pyruvate as indicators of the severity of acute circulatory failure (shock). *Circulation* 41:989, 1970.
90. Marliss EB, Ohman JL Jr, Aoki TT, Kozak GP. Altered redox state obscuring ketoacidosis in diabetic patients with lactic acidosis. *N Engl J Med* 283:978, 1970.
91. Gopinath R, Hutcheon M, Cheema-Dhadli S, Halperin M. Chronic lactic acidosis in a patient with acquired immunodeficiency syndrome and mitochondrial myopathy: Biochemical studies. *J Am Soc Nephrol* 3:1212, 1992.
92. Adrogué HJ, Madias NE. Management of life-threatening acid-base disorders. *N Engl J Med* 338:26, 1998.
93. Narins RG, Cohen JJ. Bicarbonate therapy for organic acidosis: The case for its continued use. *Ann Intern Med* 106:615, 1987.
94. Mattar JA, Weil MH, Shubin H, Stein L. Cardiac arrest in the critically ill: II. Hyperosmolal states following cardiac arrest. *Am J Med* 56:162, 1974.
95. Burnier M, Van Putten VJ, Scheippati A, Schrier RW. Effect of extracellular acidosis on ^{45}Ca uptake in isolated hypoxic proximal tubules. *Am J Physiol* 254:C839, 1988.
96. Graf H, Leach W, Arieff AI. Evidence for a detrimental effect of bicarbonate therapy in hypoxic lactic acidosis. *Science* 227:754, 1985.

97. Stacpoole PW. Lactic acidosis: The case against bicarbonate therapy. *Ann Intern Med* 105:276, 1986.
98. Fields ALA, Wolman SL, Halperin ML. Chronic lactic acidosis in a patient with cancer: Therapy and metabolic consequences. *Cancer* 47:2026, 1981.
99. Kette F, Weil MH, von Planta M, et al. Buffer agents do not reverse intramyocardial acidosis during cardiac resuscitation. *Circulation* 81:1660, 1990.
100. Weisfeld ML, Guerci AD. Sodium bicarbonate in CPR. *JAMA* 266:2121, 1991.
101. Shapiro JI. Functional and metabolic responses of isolated hearts to acidosis: Effect of sodium bicarbonate and Carbicarb. *Am J Physiol* 258:1835, 1990.
102. Bishop RL, Weisfeldt ML. Sodium bicarbonate administration during cardiac arrest: Effect on arterial pH, P_{CO_2}, and osmolality. *JAMA* 235:506, 1976.
103. Weil MH, Rackow EC, Trevino R, et al. Difference in acid-base state between venous and arterial blood during cardiopulmonary resuscitation. *N Engl J Med* 315:153, 1986.
104. Adrogué HJ, Rashad MN, Gorin AD, et al. Assessing acid-base status in circulatory failure: Differences between arterial and central venous blood. *N Engl J Med* 320:1312, 1989.
105. Urban P, Scheidegger D, Buchmann B, Barth D. Cardiac arrest and blood ionized calcium levels. *Ann Intern Med* 109:110, 1988.
106. Stacpoole PW, Wright EC, Baumgartner TG, et al. A controlled trial of dichloroacetate for treatment of lactic acidosis in adults. *N Engl J Med* 327:1564, 1992.
107. Nahas GG, Sutin KM, Fermon C, et al. Guidelines for the treatment of acidaemia with THAM. *Drugs* 55:191, 1998.
108. Cahill GF Jr. Ketosis. *Kidney Int* 20:416, 1981.
109. Foster DW, McGarry JD. The metabolic derangements and treatment of diabetic ketoacidosis. *N Engl J Med* 309:159, 1983.
110. Foster DW. From glycogen to ketones—and back. *Diabetes* 33:1188, 1984.
111. Madison LL, Mebane D, Unger RH, Lochner A. The hypoglycemic action of ketones: II. Evidence for a stimulatory feedback of ketones on the pancreatic beta cells. *J Clin Invest* 43:408, 1964.
112. Reichard GA Jr, Owen OE, Haff AC, et al. Ketone body production and oxidation in fasting obese humans. *J Clin Invest* 53:508, 1974.
113. Levy LJ, Duga J, Girgis M, Gordon EE. Ketoacidosis associated with alcoholism in nondiabetic subjects. *Ann Intern Med* 78:213, 1973.
114. Miller PD, Heinig RE, Waterhouse C. Treatment of alcoholic acidosis: The role of dextrose and phosphorus. *Arch Intern Med* 138:67, 1978.
115. Wrenn KD, Slovis CM, Minion GE, Rutkowski R. The syndrome of alcoholic ketoacidosis. *Am J Med* 91:119, 1991.
116. Lefevre AJ, Adler H, Lieber C. Effect of ethanol on ketone metabolism. *J Clin Invest* 49:1775, 1970.
117. Halperin ML, Hammeke M, Josse RG, Jungas RL. Metabolic acidosis in the alcoholic: A pathophysiologic approach. *Metabolism* 32:308, 1983.
118. Cohen JJ. Methylmalonic acidemia. *Kidney Int* 15:311, 1979.
119. Stanbury JB, Wyngaarden JB, Fredrickson DS, et al. *The Metabolic Basis of Inherited Disease*, 5th ed. New York, McGraw-Hill, 1983, chaps. 22 and 23.
120. Braden GL, Strayhorn CH, Germain MJ, et al. Increased osmolal gap in alcoholic acidosis. *Arch Intern Med* 153:2377, 1993.
121. Schelling JR, Howard RL, Winter SD, Linas SL. Increased osmolal gap in alcoholic ketoacidosis and lactic acidosis. *Ann Intern Med* 113:580, 1990.
122. Narins RG, Jones ERS, Stom MC, et al. Diagnostic strategies in disorders of fluid, electrolyte and acid-base homeostasis. *Am J Med* 72:496, 1982.
123. Csako G, Elin RJ. Unrecognized false-positive ketones from drugs containing free-sulfhydryl groups (letter). *JAMA* 269:1634, 1993.
124. Morris LR, Murphy MB, Kitabachi AE. Bicarbonate therapy in diabetic ketoacidosis. *Ann Intern Med* 150:836, 1986.

125. Hale PJ, Crase J, Nattrass M. Metabolic effects of bicarbonate in the treatment of diabetic ketoacidosis. *Br Med J* 289:1035, 1984.

126. Machiels JP, Dive A, Donckier J, Installe E. Reversible myocardial dysfunction in a patient with alcoholic ketoacidosis: A role for hypophosphatemia. *Am J Emerg Med* 16:371, 1998.

127. Warnock DG. Uremic acidosis. *Kidney Int* 34:278, 1988.

128. Dorhout Mees EJ, Machado M, Slatopolsky E, et al. The functional adaptation of the diseased kidney: III. Ammonium excretion. *J Clin Invest* 45:289, 1966.

129. Welbourne T, Weber M, Bank N. The effect of glutamine administration on urinary ammonium excretion in normal subjects and patients with renal disease. *J Clin Invest* 51:1852, 1972.

130. Schwartz WB, Hall PW, Hays R, Relman AS. On the mechanism of acidosis in chronic renal disease. *J Clin Invest* 38:39, 1959.

131. Wrong O, Davies HEF. The excretion of acid in renal disease. *Q J Med* 28:259, 1959.

132. Espinel CH. The influence of salt intake on the metabolic acidosis of chronic renal failure. *J Clin Invest* 56:286, 1975.

133. Lameire N, Matthys E. Influence of progressive salt restriction on urinary bicarbonate wasting in uremic acidosis. *Am J Kidney Dis* 8:151, 1986.

134. Wong NLM, Quamme GA, Dirks JH. Tubular handling of bicarbonate in dogs with experimental renal failure. *Kidney Int* 25:912, 1984.

135. Litzow JR, Lemann J Jr, Lennon EJ. The effect of treatment of acidosis on calcium balance in patients with chronic azotemic renal disease. *J Clin Invest* 46:280, 1967.

136. Green J, Kleeman CR. Role of bone in regulation of systemic acid-base balance. *Kidney Int* 39:9, 1991.

137. McSherry E, Morris RC Jr. Attainment and maintenance of normal stature with alkali therapy in infants and children with classic renal tubular acidosis. *J Clin Invest* 61:59, 1978.

138. Alpern RJ, Sakhaee K. Clinical spectrum of chronic metabolic acidosis: Homeostatic mechanisms produce significant morbidity. *Am J Kidney Dis* 29:291, 1997.

139. Lefebvre A, de Vernejoul MC, Gueris J, et al. Optimal correction of acidosis changes progression of dialysis osteodystrophy. *Kidney Int* 36:1112, 1989.

140. Graham NA, Hoenich NA, Tarbit M, et al. Correction of acidosis in hemodialysis patients increases the sensitivity of the parathyroid glands to calcium. *J Am Soc Nephrol* 8:627, 1997.

141. May RC, Kelly RA, Mitch WE, Mechanisms for defects in muscle protein metabolism in rats with chronic uremia: Influence of metabolic acidosis. *J Clin Invest* 79:1099, 1987.

142. Williams B, Hattersley J, Layward E, Walls J. Metabolic acidosis and skeletal muscle adaptation to low protein diets in chronic uremia. *Kidney Int* 40:779, 1991.

143. Garibotto G, Russo R, Sofia A, et al. Skeletal muscle protein synthesis and degradation in patients with chronic renal failure. *Kidney Int* 45:1432, 1994.

144. Ballmer PE, McNurlan MA, Hulter HN, et al. Chronic metabolic acidosis decreases albumin synthesis and induces negative nitrogen balance in humans. *J Clin Invest* 95:39, 1995.

145. Bailey JL, Wang X, England BK, et al. The acidosis of chronic renal failure activates muscle proteolysis in rats by augmenting transcription of genes encoding proteins of the ATP-dependent ubiquitin-proteasome pathways. *J Clin Invest* 97:1447, 1996.

146. Graham KA, Reaich D, Channon SM, et al. Correction of acidosis in CAPD decreases whole body protein degradation. *Kidney Int* 49:1396, 1996.

147. Molvilli E, Zani R, Carli O, et al. Correction of metabolic acidosis increases serum albumin concentrations and decreases kinetically evaluated protein intake in haemodialysis patients: A prospective study. *Nephrol Dial Transplant* 13:1719, 1998.

148. Nath KA, Hostetter MK, Hostetter TH. Pathophysiology of chronic tubulo-interstitial disease in rats. Interactions of dietary acid load, ammonia, and complement component C3. *J Clin Invest* 76:667, 1985.

149. Husted FC, Nolph KD, Maher JF. $NaHCO_3$ and $NaCl$ tolerance in chronic renal failure. *J Clin Invest* 56:414, 1975.

150. Molitoris BA, Froment DH, Mackenzie TA, et al. Citrate: A major factor in the toxicity of orally administered aluminum compounds. *Kidney Int* 36:949, 1989.

155. Walker JA, Sherman RA, Cody RF. The effect of oral bases on enteral aluminum absorption. *Arch Intern Med* 150:2037, 1990.
156. Hill J. Salicylate intoxication. *N Engl J Med* 288:1110, 1973.
157. Garella S. Extracorporeal techniques in the treatment of exogenous intoxications. *Kidney Int* 33:735, 1988.
158. Gabow PA, Anderson R, Potts DE, Schrier RW. Acid-base disturbances in the salicylate-intoxicated adult. *Arch Intern Med* 138:1481, 1978.
159. Tenny SM, Miller RM. The respiratory and circulatory actions of salicylate. *Am J Med* 19:498, 1955.
160. Winters RW, White JS, Hughes MC. Disturbances of acid-base equilibrium in salicylate intoxication. *Pediatrics* 23:260, 1959.
161. Eichenholz A, Mulhausen RO, Redleaf PS. Nature of acid-base disturbance in salicylate intoxication. *Metabolism* 12:164, 1963.
162. Chatton J-Y, Besseghir K, Roch-Ramel F. Salicylic acid permeability properties of the rabbit cortical collecting duct. *Am J Physiol* 259:F613, 1990.
163. Prescott LF, Balali-Mood M, Critchley JAJH, et al. Diuresis or urinary alkalinisation for salicylate poisoning? *Br Med J* 2:1383, 1982.
164. Higgins RM, Connolly JO, Hendry BM. Alkalinization and hemodialysis in severe salicylate poisoning: Comparison of elimination techniques in the same patient. *Clin Nephrol* 50:178, 1998.
165. Bennett IL Jr, Cary FH, Mitchell GI, Cooper MN. Acute methyl alcohol poisoning: A review based on experiences in an outbreak of 323 cases. *Medicine* 32:431, 1953.
166. McMartin KE, Ambre JJ, Tephly TR. Methanol poisoning in human subjects: Role for formic acid accumulation in the metabolic acidosis. *Am J Med* 68:414, 1980.
167. Eells JT, McMartin KE, Black K, et al. Formaldehyde poisoning. *JAMA* 246:1237, 1981.
168. Glasser L, Sternglanz PD, Combie J, Robinson A. Serum osmolality and its applicability to drug overdose. *Am J Clin Pathol* 60:695, 1973.
169. Gabow PA. Ethylene glycol intoxication. *Am J Kidney Dis* 11:277, 1988.
170. DiNubile MJ. Serum osmolality (letter). *N Engl J Med* 310:1609, 1984.
171. Sklar AH, Linas SL. The osmolal gap in renal failure. *Ann Intern Med* 98:480, 1983.
172. Walker JA, Schwartzbard A, Krauss EA, et al. The missing gap: A pitfall in the diagnosis of alcohol intoxication by osmometry. *Arch Intern Med* 146:1843, 1986.
173. Sweeney TE, Beuchat CA, et al. Limitations of methods of osmometry: Measuring the osmolality of body fluids. *Am J Physiol* 264:R469, 1993.
174. Burns MJ, Schwartzstein RM. General approach to drug intoxications, in Rose BD (ed): *UpToDate in Medicine.* Wellesley, MA, UpToDate, 2000.
175. Gonda A, Gault H, Churchill D, Hollomby D. Hemodialysis for methanol intoxication. *Am J Med* 64:749, 1978.
176. McCoy HG, Cipolle RJ, Ehlers SM, et al. Severe methanol poisoning: Application of a pharmacokinetic model for ethanol therapy and hemodialysis. *Am J Med* 67:804, 1979.
177. Keyvan-Larijarn H, Tannenberg AM. Methanol intoxication. *Arch Intern Med* 134:293, 1974.
178. Freed CR, Bobbitt WH, Williams RM, et al. Ethanol for ethylene glycol poisoning. *N Engl J Med* 304:976, 1981.
179. Peterson CD, Collins AJ, Himes JM, et al. Ethylene glycol poisoning: Pharmacokinetics during therapy with ethanol and hemodialysis. *N Engl J Med* 304:21, 1981.
180. Palmisano J, Gruver C, Adams ND. Absence of anion gap metabolic acidosis in severe methanol poisoning. *Am J Kidney Dis* 9:441, 1987.
181. Barceloux DG, Krenzelok EP, Olson K, Watson W. American Academy of Clinical Toxicology Practice Guidelines on the Treatment of Ethylene Glycol Poisoning. Ad Hoc Committee. *J Toxicol Clin Toxicol* 37:537, 1999.
182. Baud FJ, Galliot M, Astier A, et al. Treatment of ethylene glycol poisoning with intravenous 4-methylpyrazole. *N Engl J Med* 319:97, 1988.
183. Baud FJ, Bismuth C, Garnier R, et al. 4-methylpyrazole may be an alternative to ethanol therapy for ethylene glycol intoxication in man. *Clin Toxicol* 24:463, 1986.

184. Brent J, McMartin K, Phillips S, et al. Fomepizole for the treatment of ethylene glycol poisoning. *N Engl J Med* 340:832, 1999.
185. Borron SW, Megarbane B, Baud FJ. Fomepizole in treatment of uncomplicated ethylene glycol poisoning. *Lancet* 354:831, 1999.
186. Whalen JE, Richards CJ, Ambre J. Inadequate removal of methanol and formate using sorbent based regeneration hemodialysis delivery system. *Clin Nephrol* 11:318, 1979.
187. Gabow PA, Clay, K, Sullivan JB, Lepoff R. Organic acid in ethylene glycol intoxication. *Ann Intern Med* 105:16, 1986.
188. Bove KE. Ethylene glycol toxicity. *Am J Clin Pathol* 45:46, 1966.
189. Parry MF, Wallach R. Ethylene glycol poisoning. *Am J Med* 57:143, 1974.
190. Case Records of Massachusetts General Hospital (Case 38-1979). *N Engl J Med* 301:650, 1979.
191. Jacobsen D, Hewlett TP, Webb R, et al. Ethylene glycol intoxication: Evaluation of kinetics and crystalluria. *Am J Med* 84:145, 1988.
192. Gilmour IJ, Blanchard RJW, Perry WF. Mannitol gives false-positive biochemical estimations of ethylene glycol. *N Engl J Med* 291:51, 1974.
193. Blum JE, Coe FL. Metabolic acidosis after sulfur ingestion. *N Engl J Med* 297: 869, 1977.
194. Szerlip HM, Singer I. Hyperchloremic metabolic acidosis after chlorine inhalation. *Am J Med* 77:581, 1984.
195. Heird WC, Dell B, Driscoll JM Jr, et al. Metabolic acidosis resulting from intravenous alimentation mixtures containing synthetic amino acids. *N Engl J Med* 287:943, 1972.
196. Fraley DS, Adler S, Bruns F, Segal D. Metablic acidosis after hyperalimentation with casein hydrolysate. *Ann Intern Med* 88:352, 1978.
197. Perez GO, Oster JR, Rogers A. Acid-base disturbances in gastrointestinal disease. *Dig Dis Sci* 32:1033, 1987.
198. Teree T, Mirabal-Font E, Ortiz A, Wallace W. Stool losses and acidosis in diarrheal disease of infancy. *Pediatrics* 36:704, 1965.
199. Schwartz WB, Relman AS. Metabolic and renal studies in chronic potassium depletion resulting from overuse of laxatives. *J Clin Invest* 32:538, 1953.
200. Harris RT. Bulimarexia and related serious eating disorders with medical complications. *Ann Intern Med* 99:800, 1983.
201. Bytzer P, Stokholm M, Andersen I, et al. Prevalence of surreptitious laxative abuse in patients with diarrhea of uncertain origin: A cost benefit analysis of a screening procedure. *Gut* 30:1379, 1989.
202. Oster JR, Materson BJ, Rogers AI. Laxative abuse syndrome. *Am J Gastroenterol* 74:451, 1980.
203. Field M, Rao MC, Chang EB. Intestinal electrolyte transport and diarrheal disease. *N Engl J Med* 321:800, 879, 1989.
204. McDougal WS. Metabolic complications of urinary diversion. *J Urol* 147:1199, 1992.
205. Koch MO, McDougal WS. The pathophysiology of hyperchloremic metabolic acidosis after urinary diversion through intestinal segments. *Surgery* 98:561, 1985.
206. Cruz DN, Huot SJ. Metabolic complications of urinary diversions: An overview. *Am J Med* 102:477, 1997.
207. Mundy AR. Metabolic complications of urinary diversion. *Lancet* 353:1813, 1999.
208. D'Agostino A, Leadbetter WF, Schwartz WB. Alterations in the ionic composition of isotonic saline solution installed in the colon. *J Clin Invest* 32:444, 1953.
209. Kaveggia FF, Thompson JS, Schafer EC, et al. Hyperammonemic encephalopathy in urinary diversion with urea-splitting urinary tract infection. *Arch Intern Med* 150:2389, 1990.
210. Kleinman PK. Cholestyramine and metabolic acidosis. *N Engl J Med* 290:861, 1974.
211. Kurtzman NA. Disorders of distal acidification. *Kidney Int* 38:720, 1990.
212. Kurtzman NA. Renal tubular acidosis: A constellation of syndromes. *Hosp Pract* 22(11):131, 1987.
213. Levine DZ, Jacobson HR. The regulation of renal acid excretion: New observations from studies of distal nephron segments. *Kidney Int* 29:1099, 1986.

214. Garg LC. Respective roles of H-ATPase and H-K-ATPase in ion transport in the kidney. *J Am Soc Nephrol* 2:949, 1991.

215. Steinmetz PR. Cellular organization of urinary acidification. *Am J Physiol* 251:F173, 1986.

216. Harrington JT, Hulter HN, Cohen JJ, Madias NE. Mineralocorticoid-stimulated renal acidification: The critical role of dietary sodium. *Kidney Int* 30:43, 1986.

217. Batlle DC. Segmental characterization of defects in collecting tubule acidification. *Kidney Int* 30:546, 1986.

218. Lombard WE, Kokko JP, Jacobson HR. Bicarbonate transport in cortical and outer medullary collecting tubules. *Am J Physiol* 244:F289, 1983.

219. Cohen EP, Bastani B, Cohen MR, et al. Absence of H^+-ATPase in cortical collecting tubules of a patient with Sjögren's syndrome and distal renal tubular acidosis. *J Am Soc Nephrol* 3:264, 1992.

220. Bastani B, Haragsim L, Gluck S, Siamopoulos KC. Lack of H-ATPase in distal nephron causing hypokalemic distal RTA in a patient with Sjögren's syndrome (letter). *Nephrol Dial Transplant* 10:908, 1995.

221. Bruce LJ, Cope DL, Jones GK, et al. Familial distal renal tubular acidosis is associated with mutations in the red cell anion exchanger (band 3, AE1) gene. *J Clin Invest* 100:1693, 1997.

222. Jarolim P, Shayakul C, Prabakaran D, et al. Autosomal dominant distal renal tubular acidosis is associated in three families with heterozygosity for the R589H mutation in the AE1 (band 3) Cl^-/HCO_3^- exchanger. *J Biol Chem* 273:6380, 1998.

223. Karet FE, Gainza FJ, Gyory AZ, et al. Mutations in the chloride-bicarbonate exchanger, gene AE1 cause autosomal dominant but not autosomal recessive distal renal tubular acidosis. *Proc Natl Acad Sci U S A* 95:6337, 1998.

224. Karet FE, Finberg KE, Nelson RD, et al. Mutations in the gene encoding B1 subunit of H^+-ATPase case renal tubular acidosis with sensorineural deafness. *Nat Genet* 21:84, 1999.

225. Sansom S, Muto S, Giebisch G. Na-dependent effects of DOCA on cellular transport properties of CCDs from ADX rabbits. *Am J Physiol* 253:F753, 1987.

226. Batlle DC, Itsarayoungyuen K, Arruda JAL, Kurtzman NA. Hyperkalemic hyperchloremic metabolic acidosis in sickle cell hemoglobinopathies. *Am J Med* 72:188, 1982.

227. Batlle DC, Arruda JAL, Kurtzman NA. Hyperkalemic distal renal tubular acidosis associated with obstructive uropathy. *N Engl J Med* 304:373, 1981.

228. Rastogi S, Bayliss JM, Nascimento L, Arruda JAL. Hyperkalemic renal tubular acidosis: Effect of furosemide in humans and in rats. *Kidney Int* 28:801, 1985.

229. Sabatini S, Kurtzman NA. Enzyme activity in obstructive uropathy: Basis for salt wastage and the acidification defect. *Kidney Int* 37:79, 1990.

230. Batlle DC, von Riotte A, Schlueter W. Urinary sodium in the evaluation of hyperchloremic metabolic acidosis. *N Engl J Med* 316:140, 1987.

231. Schlueter W, Keilani T, Hizon M, et al. On the mechanism of impaired distal acidification is hyperkalemic renal tubular acidosis: Evaluation with amiloride and bumetanide. *J Am Soc Nephrol* 3:953, 1992.

232. Gil FZ, Malnic G. Effect of amphotericin B on renal tubular acidification in the rat. *Pfluegers Arch* 413:280, 1989.

233. Kurtzman NA, Gonzalez J, DeFronzo RA, Giebisch G. A patient with hyperkalemia and metabolic acidosis. *Am J Kidney Dis* 15:333, 1990.

234. Portwood RM, Weldin DW, Rector FC, Cade R. The relation of urinary CO_2 tension to bicarbonate excretion. *J Clin Invest* 38:770, 1959.

235. McSherry E, Sebastian A, Morris RC Jr. Renal tubular acidosis in infants: The several kinds, including bicarbonate-wasting classic renal tubular acidosis. *J Clin Invest* 51:499, 1972.

236. Sebastian A, McSherry E, Morris RC Jr. Renal potassium wasting in renal tubular acidosis (RTA): Its occurrence in types 1 and 2 RTA despite sustained correction of systemic acidosis. *J Clin Invest* 50:667, 1971.

237. Gill JR Jr, Bell NH, Bartter FC. Impaired conservation of sodium and potassium in renal tubular acidosis and its correction by buffer anions. *Clin Sci* 33:577, 1967.

238. Codina J, Delmas-Mata J, DuBose TD. Expression of HK2 protein is increased selectively in renal medulla by chronic hypokalemia. *Am J Physiol* 275:F433, 1998.
239. Dafnis E, Spohn M, Lonis B, et al. Vanadate causes hypokalemic distal renal tubular acidosis. *Am J Physiol* 262:F449, 1992.
240. Cogan MG, Rector FC. Proximal reabsorption during metabolic acidosis in the rat. *Am J Physiol* 242:F499, 1982.
241. Wingo CS. Effect of acidosis on chloride transport in the cortical thick ascending limb of Henle perfused in vitro. *J Clin Invest* 78:1324, 1986.
242. Sebastian A, McSherry E, Morris RC Jr. Impaired renal conservation of sodium and chloride during sustained correction of systemic acidosis in patients with type 1, classic renal tubular acidosis. *J Clin Invest* 58:454, 1976.
243. Bastani B, Underhill D, Chu N, et al. Preservation of intercalated cell H^+-ATPase in two patients with lupus nephritis and hyperkalemic distal renal tubular acidosis. *J Am Soc Nephrol* 8:1109, 1997.
244. Buckalew VM Jr, Purvis M, Shulman M, et al. Hereditary renal tubular acidosis. *Medicine* 53:229, 1974.
245. Caruana RJ, Buckalew VM Jr. The syndrome of distal (type 1) renal tubular acidosis. *Medicine* 67:84, 1988.
246. Coe FL, Parks JH. Stone disease in hereditary distal renal tubular acidosis. *Ann Intern Med* 93:60, 1980.
247. Brenner RJ, Spring DB, Sebastian A, et al. Incidence of radiographically evident bone disease, nephrocalcinosis, and nephrolithiasis in various types of renal tubular acidosis. *N Engl J Med* 307:217, 1982.
248. Preminger GM, Sakhaee K, Skurla C, Pak CYC. Prevention of renal calcium stone formation with potassium citrate therapy in patients with distal renal tubular acidosis. *J Urol* 134:20, 1985.
249. Lemann J Jr, Gray RW, Maierhoffer WJ, Cheung HS. The importance of renal net acid excretion as a determinant of fasting urinary calcium excretion. *Kidney Int* 29:743, 1986.
250. Breslau NA, Brinkley L, Hill KD, Pak CYC. Relationship of animal protein-rich diet to kidney stone formation and calcium metabolism. *J Clin Endocrinol Metab* 66:140, 1988.
251. Marone CC, Wong NLM, Sutton RAL, Dirks JH. Effects of metabolic alkalosis on calcium excretion in the conscious dog. *J Lab Clin Med* 101:264, 1983.
252. Kempson SA. Effect of metabolic acidosis on renal brush border membrane adaptation to low phosphorus diet. *Kidney Int* 22:225, 1982.
253. Kinsella J, Cujdik T, Sacktor B. Na^+-H^+ exchange activity in renal brush border membrane vesicles in response to metabolic acidosis: The role of glucocorticoids. *Proc Natl Acad Sci U S A* 81:630, 1984.
254. Rodriguez-Soriano J, Vallo A, Vastillo G, Oliveros R. Natural history of primary distal renal tubular acidosis treated since infancy. *J Pediatr* 101:669, 1982.
255. Norman ME, Feldman NI, Cohn RM, et al. Urinary citrate excretion in the diagnosis of distal renal tubular acidosis. *J Pediatr* 92:394, 1978.
256. Simpson DP. Citrate excretion: A window on renal metabolism. *Am J Physiol* 244:F223, 1983.
257. Hamm LL. Renal handling of citrate. *Kidney Int* 38:728, 1990.
258. Brennan S, Hering-Smith K, Hamm LL. Effect of pH on citrate reabsorption in the proximal tubule. *Am J Physiol* 255:F301, 1988.
260. Gault MH, Chafe LL, Morgan JM, et al. Comparison of patients with idiopathic calcium phosphate and calcium oxalate stones. *Medicine* 70:345, 1991.
261. McSherry E. Renal tubular acidosis in childhood. *Kidney Int* 20:799, 1981.
262. Preminger GM, Sakhaee K, Pak CYC. Alkali action on the urinary crystallization of calcium salts: Contrasting responses to sodium citrate and potassium citrate. *J Urol* 139:420, 1988.
263. Sakkhaee K, Nicar M, Hill K, Pak CYC. Contrasting effects of potassium citrate and sodium citrate therapies on urinary chemistries and crystallization of stone-forming salts. *Kidney Int* 24:348, 1983.

264. Lau K, Wolf C, Nussbaum P, et al. Differing effects of avid versus neutral phosphate therapy of hypercalciuria. *Kidney Int* 16:736, 1979.
265. Smith LH. Calcium-containing renal stones. *Kidney Int* 13:383, 1978.
266. Parks JH, Coe FL. A urinary calcium-citrate index for the evaluation of nephrolithiasis. *Kidney Int* 30:85, 1986.
267. Buckalew VM Jr, McCurdy DK, Ludwig GD, et al. Incomplete renal tubular acidosis. *Am J Med* 45:32, 1968.
268. Donnelly S, Kamel KS, Vasuvattakul S, et al. Might distal renal tubular acidosis be a proximal tubular cell disorder? *Am J Kidney Dis* 19:272, 1992.
269. Pun K-K, Wong C-K, Tsui E-L, et al. Hypokalemic periodic paralysis due to the Sjogren's syndrome in Chinese patients. *Ann Intern Med* 110:405, 1989.
270. Cohen EP, Bastani B, Cohen MR, et al. Absence of H^+-ATPase in cortical collecting tubules of a patient with Sjögren's syndrome and distal renal tubular acidosis. *J Am Soc Nephrol* 3:264, 1992.
271. Creamer P, Hochberg MC, Moschella SL. Clinical manifestations of Sjögren's syndrome, in Rose BD (ed): *UpToDate in Medicine*. Wellesley, MA, UpToDate, 2000.
272. Richardson RMA, Halperin ML. The urine pH: A potentially misleading diagnostic test in patients with hyperchloremic metabolic acidosis. *Am J Kidney Dis* 10:140, 1987.
273. Nash M, Torrado AD, Greifer I, et al. Renal tubular acidosis in infants and children. *J Pediatr* 80:738, 1972.
274. DuBose TD Jr, Lucci MS. Effect of carbonic anhydrase inhibition on superficial and deep nephron bicarbonate reabsorption in the rat. *J Clin Invest* 71:55, 1983.
275. Manz F, Waldherr R, Fritz HP, et al. Idiopathic de Toni-Debre-Fanconi syndrome with absence of proximal tubular brush border. *Clin Nephrol* 22:149, 1984.
276. Roth KS, Foreman JW, Segal S. The Fanconi syndrome and mechanisms of tubular transport dysfunction. *Kidney Int* 20:705, 1981.
277. Donckerwolcke RA, van Stekelenburg GJ, Tiddens HA. A case of bicarbonate-losing renal tubular acidosis with defective carboanhydrase activity. *Arch Dis Child* 45:769, 1970.
278. Sly WS, Whyte MP, Sundaram V, et al. Carbonic anhydrase II deficiency in 12 families with the autosomal recessive syndrome of osteopetrosis with renal tubular acidosis and cerebral calcification. *N Engl J Med* 313:139, 1985.
279. Coor C, Salmon RF, Quigley R, et al. Role of adenosine triphosphate (ATP) and NaK ATPase in the inhibition of proximal tubule transport with intracellular cystine loading. *J Clin Invest* 87:955, 1991.
280. Heller I, Halevy J, Cohen S, Theodor E. Significant metabolic acidosis induced by acetazolamide: Not a rare complication. *Arch Intern Med* 145:1815, 1985.
281. White MG, Asch MJ. Acid-base effects of topical mafenide acetate in the burned patient. *N Engl J Med* 284:1281, 1971.
282. Maldonado JE, Velosa JA, Kyle RA, et al. Fanconi syndrome in adults: A manifestation of a latent form of myeloma. *Am J Med* 58:354, 1975.
283. Smithline N, Kassirer JP, Cohen JJ. Light-chain nephropathy: Renal tubular dysfunction associated with light-chain proteinuria. *N Engl J Med* 294:71, 1976.
284. Fang LS. Light-chain nephropathy. *Kidney Int* 27:582, 1985.
285. Skinner R, Pearson ADJ, Price L, et al. Nephrotoxicity after ifosfamide. *Arch Dis Child* 65:732, 1990.
286. Ho PT, Zimmerman K, Wexler LH, et al. A prospective evaluation of ifosfamide-related nephrotoxicity in children and young adults. *Cancer* 76:2557, 1995.
287. Zamlauski-Tucker MJ, Morris M, Springate J. Ifosfamide metabolite chloracetaldehyde causes Fanconi syndrome in the perfused rat kidney. *Toxicol Appl Pharmacol* 129:170, 1994.
288. Sebastian A, McSherry E, Morris RC Jr. On the mechanism of renal potassium wasting in renal tubular acidosis with the Fanconi syndrome (type 2 RTA). *J Clin Invest* 50:231, 1971.
289. Fordtran JS, Morawski SG, Santa Ana CA, Rector FC Jr. Gas production after reaction of sodium bicarbonate and hydrochloric acid. *Gastroenterology* 87:1014, 1984.

290. Donckerwolcke RA, van Stekelenberg GJ, Tiddens HA. Therapy of bicarbonate-losing renal tubular acidosis. *Arch Dis Child* 45:774, 1970.
291. Garg LC, Narang N. Effects of aldosterone on NEM-sensitive ATPases in rabbit nephron segments. *Kidney Int* 34:13, 1988.
292. Jaeger P, Karlmark B, Giebisch G. Ammonia transport in rat cortical tubule: Relationship to potassium metabolism. *Am J Physiol* 245:F593, 1983.
293. Hulter HN, Ilnicki LP, Harbottle JA, Sebastian A. Impaired renal H^+ secretion and NH_3 production in mineralcorticoid-deficient, glucocorticoid-replete dogs. *Am J Physiol* 232:F136, 1977.
294. Szylman P, Better OS, Chaimowitz C, Rosler A. Role of hyperkalemia in the metabolic acidosis of isolated hypoaldosteronism. *N Engl J Med* 294:361, 1976.
295. DuBose TD Jr, Good DW. Effects of chronic hyperkalemia on renal production and proximal tubular transport of ammonium in rats. *Am J Physiol* 260:F680, 1991.
296. Sebastian A, Schambelan M, Lindenfeld S, Morris RC Jr. Amelioration of metabolic acidosis with fluorocortisone therapy in hyporeninemic hypoaldosteronism. *N Engl J Med* 297:576, 1977.
297. DeFronzo RA. Hyperkalemia and hyporeninemic hypoaldosteronism. *Kidney Int* 17:118, 1980.
298. Sebastian A, Schambelan M. Amelioration of type 4 renal tubular acidosis in chronic renal failure with furosemide. *Kidney Int* 12:534, 1977.
299. McCarron DA, Elliott WC, Rose JS, Bennett WM. Severe mixed metabolic acidosis secondary to rhabdomyolysis. *Am J Med* 67:905, 1979.
300. Mitchell JH, Wildenthal K, Johnson RL Jr. The effects of acid-base disturbances on cardiovascular and pulmonary function. *Kidney Int* 1:375, 1972.
301. Orchard CH, Kentish JC. Effects of changes in pH on the contractile function of cardiac muscle. *Am J Physiol* 258:C967, 1990.
302. Posner JB, Plum F. Spinal-fluid pH and neurologic symptoms in systemic acidosis. *N Engl J Med* 277:605, 1967.
303. Adler S, Simplaceanu V, Ho C. Brain pH in acute isocapnic metabolic acidosis and hypoxia: A ^{31}P-nuclear magnetic resonance study. *Am J Physiol* 258:F34, 1990.
304. Mitchell RA, Carman CT, Severinghaus JW, et al. Stability of cerebrospinal fluid pH in chronic acid-base disturbances in blood. *J Appl Physiol* 20:443, 1965.
305. Fulop M, Tannenbaum H, Dreyer N. Ketotic hyperosmolar coma. *Lancet* 2:635, 1973.
306. Lemann J Jr, Adams ND, Gray RW. Urinary calcium excretion in human beings. *N Engl J Med* 301:535, 1979.
307. Potter DE, Greifer I. Statural growth of children with renal disease in human beings. *Kidney Int* 14:334, 1978.
308. Cunningham J, Fraher LJ, Clemmens TL, et al. Chronic acidosis with metabolic bone disease. *Am J Med* 73:199, 1982.
309. Chesney RW, Moorthy AV, Eisman JA, et al. Increased growth after oral $1\alpha,25$-vitamin D_3 in childhood osteodystrophy. *N Engl J Med* 298:238, 1978.
310. Simmons JM, Wilson CJ, Potter DE, Holliday MA. Relation of calorie deficiency to growth failure in children on hemodialysis and the growth response to calorie supplementation. *N Engl J Med* 285:653, 1971.
311. Bleich HL, Schwartz WB. Tris buffer (Tham): An appraisal of its physiologic effects and clinical usefulness. *N Engl J Med* 274:782, 1966.
312. Schwartz WB, Waters W. Lactate versus bicarbonate: A reconsideration of the therapy of metabolic acidosis. *Am J Med* 32:831, 1962.
313. Vaziri ND, Ness R, Wellikson L, et al. Bicarbonate-buffered peritoneal dialysis: An effective adjunct in the treatment of lactic acidosis. *Am J Med* 67:392, 1977.

TWENTY

RESPIRATORY ACIDOSIS

The introduction to acid-base disorders presented in Chap. 17 should be read before proceeding with this discussion. Respiratory acidosis is a clinical disorder characterized by a reduced arterial pH (or increased H^+ concentration), an elevation in the P_{CO_2} (hypercapnia), and a variable increase in the plasma HCO_3^- concentration. Hypercapnia also constitutes the respiratory compensation to metabolic alkalosis. However, the increase in the P_{CO_2} is appropriate in this setting, since it lowers the arterial pH toward normal.

PATHOPHYSIOLOGY AND ETIOLOGY

Endogenous metabolism results in the production of approximately 15,000 mmol of CO_2 per day. Although CO_2 is not an acid, it combines with H_2O as it is added to the bloodstream, resulting in the formation of H_2CO_3:

$$CO_2 + H_2O \quad \leftrightarrow \quad H_2CO_3 \quad \leftrightarrow \quad H^+ + HCO_3^- \qquad (20\text{-}1)$$

The ensuing elevation in the H^+ concentration is then minimized because most of the excess H^+ ions combine with intracellular buffers, including hemoglobin (Hb) in red cells:

$$H_2CO_3 + Hb^- \quad \leftrightarrow \quad HHb + HCO_3^- \qquad (20\text{-}2)$$

The HCO_3^- generated by this reaction leaves the erythrocyte and enters the extracellular fluid in exchange for extracellular Cl^-.

The net effect is that metabolically generated CO_2 *is primarily carried in the bloodstream as* HCO_3^-, *with little change in the extracellular pH*. These processes are reversed in the alveoli. As HHb is oxygenated, H^+ is released. These H^+ ions combine with HCO_3^- to form H_2CO_3 and then CO_2, which is excreted.

Control of Ventilation

Before we discuss how hypercapnia can occur, it is helpful to review briefly the basic aspects of ventilatory regulation. Alveolar ventilation provides the oxygen necessary for oxidative metabolism and eliminates the CO_2 produced by these metabolic processes. It is therefore appropriate that the *main physiologic stimuli to respiration are a reduction in the arterial* P_{O_2} *(hypoxemia) and an elevation in the arterial* P_{CO_2} (Fig. 20-1).[1,2]

The CO_2 stimulus to ventilation occurs primarily in chemosensitive areas in the respiratory center in the medulla, which respond to CO_2-induced changes in the cerebral interstitial pH.[1-3] In contrast, the initial hypoxemic enhancement of ventilation is mostly mediated by chemoreceptors in the carotid bodies, which are located near the bifurcation of the carotid arteries.[1,4] In normal subjects, these regulatory processes permit adequate oxygenation to be maintained and the arter-

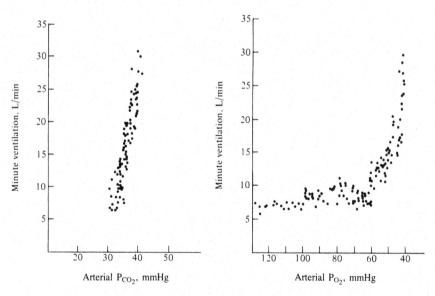

Figure 20-1   Relationship between arterial P_{CO_2} (left panel) and P_{O_2} (right panel) and the respiratory minute volume in normal subjects. (*Adapted from Hudgel DW, Control of breathing in asthma, in Weiss EB, Segal MS, Stein M (eds):* Bronchial Asthma: Mechanisms and Therapeutics, *2d ed. Boston, Little, Brown, 1984, with permission.*)

ial P_{CO_2} to be held within narrow limits (40 ± 4 mmHg), despite the large daily CO_2 load and variability in the respiratory quotient and metabolic rate.

Carbon dioxide is the major stimulus to respiration, and minute ventilation is enhanced by even minor elevations in the arterial P_{CO_2} (Fig. 20-1). For example, among most normal subjects in whom hypercapnia is induced by breathing a hypercapnic gas mixture, minute ventilation rises by 1 to 4 L for every 1 mmHg in the P_{CO_2}.[2,5]

In contrast, hypoxemia does not begin to substantially promote ventilation until the arterial P_{O_2} is less than 50 to 60 mmHg (Figs. 20-1 and 20-2). Lesser degrees of hypoxemia initially increase ventilation; however, the ensuing fall in P_{CO_2} raises the extracellular pH, which depresses respiration and blunts the hypoxemic stimulus.

The importance of pH in influencing the ventilatory response to hypoxemia is illustrated by the upper curve in Fig. 20-2. If the arterial P_{CO_2} is held at normal values (or is elevated because of intrinsic lung disease), then the limiting respiratory alkalosis does not occur and ventilation begins to be enhanced at a much higher arterial P_{O_2} of 70 to 80 mmHg (Fig. 20-2).[2] This relationship has important implications for the control of ventilation in patients with chronic respiratory acidosis (see below).

Development of Hypercapnia

Since the CO_2 stimulus to ventilation is so strong, hypercapnia and respiratory acidosis are almost always due to a reduction in effective alveolar ventilation, not

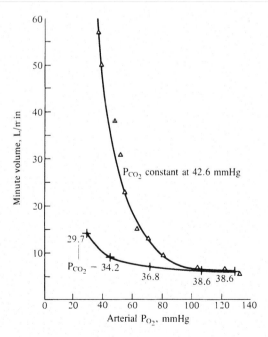

Figure 20-2 Influence of arterial P_{CO_2} on the ventilatory response to hypoxemia. In normal subjects (lower curve), lowering the partial pressure of oxygen in the inspired air increases ventilation and lowers the arterial P_{CO_2}. However, these changes are relatively minor until the arterial P_{O_2} falls below 50 mmHg. The earlier and greater degree of hyperventilation seen when the arterial P_{CO_2} is held constant (upper curve) indicates that the development of mild hypocapnic alkalosis normally limits the ventilatory response to hypoxemia. (*Adapted from Loeschcke HH, Gertz KH, Arch Ges Physiol 267:460, 1958, with permission.*)

an increase in CO_2 production. Hypoventilation can occur when there is interference with any step in the ventilatory process (Table 20-1).[5] In patients with reduced respiratory drive or neuromuscular dysfunction, for example, there tends to be a generalized fall in alveolar ventilation. In contrast, CO_2 retention in intrinsic pulmonary disease is thought to be due primarily to an *imbalance between ventilation and perfusion* (which is functionally equivalent to increasing the amount of dead space to tidal volume ratio).[6] The hypercapnia in this setting is

Table 20-1 Causes of acute and chronic respiratory acidosis

Inhibition of the medullary respiratory center
  A. Acute
    1. Drugs: opiates, anesthetics, sedatives
    2. Oxygen in chronic hypercapnia
    3. Cardiac arrest
    4. Central sleep apnea
  B. Chronic
    1. Extreme obesity (PIckwickian syndrome)
    2. Central nervous system lesions (rare)
    3. Metabolic alkalosis (although hypercapnia is an appropriate response to the rise in pH in this setting)
Disorders of the respiratory muscles and chest wall
  A. Acute
    1. Muscle weakness: crisis in myasthenia gravis, periodic paralysis, aminoglycosides, Guillain-Barré syndrome, severe hypokalemia or hypophosphatemia
  B. Chronic
    1. Muscle weakness: spinal cord injury, poliomyelitis, amyotrophic lateral sclerosis, multiple sclerosis, myxedema
    2. Kyphoscoliosis
    3. Extreme obesity
Upper airway obstruction
  A. Acute
    1. Aspiration of foreign body or vomitus
    2. Obstructive sleep apnea
    3. Laryngospasm
Disorders affecting gas exchange across the pulmonary capillary
  A. Acute
    1. Exacerbation of underlying lung disease (including increased CO_2 production with high-carbohydrate diet)
    2. Adult respiratory distress syndrome
    3. Acute cardiogenic pulmonary edema
    4. Severe asthma or pneumonia
    5. Pneumothorax or hemothorax
  B. Chronic
    1. Chronic obstructive pulmonary disease: bronchitis, emphysema
    2. Extreme obesity
Mechanical ventilation

in part beneficial in that it allows the metabolically produced CO_2 to be excreted at a lower minute ventilation, thereby diminishing the work of breathing and often reducing the feeling of breathlessness.[5]

If ventilatory function is not restored, the decrease in pH produced by CO_2 retention is minimized by the cell buffers and by increased renal H^+ secretion, both of which result in an elevation in the plasma HCO_3^- concentration. Since the renal response occurs over several days,[7] protection of the extracellular pH in acute respiratory acidosis is much less efficient than that in chronic respiratory acidosis (see Figs. 20-3 and 20-4).

Relationship between Hypercapnia and Hypoxemia

All patients with hypercapnia who are breathing room air experience a fall in alveolar and arterial P_{O_2} because the sum of partial pressures of all gases in the alveoli must equal atmospheric pressure. In most cases, *hypoxemia occurs earlier and is more prominent than hypercapnia.* Two factors contribute to this difference:

- CO_2 can diffuse across the alveolar capillary wall 20 times as quickly as O_2.
- As patients attempt to increase ventilation in relatively normal segments of the lung, more CO_2 can be excreted but *more O_2 cannot be taken up*, since the saturation of hemoglobin already approaches 100 percent in these areas.

The clinical importance of this relationship between the arterial P_{O_2} and P_{CO_2} can be illustrated by the sequence seen in patients with acute asthma.[8] The combination of mucous plugs and bronchoconstriction initially induces hypoxemia; both the fall in P_{O_2} and activation of intrapulmonary mechanoreceptors then lead to enhanced ventilation.[8,9] Thus, a mild to moderate asthmatic attack is associated with hypocapnia and respiratory *alkalosis*. With increasing severity of the attack,

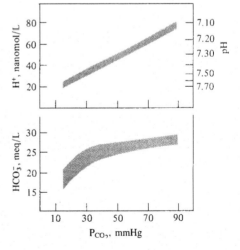

Figure 20-3 Combined significance bands for plasma pH and H^+ and HCO_3^- concentration in acute hypocapnia and hypercapnia in humans. In uncomplicated acute respiratory acid-base disorders, values for the H^+ and HCO_3^- concentrations will, with an estimated 95 percent probability, fall within the band. Observations lying outside the band indicate the presence of a complicating metabolic acid-base disturbance. (*From Arbus GS, Herbert LA, Levesque PR, et al,* N Engl J Med *280:117, 1969. By permission from the* New England Journal of Medicine.)

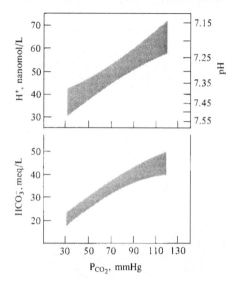

Figure 20-4 Ninety-five percent significance bands for plasma pH and H^+ and HCO_3^- concentrations in chronic hypercapnia. Note that, per change in P_{CO_2}, there is much less change in H^+ concentration and pH than in acute hypercapnia (Fig. 20-3). This reflects the effect of increased renal HCO_3^- generation. (*From Schwartz WB, Brackett NC Jr, Cohen JJ, J Clin Invest 44:291, 1965, by copyright permission of the American Society for Clinical Investigation.*)

airway resistance rises, the maximal minute ventilation falls, and consequently the P_{CO_2} rises, eventually to normal and even hypercapnic levels. Thus, the combination of hypoxemia and a "normal" P_{CO_2} of 40 mmHg represents severe disease in the acute asthmatic.[8] This principle can be applied generally to patients with intrinsic lung disease: Hypercapnia is a *late finding*, and even a small elevation in the P_{CO_2} of a few millimeters of mercury indicates *advanced pulmonary dysfunction* or a concomitant insult to ventilatory drive (e.g., narcotic use), since CO_2 is normally such a powerful stimulus to ventilation (Fig. 20-1).

Although hypoxemia-induced hyperventilation helps to delay the onset or minimize the degree of hypercapnia, there is a 16-fold variability (probably inherited) in the sensitivity to hypoxemic stimuli.[5,10,11] Those subjects who are less sensitive to hypoxemia will be more likely to develop respiratory acidosis in the presence of an appropriate cause, such as chronic bronchitis or marked obesity (see below).

Regulation of Ventilation in Chronic Respiratory Acidosis

Two general statements are often made concerning ventilatory control in the patient with chronic hypercapnia:

- The respiratory centers become less sensitive to the CO_2 and therefore the acidemic drive to ventilation.
- As a result, hypoxemia becomes the primary stimulus to respiration.

However, these conclusions are based upon observations that are subject to somewhat different interpretation.

Insensitivity to CO_2   Evidence for insensitivity to CO_2 is primarily based upon experiments that showed that patients with chronic respiratory acidosis have a *lesser increase in ventilation* than normals when the P_{CO_2} is raised by increasing the CO_2 content of inspired air (Fig. 20-5). This apparent insensitivity, however, may, at least in part, reflect the high plasma HCO_3^- concentration induced by the renal compensation in this setting.[5,12] From the law of mass action,

$$[H^+] = 24 \times \frac{P_{CO_2}}{[HCO_3^-]} \qquad (20\text{-}3)$$

it can be seen that a given rise in the P_{CO_2} will induce a smaller increase in the arterial H^+ concentration when the plasma HCO_3^- concentration is elevated. Thus, the lesser increment in ventilation in chronic respiratory acidosis and therefore the apparent insensitivity to CO_2 may simply reflect the *lesser rise in H^+ concentration.*[12,13]

Consider, for example, the response to ammonium chloride, which is metabolized to hydrochloric acid and reverses the compensatory rise in the plasma HCO_3^- concentration. In this setting, the slope of the curve between alveolar ventilation and the P_{CO_2} increases toward normal (Fig. 20-5), being limited by the mechanical properties of the diseased lung, not by the responsiveness to pH.[12] This enhanced sensitivity to CO_2 is directly related to the fall in the plasma HCO_3^- concentration, since the increase in ventilation *per increase in H^+ concentration* is the same in the control state and after the administration of ammonium chloride.[12,13]

In addition to normalizing the slope, reducing the plasma HCO_3^- concentration also leads to an increase in the baseline rate of ventilation, resulting in a fall in

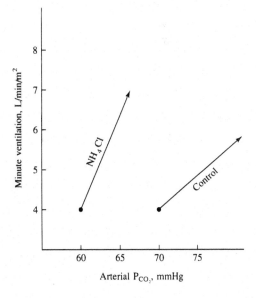

Figure 20-5 Ventilatory responses to inhalation of CO_2 in a patient with chronic hypercapnia in the control state and after the HCO_3^- concentration has been lowered by the administration of ammonium chloride. The latter therapy increases baseline ventilation (as evidenced by a lower initial P_{CO_2}) and increases the respiratory responsiveness to CO_2 toward normal. (*From Goldring RM, Turino GM, Heinemann HO, Am J Med 51:772, 1971, with permission.*)

Minute ventilation, L/min/m²

NH₄Cl

Control

Arterial P_{CO_2}, mmHg

P_{CO_2} and a rise in P_{O_2} (Fig. 20-5).[12-14] These findings indicate that the renal compensation to chronic hypercapnia has two effects: *It protects the extracellular pH, but, in so doing, it limits the stimulus to respiration, aggravating the hypoxemia and hypercapnia.* Similarly, the induction of metabolic alkalosis with diuretic therapy also suppresses ventilation, further evidence that the pH stimulus is intact.[15]

Dependence upon hypoxemia Patients with chronic respiratory acidosis do rely upon hypoxemia to stimulate ventilation.[16] This relationship, however, is based not upon insensitivity to pH, but upon two other factors. First, the renal compensation, plus the frequent concomitant use of diuretics for edema in cor pulmonale, results in a rise in the plasma HCO_3^- concentration that returns the extracellular pH toward or, in some cases, above normal. Thus, there is little or no acidemic stimulus to ventilation in many patients with chronic hypercapnia.

Second, the relationship between the P_{O_2} and ventilation is altered in the presence of a high P_{CO_2}. As shown in Fig. 20-2, hypoxemia does not importantly stimulate respiration in normals until the P_{O_2} is below 50 to 60 mmHg, because of the potent suppressive effect of concurrent hypocapnia and respiratory alkalosis. In comparison, this fall in P_{CO_2} does not occur in chronic respiratory acidosis; as a result, ventilation is enhanced as soon as the P_{O_2} falls below 80 mmHg.

Correction of hypoxemia is important clinically, since maintaining the P_{O_2} above 55 mmHg improves both survival and the quality of life in patients with chronic lung disease (see "Treatment," below).[17-19] However, oxygen must be given carefully, because rapid and excessive correction can produce a further elevation in the P_{CO_2} that, if marked, can lead to neurologic symptoms.[11,16,17]

Interestingly, a reduction in minute ventilation is not the primary factor responsible for the development of worsening hypercapnia.[11,20,21] In one study, for example, the administration of oxygen to patients with chronic lung disease and acute respiratory failure produced a 7 percent reduction in minute ventilation, which accounted for only 5 mmHg of the 23 mmHg elevation in P_{CO_2}.[11] Of greater importance were worsening of ventilation/perfusion mismatching due to attenuation of hypoxemia-induced vasoconstriction (which will increase the dead space to tidal volume ratio by increasing blood flow to poorly ventilated areas) and decreased affinity of hemoglobin for CO_2 (the Haldane effect).

Acute Respiratory Acidosis

The ability to acutely protect the extracellular pH is different in metabolic and respiratory acidosis. In the former, extracellular and intracellular buffering and compensatory hyperventilation all minimize the fall in pH (see Chap. 19). In contrast, the body is not so well adapted to handle an acute elevation in the P_{CO_2}. There is *virtually no extracellular buffering*, because HCO_3^- cannot buffer H_2CO_3:[22]

$$H_2CO_3 + HCO_3^- \rightarrow H_2CO_3 + HCO_3^- \qquad (20\text{-}4)$$

Since the renal response takes time to develop, the cell buffers, particularly hemoglobin [Eq. (20-2)] and proteins, constitute the only protection against acute hypercapnia:

$$H_2CO_3 + Buf^- \rightarrow HBuf + HCO_3^- \qquad (20\text{-}5)$$

As a result of these buffering reactions, there is an increase in the plasma HCO_3^- concentration, averaging *1 meq/L for every 10 mmHg rise in the* P_{CO_2} (Fig. 20-4).[23,24] Thus, if the P_{CO_2} is acutely increased to 80 mmHg, there will be approximately a 4-meq/L elevation in the plasma HCO_3^- concentration to 28 meq/L and a potentially serious reduction in the extracellular pH to 7.17:

$$pH = 6.10 + \log\frac{28}{0.03(80)}$$

$$= 7.17$$

This is not very efficient, since the pH would have been only slightly lower at 7.10 if there were no buffering and the plasma HCO_3^- concentration had remained at 24 meq/L. A more severe reduction in the pH to below 7.00 can occur when there is a combined respiratory and metabolic acidosis, as with acute pulmonary edema and lactic acidosis due to severe heart failure.[25]

Etiology   Common causes of acute respiratory acidosis include acute exacerbations of underlying lung disease, severe asthma or pneumonia, pulmonary edema, and suppression of the respiratory center following a cardiac arrest, a drug overdose, or the administration of oxygen to a patient with chronic hypercapnia.[11,26]

In addition, an increasingly recognized cause of hypercapnia is the *sleep apnea syndrome*.[27-29] This disorder is characterized by multiple (up to several hundred) apneic episodes per night associated with short periods of arousal (which are not apparent to the patient) due to hypoxemia and hypercapnia. Three different types of sleep apnea have been recognized: *central*, in which rare cerebral disorders interfere with the medullary control of ventilation; *obstructive*, in which there is abnormal passive collapse of the pharyngeal muscles during inspiration, such that the airway becomes occluded from the apposition of the tongue and soft palate against the posterior oropharynx; and a *mixed* central and obstructive picture.[28-30] Most patients have at least some obstructive component, which is typically manifested by loud snoring. Obesity, hypothyroidism, tonsillar enlargement, and nasal obstruction also may contribute to the development of inspiratory obstruction.[31]

The sleep apnea syndrome is associated with a variety of occasionally subtle clinical manifestations, which are due both to the repeated episodes of hypoxemia and hypercapnia and/or to the lack of uninterrupted sleep. These include headaches, daytime somnolence and fatigue, morning confusion with difficulty in concentration, personality changes, depression, persistent pulmonary and systemic hypertension, and potentially life-threatening cardiac arrhythmias.[28,29,32] Serious job-related and familial problems frequently ensue.

The diagnosis of sleep apnea should be suspected from the clinical history (particularly loud snoring and daytime somnolence) and can be confirmed by appropriate evaluation while the patient is asleep.[33] Cardiac monitoring is performed as part of the polysomnographic evaluation to check for the presence of serious arrhythmias. Effective treatment can rapidly reverse almost all of the clinical findings.[34]

Chronic hypercapnia is unusual in the sleep apnea syndrome, since the CO_2 retained during apneic episodes can be excreted when the patient is awake and ventilation is relatively normal.[5] In a minority of cases, the combination of underlying lung disease, obesity, and repetitive apneic episodes (including those due to daytime somnolence) can lead to a low total daily alveolar ventilation and persistent CO_2 retention.[35,36] This disorder is called the obesity hypoventilation syndrome.[37]

Finally, mechanical ventilation may be associated with hypercapnia if the rate of effective alveolar ventilation is inadequate. These patients, in whom ventilation is *fixed*, may also retain CO_2 if the rate of CO_2 production is increased. This sequence can occur either with the administration of $NaHCO_3$ to treat lactic acidosis during cardiopulmonary resuscitation[27,38-40] or with enteral or parenteral overfeeding.[41] In the former setting, the presence of marked hypercapnia may be missed if arterial blood is measured, since the lungs are capable of removing CO_2 from the diminished amount of blood flow that is delivered. Use of mixed venous blood is required to more closely measure acid-base status at the tissue level (see page 598).[42]

Chronic Respiratory Acidosis

The acid-base picture is different with chronic hypercapnia because of the compensatory renal response. The persistent elevation in the P_{CO_2} stimulates renal H^+ secretion, resulting in the addition of HCO_3^- to the extracellular fluid (see page 348).[7] The net effect is that, after 3 to 5 days, a new steady state is attained in which there is roughly a *3.5-meq/L increase in the plasma HCO_3^- concentration for every 10 mmHg increment in the P_{CO_2}* (Fig. 20-4).[43,44]

If, for example, the P_{CO_2} were chronically increased to 80 mmHg, the plasma HCO_3^- concentration should rise by approximately 14 meq/L, up to a level of 38 meq/L. This response is extremely effective, since the arterial pH falls only to 7.30, in contrast to 7.17, as seen above, with a similar degree of acute hypercapnia. The efficiency of the renal compensation has allowed some patients to tolerate a P_{CO_2} as high as 90 to 110 mmHg without a fall in the arterial pH to less than 7.25 and without symptoms as long as adequate oxygenation is maintained.[45]

The extent of the rise in the plasma HCO_3^- concentration in chronic respiratory acidosis is determined *solely by the increase in renal H^+ secretion*, which is presumably mediated by a fall in renal tubular cell pH induced by the extracellular acidemia. The net result is that maximal HCO_3^- reabsorptive capacity is enhanced and the plasma HCO_3^- concentration rises to a new steady state level as in

Fig. 20-4. Exogenous alkali therapy is both unnecessary (since the pH is so well protected) and ineffective, as the excess HCO_3^- is rapidly excreted in the urine without raising the final plasma HCO_3^- concentration.[46]

Etiology   Chronic respiratory acidosis is a relatively common clinical disturbance that is most often due to chronic obstructive lung disease (bronchitis and emphysema) in smokers. Despite the presence of severe intrinsic pulmonary dysfunction, it is not completely understood why some patients become hypercapnic and hypoxemic relatively early ("blue bloaters"), whereas others do not ("pink puffers"). Some *unaffected* family members of patients with chronic hypercapnia have a reduced ventilatory response to hypoxemia and, to a lesser degree, hypercapnia, presumably because of genetic variation in the sensitivity of the respiratory center.[47]

Such genetic factors can lead to the following sequence: Lung disease initially impairs net alveolar gas exchange, resulting in hypoxemia and eventually hypercapnia, both of which can stimulate ventilation and return the arterial P_{O_2} and P_{CO_2} toward normal. Persistent hypercapnia will occur relatively early (as in blue bloaters) when the ventilatory response to these stimuli is impaired. If, on the other hand, the central control of respiration is normal, persistent hypercapnia will not occur until pulmonary dysfunction is more severe (as in pink puffers).[5]

A similar problem may be present when chronic respiratory acidosis occurs in extremely obese patients (called the obesity hyperventilation or Pickwickian syndrome).[36-38] It had been assumed that the primary problem in this disorder was increased weight of the chest wall, leading to enhanced work of breathing and inspiratory muscle weakness.[48] Reversal of the hypercapnia with weight loss in some patients is consistent with this hypothesis. However, the following observations suggest that factors other than obesity also play a contributory role. First, most morbidly obese patients do not become hypercapnic, and, in those who do, there is no correlation between the degree of obesity and the ventilatory abnormalities.[49] Second, a more normal ventilatory pattern can be produced in some patients with progesterone (a direct respiratory stimulant);[29,50,51] this finding indicates that these patients can increase alveolar ventilation and raises the possibility of an associated central defect.

An abnormality in respiratory control is also suggested by the demonstration that obese hypoventilators have decreased respiratory responsiveness to both hypoxemia and hypercapnia.[49,52,53] In contrast, obese patients with normal ventilation respond normally to these stimuli.[53,54] Once again, an inherited defect in ventilatory regulation may select out those obese patients who will develop chronic hypercapnia.

Obese hypoventilators may also have a component of obstructive sleep apnea.[31] The symptoms are somewhat similar to these two conditions, as many Pickwickian patients complain of excessive daytime somnolence. However, there are also important differences, since obstructive sleep apnea alone is uncommonly associated with chronic CO_2 retention.[35]

SYMPTOMS

Severe *acute* respiratory acidosis can produce a variety of neurologic abnormalities.[55] The initial symptoms include headache, blurred vision, restlessness, and anxiety, which can progress to tremors, asterixis, delirium, and somnolence (called CO_2 narcosis). The cerebrospinal fluid (CSF) pressure is often elevated, and papilledema may be seen. These latter effects may be mediated in part by an acidemia-induced elevation in cerebral blood flow.[56] This hemodynamic change can be viewed as an appropriate response, since the increase in cerebral perfusion will tend to wash away the excess CO_2, thereby returning the cerebral pH toward normal.[56]

Both the neurologic symptoms and the increase in cerebral blood flow appear to be related to changes in the CSF (or cerebral interstitial) pH, not to the arterial pH or P_{CO_2}.[57,58] CO_2 is lipid-soluble and rapidly equilibrates across the blood-brain barrier; HCO_3^-, in comparison, is a polar compound that crosses this barrier very slowly. Thus, acute hypercapnia produces a greater fall in CSF pH than does acute metabolic acidosis;[57] this probably explains why neurologic abnormalities are less prominent in the latter disorder. Symptoms are also less common with *chronic* hypercapnia, since the renal compensation returns the arterial pH and ultimately the CSF pH toward normal.

In addition to neurologic abnormalities, arrhythmias and peripheral vasodilation may combine to produce severe hypotension if the systemic pH is reduced to below 7.10. In the patient with underlying lung disease, this problem is most often seen when respiratory acidosis is complicated by a superimposed metabolic acidosis.

Chronic respiratory acidosis is also commonly associated with cor pulmonale and peripheral edema. The cardiac output and glomerular filtration rate (GFR) are usually normal to near normal in this disorder, which generally occurs only in those patients with severe lung disease who are hypercapnic.[58] These findings suggest a direct role for CO_2 in the renal Na^+ retention in this setting, although marked hypoxemia also may contribute (see page 509).[58,59]

DIAGNOSIS

The presence of an acid pH and hypercapnia is diagnostic of respiratory acidosis. However, identifying the underlying acid-base disorder is more complicated than in metabolic acidosis or alkalosis, since the responses to acute and chronic respiratory acidosis are different. The following examples will illustrate how the confidence bands in Figs. 20-3 and 20-4 can be used in the evaluation of patients with respiratory acidosis. As will be demonstrated, there is *no substitute for an accurate and complete history*, since a given set of arterial blood values can be associated with several different disorders.

In acute hypercapnia, the plasma HCO_3^- concentration should be between 24 and 29 meq/L (Fig. 20-3). Values above or below this range indicate superimposed metabolic disorders. For example:

Case history 20-1   A previously well patient is brought into the emergency room in a moribund state. Physical examination and chest x-ray suggest acute pulmonary edema. The laboratory tests include the following:

$$Arterial\ pH = 7.02$$

$$P_{CO_2} = 60\ mmHg$$

$$[HCO_3^-] = 15\ meq/L$$

$$P_{O_2} = 40\ mmHg$$

Comment   Since the plasma HCO_3^- concentration should rise 1 meq/L for each 10 mmHg increment in P_{CO_2} in acute respiratory acidosis, an acute elevation of the P_{CO_2} to 60 mmHg should increase the plasma HCO_3^- concentration to 26 meq/L (pH of 7.24). Therefore, the findings in this patient represent a combined respiratory and metabolic acidosis, a life-threatening combination not infrequently seen in severe acute pulmonary edema in which lactic acidosis is superimposed upon the pulmonary dysfunction.[25]

The difficulties in interpretation in chronic respiratory acidosis are illustrated in Figs. 20-6 to 20-8. Consider the following set of arterial blood tests:

$$Arterial\ pH = 7.27$$

$$P_{CO_2} = 70\ mmHg$$

$$[HCO_3^-] = 31\ meq/L$$

$$P_{O_2} = 35\ mmHg$$

The 30 mmHg increase in the P_{CO_2} should be associated with a 3-meq/L elevation in the plasma HCO_3^- concentration to 27 meq/L in acute hypercapnia or an 11-meq/L increment (3.5 meq/L per 10 mmHg rise in the P_{CO_2}) to 35 meq/L in chronic hypercapnia. The observed value of 31 meq/L falls *between* the confidence bands for acute and chronic respiratory acidosis (Fig. 20-6a, point A). This can represent (1) metabolic acidosis complicating chronic hypercapnia (Fig. 20-6b); (2) acute, superimposed on chronic, respiratory acidosis (Fig. 20-6c); or (3) metabolic alkalosis and acute hypercapnia (Fig. 20-6d). *These possibilities cannot be distinguished without the respective histories*:

- A patient with chronic bronchitis develops persistent diarrhea.
- A patient with chronic hypercapnia complains of fever and increased sputum production. The chest x-ray is consistent with pneumonia.

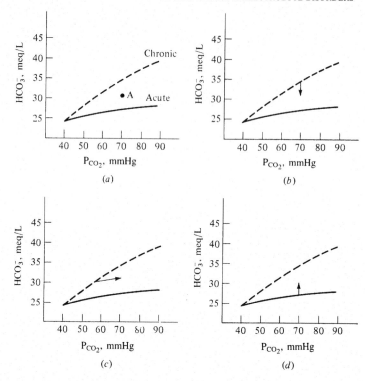

Figure 20-6 Confidence bands for acute and chronic hypercapnia have been transposed from Figs. 20-3 and 20-4. (*a*) Point A lies between the curves and can represent three different disorders. (*b*) Metabolic acidosis complicating chronic respiratory acidosis. (*c*) Acute, superimposed on chronic, hypercapnia. (*d*) Acute respiratory acidosis and metabolic alkalosis. (*Adapted from Cohen JJ, Schwartz WB, Am J Med 41:163, 1966, with permission.*)

- A patient with a history of extrinsic asthma has 5 days of vomiting as a result of theophylline toxicity and then develops an acute asthmatic attack after the theophylline is discontinued.

A different problem in interpretation is present in the following example. The initial laboratory data were as follows:

$$\text{Arterial pH} = 7.53$$

$$P_{CO_2} = 50 \text{ mmHg}$$

$$[HCO_3^-] = 40 \text{ meq/L}$$

$$P_{O_2} = 45 \text{ mmHg}$$

Oxygen was started and repeat tests were obtained:

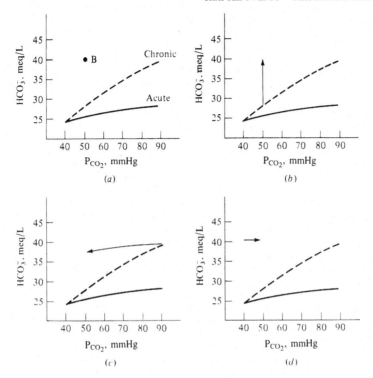

Figure 20-7 Confidence bands for acute and chronic respiratory acidosis. (*a*) Point B lies outside the confidence bands and can be due to one of three disorders. (*b*) Metabolic alkalosis complicating chronic (or acute) hypercapnia. (*c*) An acute reduction in the P_{CO_2} in a patient with chronic respiratory acidosis. (*d*) Primary metabolic alkalosis with compensatory CO_2 retention.

$$\text{Arterial pH} = 7.47$$

$$P_{CO_2} = 57 \text{ mmHg}$$

$$[HCO_3^-] = 40 \text{ meq/L}$$

$$P_{O_2} = 80 \text{ mmHg}$$

Because of the increase in P_{CO_2} oxygen was discontinued for fear of further hypercapnia and CO_2 narcosis. After appropriate therapy with NaCl, the following values were noted:

$$\text{Arterial pH} = 7.41$$

$$P_{CO_2} = 39 \text{ mmHg}$$

$$[HCO_3^-] = 24 \text{ meq/L}$$

$$P_{O_2} = 68 \text{ mmHg}$$

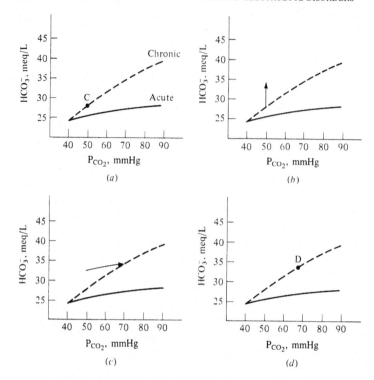

Figure 20-8   A patient with stable chronic hypercapnia (*a*, point C) develops metabolic alkalosis due to vomiting (*b*). During one episode, he aspirates some vomitus and has an acute increase in P_{CO_2} (*c*). At this point, his blood values lie within the confidence band and are indistinguishable from those seen in uncomplicated chronic respiratory acidosis (*d*, point D).

Despite the high P_{CO_2} on admission, the pH was alkaline. Most commonly, this degree of hypercapnia in an alkalemic patient is due to metabolic alkalosis complicating chronic hypercapnia (Fig. 20-7*b*). However, this can also represent acute hypocapnia superimposed on chronic respiratory acidosis (Fig. 20-7*c*) or hypercapnia as part of the normal respiratory compensation to metabolic alkalosis (Fig. 20-7*d*). This specific diagnosis cannot be made directly from the laboratory data, and the respective clinical histories are required:

- A patient with chronic obstructive pulmonary disease develops pedal edema due to cor pulmonale and is started on diuretics.
- Tracheal intubation and mechanical ventilation are begun in a patient with severe CO_2 retention. This entity is referred to as *posthypercapnic alkalosis.*
- A patient has 5 days of persistent vomiting.

The correction of the alkalemia and hypercapnia with NaCl indicates that this patient's primary problem was metabolic alkalosis due to vomiting. Although a high P_{CO_2} that increases after the administration of oxygen is most often seen with chronic respiratory acidosis, it may also occur with metabolic alkalosis, since the development of severe hypoxemia can limit the degree of compensatory hypoventilation. This is most likely to occur in patients with underlying lung disease; the postcorrection P_{O_2} of only 68 mmHg in this patient is compatible with this possibility.

It should also be noted that the further increment in P_{CO_2} after oxygen therapy is *beneficial* in this setting, as the arterial pH decreased toward normal (from 7.53 to 7.47). There was no danger of CO_2 narcosis, and oxygen could safely have been continued.

Finally, one *cannot assume that values within the confidence bands connote an uncomplicated disorder.* Suppose a patient with stable chronic hypercapnia (Fig. 20-8a, point C) develops recurrent vomiting (Fig. 20-8b) and then aspiration pneumonia (Fig. 20-8c). Although this represents a triad of chronic respiratory acidosis, metabolic alkalosis, and acute respiratory acidosis, the final blood values lie within the confidence band and cannot be distinguished from pure, severe chronic hypercapnia (Fig. 20-8d).

In summary, the confidence bands are useful guides in the interpretation of acid-base measurements. However, this interpretation cannot proceed in a vacuum and must be correlated with a complete history and physical examination.

Use of the Alveolar-Arterial Oxygen Gradient

Calculation of the alveolar-arterial (A-a) oxygen gradient may be helpful in differentiating intrinsic pulmonary disease from extrapulmonary disorders as the cause of hypercapnia. The derivation of a formula that can be used to estimate this gradient requires a brief review of the physiology of alveolar gas exchange.[60] At a barometric pressure of 1 atm (P_B equals 760 mmHg) in the inspired air at sea level, water vapor accounts for approximately 47 mmHg, nitrogen for 563 mmHg, and oxygen for the remaining 150 mmHg (Fig. 20-9). Since the pressure in the alveolus remains at 1 atm and there is no net movement of nitrogen or water vapor across the alveolar capillary, the P_{N_2} and P_{H_2O} in the alveolus are the same as those in the inspired air and equal 610 mmHg. Thus, the *sum of the partial pressures of the other gases in the alveolus must be equal to 150 mmHg*, i.e., to the partial pressure of oxygen in the inspired air ($P_{I_{O_2}}$) (Fig. 20-9).

In the alveolus, inspired O_2 enters the blood, and CO_2 leaves the blood and enters the alveolus. If the amount of CO_2 added were equal to the amount of O_2 taken up, then the alveolar P_{O_2} ($P_{A_{O_2}}$) would be less than the inspired P_{O_2} ($P_{I_{O_2}}$) by an amount equal to the alveolar P_{CO_2} ($P_{A_{CO_2}}$):

$$P_{A_{O_2}} = P_{I_{O_2}} - P_{A_{CO_2}} \tag{20-6}$$

However, more O_2 is usually taken up than CO_2 produced, since, on a normal diet, each molecule of CO_2 generated represents the utilization of 1.25 molecules of O_2, i.e., the respiratory quotient is 0.8. To account for this, Eq. (20-6) can be rewritten:

Trachea Alveoli

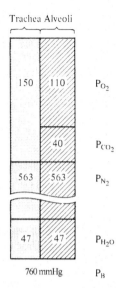

P_{O_2}

P_{CO_2}

P_{N_2}

P_{H_2O}

760 mmHg P_B

Figure 20-9 Composition of gas in the trachea at end inspiration (the same as that in the inspired air) and composition of alveolar gas. The total pressure and the partial pressures of nitrogen and water vapor are the same in both compartments; alveolar P_{O_2} goes down in proportion to the increase in alveolar P_{CO_2}. It should be noted that these values are for a patient breathing room air. If a patient is given supplemental oxygen, the alveolar P_{O_2} will be proportionately increased. (*Adapted from Snider GL, Chest 63:801, 1973, with permission.*)

$$P_{AO_2} = P_{IO_2} - 1.25P_{ACO_2} \qquad (20\text{-}7)$$

Since CO_2 diffuses across the alveolar capillary rapidly (20 times as fast as O_2), the P_{ACO_2} is essentially equal to the arterial P_{CO_2} (Pa_{CO_2}). Therefore,

$$P_{AO_2} = P_{IO_2} - 1.25Pa_{CO_2} \qquad (20\text{-}8)$$

In a subject inspiring room air (P_{IO_2} equals 150 mmHg) with a Pa_{CO_2} of 40 mmHg,

$$P_{AO_2} = 150 - (1.25 \times 40)$$
$$= 100 \text{ mmHg}$$

Not all of this oxygen enters the blood, however, since there is an alveolar-arterial (A-a) oxygen gradient averaging, on room air, 5 to 10 mmHg in subjects under the age of 30 and gradually increasing to 15 to 20 mmHg in the elderly. This gradient probably is due both to pulmonary arteriovenous shunts and to perfusion of underventilated areas of the lung. Since

$$\text{(A-a) } O_2 \text{ gradient} = P_{AO_2} - Pa_{O_2} \qquad (20\text{-}9)$$

by substituting Eq. (20-8) for P_{AO_2}, we have

$$\text{(A-a) } O_2 \text{ gradient} = P_{IO_2} - 1.25Pa_{CO_2} - Pa_{O_2} \qquad (20\text{-}10)$$

The (A-a) oxygen gradient is always increased in hypercapnic patients with intrinsic pulmonary disease and may be increased in some patients with extrapulmonary disorders.[60] However, a normal gradient essentially excludes pulmonary disease and suggests some form of central alveolar hypoventilation (including primary metabolic alkalosis) or an abnormality of the chest wall or inspiratory muscles.

TREATMENT

A complete discussion of the treatment of all of the causes of acute and chronic respiratory acidosis is beyond the scope of this chapter. Nevertheless, it is useful to review some of the general principles that are involved, particularly those related to acid-base balance.

Acute Respiratory Acidosis

Patients with acute respiratory acidosis are at risk from both hypercapnia and hypoxemia. Although the P_{O_2} can usually be raised by the administration of supplemental oxygen, reversal of the hypercapnia requires an increase in effective alveolar ventilation. This can be achieved by control of the underlying disease (as with bronchodilators and corticosteroids in asthma) or by mechanical ventilation, delivered via either a tight-fitting mask or an endotracheal tube. Indications for mechanical ventilation include refractory severe hypoxemia, symptomatic or progressive hypercapnia, and depression of the respiratory center due, for example, to a drug overdose.

Sodium bicarbonate The role of $NaHCO_3$ in the treatment of acute respiratory acidosis (without concomitant metabolic acidosis) is not well defined. Although the primary aim of therapy is to restore normal ventilation, small doses of $NaHCO_3$ (44 to 88 meq) can be infused over 5 to 10 min if the P_{CO_2} cannot be promptly controlled in a severely acidemic patient (pH less than 7.15). This regimen may be particularly beneficial in patients with severe status asthmaticus requiring mechanical ventilation.[61] In this setting, elevating the plasma HCO_3^- concentration allows the pH to be controlled at a high P_{CO_2} and, therefore, at a lower minute ventilation with lower transpulmonary pressures. The latter change may minimize the incidence of potentially serious complications such as pneumothorax or pneumomediastinum.[61]

There are, however, several potential hazards with the use of $NaHCO_3$ in acute respiratory acidosis:

- The administration of $NaHCO_3$ should be avoided, if possible, in patients with pulmonary edema, because it can increase the degree of pulmonary congestion. In general, most of these patients can be managed without $NaHCO_3$, since correction of the pulmonary edema and hypoxemia is usually sufficient to restore acid-base balance.[25,62]
- Bicarbonate therapy does not protect against the central nervous system effects of hypercapnia, since bicarbonate does not readily cross the blood-brain barrier.
- The infusion of $NaHCO_3$ can result in an increase in CO_2 generation and therefore in the P_{CO_2} by the following reaction:

$$HCO_3^- + H^+ \rightarrow H_2CO_3 \rightarrow CO_2 + H_2O$$

Normally, the CO_2 that is generated is rapidly eliminated by the lungs. However, in patients with inadequate pulmonary blood flow (especially during a cardiac arrest), the CO_2 may be retained, and the resultant elevation in the P_{CO_2} can exacerbate the tissue acidemia.[38-40,42] Thus, careful monitoring is required; furthermore, during cardiopulmonary resuscitation, measurement of the mixed venous pH may be the best indicator of the acid-base status at the tissue level (see page 452).[42]

- Metabolic alkalosis (due to the excess HCO_3^-) may ensue after the P_{CO_2} has returned to normal. This is usually not a major problem.

Tromethamine   The limitations and potential deleterious effects of bicarbonate therapy have promoted investigation into the use of alternative buffering agents, such as tromethamine (THAM; trometamol). THAM is an inert amino alcohol that buffers acids and CO_2 by virtue of its amine moiety via the following reactions:[63]

$$THAM-NH_2 + H^+ \rightarrow THAM-NH_3^+$$

$$THAM-NH_2 + H_2O + CO_2 \rightarrow THAM-NH_3^+ + HCO_3^-$$

Protonated THAM is excreted in the urine at a rate slightly higher than creatinine clearance in conjunction with either chloride or bicarbonate. Thus, THAM supplements the buffering capacity of blood without generating carbon dioxide but is less effective in patients with renal failure. Reported toxicities include hyperkalemia, hypoglycemia, and respiratory depression; the last complication probably results from the ability of THAM to rapidly increase the pH and decrease the P_{CO_2} in the central nervous system.

Published clinical experience with THAM is limited, but the drug has been used to treat severe acidemia due to sepsis, hypercapnia, diabetic ketoacidosis, and other disorders.[63] Its clinical efficacy compared to that of sodium bicarbonate in the treatment of respiratory acidosis remains unproven, and THAM is of uncertain safety.

Chronic Respiratory Acidosis

The primary goals of therapy in patients with chronic respiratory acidosis are to maintain adequate oxygenation and, if possible, to improve effective alveolar ventilation. Because of the effectiveness of the renal compensation, it is usually not necessary to treat the pH, even in patients with severe hypercapnia.[45] In addition, the frequent concurrent use of diuretics in patients with cor pulmonale can further raise the pH, occasionally to normal or even alkalemic levels.

The appropriate treatment varies with the underlying disease.[26] As a general rule, excessive oxygen and sedatives should be avoided, since they can act as respiratory depressants, producing further hypoventilation. For patients with chronic obstructive lung disease, bronchodilators and, when infection is present, antimicrobials may ameliorate the airflow characteristics of the disease.[6,64]

Dietary modification to reduce the respiratory quotient also may be helpful in selected patients by reducing CO_2 production.[65] In obese patients, weight reduction can improve alveolar ventilation, leading to an elevation in the arterial P_{O_2} and reduction in the P_{CO_2} (of as much as 10 mmHg each).[48,66] Although the loss of weight may directly improve ventilatory mechanics, carbohydrate restriction itself (to about 200 g/day) can produce a similar improvement in the absence of any change in weight.[67] The beneficial effect seen in this setting appears to involve increased central stimulation of ventilation; how this occurs, however, is not clear. (The appropriate management of the obesity hypoventilation syndrome is beyond the scope of this discussion.[34])

If severe hypoxemia persists (arterial P_{O_2} below 50 to 55 mmHg), continuous low-flow oxygen therapy is indicated to prolong survival, diminish the severity of cor pulmonale, and improve the quality of life.[17-19,26,68] The pulmonary benefits derived from correction of hypoxemia may result from improved perfusion due to reversal of pulmonary vasoconstriction and of secondary polycythemia, which increases blood viscosity. The aim of therapy is to raise the P_{O_2} to 60 to 65 mmHg (hemoglobin saturation above 90 percent), while carefully monitoring the P_{CO_2} to ascertain that ventilation has not been suppressed to a clinically important degree by partial correction of the hypoxemia.

Mechanical ventilation may be required when there is an acute exacerbation of chronic hypercapnia (as with the development of pneumonia). In this setting, care must be taken to *lower the P_{CO_2} gradually*. Rapid correction of hypercapnia to near normal levels can lead to an overshoot alkalemia and a marked rise in the pH in the central nervous system (CNS), since CO_2 can easily diffuse out of the brain. The acute increase in CNS pH can, in selected cases, lead to severe neurologic abnormalities, such as seizures and coma.[69,70] These findings typically improve if the P_{CO_2} is allowed to rise toward its previous level.

Effect of superimposed metabolic alkalosis   As described above, the influence of pH on ventilation is maintained in chronic respiratory acidosis.[12-15] Thus, the induction of metabolic alkalosis (usually due to diuretic therapy for cor pulmonale) will further depress ventilation, aggravating both the hypoxemia and the hypercapnia.[15,71] In this setting, lowering the plasma HCO_3^- concentration can reverse these abnormalities and may improve the patient's sense of well-being.[15]

Correction of a superimposed metabolic alkalosis can be achieved by discontinuing diuretic therapy and administering NaCl. This is not practical, however, in the patient who is still significantly edematous. In this circumstance, acetazolamide (250 to 375 mg once or twice a day) can both lower the plasma HCO_3^- concentration and increase the urine output by inhibiting proximal $NaHCO_3$ reabsorption (see Chap. 15). Monitoring the urine pH is a simple method of assessing the efficacy of this regimen, since a HCO_3^- diuresis leads to an elevation in the urine pH to above 7.0.

Despite its effectiveness in many patients, there are two potential problems with the use of acetazolamide. First, the plasma HCO_3^- concentration should be lowered to the level *appropriate for the degree of hypercapnia* (see Fig. 20-4). Returning the plasma HCO_3^- concentration to the normal value of 24 meq/L can lead to severe acidemia due to persistent marked hypercapnia.[14] Second, acetazolamide can produce a *transient elevation* in the P_{CO_2} (usually 3 to 7 mmHg) prior to its diuretic effect.[72] This complication, which is generally not clinically important, may be due to partial inhibition of carbonic anhydrase in the red blood cell.[14,72] This enzyme catalyzes the hydration of CO_2 to H_2CO_3, a reaction that is essential for CO_2 transport by the red cell [see Eqs. (20-1) and (20-2)] and, therefore, for the elimination of CO_2 by the lungs.

PROBLEMS

20-1 Match the clinical histories with the appropriate arterial blood values:

	pH	P_{CO_2}, mmHg	$[HCO_3^-]$, meq/L
(a)	7.37	65	37
(b)	7.22	60	26
(c)	7.35	60	32

1. A 60-year-old man with chronic bronchitis develops persistent diarrhea.
2. A 24-year-old man is markedly obese.
3. A 14-year-old girl has a severe acute asthmatic attack.
4. A 56-year-old woman with chronic bronchitis is started on diuretic therapy for peripheral edema, resulting in a 3-kg weight loss.

20-2 A 54-year-old man with a history of chronic obstructive lung disease has a 2-day episode of increasing shortness of breath and sputum production. The chest radiograph reveals a left lower-lobe pneumonia. The following laboratory data are obtained with the patient breathing room air:

$$\text{Artertial pH} = 7.25$$

$$P_{CO_2} = 70 \text{ mmHg}$$

$$[HCO_3^-] = 30 \text{ meq/L}$$

$$P_{O_2} = 30 \text{ mmHg}$$

$$\text{Urine } [Na^+] = 4 \text{ meq/L}$$

The patient is started on intravenous aminophylline and nasal oxygen and becomes less responsive. Repeat blood tests are obtained and show the following:

$$\text{Arterial pH} = 7.18$$

$$P_{CO_2} = 86 \text{ mmHg}$$

$$[HCO_3^-] = 31 \text{ meq/L}$$

$$P_{O_2} = 62 \text{ mmHg}$$

(a) What is the probable acid-base disturbance on admission?
(b) What is responsible for the increase in the P_{CO_2} in the hospital?
(c) What further therapy would you recommend?

(d) If the P_{CO_2} is rapidly lowered to 40 mmHg, what will happen to the arterial pH?

(e) If the patient is then maintained on a low-sodium diet, how long will it take for the plasma HCO_3^- concentration to return to normal?

20-3 A 65-year-old man has a history of smoking and hypertension, which is treated with a diuretic. The following arterial blood values are obtained on room air:

$$\text{Arterial pH} = 7.48$$

$$P_{CO_2} = 51 \text{ mmHg}$$

$$[HCO_3^-] = 36 \text{ meq/L}$$

$$P_{O_2} = 73 \text{ mmHg}$$

(a) What is the most likely acid-base disturbance?

(b) Does the patient have significant underlying lung disease?

REFERENCES

1. Berger AJ, Michell RA, Severinghaus JW. Regulation of respiration. *N Engl J Med* 297:92,138, 194, 1977.
2. Berger AJ. Control of breathing, in Murray J, Nadel J (eds): *Textbook of Respiratory Medicine*, 2nd ed. Philadelphia, Saunders, 1994, p. 199.
3. Fencl V, Miller TB, Papenheimer JR. Studies on the respiratory response to disturbances of acid-base balance, with deductions concerning the ionic composition of cerebral interstitial fluid. *Am J Physiol* 210:459, 1966.
4. Lugliani R, Whipp BJ, Seard C, Wasserman K. Effect of bilateral carotid-body resection on ventilatory control at rest and during exercise in man. *N Engl J Med* 285:1105, 1971.
5. Weinberger SE, Schwartzenstein RM, Weiss JW. Hypercapnia. *N Engl J Med* 321:1223, 1989.
6. American Thoracic Society. Standards for the diagnosis and care of patients with chronic obstructive pulmonary disease. *Am J Respir Crit Care Med* 152(5 Pt 2):S77, 1995.
7. Polak A, Haynie GD, Hays RM, Schwartz WB. Effects of chronic hypercapnia on electrolyte and acid-base equilibrium: I. Adaptation. *J Clin Invest* 40:1223, 1961.
8. Franklin W. Treatment of severe asthma. *N Engl J Med* 290:1469, 1974.
9. Kornbluth RS, Turino GM. Respiratory control in diffuse interstitial lung disease and diseases of the pulmonary vasculature. *Clin Chest Med* 1:91, 1980.
10. Hirshman CA, McCullough RE, Weil JV. Normal values for hypoxic and hypercapnic ventilatory drives in man. *J Appl Physiol* 38:1095, 1975.
11. Aubier M, Murciano D, Milic-Emili J, et al. Effects of the administration of O_2 on ventilation and blood gases in patients with chronic obstructive pulmonary disease during acute respiratory failure. *Am Rev Respir Dis* 122:747, 1980.
12. Heinemann HO, Goldring RM. Bicarbonate and the regulation of ventilation. *Am J Med* 57:361, 1974.
13. Goldring RM, Turino GM, Heinemann HO. Respiratory-renal adjustments in chronic hypercapnia in man: Extracellular bicarbonate concentration and the regulation of ventilation. *Am J Med* 51:772, 1971.
14. Dorris R, Olivia JV, Rodman T. Dichlorphenamide, a potent carbonic anhydrase inhibitor: Effect on alveolar ventilation, ventilation-perfusion relationships and diffusion in patients with chronic lung disease. *Am J Med* 36:79, 1964.
15. Bear R, Goldstein M, Philipson M, et al. Effect of metabolic alkalosis on respiratory function in patients with chronic obstructive lung disease. *Can Med Assoc J* 117:900, 1977.
16. Eldridge F, Gherman G. Studies of oxygen administration in respiratory failure. *Ann Intern Med* 68:569, 1968.

17. Anthonisen NR. Long-term oxygen therapy. *Ann Intern Med* 99:519, 1983.
18. Nocturnal Oxygen Trial Therapy Group. Continuous or nocturnal oxygen therapy in hypoxemic chronic obstructive lung disease: A clinical trial. *Ann Intern Med* 93:391, 1980.
19. Report of the Medical Research Council Working Party. Long term domiciliary oxygen therapy in chronic hypoxic cor pulmonale complicating chronic bronchitis and emphysema. *Lancet* 1:681, 1981.
20. Aubier M, Murciano D, Fournier M, et al. Central respiratory drive in acute respiratory failure of patients with chronic obstructive pulmonary disease. *Am Rev Respir Dis* 122:191, 1980.
21. Feller-Kopman DJ, Schwartzstein RM. The use of oxygen in patients with hypercapnia, in Rose BD (ed): *UpToDate in Medicine*. Wellesley, MA, UpToDate, 2000.
22. Giebisch GE, Berger L, Pitts RF. The extrarenal response to acute acid-base disturbances of respiratory origin. *J Clin Invest* 34:231, 1955.
23. Arbus GS, Herbert LA, Levesque PR, et al. Characterization and clinical application of the "significance band" for acute respiratory alkalosis. *N Engl J Med* 280:117, 1969.
24. Brackett NC Jr, Cohen JJ, Schwartz WB. Carbon dioxide titration curve of normal man: Effect of increasing degrees of acute hypercapnia on acid-base equilibrium. *N Engl J Med* 272:6, 1965.
25. Aberman A, Fulop M. The metabolic and respiratory acidosis of acute pulmonary edema. *Ann Intern Med* 76:173, 1972.
26. Palevsky HI, Fishman AP. Chronic cor pulmonale: Etiology and management. *JAMA* 263:2347, 1990.
27. Badr MS. Pathogenesis of obstructive sleep apnea. *Prog Cardiovasc Dis* 41:323,
28. Guilleminault C, Cummiskey J, Dement WC. Sleep apnea syndrome: Recent advances. *Adv Intern Med* 26:347, 1980.
29. Kales A, Vela-Bueno A, Kales JD. Sleep disorders: Sleep apnea and narcolepsy. *Ann Intern Med* 106:434, 1987.
30. White DP, Zwillich CW, Pickett CK, et al. Central sleep apnea: Improvement with acetazolamide therapy. *Arch Intern Med* 142:1816, 1982.
31. Stradling JR. Obstructive sleep apnoea syndrome. *Br Med J* 2:528, 1982.
32. Guilleminault C, Connolly SJ, Winkle RA. Cardiac arrhythmia and conduction disturbances during sleep in 400 patients with sleep apnea syndrome. *Am J Cardiol* 52:490, 1983.
33. Millman RP, Kramer NR. Polysomnography in the diagnostic evaluation of sleep apnea, in Rose BD (ed): *UpToDate in Medicine*, Wellesley, MA, UpToDate, 2000.
34. Martin TJ. Treatment of the obesity hypoventilation syndrome, in Rose BD (ed): *UpToDate in Medicine*. Wellesley, MA, UpToDate, 2000
35. Rapoport DM, Sorkin B, Garay SM, Goldring RM. Reversal of the "Pickwickian syndrome" by long-term use of nocturnal nasal-airway pressure. *N Engl J Med* 307:931, 1982.
36. Fishman A, Turino GM, Bergofsky EH. The syndrome of alveolar hypoventilation. *Am J Med* 23:333, 1957.
37. Suratt PM, Findley LJ. Clinical manifestations and diagnosis of obesity hyperventilation syndrome, in Rose BD (ed): *UpToDate in Medicine*. Wellesley, MA, UpToDate, 2000.
38. Bishop RL, Weisfeldt ML. Sodium bicarbonate administration during cardiac arrest: Effect on arterial pH, P_{CO_2} and osmolality. *JAMA* 235:506, 1976.
39. Ostrea EM, Odell GB. The influence of bicarbonate administration on blood pH in a "closed system": Clinical implications. *J Pediatr* 80:671, 1972.
40. Adrogué HJ, Rashad MN, Gorin AD, et al. Assessing acid-base status in circulatory failure: Differences between arterial and central venous blood. *N Engl J Med* 320:1312, 1989.
41. Covelli HD, Black JW, Olson MS, Beekman JF. Respiratory failure precipitated by high carbohydrate loads. *Ann Intern Med* 95:579, 1981.
42. Weil MH, Rackow EC, Trevino R, et al. Difference in acid-base state between venous and arterial blood during cardiopulmonary resuscitation. *N Engl J Med* 315:153, 1986.
43. Schwartz WB, Brackett NC, Cohen JJ. The response of extracellular hydrogen ion concentration to graded degrees of chronic hypercapnia: The physiologic limits of the defense of pH. *J Clin Invest* 44:291, 1965.

44. van Ypersele de Strihou C, Brasseur L, de Coninck J. "Carbon dioxide response curve" for chronic hypercapnia in man. *N Engl J Med* 275:117, 1966.
45. Neff TA, Petty TL. Tolerance and survival in severe chronic hypercapnia. *Arch Intern Med* 129:591, 1972.
46. van Ypersele de Strihou C, Gulyassy PF, Schwartz WB. Effects of chronic hypercapnia on electrolyte and acid-base equilibrium: II. Characteristics of the adaptive and recovery process as evaluated by provision of alkali. *J Clin Invest* 41:2246, 1962.
47. Mountain R, Zwillich C, Weil JV. Hypoventilation in obstructive lung disease: The role of familial factors. *N Engl J Med* 298:521, 1978.
48. Rochester DF, Enson Y. Current concepts in the pathogenesis of the obesity-hypoventilation syndrome. *Am J Med* 57:402, 1974.
49. Zwillich CW, Sutton FD, Pierson DJ, et al. Decreased hypoxic ventilatory drive in the obesity-hypoventilation syndrome. *Am J Med* 59:343, 1975.
50. Lyons HA, Huang CT. Therapeutic use of progesterone in alveolar hypoventilation associated with obesity. *Am J Med* 44:881, 1968.
51. Sutton FD, Zwillich CW, Creagh E, et al. Progesterone for outpatient treatment of Pickwickian syndrome. *Ann Intern Med* 83:476, 1975.
52. Kronenberg RS, Gabel RA, Severinghaus JW. Normal chemoreceptor function in obesity before and after ileal bypass surgery to force weight reduction. *Am J Med* 59:349, 1975.
53. Sampson MG, Grassino A. Neuromechanical properties in obese patients during CO_2 rebreathing. *Am J Med* 75:83, 1983.
54. Kronenberg RS, Drage CW, Stevenson JE. Acute respiratory failure and obesity with normal ventilatory response to carbon dioxide and absent hypoxic ventilatory drive. *Am J Med* 62:773, 1977.
55. Kilburn K. Neurologic manifestations of respiratory failure. *Arch Intern Med* 116:409, 1965.
56. Fencl V, Vale JR, Broch JA. Respiration and cerebral blood flow in metabolic acidosis and alkalosis in humans. *J Appl Physiol* 27:67, 1969.
57. Posner JB, Swanson AG, Plum F. Acid-base balance in cerebrospinal fluid. *Arch Neurol* 12:479, 1965.
58. Farber MO, Roberts LR, Weinberger MH, et al. Abnormalities of sodium and H_2O handling in chronic obstructive lung disease. *Arch Intern Med* 142:1326, 1982.
59. Reihman DH, Farber MO, Weinberger MH, et al. Effect of hypoxemia on sodium and water excretion in chronic obstructive lung disease. *Am J Med* 78:87, 1985.
60. Snider GL. Interpretation of the arterial oxygen and carbon dioxide partial pressure. *Chest* 63:801, 1973.
61. Menitove SM, Goldring RM. Combined ventilator and bicarbonate strategy in the management of status asthmaticus. *Am J Med* 74:898, 1983.
62. Fulop M, Horowitz M, Aberman A, Jaffee E. Lactic acidosis in pulmonary edema due to left ventricular failure. *Ann Intern Med* 79:180, 1973.
63. Nahas GG, Sutin KM, Fermon C, et al. Guidelines for the treatment of acidaemia with THAM. *Drugs* 55:191, 1998.
64. Ferguson GT, Make B. Overview of management of stable chronic obstructive pulmonary disease, in Rose BD (ed): *UpToDate in Medicine.* Wellesley, MA, UpToDate, 2000.
65. Donahoe M. Nutritional support in advanced lung disease. *Clin Chest Med* 18:547, 1997.
66. Tiralapur VG, Mir MA. Effect of a low calorie intake an abnormal pulmonary physiology in patients with chronic hypercapneic respiratory failure. *Am J Med* 77:987, 1984.
67. Kwan R, Mir MA. Beneficial effects of dietary carbohydrate restriction in chronic cor pulmonale. *Am J Med* 82:751, 1987.
68. Fulmer JD, Snider GL. American College of Chest Physicians (ACCP)—National Heart, Lung, and Blood Institute (NHLBI) Conference on oxygen therapy. *Arch Intern Med* 144:1645, 1984.
69. Rotheram EB Jr, Safar P, Robin ED. CNS disorder during mechanical ventilation in chronic pulmonary disease. *JAMA* 189:993, 1964.

70. Kilburn KH. Shock, seizures and coma with alkalosis during mechanical ventilation. *Ann Intern Med* 65:977, 1966.
71. Miller PD, Berns AS. Acute metabolic alkalosis perpetuating hypercapnia: A role for acetazo-lamide in chronic obstructive pulmonary disease. *JAMA* 238:2400, 1977.
72. Bell ALL, Smith CN, Andreae E. Effects of the carbonic anhydrase inhibitor "6063" (Diamox) on respiration and electrolyte metabolism of patients with respiratory acidosis. *Am J Med* 18:536, 1955.

RESPIRATORY ALKALOSIS

The introduction to acid-base disorders presented in Chap. 17 should be read before proceeding with this discussion. Respiratory alkalosis is a clinical disturbance characterized by an elevated arterial pH (or a decreased H^+ concentration), a low P_{CO_2} (hypocapnia), and a variable reduction in the plasma HCO_3^- concentration. It must be differentiated from metabolic acidosis, in which the plasma HCO_3^- concentration and P_{CO_2} also are diminished, but the pH is reduced rather than increased.

PATHOPHYSIOLOGY

A primary decrease in the P_{CO_2} occurs when effective alveolar ventilation is increased to a level beyond that needed to eliminate the daily load of metabolically produced CO_2. Before discussing the different disorders that can cause a respiratory alkalosis, it is helpful to first review how the body responds to hypocapnia. From the law of mass action,

$$[H^+] = 24 \times \frac{P_{CO_2}}{[HCO_3^-]}$$

it can be seen that the reduction in the extracellular H^+ concentration induced by hypocapnia can be minimized by lowering the HCO_3^- concentration. This protective response involves two steps: rapid cell buffering and a later decrease in net renal acid excretion. As a result of the time differential between the cellular and renal effects, the changes in acute and chronic respiratory alkalosis are different.

Acute Respiratory Alkalosis

Within 10 min after the onset of respiratory alkalosis, H^+ ions move from the cells into the extracellular fluid; they then combine with HCO_3^-, resulting in an appropriate fall in the plasma HCO_3^- concentration:

$$H^+ + HCO_3^- \rightarrow H_2CO_3 \rightarrow CO_2 + H_2O$$

These H^+ ions are primarily derived from the protein, phosphate, and hemoglobin buffers in the cells,

$$HBuf \rightarrow H^+ + Buf^-$$

and from an alkalemia-induced increase in cellular lactic acid production.[1]

In general, enough H^+ ions enter the extracellular fluid to lower the plasma HCO_3^- concentration 2 meq/L for each 10 mmHg decrease in the P_{CO_2} (see Fig. 20-3).[2] If, for example, the P_{CO_2} were reduced to 20 mmHg (20 mmHg less than normal), the plasma HCO_3^- concentration should fall by 4 meq/L to 20 meq/L (pH equals 7.63):

$$pH = 6.10 + \log \frac{20}{0.03(20)}$$

$$= 7.63$$

This cellular response is not very efficient, since the pH would have been only slightly greater, at 7.70, if there were no cell buffering and the plasma HCO_3^- concentration had remained at 24 meq/L.

Chronic Respiratory Alkalosis

In the presence of persistent hypocapnia, there is a compensatory decrease in renal H^+ secretion that begins within 2 h but is not complete for 2 to 3 days.[3-5] This response, which is presumably mediated at least in part by a parallel rise in renal tubular cell pH, is manifested by HCO_3^- loss in the urine and by decreased urinary ammonium excretion.[4,5] Both of these effects lower the plasma HCO_3^- concentration, the latter by preventing the excretion of the daily H^+ load, thereby resulting in H^+ retention.

On average, the combined effects of the cell buffers and the renal compensation result in a new steady state in which the plasma HCO_3^- concentration falls in humans approximately 4 meq/L for each 10 mmHg reduction in the P_{CO_2} (Fig. 21-1).[6] Thus, if the P_{CO_2} were chronically reduced to 20 mmHg, the plasma HCO_3^- concentration should fall by 8 meq/L, to 16 meq/L. This response effectively protects the extracellular pH, which is increased only to 7.53, as compared to 7.63 with a similar degree of acute hypocapnia.

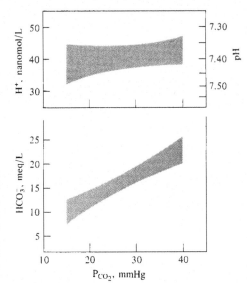

Figure 21-1 Significance bands of 95 percent probability for plasma pH and H^+ and HCO_3^- concentrations in chronic hypocapnia. Note that there is only a minimal change in the H^+ concentration and pH as the P_{CO_2} is reduced. (*From Gennari JF, Goldstein MB, Schwartz WB, J Clin Invest 51:1722, 1972, by copyright permission of the American Society for Clinical Investigations.*)

ETIOLOGY

Respiration is physiologically governed by two sets of chemoreceptors: those in the respiratory center in the brainstem and those in the carotid and aortic bodies, located at the bifurcation of the carotid arteries and in the aortic arch, respectively.[7,8]

- The central chemoreceptors are stimulated by an increase in the P_{CO_2} or by metabolic acidosis, both of which appear to be sensed as a fall in the pH of the surrounding cerebral interstitial fluid.[9]
- The peripheral chemoreceptors are primarily stimulated by hypoxemia, although they also contribute to the acidemic response.[7,8,10]

Thus, *primary* hyperventilation resulting in respiratory alkalosis can be produced by hypoxemia or anemia, a reduction in the cerebral pH (an apparently rare event, since the cerebrospinal fluid pH is usually elevated in respiratory alkalosis) or other stimuli for hyperventilation, such as pain, anxiety, stimulation of mechanoreceptors within the respiratory system, or direct stimulation of the central respiratory center (Table 21-1).[11-13]

Hypoxemia

The respiratory response to hypoxemia (which includes reduced oxygen delivery due to severe hypotension or anemia) occurs in two stages, which illustrate the interaction between the peripheral and central chemoreceptors (Fig. 21-2).[8,14,15]

Table 21-1 Causes of respiratory alkalosis

Hypoxemia
  A. Pulmonary disease: pneumonia, interstitial fibrosis, emboli, edema
  B. Congestive heart failure
  C. Hypotension or severe anemia
  D. High-altitude residence

Pulmonary disease

Direct stimulation of the medullary respiratory center
  A. Psychogenic or voluntary hyperventilation
  B. Hepatic failure
  C. Gram-negative septicemia
  D. Salicylate intoxication
  E. Postcorrection of metabolic acidosis
  F. Pregnancy and the luteal phase of the menstrual cycle (due to progesterone)
  G. Neurologic disorders: cerebrovascular accidents, pontine tumors

Mechanical ventilation

Hypoxemia initially activates the peripheral chemoreceptors, resulting in hyperventilation, hypocapnia, and mild increases in the arterial and cerebral pH. However, the cerebral alkalosis inhibits the central respiratory center, thereby limiting the degree of hyperventilation. Thus, hypoxemia does not significantly stimulate respiration acutely unless the arterial P_{O_2} falls below 50 to 60 mmHg or hypocapnia does not occur because of underlying lung disease (Fig. 21-2). In the

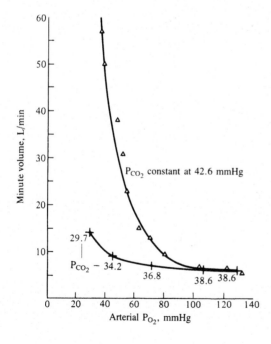

Figure 21-2 Influence of arterial P_{CO_2} on the ventilatory response to hypoxemia. In normal subjects (lower curve), lowering the partial pressure of oxygen in the inspired air increases ventilation and lowers the arterial P_{CO_2}. However, these changes are relatively minor until the arterial P_{O_2} falls below 50 mmHg. The earlier and greater degree of hyperventilation seen when the arterial P_{CO_2} is held constant (upper curve) indicates that the development of mild hypocapnic alkalosis normally limits the ventilatory response to hypoxemia. (*Adapted from Loeschcke HH, Gertz KH, Arch Ges Physiol 267:460, 1958, with permission.*)

latter setting, ventilation begins to rise rapidly when the P_{O_2} is less than 70 to 80 mmHg.

Persistent hypoxemia, on the other hand, can lead to a greater degree of hyperventilation. The initial fall in P_{CO_2} induces a compensatory reduction in the plasma HCO_3^- concentration that lowers the extracellular pH toward normal (Fig. 21-1). This response partially removes the alkalemic inhibition of ventilation, thereby allowing a greater respiratory response to hypoxemia.

Pulmonary Disease

Respiratory alkalosis is a common finding in a variety of pulmonary diseases, including pneumonia, pulmonary embolism, and interstitial fibrosis.[16-18] It may also occur in pulmonary edema, but metabolic and respiratory acidosis are much more common in this disorder.[19]

Although hyperventilation in pulmonary disease may be due in part to hypoxemia, it is frequently not corrected by the administration of oxygen.[16,17] This observation indicates that other factors contribute to the increase in ventilation. The most important appear to be mechanoreceptors located throughout the airways, lungs, and chest wall, which stimulate the respiratory center via afferent signals sent through the vagus nerves.[16,17,20]

Several different receptors may participate in this response, including *juxtacapillary* receptors in the interstitium of the alveolar wall—which can be activated by interstitial edema, fibrosis, or pulmonary vascular congestion—and *irritant* receptors in the epithelial lining of the airways, which can be activated by the inhalation of irritants and perhaps by local inflammatory processes such as pneumonia and asthma.[16,20] Although direct confirmation of the importance of these receptors in humans is limited, vagal blockade can reverse the hyperventilation associated with pulmonary disease in experimental animals.[16,20,21]

These receptors play little role in the control of ventilation in normal subjects, and their effect in pulmonary disease can be somewhat maladaptive. For example, dyspnea and breathlessness are common complaints in diffuse pulmonary interstitial fibrosis, even in patients without severe hypoxemia. These symptoms are probably due at least in part to increased ventilatory drive.[13,16]

Direct Stimulation of the Medullary Respiratory Center

Primary hyperventilation due to stimulation of the respiratory center may be found in a variety of disorders (Table 21-1). The possible mechanisms by which this occurs are variable and include the primary effect of cortical centers in psychogenic hyperventilation,[22] retained amines in hepatic failure,[23,24] bacterial toxins in gram-negative septicemia,[25] salicylates in salicylate intoxication,[26,27] progesterone in pregnancy and, to a lesser degree, the luteal phase of the menstrual cycle,[28,29] and a persistently acid cerebrospinal fluid (CSF) pH following the rapid correction of metabolic acidosis.[30,31]

In the last situation, the administration of $NaHCO_3$ raises the extracellular HCO_3^- concentration and pH. As the increase in pH is sensed by the peripheral chemoreceptors, there is a decrease in the degree of compensatory hyperventilation and a moderate elevation in the P_{CO_2}. Since CO_2 but not HCO_3^- rapidly crosses the blood-brain barrier, the brain initially senses only the higher P_{CO_2}. This produces a paradoxical fall in the CSF pH,[31] which tends to prolong the hyperventilatory state.[30]

Respiratory alkalosis is also an occasional finding in neurologic disorders. With pontine tumors, a reduction in the cerebral pH due to local lactic acid production may be responsible for increased ventilation.[32] Hypocapnia also may be seen with acute cerebrovascular accidents.

Mechanical Ventilation

The use of mechanical ventilation not uncommonly leads to respiratory alkalosis. The imposition of forced hyperventilation often results from an attempt to correct hypoxemia. If necessary, the respiratory alkalosis can be reversed by increasing the dead space or reducing either the tidal volume or the respiratory rate.

SYMPTOMS

The symptoms produced by respiratory alkalosis are related to increased irritability of the central and peripheral nervous systems and include light-headedness, altered consciousness, paresthesias of the extremities and circumoral area, cramps, carpopedal spasm that is indistinguishable from that seen with hypocalcemia, and syncope.[22,33] A variety of supraventricular and ventricular arrhythmias also may occur, particularly in critically ill patients.[34]

These abnormalities are thought to be related to the ability of alkalosis to impair cerebral function and to increase membrane excitability. Respiratory alkalosis also reduces cerebral blood flow (by as much as 35 to 40 percent if the P_{CO_2} falls by 20 mmHg),[35] which may contribute to the neurologic symptoms. In addition, some complaints may be unrelated to the change in pH. Patients with psychogenic hyperventilation, for example, frequently complain of headache, shortness of breath, chest pain or tightness, and other somatic symptoms that may be emotional in origin and not caused by the alkalemia.

The above problems primarily occur in *acute* respiratory alkalosis when the P_{CO_2} falls below 25 to 30 mmHg, a setting in which there is a substantial rise in cerebral pH. They are much less likely to be seen in chronic respiratory alkalosis (since the pH is so well protected) or in metabolic alkalosis, where there is a lesser elevation in CSF pH because of the relative inability of HCO_3^- to cross the blood-brain barrier.[11,36]

An additional finding in many patients with severe respiratory alkalosis is a reduction in the plasma phosphate concentration (measured in the laboratory as the plasma concentration of inorganic phosphorus) to as low as 0.5 to 1.5 mg/dL (normal equals 2.5 to 4.5 mg/dL).[37] This finding reflects a rapid shift of phosphate from the extracellular fluid into the cells. It may be mediated by the stimulation of glycolysis by intracellular alkalosis, resulting in increased formation of phosphorylated compounds such as glucose 6-phosphate and fructose 1,6-diphosphate.

DIAGNOSIS

The physical finding of tachypnea may be an important clue to the presence of hypocapnia, due either to primary respiratory alkalosis or to the respiratory compensation to metabolic acidosis. Once the presence of respiratory alkalosis has been confirmed by measurement of the extracellular pH, P_{CO_2}, and HCO_3^- concentration, the cause of this condition should be identified (Table 21-1). For example, respiratory alkalosis is a relatively early finding in septicemia,[25] and this diagnosis should be considered in the appropriate clinical setting when there is no other apparent cause for the hyperventilation.

Since the responses to acute and chronic hypocapnia are different, the determination of the correct acid-base disorder is more difficult than in metabolic acidosis or alkalosis. Suppose, for example, that a patient has the following arterial blood values:

$$Arterial\ pH = 7.48$$

$$P_{CO_2} = 20\ mmHg$$

$$[HCO_3^-] = 16\ meq/L$$

The alkaline pH and hypocapnia are diagnostic of respiratory alkalosis. With a P_{CO_2} of 20 mmHg, the plasma HCO_3^- concentration should be roughly 20 meq/L in acute respiratory alkalosis (a reduction of 2 meq/L per 10 mmHg fall in the P_{CO_2}) and 16 meq/L in chronic respiratory alkalosis (a reduction of 4 meq/L per 10 mmHg fall in the P_{CO_2}).

Thus, 16 to 20 meq/L describes the approximate normal range for the plasma HCO_3^- concentration in a patient with respiratory alkalosis and P_{CO_2} of 20 mmHg. Values significantly above or below this range represent superimposed metabolic alkalosis or acidosis. In this patient, the plasma HCO_3^- concentration of 16 meq/L is consistent with uncomplicated chronic respiratory alkalosis. However, it is also compatible with acute respiratory alkalosis combined with metabolic acidosis to produce the greater than expected reduction in the plasma HCO_3^- concentration. Thus, evaluation of the laboratory data must proceed in conjunction with the history and physical examination, as illustrated by the following example:

Case History 21-1   A 5-year-old child is brought into the emergency room in a stuporous condition. The only pertinent history is that he had been playing with a bottle of aspirin tablets earlier that day.

Comment   The most likely explanation for the above laboratory findings is a salicylate overdose. The acute respiratory alkalosis in this disorder is often complicated by a salicylate-induced metabolic acidosis, leading to a reduction in the plasma HCO_3^- concentration (from the expected value of 20 meq/L down to 16 meq/L).[27]

TREATMENT

In general, treatment of the alkalemia is not necessary, and therapy should be aimed at the diagnosis and correction of the underlying disorder. There is no rationale for the use of respiratory depressants or for the administration of acid, such as HCl, in an effort to normalize the pH. In severely symptomatic patients with acute respiratory alkalosis, rebreathing into a paper bag—i.e., increasing the P_{CO_2} in the inspired air—may partially correct the hypocapnia and relieve the symptoms. The extracellular pH should be monitored in this setting, since the compensatory decrease in the plasma HCO_3^- concentration will persist and may result in metabolic acidosis as the P_{CO_2} is increased toward normal. This is usually mild but rarely may require small amounts of $NaHCO_3$.

REFERENCES

1. Giebisch GE, Berger L, Pitts RF. The extrarenal response to acute acid-base disturbances of respiratory origin. *J Clin Invest* 34:231, 1955.
2. Arbus GS, Herbert LA, Levesque PR, et al. Characterization and clinical application of the "significance band" for acute respiratory alkalosis. *N Engl J Med* 280:117, 1969.
3. Gennari JF, Goldstein MB, Schwartz WB. The nature of the renal adaptation to chronic hypocapnia. *J Clin Invest* 51:1722, 1972.
4. Gledhill N, Beirne GJ, Dempsey JA. Renal response to short-term hypocapnia in man. *Kidney Int* 8:376, 1975.
5. Gougoux A, Kaehny WD, Cohen JJ. Renal adaptation to chronic hypocapnia: Dietary constraints in achieving H^+ retention. *Am J Physiol* 229:1330, 1975.
6. Krapf R, Beeler I, Hertner D, Hulter HN. Chronic respiratory alkalosis—The effect of sustained hyperventilation on renal regulation of acid-base equilibrium. *N Engl J Med* 324:1394, 1991.
7. Guyton AC. *Textbook of Medical Physiology*, 8th ed. Philadelphia, Saunders, 1991, chap. 41.
8. Berger AJ, Mitchell RA, Severinghaus JW. Regulation of respiration. *N Engl J Med* 297:92,138,194, 1977.
9. Fencl V, Miller TB, Pappenheimer JR. Studies on the respiratory response to disturbances of acid-base balance, with deductions concerning the ionic composition of cerebral interstitial fluid. *Am J Physiol* 210:459, 1966.
10. Lugliani R, Whipp BJ, Seard C, Wasserman K. Effect of bilateral carotid-body resection on ventilatory control at rest and during exercise in man. *N Engl J Med* 285:1105, 1971.
11. Mitchell RA, Carman CT, Severinghaus JW, et al. Stability of cerebrospinal fluid pH in chronic acid-base disturbances in blood. *J Appl Physiol* 20:443, 1965.
12. Dempsey JA, Foster HV, DoPico GA. Ventilatory acclimatization to moderate hypoxemia in man: The role of spinal fluid [H^+]. *J Clin Invest* 53:1091, 1974.
13. Manning HL, Schwartzstein RM. Pathophysiology of dyspnea. *N Engl J Med* 333:1547, 1995.

14. Weil JV, Byrne-Quinn E, Sadal E, et al. Hypoxic ventilatory drive in normal man. *J Clin Invest* 49:1061, 1970.

15. Lenfant C, Sullivan K. Adaptation to high altitude. *N Engl J Med* 284:1298, 1971.

16. Kornbluth RS, Turino GM. Respiratory control in diffuse interstitial lung disease and diseases of the pulmonary vasculature. *Clin Chest Med* 1:91, 1980.

17. Lourenco RV, Turino GM, Davidson LAG, Fishman AP. The regulation of ventilation in diffuse pulmonary fibrosis. *Am J Med* 38:199, 1965.

18. Szucs MM, Brooks HL, Grossman W, et al. Diagnostic sensitivity of laboratory findings in acute pulmonary embolism. *Ann Intern Med* 74:161, 1971.

19. Aberman A, Fulop M. The metabolic and respiratory acidosis of acute pulmonary edema. *Ann Intern Med* 76:173, 1972.

20. Trenchard D, Gardner D, Guz A. Role of pulmonary vagal afferent nerve fibres in the development of rapid shallow breathing in lung inflammation. *Clin Sci* 42:251, 1972.

21. Horres AD, Bernthal T. Localized multiple minute pulmonary embolism and breathing. *J Appl Physiol* 16:842, 1961.

22. Rice RL. Symptom patterns of the hyperventilation syndrome. *Am J Med* 8:691, 1950.

23. Karetzky MS, Mithoefer JC. The cause of hyperventilation and arterial hypoxia in patients with cirrhosis of the liver. *Am J Med Sci* 254:797, 1967.

24. Record O, Iles RA, Cohen RD, Williams R. Acid-base and metabolic disturbances in fulminant hepatic failure. *Gut* 16:144, 1975.

25. Simmons DH, Nicoloff J, Guze LB. Hyperventilation and respiratory alkalosis as signs of gram-negative bacteremia. *JAMA* 174:2196, 1960.

26. Tenny SM, Miller RM. The respiratory and circulatory actions of salicylate. *Am J Med* 19:498, 1955.

27. Gabow PA, Anderson R, Potts DE, Schrier RW. Acid-base disturbances in the salicylate-intoxicated adult. *Arch Intern Med* 138:1481, 1978.

28. Lim VS, Katz AI, Lindheimer MD. Acid-base regulation in pregnancy. *Am J Physiol* 231:1764, 1976.

29. Takano N, Kaneda T. Renal contribution to acid-base regulation during the menstrual cycle. *Am J Physiol* 244:F320, 1983.

30. Rosenbaum BJ, Coburn JW, Shinaberger JH, Massry SG. Acid-base status during the interdialytic period in patients maintained with chronic hemodialysis. *Ann Intern Med* 71:1105, 1969.

31. Posner JB, Plum F. Spinal-fluid pH and neurologic symptoms in systemic acidosis. *N Engl J Med* 277:605, 1967.

32. Plum F. Mechanisms of central hyperventilation. *Ann Neurol* 11:636, 1982.

33. Saltzman H, Heyman A, Sieker HO. Correlation of clinical and physiologic manifestations of sustained hyperventilation. *N Engl J Med* 268:1431, 1963.

34. Ayres SM, Grace WJ. Inappropriate ventilation and hypoxemia as causes of cardiac arrhythmias: The control of arrhythmias without antiarrhythmic drugs. *Am J Med* 46:495, 1969.

35. Wasserman AJ, Patterson JL. The cerebral vascular response to reduction in arterial carbon dioxide tension. *J Clin Invest* 40:1297, 1961.

36. Posner JB, Swanson AG, Plum F. Acid-base balance in cerebrospinal fluid. *Arch Neurol* 12:479, 1965.

37. Knochel JP. The pathophysiology and clinical characteristics of severe hypophosphatemia. *Arch Intern Med* 137:203, 1977.

TWENTY-TWO

INTRODUCTION TO DISORDERS
OF OSMOLALITY

Hyponatremia and hypernatremia are common clinical problems. Although it is the plasma Na^+ concentration that is abnormal, these disorders reflect abnormalities in water balance that may or may not be accompanied by changes in Na^+ balance. The review presented below, which is essential for understanding the approach to patients with hyponatremia or hypernatremia, is discussed in greater detail in Chaps. 7 and 9.

WATER DISTRIBUTION AND OSMOTIC PRESSURE

The total body water (TBW) makes up about 60 percent of lean body weight in men and 50 percent in women. It is primarily distributed between the intracellular (60 percent of body water) and extracellular (40 percent of body water) compartments. In addition, roughly one-fifth of the extracellular fluid is confined to the intravascular space (the plasma water). Thus, in an average 70-kg man, the total body water is approximately 42 liters, of which 25 liters is intracellular and 17 liters is extracellular. Within the extracellular compartments, 3 liters is in the vascular space.

Osmotic forces are the primary determinants of the distribution of water between these compartments. Each compartment has one major solute that, because it is restricted primarily to that compartment, acts to hold water within the compartment. Thus, Na^+ *salts* (extracellular osmoles), K^+ *salts* (intracellular osmoles), and the *plasma proteins* (intravascular osmoles) help to maintain the volumes of the extracellular, intracellular, and intravascular spaces. In contrast to Na^+ and K^+, urea rapidly crosses cell membranes and equilibrates throughout the total body water. As a result, urea does not affect the distribution of water between the cells and the extracellular fluid and is therefore called an *ineffective* osmole.

The extracellular and intracellular fluids (ECF and ICF) are in *osmotic equilibrium*, since the cell membranes are freely permeable to water. (The renal medulla is one exception.) If an osmotic gradient is established, *water will flow from the compartment of low osmolality to that of high osmolality until the osmotic pressures are equalized.*

PHYSIOLOGIC EFFECTS OF CHANGES IN PLASMA OSMOLALITY

The effects of variations in the effective plasma osmolality on internal water distribution can be illustrated by the responses to NaCl, water, and an isotonic solution of NaCl and water (Fig. 22-1). (The methods used to calculate the new steady state are discussed on page 243.) Since Na^+ is essentially limited to the ECF, the administration of NaCl without water augments ECF osmolality, resulting in water movement *out of* the cells (Fig. 22-1b). Equilibrium is characterized by hypernatremia and equal increases in the osmolality of the ECF (due to the excess NaCl) and the ICF (due to water loss). In addition, the redistribution of water enhances the extracellular volume and reduces the intracellular volume.

Thus, *the osmotic effect of the administered NaCl is distributed throughout the total body water, even though NaCl itself is largely restricted to the ECF.* In this example, one might have expected the addition of 210 meq of Na^+ to 17 liters of ECF to increase the plasma Na^+ concentration by 12.5 meq/L ($210 \div 17 = 12.5$). However, the plasma Na^+ concentration rises by only 5 meq/L, because the osmotic water movement out of the cells lowers the plasma Na^+ concentration by dilution.

The results are different when only water is given. In this setting, there is an initial fall in ECF osmolality, thereby promoting water movement *into* the cells (Fig. 22-1c). The new steady state is characterized by a reduction in ECF and ICF osmolality, hyponatremia, and expansion of both the extracellular and intracellular volumes.

In contrast, the effect of an isotonic NaCl solution is limited to expansion of the ECF volume (Fig. 22-1d). Since there is no change in osmolality, there is no shifting of water and the composition of the ICF is unchanged.

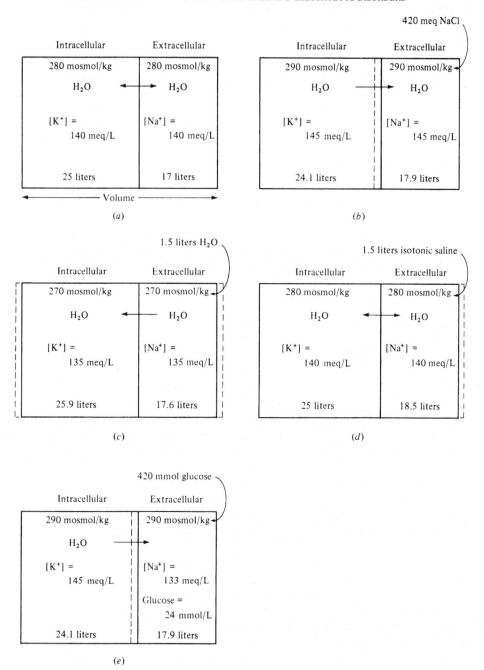

Figure 22-1 Osmolality of the body fluids and the distribution of water between the intracellular fluid and the extracellular fluid in the control state (*a*) and after the addition of NaCl (*b*), H_2O (*c*), isotonic NaCl and H_2O (*d*), or glucose (*e*) to the extracellular fluid. For simplicity, it is assumed that the only extracellular and intracellular osmoles are Na^+ salts and K^+ salts, respectively.

These examples illustrate two important clinical points. First, an increase in effective ECF osmolality results in cellular dehydration (Fig. 22-1*b*), and a decrease in effective ECF osmolality results in cellular overhydration (Fig. 22-1*c*). As will be seen, it is this flow of water out of and into brain cells that is primarily responsible for the symptoms that may be associated with hypernatremia and hyponatremia, respectively. These water shifts do not occur and the symptoms of hyperosmolality are absent when the plasma osmolality is elevated by a gradual increase in urea concentration, as occurs in renal failure. Urea, in contrast to Na^+, readily crosses the cell membrane, and osmotic equilibrium is reached by urea entry into cells rather than water movement out of cells.

Second, it can be seen that the plasma Na^+ concentration, which is a function of the *ratio* of the amounts of solute and water present, does not necessarily correlate with volume, which is a function of the *total* amount of Na^+ and water present. In each of the examples in Fig. 22-1, the extracellular volume is increased, yet the plasma Na^+ concentration is high, low, and normal, respectively. The different physiologic responses to these three states will be discussed below (see "Osmoregulation versus Volume Regulation").

MEANING OF PLASMA SODIUM CONCENTRATION

An understanding of what the plasma Na^+ concentration represents, including its differences from the extracellular volume, is essential in the approach to patients with hyponatremia or hypernatremia. Although it may appear logical to consider alterations in the plasma Na^+ concentration as indicating abnormal Na^+ balance, they are almost always a reflection of *abnormal water balance*.

Plasma Sodium Concentration and Plasma Osmolality

The osmolality of a solution is determined by the number of solute particles per kilogram of water. Since Na^+ salts (particularly NaCl and $NaHCO_3$), glucose, and urea (measured as the blood urea nitrogen, or BUN) are the primarily extracellular (and plasma) osmoles, the plasma osmolality (P_{osm}) can be approximated from

$$P_{osm} \cong 2 \times \text{plasma } [Na^+] + \frac{[\text{glucose}]}{18} + \frac{BUN}{2.8} \qquad (22\text{-}1)$$

where 2 reflects the osmotic contribution of the anion accompanying Na^+ and 18 and 2.8 represent the conversion of the plasma glucose concentration and the BUN from units of milligrams per deciliter (mg/dL) into millimoles per liter (mmol/L).

Although urea contributes to the absolute value of the P_{osm}, it does not act to hold water within the extracellular space because of its membrane permeability. As a result, urea is an ineffective osmole and does not contribute to the effective P_{osm}:

$$\text{Effective } P_{osm} \cong 2 \times \text{plasma } [Na^+] + \frac{[glucose]}{18} \qquad (22\text{-}2)$$

In humans, the normal values for these parameters are

$$P_{osm} = 275\text{–}290 \text{ mosmol/kg}$$

$$\text{Effective } P_{osm} = 270\text{–}285 \text{ mosmol/kg}$$

$$\text{Plasma } [Na^+] = 137\text{–}143 \text{ meq/L}$$

$$\text{Plasma [glucose]} = 60\text{–}100 \text{ mg/dL (fasting)}$$

$$BUN = 10\text{–}20 \text{ mg/dL}$$

Under normal conditions, glucose and urea contribute less than 10 mosmol/kg, and the plasma Na^+ concentration is the main determinant of the P_{osm}:

$$P_{osm} \cong 2 \times \text{plasma } [Na^+] \qquad (22\text{-}3)$$

Thus, *hypernatremia represents hyperosmolality and, in most instances, hyponatremia reflects hypoosmolality.* A common exception to this general relationship occurs with hyperglycemia due to uncontrolled diabetes mellitus. The elevation in the plasma glucose concentration raises the effective P_{osm}, pulling water out of the cells and lowering the plasma Na^+ concentration by dilution (Fig. 22-1e). This is clinically important, because therapy should be directed toward hyperosmolality and not, as suggested by the reduced plasma Na^+ concentration, hypoosmolality.

Plasma Sodium Concentration and Total Body Osmolality

If the plasma Na^+ concentration is a reflection of the P_{osm} and the P_{osm} is in equilibrium with the total body osmolality, then (see page 247)

$$\text{Plasma } [Na^+] \propto \text{total body osmolality} \qquad (22\text{-}4)$$

Since

$$\text{Total body osmolality} = \frac{\text{extracellular} + \text{intracellular solutes}}{\text{TBW}}$$

and Na^+ and K^+ salts (including the accompanying anions) are the primary extracellular and intracellular solutes, respectively, Eq. (22-4) can be converted to

$$\text{Plasma } [Na^+] \cong \frac{Na_e^+ + K_e^+}{\text{TBW}} \qquad (22\text{-}5)$$

where Na_e^+ and K_e^+ refer to the total "exchangeable" quantities of these ions (Fig. 22-2).[1] The exchangeable portion is used because about 30 percent of the body Na^+ and a small fraction of the body K^+ are bound in areas such as bone where they are "nonexchangeable" and therefore are *osmotically inactive.*

The importance of the variables in Eq. (22-5) can be appreciated from the examples in Fig. 22-1. Increasing the Na_e^+ with NaCl elevates the plasma Na^+ concentration; raising the TBW lowers the plasma Na^+ concentration; and

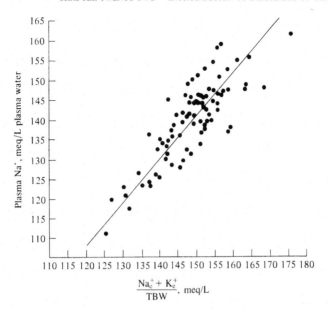

Figure 22-2 Relation between the plasma water Na^+ concentration and the ratio of $(Na_e^+ + K_e^+)/TBW$. (*Adapted from Edelman I, Leibman J, O'Meara M, Birkenfeld L. J Cin Invest 37:1236, 1958, by copyright permission of the American Society for Clinical Investigation.*)

increasing Na_e^+ and TBW proportionately with isotonic saline has no effect on the plasma Na^+ concentration.

The effect of K^+ is less apparent but can be clinically important. If, for example, K^+ is lost from the extracellular fluid (as a result of renal or gastrointestinal losses), the extracellular K^+ concentration will fall. This will create a concentration gradient favoring the movement of K^+ out of the cells. Since large proteins and organic phosphates are the major intracellular anions and cannot easily leave the cells, electroneutrality is preserved in one of three ways, each of which will lower the plasma Na^+ concentration:

- Extracellular Na^+ will enter the cells, directly lowering the plasma Na^+ concentration.
- Intracellular Cl^- will leave the cells (primarily red blood cells). The loss of KCl will lower the cell osmolality, resulting in H_2O movement out of the cells and thereby reducing the plasma Na^+ concentration by dilution.
- Extracellular H^+ ions will dissociate from extracellular buffers and enter the cells, where they will combine with cell buffers. This movement of H^+ is osmotically neutral, but the loss of cell K^+ will lower the cell osmolality and induce osmotic H_2O movement out of the cells.

In some patients with diuretic-induced hyponatremia, for example, it is the reduction in exchangeable K^+, not Na^+, that is primarily responsible for the fall in the plasma Na^+ concentration.[2] Furthermore, administration of KCl alone will raise both the plasma K^+ and Na^+ concentrations.

A more common clinical example of the osmotic importance of K^+ is seen with fluid replacement for volume depletion. In diabetic ketoacidosis, for example, the elevation in the plasma glucose concentration raises the effective P_{osm}. As a result, hypotonic fluids, such as half-isotonic saline, are often administered both to reexpand volume and to lower the P_{osm}. This solution, which contains 77 meq each of Na^+ and Cl^-, is essentially composed of two solutions: 500 mL of isotonic saline (77 meq of Na^+ in 500 mL or 154 meq/L) and 500 mL of free water. However, patients with diabetic ketoacidosis are also K^+-depleted, and 40 meq of KCl is frequently added to the replacement fluid. This raises the $(Na^+ + K^+)$ concentration to 117 meq/L. Consequently, each liter now contains 760 mL of isotonic fluid (117 meq in 760 mL or 154 meq/L) and only 240 mL of free water. Administration of this solution at 200 mL/h will supply 50 mL/h of free water, which is roughly equivalent to the rate of insensible water losses from the skin and respiratory tract. Thus, there will be no free-water retention and no lowering of the P_{osm}.

Hyponatremia and Hypernatremia

From Eq. (22-5), it can be seen that hyponatremia or hypernatremia can be induced by alterations in Na^+, K^+, or water balance. In the clinical setting, however, these disorders are *almost always due to changes in water balance*. Hyponatremia, for example, almost always results from the retention of ingested or administered water. Although $(Na^+ + K^+)$ loss in excess of water also can lower the plasma Na^+ concentration, this is a rare event, occurring in some patients with thiazide diuretic-induced hyponatremia (see Chap. 23).

Hypernatremia, on the other hand, usually results from water loss in excess of solute and less often from the administration of a hypertonic Na^+ solution (see Chap. 24). The toxicity of hyperkalemia (high plasma K^+ concentration) prevents the retention of enough K^+ to raise the plasma Na^+ concentration.

As will be described below, different protective mechanisms normally prevent alterations in the plasma Na^+ concentration. Water retention leading to hyponatreamia does not usually occur because the excess water can be excreted in the urine via suppression of the secretion of antidiuretic hormone. Water loss leading to hypernatremia does not usually occur because stimulation of thirst will promote water intake to replace the lost fluid.

Diarrheal states A clinical illustration of the multiple factors that can influence the plasma Na^+ concentration occurs in patients with diarrhea. Although diarrheal fluid is roughly isosmotic to plasma, the ionic composition is variable.[3,4] In secretory diarrheas (such as cholera), the $(Na^+ + K^+)$ concentration of the diarrheal fluid is similar to that of the plasma.[3] Thus, loss of this fluid will produce volume and K^+ depletion but will not directly alter either the P_{osm} or the plasma Na^+ concentration.

The findings are different with osmotic diarrheas, as occur with lactulose therapy, malabsorption, and some infectious enteritides. In this setting, the fecal $(Na^+ + K^+)$ concentration is usually between 30 and 110 meq/L, with nonreabsorbed solutes (such as lactulose) accounting for most of the remaining osmoles.[3,4] As a result, the plasma Na^+ concentration will tend to rise, since water is lost in excess of Na^+ and K^+ even though the fluid is isosmotic to plasma.[5]

Diarrheal syndromes also have other effects on water balance, as they may be associated with fever, metabolic acidosis, and volume depletion. Fever increases water loss as sweat, and metabolic acidosis leads to compensatory hyperventilation, which enhances water loss from the lungs. On the other hand, volume depletion is a potent stimulus to thirst and antidiuretic hormone (ADH) secretion, resulting in water retention due to the combined effects of increased intake and reduced excretion.

In most patients with diarrhea, the increments in free-water loss and water retention are of roughly the same magnitude, resulting in little change in the plasma Na^+ concentration. In infants, however, water intake may not be increased, since access to water is often limited. As a result, enteric infections with fever can lead to negative water balance and hypernatremia, particularly when gastrointestinal water loss also is present as a result of an osmotic diarrhea.[6] Conversely, the hypovolemic adult is often able to satisfy thirst, possibly leading to positive water balance with consequent hyponatremia.

REGULATION OF PLASMA OSMOLALITY

The relationship of the plasma Na^+ concentration to water balance is also illustrated by the manner in which the plasma Na^+ concentration and P_{osm} are normally regulated: namely, by alterations in the intake and excretion of water, not of Na^+.

Each day, there is a variable degree of water intake and loss that can lead to changes in the P_{osm} (see Chap. 9). Water intake is derived from three sources: drinking, the water content of food, and water of oxidation (e.g., carbohydrates are metabolized to CO_2 and water; Table 22-1). The retention of this water tends to lower the P_{osm}. On the other hand, water is lost in the urine and feces as well as from the skin and respiratory tract as insensible and sweat losses. This loss of water tends to raise the P_{osm}.

Under normal circumstances, there is a balance between net water intake and excretion such that the P_{osm} is maintained within narrow limits. This regulatory response is mediated by osmoreceptors in the hypothalamus which sense changes in the P_{osm} of as little as 1 percent and which affect both water intake via thirst and water excretion via the secretion of ADH from the posterior lobe of the pituitary (see Chap. 6). In the kidney, ADH augments the water permeability of the collecting tubules, resulting in increased water reabsorption and the excretion of a hyperosmotic urine (high U_{osm} and specific gravity). When ADH is absent, water reabsorption falls, and a dilute urine is excreted (low U_{osm} and

Table 22-1 Typical daily water balance in a normal human[a]

Source	Water intake, mL/day	Source	Water output, mL/day
Ingested water	1400	Urine	1500
Water content of food	850	Skin	500
Water of oxidation	350	Respiratory tract	400
		Stool	200
Total	2600		2600

[a] These values assume a low rate of sweat production. With exercise and/or hot weather, however, water losses from the skin as sweat can increase markedly, occasionally exceeding 5 L/day. In this setting, the ensuing rise in plasma osmolality enhances thirst, resulting in an appropriate increase in water intake.

specific gravity), since the collecting tubules are now relatively impermeable to water.

The osmoreceptors regulate the P_{osm} in the following manner. After a water load, there is a fall in the P_{osm}, which inhibits ADH secretion. This promotes the urinary excretion of the excess water, thereby returning the P_{osm} to normal. If, on the other hand, a patient becomes hyperosmolal (as with hypernatremia due to insensible water losses), thirst and ADH release are stimulated. The combination of enhanced water intake and renal water conservation results in water retention and an appropriate reduction in the P_{osm}. (In contrast, the osmoreceptors are not stimulated by hyperosmolality due to an elevation in the BUN, since urea is an ineffective osmole.)

This regulatory system can be disrupted either by neurologic disorders, which interfere with hypothalamic or posterior pituitary function, or by renal disorders, which can impair concentrating or diluting ability. In addition, there are non-osmolal factors that can influence hypothalamic function and *override* the effects of osmolality. In particular, volume depletion is a potent stimulus to ADH release and thirst (see Chap. 6).[7-9] As a result, patients who are hypovolemic may have persistent thirst and ADH secretion, even in the presence of hyponatremia. In this setting, volume and tissue perfusion are maintained at the expense of the P_{osm}.

Osmoregulation versus Volume Regulation

It is important to understand the differences between osmoregulation and volume regulation (Table 22-2). As described above, the P_{osm} is determined by the *ratio* of solutes (primarily Na^+ and K^+ salts) and water, whereas the extracellular volume is determined by the *absolute amounts* of Na^+ and water that are present. Two simple examples can illustrate the frequent dissociation between these parameters. Exercising on a hot day leads to the loss of dilute fluid as sweat. The net effect is a *rise* in the plasma Na^+ concentration but a *fall* in the extracellular volume. On the

Table 22-2   Differences between osmoregulation and volume regulation

	Osmoregulation	Volume regulation
What is being sensed	Plasma osmolality	Effective circulating volume
Sensors	Hypothalamic osmoreceptors	Carotid sinus
		Afferent arteriole
		Atria
Effectors	Antidiuretic hormone	Renin-angiotensin-aldosterone
	Thirst	system
		Sympathetic nervous system
		Natriuretic peptides, including
		atrial natriuetic peptide and
		urodilatin
		Pressure natriuresis
		Antidiuretic hormone
What is affected	Water excretion and, via	Urinary sodium excretion
	thirst, water intake	

other hand, water retention due to persistent ADH release will lead to a *reduction* in the plasma Na^+ concentration but an *increase* in volume. Thus, knowledge of the plasma Na^+ concentration gives *no predictable information* on volume status.

The preceding discussion has emphasized the roles of the hypothalamic osmoreceptors, ADH, and thirst in the regulation of the P_{osm}, which is achieved primarily by changes in water balance. Volume regulation, on the other hand, attempts to maintain tissue perfusion. Different sensors and effectors are involved in this process, as it is urinary Na^+ excretion, not osmolality, that is being regulated (Table 22-2). The rate of Na^+ excretion is primarily regulated by aldosterone, angiotensin II, and perhaps natriuretic peptides; changes in the plasma Na^+ concentration have little effect unless there are associated changes in volume (see Chap. 8). Thus, the urine Na^+ concentration should be less than 25 meq/L when hyponatremia is due to net Na^+ loss (volume depletion) and greater than 40 meq/L when it is due to primary water retention (volume expansion). As a result, measurement of the urine Na^+ concentration is an important component of the diagnostic approach to hyponatremia (see Chap. 23).

The independent roles of the osmoregulatory and volume regulatory pathways can be illustrated by the different responses elicited by NaCl, water, and isotonic NaCl and water (as in Fig. 22-1):

- Isotonic saline enhances the extracellular volume without change in the P_{osm} (Fig. 22-1*d*). Thus, only the volume receptors are activated, resulting in NaCl (and water) loss in the urine due to inhibition of the renin-angiotensin-aldosterone system and perhaps also to increased secretion of atrial natriuretic peptide (or related peptides; see page 190).

- A water load lowers the P_{osm} (Fig. 22-1c). This leads sequentially to the inhibition of ADH release, the formation of a dilute urine, and the rapid excretion of the excess water. This response is normally so efficient that volume is only transiently increased and there is little change in the volume regulatory hormones (such as atrial natriuretic peptide) or in NaCl excretion.[10]
- The administration of NaCl without water increases the extracellular volume (Fig. 22-1b) and leads to renal NaCl loss. In addition, the increase in P_{osm} stimulates ADH release and thirst. These changes result in water retention, which both reduces osmolality toward normal and augments volume, further promoting the renal excretion of the NaCl load. The net effect is the excretion of the excess Na^+ in a relatively concentrated urine, a composition similar to net intake.

Volume Depletion versus Dehydration

A common mistake in terms of terminology is the assumption that dehydration and volume depletion (or hypovolemia) are synonymous.[11] Volume depletion refers to extracellular volume depletion from any cause, most often due to salt and water loss. In contrast, dehydration refers to the presence of hypernatremia due to pure water loss; such patients are also hypovolemic.

URINE OSMOLALITY AND SPECIFIC GRAVITY

Estimating the ability to concentrate or dilute the urine can be helpful in the diagnosis of patients with hypernatremia or hyponatremia. This can be done by measuring the urine osmolality or, if an osmometer is not available, the specific gravity of the urine. In general, the urinary specific gravity correlates reasonably well with the U_{osm}, according to the following approximate relationship:

Specific gravity	Osmolality
1.000	0
1.010	350
1.020	700
1.030	1050

However, this relationship is changed when larger molecules are present in the urine, as occurs during a glucose osmotic diuresis or after the administration of radiocontrast media. In these settings, use of the specific gravity can be misleading, since it will be elevated out of proportion to any change in the U_{osm}.

RELATION BETWEEN INTAKE AND OUTPUT

In the treatment of patients with hyponatremia or hypernatremia, attention is appropriately paid to comparing net fluid intake to urinary output, since changing the state of water balance can return the plasma Na^+ concentration toward normal. For example, hyponatremic patients who are not volume-depleted can be treated with fluid restriction. If intake is kept below output, there will be a net loss of water and an elevation in the plasma Na^+ concentration.

It must be emphasized, however, that the *composition of the fluids given and those excreted is often markedly different.* Thus, merely comparing intake and output may be insufficient to accurately predict the effects of therapy. If, for example, urinary NaCl and water loss is induced by a diuretic and the fluid losses are replaced by an equal volume of water, the patient will be in water balance. However, loss of the unreplaced solute will induce hypoosmolality and hyponatremia.

A more complex evaluation of fluid balance can be illustrated by the following case history:

Case history 22-1   A 58-year-old woman with an oat-cell carcinoma of the lung is admitted for progressive lethargy and confusion. The physical examination shows no focal neurologic findings and a weight of 60 kg. Laboratory data reveal

$$\text{Plasma } [Na^+] = 102 \, \text{meq/L}$$

$$P_{osm} = 230 \, \text{mosmol/kg}$$

$$\text{Urine } [Na^+] = 70 \, \text{meq/L}$$

$$U_{osm} = 420 \, \text{mosmol/kg}$$

A diagnosis of inappropriate ADH secretion due to the lung tumor is made (see Chap. 23). In view of the severe hyponatremia, the patient is treated with water restriction, hypertonic saline (Na^+ concentration equals 513 meq/L; osmolality equals 1026 mosmol/kg) and furosemide.

Overnight, the patient is given 1700 mL of hypertonic saline and excretes 3300 mL of urine with an osmolality of 300 mosmol/kg and Na^+ and K^+ concentrations of 95 and 35 meq/L, respectively. Repeat blood tests in the morning reveal a plasma Na^+ concentration of 123 meq/L and a plasma osmolality of 271 mosmol/kg.

Comment   At first glance, it seems unlikely that a negative fluid balance of only 1600 mL can result in such a marked rise in the plasma Na^+ concentration and osmolality. However, a more complete evaluation of intake and output shows how this change occurred.[4a]* The patient weighed 60 kg on admission, approximately one-half of which was water. Thus, her TBW on admission was 30 liters. Since the osmolality in all fluid compartments is equal,

$$\text{Total body osmoles} = \text{TBW} \times P_{osm}$$

Since the effective P_{osm} is roughly equal to $2 \times$ plasma $[Na^+]$,

$$\text{Total effective osmoles} = \text{TBW} \times 2 \times \text{plasma } [Na^+]$$

$$= 30 \times 204$$

$$= 6120 \,\text{mosmol} \qquad (22\text{-}6)$$

With the loss of 1600 mL of water, her TBW fell to 28.4 liters. If her total osmoles were still 6120, then, by rearranging Eq. (22-6),

$$\text{Plasma } [Na^+] = \text{total osmoles} \div (2 \times \text{TBW})$$

$$= 6120 \div 56.8$$

$$= 108 \,\text{meq/L} \qquad (22\text{-}7)$$

This is clearly much different from the measured value of 123 mosmol/kg. The error lies in the assumption that the patient's total osmoles were unchanged. The total osmolar intake was 1745 mosmol (1700 mL at 1026 mosmol/kg) and total $(Na^+ + K^+)$ loss was 860 mosmol [3.3 L $\times$ 130 meq/L $\times$ 2 (to account for accompanying anions)]. Thus, there was a 885-mosmol *increase* in total osmoles, from 6120 up to 6980 mosmol. As a result, from Eq. (22-7),

$$\text{Plasma } [Na^+] = 6980 \div 56.8$$

$$= 123 \,\text{meq/L}$$

This value is identical to the measured value.

PROBLEMS

22-1 A patient has the following laboratory data:

$$\text{Plasma } [Na^+] = 125 \,\text{meq/L}$$

$$[\text{Glucose}] = 108 \,\text{mg/dL}$$

$$\text{BUN} = 140 \,\text{mg/dL}$$

(a) Calculate the plasma osmolality.
(b) Would this patient have symptoms of hyperosmolality?

---

* The calculations in this example are similar to those involved in the calculation of the new steady states in Fig. 22-1 (see page 684).

22-2 Suppose a patient can excrete only urine that is isosmotic to plasma. If the patient's intake were limited to the administration of isotonic saline (Na^+ concentration equals 154 meq/L, the same as the Na^+ concentration in the plasma water):

(a) What would happen to the plasma osmolality and Na^+ concentration?

(b) Would the slow infusion of half-isotonic saline (Na^+ concentration of 77 meq/L) supplemented with 77 meq/L of K^+ (as KCl) have different effects on the plasma osmolality and Na^+ concentration and on the extracellular volume?

REFERENCES

1. Edelman IS, Leibman J, O'Meara MP, Birkenfeld L. Interrelations between serum sodium concentration, serum osmolarity and total exchangeable sodium, total exchangeable potassium and total body water. *J Clin Invest* 37:1236, 1958.

2. Fichman MP, Vorherr H, Kleeman CR, Telfer N. Diuretic-induced hypantremia. *Ann Intern Med* 75:853, 1971.

3. Shiau Y-F, Feldman GM, Resnick MA, Coff PM. Stool electrolyte and osmolality measurements in the evaluation of diarrheal disorders. *Ann Intern Med* 102:773, 1985.

4. Teree T, Mirabal-Font E, Ortiz A, Wallace W. Stool losses and acidosis in diarrheal disease of infancy. *Pediatrics* 36:704, 1965.

5. Rose BD. New approach to disturbances in the plasma sodium concentration. *Am J Med* 81:1033, 1986.

6. Bruck E, Abal G, Aceto T. Pathogenesis and pathophysiology of hypertonic dehydration with diarrhea. *Am J Dis Child* 115:122, 1968.

7. Leaf A, Mamby AR. An antidiuretic mechanism not regulated by extracellular fluid tonicity. *J Clin Invest* 31:60, 1952.

8. Robertson GL. Physiology of ADH secretion. *Kidney Int* 32(suppl 21):S-20, 1987.

9. Schrier RW, Bichet DG. Osmotic and nonosmotic control of vasopressin release and the pathogenesis of impaired water excretion in adrenal, thyroid, and edematous disorders. *J Lab Clin Med* 98:1, 1981.

10. Shore AC, Markandu ND, Sagnella GA, et al. Endocrine and renal response to water loading and water restriction in normal man. *Clin Sci* 75:171, 1988.

11. Mange K, Matsuura D, Cizman B, et al. Language guiding therapy: The case of dehydration versus volume depletion. *Ann Intern Med* 127:848, 1997.

TWENTY-THREE

HYPOOSMOLAL STATES— HYPONATREMIA

The introduction to disorders of water balance presented in Chap. 22 should be read before proceeding with this discussion.

PATHOPHYSIOLOGY

The plasma Na^+ concentration is the main determinant of the plasma osmolality (P_{osm}). As a result, hyponatremia, defined as a plasma Na^+ concentration below 135 meq/L, usually reflects hypoosmolality. This is an important relationship because the low P_{osm} results in water movement into the cells; it is this cellular overhydration, particularly in brain cells, that is primarily responsible for the symptoms that may be associated with this disorder (see "Symptoms," below).

The basic mechanisms by which hyponatremia and hypoosmolality occur can be most easily understood if we ask two separate questions:

- How do patients develop hyponatremia?
- Why do they stay hyponatremic?

Generation of Hyponatremia

From the relationship between the plasma Na^+ concentration and the osmolality of the body fluids (see Fig. 22-2),

$$\text{Plasma } [Na^+] \cong \frac{Na_e^+ + K_e^+}{\text{total body water}} \tag{23-1}$$

it can be seen that either solute (Na^+ or K^+) loss or water retention can produce hyponatremia. However, solute loss, as with vomiting or diarrhea, usually occurs in a fluid that is isosmotic to plasma.[1] Isosmotic fluid loss cannot directly lower the plasma Na^+ concentration, but hyponatremia will ensue if these losses are replaced with ingested or administered water. Thus, *water retention leading to an excess of water in relation to solute is the common denominator in almost all hypoosmolal states.* The corollary of this relationship is that hypoosmolality generally cannot be produced if there is no water intake.

Perpetuation of Hyponatremia

The primary response to a fall in the P_{osm}, as occurs in normal subjects after the ingestion of a water load, is to diminish the secretion and synthesis of antidiuretic hormone (ADH; also called vasopressin), a response that is mediated in part by decreased ADH-specific messenger RNA.[2,3] This results sequentially in decreased water reabsorption in the collecting tubules, the production of a dilute urine, and the rapid excretion of the excess water (more than 80 percent within 4 h). This is a dose-dependent effect, so the final urine osmolality (U_{osm}) is determined by how much ADH release is inhibited.

As depicted in Fig. 23-1, ADH secretion essentially ceases when the P_{osm} falls below 275 mosmol/kg, a setting in which the plasma Na^+ concentration should be about 135 meq/L. In the absence of ADH, the U_{osm} can fall to 40 to 100 mosmol/kg (specific gravity equals 1.001 to 1.003), with a maximum water excretory capacity that can exceed 10 L/day of solute-free water on a regular diet.

Since the capacity for water excretion is normally so great, water retention resulting in hyponatremia typically occurs only when there is *a defect in renal water excretion.* A rare exception to this rule is seen in patients with primary polydipsia who drink such large volumes of fluid that they overwhelm even the normal excretory capacity.

The excretion of free water is dependent upon two factors:

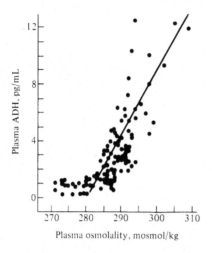

Figure 23-1 Relationship of plasma ADH concentration to plasma osmolality in normal humans in whom the plasma osmolality was changed by varying the state of hydration. ADH secretion is almost totally suppressed when the plasma osmolality falls below 275 to 280 mosmol/kg. (*Adapted from Robertson GL, Aycinena P, Zerbe RL, Am J Med 72:339, 1982, with permission.*)

- The generation of free water and a dilute urine by NaCl reabsorption without water in the diluting segments in the ascending limb of the loop of Henle and, to a lesser degree, the distal tubule.
- The excretion of this water by keeping the collecting tubules impermeable to water (see Chap. 4).

Therefore, a reduction in free-water excretion, which is required for the development of hyponatremia in most patients, must involve an abnormality in one or both of these steps (Table 23-1). Virtually all hyponatremic patients (except for those with renal failure and primary polydipsia) have an excess of ADH, most often due to the syndrome of inappropriate ADH secretion (SIADH) or to effective circulating volume depletion.[4,5]

This decrease in free-water excretion is manifested by a U_{osm} that is inappropriately high (U_{osm} greater than 100 mosmol/kg and usually greater than 300 mosmol/kg), considering the presence of hypoosmolality. The impairment in

Table 23-1 Pathophysiologic factors that diminish renal water excretion

Diminished generation of free water in the loop of Henle and distal tubule
    A. Decreased fluid delivery to these segments
        1. Effective circulating volume depletion
        2. Renal failure
    B. Inhibition of NaCl reabsorption by diuretics
Enhanced water permeability of the collecting tubules due to the presence of ADH
    A. Syndrome of inappropriate ADH secretion
    B. Effective circulating volume depletion
    C. Adrenal insufficiency
    D. Hypothyroidism

water excretion does not have to be very severe. Suppose a patient has a daily solute intake of 400 mosmol and a net water intake (intake minus insensible loss) of 2 liters. To excrete this load and remain in the steady state, the average U_{osm} will be 200 mosmol/kg. If this patient were unable to reduce the U_{osm} below 222 mosmol/kg (a level still hypoosmotic to plasma), the 400 mosmol of solute would be excreted in only 1800 mL of water, resulting in the daily retention of 200 mL of water and a gradual fall in the plasma Na^+ concentration.

In theory, shutting off thirst should protect against progressive hyponatremia in this setting. However, this does not occur, because most fluid is ingested out of habit or for cultural reasons (e.g., coffee or soda with meals or as snacks), not because of osmotic stimulation of thirst (see Chap. 9).

ETIOLOGY

Since hyponatremia with hypoosmolality is caused by the retention of solution-free water, the differential diagnosis of this disturbance consists primarily of those conditions that limit water excretion (Table 23-2).[5]

Table 23-2 Etiology of hyponatremia and hypoosmolality

Disorders in which renal water excretion is impaired
  A. Effective circulating volume depletion
    1. Gastrointestinal losses: vomiting, diarrhea, tube drainage, bleeding, intestinal obstruction
    2. Renal losses: diuretics, hypoaldosteronism, Na^+-wasting nephropathy
    3. Skin losses: ultramarathon runners, burns, cystic fibrosis
    4. Edematous states: heart failure, hepatic cirrhosis, nephrotic syndrome with marked hypoalbuminemia
    5. K^+ depletion
  B. Diuretics
    1. Thiazides in almost all cases
    2. Loop diuretics
  C. Renal failure
  D. Nonhypovolemic states of ADH excess
    1. Syndrome of inappropriate ADH secretion
    2. Cortisol deficiency
    3. Hypothyroidism
  E. Decreased solute intake
  F. Cerebral salt wasting
Disorders in which renal water excretion is normal
  A. Primary polydipsia
  B. Reset osmostat: effective volume depletion, pregnancy, psychosis, quadriplegia, malnutrition

Effective Circulating Volume Depletion

The term *effective circulating volume* refers to that fluid which is effectively perfusing the tissues (see Chap. 8). Effective volume depletion may be associated with either reduction or expansion of the extracellular volume. True volume depletion, i.e., depletion of both the intravascular and interstitial compartments, can be produced by fluid loss from the gastrointestinal tract, kidneys, or skin (Table 23-2). In addition, decreased tissue perfusion also may be present in some edematous states—for example, as a result of a primary reduction in the cardiac output in heart failure or decreased vascular resistance in cirrhosis (see Chap. 16).

Effective volume depletion predisposes toward the development of hyponatremia through its effects on renal water excretion, thirst, and K^+ balance (Fig. 23-2). Regardless of the underlying disorder, volume depletion can impair water excretion in two ways:

- Hypovolemia, acting via the carotid sinus baroreceptors, is a potent stimulus to ADH secretion (see Fig. 6-8), resulting in augmented water permeability in the collecting tubules. For example, almost all hyponatremic patients with advanced heart failure or cirrhosis have elevated circulating ADH levels.[5-8] This can be called *appropriate ADH secretion*, since the retained water attempts to restore normovolemia. Furthermore, the hypersecretion of ADH can be reversed if perfusion is increased, as with the administration of an angiotensin converting enzyme (ACE) inhibitor to some patients with heart failure.[9]

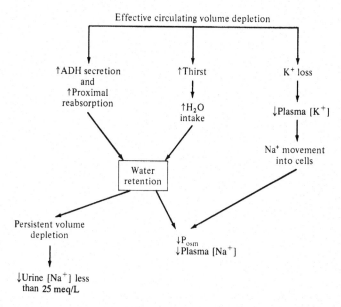

Figure 23-2   Pathophysiology of the development of hyponatremia in effective circulating volume depletion.

- The combination of a fall in glomerular filtration rate (GFR) and an increase in proximal tubular Na^+ and water reabsorption diminishes fluid delivery to the diluting segments. As a result, the amount of free water that can be generated is limited,[10] even if ADH release is suppressed.[11] It seems likely that this intrarenal effect is generally less important than the rise in ADH, since the administration of an ADH antagonist largely reverses the defect in water excretion in experimental heart failure, cirrhosis, and adrenal insufficiency without improving tissue perfusion.[12-14]

Not surprisingly, the tendency to increase ADH release and to reduce loop delivery is related to the degree of volume depletion. Thus, increasing severity of heart failure or cirrhosis is associated with a progressive rise in the release of ADH and of the two other "hypovolemic" hormones, renin and norepinephrine.[15-18] The net effect is that *hyponatremia does not occur in the absence of advanced disease*.[15-18] Patients with heart failure who have a plasma Na^+ concentration below 137 meq/L have a significant reduction in survival compared to similar patients who are normonatremic.[19] It is important to remember in this regard that the capacity to excrete water is normally so great that even *a minor reduction in the plasma Na^+ concentration reflects a severe impairment in water excretion* (unless intake is markedly enhanced).

The *volume of water that is retained is related to both the severity of the reduction in water excretion and the intake of water*. Increased intake may contribute to the development of hyponatremia in this setting, since volume depletion can directly stimulate thirst.[20] An interesting example of this relationship between intake and excretion has been described in ultramarathon runners, who have estimated sweat losses of 10 to 14 liters of fluid containing 20 to 100 meq/L of Na^+ and K^+. These losses are almost entirely replaced by carbohydrate-containing solutions that have a much lower solute content. The net effect is water retention and, in some cases, symptomatic hyponatremia, with a fall in the plasma Na^+ concentration below 120 meq/L.[21]

Another example is the replacement of severe diarrheal losses due to cholera (which is associated with a sodium concentration in stool of 120 to 140 meq/L) with an oral rehydration solution with reduced osmolarity. Compared with standard (i.e., higher sodium concentration) oral rehydration therapy, the use of a lower-solute solution may result in an increased incidence of hyponatremia.[22]

Lastly, concurrent K^+ depletion also represents the loss of effective solute and can contribute to the development of hyponatremia. This effect is due to a *transcellular cation exchange*, in which K^+ leaves the cells to replete the extracellular stores and electroneutrality is in part maintained by Na^+ movement into the cells. In otherwise normal subjects, the fall in the P_{osm} is transient, since ADH secretion is suppressed (Fig. 23-1), leading to enhanced water excretion and normalization of the P_{osm} and Na^+ concentration. If ADH release is increased because of volume depletion, however, the hyponatremia may persist. In this setting, the administration of KCl alone can reverse the cation exchange and partially correct the fall in the plasma Na^+ concentration.[23-25]

Diuretics

Hyponatremia is a relatively common, though usually mild, complication of diuretic therapy. However, acute severe hyponatremia may occur as an idiosyncratic reaction,[24-29] particularly in patients who also drink large volumes of water.[26,30] A careful analysis of 13 patients with a history of acute thiazide-induced hyponatremia evaluated these patients and controls after rechallenge with 50 mg of hydrochlorothiazide.[26] Only those with prior hyponatremia developed a reduction in the plasma Na^+ concentration, which appeared to be due primarily to *increased water intake* rather than a greater natriuretic or diuretic response.

Three mechanisms in addition to fluid intake may also contribute to diuretic-induced hyponatremia: volume depletion (by mechanisms similar to those in Fig. 23-2), K^+ depletion, and direct inhibition of urinary dilution by diminished NaCl reabsorption in the loop of Henle and distal tubule.[29] Concurrent measurement of the blood urea nitrogen (BUN) and plasma uric acid concentration can help to distinguish between these mechanisms in an individual patient.[31] Increased water intake and transient volume expansion lead to increases in the urinary excretion of urea and uric acid and the development of hypouremia (with the BUN often falling below 10 mg/dL) and hypouricemia (with the plasma uric acid level often falling below 4 mg/dL). In comparison, volume depletion leads to elevations in both of these parameters.

One, at first surprising, observation is that *almost all cases of diuretic-induced hyponatremia are due to thiazide, not loop, diuretics.*[24-30] This difference in susceptibility may be related to the different sites of action of these drugs within the nephron (see Chap. 15), which lead to varying effects on urinary concentrating ability.[32] A concentrated urine is produced by equilibration of the fluid in the collecting tubules with the hyperosmotic medullary interstitium (see Chap. 4). The loop diuretics interfere with this process by inhibiting NaCl reabsorption in the medullary thick ascending limb, thereby diminishing the interstitial osmolality.[32] Thus, loop diuretics can induce volume depletion, leading to the release of ADH and a subsequent increase in the permeability of the collecting tubules to water; however, the *degree of water retention and therefore the tendency to hyponatremia are limited by the lack of medullary hypertonicity.* As will be described below, this ability of the loop diuretics to diminish ADH-induced free-water reabsorption can actually be used to treat hyponatremia in SIADH.

The thiazides, in comparison, act in the cortex in the distal tubule and do not interfere with urinary concentration or the ability of ADH to promote water retention.[32] Furthermore, use of thiazide diuretics represents virtually the only clinical setting in which hyponatremia can be produced in part by the *loss of effective solute $(Na^+ + K^+)$ in excess of water*. This effect results from the combination of diuretic-induced Na^+ plus K^+ loss and ADH-induced water retention. In one study of seven patients, for example, the urine Na^+ plus K^+ concentration at presentation averaged 156 meq/L while the plasma levels were below 110 meq/L.[27] These losses will directly lower the plasma Na^+ concentration, independent of the level of water intake.

Rechallenge studies have shown that the plasma Na^+ concentration begins to fall within 6 to 24 h in susceptible subjects;[26,27] furthermore, the hyponatremia occurs within 2 weeks of the onset of therapy in most cases.[29] These findings are not surprising, since the maximum response to a given dose of a diuretic is seen with the first dose, and all fluid and electrolyte complications begin to develop within the first few days (see page 453). After the first few weeks, a *new steady state* is established in which intake and excretion are again equal;[33] any further change in the plasma Na^+ concentration will occur only if there is some superimposed problem, such as vomiting, diarrhea, or an increase in water intake or drug dose.

Renal Failure

Progressive renal disease impairs urinary dilution, as manifested by an inability to maximally lower the urine osmolality after a water load.[34,35] This defect is largely related to the associated osmotic diuresis; if dietary intake is similar to that in normals, then patients with fewer functioning nephrons must, to maintain balance, increase the rate of solute excretion in the remaining nephrons. Nevertheless, relative water excretion (as measured by the rate of free-water excretion divided by the glomerular filtration rate) is not diminished in mild-to-moderate disease.[34] Thus, nonoliguric patients are usually able to maintain a near normal plasma Na^+ concentration as long as water intake is not excessive. However, water retention and hyponatremia are common when the GFR falls to very low levels.

Syndrome of Inappropriate ADH Secretion

SIADH is a common problem that can be seen in a wide variety of clinical states (Table 23-3). It is characterized by the nonphysiologic release of ADH (i.e., not due to the usual stimuli or hyperosmolality or hypovolemia) and by the relatively unusual finding of *impaired water excretion at a time when Na^+ excretion is normal*. Understanding the implications of this relationship is essential if effective therapy is to be instituted (see "Treatment," below).[36]

Pathogenesis   The fluid and electrolyte consequences of persistent ADH activity are depicted in Fig. 23-3.[89] Because of the hormonal effect to enhance renal water reabsorption, ingested water is retained, resulting in dilution (hyponatremia and hypoosmolality) and expansion of the body fluids.[90] Edema does not occur, however, because the volume receptors become activated, leading to an appropriate increase in urinary Na^+ and water excretion that may be mediated in part by enhanced release of atrial natriuetic peptide.[91]

The net effect is that the combination of water retention and secondary solute (sodium plus potassium) loss can account for essentially all of the fall in the plasma sodium concentration in SIADH.[90,92] These changes occur in the following sequence.[90] The hyponatremia is initially mediated by ADH-induced water retention. The ensuing volume expansion activates secondary natriuretic mechanisms, resulting in sodium and water loss. The net effect is that, with

Table 23-3 Causes of SIADH according to probable major mechanism of action

Increased hypothalmic production of ADH

  A. Neuropsychiatric disorders[a]
    1. Infections: meningitis, encephalitis, abscess, herpes zoster
    2. Vascular: thrombosis, subarachnoid or subdural hemorrhage, temporal arteritis
    3. Neoplasma: primary or metastatic
    4. Psychosis[37]
    5. Other: human immunodeficiency virus infection,[38] Guillain-Barré syndrome, acute intermittent porphyria, autonomic neuropathy, hypothalamic sarcoidosis, post-transsphenoidal pituitary surgery[39,40]

  B. Drugs
    1. Intravenous cyclophosphamide (increased sensitivity may also contribute)[41-56]
    2. Carbamazepine (though increased sensitivity is probably important)[44,45]
    3. Vincristine or vinblastine[46,47]
    4. Thiothixene[48]
    5. Thioridazine[49]
    6. Haloperidol[50]
    7. Amitriptyline[51]
    8. Fluoxetine or sertraline[52-54]
    9. Monoamine oxidase inhibitors[55]
    10. Bromocriptine[56]
    11. Lorcainide[57]

  C. Pulmonary disease
    1. Pneumonia[a]: viral, bacterial, or fungal[58,59]
    2. Tuberculosis[60,61]
    3. Acute respiratory failure[62]
    4. Other: asthma, atelectasis, pneumothorax[58,63]

  D. Postoperative patient[58,64,65] [a]

  E. Severe nausea[66,67]

  F. Idiopathic[68]

Ectopic (nonhypothalamic) production of ADH

  A. Carcinoma: small cell of lung,[a] bronchogenic, duodenum, pancreas, thymus, olfactory neuroblastoma[69-72]

Potentiation of ADH effect

  A. Chlorpropamide[73-77]
  B. Carbamazepine[78-81]
  C. Psychosis[37]
  D. Intravenous cyclophosphamide[42]
  E. Tolbutamide[63]

Exogenous administration of ADH

  A. Vasopressin[82,83]
  B. Oxytocin[84-86]

Possible production of another antidiuretic compound (or increased sensitivity to very low levels of ADH)

  A. Prolactinoma[87]
  B. Waldenstrom's macroglobulinemia[88]

---

[a] Most common causes.

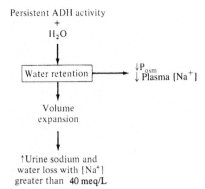

Persistent ADH activity
+
H_2O

Water retention ⟶ $\downarrow P_{osm}$
$\downarrow$ Plasma $[Na^+]$

Volume
expansion

↑Urine sodium and
water loss with $[Na^+]$
greater than **40 meq/L**

Figure 23-3 Pathophysiology of hyponatremia in the syndrome of inappropriate ADH secretion.

chronic SIADH, sodium loss is as or more prominent than water retention. Severe hyponatremia may also be associated with potassium loss; since potassium is as osmotically active as sodium, the loss of potassium can contribute to the reductions in the plasma osmolality and sodium concentration.[90] This potassium is derived from the cells and probably represents part of the volume regulatory response. Cells that increase in size as a result of water entry in hyponatremia lose potassium and other solutes in an attempt to restore cell volume (see "Symptoms," below).

If the levels of ADH release and Na^+ and water intake remain relatively constant, a new steady state will be reached within 1 to 2 weeks in which *Na^+ excretion is equal to intake* (resulting in a urine Na^+ concentration that is typically above 40 meq/L), the *plasma Na^+ concentration is reduced, due both to water retention and to Na^+ loss,*[90,92]* *and the *degree of hyponatremia is stable,* as water intake and excretion are also equal.[93,94] A further reduction in the plasma Na^+ concentration will occur only if there is an increase in either the secretion of ADH or water intake.

The stabilization of the plasma Na^+ concentration in this setting is associated with a reduction in the urine osmolality that appears to reflect partial resistance of the collecting tubules to ADH.[93,94] This escape from ADH-induced antidiuresis appears to be mediated by decreased expression of aquaporin-2, the ADH-sensitive water channel in the collecting tubules;[97,98] the regulation of aquaporin-2 in this setting appears to be unrelated to plasma or tissue osmolality.[98]

It is important to emphasize that the ingestion of water is an essential step in the development of hyponatremia in SIADH. If water intake is restricted, water retention and Na^+ loss do not occur, and *there is no fall in the plasma Na^+ concentration.*[89,93]

---

* It has been suggested that Na^+ movement into the cells, where it becomes bound and osmotically inactive, might also contribute to the reduction in the plasma Na^+ concentration in SIADH.[95] This hypothesis, however, is unproven, and it is likely that water retention and Na^+ loss are sufficient to explain the hyponatremia in most cases.[92,96]

ADH secretion Although it might be thought that ADH is secreted at random in SIADH, this occurs in only a minority of patients, as four distinct patterns of ADH release have been identified (Fig. 23-4). Furthermore, no correlation can be made between these patterns and the underlying cause of SIADH.[20]

- Type A is characterized by erratic changes in ADH secretion that are independent of the P_{osm}. In this setting, ADH release is occurring randomly or in response to volume stimuli, as all osmotic regulation appears to be lost.
- Type B represents a "reset osmostat," in which ADH secretion varies appropriately with the P_{osm}, but the curve is shifted leftward (see "Reset Osmostat," below). In this situation, the plasma Na^+ concentration is relatively stable (usually between 125 and 130 meq/L), the urine can be appropriately diluted after a water load, and progressive hyponatremia does not occur.
- Type C is characterized by normal ADH release when the P_{osm} is normal or elevated but an inability to reduce ADH secretion below a certain level with a water load. This defect reflects selective loss of the ability of hypoosmolality to suppress ADH release.
- Type D is the least common, being associated with normal ADH secretion. Either increased sensitivity to ADH (as occurs, for example, with chlorpropamide)[75-77] or some other antidiuretic factor must be present in these patients.[87]

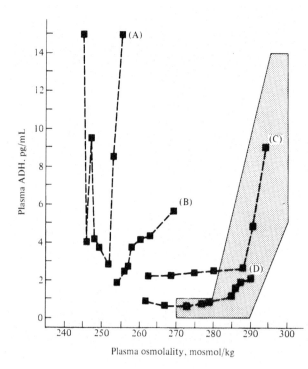

Figure 23-4 The relationship between plasma ADH levels and plasma osmolality in patients with SIADH. The plasma osmolality is increased in these initially hypoosmolar patients by the administration of hypertonic saline. The shaded area represents the normal range. (*From Robertson GL, Shelton RL, Athar S*, Kidney Int *10:25, 1976. Reprinted by permission from* Kidney International.)

Plasma ADH. pg/mL

Plasma osmolality, mosmol/kg

Acid-base and K$^+$ balance   Although the retention of water lowers the plasma Na$^+$ concentration by dilution, it does not reduce either the plasma HCO$_3^-$ concentration or, in most cases, the plasma K$^+$ concentration.[89] The maintenance of acid-base balance in the face of hypotonic volume expansion appears to be mediated both by the movement of H$^+$ ions into cells[99,100] and by increased renal H$^+$ excretion,[101] both of which prevent a dilutional fall in the plasma HCO$_3^-$ concentration. To the degree that a dilutional acidosis does at first occur, this effect will be minimized by the entry of excess H$^+$ ions into the cells, where they combine with the cell buffers.[99,100] The associated increase in urinary H$^+$ excretion[101] may reflect direct stimulation of distal H$^+$ secretion by ADH.[102]

Dilutional hypokalemia is prevented in SIADH primarily by the movement of K$^+$ out of the cells. Some of this K$^+$ transport may reflect a transcellular cation exchange, since electroneutrality must be maintained as H$^+$ ions enter the cells to be buffered.[99] However, renal K$^+$ excretion may increase and mild hypokalemia may ensue if the P$_{osm}$ falls below 240 mosmol/kg (plasma Na$^+$ concentration less than 115 meq/L).[101] A hyponatremia-induced elevation of aldosterone secretion may contribute to this process.[103,104]

Etiology   SIADH can be produced by enhanced hypothalamic secretion, ectopic (nonhypothalamic) hormone production, the potentiation of ADH effect, or the administration of exogenous ADH or oxytocin (Table 23-3). A variety of *neuropsychiatric disorders* can promote ADH release, either directly or by activation of cortical neurons that can stimulate the hypothalamus.[37,89,105] As examples, SIADH may occur in over 20 percent of patients with a subarachnoid hemorrhage[106] and in 20 to 35 percent of patients after transsphenoidal pituitary surgery [in whom adrenal insufficiency due to impaired adrenocorticotropic hormone (ACTH) release may also contribute].[39,40] In psychotic patients, on the other hand, there is often a more complex derangement in water handling, as ADH release, the renal response to ADH, and water intake all may be increased.[37,107]

Hyponatremia is also seen in up to 40 percent of patients with human immunodeficiency virus infection.[38] Volume depletion and adrenal insufficiency are responsible in some cases, but most patients appear to have SIADH.[38,108] *Pneumocystis carinii* pneumonia, malignancy, and central nervous system disease all may play a role.

Although *drugs* can cause SIADH, most of the agents listed in Table 23-3 are only rarely associated with the development of hyponatremia.[109] There are, however, certain drugs that deserve emphasis. Particular care must be taken with cyclophosphamide, an alkylating agent that can increase the sensitivity to ADH and perhaps its release when given intravenously in high doses, but not when taken orally in low doses.[41-43] A high fluid intake is generally recommended in order to limit drug contact with the bladder and prevent the development of hermorrhagic cystitis. However, the combination of increased ADH effect and enhanced water intake can lead to *severe, occasionally fatal hyponatremia* within 24 h.[41,43] This complication can be minimized by using isotonic saline rather than water to maintain a high urine output.

Chlorpropamide, an oral hypoglycemic agent that is now rarely used, is the most predictable cause of drug-induced SIADH. When used in diabetes mellitus, it lowers the plasma Na^+ concentration in roughly 4 to 6 percent of patients.[73,74] This problem is most likely to occur in patients over the age of 60 who are also taking a thiazide diuretic.[74] Some other hypoglycemic drugs, such as tolazamide and acetohexamide, have opposite effects, as they induce a small *increase* in water excretion (by an unknown mechanism).[110]

Chlorpropamide appears to act primarily by potentiating the effect of ADH, not by enhancing its secretion.[75-77] How this occurs is incompletely understood. In experimental animals, chlorpropamide directly increases NaCl reabsorption in the medullary thick ascending limb, an effect that would enhance medullary interstitial osmolality and therefore the ability of ADH to raise the U_{osm}.[76,77] It has also been proposed that chlorpropamide may act directly on the collecting tubule cells, increasing water permeability via an effect that is independent of ADH; how this might occur is not known.[111]

Although chlorpropamide increases the action of ADH, some circulating ADH must be present for this potentiation to occur.[77] As depicted in Fig. 23-1, some normal subjects maintain low basal levels of ADH ($< 2\,pg/mL$) despite the presence of hypoosmolality; it is possible that it is these individuals who are most likely to become hyponatremic with chlorpropamide.[73] The concurrent use of another drug that increases ADH secretion (such as a thiazide diuretic) will also increase the risk of hyponatremia.[73,112]

Nonsteroidal anti-inflammatory drugs also can potentiate the effect of ADH. This is mediated by a reduction in renal prostaglandin synthesis, since prostaglandins normally antagonize the action of ADH (see page 172). Despite this effect, spontaneous hyponatremia is a rare event, probably because ADH secretion is reduced, either because of a direct effect of prostaglandin synthesis inhibition[113] or because of the initial fall in P_{osm} if some water is retained. These agents may, however, exacerbate the tendency to hyponatremia in patients who are volume-depleted or have SIADH.

Pulmonary diseases—particularly pneumonia but including acute asthma, atelectasis, empyema, pneumothorax, tuberculosis, and acute respiratory failure—can lead to SIADH.[58-63] The mechanism by which this occurs is uncertain, but a decrease in pulmonary venous return, leading to activation of the volume receptors, may be involved;[114] the finding of a low urine Na^+ concentration in some patients is compatible with this hypothesis.[59,115]

Pulmonary disease also may in some way increase central release of ADH. This has been best documented in tuberculosis, where many patients have a reset osmostat pattern. Furthermore, ethanol has been shown to increase water excretion, presumably by inhibiting the hypothalamic secretion of ADH.[60,61]

In the patient who has undergone *major surgery*, inappropriate ADH secretion is common and persists for 2 to 5 days.[58,64] This response appears to be mediated by pain afferents that directly stimulate the hypothalamus.[65] An additional mechanism may also be operative in patients undergoing mitral commissurotomy to relieve mitral stenosis; in this setting, the acute reduction in left atrial pressure may activate the atrial volume receptors and contribute to enhanced ADH release.[116]

Ectopic tumor production of ADH has been reported with a variety of different neoplasms, particularly small cell (oat cell) carcinoma of the lung (Table 23-3). Direct evidence for tumor hormonal synthesis has come from the demonstration that these tumors contain and can synthesize both ADH and its carrier neurophysin, which are derived from a common precursor.[69-72]

Oxytocin is a second hormone synthesized in the hypothalamus and released from the neurohypophysis. Its primary effects are on uterine function and lactation, but oxytocin also possesses significantly antidiuretic activity. The use of intravenous infusions of this hormone in dextrose and water to stimulate labor in pregnant women has resulted in water retention, severe hyponatremia, and seizures in both the mother and the fetus.[84-86] This complication can be prevented by limiting the amount of water given and using isotonic saline rather than dextrose and water. Hyponatremia can also be induced by the administration of exogenous ADH to control gastrointestinal bleeding or dDAVP for polyuria in central diabetes insipidus or bleeding due to platelet dysfunction (see Chap. 24).[82,83]

Rarely, no cause for SIADH can be identified.[68] Although some of these patients have remained idiopathic for many years, careful and repeated monitoring for the presence of an occult tumor (particularly pulmonary) is essential.[68,71] In addition, temporal arteritis should be considered in elderly patients with an otherwise unexplained elevation in the erythrocyte sedimentation rate.[117]

In summary, SIADH can be produced by a variety of disorders. It is characterized by the following features: (1) hyponatremia and hypoosmolality; (2) a U_{osm} that is inappropriately high (greater than 100 mosmol/kg); (3) a urine Na^+ concentration greater than 40 meq/L, unless the patient is volume-depleted for some other reason; (4) normovolemia; (5) normal renal, adrenal, and thyroid function; and (6) normal acid-base and K^+ balance.

Another frequent, although not pathognomonic, finding is hypouricemia due to enhanced urinary urate excretion.[118] The initial volume expansion induced by water retention may reduce proximal Na^+ and urate reabsorption. In comparison, sodium and urate reabsorption are enhanced and hyperuricemia is common in hyponatremic patients who are effectively volume-depleted.

Cerebral Salt Wasting

Rarely, patients with cerebral disease (most often subarachnoid hemorrhage) develop hyponatremia with all of the other associated findings of SIADH (including hypouricemia), except that they are volume-depleted and the high urine Na^+ concentration is due to urinary Na^+ wasting, not volume expansion.[119-123]

The etiology of this cerebral salt-wasting syndrome is incompletely understood. One possibility is the release of a hormone from the damaged brain that causes both salt and urate wasting.[124] Brain natriuretic peptide may be such a hormone. One study prospectively evaluated 10 patients with aneurysmal subarachnoid hemorrhage and compared them to 10 patients undergoing elective cra-niotomy for cerebral tumors and 40 controls.[123] The patients with subarachnoid hemorrhage had increases in the mean plasma concentration of brain natriuretic peptide. The plasma concentration of atrial natriuretic peptide was normal, while that of aldosterone was reduced in the patients with subarachnoid hemorrhage. The fall in aldosterone may have been mediated in part by the natriuretic peptides.

Adrenal Insufficiency

Hyponatremia is a common complication of adrenal insufficiency. Although volume depletion due to diarrhea, vomiting, or renal Na^+ loss (resulting from marked lack of aldosterone) may contribute to the fall in the plasma Na^+ con-centration,[125] *cortisol deficiency* appears to play a major role, as cortisol replace-ment rapidly increases the rate of water excretion and raises the plasma Na^+ concentration toward normal.[126-128]

The deleterious effect of cortisol deficiency is largely related to increased release of ADH, as evidenced by the ability of an ADH antagonist to almost completely reverse the defect in water excretion.[13] The hypersecretion of ADH in this setting is in part due to effective volume depletion, since the systemic blood pressure, cardiac output, and ultimately renal blood flow are reduced by an unknown mechanism.[129] In addition, ADH is an important ACTH secretagogue that is cosecreted with corticotropin releasing hormone (CRH) by the cells in the paraventricular nucleus.[130-132] Thus, cortisol feeds back negatively on both CRH and ADH release, an inhibitory effect that is removed with cortisol insufficiency.[130,133]

Hypothyroidism

Significant hyponatremia is an unusual complication of hypothyroidism. Why this occurs is not well understood. The cardiac output and GFR are frequently reduced in such patients,[134,135] changes that can lead both to the release of ADH and to diminished delivery to the diluting segments.[134-138] The latter may be particularly important in those patients in whom hyponatremia has led to appropriate suppression of ADH release.[137] Normal water balance can be restored by the administration of thyroid hormone.

Reset Osmostat

As described above, patients with a reset osmostat have normal osmoreceptor responses to changes in the P_{osm}, but the threshold for ADH release (and usually thirst) is reduced (Fig. 23-4, pattern B).[20] As a result, the *plasma Na^+ concentration is below normal but stable* (usually between 125 and 130 meq/L), since the ability to excrete water is maintained.

Patients with a reset osmostat fulfill all the criteria for SIADH, and the only clue to the diagnosis is the presence of stable mild hyponatremia.[20] A reset osmostat has also been described in a number of particular settings. These include hypovolemic states (in which the baroreceptor stimulus to ADH release is superimposed upon normal osmoreceptor function; see Fig. 6-10),[20] quadriplegia (in which effective volume depletion may be induced by venous pooling in the legs),[139] psychosis,[140] and chronic malnutrition.[141] In the last setting, defective cellular metabolism may be responsible for the abnormal osmoreceptor function. Correction of the underlying problem and hyperaliminentation have been effective in returning the plasma Na^+ concentration toward normal.[141]

A reset osmostat is also present in almost all *pregnant women*, in whom the plasma Na^+ concentration falls by about 5 meq/L.[142,143] This change occurs within the first 2 months of pregnancy and is then stable until delivery. Increased secretion of human chronic gonadotropin (hCG) may play a central role in this response,[142,143] perhaps acting via the release of the ovarian hormone relaxin.[144]

It has been proposed that these hormonal changes may directly affect the osmoreceptor or may act directly by contributing to the systemic vasodilatation of pregnancy, thereby inducing relative volume depletion. Two observations in experimental animals and in women suggest a direct action on the osmoreceptor: (1) Persistent volume expansion during pregnancy does not raise the plasma Na^+ concentration, as would be expected if hypovolemia were involved; and (2) the administration of hCG to normal women during the luteal phase of the menstrual cycle[145,146] or the chronic administration of relaxin to rats[144] can lower the plasma Na^+ concentration and reset the thresholds for ADH release and thirst despite maintenance of a high-Na^+ diet.

Primary Polydipsia

Patients with primary polydipsia have a primary increase in water intake and typically complain of polyuria or excessive thirst. This disorder is particularly prevalent in psychosis, affecting as many as 7 percent of patients with schizophrenia.[37,147,148] Many of these patients have an exaggerated weight gain during the day (due to transient retention of some of the excess water). In addition to the underlying psychosis, the sensation of a dry mouth in patients taking phenothiazines may contribute to the increase in water intake.[149] Primarily polydipsia may also occur with hypothalamic disorders (such as sarcoidosis), in which the regulation of thirst may be directly affected.[150]

It is presumed that a *central defect in thirst regulation* plays an important role in the pathogenesis of polydipsia.[29,148] In some cases, for example, the osmotic threshold for thirst is reduced *below* the threshold for the release of ADH.[151]

The plasma Na^+ concentration is usually normal or only slight reduced in this disorder, since the excess water can be readily excreted.[147,152] In rare instances, however, water intake exceeds 10 to 15 L/day and overwhelms renal excretory capacity, resulting in potentially fatal hyponatremia.[147-149,153-156] One patient, for example, was able to lower her plasma Na^+ concentration to 84 meq/L, even though her GFR was normal and her urine was maximally dilute (U_{osm} equal to 74 mosmol/kg, specific gravity of 1.001).[153] Symptomatic hyponatremia can also be induced by an acute 3- to 4-liter water load in anxious patients, as has been rarely reported prior to a radiologic examination or urine drug testing.[157]

The tendency to hyponatremia in patients with primary polydipsia is increased if there is a concurrent impairment in water excretion. This combination can be seen in patients who are also taking a diuretic;[30,156] in psychotic patients, in whom the underlying cerebral dysfunction and, in selected cases, antipsychotic drugs (listed in Table 23-3) can lead to increased ADH release as well as enhanced water intake;[37,158] or with nausea- or stress-induced ADH secretion.[157]

Another interesting example of this phenomenon has been described in drinkers of beer in excessive amounts, in whom the ability to excrete water is reduced by *poor dietary intake*.[159] A normal subject may excrete 750 mosmol/day of solute, consisting mostly of NaCl, KCl, NH_4Cl, and urea (which is derived from the metabolism of proteins). If the minimum U_{osm} is 50 mosmol/kg, then the maximum daily urine volume will be 15 liters: 750 mosmol/day ÷ 50 mosmol/kg = 15 L/day. However, the daily solute load can fall to 250 mosmol or less in beer drinkers, who may ingest only small amounts of Na^+, K^+, and protein. In this setting, the maximum urine volume is only 5 liters (250 ÷ 50 = 5 L/day), and hyponatremia will ensue if more than this amount of fluid (primarily as beer) is ingested.

Pseudohyponatremia

In some patients, a decrease in the plasma Na^+ concentration is associated with a normal or increased effective P_{osm}, rather than with hypoosmolality. This has been called pseudohyponatremia (Table 23-4).[160] These disorders highlight the importance of measuring the P_{osm} in patients with hyponatremia, since *therapy should generally not be directed toward the fall in the plasma Na^+ concentration*.

Hyponatremia with normal P_{osm}

A fall in the plasma Na^+ concentration without change in the P_{osm} can occur when there is a reduction in the fraction of plasma that is composed of the plasma

Table 23-4   Etiology of pseudohyponatremia

Low plasma Na^+ concentration with normal P_{osm}
  A. Severe hyperlipidemia
  B. Severe hyperproteinemia
  C. Post-transurethral resection of prostate or bladder or ultrasonic lithotripsy
Low plasma Na^+ concentration with elevated P_{osm}
  A. Hyperglycemia
  B. Administration of hypertonic mannitol
  C. Administration of intravenous immune globulin with maltose accumulation in patients with renal failure

water; this is the classic form of pseudohyponatremia. Each liter of plasma normally contains about 930 mL of water, with the plasma proteins and lipids occupying the remaining 70 mL. However, the plasma water may fall to as low as 720 mL per liter of plasma in states of severe hyperlipidemia (as in uncontrolled diabetes mellitus) or hyperproteinemia (as in multiple myeloma).[160-162] The P_{osm} will be unaffected in this setting, since the lipids exist in a separate phase and an osmometer measures only the activity of the plasma water.* However, the plasma Na^+ concentration, *measured per liter of plasma, not of plasma water*, will be artifactually reduced to 110 meq/L (154 meq/L of plasma water × 0.72 liter of plasma water per liter of plasma).

This form of pseudohyponatremia, which requires no therapy related to the hyponatremia, is easily diagnosed by the presence of lactescent serum (with hyperlipidemia) and a normal P_{osm}. Use of an ion-selective electrode, rather than a flame photometer, may confirm that the plasma water Na^+ concentration is normal. However, even this modality may not be accurate if the plasma or serum specimen is diluted, because a 1:100 dilution of the total plasma will produce more than a 1:100 dilution of the plasma water.[160] Suppose, for example, that the plasma water (with a Na^+ concentration of 150 meq/L) is 80 percent of the plasma; in this setting, each liter of plasma will have 120 meq of Na^+. If this is now diluted to a total volume of 100 liters, there will be only 120 meq of Na^+ present and, correcting for dilution, the true Na^+ concentration will appear to be 120 meq/L.

Isosmotic or slightly hypoosmotic reduction in the plasma Na^+ concentration also can occur in patients undergoing transurethral resection of the prostate or bladder. These procedures may be associated with the use of as much as 20 to 30 liters of nonconductive flushing solutions containing glycine, sorbitol, or mannitol[163-165] Variable quantities of this fluid are absorbed, both by entry into damaged blood vessels and by leakage into the retroperitoneal space. Some patients absorb 3 liters or more, leading to a dilutional reduction in the plasma Na^+ concentration, which may fall below 100 meq/L. A similar problem can occur with the use of glycine-containing irrigation solutions during hysteroscopic surgery in women.[166,167]

The incidence of hyponatremia following transurethral resection has been reported to be approximately 7 percent.[168] Risk factors include prolonged surgery, large tissue resection, and excess height of the reservoir of the irrigant solution, which is therefore introduced under high pressure.[163,164]

The degree of hyponatremia is related to both the quantity of fluid absorbed and the rate of absorption. Severe hyponatremia generally requires a rate of fluid absorption in excess of 200 mL/10 min. The fall in the plasma sodium concentration is greatest when the fluid is first absorbed and is limited to the extracellular

---

* Proteins make only a minimal contribution to the P_{osm}, because they are very large molecules. The normal plasma protein concentration of 7 g/dL (or 70 g/L), for example, represents only 1.3 mosmol/kg. Thus, doubling the plasma protein concentration will produce a minimal increase in osmolality but will reduce the fraction of plasma that is water and therefore will lower the measured plasma Na^+ concentration

space. Within a few minutes, however, the plasma sodium concentration begins to rise even before the fluid is excreted, probably because of glycine and water entry into the cells.[166] At 2 to 4 h, glycine is almost equally distributed between the extracellular and intracellular compartments. At this time, glycine is acting as an ineffective osmole, raising the plasma osmolality (similar to the effect of urea in renal failure) without affecting water distribution between the fluid compartments.[166] This degree of hyponatremia represents true hyponatremia even though the plasma osmolality is usually near normal.

The plasma osmolality in these patients is variable.[166] The mannitol solution is isosmotic, whereas both the glycine and sorbitol solutions have an osmolality between 165 and 200 mosmol/kg.[164] Thus, the initial plasma osmolality will be normal or only modestly reduced.[163-165] However, both glycine and sorbitol are rapidly metabolized and also may be excreted in the urine, leaving free water behind. As a result, there will be a tendency for the plasma osmolality to fall unless the rate of excretion of the excess fluid is at least equal to the rate of solute metabolism and excretion.

Confusion, disorientation, twitching, seizures, and hypotension all may be seen in these patients, although why these symptoms occur is not clear. The very low plasma sodium concentration itself, the varying degree of hypoosmolality, glycine toxicity, and the accumulation of ammonia (from the metabolism of glycine) all may contribute in individual patients.[163-165,169] Experimental studies suggest that hypoosmolality may not be of primary importance, since the outcome is not improved by preventing the fall in plasma osmolality with mannitol.[170]

The diagnosis of this disorder is strongly suggested from the clinical history and can be confirmed early in the course by documenting the presence of an osmolal gap, which is the difference between the plasma osmolality measured in the laboratory and the plasma osmolality calculated from the following formula (see page 247):

$$\text{Calculated } P_{osm} = 2 \times \text{plasma Na} + \frac{[\text{glucose}]}{18} + \frac{\text{BUN}}{2.8}$$

There is little if any osmolal gap in normal subjects, as there is usually a close correlation between the measured and calculated values. In comparison, the osmolal gap can exceed 30 to 60 mosmol/kg following transurethral resection as a result of the accumulation of glycine, sorbitol, or mannitol.[164,165] The osmolal gap is also increased when there is a disparity between the P_{osm} and the plasma Na^+ concentration with hyperlipidemia, hyperproteinemia, or the administration of mannitol (see below). Other drugs, such as ethanol, methanol, and ethylene glycol, also can achieve significant osmolal concentrations in the blood, resulting in an osmolal gap (see page 607). However, these alcohols are ineffective osmoles (like urea) and do not affect water distribution or the plasma Na^+ concentration.[171]

Optimal therapy of *symptomatic* hyponatremia following transurethral resection or hysteroscopy is unclear. Hypertonic saline can be given if the plasma osmolality is reduced, but it has an uncertain role when the plasma osmolality is in the normal range.[163] The benefits of raising the plasma Na^+ concentration in this setting may be counterbalanced by a rise in the plasma osmolality above normal. Hemodialysis has been used in patients with end-stage renal disease who have no other means to excrete the excess solute and water.[165] In comparison, no specific therapy is necessary in the absence of symptoms. Renal excretion of the excess fluid and metabolism and excretion of the excess solute will rapidly correct the hyponatremia as long as renal function is near normal.

Hyponatremia with increased P_{osm}   If a solute that penetrates cells poorly, such as glucose, is added to the extracellular fluid, the P_{osm} will rise. This will create a transcellular osmotic gradient, resulting in water movement out of the cells and a reduction in the plasma Na^+ concentration by dilution (see Fig. 22-1e). Conversely, as insulin therapy drives glucose into the cells, water will follow, and the plasma Na^+ concentration will rise.

Physiologic calculations suggest that the plasma sodium concentration should fall by 1 meq/L for every 62-mg/dL (3.5-mmol/L) rise in the plasma concentration of glucose or mannitol (which have the same molecular weight).[172] However, this standard correction factor was not verified experimentally. In an attempt to address this issue, hyperglycemia was induced in six healthy subjects by the administration of somatostatin (to block endogenous insulin secretion) and a hypertonic dextrose solution.[173] A nonlinear relationship was observed between the changes in the glucose and sodium concentrations. The 1 : 62 ratio applied when the plasma glucose concentration was less than 400 mg/dL. At higher glucose concentrations, there was greater reduction in the plasma sodium concentration. An overall ratio of 1 : 42 (a 2.4-meq/L reduction in the plasma sodium concentration for every 100-mg/dL elevation in the plasma glucose) provided a better estimate of this association than the usual 1 : 62 ratio.

Two other causes of hyponatremia with an increased P_{osm} are the administration of hypertonic mannitol and of intravenous immune globulin.[174,175] Although measurement of the plasma mannitol concentration is not available in most laboratories, the presence of significant amounts of mannitol in the blood can be estimated from calculation of the osmolal gap. Intravenous immune globulin is often given in a 10 percent maltose solution. Maltose is normally metabolized by maltase in the proximal tubule. In patients with renal failure, however, maltose can accumulate in the extracellular fluid, raising the plasma osmolality and lowering the plasma sodium concentration by dilution.[175]

Hyponatremia and azotemia   Patients with renal failure have a high P_{osm} as a result of the increase in the BUN. However, urea is an ineffective osmole, and the effective P_{osm} ($2 \times$ plasma $[Na^+] + [glucose]/18$) is generally normal or reduced. As an example, consider a patient with the following plasma values:

$$\text{Plasma } [Na^+] = 115 \, meq/L$$
$$[Glucose] = 90 \, mg/dL$$
$$BUN = 140 \, mg/dL$$
$$P_{osm} = 285 \, mosmol/kg$$

Despite the normal P_{osm}, the effective P_{osm} is markedly reduced at 235 mosmol/kg. Thus, this patient has true hyponatremia, not pseudohyponatremia, and may become symptomatic.

SYMPTOMS

The symptoms directly attributable to true hyponatremia primarily reflect *neurologic dysfunction induced by hypoosmolality*.[176-178] As the P_{osm} falls, an osmolal gradient is created across the blood-brain barrier, resulting in water movement into the brain (as well as into other cells). The degree of cerebral overhydration appears to correlate with the severity of symptoms. As depicted in Fig. 23-5, a rapid reduction in the plasma Na^+ concentration to 119 meq/L in rabbits produces a marked increase in brain water content, severe symptoms, and death. In comparison, a similar degree of slowly developing hyponatremia results in a lesser degree of cerebral edema and a lesser likelihood of neurologic symptoms.[176,178,179]

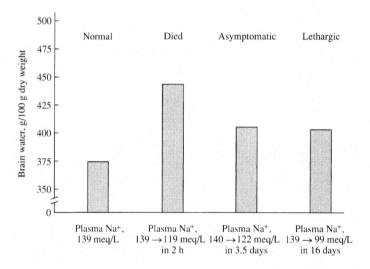

Figure 23-5 Brain water content in normal and three groups of hyponatremic rabbits. When the plasma Na^+ concentration is acutely lowered to 119 meq/L in 2 h, brain water content increases to 17 percent above normal and is associated with severe symptoms and death. In contrast, slowly lowering the plasma Na^+ concentration to the same level over $3\frac{1}{2}$ days results in a smaller elevation in brain water (7 percent) and no symptoms. Finally, gradually reducing the plasma Na^+ concentration to extremely low levels (99 meq/L) produces a small increment in brain water and only mild neurologic symptoms. (*From Arieff AI, Llach F, Massry SG, Medicine 55:121, 1976, with permission.*)

The mechanism of osmotic water movement into the brain has been partially elucidated by studies in mice without the genes for aquaporin-4, a water channel expressed at the interface between the brain and blood, and between the brain and cerebrospinal fluid.[180] Compared with wild-type mice, knockout mice exhibit considerably less brain edema, morbidity, and mortality after the induction of acute hyponatremia, suggesting that aquaporin-4 mediates a substantial portion of osmotic water transport into the brain.

Osmotic Adaptation

The adaptation to hyponatremia depicted in Fig. 23-5 involves two steps. First, the initial cerebral edema elevates the hydrostatic pressure in the cerebral interstitial fluid. This creates a favorable gradient for fluid movement from the cerebral interstitium into the cerebrospinal fluid, thereby decreasing the amount of cerebral swelling.[178,181]

Second, solutes move out of the cells, since a net decrease in cell osmolality promotes osmotic water loss, thereby diminishing cell swelling.[178,182-184] The initial cellular adaptation consists of the loss of K^+ and Na^+, processes that occur quickly via the activation of quiescent channels in the cell membrane.[178] This is followed over a period of hours to days by the loss of organic solutes such as myoinositol and the amino acids glutamine, glutamate, and taurine.[182-184] A report in humans using proton nuclear magnetic resonance (NMR) spectroscopy found a somewhat different pattern, with myoinositol and choline compounds being the primary organic solutes lost.[185] (Myoinositol appears to be the primary osmolyte *taken up* by the brain as part of the protective response in patients with hypernatremia.)

As shown in Fig. 23-6, these solutes (called *osmolytes*) account for approximately one-third of the cell solute loss in chronic hyponatremia.[182,183] Furthermore, the degree of osmolyte loss is directly related to the severity of the hyponatermia.[184]

Although there is a quantitatively greater loss of cation than of osmolyte, the percentage loss of these solutes is very different: less than 10 percent for K^+ plus Na^+ versus approximately 60 percent for the osmolytes. This observation suggests a specific function for the osmolytes. In addition to maintaining cell volume, osmolytes have the advantage of *not interfering* with protein function, in contrast to the potentially deleterious effects of large changes in the cellular K^+ plus Na^+ concentration.[186] Thus, osmolyte loss is a specific response of the cell that occurs more slowly than cation loss because the synthesis of new transporters is required.[178] (Similar changes, although in the opposite direction, occur in hypernatremia; see Chap. 24.)

The net effect of the osmotic adaptation is that the severity of neurologic symptoms is related to the *rapidity as well as the degree of the reduction in the plasma Na^+ concentration.*[177,187-189] The changes induced by acute hyponatremia (developing over 1 to 3 days) may result in permanent neurologic damage and are primarily due to cerebral overhydration. This problem is most likely to occur in

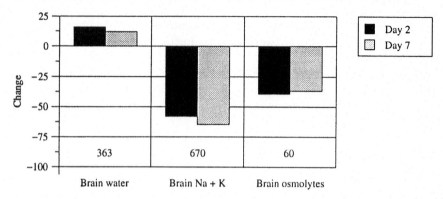

Figure 23-6   Changes in brain water, sodium plus potassium content, and three organic solutes—inositol, glutamine, and taurine—after onset of severe hyponatremia in rats (plasma sodium concentration less than 110 meq/L). The numbers at the bottom represent the baseline values. The return of brain water toward normal at day 7 is due to loss of sodium, potassium, and the organic solutes (called osmolytes). Although the absolute osmolyte loss is less than that of sodium plus potassium, the fractional loss is much greater—36 or 60, or 60 percent, versus 60 or 670, or less than 10 percent. (*Data from Verbalis JG, Gullans SR, Brain Res 567:274, 1991, with permission.*)

postoperative patients given large quantities of hypotonic fluid or those with acute thiazide-induced hyponatremia.[27,177,190,191]

In comparison, symptoms are unusual in chronic hyponatremia unless there is a marked reduction in the plasma Na^+ concentration. The findings in this setting appear to be mediated by the low plasma Na^+ concentration (rather than by cerebral edema), perhaps reflecting the importance of Na^+ in neural function. This is illustrated in the far right panel in Fig. 23-5 and may also account for some of the neurologic findings in glycine-induced hyponatremia.[163]

Neurologic Abnormalities

The neurologic symptoms induced by hyponatremia are similar to those in other metabolic encephalopathies.[27,176,177,187] In general, the patient begins to complain of nausea and malaise as the plasma Na^+ concentration falls acutely below 125 meq/L. Between 115 and 120 meq/L, headache, lethargy, and obtundation may appear, although many patients with chronic hyponatremia will have few if any symptoms. The more severe changes of seizures and coma are not usually seen until the plasma Na^+ concentration is less than 110 to 115 meq/L.[27,177,184,185] Focal neurologic findings are uncommon but may occur in patients with an underlying defect such as an old cerebral infarct.[193]*

---

* When SIADH is due to a central nervous system disorder, it may be difficult to determine whether the neurologic disease or the low plasma Na^+ concentration is reponsible for the symptoms. The inciting factor can be assessed more accurately by observing the response to correction of the hyponatremia.

There is substantial interpatient variability in the susceptibility to symptoms from acute hyponatremia. For reasons that may be related to differences in cerebral metabolism,[194] *women, particularly premenopausal women,* appear to be at much greater risk of developing severe neurologic symptoms and of irreversible neurologic damage than men.[190] The possibility that sex hormones are an important determinant of risk is also supported by the absence of a gender difference in the risk of symptomatic hyponatremia in prepubertal children.[195]

Acute, symptomatic hyponatremia can lead to permanent neurologic deficits or death.[27,177,190] In one series, for example, 15 previously healthy young women with postoperative SIADH were given an excessive quantity of intravenous water. The net result was a reduction in the plasma Na^+ concentration from 138 to 108 meq/L over a 48-h period; 4 of the women died, and the remainder had permanent neurologic deficits (Fig. 23-7).[177] A more recent study suggests that the majority of premenopausal women who develop symptomatic hyponatremia do not fully recover; thus, prevention is of primary importance.[190] In comparison, the symptoms are more often reversible in men.

There is an additional mechanism that may cause neurologic symptoms in the patient with hyponatremia: *overly rapid elevation* of the plasma Na^+ concentration. This issue will be discussed below, in the section on treatment.

When volume depletion is present, patients may also complain of the symptoms of hypovolemia, such as weakness, fatigue, muscle cramps, and postural dizziness (see Chap. 14). In contrast, signs of extracellular volume expansion such as edema are not seen in patients with water retention due to SIADH or primary polydipsia, since roughly two-thirds of the retained water is stored in the cells and persistent hypervolemia is prevented by increased Na^+ and water excretion, as Na^+ handling is intact.[89,90,92]

Figure 23-7 Clinical course in 7 women with acute, severe postoperative hyponatremia and seizures and coma. All of the women initially awoke when the plasma Na^+ concentration was raised from 105 to 131 meq/L in 41 h. After a further 58 h, seizures and recurrent coma developed despite maintenance of the plasma Na^+ concentration above 128 meq/L. (*From Arieff AI, New Engl J Med 314:1529, 1986. Reprinted by permission from the* New England Journal of Medicine.)

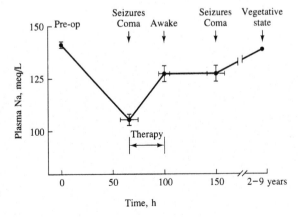

DIAGNOSIS

As with other electrolyte and acid-base disturbances, the history (possibly vomiting, diarrhea, diuretic therapy, or one of the causes of SIADH) and physical examination (perhaps findings of true volume depletion or edema) can provide important clues to the correct diagnosis. In addition, the initial laboratory evaluation should include measurement of the P_{osm}; the plasma concentrations of Na^+, K^+, Cl^-, HCO_3^-, urea, and glucose; the urine Na^+ concentration and osmolality; and, if the HCO_3^- concentration is abnormal, the extracellular pH. Tables 23-5 and 23-6 illustrate how these tests can be used to identify the cause of the hyponatremia.

Plasma Osmolality

The first step in the approach to the patient with hyponatremia is to confirm the presence of hypoosmolality (Table 23-5). If the effective P_{osm} (measured P_{osm} minus BUN/2.8) is normal or elevated, evaluation for one of the causes of pseudohyponatremia should be carried out.

Urine Osmolality

Once it is demonstrated that the patient is hypoosmolal, measurement of the U_{osm} can be used to determine whether water excretion is normal or impaired. A value below 100 mosmol/kg (specific gravity ≤ 1.003) indicates that ADH secretion is almost completely and appropriately suppressed, a finding seen with either primary polydipsia or a reset osmostat (if water intake has reduced the P_{osm} below the new threshold for ADH release). These disorders can be distinguished by the *response to water restriction*. The urine will remain dilute until the plasma

Table 23-5 Major steps in the initial evaluation of hyponatremia

Plasma osmolality
- A. Low: true hyponatremia
- B. Normal or elevated: pseudohyponatremia or renal failure

Urine osmolality
- A. Less than 100 mosmol/kg: primary polydipsia or reset osmostat
- B. Greater than 100 mosmol/kg: other causes of true hyponatremia in which water excretion is impaired

Urine sodium concentration
- A. Less than 25 meq/L: effective circulating volume depletion (including heart failure and hepatic cirrhosis), by dilution in primary polydipsia if the urine output is very high
- B. Greater than 40 meq/L: SIADH, renal failure, reset osmostat, diuretics (when drug still acting), adrenal insufficiency, some patients with vomiting (in whom there is obligatory $NaHCO_3$ loss in the urine; see page 565), osmotic diuretics (with pseudohyponatremia due to glucose or mannitol)

Table 23-6   Acid-base and potassium disturbances in hyponatremia

Metabolic acidosis	Normal pH	Metabolic alkalosis
Plasma K^+ concentration may be normal or elevated	Plasma K^+ concentration usually normal	Plasma K^+ concentration may be normal or reduced
Renal failure	SIADH	Vomiting
Adrenal insufficiency	Primary polydipsia (may see hypokalemia)	Nasogastric suction
	Edematous states (no diuretics)	Diuretics
	Pure cortisol deficiency	
Plasma K^+ concentration may be normal or reduced	Hypothyroidism	
Diarrhea or drainage of intestinal secretions		

Na^+ concentration is normal in primary polydipsia.[155] In contrast, the U_{osm} will rise progressively with a reset osmostat, since a small elevation in the plasma Na^+ concentration will stimulate the release of ADH. By using these criteria, many psychotic patients initially thought to have primarily polydipsia were shown to have a reset osmostat.[140]

In the vast majority of hyponatremic patients, however, water excretion is impaired and the U_{osm} exceeds 100 mosmol/kg. It is important to emphasize that a U_{osm} of 100 to 200 mosmol/kg may be hypoosmotic to plasma but is still inappropriately high. This can be illustrated by a simple example. Raising the U_{osm} from a maximally dilute level of 60 mosmol/kg up to 180 mosmol/kg requires the removal of two-thirds of the water. Thus, a patient with a dilute U_{osm} of 180 mosmol/kg will be able to excrete only one-third the normal amount of free water and, therefore, will be much more likely to develop hyponatremia.

Urine Sodium Concentration

The differential diagnosis of hyponatremia, hypoosmolality, and an inappropriately high U_{osm} usually narrows down to effective circulating volume depletion, SIADH, adrenal insufficiency, and rarely hypothyroidism. In addition to assessment of adrenal and thyroid function, the urine Na^+ concentration is usually helpful in differentiating among these disorders (Table 23-5). The urine Na^+ concentration should be less than 25 meq/L in hypovolemic states, but greater than 40 meq/L in SIADH (where Na^+ excretion is equal to intake), with a reset osmostat, and in Na^+-wasting conditions such as diuretic therapy, renal disease, and adrenal insufficiency.[196] The inappropriate Na^+ losses in the last disorder are due to hypoaldosteronism. In contrast, renal Na^+ handling is normal in pure cortisol deficiency (as seen in hypopituitarism), and the urine Na^+ concentration may be below 25 meq/L.[128]

In those patients in whom the findings are equivocal, the response of the U_{osm} and urine Na^+ concentration to the administration of NaCl can be used to establish the correct diagnosis. This can be illustrated by the following case history:

> **Case history 23-1**   A 49-year-old man with small cell carcinoma of the lung develops severe vomiting after the institution of chemotherapy. On admission, the estimated jugular venous pressure is below $5\,cmH_2O$, the skin turgor is reduced, and the following laboratory tests are obtained:

$$\text{Plasma }[Na^+] = 114\,meq/L$$

$$P_{osm} = 243\,mosmol/kg$$

$$\text{Urine }[Na^+] = 6\,meq/L$$

$$U_{osm} = 498\,mosmol/kg$$

The clinical and laboratory findings are consistent with true volume depletion. It is also possible, however, that the patient has underlying SIADH due to his malignancy. The patient is initially treated with isotonic NaCl, and the next morning the plasma Na^+ concentration has increased to 122 meq/L. At this time, the urine Na^+ concentration and osmolality can be used to distinguish among three possibilities:

- Hypovolemic alone was responsible for the hyponatremia, and the patient is still volume-depleted. As a result, the urine Na^+ concentration will still be low and the U_{osm} still elevated because of the nonosmotic release of ADH.
- Hypovolemia alone was responsible for the hyponatremia, and the patient is now euvolemic. In this setting, the U_{osm} will be below 100 mosmol/kg, since there is no longer any stimulus to ADH secretion. Urinary Na^+ excretion will be elevated, but the urine Na^+ concentration may, by dilution, still be less than 25 meq/L.
- Both hypovolemia and SIADH contributed to the hyponatremia, and the patient is now euvolemic. This will be manifested by a urine Na^+ concentration above 40 meq/L and a persistently elevated U_{osm}, since there is continued ADH release.

Extracellular pH and Potassium Concentration

Abnormalities in acid-base and K^+ homeostasis are occasionally associated with hyponatremic disorders, and their presence can be helpful in establishing the correct diagnosis (Table 23-6). For example, the presence of metabolic alkalosis and hypokalemia should lead one to suspect vomiting or diuretic therapy, whereas hyperkalemia and metabolic acidosis in a patient with relatively normal renal function is highly suggestive of adrenal insufficiency.

Hypokalemia may also occur in patients with primary polydipsia by a mechanism that is directly related to the high urine output.[140] In the presence of K^+ depletion, normal subjects can lower the urine K^+ concentration to a minimum of 5 to 15 meq/L.[197] If, however, the urine output is 10 L/day or more, then there will be an *obligatory* K^+ loss that can exceed 50 to 100 meq and promote the development of hypokalemia.

TREATMENT

There are two basic principles involved in the treatment of hyponatremia: raising the plasma Na^+ concentration at a safe rate and treating the underlying cause (such as giving cortisol in adrenal insufficiency). In general, hyponatremia is corrected acutely by giving Na^+ to patients who are volume-depleted and by restricting water intake in patients who are normovolemic or edematous (Table 23-7). However, more vigorous therapy (usually requiring hypertonic saline) is indicated when symptoms are present or the plasma Na^+ concentration is less than 110 meq/L, since these are the settings in which irreversible neurologic damage and death can occur. Although the dangers of acute, severe hyponatremia are clear (Fig. 23-7), attention must also be paid to the rate of correction, particularly in asymptomatic patients.

Sodium Deficit

The amount of Na^+ required to raise the plasma Na^+ concentration to a desired value can be estimated from the following formula:

$$Na^+ \text{ deficit} = \text{volume of distribution of plasma } [Na^+] \times Na^+ \text{ deficit per liter}$$

$$(23\text{-}2)$$

Although Na^+ itself is restricted to the extracellular fluid, changes in the plasma Na^+ concentration reflect changes in osmolality and are distributed through the total body water (see Fig. 22-1). The total body water is approximately 60 and 50 percent of *lean* body weight in men and women, respectively. Thus, from Eq. (23-2), the approximate amount of Na^+ (in milliequivalents) required to

Table 23-7 Basic therapeutic regimen in the different causes of hyponatremia

NaCl	H_2O restriction
True volume depletion	SIADH
Diuretics	Edematous states
Adrenal insufficiency	Renal failure
	Primary polydipsia

raise the plasma Na^+ concentration to a safe level of 120 meq/L in women is roughly equal to:

$$Na^+ \text{ deficit} = 0.5 \times \text{lean body weight (kg)} \times (120 - \text{plasma } [Na^+]) \qquad (23\text{-}3)$$

Suppose a 60-kg woman is started on a thiazide diuretic and 5 days later presents with lethargy, confusion, decreased skin turgor, and a plasma Na^+ concentration of 108 meq/L. The amount of Na^+ required to raise the plasma Na^+ concentration to 120 meq/L is approximately 360 meq:

$$
\begin{aligned}
Na^+ \text{ deficit} &= 0.5 \times 60 \times (120 - 108) \\
&= 360 \text{ meq}
\end{aligned}
\qquad (23\text{-}4)
$$

Since 3 percent saline contains 513 meq of Na^+ per liter, 700 mL of this solution will provide the required Na^+. The plasma Na^+ concentration will increase by one of two mechanisms: retention of the Na^+ in patients who are hypovolemic, or initial retention of the Na^+ followed by the excretion of water in SIADH. In the latter disorder, volume regulation is intact, and the administered Na^+ will be excreted in the urine as a result of the associated volume expansion. It is the water loss induced by excretion of the extra sodium that is responsible for the steady state elevation in the plasma sodium concentration (see below).

Three issues related to Eq. (23-3) deserve emphasis:

- It applies only to the administration of Na^+ without or in marked excess of water (i.e., hypertonic but not isotonic saline). Isotonic saline will, however, eventually correct hyponatremia due to true volume depletion. In this setting, restoration of normovolemia will eliminate the hypovolemic stimulus to ADH release, thereby allowing the excess water to be excreted in a maximally dilute urine (see "True Volume Depletion," below).
- It is only an estimate, and serial measurements of the plasma Na^+ concentration (beginning at 2 to 3 h are necessary to assess the efficiency of treatment.
- It does not include any isosmotic losses that may also be present. For example, a patient with diarrhea may lose 5 liters of isosmotic fluid and then become hyponatremic by drinking and retaining 3 liters of water. Equation (23-3) estimates the amount of Na^+ required to counteract the dilutional effect of the 3 liters of free water; a 2-liter isosmotic Na^+ and water deficit will still remain.

The adequacy of *volume* repletion can be determined by following the skin turgor, jugular venous pressure, and urine Na^+ concentration. If, for example, this woman had an initial urine Na^+ concentration of 2 meq/L, and, after the administration of 400 meq of NaCl, the urine Na^+ concentration were only 7 meq/L, then hypovolemia persists and further replacement therapy is indicated. A urine Na^+ concentration above 40 meq/L usually indicates that normovolemia has been restored.

Rate of Correction

Despite the dangers of acute, severe hyponatremia, experimental and clinical studies suggest that overly rapid correction may also be harmful, leading within one to several days to central demyelinating lesions, particularly in the pons (a disorder called central pontine myelinolysis or osmotic demyelination).[179,188,191,192,198-205] This severe neurologic disorder is characterized by paraparesis or quadriparesis, dysarthria, dysphagia, and coma; seizures also may occur but are less common.[199,202,204,205] It may, for example, have contributed to the late deterioration in mental function in the women depicted in Fig. 23-7.

The diagnosis of osmotic demyelination is generally suspected from the clinical findings and can usually be confirmed by computed tomography (CT) scanning or, more accurately, by magnetic resonance imaging.[204,206] These lesions, however, may not be detectable radiologically for as long as 4 weeks; thus, an initially negative study in a patient who develops neurologic symptoms *after* the treatment of hyponatremia does not exclude the presence of osmotic demyelination.[199,206]

The mechanism by which rapid elevation in the plasma Na^+ concentration induces demyelinating lesions is unclear. The risk is greatest in patients with severe chronic hyponatremia, a setting in which the cerebral adaptation has returned brain volume toward normal. In this setting, an acute elevation in the plasma Na^+ concentration may lead to osmotic shrinkage of axons, severing their connections with the surrounding myelin sheaths.[199]* Brain cells adapted to hyponatremia may be at particular risk, since they have inserted transporters to lose osmolytes; they may therefore be less able to switch to taking up these organic solutes.[178]

The net effect is that the adaptive loss of solutes from the cells both *minimizes early symptoms and creates a problem for therapy*: Rapid correction can now lead to cerebral dehydration and demyelination, changes that are not seen if chronic asymptomatic hyponatremia is not corrected.[179,200] The risk of posttherapy osmotic demyelination is much less in patients with acute hyponatremia (developing over 1 to 3 days) who still have cerebral edema.[179,188,208]

Although the incidence of osmotic demyelination is probably low,[203,209,210] those patients who develop this disorder generally have one or more of the following risk factors: (1) more than a 12-meq/L elevation in the plasma Na^+ concentration in the first day, (2) overcorrection of the plasma Na^+ concentration to above 140 meq/L within the first 2 days, or (3) hypoxic or anoxic episodes prior to therapy.[188,200-205] Hypercatabolism or malnutrition due to burns or chronic alcoholism also appears to predispose to osmotic demyelination.[207]

A definitive recommendation for the treatment of severe hyponatremia cannot be made with certainty. Experimental and clinical observations suggest that the *degree of correction over the first 24 h* (less than 10 to 12 meq/L being safest) is much more important than the rate over a given hour or period of

---

* A similar neurologic lesion can be seen with severe and prolonged hyperosmolality due to hypernatremia or hyperglycemia, particularly in patients with burns.[207] This observation is consistent with the central role of osmotic shrinkage during rapid correction of hyponatremia.

hours.[204,205,211,212] It therefore seems advisable to raise the plasma Na^+ concentration in *asymptomatic* patients by *less than 10 to 12 meq/L on the first day and less than 18 meq/L over the first 2 days*.[203-205] Even at this "safe" rate, however, an occasional patient will develop neurologic symptoms.[202,204] It is probably wise therefore to correct the hyponatremia at less than the maximum rate (less than 10 meq/day) in asymptomatic patients.

An exception to the above recommendation occurs in patients who already have seizures or other severe neurologic symptoms directly induced by the low plasma Na^+ concentration. In this setting, the risk of untreated hyponatremia and cerebral edema is greater than the potential harm of overly rapid correction; as a result, hypertonic saline should be given to raise the plasma Na^+ concentration more quickly (1.5 to 2 meq/L/h for 3 to 4 h or until the severe neurologic symptoms have abated).[188,191] Even with this initial rapid rate of correction, the elevation in the plasma Na^+ concentration should not exceed 10 to 12 meq in the first 24 h, since partial osmotic adaptation will already have occurred.[188,199,205] As noted previously, young women with symptomatic hyponatremia are at high risk for irreversible symptoms, independent of the type of therapy given.[190]

As an example, the woman in the case described above requires initial therapy with approximately 700 mL of hypertonic saline to raise her plasma Na^+ concentration from 108 to 120 meq/L. Administration of this fluid over 24 h at a rate of 30 mL/h should achieve the desired goal: correcting the hyponatremia at a rate of 12 meq/L in the first day. However, the initial infusion rate may be increased to 50 to 75 mL/h for the first 3 to 4 h, since the patient does have mild neurologic symptoms. Careful monitoring is required during this period, however, since the calculations in Eqs. (23-3) and (23-4) are based on only a rough estimate of the total body water.[200]

Although rapid correction generally results from the administration of hypertonic saline, there are *two settings in which this problem can occur with water restriction alone*: primary polydipsia and volume depletion after euvolemia has been restored. In each of these conditions, ADH release is appropriately suppressed by the hyponatremia, thereby allowing the excess water to be rapidly excreted in a dilute urine.[213]

An unresolved and fortunately infrequent issue is the potential benefit of administering water to lower the plasma Na^+ concentration in patients with severe hyponatremia who have been corrected too rapidly. One study in rats addressed this problem. A marked reduction in the incidence and severity of brain lesions was noted if overly rapid correction (25 meq/L or more over several hours) was partially reversed after 12 h, so that the net daily elevation in the plasma sodium concentration was less than 20 meq/L.[212] This benefit was seen only if therapy was begun before the onset of neurologic symptoms; improvement was much less likely in animals with symptomatic demyelination.

The same authors described one patient with severe thiazide-induced hyponatremia whose neurologic status deteriorated after the plasma Na^+ concentration had been increased from 106 to 127 meq/L in the first 24 h.[214] The plasma Na^+ concentration was then lowered by 16 meq/L over the ensuing 14 h by the administration of dDAVP and hypotonic fluids. This maneuver was well tolerated, and the plasma Na^+ concentration was then gradually normalized, with complete neurologic recovery. More data are needed before this approach can be recommended.

True Volume Depletion

True volume depletion due to gastrointestinal or renal losses represents the main indication for the use of NaCl in the treatment of hyponatremia. Isotonic saline or oral NaCl and water can be used in patients with asymptomatic or mild reductions in the plasma Na^+ concentration. This regimen will correct the hyponatremia in two stages:

- The plasma Na^+ concentration will initially rise slowly, since the administered fluid has a higher Na^+ concentration than the plasma. If, for example, the plasma Na^+ concentration is 114 meq/L (40 meq/L less than that in isotonic saline) and the total body water is 40 kg, then each liter of saline will supply 40 meq of extra Na^+, which will effectively be distributed through 40 L. The net result is an *elevation in the plasma Na^+ concentration of only 1 meq/L.*
- Once the hypovolemia is corrected, ADH release will be suppressed, leading to the production of a maximally dilute urine, rapid excretion of the excess water, and correction of the hyponatremia. Careful monitoring is required at this time to prevent overly rapid correction and possible osmotic demyelination.[213]

Hypertonic saline should be given only for symptomatic reductions in the plasma Na^+ concentration. There is, however, little rationale for the administration of dilute solutions, such as half-isotonic saline. Although this solution will correct the volume deficit, it will also initially exacerbate the hyponatremia.

Effect of potassium   Correction of K^+ depletion, if present, is another important component of therapy. The administration of K^+ in this setting will directly increase the P_{osm} and raise the plasma Na^+ concentration (unless given in an isosmotic solution).[24,25,36] The exogenous K^+ will primarily enter the cells, which contain 98 percent of the body K^+. In this setting, electroneutrality will be maintained in one of three ways, each of which will act to correct the hyponatremia:

- Intracellular Na^+ will leave the cells, directly increasing the plasma Na^+ concentration.
- Extracellular Cl^- will enter the cells (primarily red blood cells). The addition of KCl will increase the cell osmolality, resulting in H_2O movement into the cells, thereby raising the plasma Na^+ concentration.
- Intracellular H^+ ions will dissociate from intracellular buffers and move into the extracellular fluid, where they will combine with extracellular

buffers. This movement of H^+ is osmotically neutral, but the extra cell K^+ will raise the cell osmolality and induce osmotic H_2O movement into the cells.

The net effect is that K^+ *is as effective as* Na^+ in correcting hyponatremia. Thus, administered K^+ must be included when calculating the amount of Na^+ to be given to increase the plasma Na^+ concentration at a safe rate. In some patients with severe hypokalemia, for example, the amount of K^+ given during the first day (200 to 400 meq) may be sufficient to raise the plasma Na^+ concentration by close to the maximum rate. In this setting, also giving Na^+ can lead to overly rapid correction.

Edematous States

Treatment is different in edematous patients with hyponatremia. Therapy must be aimed at water removal, since the administration of Na^+ will increase the severity of the edema. If one assumes that the water content of food is approximately equal to the insensible water loss from the skin and respiratory tract (see Table 22-1), then negative water balance can be achieved by restricting water intake to a volume that is *less* than the urine output. For example, the patient will continue to retain water if daily fluid intake is held to 800 mL but output is only 500 mL.

Although water restriction is the initial therapy of choice in edematous states, this may be very difficult to achieve in patients with advanced heart failure. In this setting, the combination of the low cardiac output and the high circulating levels of angiotensin II often stimulates thirst. As a result, one of the major complaints of such a patient is intense and persistent thirst; achieving effective water restriction may be extremely difficult. Fortunately, the plasma Na^+ concentration falls gradually in this setting, and symptomatic hyponatremia is a rare event.

Thus, it is reasonable to allow asymptomatic hyponatremia to persist in patients with advanced heart failure and to limit the recommendations to preventing excess water intake. In patients who develop symptoms, the plasma Na^+ concentration can be raised by the use of a loop diuretic in combination with hypertonic saline or, in extreme cases, by peritoneal dialysis or hemodialysis. With the former regimen, Na^+ and water loss is induced by the diuretic, and only the Na^+ loss is then replaced; the net effect is negative water balance and a rise in the plasma Na^+ concentration.

Some hyponatremic patients with advanced heart failure benefit from the combination of a loop diuretic and unloading therapy with an ACE inhibitor.[215-217] These agents, neither of which may be effective alone, appear to have a synergistic interaction. At least two factors contribute to this response: (1) The loop diuretic increases water delivery to the collecting tubules by impairing transport in the thick ascending limb, and (2) ACE inhibitors can then diminish water reabsorption in the collecting tubules by reversing the excessive release of ADH (via the increase in cardiac output)[9,217] and perhaps also by antagonizing the tubular action of ADH, an effect that appears to be mediated by stimulation of local prostaglandin release.[218]

Other modalities Given the often refractory nature of the hyponatremia in heart failure and cirrhosis, other therapies have been evaluated. Even if effective, however, these agents will only correct a laboratory abnormality without inducing any tangible benefit in asymptomatic patients. The tetracycline derivative demeclocycline increases free-water excretion by inducing ADH resistance (see below).[219-222] The use of this agent has been limited, however, because hepatic drug metabolism is reduced in heart failure and cirrhosis, resulting in increased plasma drug levels and frequent nephrotoxicity.[221,222]

A more direct form of therapy is the administration of a specific antagonist to the V_2 receptor, which mediates the antidiuretic effects of ADH. These agents are effective in a variety of animal models of hyponatremia,[12,13] and oral V_2 receptor antagonists are undergoing clinical trials.[223-225]

Syndrome of Inappropriate ADH Secretion

Treatment of SIADH is potentially more complicated than treatment of the other causes of hyponatremia and may be different in the acute and chronic settings (Table 23-8).

Acute Hyponatremia in SIADH is due initially to water retention and then in part to Na^+ loss induced by the ensuing volume expansion.[90,92] The simplest therapy is restricting water intake while maintaining that of NaCl. If this is ineffective or if severe hyponatremia is present, the combination of hypertonic saline and a loop diuretic can be used to raise the plasma Na^+ concentration.[36,226]

A few simple calculations can demonstrate the general role of NaCl administration and loop diuretics in the treatment of SIADH. It is essential to appreciate that water excretion is impaired in this disorder as a result of the continued presence of ADH, but that *Na^+ handling and therefore volume regulation are intact.* These principles can be illustrated by the following case history:

Table 23-8 Treatment of SIADH

Acute
   Water restriction
   Hypertonic saline or NaCl tablets
   Loop diuretic
Chronic
   Water restriction
   High-salt, high-protein diet
   Loop diuretic
   Other: demeclocycline, lithium, or urea

Case history 23-2 A 58-year-old woman with a small cell carcinoma of the lung is admitted because of slight obtundation. Her weight is 60 kg. The following laboratory data are obtained, which are consistent with SIADH:

$$Plasma~[Na^+] = 115~meq/L$$

$$P_{osm} = 240~mosmol/kg$$

$$U_{osm} = 680~mosmol/kg$$

$$Urine~volume = 1000~mL/day$$

$$Urine~[Na^+] = 62~meq/L$$

If this patient is given 1000 mL of isotonic saline (Na^+ and Cl^- concentration each equals 154 meq/L, osmolality equals 308 mosmol/kg), the plasma Na^+ concentration will initially increase because the solution has a higher osmolality than the patient. However, the steady state effect will be different. The excess NaCl will be excreted in the urine in a volume of only 453 mL (308 mosmol ÷ 680 mosmol/kg = 453 mL), since the U_{osm} will be relatively constant (Table 23-9). As a result, all of the solute is excreted, more than one-half of the water is retained, and there will be a *further reduction in the plasma Na^+ concentration.*[36]

The effect of this water retention can be estimated from the equations derived on page 694:

$$Total~body~osmoles = total~body~water~(TBW) \times P_{osm}$$

Since the effective P_{osm} is roughly equal to $2 \times$ plasma $[Na^+]$,

Table 23-9 Effect of isotonic saline, hypertonic saline, and hypertonic saline with loop diuretic in SIADH with a urine osmolality of 680 mosmol/kg

	NaCl, mosmol	H_2O, mL
Isotonic saline		
In	308	1000
Out	308	453
Net	0	+547
Hypertonic saline		
In	1026	1000
Out	1026	1500
Net	0	−500
Hypertonic saline + loop diuretic ($U_{osm} = 300$ mosmol/kg)		
In	1026	1000
Out	1026	3400
Net	0	−2400

$$\text{Total effective osmoles} = \text{TBW} \times 2 \times \text{plasma } [\text{Na}^+]$$

$$= 0.5 \times 60 \times 2 \times 115$$

$$= 6900 \,\text{mosmol} \qquad (23\text{-}5)$$

The retention of 550 mL of water will raise the TBW to 30.55 L, while the total effective osmoles will be unchanged, since all of the excess solute is excreted. The new plasma Na^+ concentration can be estimated from rearranging Eq. (23-5):

$$\text{Plasma } [\text{Na}^+] = \text{total effective osmoles} \div (2 \times \text{TBW})$$

$$= 6900 \div 61.1$$

$$= 113 \,\text{meq/L} \qquad (23\text{-}6)$$

Thus, each liter of isotonic saline will lower the plasma Na^+ concentration by about 2 meq/L in this setting. To correct the hyponatremia, the *effective osmolality of the fluid given must be greater than that of the urine.* Table 23-9 illustrates the effect of giving 1000 mL of 3% saline to this patient. Although the plasma Na^+ concentration will initially rise, because of the direct effect of the administered fluid, the new steady state will be characterized by excretion of the administered Na^+ and the net loss of 500 mL of water, resulting in a new TBW of 29.5 liters. From Eq. (23-6),

$$\text{Plasma } [\text{Na}^+] = 6900 \div 5$$

$$= 117 \,\text{meq/L}$$

The net effect is that even hypertonic saline may not be so effective when the U_{osm} is very high.* What is required in this situation is a reduction in the U_{osm}, which can be achieved by the administration of a loop diuretic, such as furosemide.[36,226-228] If, for example, the U_{osm} were lowered to 300 mosmol/kg (due to an impairment of NaCl reabsorption in the medullary thick ascending limb, the first step in countercurrent multiplication; see Chap. 4), then the infused NaCl will now be excreted in 3400 mL of urine (Table 23-9), resulting in a reduction in the TBW to 27.6 liters. Thus,

$$\text{Plasma } [\text{Na}^+] = 6900 \div 55.2$$

$$= 125 \,\text{meq/L}$$

The above calculations may underestimate the true effect, since unreplaced fluid loss will lead to volume depletion. This will activate the volume regulatory systems (such as increased secretion of renin), resulting in retention of some of the administered Na^+ and a more prominent rise in the plasma Na^+ concentration.

---

* The assumption that the U_{osm} will remain constant in this setting is probably not accurate, as the marked solute load will lead to an osmotic diuresis that should make the urine somewhat less concentrated. The basic principle, however, will still apply, since the U_{osm} will not fall dramatically.

Chronic SIADH is frequently a transient phenomenon that resolves after discontinuation of the offending drug or recovery from the underlying disease process (such as meningitis, pneumonia, or active tuberculosis). However, normalization of the plasma Na^+ concentration does not necessarily indicate recovery, since inducing negative water balance will raise the plasma Na^+ concentration independent of ADH levels. Thus, the simplest regimen is to slowly increase water intake once normonatremia is achieved, particularly if it appears that the causative factor has been corrected. If hyponatremia recurs while the U_{osm} remains high, then SIADH persists and water restriction should be reintroduced.

Chronic SIADH can also occur, particularly in patients with ectopic hormone production. The mainstay of therapy in this setting is water restriction. If this is ineffective, further treatment must be aimed at increasing water excretion, either by enhancing solute excretion or by antagonizing the effect of ADH (Table 23-8). In normal subjects, water intake is the major determinant of the urine volume, via its effect on ADH release. In SIADH, however, ADH secretion and therefore the U_{osm} are relatively fixed; as a result, the *urine output is primarily determined by the rate of solute excretion.* Thus, in the above patient with a U_{osm} that is relatively fixed at 680 mosmol/kg, the daily urine output will be 1000 mL if 680 mosmol of solute is excreted, but 1500 mL if 1020 mosmol of solute is excreted. This increase in solute output can be achieved by putting the patient on a high-salt, high-protein diet (the unused protein will be excreted as urea) or, if available, by giving 30 to 60 g of urea per day.[229,230] Urea has few side effects other than some gastroinestinal discomfort as long as renal function is normal; however, this modality is rarely used in the United States.

As an alternative, the U_{osm} can be lowered by antagonizing the effect of ADH. This can be achieved by the administration of 20 to 40 mg/day of furosemide in divided doses (with NaCl to prevent hypovolemia)[227,228] or of demeclocycline or lithium.[219,231,232] In contrast to furosemide, which acts in the loop of Henle, demeclocycline and lithium directly interfere with the effect of ADH on the collecting tubules.[233,234] The mechanism by which this occurs is incompletely understood. Lithium, for example, enters the collecting tubule cells through Na^+ channels in the luminal membrane (see page 755).[235] The ensuing intracellular accumulation presumably impairs the response to ADH, perhaps by reducing expression of the aquaporin-2 water channel or by reducing ADH receptor density.[236,237]

In general, demeclocycline (in a dose of 300 to 600 mg twice a day) is more effective and better tolerated than lithium,[238] although the latter is preferred in children because tetracyclines can interfere with bone development.[239]

The choice of which regimen to use is in part dependent upon the U_{osm}. Patients with a U_{osm} below 400 mosmol/kg can usually be treated by dietary means alone. Once the U_{osm} exceeds 600 to 700 mosmol/kg, however, free-water excretion falls to very low levels, and a loop diuretic (which is probably safer) or demeclocycline may be required to maintain the plasma Na^+ concentration at a safe level.

A possible future alternative is the administration of a V_2 receptor antagonist to produce a selective water diuresis.[233-225] In one study, for example, 11 patients with SIADH were administered a vasopressin antagonist and underwent a water diuresis that was independent of urinary solute excretion.[224] The plasma Na^+ concentration rose by 3 meq/L over a 6-h period. There is, however, a potential risk if the ADH effect is completely eliminated: a marked increase in water excretion, resulting in overly rapid correction of the hyponatremia.

Reset osmostat   A reset osmostat is a variant of SIADH in which ADH secretion and thirst are regulated normally around a lower plasma osmolality (Fig. 23-4). The new plasma Na^+ concentration is usually between 125 and 135 meq/L, and the patients are asymptomatic. The presence of a reset osmostat should be suspected when multiple measurements reveal stable hyponatremia; it can be confirmed by demonstrating normal excretion of a water load.[141]

Correcting the hyponatremia in the reset osmostat is not necessary and, if attempted, is difficult to sustain. Raising the plasma Na^+ concentration above the new baseline will both stimulate ADH release and make the patient very thirsty, since the thirst threshold is also reset.[141] Treatment must be aimed at correcting the underlying disorder, such as tuberculosis or malnutrition.

Other Disorders

Somewhat different considerations may apply to the treatment of other causes of hyponatremia. Patients with *primary adrenal insufficiency* are both cortisol- and aldosterone-deficient. The administration of cortisol will rapidly increase water excretion and return the plasma Na^+ concentration toward normal.[126,127] A mineralocorticoid (such as fludrocortisone) is frequently required to correct the urinary Na^+ wasting and hyperkalemia that are commonly present. Mineralocorticoid alone will not normalize renal water excretion and is not necessary in patients with hypopituitarism in whom aldosterone secretion is relatively normal.[128] Hormone replacement will also correct the hyponatremia in patients with *hypothyroidism*.[134-137]

The imposition of water restriction will rapidly return the plasma Na^+ concentration to normal in patients with *primary polydipsia*, since water excretory capacity is intact. However, hypertonic saline may be required initially in patients with severe neurologic symptoms.[208] These patients generally have acute hyponatremia and are at less risk for osmotic demyelination;[208] nevertheless, careful monitoring of the plasma Na^+ concentration is still required, and allowing a controlled increase in water intake may be necessary in selected cases. It may also be helpful to alter the drug regimen when phenothiazines stimulate thirst by causing the sensation of a dry mouth.[149]

PROBLEMS

23-1 A 45-year-old woman is started on hydrochlorothiazide and a low-sodium diet for the treatment of hypertension. After 1 week, she complains of weakness, muscle cramps, and postural dizziness. On physical examination, the patient is found to be alert and oriented. The blood pressure is 130/86 (the pretreatment level was 150/100). The skin turgor is decreased, and the jugular venous pressure is less than $5\,cmH_2O$. The laboratory data are

$$\text{Plasma } [Na^+] = 119\,meq/L$$
$$[K^+] = 2.1\,meq/L$$
$$[Cl^-] = 71\,meq/L$$
$$[HCO_3^-] = 34\,meq/L$$
$$P_{osm} = 252\,mosmol/kg$$
$$U_{osm} = 540\,mosmol/kg$$
$$\text{Urine } [Na^+] = 4\,meq/L$$

Which of the following has contributed to the development of hyponatremia?

(a) Hydrochlorothiazide
(b) Volume depletion
(c) Increased ADH secretion
(d) Water retention
(e) K^+ depletion

The appropriate therapy should include which of the following?

(a) Water restriction alone
(b) Potassium citrate
(c) Potassium chloride
(d) Half-isotonic (0.45%) saline
(e) Isotonic (0.9%) saline

23-2 A 52-year-old man with hypertension treated with unknown medications is admitted to the hospital in a comatose state, responding only to deep pain. On physical examination, the blood pressure is found to be 200/120. The skin turgor is reduced, and the neck veins are flat. After appropriate studies, the diagnosis of an intracerebral hemorrhage is made. To minimize the degree of brain swelling, the patient is given a total of 25 g of mannitol. Only 100 mL of other fluids is given. The laboratory data at this time include

$$\text{Plasma } [Na^+] = 120\,meq/L$$
$$[K^+] = 3.3\,meq/L$$
$$[Cl^-] = 78\,meq/L$$
$$[HCO_3^-] = 29\,meq/L$$
$$P_{osm} = 253\,mosmol/kg$$
$$U_{osm} = 240\,mosmol/kg$$
$$\text{Urine } [Na^+] = 46\,meq/L$$

What is the most likely cause of the hyponatremia?

(a) Pseudohyponatremia due to mannitol
(b) Volume depletion
(c) SIADH

23-3 Match the correct therapy with the appropriate clinical setting:

1. A 41-year-old man with end-stage renal failure, mild peripheral edema, and a plasma Na^+ concentration of 125 meq/L
2. A 53-year-old woman with an oat cell carcinoma of the lung, a plasma Na^+ concentration of 107 meq/L, and a urine osmolality of 640 mosmol/kg
3. A 27-year-old woman with chronic diarrhea, decreased skin turgor, and a plasma Na^+ concentration of 126 meq/L
4. A 38-year-old man with multiple myeloma, a plasma Na^+ concentration of 127 meq/L, and a plasma osmolality of 286 mosmol/kg
5. A 58-year-old diabetic man with congestive heart failure, a plasma Na^+ concentration of 124 meq/L, and a plasma osmolality of 268 mosmol/kg
6. A 49-year-old woman with carcinoma of the lung, a stable plasma Na^+ concentration of 118 meq/L, and a urine osmolality of 290 mosmol/kg

(a) Water restriction with normal sodium intake
(b) Water and sodium restriction
(c) No therapy required
(d) Isotonic saline
(e) Hypertonic saline
(f) Hypertonic saline plus a loop diuretic

23-4 A 60-year-old man weighing 70 kg has an oat cell carcinoma of the lung and is admitted to the hospital with a 2-week history of progressive lethargy and obtundation. The physical examination is within normal limits except for the obtundation. The following laboratory studies are obtained

$$\text{Plasma } [Na^+] = 105 \text{ meq/L}$$

$$[K^+] = 4 \text{ meq/L}$$

$$[Cl^-] = 72 \text{ meq/L}$$

$$[HCO_3^-] = 21 \text{ meq/L}$$

$$P_{osm} = 222 \text{ mosmol/kg}$$

$$U_{osm} = 604 \text{ mosmol/kg}$$

$$\text{Urine } [Na^+] = 78 \text{ meq/L}$$

(a) What is the most likely diagnosis?
(b) How and at what initial rate would you raise the plasma Na^+ concentration?

23-5 Uric acid reabsorption in the proximal tubule is related to Na^+ reabsorption (see Chap. 3). Considering the effects of volume on Na^+ reabsorption, how might the plasma uric acid concentration be used to help differentiate between hyponatremia due to SIADH and volume depletion?

REFERENCES

1. Shiau Y-F, Feldman GM, Resnick MA, Coff PM. Stool electrolyte and osmolality measurements in the evaluation of diarrheal disorders. *Ann Intern Med* 102:773, 1985.
2. Robertson GL. Physiology of ADH secretion. *Kidney Int* 32(suppl 21):S-20, 1987.
3. Robinson AG, Roberts MM, Evron WA, et al. Hyponatremia in rats induces downregulation of vasopressin synthesis. *J Clin Invest* 86:1023, 1990.
4. Gross PA, Kettler M, Hausmann C, Ritz E. The chartered and unchartered waters of hyponatremia. *Kidney Int* 32(suppl 21):S-67, 1987.
5. Anderson RJ, Chung H-M, Kluge R, Schrier RW. Hyponatremia: A prospective analysis of its epidemiology and the pathogenetic role of vasopressin. *Ann Intern Med* 102:164, 1985.

6. Szatalowicz VL, Arnold PE, Chaimovitz C, et al. Radioimmunoassay of plasma arginine vasopressin in hyponatremic patients with congestive heart failure. *N Engl J Med* 305:263, 1981.

7. Bichet D, Szatalowicz V, Chaimovitz C, Schrier RW. Role of vasopressin in abnormal water excretion in cirrhotic patients. *Ann Intern Med* 96:413, 1982.

8. Schrier RW, Bichet DG. Osmotic and nonosmotic control of vasopressin release and the pathogenesis of impaired water excretion in adrenal, thyroid, and edematous disorders. *J Lab Clin Med* 98:1, 1981.

9. Bichet DG, Kortas C, Mettauer B, et al. Modulation of platelet and plasma vasopressin by cardiac function in patients with heart failure. *Kidney Int* 29:1188, 1986.

10. Anderson RJ, Cadnapaphornchai P, Harbottle JA, et al. Mechanism of effect of thoracic inferior vena cava constriction on renal water excretion. *J Clin Invest* 54:1473, 1974.

11. Valtin HV, Edwards BR. GFR and the concentration of urine in the absence of vasopressin: Berliner-Davidson re-explored. *Kidney Int* 31:634, 1987.

12. Ishikawa S-E, Saito T, Okada K, et al. Effect of vasopressin antagonist on water excretion in inferior vena cava constriction. *Kidney Int* 30:49, 1986.

13. Clairia J, Jimenez W, Arroyo V, et al. Blockade of the hydroosmotic effect of vasopressin normalizes water excretion in cirrhotic rats. *Gastroenterology* 97:1294, 1989.

14. Ishikawa S-E, Schrier RW. Effect of arginine vasopressin antagonist on renal water excretion in glucocorticoid and mineralocorticoid deficient rats. *Kidney Int* 22:587, 1982.

15. Dzau VJ, Paker M, Lilly LS, et al. Prostaglandins in severe congestive heart failure: Relation to activation of the renin-angiotensin system and hyponatremia. *N Engl J Med* 310:347, 1984.

16. Mettauer B, Rouleau J-L, Bichet D, et al. Sodium and water excretion abnormalities in congestive heart failure. *Ann Intern Med* 105:161, 1986.

17. Papadakis MA, Fraser CL, Arieff AI. Hyponatraemia in patients with cirrhosis. *Q J Med* 76:675, 1990.

18. Perez-Ayuso RM, Arroyo V, Campos J, et al. Evidence that renal prostaglandins are involved in renal water metabolism in cirrhosis. *Kidney Int* 26:72, 1984.

19. Lee WH, Packer M. Prognostic importance of serum sodium concentration and its modification by converting enzyme inhibition in patients with severe congestive heart failure. *Circulation* 73:257, 1986.

20. Robertson GL, Aycinena P, Zerbe RL. Neurogenic disorders of osmoregulation. *Am J Med* 72:339, 1982.

21. Frizzell RT, Lang GJ, Lowance DC, Lathan SR. Hyponatremia and ultramarathon running. *JAMA* 255:772, 1985.

22. Alam NH, Majumder RH, Fuchs GJ, and the CHOICE study group. Efficacy and safety of oral rehydration solution with reduced osmolarity in adults with cholera: A randomised double-blind clinical trial. *Lancet* 354:296, 1999.

23. Laragh JH. The effect of potassium chloride on hyponatremia. *J Clin Invest* 33:807, 1954.

24. Fichman MP, Vorherr H, Kleeman CR, Telfer N. Diuretic-induced hyponatremia. *Ann Intern Med* 75:853, 1971.

25. Kamel KS, Bear RA. Treatment of hyponatremia: A quantitative analysis. *Am J Kidney Dis* 21:439, 1993.

26. Friedman E, Shadel M, Halkin H, Farfel Z. Thiazide-induced hyponatremia: Reproducibility by single-dose challenge and an analysis of pathogenesis. *Ann Intern Med* 110:24, 1989.

27. Ashraf N, Locksley R, Arieff AI. Thiazide-induced hyponatremia associated with death or neurologic damage in outpatients. *Am J Med* 70:1163, 1981.

28. Ashouri OS. Severe-diuretic-induced hyponatremia in the elderly. *Arch Intern Med* 146:1355, 1986.

29. Sonnenblick M, Friedlander Y, Rosin AJ. Diuretic-induced severe hyponatremia: Review and analysis of 129 reported patients. *Chest* 103:601, 1993.

30. Kennedy RM, Earley L. Profound hyponatremia resulting from a thiazide-induced decrease in urinary diluting capacity in a patient with primarily polydipsia. *N Engl J Med* 282:1185, 1970.

31. Decaux G, Schlesser M, Loffernils M, et al. Uric acid, anion gap and urea concentration in the diagnostic approach to hyponatremia. *Clin Nephrol* 42:102, 1994.

32. Szatalowicz VL, Miller PD, Lacher JW, et al. Comparative effects of diuretics on renal water excretion in hyponatremic oedematous disorders. *Clin Sci* 62:235, 1982.

33. Maronde R, Milgrom M, Vlachakis ND, Chan L. Response of thiazide-induced hypokalemia to amiloride. *JAMA* 249:237, 1983.

34. Kleeman CR, Adams DA, Maxwell MH. An evaluation of maximal water diuresis in chronic renal disease: I. Normal solute intake. *J Lab Clin Med* 58:169, 1961.

35. Tannen RL, Regal EM, Dunn MJ, Schrier RW. Vasopressin-resistant hypothenuria in advanced chronic renal disease. *N Engl J Med* 280:1135, 1969.

36. Rose BD. New approach to disturbances in the plasma sodium concentration. *Am J Med* 81:1033, 1986.

37. Goldman MB, Luchins DJ, Robertson GL. Mechanisms of altered water metabolism in psychotic patients with polyuria and hyponatremia. *N Engl J Med* 318:397, 1988.

38. Glassock RJ, Cohen AH, Danovitch G, Parsa KP. Human immunodeficiency virus (HIV) and the kidney. *Ann Intern Med* 112:35, 1990.

39. Sane T, Rantakari K, Poranen A. Hyponatremia after transsphenoidal surgery for pituitary tumors. *J Clin Endocrinol Metab* 79:1395, 1994.

40. Olson BR, Rubino D, Gumowski J, Oldfield EH. Isolated hyponatremia after transsphenoidal pituitary surgery. *J Clin Endocrinol Metab* 80:85, 1995.

41. DeFronzo RA, Braine H, Calvin OM, Davis PJ. Water intoxication in man after cyclophosphamide therapy: Time course and relation to drug activation. *Ann Intern Med* 78:861, 1973.

42. Bressler RB, Huston DP. Water intoxication following moderate dose intravenous cyclophosphamide. *Arch Intern Med* 145:548, 1985.

43. Harlow PJ, Declerck YA, Shore NA, et al. A fatal case of inappropriate ADH secretion induced by cyclophosphamide therapy. *Cancer* 44:896, 1979.

44. Smith NJ, Espir MLE. Raised plasma arginine vasopressin concentration in carbamazepine-induced water intoxication. *Br Med J* 2:804, 1977.

45. Kimura T, Matsui K, Sato T, Yoshinaga K. Mechanism of carbamazepine (Tegretol)-induced antidiuresis: Evidence for release of antidiuretic hormone and impaired excretion of a water load. *J Clin Endocrinol Metab* 38:356, 1974.

46. Robertson GL, Bhoopalam N, Zelkowitz LJ. Vincristine neurotoxicity and abnormal secretion of antidiuretic hormone. *Arch Intern Med* 132:717, 1973.

47. Ravi Kumar TS, Grace TB. The syndrome of inappropriate antidiuretic hormone secretion secondary to vinblastine-bleomycin therapy. *J Surg Oncol* 24:242, 1983.

48. Ajlouni K, Kern MW, Teres JF, et al. Thiothixene-induced hyponatremia. *Arch Intern Med* 134:1103, 1974.

49. Vincent FM, Emery S. Antidiuretic hormone syndrome and thioridazine. *Ann Intern Med* 89:147, 1978.

50. Peck V, Shenkman L. Haloperidol-induced syndrome of inappropriate secretion of antidiuretic hormone. *Clin Pharmacol Ther* 26:442, 1979.

51. Luzecky MH, Burman KD, Schultz ER. The syndrome of inappropriate antidiuretic hormone secretion associated with amitriptyline administration. *South Med J* 67:495, 1974.

52. Jackson C, Carson W, Markowitz J, Mintzer J. SIADH associated with fluoxetine and sertraline therapy. *Am J Psychiatry* 152:809, 1995.

53. ten Holt WL, van Iperen CE, Schrijver G, et al. Severe hyponatremia during therapy with fluoxetine. *Arch Intern Med* 156:681, 1996.

54. Liu BA, Mittmann N, Knowles SR, et al. Hyponatremia and the syndrome of inappropriate secretion of antidiuretic hormone associated with the use of selective serotonin reuptake inhibitors: A review of spontaneous reports. *Can Med Assoc J* 155:519, 1996.

55. Peterson JC, Pollack RW, Mahoney JJ, Fuller TJ. Inappropriate antidiuretic hormone secondary to a monoamine oxidase inhibitor. *JAMA* 239:1422, 1978.

56. Marshall AW, Jakobovitz AW, Morgan MY. Bromocriptine-associated hyponatremia in cirrhosis. *Br Med J* 285:1534, 1982.

57. Somani P, Temesy-Armos PN, Leighton RF, et al. Hyponatremia in patients treated with lorcainide, a new antiarrhythmic drug. *Am Heart J* 108:1443, 1984.

58. Anderson RJ. Hospital-associated hyponatremia. *Kidney Int* 29:1237, 1986.

59. Thomas TH, Morgan DB, Swaminathan R, et al. Severe hyponatraemia: A study of 17 patients. *Lancet* 1:621, 1978.

60. Hill AR, Uribarri J, Mann J, Berl T. Altered water metabolism in tuberculosis: Role of vasopressin. *Am J Med* 88:357, 1990.

61. Shalhoub RJ, Antoniou LD. The mechanism of hyponatremia in pulmonary tuberculosis. *Ann Intern Med* 70:943, 1969.

62. Szatalowicz VL, Goldberg JP, Anderson RJ. Plasma antidiuretic hormone in acute respiratory failure. *Am J Med* 72:583, 1982.

63. Baker JW, Yerger S, Segar WE. Elevated plasma antidiuretic hormone levels in status asthmaticus. *Mayo Clin Proc* 51:31, 1976.

64. Fieldman NR, Forsling ML, Le Quesne LP. The effect of vasopressin on solute and water excretion during and after surgical operations. *Ann Surg* 201:383, 1985.

65. Ukai M, Moran W Jr, Zimmerman B. The role of visceral afferent pathways on vasopressin secretion and urinary excretory patterns during surgical stress. *Ann Surg* 168:16, 1968.

66. Coslovsky R, Bruck R, Estrov Z. Hypo-osmolal syndrome due to prolonged nausea. *Arch Intern Med* 144:191, 1984.

67. Rowe JW, Shelton RL, Helderman JH, et al. Influence of the emetic reflex on vasopressin release in man. *Kidney Int* 16:729, 1979.

68. Martinez-Maldonado M. Inappropriate antidiuretic hormone secretion of unknown origin. *Kidney Int* 17:554, 1980.

69. Hamilton BPB, Upton GV, Amatruda TT. Evidence for the presence of neurophysin in tumors producing the syndrome of inappropriate antidiuresis. *J Clin Endocrinol Metab* 35:764, 1972.

70. George JM, Capen CC, Phillips AS. Biosynthesis of vasopressin in vitro and ultrastructure of a bronchogenic carcinoma. *J Clin Invest* 51:141, 1972.

71. Yamaji T, Ishibashi M, Hori T. Propressophysin in human blood: A possible marker of ectopic vasopressin production. *J Clin Endocrinol Metab* 59:505, 1984.

72. Osterman J, Calhoun A, Dunham M, et al. Chronic syndrome of inappropriate antidiuretic hormone secretion and hypertension in a patient with olfactory neuroblastoma: Evidence of ectopic production of arginine vasopressin by the tumor. *Arch Intern Med* 146:1731, 1986.

73. Weissman P, Shenkman L, Gregerman RI. Chlorpropamide hyponatremia: Drug-induced inappropriate antidiuretic-hormone activity. *N Engl J Med* 284:65, 1971.

74. Kadowaki T, Hagura R, Kajinuma H, et al. Chlorpropamide-induced hyponatremia: Incidence and risk factors. *Diabetes Care* 6:468, 1983.

75. Moses AM, Fenner R, Schroeder ET, Coulson R. Further studies on the mechanism by which chlorpropamide alters the action of vasopressin. *Endocrinology* 111:2025, 1982.

76. Welch WJ, Ott CE, Lorenz JN, Kotchen TE. Effects of chlorpropamide on loop of Henle function and plasma renin. *Kidney Int* 30:712, 1986.

77. Kusano E, Braun-Werness JL, Vick DJ, et al. Chlorpropamide action on renal concentrating mechanism in rats with hypothalamic diabetes insipidus. *J Clin Invest* 72:1298, 1983.

78. Meinder AE, Cejka V, Robertson GL. The antidiuretic effect of carbamazepine in man. *Clin Sci Mol Med* 47:289, 1974.

79. Gold PW, Robertson GL, Ballenger JC, et al. Carbamazepine diminishes the sensitivity of the plasma arginine vasopressin response to osmotic stimulation. *J Clin Endocrinol Metab* 57:952, 1983.

80. Flegel KM, Cole CH. Inappropriate antidiuresis during carbamazepine treatment. *Ann Intern Med* 87:722, 1977.

81. Hagen GA, Frawley TF. Hyponatremia due to sulfonylurea compounds. *J Clin Endocrinol Metab* 31:570, 1970.

82. Shepherd LL, Hutchinson RJ, Worden EK, et al. Hyponatremia and seizures after intravenous administration of desmopressin acetate for surgical hemostasis. *J Pediatr* 114:470, 1989.

83. Humphries JE, Siragy H. Significant hyponatremia following DDAVP administration in a healthy adult. *Am J Hematol* 44:12, 1993.
84. Pittman JG. Water intoxication due to oxytocin. *N Engl J Med* 268:481, 1963.
85. Schwartz RH, Jones RWA. Transplacental hyponatraemia due to oxytocin. *Br Med J* 1:152, 1978.
86. Feeney JG. Water intoxication and oxytocin. *Br Med J* 285:243, 1982.
87. Kern PA, Robbins RJ, Bichet D, et al. Syndrome of inappropriate antidiuresis in the absence of arginine vasopressin. *J Clin Endocrinol Metab* 62:148, 1986.
88. Braden GL, Mikolich DJ, White CF, et al. Syndrome of inappropriate antidiuresis in Waldenstrom's macroglobulinemia. *Am J Med* 80:1242, 1986.
89. Bartter FC, Schwartz WB. The syndrome of inappropriate secretion of antidiuretic hormone. *Am J Med* 42:790, 1967.
90. Verbalis JG. Pathogenesis of hyponatremia in an experimental model of the syndrome of inappropriate antidiuresis. *Am J Physiol* 267:R1617, 1994.
91. Cogan E, Debieve M-F, Pepersack T, Abramow M. Natriuresis and atrial natriuretic factor secretion during inappropriate antidiuresis. *Am J Med* 84:409, 1988.
92. Cooke CR, Turin MD, Walker WG. The syndrome of inappropriate antidiuretic hormone secretion: Pathophysiologic mechanisms in solute and volume regulation. *Medicine* 58:240, 1979.
93. Leaf A, Bartter FC, Santos RF, Wrong O. Evidence in man that urinary electrolyte loss induced by Pitressin is a function of water retention. *J Clin Invest* 32:868, 1953.
94. Jaenike JR, Waterhouse C. The renal response to sustained administration of vasopressin and water in man. *J Clin Endocrinol Metab* 21:231, 1961.
95. Nolph KD, Schrier RW. Sodium, potassium and water metabolism in the syndrome of inappropriate antidiuretic hormone secretion. *Am J Med* 49:533, 1970.
96. Gross PA, Anderson RJ. Effects of DDAVP and AVP on sodium and water balance in conscious rat. *Am J Physiol* 243:R512, 1982.
97. Ecelbarger CA, Nielsen S, Olson BR, et al. Role of renal aquaporins in escape from vasopressin-induced antidiuresis in rat. *J Clin Invest* 99:1852, 1997.
98. Murase T, Ecelbarger CA, Baker EA, et al. Kidney aquaporin-2 expression during escape from antidiuresis is not related to plasma or tissue osmolality. *J Am Soc Nephrol* 10:2067, 1999.
99. Garella S, Tzamaloukas AH, Chazan JA. Effect of isotonic volume expansion on extracellular bicarbonate stores in normal dogs. *Am J Physiol* 225:628, 1973.
100. Garella S, Chang BS, Kahn SI. Dilution acidosis and contraction alkalosis: Review of a concept. *Kidney Int* 8:279, 1975.
101. Lowance DC, Garfinkel HB, Mattern WD, Schwartz WB. The effect of chronic hypotonic volume expansion of the renal regulation of acid-base equilibrium. *J Clin Invest* 51:2928, 1972.
102. Bichara M, Mercier O, Houillier P, et al. Effect of antidiuretic hormone on urinary acidification and on tubular handling of bicarbonate in the rat. *J Clin Invest* 80:621, 1987.
103. Cohen JJ, Hulter HN, Smithline N, et al. The critical role of the adrenal gland in the renal regulation of acid-base equilibrium during chronic hypotonic expansion: Evidence that chronic hyponatremia is a potent stimulus to aldosterone secretion. *J Clin Invest* 58:1201, 1976.
104. Taylor RE Jr, Glass GT, Radke KJ, Schneider EG. Specificity of effect of osmolality on aldosterone secretion. *Am J Physiol* 252:E118, 1987.
105. Dubovsky SL, Gravon S, Berl T, Schrier RW. Syndrome of inappropriate secretion of antidiuretic hormone with exacerbated psychosis. *Ann Intern Med* 79:551, 1973.
106. Wijdicks EF, Vermeulen M, Hijdra A, van Gign J. Hyponatremia and cerebral infarction in patients with ruptured intracranial aneurysms: Is fluid restriction harmful? *Ann Neurol* 17:137, 1985.
107. Goldman MB, Robertson GL, Luchins DJ, et al. Psychotic exacerbations and enhanced vasopressin secretion in schizophrenic patients with hyponatremia and polydipsia. *Arch Gen Psychiatry* 54:443, 1997.

108. Vitting KE, Gardenswartz MH, Zabetakis PM, et al. Frequency of hyponatremia and nonosmolar vasopressin release in the acquired immune deficiency syndrome. *JAMA* 263:973, 1990.

109. Moses AM, Miller M. Drug-induced dilutional hyponatremia. *N Engl J Med* 291:1234, 1974.

110. Moses AM, Howanitz J, Miller M. Diuretic action of three sulfonylurea drugs. *Ann Intern Med* 78:541, 1973.

111. Rocha AS, Ping WC, Kudo LH. Effect of chlorpropamide on water and urea transport in the inner medullary collecting duct. *Kidney Int* 39:79, 1991.

112. Zalin AM, Hutchinson CE, Jong M, Matthews K, Hyponatremia during treatment with chlorpropamide and Moduretic (amiloride plus hydrochlorothiazide). *Br Med J* 289:659, 1984.

113. Ishikawa S-E, Saito T, Yoshida S. The effect of prostaglandins on the release of arginine vasopressin from the guinea pig hypothalamo-neurohypophyseal complex in organ culture. *Endocrinology* 108:193, 1981.

114. Benson H, Akbarian M, Adler LN, Abelmann WH. Hemodynamic effects of pneumonia. I. Normal and hypodynamic responses. *J Clin Invest* 49:791, 1970.

115. Miller AC: Hyponatraemia in legionnaires' disease. *Br Med J* 284:558, 1982.

116. Bruce RA, Merendina KA. Observations on hyponatremia following mitral valve surgery. *Surg Gynecol Obstet* 100:293, 1955.

117. Gentric A, Baccino E, Mottier D, et al. Temporal arteritis revealed by a syndrome of inappropriate secretion of antidiuretic hormone. *Am J Med* 85:559, 1988.

118. Beck LH. Hypouricemia in the syndrome of inappropriate secretion of antidiuretic hormone. *N Engl J Med* 301:528, 1979.

119. Ishikawa S-E, Saito T, Kaneko K, et al. Hyponatremia responsive to fludrocortisone acetate in elderly patients after head injury. *Ann Intern Med* 106:187, 1987.

120. Al-Mufti H, Arieff AI. Hyponatremia due to cerebral salt-wasting syndrome: Combined cerebral and distal tubular lesion. *Am J Med* 77:740, 1984.

121. Kamoi K, Toyama M, Ishibashi M, et al. Hyponatremia and osmoregulation of vasopressin secretion in patients with intracranial bleeding. *J Clin Endocrinol Metab* 80:2906, 1995.

122. Atkin SL, Coady AM, White MC, et al. Hyponatraemia secondary to cerebral salt wasting syndrome following routine pituitary surgery. *Eur J Endocrinol* 135:245, 1996.

123. Berendes E, Walter M, Cullen P, et al. Secretion of brain natriuretic peptide in patients with aneurysmal subarachnoid hemorrhage. *Lancet* 349:245, 1997.

124. Maesaka J, Venkatesan J, Piccione M, et al. Abnormal urate transport in patients with intracranial disease. *Am J Kidney Dis* 19:10, 1992.

125. Gill JR Jr, Gann DS, Bartter FC. Restoration of water diuresis in Addisonian patients by expansion of the volume of extracellular fluid. *J Clin Invest* 41:1078, 1962.

126. Ahmed AB, George BC, Conyalez-Auvert C, Dingman JF. Increased plasma arginine vasopressin in clinical adrenocortical insufficiency and its inhibition by glucosteroids. *J Clin Invest* 46:111, 1967.

127. Green HH, Harrington AR, Valtin H. On the role of antidiuretic hormone in the inhibition of acute water diuresis in adrenal insufficiency and the effects of gluco- and mineralocorticoids in reversing the inhibition. *J Clin Invest* 49:1724, 1970.

128. Oelkers W. Hyponatremia and inappropriate secretion of vasopressin (antidiuretic hormone) in patients with hypopituitarism. *N Engl J Med* 321:492, 1989.

129. Linas SL, Berl T, Robertson GL, et al. Role of vasopressin in impaired water excretion of glucocorticoid deficiency. *Kidney Int* 18:58, 1980.

130. Wolfson B, Manning RW, Davis LG, et al. Co-localization of corticotropin releasing factor and vasopressin in RNA in neurons after adrenalectomy. *Nature* 315:59, 1985.

131. Papanek PE, Raff H. Physiological increases in cortisol inhibit basal vasopressin release in conscious dogs. *Am J Physiol* 266:R1744, 1994.

132. Kalogeras KT, Nieman LK, Friedman TC, et al. Inferior petrosal sampling in healthy human subjects reveals a unilateral corticotropin-releasing hormone-mediated arginine vasopressin release associated with ipsilateral adrenocorticotropin secretion. *J Clin Invest* 97:2045, 1996.

133. Raff H. Glucocorticoid inhibition of neurohypophysial vasopressin secretion. *Am J Physiol* 252:R635, 1987.

134. DeRubertis FR Jr, Michelis MF, Bloom ME, et al. Impaired water excretion in myxedema. *Am J Med* 51:41, 1971.

135. Kreisman SH, Hennessey JV. Consistent reversible elevations of serum creatinine levels in severe hypothyroidism. *Arch Intern Med* 159:79, 1999.

136. Skowsky WR, Kikuchi TA. The role of vasopressin in the impaired water excretion of myxedema. *Am J Med* 64:613, 1978.

137. Iwasaki Y, Oiso Y, Yamauchi K, et al. Osmoregulation of plasma vasopressin in myxedema. *J Clin Endocrinol Metab* 70:534, 1990.

138. Hanna FW, Scanlon MR. Hyponatraemia, hypothyroidism, and role of arginine-vasopressin. *Lancet* 350:755, 1997.

139. Leehey DJ, Picache AA, Robertson GL. Hyponatremia in quadriplegic patients. *Clin Sci* 75:441, 1988.

140. Hariprasad MK, Eisinger RP, Nadler IM, et al. Hyponatremia in psychogenic polydipsia. *Arch Intern Med* 140:1639, 1980.

141. DeFronzo RA, Goldberg M, Agus ZS. Normal diluting capacity in hyponatremic patients: Reset osmostat or a variant of the syndrome of inappropriate antidiuretic hormone secretion. *Ann Intern Med* 84:538, 1976.

142. Lindheimer MD, Marron WM, Davidson JM. Osmoregulation of thirst and vasopressin release in pregnancy. *Am J Physiol* 257:F159, 1989.

143. Davison JM, Shiells EA, Phillips PR, Lindheimer MD. Serial evaluation of vasopressin release and thirst in human pregnancy: Role of human chorionic gonadotropin in the osmoregulatory changes in gestation. *J Clin Invest* 81:798, 1988.

144. Danielson LA, Sherwood OD, Conrad KP. Relaxin is a potent renal vasodilator in conscious rats. *J Clin Invest* 103:525, 1999.

145. Barron WM, Durr JA, Schrier RW, Lindheimer MD. Role of hemodynamic factors in osmoregulatory alterations of rat pregnancy. *Am J Physiol* 257:R909, 1989.

146. Davison JM, Shiells EA, Philips P, Lindheimer MD. Influence of humoral and volume factors on altered osmoregulation of normal human pregnancy. *Am J Physiol* 258:F900, 1990.

147. Jose CJ, Perez-Cruet J. Incidence and morbidity of self-induced water intoxication in state mental hospital patients. *Am J Psychiatry* 136:221, 1979.

148. Illowsky BP, Kirch DG. Polydipsia and hyponatremia in psychotic patients. *Am J Psychiatry* 145:675, 1988.

149. Rao KJ, Miller M, Moses A. Water intoxication and thioridazine. *Ann Intern Med* 82:61, 1975.

150. Stuart CA, Neelon FA, Levovitz HE. Disordered control of thirst in hypothalamic-pituitary sarcoidosis. *N Engl J Med* 303:1078, 1980.

151. Thompson CJ, Edwards CR, Baylis PH. Osmotic and non-osmotic regulation of thirst and vasopressin secretion in patients with compulsive water drinking. *Clin Endocrinol (Oxf)* 35:221, 1991.

152. Miller M, Kalkos T, Moses AM, et al. Recognition of partial defects in antidiuretic hormone secretion. *Ann Intern Med* 73:721, 1970.

153. Langgard H, Smith WO. Self-induced water intoxication without predisposing illness. *N Engl J Med* 266:378, 1962.

154. Rendell M, McGrane D, Cuesta M. Fatal compulsive water drinking. *JAMA* 240:2557, 1978.

155. Gillum DM, Linas SL. Water intoxication in a psychotic patient with normal water excretion. *Am J Med* 77:773, 1984.

156. Levine S, McManus BM, Blackbourne BD, Roberts WC. Fatal water intoxication, schizophrenia, and diuretic therapy for systemic hypertension. *Am J Med* 82:153, 1987.

157. Klonoff DC, Jurow AH. Acute water intoxication as a complication of urine drug testing in the workplace. *JAMA* 265:84, 1991.

158. Goldman MB, Robertson GL, Luchins DJ, et al. Psychotic exacerbations and enhanced vasopressin secretion in schizophrenic patients with hyponatremia and polydipsia. *Arch Gen Psychiatry* 54:443, 1997.

159. Hilden T, Svendsen TL. Electrolyte disturbances in beer drinkers. *Lancet* 2:245, 1975.

160. Weinberg LS. Pseudohyponatremia: A reappraisal. *Am J Med* 86:315, 1989.
161. Albrink M, Hold PM, Man EB, Peters JP. The displacement of serum water by the lipids of hyperlipemic serum. A new method for the rapid determination of serum water. *J Clin Invest* 34:1483, 1955.
162. Tarail R, Buchwald KW, Holland JF, Selawry OS. Misleading reductions of serum sodium and chloride: Association with hyperproteinemia in patients with multiple myeloma. *Proc Soc Exp Biol Med* 110:145, 1962.
163. Sunderrajan S, Bauer JH, Vopat RL, et al. Posttransurethral prostatic resection hyponatremic syndrome: Case report and review of the literature. *Am J Kidney Dis* 4:80, 1984.
164. Rothenberg DM, Berns AS, Ivankovich AD. Isotonic hyponatremia following transurethral prostate resection. *J Clin Anesth* 2:48, 1990.
165. Campbell HT, Fincher ME, Sklar AH. Severe hyponatremia without severe hypoosmolality following transurethral resection of the prostate (TURP) in end-stage renal disease. *Am J Kidney Dis* 12:152, 1988.
166. Gonzalez R, Brensilver JM, Rovinsky JJ. Posthysteroscopic hyponatremia. *Am J Kidney Dis* 23:735, 1994.
167. Istre O, Bjoennes J, Naess R, et al. Postoperative cerebral oedema after transcervical endometrial resection and uterine irrigation with 1.5% glycine. *Lancet* 344:1187, 1994.
168. Rhymer JC, Bell TJ, Perry KC, Ward JP. Hyponatremia following transurethral resection of the prostate. *Br J Urol* 57:450, 1985.
169. Ryder KW, Olson JF, Kahnoski RJ, et al. Hyperammonemia after transurethral resection of the prostate: A report of 2 cases. *J Urol* 132:995, 1984.
170. Bernstein GT, Loughlin KR, Gittes RF. The physiologic basis of the TUR syndrome. *Surg Res* 46:135, 1989.
171. Robinson AG, Loeb JN. Ethanol ingestion: Commonest cause of elevated plasma osmolality? *N Engl J Med* 284:1253, 1971.
172. Katz M. Hyperglycemia-induced hyponatremia: Calculation of expected serum sodium depression (letter). *N Engl J Med* 289:843, 1973.
173. Hillier TA, Abbott RD, Barett EJ. Hyponatremia: Evaluating the correction factor for hyperglycemia. *Am J Med* 106:399, 1999.
174. Aviram A, Pfau A, Czackes JW, Ullman TD. Hyperosmolality with hypoantremia caused by inappropriate administration of mannitol. *Am J Med* 42:648, 1967.
175. Palevsky PM, Rendulic D, Diven WF. Maltose-induced hyponatremia. *Ann Intern Med* 118:526, 1993.
176. Pollock AS, Arieff AI. Abnormalities of cell volume regulation and their functional consequences. *Am J Physiol* 239:F195, 1980.
177. Arieff AI. Hyponatremia, convulsions, respiratory arrest, and permanent brain damage after selective surgery in healthy women. *N Engl J Med* 314:1529, 1986.
178. Strange K. Regulation of solute and water balance and cell volume in the central nervous system. *J Am Soc Nephrol* 3:12, 1992.
179. Sterns RH, Thomas DJ, Herndon RM. Brain dehydration and neurologic deterioration after correction of hyponatremia. *Kidney Int* 35:69, 1989.
180. Manley GT, Fujimura M, Ma T, et al. Aquaporin-4 deletion in mice reduces brain edema after acute water intoxication and ischemic stroke. *Nat Med* 6:159, 2000.
181. Melton JE, Patlak CS, Pettigrew KD, Cserr HF. Volume regulatory loss of Na, Cl, and K from rat brain during acute hyponatremia. *Am J Physiol* 252:F661, 1987.
182. Verbalis JG, Gullans SR. Hyponatremia causes large sustained reductions in brain content of multiple organic osmolytes in rats. *Brain Res* 567:274, 1991.
183. Lien Y, Shapiro JI, Chan L. Study of brain electrolytes and organic osmolytes during correction of chronic hyponatremia: Implications for the pathogenesis of central pontine myelinolysis. *J Clin Invest* 88:303, 1991.
184. Sterns RH, Baer J, Ebersol S, et al. Organic osmolytes in acute hyponatremia. *Am J Physiol* 264:F833, 1993.
185. Videen JS, Michaelis T, Pinto P, Ross BD. Human cerebral osmolytes during chronic hyponatremia: A protein magnetic resonance spectroscopy study. *J Clin Invest* 95:788, 1995.

186. Somero GN. Protons, osmolytes, and fitness of internal milieu for protein function. *Am J Physiol* 251:R197, 1986.
187. Arieff AI, Llach F, Massry SG. Neurological manifestations and morbidity of hyponatremia: Correlation with brain water and electrolytes. *Medicine* 55:121, 1976.
188. Berl T. Treating hyponatremia: Damned if we do and damned if we don't. *Kidney Int* 37:1006, 1990.
189. Ellis SJ. Severe hyponatraemia: Complications and treatment. *Q J Med* 88:905, 1995.
190. Ayus JC, Wheeler JM, Arieff AI. Postoperative hyponatremic encephalopathy in menstruant women. *Ann Intern Med* 117:891, 1992.
191. Cluitmans FHM, Meinders AE. Management of hyponatremia: Rapid or slow correction? *Am J Med* 88:161, 1990
192. Singer I, Oster JR. Hyponatremia, hyposmolality, and hypotonicity. *Arch Intern Med* 159:333, 1999.
193. Gilbert GJ. Neurologic manifestations of hyponatremia. *N Engl J Med* 274:1153, 1966.
194. Fraser CL, Kucharczyck J, Arieff AI, et al. Sexual differences result in increased morbidity from hyponatremia in female rats. *Am J Physiol* 256:R880, 1989.
195. Arieff AI, Ayus JC, Fraser CL. Hyponatraemia and death or permanent brain damage in children. *Br Med J* 304:1218, 1992.
196. Chung H-M, Kluge R, Schrier R, et al. Clinical assessment of extracellular fluid volume in hyponatremia. *Am J Med* 83:905, 1987.
197. Womersley RA, Darragh JH. Potassium and sodium restriction in the normal human. *J Clin Invest* 34:456, 1955.
198. Kleinschmidt-DeMasters BK, Norenberg MD. Rapid correction of hyponatremia causes demyelination: Relation to central pontine myelinolysis. *Science* 211:1068, 1981.
199. Sterns RH. The treatment of hyponatremia: First, do no harm. *Am J Med* 88:557, 1990.
200. Verbalis JG, Martinez AJ. Neurological and neuropathological sequelae of correction of chronic hyponatremia. *Kidney Int* 39:1274, 1991.
201. Ayus JC, Krothapalii RK, Arieff AI. Treatment of symptomatic hyponatremia and its relation to brain damage: A prospective study. *N Engl J Med* 317:1190, 1987.
202. Sterns RH, Riggs JE, Schochet SS Jr. Osmotic demyelination syndrome following correction of hyponatremia. *N Engl J Med* 314:1535, 1986.
203. Sterns RH, Cappuccio JD, Silver SM, Cohen EP. Neurologic sequelae after treatment of severe hyponatremia: A multicenter perspective. *J Am Soc Nephrol* 4:1522, 1994.
204. Karp BI, Laureno R. Pontine and extrapontine myelinolysis: A neurologic disorder following rapid correction of hyponatremia. *Medicine* 72:359, 1993.
205. Laureno R, Karp BI. Myelinolysis after correction of hyponatremia. *Ann Intern Med* 126:57, 1997.
206. Brunner JE, Redmond JM, Haggar AM, et al. Central pontine myelinolysis and pontine lesions after rapid correction of hyponatremia: A prospective magnetic resonance imaging study. *Ann Neurol* 27:61, 1990.
207. McKee AC, Winkelman MD, Banker BQ. Central pontine myelinolysis in severely burned patients: Relationship to serum hyperosmolality. *Neurology* 38:1211, 1988.
208. Cheng J-C, Zikos D, Skopicki HA, et al. Long-term neurologic outcome in psychogenic water drinkers with severe symptomatic hyponatremia: The effect of rapid correction. *Am J Med* 88:561, 1990.
209. Sterns RH. Severe symptomatic hyponatremia: Treatment and outcome. A study of 64 cases. *Ann Intern Med* 107:656, 1987.
210. Narins RG. Therapy of hyponatremia: Does haste make waste? *N Engl J Med* 314:1573, 1986.
211. Soupart A, Penninckx R, Stenuit A et al. Treatment of chronic hyponatremia in rats by intravenous saline: Comparison of rate versus magnitude of correction. *Kidney Int* 41:1667, 1992.
212. Soupart A, Penninckx R, Crenier L, et al. Prevention of brain demyelination in rats after excessive correction of chronic hyponatremia by serum sodium lowering. *Kidney Int* 45:193, 1994.

213. Oh MS, Uribarri J, Barrido D, et al. Danger of central pontine myelinolysis in hypotonic dehydration and recommendation for treatment. *Am J Med Sci* 298:41, 1989.
214. Soupart A, Ngassa M, Decaux G. Therapeutic relowering of the serum sodium in a patient after excessive correction of hyponatremia. *Clin Nephrol* 51:383, 1999.
215. Dzauy VJ, Hollenberg NK. Renal response to captopril in severe heart failure: Role of furosemide in natriuresis and reversal of hyponatremia. *Ann Intern Med* 100:777, 1984.
216. Packer M, Medina N, Yushak M. Correction of dilutional hyponatremia in severe chronic heart failure by converting-enzyme inhibition. *Ann Intern Med* 100:782, 1984.
217. Riegger GA, Kochsiek K. Vasopressin, renin and norepinephrine levels before and after captopril administration in patients with congestive heart failure due to dilated cardiomyopathy. *Am J Cardiol* 58:300, 1986.
218. Rouse D, Dalmeida W, Williamson FC, Suki WN. Captopril inhibits the hydroosmotic effect of ADH in the cortical collecting tubule. *Kidney Int* 32:845, 1987.
219. Cox MM, Guzzo J, Morrison G, Singer I. Demeclocycline and therapy of hyponatremia. *Ann Intern Med* 86:113, 1977.
220. DeTroyer A, Pilloy W, Broeckaert I, Demanet JC. Demeclocycline treatment of water retention in cirrhosis. *Ann Intern Med* 85:336, 1976.
221. Miller PD, Linas SL, Schrier RW. Plasma demeclocycline levels and nephrotoxicity: Correlation in hyponatremic cirrhotic patients. *JAMA* 243:2513, 1980.
222. Perez-Ayuso RM, Arroyo V, Campos J, et al. Effect of demeclocycline on renal function and urinary prostaglandin E_2 and kallikrein in hyponatremic cirrhotics. *Nephron* 36:30, 1984.
223. Palm C, Gross P. V_2-vasopressin receptor antagonists—Mechanism of effect and clinical implications in hyponatraemia. *Nephrol Dial Transplant* 14:2559, 1999.
224. Saito T, Ishikawa S, Abe K, et al. Acute aquaresis by the nonpeptide arginine vasopressin (AVP) antagonist OPC-31260 improves hyponatremia in patients with syndrome of inappropriate secretion of antidiuretic hormone (SIADH). *J Clin Endocrinol Metab* 82:1054, 1997.
225. Serradeil-Le Gal C, Lacour C, Valette G, et al. Characterization of SR 121463A, a highly potent and selective vasopressin V_2 receptor antagonist. *J Clin Invest* 98:2729, 1996.
226. Hantman D, Rossier B, Zohlman R, Schrier RW. Rapid correction of hyponatremia in the syndrome of inappropriate secretion of antidiuretic hormone: an alternative to hypertonic saline. *Ann Intern Med* 78:870, 1973.
227. Decaux G, Waterlot Y, Genette F, Mockel J. Treatment of the syndrome of inappropriate secretion of antidiuretic hormone with furosemide. *N Engl J Med* 304:329, 1981.
228. Decaux G, Waterlot Y, Genette F, et al. Inappropriate secretion of antidiuretic hormone treated with frusemide. *Br Med J* 285:89, 1982.
229. Decaux G, Brimioulle S, Genette F, Mockel J. Treatment of the syndrome of inappropriate secretion of antidiuretic hormone by urea. *Am J Med* 69:99, 1980.
230. Decaux G, Prospert F, Penninckx R, et al. 5-year treatment of chronic syndrome of inappropriate secretion of antidiuretic hormone with oral urea. *Nephron* 63:468, 1993.
231. DeTroyer A, Demanet JC. Correction of antidiuresis by demeclocycline. *N Engl J Med* 293:915, 1975.
232. White M, Fetner CD. Treatment of the syndrome of inappropriate secretion of antidiuretic hormone with lithium carbonate. *N Engl J Med* 292:390, 1975.
233. Singer I, Rotenberg D. Demeclocycline-induced nephrogenic diabetes insipidus. *Ann Intern Med* 79:679, 1973.
234. Boton R, Gaviria M, Batlle DC. Prevalence, pathogenesis, and treatment of renal dysfunction associated with chronic lithium therapy. *Am J Kidney Dis* 10:329, 1987.
235. Batlle DC, von Riotte AB, Gaviria M, Grupp M. Amelioration of polyuria by amiloride in patients receiving long-term lithium therapy. *N Engl J Med* 312:408, 1985.
236. Marples D, Christensen S, Christensen EI, et al. Lithium-induced downregulation of aquaporin-2 water channel expression in rat kidney medulla. *J Clin Invest* 95:1838, 1995.
237. Hensen J, Haenelt M, Gross P. Lithium induced polyuria and renal vasopressin receptor density. *Nephrol Dial Transplant* 11:622, 1996.

238. Forrest JN Jr, Cox M, Hong C, et al. Superiority of demeclocycline over lithium in the treatment of chronic syndrome of inappropriate secretion of antidiuretic hormone. *N Engl J Med* 298:173, 1978.
239. Baker RS, Hurley RM, Feldman W. Treatment of recurrent syndrome of inappropriate secretion of antidiuretic hormone with lithium. *J Pediatr* 90:480, 1977.

TWENTY-FOUR

HYPEROSMOLAL STATES— HYPERNATREMIA

The introduction to disorders of water balance presented in Chap. 22 should be read before proceeding with this discussion.

PATHOPHYSIOLOGY

Hypernatremia represents hyperosmolality. Since Na^+ is an effective osmole, the increase in plasma osmolality (P_{osm}) induced by the rise in the plasma Na^+ concentration creates an osmotic gradient that results in water movement out of the cells into the extracellular fluid. It is this cellular dehydration in the brain that is primarily responsible for the neurologic symptoms that may be seen with this disorder (see "Symptoms," below).

   A similar syndrome can be produced when the P_{osm} is elevated by hyperglycemia. Hyperosmolality can also result from the accumulation of a cell-permeable (or osmotically *ineffective*) solute, such as urea (as in renal failure) or ethanol;[1] in these settings, there is *no water shift* in the steady state, since osmotic equilibrium is reached by solute entry into cells. As a result, symptoms of hyperosmolality do not occur.

Since it is the effective P_{osm} that is clinically important, the contribution of urea (measured as blood urea nitrogen, or BUN) to the P_{osm} should be excluded. In general, the effective P_{osm} can be calculated from (see page 247)

$$\text{Effective } P_{osm} = \text{measured } P_{osm} - \frac{\text{BUN}}{2.8} \qquad (24\text{-}1)$$

or estimated from

$$\text{Effective } P_{osm} \cong 2 \times \text{plasma } [Na^+] + \frac{[\text{glucose}]}{18} \qquad (24\text{-}2)$$

The normal value for the effective P_{osm} is 270 to 285 mosmol/kg. The BUN and glucose concentration are divided by 2.8 and 18 to convert from units of mg/dL to mmol/L.

Generation of Hypernatremia

From the relationship between the plasma Na^+ concentration and the osmolality of the body fluids (see Fig. 22-2),

$$\text{Plasma } [Na^+] \cong \frac{Na_e^+ + K_e^+}{\text{total body water}} \qquad (24\text{-}3)$$

it can be seen that hypernatremia can result from *water loss or Na^+ retention* (Table 24-1). The serious toxicity of hyperkalemia prevents the retention of enough K^+ to significantly raise the plasma Na^+ concentration.

To cause hypernatremia, water loss in excess of $(Na^+ + K^+)$ must occur. Free water can be lost from the skin and respiratory tract and in a dilute urine. The latter requires either decreased secretion of antidiuretic hormone [central diabetes insipidus (CDI)] or end-organ resistance to its effect [nephrogenic diabetes insipidus (NDI)].

The effect of gastrointestinal water loss, as occurs with diarrhea, is more variable and illustrates the importance of the relationship in Eq. (24-3).[2] The fluid that is lost in secretory diarrheas, such as cholera, is isosmotic to plasma and is almost entirely composed of Na^+ and K^+ salts.[3] The loss of this fluid will produce volume depletion but will not directly affect the plasma Na^+ concentration. The findings are different, however, in osmotic diarrheas, such as those seen with lactulose (to treat hepatic encephalopathy), charcoal-sorbitol (to treat a drug overdose), malabsorption, and some infectious enterides. In these settings, the diarrheal fluid is also isosmotic to plasma, but has a $(Na^+ + K^+)$ concentration of only 30 to 110 meq/L, with the nonreabsorbed solute accounting for most of the remaining osmoles.[3-6] Thus, water is lost in excess of $(Na^+ + K^+)$, which will tend to raise the plasma Na^+ concentration.

Similar considerations apply to increased urinary solute losses induced by diuretic drugs or osmotic diuretics (such as glucose or mannitol). In these settings,

Table 24-1 Etiology of hypernatremia

Water loss
  A. Insensible loss
     1. Increased sweating: fever, exposure to high temperatures, exercise
     2. Burns
     3. Respiratory infections
  B. Renal loss
     1. Central diabetes insipidus
     2. Nephrogenic diabetes insipidus
     3. Osmotic diuresis: glucose, urea, mannitol
  C. Gastrointestinal loss
     1. Osmotic diarrhea: lactulose, malabsorption, some infectious enteritides
  D. Hypothalamic disorders
     1. Primary hypodipsia
     2. Reset osmostat due to volume expansion in primary mineralocorticoid excess
     3. Essential hypernatremia with loss of osmoreceptor function
  E. Water loss into cells
     1. Seizures or severe exercise
     2. Rhabdomyolysis
Sodium retention
  A. Administration of hypertonic NaCl or $NaHCO_3$
  B. Ingestion of sodium.

the plasma Na^+ concentration will tend to increase because the $Na^+ + K^+$ concentration is less than that of the plasma.[2]

Thirst and the Maintenance of Hypernatremia

The normal defense against the development of hypernatremia is the stimulation of both antidiuretic hormone (ADH) release and thirst by the hypothalamic osmoreceptors (see Chap. 6). The combination of decreased water excretion and increased water intake results in water retention and return of the plasma Na^+ concentration to normal. The secretion of ADH generally begins when the P_{osm} exceeds 275 to 285 mosmol/kg (see Fig. 23-1), whereas the threshold for thirst appears to be somewhat higher (approximately 2 to 5 mosmol/kg).[7,8] Osmoregulation is normally so efficient that the P_{osm} is *maintained within a range of 1 to 2 percent* (usually between 280 and 290 mosmol/kg), despite wide variations in Na^+ and water intake.

Although ADH release may occur earlier, it is *thirst that provides the ultimate protection against hypernatremia.*[9] In patients with CDI who secrete little or no ADH, for example, renal water reabsorption falls, and the urine output can exceed 10 to 15 L/day. Nevertheless, water balance is maintained because water intake is augmented to match output. Conversely, even with maximum ADH secretion, the kidney may be unable to retain enough water to offset insensible losses from the skin and respiratory tract in a patient with hypodipsia (diminished thirst).[10] Thus, hypernatremia due to water loss occurs only in patients who have hypodipsia (an extremely rare disorder), in adults with altered mental status, and in infants, who may have an intact thirst mechanism but are unable to ask for water.[11,12] A plasma Na^+ concentration greater than 150 meq/L is *virtually never seen in an alert adult with a normal thirst mechanism and access to water.*

In adults, *hypernatremia developing outside the hospital most often occurs in patients over the age of 60.*[12,13] In addition to an increased frequency of concurrent illness and diminished mental status, increasing age is also associated with diminished osmotic stimulation of thirst, even though the release of ADH is maintained.[14,15] Careful study of ADH-secreting neurons in the brain in elderly subjects has actually shown an increase in activity, which may reflect a compensatory response to the age-related loss of ADH receptors in the kidney.[16]

Although most otherwise healthy older patients maintain normal water balance, their response to a given stress may be impaired, increasing the likelihood of their becoming hypernatremic. Mentally handicapped patients are also at increased risk of negative water balance and hypernatremia.[17]

ETIOLOGY

The major causes of hypernatremia are listed in Table 24-1 according to their probable underlying mechanism.

Insensible and Gastrointestinal Water Loss

Insensible fluid losses from the skin and respiratory tract are hypoosmotic to plasma and average 800 to 1000 mL/day in adults. Any condition that increases these losses—such as fever, respiratory infections, burns, or exposure to high temperatures—predisposes toward the development of hypernatremia. Gastrointestinal water losses, due to an osmotic diarrhea, can also produce a similar effect.[3,5,6] Lactulose, for example, is used to treat hepatic encephalopathy. It is given in a hyperosmotic solution, resulting in the flow of water into the gastrointestinal tract. When these losses are large, as manifested by water diarrhea, hypernatremia can ensue.[5] The decreased thirst induced by the diminished mental status in these patients plays an essential permissive role.

Hypernatremia following a diarrheal illness was once a relatively common problem in infants.[18,19] Increased insensible (due to fever) and gastrointestinal losses occur in this setting, and the degree of dehydration does not have to be very large in an infant to produce a substantial elevation in the plasma Na^+ concentration. Hyperglycemia may also be seen, further elevating the effective P_{osm}.[19] This increase in the plasma glucose concentration (to as high as 300 to 500 mg/dL) appears to be a stress response, perhaps mediated by catecholamines, and is corrected with rehydration. In recent years, the incidence of hypernatremic dehydration following gastroenteritis in infants has fallen, primarily because of the use of low-solute feedings (Na^+ plus K^+ concentration about 95 meq/L), which supply more free water to replace the insensible losses.[11,20,21]

Diabetes Insipidus

Diabetes insipidus is characterized by the complete or partial failure of ADH secretion (CDI) or of the renal response to ADH (NDI). As a result, renal water reabsorption falls, and a diuresis of dilute urine ensues (3 to 20 L/day). It must be emphasized again that the majority of these patients maintain water balance with a near normal plasma Na^+ concentration because their thirst mechanism is intact.[22,23] Their major complaints are polyuria and polydipsia, not the symptoms of hypernatremia.

The outcome is different, however, if the hypothalamic disorder producing CDI also interferes with thirst. In this setting, even a partial defect in ADH release can lead to water loss and potentially severe hypernatremia.[22,24] For example, a patient with partial CDI may be able to maximally concentrate his or her urine (U_{max}) to 400 mosmol/kg. This is hyperosmotic to plasma but less than the normal U_{max} of 800 to 1400 mosmol/kg. If this patient excreted 800 mosmol/day of solute (primarily Na^+ and K^+ salts and urea), the solute load would be excreted in the urine in a minimum of 2000 mL of water (800 mosmol of solute in 2000 mL of water equals 400 mosmol/kg). In contrast, the obligatory renal water loss would be only 800 mL if the U_{max} were normal at 1000 mosmol/kg (800 mosmol in 800 mL of water equals 1000 mosmol/kg). Thus, the reduction in renal concentrating ability can result in an extra 1200 mL of water lost in the urine per day. In a hypodipsic patient, this added loss might not be replaced, leading to the development of hypernatremia.

Central diabetes insipidus   ADH is synthesized in the supraoptic and paraventricular nuclei in the hypothalmus. It then streams down the axons of the supraopticohypophyseal tract and is stored in and subsequently released from the posterior lobe of the pituitary (neurohypophysis) (Fig. 24-1).[25,26] Impaired secretion of ADH can be induced by a variety of clinical disorders that disrupt the osmoreceptors, the hypothalamic nuclei, or the supraopticohypophyseal tract (Table 24-2).[27,28] In contrast, damage to the tract below the median eminence or removal of the posterior pituitary usually produces only a *transient* period of diabetes insipidus.[28] In these settings, ADH can still be secreted into the systemic circulation via the portal capillaries in the median eminence (Fig. 24-1).

Among the causes of CDI (Table 24-2), approximately 75 percent of cases are due to idiopathic DI, neurosurgery (particularly for craniopharyngioma), head trauma, and primary or secondary malignancies or infiltrative diseases, such as Langerhans cell histiocytosis (histiocytosis X).[28-31] Idiopathic CDI accounts for approximately 30 percent of cases, being associated with destruction of the hormone-secreting cells in the hypothalamic nuclei. It has been suggested that an autoimmune process is involved in many, if not most, patients.[32] In some

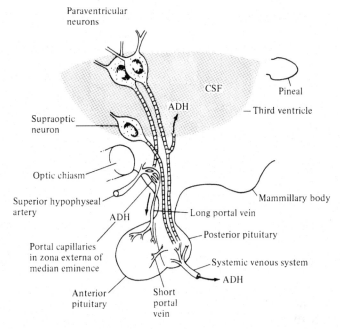

Figure 24-1   Diagram of the mammalian hypothalamus and pituitary gland depicting pathways for the secretion of ADH. The hormone is formed in the supraoptic and paraventricular nuclei, transported in granules along their axons, and then secreted at three sites: the posterior pituitary gland, the portal capillaries of the median eminence, and the cerebrospinal fluid (CSF) of the third ventricle. (*Adapted from Zimmerman EA, Robinson AG,* Kidney Int *10:12, 1976. Reprinted by permission from* Kidney International.)

Table 24-2   Etiology of central diabetes insipidus

Idiopathic—may be familial
Neurosurgery
   A. Craniopharyngioma
   B. Transsphenoidal surgery
Head trauma
Hypoxic or ischemic encephalopathy
   A. Cardiopulmonary arrest
   B. Shock
   C. Sheehan's syndrome
Neoplastic
   A. Primary: craniopharyngioma, pinealoma, cyst
   B. Metastatic: breast, lung
Miscellaneous
   A. Histiocytosis X
   B. Sarcoidosis
   C. Anorexia nervosa
   D. Cerebral aneurysm
   E. Encephalitis or meningitis

individuals, antibodies directed against the vasopressin-producing cells may be responsible for the progressive decline in ADH release.[33]

The autoimmune process is characterized by lymphocytic inflammation of the pituitary stalk and posterior pituitary that resolves after destruction of the target neurons.[32] Magnetic resonance imaging (MRI) performed when active inflammation is still present often reveals thickening and/or enlargement of these structures. The destructive process may also lead to concurrent abnormalities in anterior pituitary function, with decreased release of growth hormone and adrenocorticotropic hormone (ACTH) in some cases.[34]

Rarely, idiopathic CDI is a familial disorder, usually with autosomal dominant inheritance. The defect in at least some cases involves a point mutation in the gene encoding for preprovasopressin-neurophysin II, the precursor of ADH.[35,36] The precursor that is produced cannot be normally cleaved or transported and accumulates locally, leading to death of the ADH-producing cells.[37] This sequence probably accounts for three characteristic findings in this disorder: (1) the development of marked polyuria even though only one of the two hormone-producing genes is defective; (2) delayed onset of polyuria for months to years, with an age of onset that ranges from 1 to 28 years,[38] and a bright spot visible on MRI (perhaps due to the accumulated precursor) that is not seen in patients with nonfamilial idiopathic CDI.[37]

Neurosurgery (usually transsphenoidal) or trauma to the hypothalamus or tract is another common cause of central DI.[29-39] However, a somewhat different response has been detected with transfrontal surgery for a craniopharyngioma. In this setting, the polyuria appears to result from the release of an ADH precursor from the hypothalamus that competes for but does not activate the antidiuretic V_2 receptors.[39] These patients initially have high ADH levels by immunoassay but have little or no biological activity and a diminished response to exogenous hormone replacement. Thus, they behave as if they have nephrogenic DI, although the polyuria is typically transient.

Damage to the hypothalamus or tract can produce a typical *triphasic* response (Fig. 24-2).

- There is an initial polyuric phase that typically begins within 24 h, lasts 4 to 5 days, and probably represents inhibition of ADH release due to hypothalamic dysfunction.[29,40]
- From days 6 to 11, however, there is an antidiuretic phase that represents slow release of stored hormone from the degenerating posterior pituitary. During this time, excessive water intake can produce hyponatremia in a manner similar to that in the syndrome of inappropriate ADH secretion (SIADH; see Chap. 23).
- The second stage is often followed by permanent CDI once the neurohypophyseal stores are depleted, although some patients have only transient SIADH (also called isolated second phase) and then appear to recover without developing late polyuria.[41,42] Adrenal insufficiency due to ACTH deficiency may contribute to the hyponatremia in this setting.[41]

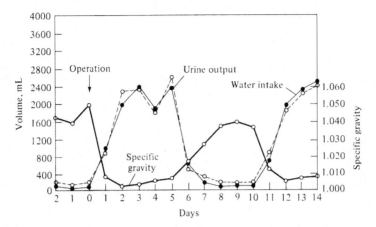

Figure 24-2   Typical triphasic cycle produced by section of the hypophyseal stalk and damage to the median eminence. The interphase of excess ADH secretion extends from day 6 to day 10 or 11. (*From Hollinshead WH*, Mayo Clin Proc *39:92, 1964, with permission.*)

It must be emphasized, however, that polyuria following neurosurgery is most often *not* due to CDI.[29] More common causes in this setting include excretion of excess fluid administered during surgery and an osmotic diuresis resulting from treatment aimed at minimizing cerebral edema with mannitol or corticosteroids (which can lead to hyperglycemia and glucosuria). These conditions can be distinguished by measuring the urine osmolality and the response to water restriction and the administration of exogenous ADH (see "Polyuria," below).

Hypoxic encephalopathy or severe ischemia, as occurs following cardiopulmonary arrest or shock, can also lead to diminished ADH release.[28,43] Although marked polyuria can occur in these settings, the functional impairment is mild and subclinical in some cases. As an example, overt diabetes insipidus is unusual in patients with Sheehan's syndrome (postpartum panhypopituitarism) despite frequent atrophy of the posterior pituitary and hypothalamic nuclei. Nevertheless, ADH secretion in response to raising the P_{osm} is frequently subnormal.[44]

Hemodynamic factors can also lead to transient CDI by a second mechanism. Polyuria is occasionally seen after correction of a supraventricular tachycardia. In this setting, both a natriuresis and a water diuresis occur, which may be due to enhanced release of atrial natriuretic peptide and diminished secretion of ADH, respectively.[45] Increases in left atrial and systemic blood pressures may activate local volume receptors, thereby leading to these transient hormonal changes.

Patients with Langerhans cell histiocytosis (histiocytosis X) are at particularly high risk for CDI.[31] As many as 40 percent develop polyuria within the first 4 years, especially if there is multisystem involvement and proptosis.

A similar infiltrative disease can occur with sarcoidosis, which can also cause polyuria due to NDI (induced by hypercalcemia) or primary polydipsia.[46] Other infiltrative disorders that may rarely cause CDI include Wegener's granulomatosis and autoimmune hypophysitis.[47-49]

Polyuria without hypernatremia is also a common finding in anorexia nervosa. ADH release in response to an elevation in the P_{osm} is erratic or subnormal in this disorder, which may also be associated with a primary increase in thirst.[50] These abnormalities are presumably due to the associated cerebral dysfunction.

Nephrogenic diabetes insipidus Nephrogenic diabetes insipidus (NDI) is a congenital or acquired disorder in which hypothalamic function and ADH release are normal, but the ability to concentrate the urine is reduced because of diminished or absent renal responsiveness to ADH.[51,52] Concentration of the urine normally involves two basic steps: (1) creation of a hyperosmotic medullary interstitium (to a maximum of 800 to 1400 mosmol/kg), primarily by NaCl reabsorption without water in the ascending limb of the loop of Henle (a process called countercurrent multiplication); and (2) osmotic equilibration of the urine in the collecting tubules with the medullary interstitium (see Chap. 4). ADH is essential for the second step since it markedly increases the water permeability of the collecting tubules (see Chap. 6).

Thus, NDI must be associated with an abnormality in either countercurrent function or the ability to respond to ADH. The various causes of NDI are listed in Table 24-3.

Hereditary NDI   Congenital NDI is an uncommon condition that is transmitted in an X-linked recessive fashion with varying degrees of penetrance in heterozygous females.[53-55] Thus, males tend to have the complete disorder, whereas the

Table 24-3   Causes of nephrogenic diabetes insipidus

Congenital
Hypercalcemia
Hypokalemia
Drugs
   1.   Lithium
   2.   Demeclocycline
   3.   Streptozotocin
Sjögren's syndrome
Amyloidosis
Osmotic diuresis: glucose, mannitol, urea
Loop diuretics
Acute and chronic renal failure
Hypercalcemia
Hypokalemia
Sickle cell anemia
Pregnancy
Ifosfamide
Propoxyphene overdose
Methoxyflurane

manifestations range from the carrier state to marked polyuria in females. Two factors contribute to the variable manifestations in females: One-half the cells will be normal by the Lyon hypothesis, and the genetic defect is of variable severity. Thus, some women may be asymptomatic in day-to-day life but develop moderate to severe polyuria during pregnancy when vasopressinases released from the placenta increase the metabolic clearance of endogenous ADH (see below).

The defect in most patients with congenital NDI appears to involve different mutations in the V_2-receptor gene.[54-57] These mutations can lead to decreased hormone binding, impaired intracellular transport or coupling to the adenylyl cyclase system, or diminished synthesis or accelerated degradation of the receptor.[54] The V_2 receptor mediates the antidiuretic response to ADH and also promotes peripheral vasodilation and the release from endothelial cells of factor VIII and von Willebrand's factor, all of which are impaired in congenital NDI.[58,59] In comparison, the V_1 receptor, which causes vasoconstriction and increased renewal prostaglandin release, functions normally in this disorder.[58]

A second, autosomal recessive form of hereditary nephrogenic DI has been described that further elucidates our understanding of the mechanism of action of ADH. In this disorder, the V_2 receptor and vasodilator and coagulation responses to ADH are intact. The defect lies in the genes for the aquaporin-2 water channels.[60,61] These channels are normally stored in the cytosol; under the influence of ADH, they move to and fuse with the luminal membrane, thereby allowing water to be reabsorbed down the favorable concentration gradient.[62,63] The mutations may lead to either impaired trafficking of the water channels, which do not fuse with the luminal membrane, or decreased channel function.[60,61]

The major causes of acquired NDI that are sufficiently severe to produce polyuria in adults are *lithium toxicity, hypercalcemia*, and the *osmotic diuresis* associated with uncontrolled diabetes mellitus. Polyuria is a common problem within lithium therapy, appearing as early as 8 to 12 weeks and ultimately occurring in approximately 20 percent of patients.[64-66*] In addition, a subclinical impairment in concentrating ability is present in another 30 percent of cases. Although generally reversible, the concentrating defect may be permanent after prolonged drug usage.[64,66]

Lithium appears to act by accumulating within the collecting tubule cells, after entering the cells through the Na^+ channels in the luminal membrane (see Fig. 5-2).[67] It then interferes with the ability of ADH to increase water permeability. How this occurs is incompletely understood, but a number of different mechanisms may be involved: Decreased stimulation of adenylate cyclase (mediated in part by enhanced activity of G_i, the inhibitory guanine regulatory protein that reduces the activity of adenylate cyclase),[68] reduced density of ADH receptors,[69] and a post-cyclic AMP defect that may be mediated by downregulation of aquaporin-2.[70]

---

* Some patients have a modest rise in the U_{osm} after the administration of ADH, suggesting that a mild impairment in ADH release may also contribute to the polyuria.[64]

A more predictable resistance to ADH occurs with the use of demeclocycline, a tetracycline derivative.[71] The duration of administration of this drug is usually too short for polyuria to be a serious problem. However, the increase in free-water excretion induced by demeclocycline has led to its use in occasional patients with refractory hyponatremia (see Chap. 23).[72]

Hypercalcemia and hypokalemia Hypercalcemia and hypokalemia produce a form of NDI that is generally reversible within 1 to 12 weeks after correction of the electrolyte disturbance.[73-75] With *hypercalcemia*, the concentrating defect may become clinically apparent when the plasma Ca^{2+} concentration exceeds 11 mg/dL.[74] It was originally suggested that calcium deposition in the medulla with secondary tubulointerstitial injury may play an important role.[76] More recent studies suggest an important role for impaired regulation of aquaporin-2[77] and for activation of the normal calcium-sensing receptor by the elevation in the plasma calcium concentration.[78]

- Calcium-sensing receptors are expressed on the *basolateral* membrane in the thick ascending limb of the loop of Henle. Activation of these receptors by calcium reduces sodium chloride and calcium reabsorption in the thick ascending limb, an effect that appears to be mediated by the generation of a P450 arachidonic acid metabolite (possibly 20-HETE), which then induces closure of the luminal potassium channel.[79] Inhibition of loop reabsorption impairs generation of the medullary osmotic gradient that is essential for urinary concentration.
- Calcium-sensing receptors are expressed on the *luminal* membrane of the cells of the inner medullary collecting duct. Diminished calcium reabsorption in the loop of Henle in hypercalcemia results in more calcium being delivered to and binding with calcium-sensing receptors in the collecting duct. Activation of these receptors reduces the antidiuretic hormone–induced increase in water permeability.[80]

The concentrating defect seen with *hypokalemia* requires a K^+ deficit of 300 to 400 meq, a setting in which the plasma K^+ concentration should be under 3.0 meq/L (see Fig. 12-1).[75] Collecting tubule responsiveness to ADH is diminished by hypokalemia,[81,82] an effect that may be mediated in part by a reduction in cyclic AMP generation.[83] Hypokalemia may also impair countercurrent function by interfering with NaCl transport in the thick ascending limb.[84,85]

The polyuria seen with these electrolyte disorders has been largely attributed to the associated defects in concentrating ability. However, hypokalemia and perhaps hypercalcemia also may directly stimulate thirst.[86-88] How this might occur is not known.

Osmotic and nonosmotic diuretics An osmotic diuresis refers to enhanced urinary water loss induced by the presence of large amounts of nonreabsorbed solute in the tubular lumen.[89] The increase in urine output induced by the excess solutes results in a dilutional fall in the urine $(Na^+ + K^+)$ concentration to a level below that in the plasma.[90] From Eq. (24-3), this *loss of water in excess of $(Na^+ + K^+)$* will directly raise the plasma Na^+ concentration unless there is a concomitant increase in fluid intake.

Uncontrolled diabetes mellitus with glucosuria is the most common cause of an osmotic diuresis, although a similar problem can also occur in patients given either high-protein tube feedings (resulting in the formation of urea from hepatic protein metabolism) or prolonged infusions of hypertonic mannitol.[90-92] The plasma Na^+ concentration is variable at presentation in uncontrolled diabetes, since the effect of the osmotic diuresis is counteracted by hyperglycemia-induced water movement out of the cells (see Chap. 25).[93] However, hypernatremia is not uncommon after insulin therapy has been initiated, as both glucose and water reenter the cells.

Loop diuretics, such as furosemide and bumetanide, impair urinary concentration by inhibiting NaCl reabsorption in the thick ascending limb. However, these agents are short-acting, and the water losses can be replaced by oral intake. As a result, hypernatremia is an unusual consequence of diuretic therapy.

Other An inability to concentrate the urine maximally is an early finding in most forms of renal failure. Several factors contribute to this problem, including the osmotic diuresis resulting from increased solute excretion in the remaining functioning nephrons,[94,95] decreased tubular responsiveness to ADH,[96] and interference with the countercurrent mechanism in disorders affecting the renal medulla, such as chronic pyelonephritis and analgesic abuse nephropathy.[97] The net effect is that, as the renal failure becomes more severe, the U_{max} falls, becoming isosmotic or even slightly hypoosmotic to plasma.[98] However, the degree of *polyuria is usually limited by the reduction in functioning renal mass.* A more severe concentrating defect (U_{max} less than 150 mosmol/kg) with marked polyuria may transiently follow the relief of urinary tract obstruction, but this is clearly a rare occurrence.[99]

Diminished concentrating ability is an early and uniform finding in patients with sickle cell anemia.[100,101] The low partial pressure of oxygen and high osmolality of the renal medulla favor sickling in the vasa recta, thereby impairing countercurrent function.[102] The net effect is that, by the age of 10, the U_{max} is only 400 to 500 mosmol/kg, less than half the normal value.[103,104] These changes occur later and are less severe in patients with sickle cell (SC) trait or hemoglobin SC disease.[100] Transfusions with hemoglobin A can initially reverse the concentrating defect, presumably by restoring vasa recta flow.[103,104] However, this beneficial response is lost by age 15, at which time chronic medullary ischemia has produced irreversible interstitial fibrosis and tubular atrophy.

On rare occasions, amyloidosis[105] and Sjögren's syndrome[106] are associated with NDI and polyuria. Biopsy specimens reveal, respectively, amyloid deposits in and lymphocytic infiltration around the collecting tubules. These changes presumably interfere with tubular function and are responsible for the concentrating defect.

Another cause of NDI is the chemotherapeutic agent ifosfamide, which is a potent tubular toxin.[107] Both proximal and distal nephron injury are common problems with this drug. Thus, in addition to decreased concentrating ability, one or more of the following tubular abnormalities also may be seen: type 1 or type 2 renal tubular acidosis, phosphate wasting and hypophosphatemia (possibly leading to rickets in children), renal glucosuria, and aminoaciduria. Two other drugs that are infrequently associated with NDI are cidofovir and foscarnet, which are used to treat cytomegalovirus infection in HIV-infected patients.[108,109]

Finally, an unusual form of NDI and polyuria has been described in selected women during the second half of pregnancy.[110,111] Normal pregnancy is associated with high circulating levels of vasopressinase (probably released from the placenta), leading to rapid degradation of endogenous or exogenous ADH.[112] In the great majority of patients, this change is not clinically important and leads to no symptoms. Those women who develop polyuria may have higher than normal vasopressinase activity or, possibly, subclinical central or perhaps congenital NDI that is unmasked during pregnancy. Although these patients are resistant to vasopressin, the polyuria can be controlled by the administration of dDAVP, which appears to be resistant to the vasopressinase, perhaps because it has a different N-terminus.[111,112] The polyuria is transient in all patients, resolving spontaneously within a few weeks after delivery.

Polyuria in diabetes insipidus   Several factors contribute to the degree of polyuria in CDI and NDI, including the severity of the concentrating defect, the rate of solute excretion, and the patient's volume status. The interrelationship between the U_{max} and solute excretion can be illustrated by the following examples. Suppose the daily rate of solute excretion is 750 mosmol (composed mostly of Na^+ and K^+ salts and urea). If the U_{max} is 300 mosmol/kg (similar to the P_{osm}), then the minimum urine output will be 2.5 L/day (750 mosmol/day $\div 300$ mosmol/kg = 2.5 L/day). In comparison, the minimum urine output will exceed 7.5 L/day if the U_{max} is 100 mosmol/kg or less. In general, such a severe concentrating defect is seen only in complete CDI, congenital NDI, lithium nephrotoxicity, or occasional patients with hypercalcemia. Most other cases of acquired NDI are associated with a U_{max} that is greater than 300 mosmol/kg. In this setting, *nocturia* may be the primary complaint, since the urine normally becomes most concentrated overnight, when there is no fluid intake.

When the U_{osm} is relatively fixed, as it is in diabetes insipidus, the *rate of solute excretion* becomes the primary determinant of the urine output.* If, for example, the U_{osm} is 100 mosmol/kg, then the daily urine volume will be 8 liters if 800 mosmol is excreted but only 4 liters if 400 mosmol is excreted. This has potential therapeutic importance, since a low-sodium, low-protein diet can limit the degree of polyuria by diminishing solute excretion.

---

* This is in contrast to normal subjects, in whom the major factor affecting the urine output is water intake via its effect on ADH secretion and subsequently the U_{osm}.

Effective circulating volume depletion also can limit the urine volume. Since collecting tubule water reabsorption is diminished in diabetes insipidus, the urine output in this condition is directly related to the volume of water delivered to these segments. The kidney responds to volume depletion in part by lowering the glomerular filtration rate and by increasing proximal Na^+ and water reabsorption (see Chap. 8).[113] As a result, distal delivery and, consequently, the urine output will fall.

This effect of hypovolemia constitutes the rationale for the use of diuretics and a low-sodium diet in the therapy of CDI or NDI (see "Treatment," below). It also explains why cortisol deficiency— which is associated with reductions in systemic blood pressure, cardiac output, and renal blood flow[114] and increased release of ADH from the paraventricular nuclei (see page 710)—limits the urine output in diabetes insipidus. Thus, patients with coexistent anterior and posterior pituitary insufficiency may not initially complain of polyuria. However, the underlying CDI will be unmasked and polyuria will ensue when cortisol replacement is given.[115]

Hypothalamic Dysfunction

Chronic hypernatremia in an alert patient with access to water is indicative of hypothalamic disease affecting thirst. Two somewhat different syndromes have been described which are most often due to tumors, granulomatous diseases such as sarcoidosis, and vascular disease.[7,9] In one disorder, there is a defect in thirst with or without concomitant CDI.[9,10,116,117] In general, *forced water intake* is sufficient to return the plasma Na^+ concentration to normal in this disorder, although partial CDI, if present, may also have to be treated (see below).

In other hypodipsic patients, water loading is ineffective in lowering the plasma Na^+ concentration, as the administered water is excreted in the urine.[118-119] This diuretic response to water, presumably mediated by inhibition of ADH secretion, initially suggested that the osmoreceptors in the hypothalamus were reset to recognize the elevated plasma Na^+ concentration as normal. This syndrome has been called *essential hypernatremia.*

Although rare, essential hypernatremia affords an interesting clinical opportunity to study the independent effects of osmolality and volume of ADH secretion. If the osmostat has been reset upward, its characteristics should be similar to those of the normal osmostat:

- Inhibition of ADH release and the excretion of a dilute urine after a water load
- Stimulation of ADH release and the excretion of a concentrated urine after water restriction
- Maintenance of the new "normal" plasma Na^+ concentration within arrow limits ($\pm$ 1 to 2 percent)

Patients with essential hypernatremia satisfy the first two criteria, but usually display wide variations in the plasma Na^+ concentration, which can range between 150 and 180 meq/L.[118-121]

The latter findings suggests that the *osmoreceptors are relatively insensitive, rather than being reset at a higher level.* The appropriate responses to variations in water intake in this setting might be mediated by the volume receptors, rather than reflecting intact osmoreceptor function. As an example, water loading increases the effective circulating volume, which could inhibit ADH secretion and allow the excess water to be excreted. Conversely, water restriction decreases volume, which could augment ADH secretion.

To test this hypothesis, hypertonic saline can be administered. This increases both the P_{osm} and volume, respectively stimulating and inhibiting ADH release. In a normal subject, the osmotic effect predominates, causing ADH secretion and an increase in U_{osm}.[7,122] However, the U_{osm} typically falls in patients with essential hypernatremia, indicating reduced ADH release despite the rise in P_{osm} (Fig. 24-3).

These findings suggest that essential hypernatremia represents selective damage to the osmoreceptors, resulting in hypodipsia, hypernatremia, and volume-mediated ADH release.[7,119,121] This hypothesis has been directly confirmed in at least one patient, in whom plasma ADH levels increased normally with the induction of hypotension but showed little change with an elevation in the P_{osm}.[121] The normal response to volume again illustrates that the osmoreceptor cells are distinct from the hormone-producing cells.

Hypernatremia due to true resetting of the osmostat has been reported only in states of *primary mineralocorticoid excess* such as primary hyperaldosteronism.[7] The chronic mild hypervolemia induced by the mineralocorticoid effect retards ADH secretion. This shifts the osmotic threshold for ADH release upward by 5 to

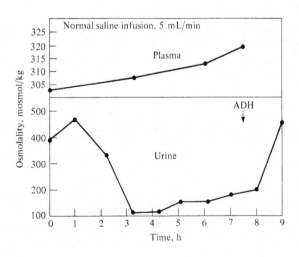

Figure 24-3 Response to saline infusion in a patient with essential hypernatremia. After overnight dehydration, an infusion of approximately 500 mL of saline results in urinary dilution (U_{osm} is 102 mosmol/kg). With continued saline infusion, a sustained water diuresis is observed despite a rising plasma osmolality (301 to 320 mosmol/kg). The ability of exogenous ADH to terminate the water diuresis suggests that endogenous ADH release has been inhibited despite the rise in P_{osm}. (*From DeRubertis FR, Michelis MF, Beck N, et al, J Clin Invest 50:97, 1971, by copyright permission of the American Society for Clinical Investigation.*)

10 mosmol/kg (see Fig. 6-10). As a result, the normal plasma Na^+ concentration in these disorders is slightly elevated at about 145 meq/L. Normal osmoregulation can be restored by removing the source of hormone secretion or by lowering the effective circulating volume with diuretics.[7]

Water Loss into Cells

Transient hypernatremia (in which the plasma Na^+ concentration can rise by as much as 10 to 15 meq/L) can be induced by severe exertion, as with exercise or seizures.[123,124] This effect is presumed to result from an increase in intracellular osmolality, which promotes water movement into the cells. Lactic acidosis also occurs in this setting, and it may be the breakdown of glycogen into smaller molecules (such as lactate) that is responsible for the cellular hyperosmolality.[123] A similar effect can also be seen in rare cases of rhabdomyolysis.[125]

Sodium Overload

Although hypernatremia is generally a problem of water loss, it can also be induced by the ingestion or infusion of hypertonic Na^+ solutions. This problem can occur in infants given high-Na^+ feedings (either accidentally or purposefully) or hypertonic $NaHCO_3$,[126-129] after the use of $NaHCO_3$ during cardiopulmonary resuscitation,[130] or after massive salt ingestion, as might occur with the ingestion of a hypertonic saline emetic or gargle.[131] For example, the inadvertent administration of only 1 tablespoon of NaCl to a newborn can raise the plasma Na^+ concentration by as much as 70 meq/L.[127] These patients are volume overloaded and generally have a high urine Na^+ concentration, in contrast to the low values seen with hypovolemia due to water loss.[129]

SYMPTOMS

The symptoms of hypernatremia (hyperosmolality) are primarily neurologic. Lethargy, weakness, and irritability are the earliest findings, which can then progress to twitching, seizures, coma, and death in severe cases.[132,133] These symptoms are related less to the absolute level of the plasma Na^+ concentration than to the movement of water out of the brain cells down the osmotic gradient created by the rise in the effective P_{osm} (Fig. 24-4). Studies in experimental animals and in humans have revealed that this decrease in brain volume causes rupture of the cerebral veins, resulting in focal intracerebral and subarachnoid hemorrhages and neurologic dysfunction that may be irreversible.[126,133-136] A lumbar puncture at this time may reveal blood in the cerebrospinal fluid.

A clinically significant acute water shift appears to require at least a 30- to 35-mosmol/kg osmolal gradient between the plasma and the brain.[137,138] This gradient, which is derived from animal studies, correlates well with the findings in humans. In children with acute hypernatremia, for example, seizures and

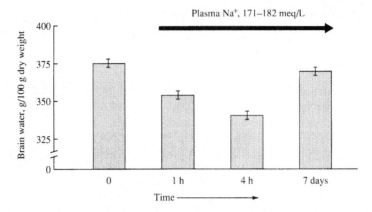

Figure 24-4   Effect of sustained hypernatremia on brain water content in rabbits. Brain water was significantly reduced by 1 to 4 h but returned to normal within 1 week. No values were obtained between 4 h and 1 week. (*From Pollock AS, Arieff AI, Am J Physiol 239:F195, 1980, with permission.*)

potentially permanent neurologic damage are most likely to occur when the plasma Na^+ concentration exceeds 158 meq/L.[135] This 17-meq/L elevation above normal represents, if the anion accompanying Na^+ is included, approximately a 34-mosmol/kg rise in the P_{osm}. However, there is wide interpatient variability in the likelihood of irreversible neurologic dysfunction. For example, some infants have apparently complete recovery from acute elevations in the plasma Na^+ concentration to above 200 meq/L.[129]

Osmotic Adaptation

The cerebral dehydration induced by hypernatremia is transient. Within several hours, the brain begins to adapt to the hyperosmolal state with an increase in brain cell osmolality, resulting in water movement back into the brain and the return of brain volume toward normal (Fig. 24-4).[139-141] Two factors are involved in this initial protective response:

- First, the cerebral contraction induced by hypernatremia lowers the hydraulic pressure in the cerebral interstitial fluid, creating a gradient that favors the bulk movement of fluid from the cerebrospinal fluid into the dehydrated brain, thereby increasing the interstitial volume.[142-144]
- Second, the cells take up Na^+, K^+, Cl^-, and organic solutes, and this leads to an elevation in cell osmolality that pulls water into the cells, thereby returning cell volume toward normal.[139,142]

Similar changes, but in the opposite direction, occur in hyponatremia (see page 669).

If uptake of Na^+ and K^+ were the only cell adaptation, the associated elevation in cell cation concentration could have deleterious effects on the activity of cell proteins.[145] This is minimized by the accumulation of organic solutes called *osmolytes*, which do not interfere with protein function as their concentration rises.[145] Within the brain, increases in the amino acids glutamine and glutamate and in inositol appear to constitute most of the osmolyte response to hypernatremia in animals,[146,147] accounting for approximately 35 percent of the rise in brain cell osmoles.[147]

Inositol accumulation is primarily mediated by uptake from the extracellular fluid via an increased number of inositol transporters in the cell membrane.[139,148] It is not clear whether enhanced uptake or intracellular release from cell proteins is responsible for the accumulation of glutamine and glutamate. This requirement of the synthesis of new transporters explains why osmolyte uptake occurs more slowly than cation uptake, since the latter is probably mediated by the activation of quiescent channels in the cell membrane.[139]

One study of an infant with an initial plasma sodium concentration of 195 meq/L confirmed the general applicability of these observations to humans.[149] The patient was first studied, using proton nuclear magnetic resonance (NMR) spectroscopy, on day 4, when the plasma sodium concentration had fallen to 156 meq/L. At this time, there was a 17-mosmol/kg increase in brain osmolyte concentration, due primarily to the accumulation of inositol. The excess brain osmolyte concentration fell to 6 mosmol/kg on day 7 and was normal by day 36.

One question that remains unresolved in the process of osmotic adaptation in hypernatremia is how the alterations in osmolality are sensed by the cells and then lead to the desired changes in solute balance. There is evidence that hyperosmolality, perhaps via stress on the cytoskeleton as the cell volume falls, activates a specific protein kinase.[150] This kinase, via protein phosphorylation, may then lead to activation of transporters, such as the sodium-inositol cotransporter, that promote solute uptake into the cells.

Clinical consequences   The near normalization of brain water content has two important clinical consequences. First, patients with *chronic* hypernatremia may be relatively asymptomatic, despite a plasma Na^+ concentration as high as 170 to 180 meq/L.[151] Thus, the severity of the neurologic symptoms is related to both the degree and, more importantly, the *rate of rise in the effective P_{osm}*. Symptoms appear to be primarily related to cerebral dehydration, which is more prominent with acute hypernatremia. Second, overly rapid correction of chronic hypernatremia can cause the now near normal brain water to increase above normal, leading to *cerebral edema* and possible neurologic deterioration (see "Treatment," below).

Other Findings

Underlying neurologic disease frequently precedes the onset of hypernatremia, and it may be difficult to tell initially whether the neurologic abnormalities are, in fact, due to the increase in the plasma Na^+ concentration. For example, patients with CDI, primary hypodipsia, and essential hypernatremia have hypothalamic lesions that may be due to tumors. Also, patients with decreased mentation due to dementia or cerebrovascular disease are particularly prone to develop hypernatremia because of their decreased access to water.[13] The relative roles of hyperosmolality and the underlying disease can be evaluated more accurately after the restoration of a normal plasma Na^+ concentration.

In addition to the neurologic changes, hypernatremic patients may show signs of volume expansion or volume depletion, depending upon the underlying disease mechanism. Patients with Na^+ overload may have peripheral and/or pulmonary edema; in comparison, patients with an osmotic diuresis or enteric infections (who have lost both Na^+ and water) may have marked extracellular volume depletion, manifested by a jugular venous pressure below $5\,cmH_2O$, decreased skin turgor, and postural hypotension. These findings occur later when only water is lost (as with diabetes insipidus or unreplaced insensible losses), since roughly two-thirds of the water deficit comes from the cells. The plasma Na^+ concentration usually exceeds 160 to 165 meq/L in these settings before signs of hypovolemia are detected.

As noted above, hypernatremia is uncommon in either form of diabetes insipidus because of the effectiveness of thirst. These patients complain of polyuria, nocturia, and polydipsia rather than symptoms of hyperosmolality. Most normal subjects form a highly concentrated urine only while sleeping at night, since no water is taken in during this time. As a result, nocturia may be the only symptom in patients with a mild to moderate concentrating defect, as occurs, for example, with moderate renal insufficiency. The underlying partial diabetes insipidus is usually masked during the day, when there is no need form maximum ADH effect.

For reasons that are unclear, patients with central diabetes insipidus often have a predilection for iced water to satisfy their thirst.[152] It is possible that this represents activation of a cold-sensitive oropharyngeal receptor, since sucking ice chips can acutely lower ADH levels in normal subjects—a response that is not seen with exposure to water at 25°C or to hypertonic saline.[152]

Untreated patients with chronic polyuria may also develop functional dilatation of the bladder, hydroureter, and hydronephrosis because of voluntary suppression of urination in an attempt to minimize urinary frequency. This can result in a marked increase in bladder capacity such that the patient may void as much as 1000 mL at a time.

DIAGNOSIS

Since polyuric states can, if accompanied by diminished thirst, lead to an elevation in the plasma Na^+ concentration, the diagnostic approach to both hypernatremia and polyuria will be considered in this section.

Hypernatremia

Hypernatremia generally occurs in adults with an altered mental status or in infants, since there are the settings in which thirst is most often impaired. An awake, alert patient with hypernatremia, on the other hand, can be assumed to have a hypothalamic lesion affecting the thirst center. Although the history may be helpful (possibly polyuria, polydipsia, diabetes mellitus), neurologic abnormalities induced by the hyperosmolality or by underlying cerebral disease frequently limit the information that can be attained at presentation. In this setting, measurement of the U_{osm} can be particularly helpful.

To understand the meaning of this measurement, it is helpful to first review the response of a normal subject to the induction of hypernatremia by water restriction or the administration of hypertonic saline. As the P_{osm} rises, ADH release is stimulated (Fig. 24-5), resulting in enhanced renal water reabsorption and an elevation in the U_{osm} to a maximum value of 800 to 1400 mosmol/kg (specific gravity equals 1.023 to 1.035). This limit represents *maximum ADH effect on the kidney* and is reached when the P_{osm} is 285 to 295 mosmol/kg. In this setting, the administration of *exogenous ADH will not induce a further increase in the* U_{osm}.[23]

Patients with hypernatremia (plasma Na^+ concentration above 150 meq/L) already have a P_{osm} greater than 295 mosmol/kg, the level at which the urine should be maximally concentrated. Thus, two conclusions can be drawn from the U_{osm} in this setting:

- There is at least a partial defect in ADH release or effect if the U_{osm} is less than 800 mosmol/kg.

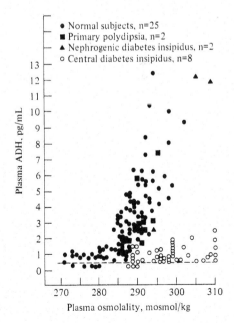

Figure 24-5 Relationship of plasma ADH levels to plasma osmolality in normal subjects and patients with polyuria of diverse etiologies. ADH secretion is reduced only in central diabetes insipidus. (*From Robertson GL, Mahr EA, Atkar S, Sinka T, J Clin Invest 52:2340, 1973, by copyright permission of the American Society for Clinical Investigation.*)

- Exogenous ADH (given as 5 units of aqueous vasopressin subcutaneously or 10 μg of dDAVP by nasal insufflation) will increase the U_{osm} only if endogenous secretion is impaired, as occurs in CDI.[23]

These responses can be used to evaluate the hypernatremic patient (Table 24-4):

- Concentrating ability should be normal in subjects with Na^+ overload, enhanced insensible loss, and primary hypodipsia without CDI. In these conditions, the U_{osm} should exceed 800 mosmol/kg if there is no underlying concentrating defect, and will be unaffected by vasopressin. The urine Na^+ concentration is generally below 25 meq/L when hypernatremia is due to water loss but often well above 100 meq/L when hypernatremia is due to Na^+ overload.[129] Both the concentrated urine and the increased rate of Na^+ excretion contribute to the high urine Na^+ concentration in this setting.
- Either severe CDI or NDI is present if the urine is hypoosmotic to plasma (U_{osm} less than 300 mosmol/kg, specific gravity less than 1.010). These disorders can be differentiated by the administration of ADH, which will produce at least a 50 percent increase in the U_{osm} and a marked fall in urine volume in CDI but will have little or no effect in NDI (see below).[23]
- Many patients fall in an intermediate area, with the U_{osm} ranging from 300 to 800 mosmol/kg (specific gravity of 1.010 to 1.023). This can reflect volume depletion in severe CDI, partial CDI, partial NDI, or an osmotic diuresis. Exogenous ADH is effective only in the first two conditions, augmenting the U_{osm} by at least 60 mosmol/kg and frequently by much more.[23]

Table 24-4 Urine osmolality and response to ADH in patients with hypernatremia

Urine osmolality	Response to vasopressin
Less than 300 mosmol/kg	
CDI	+
NDI	−
300 to 800 mosmol/kg	
Volume depletion in CDI	+
Partial CDI	+
Partial NDI	−
Osmotic diuresis	−
Greater than 800 mosmol/kg	
Insensible or gastrointestinal water losses	−
Primary hypodipsia	−
Na^+ overload	−
Variable	
Essential hypernatremia	Variable

Two factors need to be considered when evaluating the U_{osm} in patients with hypernatremia: (1) the effect of concurrent volume depletion, and (2) the frequently limited clinical utility of finding values in the intermediate range. Volume depletion alone can raise the U_{osm} in severe CDI to as high as 400 mosmol/kg or more.[113,153] The ability to concentrate the urine in this setting is related to two factors: The distal nephron, particularly the inner medullary collecting tubule, has some permeability to water even in the absence of ADH,[154] and the combination of a fall in glomerular filtration rate and a rise in proximal reabsorption induced by hypovolemia can markedly diminish distal water delivery. Since delivery is so low, the reabsorption of even a small amount of water in the inner medulla can substantially raise the U_{osm} and lower the urine volume. This effect is more prominent in patients with partial CDI, since volume depletion can increase in ADH release (although to a lesser degree than in normal subjects) (see Fig.   24-5). This provides an additional mechanism for raising the U_{osm} and lowering the urine volume, possibly masking the underlying polyuria. These changes are readily reversed with volume repletion.

Many individuals without hypernatremia have modest reductions in concentrating ability (U_{max} between 350 and 700 mosmol/kg). Included in this group are patients with underlying renal disease and elderly subjects.[94,95,155] These patients are not polyuric, and loss of this mildly hyperosmotic urine will not substantially raise the plasma Na^+ concentration. However, the ability of the kidney to conserve water is impaired in this setting, an abnormality that can play a contributory role in the presence of some other insult, such as unreplaced insensible losses.

The U_{osm} in essential hypernatremia is variable and depends upon the state of hydration: high if water-restricted, low if water-loaded. The presence of this rare syndrome of selective osmoreceptor dysfunction should be suspected in a persistently hypernatremic patient who is alert and in whom the administration of water is relatively ineffective in lowering the plasma Na^+ concentration.

Polyuria

Polyuria is a relatively common clinical problem. It is arbitrarily defined as a urine volume above 3 liters per day and must be distinguished from urinary frequency, a more frequent complaint in which there are multiple voids of relatively small volume and the urine volume is within the normal range.

The diagnostic approach to this problem can be simplified by considering polyuria in the outpatient and inpatient settings separately. The differential diagnosis in outpatients includes *inappropriate* water loss due to CDI or NDI (particularly uncontrolled diabetes mellitus) and *appropriate* water loss due to increased water intake (primary polydipsia; see Chap. 23) (Table 24-5).[23]

The history may be helpful in identifying a possible cause for the polyuria. Examples include NDI due to lithium or uncontrolled diabetes and CDI due to neurologic disease. Sarcoidosis can cause all three disorders associated with a

Table 24-5   Major causes of polyuria

	Appropriate	Inappropriate
Water diuresis ($U_{osm} < 250$ mosmol/kg)	Primary polydipsia Intravenous infusion of dilute solutions	Central diabetes insipidus Nephrogenic diabetes insipidus
Solute diuresis ($U_{osm} > 300$ mosmol/kg)	Saline loading Postobstructive diuresis	Hyperglycemia High-protein tube feedings Na^+-wasting nephropathy (rare)

water diuresis: CDI or primary polydipsia due to granulomatous infiltration of the hypothalamus and NDI due to hypercalcemia.[46]

There are several other clues in the history and laboratory data that may point toward the correct diagnosis.

- Patients with CDI frequently have a predilection for very cold or iced water, a finding that does not seem to be present in other polyuric disorders.[152] In addition, CDI typically begins abruptly, so that the patient can date the exact onset of the disease. A more gradual onset suggests NDI or primary polydipsia.
- Severe polyuria with a urine output exceeding 4 to 5 L/day is seen only with primary polydipsia or a severe concentrating defect (U_{max} less than 200 to 250 mosmol/kg). In general, the latter occurs primarily with CDI, lithium toxicity, or congenital NDI. Marked polyuria can occur but is unusual in the other causes of acquired NDI.
- Measurement of the plasma Na^+ concentration may be helpful in selected cases. Primary polydipsia is a disorder of water excess, so the plasma Na^+ concentration is typically in the low-normal range (135 to 140 meq/L) and can, in rare cases in which there is massive water intake, be associated with true hyponatremia.[23,156] In comparison, diabetes insipidus is a disorder of water loss, and the plasma Na^+ concentration tends to be in the high-normal range (140 to 145 meq/L).[23] Although there is substantial overlap between the plasma Na^+ concentrations in these conditions, a clearly high or low value can point toward the likely diagnosis.

Water-restriction test   The definitive diagnosis can be made by inducing hyperosmolality with complete water restriction, thereby stimulating endogenous ADH release (Fig. 24-5) and raising the U_{osm}.[23] The urine volume, U_{osm}, and body weight are measured hourly, and the P_{osm} and plasma Na^+ concentration every 2 h. Water restriction is continued until the U_{osm} reaches a plateau (defined as less than a 30-mosmol/kg increase in the U_{osm} in two consecutive hourly specimens) or until the P_{osm} reaches 295 to 300 mosmol/kg.* At the latter level, the plasma ADH concentration is usually greater than 3 to 5 pg/mL (Fig. 24-5), which should lead to maximum ADH effect on the kidney in subjects with normal renal function.[157] At this point, exogenous ADH [10 µg of desmopressin (dDAVP) by nasal insufflation or 1 to 2 µg subcutaneously or intravenously] is given and the hourly measurements continued. (The subcutaneous administration of aqueous vasopressin is now rarely used.)

Accurate interpretation of the water-restriction test generally requires that desmopressin *not be given* before the U_{osm} has stabilized or the P_{osm} has reached 295 mosmol/kg. Below this level, maximum *endogenous* ADH effect may not be present and an antidiuretic response to desmopressin is of no diagnostic benefit, since it will raise the U_{osm} even in normal subjects. One exception to this rule is in the patient in whom NDI is strongly suspected (e.g., gradual onset of polyuria in a patient on chronic lithium therapy). In this setting, simply giving desmopressin without water restriction may be sufficient to establish the diagnosis if the patient shows little or no response using the criteria described in the next section.

The different patterns of response during the water-restriction test are illustrated in Fig. 24-6. In normal subjects, the urine becomes maximally concentrated, the urine volume falls to less than 0.5 mL/min, and the administration of desmopressin is without effect. Patients with complete or partial CDI or NDI respond to induced hyperosmolality and desmopressin in the same manner as when endogenous ADH is released in response to spontaneously developing hypernatremia and hyperosmolality (Table 24-4). Urinary concentration is impaired; therefore, the urine osmolality does not rise to the level seen in normal subjects.

A major positive response to desmopressin is seen only with CDI. The elevation in urine osmolality ranges from 100 to 800 percent in complete and 15 to 50 percent in partial CDI, typically to values above the plasma osmolality.[23,159] This increase in urinary concentration is associated with an equivalent fall in urine output.

Many patients with NDI are partially, not completely, resistant to ADH. As a result, the administration of desmopressin (which produces a supraphysiologic antidiuretic response) may result in a modest (up to 45 percent) elevation in urine osmolality.[23,159] Although this value is similar to that seen with partial CDI, the absolute numbers are quite different. Patients with partial CDI usually have a urine osmolality of 300 mosmol/kg or higher after water restriction, while patients with symptomatic NDI typically have a persistently dilute urine after water restriction with an osmolality that rises, but remains well below isosmotic, after desmopressin. As noted above, the history may also be helpful in distinguish-

---

*Accurate measurement of the P_{osm} is an essential part of this test. A potential error of as much as 8 mosmol/kg can occur if the blood specimen is stored for 1 to 4 h after it has been obtained.[158] In this setting, persistent glycolytic activity in erythrocytes and leukocytes can result in the production of lactic acid and its release into the plasma. This problem can be prevented by refrigeration at 0°C or by separation of the plasma from the cells within 20 min.

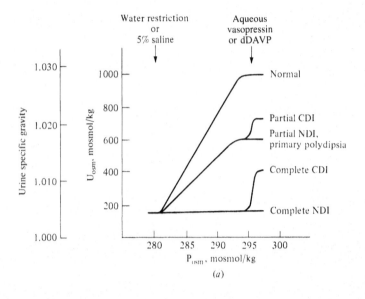

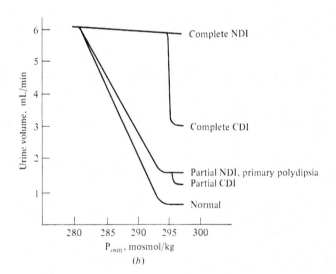

Figure 24-6   Effect of the induction of hyperosmolality, either by water restriction or by hypertonic saline, and exogenous ADH (vasopressin) on (*a*) urine osmolality and (*b*) urine volume in normal subjects and in polyuric states. In normal subjects, there is maximum ADH effect on the kidney as the P_{osm} reaches 285 to 295 mosmol/kg, resulting in a U_{osm} greater than 800 mosmol/kg and a urine volume less than 0.5 mL/min. Exogenous ADH will be without effect. In patients with complete central diabetes insipidus (CDI) or nephrogenic diabetes insipidus (NDI), the urine will remain hypoosmotic to plasma with a high urine volume. ADH will increase the U_{osm} and lower the urine volume only in CDI. Patients with partial CDI (or complete CDI with volume depletion) or NDI show an intermediate response, and only the former will respond to ADH. Since primary polydipsia may induce a form of acquired NDI, these tests may not differentiate this condition from other mild forms of NDI.

ing between these disorders. NDI is a rare cause of true polyuria in adults in the absence of lithium use, hypercalcemia, or rarely tubular damage in patients with amyloidosis or Sjögren's syndrome.

As depicted in Fig. 24-6, the U_{max} achieved in CDI (after vasopressin) and primary polydipsia is less than that in normal subjects. In both of these disorders, ADH secretion is reduced (due, in primary polydipsia, to the chronic water loading). In addition, chronic overhydration in primary polydipsia appears to down-regulate ADH release, so that plasma ADH levels in response to an elevation in the plasma osmolality are subnormal.[160] Since the lack of ADH impairs urea accumulation in the medullary interstitium, interstitial osmolality and, therefore, the U_{max} are diminished (see page 127). This defect is readily correctible by the chronic administration of desmopressin in CDI or by the restriction of water intake in primary polydipsia. Thus, both conditions represent *reversible forms of acquired NDI.*

Primary polydipsia can usually be differentiated from other causes of NDI by the history and laboratory data and, since ADH secretion is normal (Fig. 24-5), from partial CDI by its lack of response to desmopressin.

Patients undergoing the water-restriction test must be monitored carefully, since complications can occur. In some patients with complete CDI, for example, the urine output can reach 700 to 800 mL/h. In this setting, severe volume depletion and vascular collapse can occur if water deprivation is allowed to continue beyond the above limits (stable U_{osm} or P_{osm} of 295 mosmol/kg). In general, the maximum weight loss should not exceed 3 to 5 percent of body weight. A loss of 1.0 to 2.5 kg is usually sufficient, requiring 4 to 12 h of water restriction. A longer period may be necessary in patients with primary polydipsia, who may be water-overloaded at the start of the test. These patients must be observed carefully, since they can discover bizarre ways in which to ingest water, e.g., from a flower vase.

Results similar to those of the water-restriction test can be obtained by inducing hyperosmolality with an intravenous infusion of hypertonic saline. This has been called the Hickey-Hare test. Five percent saline (Na^+ concentration of 855 meq/L) is infused at the rate of 0.05 mL/kg/min for no more than 2 h, and the urine volume and U_{osm} are followed.[122] This method is used less frequently than water restriction because of the danger of circulatory overload. It does, however, have the advantage of being shorter than the water-restriction test, and it may be particularly useful in essential hypernatremia, where hypertonic saline may produce a paradoxical fall in the U_{osm}, since ADH secretion is governed primarily by volume, not osmolality (Fig. 24-3).

Although the response to water restriction or hypertonic saline has been the standard approach to patients with polyuria, these tests are indirect, since the U_{osm} is used as an index of ADH secretion or effect. The accuracy of the water restriction test has been evaluated directly by concomitant measurement of plasma ADH levels.[159] The water-restriction test established the correct diagnosis in 80 percent of patients, with the *major error occurring in the distinction between the partial CDI and primary polydipsia.* Some patients with partial CDI appear to have increased sensitivity to ADH,[159] possibly because of compensatory upregulation of hormone receptors.[161] As a result, they are polyuric at the normal P_{osm} of 280 to 290 mosmol/kg, when ADH secretion is low, but have a maximally concentrated urine at a P_{osm} of 295 mosmol/kg, when their ADH levels are higher but still subnormal. The administration of desmopressin will produce no further effect in this setting, and an incorrect diagnosis of primary polydipsia will be made.

Distinguishing between partial CDI and primary polydipsia is essential from the viewpoint of therapy: The administration of desmopressin will relieve the polyuria and polydipsia in CDI but can produce *potentially life-threatening hyponatremia* in primary polydipsia, since the excess water now cannot be excreted. Measurement of plasma ADH levels is less easily available and of variable utility. Normal values indicate primary polydipsia,[159] but, as noted above, there is frequent downregulation of ADH release in this disorder, so that subnormal values similar to those in partial CDI are often seen.[160]

Thus, when the results of the water-restriction test are not definitive, the clinical clues described previously (acute versus gradual onset, presence of psychiatric illness) can be used to suggest the correct diagnosis. In appropriate patients in whom primary polydipsia seems less likely from the history, it is reasonable to institute a trial of desmopressin (see "Treatment," below). Patients with CDI will note immediate relief of the polyuria and the polydipsia. The urine output will also fall in primary polydipsia, but stimulation of thirst will persist and the excess water taken in may be retained. As a result, careful monitoring of the plasma Na^+ concentration is required if intake remains high.

Another possible error with the water-restriction test occurs in polyuria developing during pregnancy. As noted above, this disorder, which has been called gestational diabetes insipidus, is typically due to the release of vasopressinases from the placenta).[110,111] In this setting, the patient will be resistant to aqueous vasopressin (mistakenly suggesting NDI) but will respond to desmopressin.[112]

Polyuria in hospitalized patients   The approach to polyuria must be modified when it develops in the hospital. In this setting, the increase in urine output frequently reflects a *solute (or osmotic) diuresis* due to the administration of large amounts of saline solutions, the use of hypertonic, high-protein enteral feedings,[51] or the relief of urinary tract obstruction.[162,163] It is useful to evaluate such patients by asking two questions (Table 24-5):

- Does the polyuria reflect a solute or a water diuresis?
- Is the diuresis appropriate or inappropriate?

Water transport in the kidney occurs by two passive mechanisms: It follows the reabsorption of NaCl in the proximal tubule and loop of Henle, and, in the presence of ADH, it is reabsorbed down a favorable osmotic gradient in the collecting tubules (see Chap. 4). Thus, polyuria, which represents an increase in water excretion, can occur during a solute diuresis, when NaCl reabsorption is reduced, or during a pure water diuresis due to diminished activity of ADH.

If polyuria is arbitrarily defined as a urine output exceeding 3 to 4 L/day, the distinction between a solute and a water diuresis can usually be made by measuring the U_{osm}. A U_{osm} below 250 mosmol/kg generally indicates a water diuresis, and the patient should undergo a water-restriction test to differentiate diabetes insipidus from increased water intake (including fluids administered intravenously). One exception to this general rule occurs in patients given large volumes of half- isotonic saline. In this setting, there will be both a water diuresis (due to the dilute fluid) and a Na^+ diuresis that will be apparent from the high rate of Na^+ excretion.

An isosmotic or hyperosmotic urine (U_{osm} greater than 300 mosmol/kg), on the other hand, is generally indicative of a solute or osmotic diuresis. Although partial CDI or NDI can also result in a similar U_{osm}, such a moderate concentrating defect will not lead to marked polyuria if solute excretion is normal. The normal range of solute excretion (composed primarily of Na^+ and K^+ salts and urea) on a typical western diet is 600 to 900 mosmol/day. If the U_{max} is 300 mosmol/kg, then the maximum urine output will be only 2 to 3 L/day (900 mosmol/day $\div$ 300 mosmol/kg $=$ 3 L/day). A value greater than this can be achieved only if solute excretion is increased or if the U_{osm} is reduced.

In patients with a solute diuresis, hyperglycemia and high-protein feedings can be excluded by the history and laboratory data. In uncertain cases, measuring the urine Na^+, glucose, and urea concentrations can be used to identify the major solute that is being excreted. When Na^+ is the primary solute, the polyuria is *almost always appropriate*, being induced by volume expansion due to the administration of excessive amounts of saline or the release of bilateral urinary tract obstruction.

Some patients, for example, may have a urine output in excess of 10 L/day because of the initial infusion of 1 to 2 liters of saline followed by orders to replace the urine output with an equivalent volume of saline. As a result, the urine output gradually increases, since the patient remains volume-expanded. Similarly, a postobstructive diuresis is almost always appropriate, representing the excretion of fluid retained during the period of obstruction.[162,163] The correct therapy in either of these settings is to limit fluid intake to a maintenance level, thereby allowing the patient to develop negative fluid balance. The polyuria will cease when the excess fluid has been excreted.

An *inappropriate* sodium diuresis as a cause of polyuria is much less common and should be suspected if the patient develops hypotension, reduced skin turgor, or decreased renal function. Although Na^+ wasting can occur with renal insufficiency or the uncommon disorder cerebral salt wasting, polyuria is an unusual complaint in these disorders, since the obligatory urine output is generally less than 2 L/day.[164] The kidney has an important protective mechanism that prevents more severe salt wasting: tubuloglomerular feedback, which is mediated by the cells of the macula densa. Through this phenomenon, increased sodium chloride delivery to the macula densa (due to decreased proximal and/or loop reabsorption) results in afferent arteriolar constriction and a fall in the glomerular filtration rate, thereby limiting the degree of sodium chloride loss (see Chap. 2).

These observations imply that when severe salt wasting, appropriate or inappropriate, does occur, there must be an impairment in tubuloglomerular feedback. This can be achieved by volume expansion (which permits appropriate salt wasting), the administration of loop diuretics (which prevents sensing of the increase in Cl^- delivery by blocking the Na^+-K^+-$2Cl^-$ cotransporter in the luminal membrane of the macula densa cells), and glucosuria in uncontrolled diabetes mellitus (via an uncertain mechanism).[165,166]

One rare setting in which inappropriate salt wasting can be severe enough to produce polyuria is after the administration of dopamine to some hypotensive patients with sepsis.[167,168] The urine output can exceed 300 to 500 mL/h in this setting. How sepsis might potentiate the normal natriuretic effect of dopamine (see Chap. 6) and why it occurs so infrequently are not known.

Clinical Example

The sequential approach to the polyuric patient can be illustrated by the following case history.

> **Case history 24-1** A 60-year-old man has a cardiac arrest and is resuscitated. Although circulatory function is restored, the patient remains comatose. The urine output is noticed to increase to 300 to 400 mL/h within the first day. At this time, the laboratory data reveal the following:
>
> $$Plasma [Na^+] = 144 \, meq/L$$
>
> $$P_{osm} = 290 \, mosmol/kg$$
>
> $$U_{osm} = 120 \, mosmol/kg$$
>
> A water-restriction test is begun. When the P_{osm} is 296 mosmol/kg, the U_{osm} is only 130 mosmol/kg, but it rises to 370 mosmol/kg after the administration of desmopressin. A diagnosis of CDI is made, and the patient is begun on desmopressin therapy and enteral hyperalimentation. The urine output is initially well controlled, but it increases to over 150 mL/h on the fourth day and is now refractory to desmopressin. At this time, examination of the urine reveals the following:
>
> $$U_{osm} = 500 \, mosmol/kg$$
>
> $$[Na^+] = 30 \, meq/L$$
>
> $$[K^+] = 33 \, meq/L$$
>
> $$[Glucose] = 0$$
>
> $$[Urea \, nitrogen] = 840 \, mg/dL$$
>
> **Comment** The low U_{osm} when the patient is initially polyuric indicates the presence of a water diuresis. The subsequent response to the water-restriction test is consistent with CDI, presumably induced by hypoxic encephalopathy.

The recurrent polyuria, in comparison, is refractory to desmopressin, a finding not consistent with CDI. However, the high U_{osm} of 500 mosmol/kg indicates that this is a solute diuresis, probably due to the high-protein enteral alimentation. This diagnosis was confirmed by analysis of the urine, which demonstrated that urea was the major urinary osmole; a urea nitrogen concentration of 840 mg/dL represents a concentration of 300 mmol/L or 300 mosmol/kg.* Treatment of the polyuria now requires a decrease in protein intake, not administration of higher doses of vasopressin.

TREATMENT

General Principles

Rapid correction of hypernatremia can induce *cerebral edema, seizures, permanent neurologic damage, and death.*[141,169] This potential complication is a direct result of the beneficial increase in brain volume toward normal that initially protects against the symptoms of hypernatremia (see Fig. 24-4). In this setting, a rapid reduction in the P_{osm} results in water entry into the brain down an osmotic gradient, thereby increasing brain volume to above normal levels. The brain cells can lose the excess K^+ and Na^+ taken up during osmotic adaptation relatively quickly, thereby minimizing the risk of cerebral edema. However, this protection is not complete, since the loss of excess osmolytes occurs more slowly, perhaps because of the time required to stop synthesizing new transporters (such as the Na^+-inositol cotransporter) and to remove previously inserted transporters from the cell membrane.[139,148]

To minimize this risk, the current recommendation is that the *plasma Na^+ concentration be slowly lowered* unless the patient has symptomatic hypernatremia (see below). The potential danger of more rapid correction is illustrated by the following example.

Case history 24-2   A slightly somnolent 19-year-old woman is found to have a plasma Na^+ concentration of 183 meq/L. Her past history reveals 3 years of progressive panhypopituitarism, which was being treated with hydrocortisone and thyroid hormone replacement. The patient is given large volumes of dextrose and water in an attempt to correct the hypernatremia. During the first 6 h, the plasma Na^+ concentration falls to 154 meq/L, but the patient becomes unresponsive. A lumbar puncture reveals an opening pressure of 30 cmH_2O (normal is 10 to 20 cmH_2O), clear fluid, and no cells. Over the next 36 h, the patient's mental status gradually returns to normal.

---

*The urea nitrogen concentration in mg/dL must be divided by 2.8 to convert to mmol/L or mosmol/kg (see page 15). Thus

$$[\text{Urea nitrogen}] = 840 \text{ mg/dL} \div 2.8$$

$$= 300 \text{ mosmol/kg}$$

Water Deficit

Most cases of hypernatremia are due to water loss. Gradual correction of this problem with fluid replacement requires calculation of the water deficit. The formula to estimate this deficit can be derived in the following way. The quantity of osmoles in the body is equal to the osmolal space [the total body water (TBW)] times the osmolality of the body fluids:

$$\text{Total body osmoles} = \text{TBW} \times P_{osm}$$

Since the P_{osm} is primarily determined by the plasma Na^+ concentration,

$$\text{Total body osmoles} \propto \text{TBW} \times \text{plasma } [Na^+] \qquad (24\text{-}4)$$

If hypernatremia results only from water loss, then

$$\text{Current total body osmoles} = \text{normal total body osmoles}$$

or, if the normal plasma Na^+ concentration is 140 meq/L,

$$\text{Current body water (CBW)} \times \text{plasma } [Na^+] = \text{normal body water (NBW)} \times 140$$

Solving this equation for normal body water,

$$\text{NBW} = \text{CBW} \times \frac{\text{plasma } [Na^+]}{140} \qquad (24\text{-}5)$$

The water deficit can then be estimated from

$$\text{Water deficit} = \text{NBW} - \text{CBW}$$

or, by substituting for NBW from Eq. (24-5),

$$\text{Water deficit} = \left(\text{CBW} \times \frac{\text{plasma } [Na]^+}{140} \right) - \text{CBW}$$
$$= \text{CBW} \times \left(\frac{\text{plasma } [Na^+]}{140} - 1 \right) \qquad (24\text{-}6)$$

The total body water is normally about 60 and 50 percent of lean body weight in men and women, respectively. However, it is probably reasonable to use values about 10 percent lower in hypernatremic patients who are water-depleted. Thus, in women, Eq. (24-6) becomes

$$\text{Water deficit} = 0.4 \times \text{lean body weight} \times \left(\frac{\text{plasma } [Na^+]}{140} - 1 \right) \qquad (24\text{-}7)$$

This formula estimates the amount of positive water balance required to return the plasma Na^+ concentration to 140 meq/L. It does not include any additional *isosmotic fluid deficit*, a condition that is frequently present when both Na^+ and water have been lost, as occurs with an osmotic diuresis.

The patient described in Case History 24-2 can be used as an example of the approach to therapy. If her lean body weight were 50 kg, then

$$\text{Water deficit} = 0.4 \times 50 \times \left(\frac{183}{140} - 1\right)$$

$$= 6\,\text{liters}$$

Although no definitive trials have been performed, observations in children suggest that the *maximum safe rate at which the plasma Na$^+$ concentration should be lowered (in the absence of hypernatremic symptoms) is 0.5 meq/L per hour* or 12 meq/L per day,[170] a rate equivalent to that in severe hyponatremia (see page 725). Thus, administration of 6 liters of free water to lower the plasma Na$^+$ concentration by 43 meq/L should occur over a minimum of 86 h, which represents a rate of fluid administration of 70 mL/h. Since the aim is to induce positive water balance, estimated insensible losses (usually 30 to 50 mL/h) must be replaced raising the infusion rate of free water to about 110 mL/h.

Although not applicable to this patient, high levels of urinary or gastrointestinal losses must also be considered in the replacement calculations. It is important in this regard to return to the idea that the plasma Na$^+$ concentration is affected only by Na$^+$, K$^+$, and the total body water. For example, a patient with hypernatremia and lithium-induced nephrogenic diabetes insipidus may put out 150 mL/h of isosmotic urine (urine osmolality equals 325 mosmol/kg) because, as noted above, volume depletion ameliorates the polyuria. At first glance, it may appear that there is no free water in the urine and therefore that the urinary losses do not have to be replaced in order to correct the hypernatremia (even though replacement is indicated for prevention of volume and potassium depletion). However, as described in Chap. 9, urinary urea and ammonium may make up much of the urine osmolality even though their loss does not affect the plasma Na$^+$ concentration. Thus, it is the urine (Na$^+$ + K$^+$) concentration that must be evaluated, not the total urine osmolality. If this value is 60 meq/L in a patient with a plasma (Na$^+$ + K$^+$) concentration of 150 meq/L, then the effective urine osmolality is basically 40 percent that of the plasma even though the total urine output is free water and must be added to the above calculations to correct the hypernatremia. The polyuria and therefore the water replacement requirements are likely to increase as the hypovolemia is corrected.

The type of fluid administered to replace these losses is variable, depending upon the patient's clinical state and the cause of the hypernatremia:

- Free water can be given orally or intravenously (as dextrose in water)* in patients with hypernatremia due to pure water loss.

---

* The osmotic contribution of dextrose usually can be ignored, since it is rapidly metabolized in nondiabetics to carbon dioxide and water. Thus, although 5 percent dextrose in water has an osmolality of 278 mosmol/kg, it is equivalent to free water in the body. However, intravenous administration of large volumes of dextrose in water can, in some patients, lead to marked hyperglycemia, since the quantity of glucose given can exceed the maximum amount that can normally be metabolized.[171] This problem can be avoided by giving free water orally, by minimizing the urine output in CDI with desmopressin (see below), or by careful monitoring of the plasma glucose concentration.

- An infusion of quarter-isotonic saline is preferable if Na^+ depletion is also present, as typically occurs with concurrent vomiting, diarrhea, or diuretic use. One liter of this solution is a combination of 750 mL of free water and 250 mL of isotonic saline. Thus, about 150 mL/h of quarter-isotonic saline must be administered to provide 110 mL/h of free water.
- Isotonic saline should be used initially if the patient is hypotensive. In this setting, restoration of tissue perfusion is the most urgent requirement; this can be best achieved with isotonic saline. This solution may also lower the plasma Na^+ concentration, since it is hypoosmotic to the hypernatremic patient. More dilute solutions can be substituted once tissue perfusion is adequate.
- The contribution of K^+ salts must be taken into account when calculating the tonicity of the fluid that is to be given. As an example, quarter-isotonic saline to which 40 meq of K^+ has been added is osmotically equivalent to half-isotonic saline.

It must be emphasized that Eq. (24-7) is only an approximation of the water deficit and that serial measurements of the plasma Na^+ concentration are required to ascertain that the desired rate of correction is being achieved. For example, the total body water may be substantially less than 40 to 50 percent of lean body weight in elderly patients who are cachectic. In this setting, the calculated TBW and water deficit will be falsely elevated, possibly leading to an overly rapid reduction in the plasma Na^+ concentration.

Central Diabetes Insipidus

The most physiologic therapy of CDI is to give exogenous ADH (Table 24-6). This is typically achieved by the administration of desmopressin (dDAVP), a two-

Table 24-6 Drug therapy of central diabetes insipidus according to probable mechanism of action

ADH preparations
   A. dDAVP nasal spray (desmopressin)
   B. Aqueous vasopressin
   C. Lysine-vasopressin nasal spray
   D. Vasopressin tannate in oil
Drugs that potentiate ADH effect
   A. Chlorpropamide
   B. Carbamazepine
   C. Nonsteroidal anti-inflammatory drugs
Drugs that increase ADH secretion
   A. Clofibrate
Drugs not requiring ADH
   A. Thiazide diuretics

amino-acid substitute of arginine vasopressin. In contrast to older vasopressin preparations, desmopressin has more antidiuretic activity, has no vasopressor effect, and has to be taken only once or twice a day (in 5- to 20-µg doses by nasal insufflation) because of a longer duration of action.[172] In addition, chronic use of the other ADH preparations, but not desmopressin, can lead to anti-vasopressin antibody production and a secondary increase in urine output that now appears to be partially ADH-resistant.[173]

An oral tablet preparation of desmopressin is available in 0.1- and 0.2-mg sizes. The absorption of desmopressin in normal persons is decreased by 40 to 50 percent when taken with meals.[174] This usually has little effect on the antidiuretic action, but administering the drug in the fasting state may be tried if there is a poor response to the usual doses taken with meals.

The oral form has about one-tenth to one-twentieth the potency of the nasal form because only about 5 percent is absorbed from the gut. Thus, a 0.1-mg tablet is the equivalent of 2.5 to 5 µg of the nasal spray. However, because the oral dose cannot be precisely predicted from a previous nasal dose, transferring from nasal to oral therapy will usually require some retitration.

The oral form of desmopressin is typically preferred because of ease of administration. The initial dose is 0.05 mg (one-half a 0.1-mg tablet) at bedtime, with subsequent titration according to response. The usual daily maintenance dose ranges from 0.1 to 0.8 mg in two or three divided doses but may be as high as 1.2 mg/day.

There are few long-term data on the use of oral desmopressin. In one study, eight children with central DI were treated and followed for up to 3.5 years.[175] There was no attenuation of the antidiuretic effect, and no side effects or antibody formation was noted. In another report, 10 adults had satisfactory maintenance of the antidiuretic effect over 1 year with doses of 0.3 to 0.6 mg/day given in two to three doses per day; doses larger than 0.2 mg—e.g., 0.4 versus 0.2 mg—had no greater effect, but probably lasted longer.[176]

It is important to be aware that there is potential risk to the administration of desmopressin in CDI. Patients with this disorder are polyuric but not in danger of marked fluid loss and hypernatremia as long as their thirst mechanism is intact. However, once desmopressin is given, the patient has *nonsuppressible* ADH activity and is at risk of developing water retention and hyponatremia. As a result, the *minimum dose must be used to allow the maintenance of an adequate urine output.* This can be achieved by giving the first dose in the late evening to control the most troubling symptom, nocturia. The necessity for and size of a daytime dose can then be determined from the effectiveness of the evening dose. If, for example, polyuria does not recur until noon, then half the evening dose may be sufficient at that time.

Non-ADH therapy   Although desmopressin is the treatment of choice for CDI, other drugs can also be given to lower the urine output (Table 24-6). For example, the induction of mild volume depletion with a low-sodium diet and a thiazide diuretic (such as hydrochlorothiazide, 12.5 to 25 mg once or twice daily) is often extremely effective in diabetes insipidus, being primarily used in patients with NDI. Although it seems paradoxical to treat polyuria with a diuretic, as little as a 1.0- to 1.5-kg weight loss can reduce the urine output by more than 50 percent, from, for example, almost 10 L to below 3.5 L per day.[177] Addition of the K^+-sparing diuretic amiloride can enhance the response, while also minimizing thiazide-induced hypokalemia.[178]

This response is primarily due to diuretic-induced hypovolemia. Volume depletion is associated with enhanced proximal NaCl and water reabsorption (see Chap. 8). As a result, less water is delivered to the collecting tubules (the site of ADH action),[113] and therefore less water is excreted.[176] (Note that a *loop diuretic should not be used* in this setting, since it will further impair concentrating ability by inhibiting the first step in the countercurrent mechanism: The reabsorption of NaCl without water in the thick ascending limb of the loop of Henle; see Chap. 4.)

The addition of moderate dietary protein restriction can also contribute to control of the polyuria. The combination of sodium and protein restriction reduces the rate of solute excretion, which, as described above, will diminish the urine output in diabetes insipidus.

The action of diuretics and diet is *independent* of ADH. In contrast, the other drugs used in the treatment of CDI act by potentiating the effect of ADH or by increasing its secretion (Table 24-6). These drugs generally require at least some ADH to be present and are not effective in those patients who secrete no ADH, as may occur after neurosurgery.[29]

Chlorpropamide is an oral hypoglycemic agent (now largely replaced by other hypoglycemic drugs) that enhances the action of ADH.[179-181] Two different mechanisms may contribute to this response: increased efficiency of the countercurrent mechanism by enhanced NaCl reabsorption in the thick ascending limb of the loop of Henle[182,183] and a direct elevation in collecting tubule water permeability.[184] These unique effects of chlorpropamide allow it to be given alone or in conjunction with desmopressin, since it will potentiate the antidiuretic response.

The usual dose of chlorpropamide is 125 to 250 mg, once or twice a day. Higher doses (up to 1250 mg/day) can increase the antidiuresis,[180] but they also increase the risk of hypoglycemia and should not be used. If hypoglycemia does develop, a problem that is particularly likely to occur in patients with associated anterior pituitary insufficiency, the dose can be reduced or a thiazide can be added, since the latter tends to raise the plasma glucose concentration (Fig. 24-7).[179,185] Occasionally, chlorpropamide has to be discontinued because of severe or recurrent hypoglycemia.

Both *clofibrate* (now rarely used in the treatment of hyperlipidemia; 500 mg every 6 h)[186,187] and *carbamazepine* (used in the treatment of seizures and tic douloureux; 100 to 300 mg, twice daily) also can effectively lower the urine output in partial CDI.[180,188,189] Clofibrate appears to enhance ADH secretion,[186] whereas carbamazepine seems to increase the effect of ADH[189,190] and perhaps augment its secretion cases.[191]

Like thiazide diuretics, carbamazepine and clofibrate can produce more than a 50 percent reduction in urine output in responsive patients. If, however, this

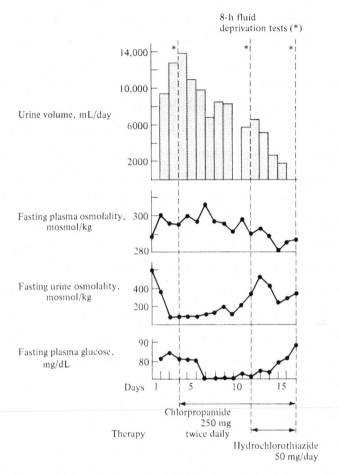

Figure 24-7 Serial observation in control and treatment periods in a patient with partial CDI. Note the additive antidiuretic effects of chlorpropamide and hydrochlorothiazide, and the ability of the latter drug to protect against a fall in the plasma glucose concentration induced by chlorpropamide. (*From Webster B, Bain J, J Clin Endocrinol Metab 30:215, 1970. Used by permission from the* Journal of Clinical Endocrinology and Metabolism *and from Lippincott.*)

represents a decrease in output from 12 to 6 L/day, then the patient, although much improved, will still complain of polyuria. In this setting, combination therapy can be used. Additive antidiuretic effects can often be achieved by choosing agents that have different mechanisms of action. For example, a thiazide diuretic and chlorpropamide can be used together or in conjunction with desmopressin with excellent results (Fig. 24-7).[179] Carbamazepine and chlorpropamide also can be an effective combination.[180]

As discussed in Chap. 23, the antidiuretic properties of thiazide diuretics, chlorpropamide, and carbamazepine can lead to water retention and hyponatremia. This is particularly true in patients with primary polydipsia. Thus, one must be certain to exclude the latter disorder as the cause of polyuria before beginning therapy for CDI. Less commonly, chloropropamide can induce symptomatic hyponatremia in patients with partial CDI.[179] Since the symptoms of hyponatremia can mimic those of hypernatremia and the therapy is diametrically opposite (water restriction versus water loading), it is important to establish the correct diagnosis and not to assume the presence of hypernatremia (which does not occur in diabetes insipidus if thirst is intact) because of the history of CDI.

Administration of a nonsteroidal anti-inflammatory drug (NSAID) represents another possible mechanism by which the ADH effect can be enhanced. Renal prostaglandins normally impair the response to ADH, in part by diminishing the generation of cyclic AMP (see page 172);[192,193] as a result, inhibiting prostaglandin synthesis with one of these agents can lead to a significant potentiation of the response to ADH.[194] Because of the efficacy of the modalities described above, there is little experience with the use of NSAIDs in CDI; they have, however, been helpful in many patients with NDI.

Nephrogenic Diabetes Insipidus

Chronic therapy for NDI should be reserved for those patients with symptomatic polyuria in whom the renal defect is not rapidly correctable. This represents a very small group of patients, such as those with congential NDI, lithium toxicity, or rarely amyloidosis or Sjögren's syndrome.[57,64,66] Specific treatment is not required when the concentrating defect is reversible (drugs, osmotic diuresis, hypercalcemia, hypokalemia) or when polyuria is not a problem (renal failure, sickle cell anemia).

Since patients with NDI do not usually have a major response to ADH, desmopressin or drugs depending upon ADH for their action are ineffective. The major form of therapy in this disorder is the use of a *thiazide diuretic and a low-sodium, low-protein diet*, as described above in the treatment of CDI.[177,195] In addition, the K^+-sparing diuretic amiloride may produce additional benefit by two mechanisms: (1) It can enhance the initial natriuresis by acting at a different site (cortical collecting tubule versus distal tubule and connecting segment with a thiazide),[178] and (2) it is specifically indicated in patients with mild to moderate lithium toxicity.[67] Filtered lithium enters the collecting tubule cells through Na^+ channels in the luminal membrane; this pathway is blocked by amiloride. However, this effect of amiloride will be beneficial only if the lithium is continued and only if the collecting tubule injury is at least partially reversible. (Reversibility is usually present if the maximum urine osmolality that can be achieved is above 200 to 250 mosmol/kg.)

There is some risk, however, in using diuretics in patients who must continue to take lithium. Although the ensuing volume depletion can reduce the urine output,[66,67] it also increases the proximal reabsorption of Na^+ and secondarily of lithium, resulting in decreased excretion and potential lithium toxicity.[196] Careful monitoring of the plasma lithium concentration is therefore required in this setting.

One other modality that has been effective in some patients with congenital NDI or lithium toxicity is the administration of a NSAID, which increases urinary concentrating ability and lowers the urine volume[197-200] by impairing renal prostaglandin synthesis.[192] These agents can increase the U_{osm}, even in the absence of ADH.[193]

In children with congenital NDI, for example, the administration of a NSAID can raise the maximum U_{osm} by up to 100 percent, thereby reducing the urine volume by 50 percent.[197-200] This beneficial effect is additive to that of a thiazide diuretic, potentially resulting in more than a two-thirds decline in urine output from the pretreatment level.[178,200] However, a similar response with fewer side effects can often be achieved with the combination of a thiazide and amiloride.[178]

It should not be assumed, however, that all NSAIDs are equally effective. In some patients, ibuprofen has been without benefit despite a good antidiuretic response to indomethacin.[198] In addition, sulindac may be less effective in this setting, since it appears to relatively spare renal prostaglandin synthesis.[201]

There may be a role for desmopressin in patients with persistent symptomatic polyuria after institution of the above regimen. Most patients with NDI have partial rather than complete resistance to ADH. Thus, attaining supraphysiologic hormone levels may increase the renal effect of ADH to a clinically important degree. For example, three patients described in two reports evaluating the water-restriction test in polyuric patients found that exogenous ADH raised the urine osmolality by 40 to 45 percent, which should produce a similar decline in urine volume.[23,159]

Hypothalamic Dysfunction

The proper treatment of patients with hypothalamic dysfunction depends upon the pattern of ADH secretion. Patients with primary hypodipsia but without CDI can be simply treated with forced water intake.[9,10] The patient can be instructed to drink 1500 to 2000 mL of water per day, regardless of thirst. There is no risk of water overload in this setting, since the ability to excrete water is generally not impaired.

Correction of the hypernatremia is somewhat more difficult in hypodipsic patients who also have partial CDI or essential hypernatremia. In these conditions, water loading will diminish ADH secretion, resulting in polyuria, excretion of the ingested water, and persistent elevation of the plasma Na^+ concentration.[118-121] Chlorpropamide has been effective in many of these patients,[116,118-121] probably by enhancing the action of the small amount of ADH being released.[118] There is, however, some risk of *hyponatremia* in this setting, since the osmoreceptor defect may prevent complete suppression of ADH release after a water load.[7]

In addition to these regimens, an integral part of the therapeutic approach to patients with CDI or hypothalamic disease is a neurologic evaluation to determine the underlying cause. Some tumors, for example, may respond to radiotherapy.

Sodium Overload

Therapy in patients with primary Na^+ overload is best aimed at removing the excess Na^+. When renal function is normal, the Na^+ load will usually be excreted rapidly in the urine. This process can be facilitated by inducing a Na^+ and water diuresis with diuretics and replacing the urine output solely with water. Intravenous dextrose in water can also be used in those patients who present with marked hypernatremia. However, careful monitoring is necessary, since these patients are volume-expanded and the excess fluid may lead to pulmonary congestion in susceptible cases.

In patients with poor renal function or in infants, peritoneal dialysis with an electrolyte-free, hypertonic (8%) dextrose and water solution can initially be used to remove the excess Na^+.[127] Water retention is minimized, since the dialysis solution is hyperosmotic to plasma. The rate of dialysis should be adjusted to prevent an overly rapid fall in the plasma Na^+ concentration and the possible development of cerebral edema.

PROBLEMS

24-1 A 45-year-old woman with sarcoidosis complains of drinking 8 to 10 liters of water per day. The results of laboratory studies are as follows:

$$\text{Plasma } [Na^+] = 134 \, meq/L$$

$$P_{osm} = 274 \, mosmol/kg$$

$$U_{osm} = 80 \, mosmol/kg$$

(a) What is the most likely diagnosis?
(b) How would you establish the correct diagnosis?

24-2 An 80-year-old partially senile woman treated with hydrochlorothiazide for hypertension is admitted from a nursing home with a 4-day history of a viral-like illness, diarrhea, and increasing confusion. Physical examination reveals a 50-kg woman with decreased skin turgor and mentation, but a normal blood pressure. The laboratory findings include the following:

$$\text{Plasma } [Na^+] = 174 \, meq/L$$

$$\text{Urine } [Na^+] = 5 \, meq/L$$

$$U_{osm} = 606 \, mosmol/kg$$

Which of the following are the most important factors in the development of the hypernatremia?

(a) Diarrhea
(b) Decreased thirst
(c) Diabetes insipidus
(d) Diuretic therapy
(e) Insensible losses

Is the low urine Na^+ concentration surprising in a patient with hypernatremia? What is the most appropriate initial therapy for the hypernatremia?

(a) Isotonic saline at 100 mL/h
(b) Five percent dextrose in water at 200 mL/h
(c) Quarter-isotonic saline at 100 mL/h
(d) Quater-isotonic saline at 200 mL/h
(e) Five percent dextrose in water at 500 mL/h

24-3 A 40-year-old male alcoholic is brought into the hospital in a comatose state. He is found to have a skull fracture. It is noted that his weight is 70 kg and his urine output is 175 mL/h. The following laboratory data are obtained:

$$\text{Plasma } [\text{Na}^+] = 168 \, \text{meq/L}$$

$$[\text{K}^+] = 4 \, \text{meq/L}$$

$$[\text{Cl}^-] = 130 \, \text{meq/L}$$

$$[\text{HCO}_3^-] = 25 \, \text{meq/L}$$

$$\text{P}_{\text{osm}} = 350 \, \text{mosmol/kg}$$

$$\text{U}_{\text{osm}} = 80 \, \text{mosmol/kg}$$

The diagnosis of central diabetes insipidus is considered.

(a) How would you confirm this diagnosis?

(b) What is the approximate water deficit?

(c) How much free water should be given and at what rate to lower the plasma Na^+ concentration to normal (assuming that the urine output has fallen to low levels)?

The diagnosis of central diabetes insipidus is made, and the patient has a good response to vasopressin tannate in oil. Two days later, the plasma Na^+ concentration has fallen to 124 meq/L.

(d) What is responsible for the late development of hyponatremia?

REFERENCES

1. Robinson AG, Loeb JN. Ethanol ingestion: Commonest cause of elevated plasma osmolality? *N Engl J Med* 284:1253, 1971.
2. Rose BD. New approach to disturbances in the plasma sodium concentration. *Am J Med* 81:1033, 1986.
3. Shiau Y-F, Feldman GM, Resnick MA, Coff PM. Stool electrolyte and osmolality measurements in the evaluation of diarrheal disorders. *Ann Intern Med* 102:773, 1985.
4. Teree T, Mirabal-Font E, Ortiz A, Wallace W. Stool losses and acidosis in diarrheal disease of infancy. *Pediatrics* 36:704, 1965.
5. Nelson DC, McGrew WRG, Hoyumpa AM. Hypernatremia and lactulose therapy. *JAMA* 249:1295, 1983.
6. Allerton JP, Strom JA. Hypernatremia due to repeated doses of charcoal-sorbitol. *Am J Kidney Dis* 17:581, 1991.
7. Robertson GL, Aycinena P, Zerbe RL. Neurogenic disorders of osmoregulation. *Am J Med* 72:339, 1982.
8. Davison JM, Shiells EA, Phillips PR, Lindheimer MD. Serial evaluation of vasopressin release and thirst in human pregnancy: Role of human chorionic gonadotropin in the osmoregulatory changes of gestation. *J Clin Invest* 81:798, 1988.
9. Robertson GL. Abnormalities of thirst regulation. *Kidney Int* 25:460, 1984.
10. Hammond DN, Moll GW, Robertson GL, Chelmicka-Schorr E. Hypodipsic hypernatremia with normal osmoregulation of vasopressin. *N Engl J Med* 315:433, 1986.
11. Moritz ML, Ayus JC. The changing pattern of hypernatremia in hospitalized children. *Pediatrics* 104:435, 1999.
12. Palevsky PM, Bhagrath R, Greenberg A. Hypernatremia in hospitalized patients. *Ann Intern Med* 124:197, 1996.
13. Snyder NA, Feigal DW, Arieff AI. Hypernatremia in elderly patients: A heterogeneous, morbid, and iatrogenic entity. *Ann Intern Med* 107:309, 1987.
14. Phillips PA, Bretherton M, Johnston CI, Gray L. Reduced osmotic thirst in healthy elderly men. *Am J Physiol* 261:R166, 1991.

15. Dyke MM, Davis KM, Clark BA, et al. Effects of hypertonicity on water intake in the elderly: An age-related failure. *Geriatr Nephrol Urol* 7:11, 1997.

16. Lucassen PJ, Salehi A, Pool CW, et al. Activation of vasopressin neurons in aging and Alzheimer's disease. *J Neuroendocrinol* 66:673, 1994.

17. Macdonald NJ, McConnell KN, Stephen MR, Dunnigan MG. Hypernatremic dehydration in patients in a large hospital for the mentally handicapped. *Br Med J* 299:1426, 1989.

18. Bruck E, Abal G, Aceto T. Pathogenesis and pathophysiology of hypertonic dehydration with diarrhea. *Am J Dis Child* 115:122, 1968.

19. Finberg L. Hypernatremic (hypertonic) dehydration in infants. *N Engl J Med* 289:196, 1973.

20. Finberg L. Dehydration and osmolality. *Am J Dis Child* 135:997, 1981.

21. Pizzaro D, Castillo B, Posada G, et al. Efficiency comparison of oral rehydration solutions containing 90 or 75 millimoles of sodium per liter. *Pediatrics* 79:190, 1987.

22. Thompson CJ, Baylis PH. Thirst in diabetes insipidus: Clinical relevance of quantitative assessment. *Q J Med* 65:853, 1987.

23. Miller M, Kalkos T, Moses AM, et al. Recognition of partial defects in antidiuretic hormone secretion. *Ann Intern Med* 73:721, 1970.

24. McIver B, Connacher A, Whittle I, et al. Adipsic hypothalamic diabetes insipidus after clipping of anterior communicating artery aneurysm. *Br Med J* 303:1465, 1991.

25. Zimmerman EA, Robinson AG. Hypothalamic neurons secreting vasopressin and neurophysin. *Kidney Int* 10:12, 1976.

26. Zimmerman EA, Nilaver G, Hou-Yu A, Silverman AJ. Vasopressinergic and oxytocinergic pathways in central nervous system. *Fed Proc* 43:91, 1984.

27. Baylis PH, Gaskill MB, Robertson GL. Vasopressin secretion in primary polydipsia and cranial diabetes insipidus. *Q J Med* 50:345, 1981.

28. Leaf A. Neurogenic diabetes insipidus. *Kidney Int* 15:572, 1979.

29. Seckl J, Dunger D. Postoperative diabetes insipidus: Correct interpretation of water balance and electrolye data essential. *Br Med J* 298:2, 1989.

30. Kimmel DW, O'Neill BP. Systemic cancer presenting as diabetes insipidus: Clinical and radiographic features of 11 patients with a review of metastatic-induced diabetes insipidus. *Cancer* 52:2355, 1983.

31. Dunger DB, Broadbent V, Yeoman E, et al. The frequency and natural history of diabetes insipidus in children with Langerhans-cell histiocytosis. *N Engl J Med* 321:1157, 1989.

32. Imura H, Nakao K, Shimatsu A, et al. Lymphocytic infundibuloneurohypophysitis as a cause of central diabetes insipidus. *N Engl J Med* 329:683, 1993.

33. De Bellis A, Colao A, Di Salle F, et al. A longitudinal study of vasopressin cell antibodies, posterior pituitary function, and magnetic resonance imaging evaluations in subclinical autoimmune central diabetes insipidus. *J Clin Endocrinol Metab* 84:3047, 1999.

34. Czernichow P, Pomarede R, Basmaciogullari A, et al. Diabetes insipidus in children: III. Anterior pituitary dysfunction in idiopathic types. *J Pediatr* 106:41, 1985.

35. Ito M, Mori Y, Oiso Y, Saito H. A single base substitution in the coding region for neurophysin II associated with familial central diabetes insipidus. *J Clin Invest* 87:725, 1991.

36. Rittig S, Robertson GL, Siggaard C, et al. Identification of 13 new mutations in the vasopressin-neurophysin II gene in 17 kindreds with familial autosomal dominant neurohypophyseal diabetes insipidus. *Am J Hum Genet* 58:107, 1996.

37. Ito M, Lameson JL, Ito M. Molecular basis of autosomal dominant neurohypophyseal diabetes insipidus: Cellular toxicity caused by the accumulation of mutant vasopressin precursors within the endoplasmic reticulum. *J Clin Invest* 99:1897, 1997.

38. Repaske DR, Medlej R, Gültekin EK, et al. Heterogeneity in clinical manifestations of autosomal dominant neurohypophyseal diabetes insipidus caused by a mutation encoding Ala-1 to Val in the signal peptide of the arginine vasopressin/neurophysin II copeptin precursor. *J Clin Endocrinol Metab* 82:51, 1997.

39. Seckl JR, Dunger DB, Bevan JS, et al. Vasopressin antagonist in early postoperative diabetes insipidus. *Lancet* 335:1353, 1990.

40. Hensen J, Henig A, Fahlbusch R, et al. Prevalence, predictors and patterns of postoperative polyuria and hyponatraemia in the immediate course after transsphenoidal surgery for pituitary adenomas. *Clin Endocrinol (Oxf)* 50:431, 1999.

41. Sane T, Rantakari K, Poranen A. Hyponatremia after transsphenoidal surgery for pituitary tumors. *J Clin Endocrinol Metab* 79:1395, 1994.

42. Olson BR, Rubino D, Gumowski J, Oldfield EH. Isolated hyponatremia after transsphenoidal pituitary surgery. *J Clin Endocrinol Metab* 80:85, 1995.

43. Wickramasinge LSP, Chazan BI, Mandal AR, et al. Cranial diabetes insipidus after upper gastrointestinal hemorrhage. *Br Med J* 296:969, 1988.

44. Bakiri F, Benmiloud M, Vallotton MB. Arginine-vasopressin in postpartum hypopituitarism: Urinary excretion and kidney response to osmolar load. *J Clin Endocrinol Metab* 58:511, 1984.

45. Canepa-Anson R, Williams S, Marshall J, et al. Mechanism of polyuria and natriuresis in atrioventricular nodal tachycardia. *Br Med J* 289:866, 1984.

46. Stuart CA, Neelon FA, Lebovitz HE. Disordered control of thirst in hypothalamic-pituitary sarcoidosis. *N Engl J Med* 303:1078, 1980.

47. Weiman E, Molenkamp G, Bohles HJ. Diabetes insipidus due to hypophysitis. *Horm Res* 47:81, 1997.

48. Bruch J. Visual vignette. *Endocr Pract* 3:96, 1997.

49. Nishioka H, Ito H, Fukushima C. Recurrent lymphocytic hypophysitis: Case report. *Neurosurgery* 41:684, 1997.

50. Gold PW, Kaye W, Robertson GL, Ebert M. Abnormalities in plasma and cerebrospinal-fluid arginine vasopressin in patients with anorexia nervosa. *N Engl J Med* 308:117, 1983.

51. Jamison RL, Oliver RE. Disorders of urinary concentration and dilution. *Am J Med* 72:308, 1982.

52. Singer I, Forrest JN. Drug-induced states of nephrogenic diabetes insipidus. *Kidney Int* 10:82, 1976.

53. Bode HH, Crawford JD. Nephrogenic diabetes insipidus in North America: The Hopewell hypothesis. *N Engl J Med* 280:750, 1969.

54. Bichet DG, Oksche A, Rosenthal W. Congenital nephrogenic diabetes insipidus. *J Am Soc Nephrol* 8:1951, 1997.

55. Van Lieburg AF, Knoers NV, Monnens LA. Clinical presentation and follow-up of 30 patients with congenital nephrogenic diabetes insipidus. *J Am Soc Nephrol* 10:1958, 1999.

56. Lolait SJ, O'Carroll A, McBride OW, et al. Cloning and characterization of a vasopressin V_2 receptor and possible link to nephrogenic diabetes insipidus. *Nature* 357:336, 1992.

57. Holtzman EJ, Harris HW Jr, Kolakowski LF Jr, et al. Brief report: A molecular defect in the vasopressin V_2-receptor gene causing nephrogenic diabetes insipidus. *N Engl J Med* 328:1534, 1993.

58. Bichet DG, Razi M, Lonergan M, et al. Hemodynamic and coagulation responses to 1-desamino [8-D-arginine] vasopressin in patients with congenital nephrogenic diabetes insipidus. *N Engl J Med* 318:881, 1988.

59. Bichet DG, Razi M, Arthus M-F, et al. Epinephrine and dDAVP administration in patients with congenital nephrogenic diabetes insipidus. Evidence for a pre-cyclic AMP V_2 receptor defective mechanism. *Kidney Int* 36:859, 1989.

60. Deen PM, Croes H, van Aubel RA, et al. Water channels encoded by mutant aquaporin-2 genes in nephrogenic diabetes insipidus are impaired in their cellular trafficking. *J Clin Invest* 95:2291, 1995.

61. Hochberg Z, van Lieburg A, Even L, et al. Autosomal recessive nephrogenic diabetes insipidus caused by an aquaporin-2 mutation. *J Clin Endocrinol Metab* 82:686, 1997.

62. Yamamoto T, Sasaki S. Aquaporins in the kidney: Emerging new aspects. *Kidney Int* 54:1041, 1998.

63. Nielsen S, Kwon T-H, Christensen BM, et al. Physiology and pathophysiology of renal aquaporins. *J Am Soc Nephrol* 10:647, 1999.

64. Boton R, Gaviria M, Batlle DC. Prevalence, pathogenesis, and treatment of renal dysfunction associated with chronic lithium therapy. *Am J Kidney Dis* 10:329, 1987.

65. Baylis PH, Heath DA. Water disturbances in patients treated with oral lithium carbonate. *Ann Intern Med* 88:607, 1978.
66. Simon NM, Garber E, Arieff AJ. Persistent nephrogenic diabetes insipidus after lithium carbonate. *Ann Intern Med* 86:446, 1977.
67. Batlle DC, von Riotte AB, Gaviria M, Grupp M. Amelioration of polyuria by amiloride in patients receiving long-term lithium therapy. *N Engl J Med* 312:408, 1985.
68. Yamaki M, Kusano E, Tetsuka T, et al. Cellular mechanism of lithium-induced nephrogenic diabetes insipidus in rats. *Am J Physiol* 261:F505, 1991.
69. Hensen J, Haenelt M, Gross P. Lithium induced polyuria and renal vasopressin receptor density. *Nephrol Dial Transplant* 11:622, 1996.
70. Marples D, Christensen S, Christensen EI, et al. Lithium-induced downregulation of aquaporin-2 water channel expression in rat kidney medulla. *J Clin Invest* 95:1838, 1995.
71. Singer I, Rotenberg D. Demeclocycline-induced nephrogenic diabetes insipidus. *Ann Intern Med* 76:679, 1973.
72. Forrest JN Jr, Cox M, Hong C, et al. Superiority of demeclocycline over lithium in the treatment of chronic syndrome of inappropriate secretion of antidiuretic hormone. *N Engl J Med* 298:173, 1978.
73. Schwartz WB, Relman AS. Effects of electrolyte disorders on renal structure and function. *N Engl J Med* 276:383,452, 1967.
74. Zeffren JL, Heinemann HO. Reversible defect in renal concentrating mechanism in patients with hypercalcemia. *Am J Med* 33:54, 1962.
75. Rubini M. Water excretion in potassium-deficient man. *J Clin Invest* 40:2215, 1961.
76. Rosen S, Greenfeld Z, Bernheim J, et al. Hypercalcemic nephropathy: Chronic disease with predominant medullary inner stripe injury. *Kidney Int* 37:1067, 1990.
77. Earm JH, Christensen BM, Frokiaer J, et al. Decreased aquaporin-2 expression and apical plasma membrane delivery in kidney collecting ducts of polyuric hypercalcemic rats. *J Am Soc Nephrol* 9:2181, 1998.
78. Hebert SC. Extracellular calcium-sensing receptor: Implications for calcium and magnesium handling in the kidney. *Kidney Int* 50:2129, 1996.
79. Wang WH, Lu M, Hebert SC. Cytochrome P-450 metabolites mediate extracellular Ca^{2+}-induced inhibition of apical K^+ channels in the TAL. *Am J Physiol* 271:C103, 1996.
80. Sands JM, Naruse M, Baum M, et al. Apical extracellular calcium/polyvalent cation-sensing receptor regulates vasopressin-elicited water permeability in rat kidney inner medullary collecting duct. *J Clin Invest* 99:1399, 1997.
81. Manitius A, Levitin H, Beck D, Epstein FH. On the mechanism of impairment of renal concentrating ability in potassium deficiency. *J Clin Invest* 39:684, 1960.
82. Raymond KH, Lifschitz MD, McKinney TD. Prostaglandins and the urinary concentrating defect in potassium-depleted rabbits. *Am J Physiol* 253:F1119, 1987.
83. Jin K, Summer SN, Berl T. The cyclic AMP system in the inner medullary collecting duct of the potassium depleted rat. *Kidney Int* 26:384, 1984.
84. Bennett CM. Urine concentration and dilution in hypokalemic and hypercalcemic dogs. *J Clin Invest* 49:1447, 1970.
85. Luke RG, Wright FS, Fowler N, et al. Effects of potassium depletion on renal tubular chloride transport in the rat. *Kidney Int* 14:414, 1978.
86. Berl T, Linas SL, Aisenbrey GA, Anderson RJ. On the mechanism of polyuria in potassium depletion: The role of polydipsia. *J Clin Invest* 60:620, 1977.
87. Levi M, Peterson L, Berl T. Mechanism of concentrating defect in hypercalcemia. Role of polyuria and prostaglandins. *Kidney Int* 23:489, 1983.
88. Fourman P, Leeson PM. Thirst and polyuria. *Lancet* 1:268, 1959.
89. Seely JF, Dirks JH. Micropuncture study of hypertonic mannitol diuresis in the proximal and distal tubule of the dog kidney. *J Clin Invest* 48:2330, 1969.
90. Seldin DW, Tarail R. The metabolism of glucose and electrolytes in diabetic acidosis. *J Clin Invest* 29:552, 1950.
91. Gault MH, Dixon ME, Doyle M, Cohen WM. Hypernatremia, azotemia, and dehydration due to high-protein tube feeding. *Ann Intern Med* 68:778, 1968.

92. Gipstein RM, Boyle JD. Hypernatremia complicating prolonged mannitol diuresis. *N Engl J Med* 272:1116, 1965.
93. Arieff AI, Carroll HJ. Nonketotic hyperosmolar coma with hyperglycemia: Clinical features, pathophysiology, renal function, acid-base balance, plasma-cerebrospinal fluid equilibria and the effects of therapy in 37 cases. *Medicine* 51:73, 1972.
94. Dorhout Mees EJ. Relation between maximal urine concentration, maximal water reabsorption capacity, and mannitol clearance in patients with renal disease. *Br Med J* 1:1159, 1959.
95. Kleeman CR, Adams DA, Maxwell MH. An evaluation of maximal water diuresis in chronic renal disease: I. Normal solute intake. *J Lab Clin Med* 58:169, 1961.
96. Fine LG, Schlondorff D, Trizna W, Gilbert RM. Functional profile of the isolated uremic nephron: Impaired water permeability and adenylate cyclase responsiveness of the cortical collecting tubule to vasopressin. *J Clin Invest* 61:1519, 1978.
97. Gilbert RM, Weber H, Turchin L, et al. A study of the intrarenal recycling of urea in the rat with chronic experimental pyelonephritis. *J Clin Invest* 58:1348, 1976.
98. Tannen RL, Regal EM, Dunn MJ, Schrier RW. Vasopressin-resistant hypothenuria in advanced chronic renal disease. *N Engl J Med* 280:1135, 1969.
99. Earley LE. Extreme polyuria in obstructive uropathy. *N Engl J Med* 255:600, 1956.
100. Jong D, Statius van Eps LW. Sickle cell nephropathy: New insights into its pathophysiology. *Kidney Int* 27:711, 1985.
101. Pham PT, Pham PC, Wilkinson AH, Lew SQ. Renal abnormalities in sickle cell disease [in process citation]. *Kidney Int* 57:1, 2000.
102. Statius van Eps LW, Pinedo-Veels CE, de Vries GH, de Koning J. Nature of concentrating defect in sickle-cell nephropathy: Microradioangiographic studies. *Lancet* 1:450, 1970.
103. Keitel HG, Thompson D, Itano HA. Hyposthenuria in sickle cell anemia: A reversible renal defect. *J Clin Invest* 35:998, 1956.
104. Statius van Eps LW, Schouten H, la Porte-Wijsman LW, Struyker-Budier AM. The influence of red blood cell transfusion on the hyposthenuria and renal hemodynamics of sickle cell anemia. *Clin Chim Acta* 17:449, 1967.
105. Carone FA, Epstein FH. Nephrogenic diabetes insipidus caused by amyloid disease: Evidence in man of the role of the collecting ducts in concentrating urine. *Am J Med* 29:539, 1960.
106. Shearn MA, Tu W. Nephrogenic diabetes insipidus and other defects of renal tubular function in Sjögren's syndrome. *Am J Med* 39:312, 1965.
107. Skinner R, Pearson ADJ, Price L, et al. Nephrotoxicity after ifosfamide. *Arch Dis Child* 65:732, 1990.
108. Schliefer K, Rockstroh JK, Spengler U, et al. Nephrogenic diabetes insipidus in a patient taking cidofovir. *Lancet* 350:413, 1997.
109. Navarro JF, Quereda C, Quereda C, et al. Nephrogenic diabetes insipidus and renal tubular acidosis secondary to foscarnet therapy. *Am J Kidney Dis* 27:431, 1996.
110. Barron WH, H CL, Ulland LA, et al. Transient vasopressin-resistant diabetes insipidus of pregnancy. *N Engl J Med* 310:442, 1984.
111. Durr JA, Haggard JG, Hunt JM, Schrier RW. Diabetes insipidus in pregnancy associated with abnormally high circulating vasopressinase activity. *N Engl J Med* 316:1070, 1987.
112. Davison JM, Sheills EA, Philips PR. Metabolic clearance of vasopressin and an analogue resistant to vasopressinase in human pregnancy. *Am J Physiol* 264:F348, 1993.
113. Valtin HV, Edwards BR. GFR and the concentration of urine in the absence of vasopressin: Berliner-Davidson re-explored. *Kidney Int* 31:634, 1987.
114. Linas SL, Berl T, Robertson GL, et al. Role of vasopressin impaired water excretion of glucocorticoid deficiency. *Kidney Int* 18:58, 1980.
115. Martin MM. Coexisting anterior pituitary and neurohypophyseal insufficiency. *Arch Intern Med* 123:409, 1969.
116. Bode HH, Harley BM, Crawford JD. Restoration of normal drinking behavior by chlorpropamide in patients with hypodipsia and diabetes insipidus. *Am J Med* 51:304, 1971.
117. Hays RM, McHugh PR, Williams HE. Absence of thirst in association with hydrocephalus. *N Engl J Med* 269:227, 1963.

118. Sridhar DB, Calbert GD, Ibbertson HK. Syndrome of hypernatremia, hypodipsia, and partial diabetes insipidus: A new interpretation. *J Clin Endocrinol Metab* 38:890, 1974.
119. DeRubertis FR, Michelis MF, Beck N, et al. Essential hypernatremia due to ineffective osmotic and intact volume regulation of vasopressin secretion. *J Clin Invest* 50:97, 1971.
120. DeRubertis FR, Michelis MF, Davis BB. Essential hypernatremia. *Arch Intern Med* 134:889, 1974.
121. Halter JB, Goldberg AP, Robertson GL, Porte D Jr. Selective osmoreceptor dysfunction in the syndrome of chronic hypernatremia. *J Clin Endocrinol Metab* 44:609, 1977.
122. Moses AM, Streeten DHP. Differentiation of polyuric states by measurement of responses to changes in plasma osmolality induced by hypertonic saline infusions. *Am J Med* 42:368, 1967.
123. Lindinger M, Heigenhauser GJF, McKelvie RS, Jones NL. Blood ion regulation during repeated maximal exercise and recovery in humans. *Am J Physiol* 262:R126, 1992.
124. Welt LG, Orloff J, Kydd M, Oltman JE. An example of cellular hyperosmolarity. *J Clin Invest* 29:935, 1950.
125. Marsden PA, Halperin ML. Pathophysiological approach to patients presenting with hypernatremia. *Am J Nephrol* 5:229, 1985.
126. Finberg L, Kiley J, Luttrell CN. Mass accidental salt poisoning in infancy. *JAMA* 184:187, 1963.
127. Miller NL, Finberg L. Peritoneal dialysis for salt poisoning. *N Engl J Med* 263:1347, 1960.
128. Simmons MA, Adcock EI, Bard H, Battageia F. Hypernatremia, intracranial hemorrhage and NaHCO$_3$ administration in neonates. *N Engl J Med* 291:6, 1974.
129. Meadow R. Non-accidental salt poisoning. *Arch Dis Child* 68:448, 1993.
130. Mattar JA, Weil MH, Shubin H, Stein L. Cardiac arrest in the critically ill: II. Hyperosmolal states following cardiac arrest. *Am J Med* 56:162, 1974.
131. Moder KG, Hurley DL. Fatal hypernatremia from exogenous salt intake: Report of a case and review of the literature. *Mayo Clin Proc* 65:1587, 1990.
132. Ross EJ, Christie SBM. Hypernatremia. *Medicine* 48:441, 1969.
133. Arieff AI, Guisado R. Effects of the central nervous system of hypernatremic and hyponatremic states. *Kidney Int* 10:104, 1976.
134. Finberg L, Luttrell E, Redd H. Pathogenesis of lesions in the nervous system in hypernatremic states: II. Experimental studies of gross anatomic changes and alterations of chemical composition of the tissues. *Pediatrics* 23:46, 1959.
135. Morris-Jones PH, Houston IB, Lord MB, Manc MD. Prognosis of the neurological complications of acute hypernatraemia. *Lancet* 2:1385, 1967.
136. Macaulay D, Watson M. Hypernatraemia in infants as a cause of brain damage. *Arch Dis Child* 42:485, 1967.
137. Stern WE, Coxon RV. Osmolality of brain tissue and its relation to brain bulk. *Am J Physiol* 206:1, 1964.
138. Guisado R, Arieff AI, Massry SG. Effects of glycerol infusions on brain water and electrolytes. *Am J Physiol* 227:865, 1974.
139. Strange K. Regulation of solute and water balance and cell volume in the central nervous system. *J Am Soc Nephrol* 3:12, 1992.
140. Holliday MA, Kalyci MN, Harrah J. Factors that limit brain volume changes in response to acute and sustained hyper- and hyponatremia. *J Clin Invest* 47:1916, 1968.
141. Pollock AS, Arieff AI. Abnormalities of cell volume regulation and their functional consequences. *Am J Physiol* 239:F195, 1980.
142. Kleeman CR. Metabolic coma. *Kidney Int* 36:1142, 1989.
143. Pullen RGL, DePasquale M, Cserr HF. Bulk flow of cerebrospinal fluid into brain in response to acute hyperosmolality. *Am J Physiol* 253:F538, 1987.
144. DePasquale M, Patlak CS, Cserr HF. Brain ion and volume regulation during acute hypernatremia in Brattleboro rats. *Am J Physiol* 256:F1059, 1989.
145. Somero GN. Protons, osmolytes, and fitness of internal milieu for protein function. *Am J Physiol* 251:R197, 1986.
146. Heilig CW, Stromski ME, Blumenfeld JB, et al. Characterization of the major brain osmolytes that accumulate in salt-loaded rats. *Am J Physiol* 257:F1108, 1989.

147. Lien Y-HH, Shapiro JI, Chan L. Effect of hypernatremia on organic brain osmoles. *J Clin Invest* 85:1427, 1990.

148. Paredes A, McManus M, Kwon HM, Strange K. Osmoregulation of Na^+ inositol cotransporter activity and mRNA levels in brain glial cells. *Am J Physiol* 263:C1282, 1992.

149. Lee JH, Arcinue E, Ross BD. Brief report: Organic osmolytes in the brain of an infant hypernatremia. *N Engl J Med* 331:439, 1994.

150. Galcheva-Gargova Z, Derijard B, Wu IH, Davis RJ. An osmosensing signal transduction pathway in mammalian cells. *Science* 265:806, 1994.

151. Kastin AJ, Lipsett MB, Ommaya AK, Moser JM Jr. Asymptomatic hypernatremia. *Am J Med* 38:306, 1965.

152. Salata RA, Verbalis JG, Robinson AG. Cold water stimulation of oropharygeal receptors in man inhibits release of vasopressin. *J Clin Endocrinol Metab* 65:561, 1987.

153. Berliner RW, Davidson DG. Production of hypertonic urine in the absence of pituitary antidiuretic hormone. *J Clin Invest* 36:1416, 1957.

154. Sands JB, Nonoguchi H, Knepper MA. Vasopressin effects on urea and H_2O transport in inner medullary collecting ducts subsegments. *Am J Physiol* 253:F823, 1987.

155. Sporn IN, Lancestremere RG, Papper S. Differential diagnosis of oliguria in aged patients. *N Engl J Med* 267:130, 1962.

156. Gillum DM, Linas SL. Water intoxication in a psychotic patient with normal water excretion. *Am J Med* 77:773, 1984.

157. Andersen LJ, Andersen JL, Schutten HJ, et al. Antidiuretic effect of subnormal levels of arginine vasopressin in normal humans. *Am J Physiol* 259:R53, 1990.

158. Redetzki HM, Hughes JR, Redetzki JE. Differences between serum and plasma osmolalities and their relationship to lactic acid values. *Proc Soc Exp Biol Med* 139:315, 1972.

159. Zerbe RL, Robertson GL. A comparison of plasma vasopressin measurements with a standard indirect test in the differential diagnosis of polyuria. *N Engl J Med* 305:1539, 1981.

160. Moses AM, Clayton B. Impairment of osmotically stimulated AVP release in patients with primary polydipsia. *Am J Physiol* 265:R1247, 1993.

161. Dunger DB, Seckl JR, Lightman SL. Increased renal sensitivity to vasopressin in 2 patients with essential hypernatremia. *J Clin Endocrinol Metab* 64:185, 1987.

162. Howard SS. Post-obstructive diuresis: A misunderstood phenomenon. *J Urol* 110:537, 1973.

163. Bishop MC. Diuresis and renal functional recovery in chronic retention. *Br J Urol* 57:1, 1985.

164. Coleman AJ, Arias M, Carter NW, et al. The mechanism of salt-wasting in chronic renal disease. *J Clin Invest* 45:1116, 1966.

165. Blantz RC, Pelayo JC. A functional role for the tubuloglomerular feedback mechanism. *Kidney Int* 25:739, 1984.

166. Moore LC, Casellas D. Tubuloglomerular feedback dependence of autoregulation in rat juxtaglomerular afferent arterioles. *Kidney Int* 37:1402, 1990.

167. Flis RS, Scoblionco DP, Bastl CP, Popovtzer MM. Dopamine-related polyuria in patients with gram-negative infection. *Arch Intern Med* 137:1547, 1977.

168. Polansky D, Eberhard N, McGrath R. Dopamine and polyuria (letter). *Ann Intern Med* 107:941, 1987.

169. Hogan G, Dodge PR, Gill S, et al. Pathogenesis of seizures occurring during restoration of plasma tonicity to normal in animals previously chronically hypernatremic. *Pediatrics* 43:54, 1969.

170. Blum D, Brasseur D, Kahn A, Brachet E. Safe oral rehydration of hypertonic dehydration. *J Pediatr Gastroenterol Nutr* 5:232, 1986.

171. Freidenberg GR, Kosnik EJ, Sotos JF. Hyperglycemic coma after suprasellar surgery. *N Engl J Med* 303:863, 1980.

172. Richardson DW, Robinson AG. Desmopressin. *Ann Intern Med* 103:228, 1985.

173. Vokes TJ, Gaskill MB, Robertson GL. Antibodies to vasopressin in patients with diabetes insipidus. Implications for diagnosis and therapy. *Ann Intern Med* 108:190, 1988.

174. Rittig S, Jensen AR, Jensen KT, et al. Effect of food intake on the pharmacokinetics and antidiuretic activity of oral desmopressin (DDAVP) in hydrated normal subjects. *Clin Endocrinol* 48:235, 1998.

175. Fjellestad-Paulsen A, Laborde K, Kindermans C, et al. Water-balance hormones during long-term follow-up of oral DDAVP treatment in diabetes insipidus. *Acta Paediatr* 82:752, 1993.

176. Lam KSL, Wat MS, Choi KL, et al. Pharmacokinetics, pharmacodynamics, long-term efficacy and safety of oral 1-deamino-8-D-arginine vasopressin in adult patients with central diabetes insipidus. *Br J Clin Pharmacol* 42:379, 1996.

177. Earley LE, Orloff J. The mechanism of antidiuresis associated with the administration of hydrochlorothiazide to patients with vasopressin-resistant diabetes insipidus. *J Clin Invest* 41:1988, 1962.

178. Knoers N, Monnens LAH. Amiloride-hydrochlorothiazide versus indomethacin-hydrochlorothiazide in the treatment of nephrogenic diabetes insipidus. *J Pediatr* 117:499, 1990.

179. Webster B, Bain J. Antidiuretic effect and complications of chlorpropamide therapy in diabetes insipidus. *J Clin Endocrinol Metab* 30:215, 1970.

180. Rado J. Combination of carbamazepine and chlorpropamide in the treatment of "hyporesponder" pituitary diabetes insipidus. *J Clin Endocrinol Metab* 38:1, 1974.

181. Moses AM, Fenner R, Schroeder ET, Coulson R. Further studies on the mechanism by which chlorpropamide alters the action of vasopressin. *Endocrinology* 111:2025, 1982.

182. Welch WJ, Ott CE, Lorenz JN, Kotchen TE. Effects of chlorpropamide on loop of Henle function and plasma renin. *Kidney Int* 30:712, 1986.

183. Kusano E, Braun-Werness JL, Vick DJ, et al. Chlorpropamide action on renal concentrating mechanism in rats with hypothalamic diabetes insipidus. *J Clin Invest* 72:1298, 1983.

184. Rocha AS, Ping WC, Kudo LH. Effect of chlorpropamide on water and urea transport in the inner medullary collecting duct. *Kidney Int* 39:79, 1991.

185. Houston MC. The effects of antihypertensive drugs on glucose intolerance in hypertensive non-diabetics and diabetics. *Am Heart J* 115:640, 1988.

186. Moses AM, Howanitz J, van Gemert M, Miller M. Clofibrate-induced antidiuresis. *J Clin Invest* 52:535, 1973.

187. Hamuth YA, Gelb M. Clofibrate treatment of idiopathic diabetes insipidus. *JAMA* 224:1041, 1973.

188. Wales JK. Treatment of diabetes insipidus with carbamazepine. *Lancet* 2:948, 1975.

189. Meinder AE, Cejka V, Robertson GL. The antidiuretic effect of carbamazepine in man. *Clin Sci Mol Med* 47:289, 1974.

190. Gold PW, Robertson GL, Ballenger JC, et al. Carbamazepine diminishes the sensitivity of the plasma arginine vasopressin response to osmotic stimulation. *J Clin Endocrinol Metab* 57:952, 1983.

191. Kimura T, Matsui K, Sato T, Yoshinaga K. Mechanism of carbamazepine (Tegretol)-induced antidiuresis: Evidence for release of antidiuretic hormone and impaired excretion of a water load. *J Clin Endocrinol Metab* 38:356, 1974.

192. Stokes JB. Integrated actions of renal medullary prostaglandins in the control of water excretion. *Am J Physiol* 240:F471, 1981.

193. Walker RM, Brown RS, Stoff JS. Role of renal prostaglandins during antidiuresis and water diuresis in man. *Kidney Int* 21:365, 1981.

194. Berl T, Raz A, Wald H, et al. Prostaglandin synthesis inhibition and the action of vasopressin: Studies in man and rat. *Am J Physiol* 232:F529, 1977.

195. Cutler RE, Kleeman CR, Maxwell MH, Dowling JT. Physiologic studies in nephrogenic diabetes insipidus. *J Clin Endocrinol Metab* 22:827, 1962.

196. Peterson V, Hvidt S, Thomsen K, Schou M. Effect of prolonged thiazide treatment on renal lithium clearance. *Br Med J* 3:143, 1974.

197. Usberti M, Dechaux M, Guillot M, et al. Renal prostaglandin E_2 in nephrogenic diabetes insipidus: Effects of inhibition of prostaglandin synthesis by indomethacin. *J Pediatr* 97:476, 1980.

198. Libber S, Harrison H, Spector D. Treatment of nephrogenic diabetes insipidus with prostaglandin synthesis inhibitors. *J Pediatr* 108:305, 1986.

199. Allen HM, Jackson RL, Winchester MD. Indomethacin in the treatment of lithium-induced nephrogenic diabetes insipidus. *Arch Intern Med* 149:1123, 1989.

200. Monnens J, Jonkman A, Thomas C. Response to indomethacin and hydrochlorothiazide in nephrogenic diabetes insipidus. *Clin Sci* 66:709, 1984.
201. Patrono C, Dunn MJ. The clinical significance of inhibition of renal prostaglandin synthesis. *Kidney Int* 32:1, 1987.

TWENTY-FIVE

HYPEROSMOLAL STATES— HYPERGLYCEMIA

PATHOPHYSIOLOGY

Hyperglycemia due to poorly controlled diabetes mellitus is a common clinical problem. In addition to producing a hyperosmolal state similar to hypernatremia, hyperglycemia may also be associated with severe metabolic acidosis (ketoacidosis) and volume depletion, both of which can jeopardize the life of the patient.

Although a complete discussion of the regulation of carbohydrate and fat metabolism is beyond the scope of this chapter, a review of the roles of insulin, glucagon, and other hormones is essential to understand the pathophysiology of this disorder. As will be seen, both *insulin deficiency* and *glucagon excess* play a major role in the increases in glucose and ketoacid levels—glucagon by altering hepatic metabolism to promote glucose and ketoacid production, and insulin deficiency by both affecting hepatic function and increasing the supply of substrates to the liver to allow these processes to occur.[1-4]

Glucose Metabolism

The glucose concentration in the extracellular fluid is determined by the relationship between production and utilization. Net glucose production is influenced by three factors: dietary intake, glycogenolysis, and hepatic gluconeogenesis, using lactate, amino acids (primarily alanine), and glycerol as substrates (Fig. 25-1). The glucose that is produced can then be utilized for energy or stored, for future use, in the liver and skeletal muscle as glycogen.

In the normal subject, the extracellular supply of glucose is carefully regulated, with the plasma glucose concentration being maintained within narrow limits (60 to 100 mg/dL, fasting). Insulin and glucagon, which are secreted from the pancreas, play a central role in this process by affecting both glucose production and glucose utilization (Fig. 25-1).[3,5-7] Following a glucose meal, the ensuing elevation in the plasma glucose concentration produces a similar change in the pancreatic beta cell as glucose enters the cell via GLUT2 and GLUT1 transporters in the cell membrane, the expression of which is increased by chronic exposure to high glucose concentration.[8,9]

The enzyme glucokinase, which phosphorylates glucose to glucose 6-phosphate, may act as the *glucose sensor* within the cell.[10] In mice, deletion of one of

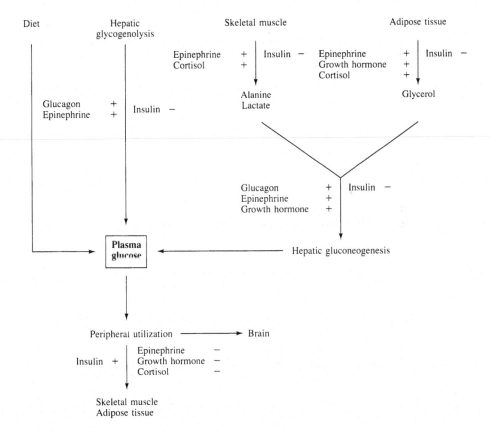

Figure 25-1   Hormonal regulation of carbohydrate and fat metabolism. Insulin and glucagon are most important in this process: the former by increasing the utilization of glucose; the latter by increasing its rate of production.

the glucokinase genes reduces the glucose sensitivity of insulin secretion, and deletion of both genes causes perinatal death due to severe hyperglycemia.[11,12] In humans, mutations in this enzyme can lead to one of the forms of maturity-onset diabetes of the young.[13]

The metabolism of glucose increases cellular adenosine triphosphate (ATP) concentrations and closes potassium-dependent ATP (KATP) channels in the beta cell membrane, causing membrane depolarization, an influx of calcium, and insulin release.[10] The KATP channel plays an important role in this process. This channel is a functional complex of the sulfonylurea 1 receptor (SUR1) and an inward rectifier potassium channel subunit, Kir6.2.[14] The administration of a sulfonylurea is one of the major therapies for treating type 2 diabetes, acting to increase insulin secretion.[15] In addition, mutations in either the SUR1 gene or the Kir6.2 gene lead to the loss of KATP activity; thus, the cell is persistently depolarized, resulting in calcium influx and the release of insulin, producing a syndrome called persistent hyperinsulinemic hypoglycemia of infancy.[16]

Insulin acts to restore normoglycemia by three effects: It decreases hepatic glucose production by diminishing both glycogenolysis and gluconeogenesis; it increases glucose uptake by skeletal muscle and adipose tissue by translocating glucose transporters from an intracellular pool to the cell surface;[17] and it diminishes the hepatic delivery of the gluconeogenetic precursors, alanine and glycerol, by its antiproteolytic and antilipolytic effects.[5-7] Insulin also inhibits glucagon secretion by direct inhibition of the glucagon gene in the pancreatic alpha cells,[18] which further diminishes hepatic glucose production.[1,3]

Glucagon, in comparison, has a primary effect on *hepatic* glucose metabolism, altering the ratio between glycolysis and gluconeogenesis.[1,4] The major regulatory compound in this process is *fructose 2,6-bisphosphate* (fructose 2,6-P_2), which normally increases the activity of 6-phosphofructo-1-kinase (PF-1-K) and impairs the activity of fructose 1,6-bisphosphatase; both of the latter enzymes are part of one bifunctional enzyme (Fig. 25-2).[1,19] PFK drives the reaction

$$\text{Fructose 6-phosphate} \leftrightarrow \text{fructose 1,6-bisphosphate} \qquad (25\text{-}1)$$

to the right, thereby promoting the conversion of glucose into pyruvate (glycolysis).[1,4] The last step in this sequence, the conversion of phosphoenolpyruvate to pyruvate, is further enhanced, since fructose 1,6-bisphosphate directly increases the activity of pyruvate kinase (Fig. 25-2).[19] In comparison, fructose 1,6-bisphosphatase drives Eq. (25-1) to the left, leading to gluconeogenesis, and pyruvate (derived in part from alanine and lactate) can be converted to glucose.

Glucagon, one of the counterregulatory hormones, is normally secreted in response to a fall in the plasma glucose concentration, which directly increases glucagon gene expression.[20] After it reaches the liver via the portal vein, glucagon (acting via the generation of cyclic adenosine monophosphate, or AMP) rapidly *reduces hepatic fructose 2,6-P_2 formation* by decreasing the activity of 6-phosphofructo-2-kinase (PF-2-K), the enzyme that catalyzes the production of fructose 2,6-P_2 from fructose 6-phosphate (Fig. 25-2).[19] As a result, there is a concurrent inactivation of PFK and disinhibition of fructose 1,6-bisphosphatase. Thus, Eq.

Figure 25-2 Schematic representation of the regulation of hepatic gluconeogenesis (arrows that point upward) and glycolysis (arrows that point downward). For simplicity, only the important regulatory reactions are shown. Fructose 2,6-bisphosphate (fructose 2,6-P$_2$) plays a central role in this process by increasing the activity of phosphofructokinase (PFK), thereby promoting glycolysis by enhancing the conversion of fructose 6-phosphate to fructose 1,6-bisphosphate. The circles with positive or negative signs represent the reactions that are affected by glucagon. The most important is diminished formation of fructose 2,6-P$_2$, thereby impairing glycolysis and facilitating gluconeogenesis by allowing pyruvate to be converted into glucose. Glucagon also induces a second block in the glycolytic pathway, as the pyruvate kinase (PK)–mediated conversion of phosphoenolpyruvate to pyruvate is diminished. The sites of entry of the gluconeogenetic precursors, alanine, lactate, and glycerol, are also shown.

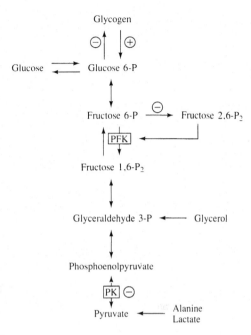

(25-1) moves to the left, a change that enhances gluconeogenesis, appropriately raising the plasma glucose concentration toward normal. Glucagon also promotes glycogen breakdown, further increasing hepatic glucose production.[1]

Insulin tends to counteract the hepatic effect of glucagon, increasing PF-2-K activity.[19] This leads to the formation of fructose 2,6-bisphosphate and the promotion of glycolysis.

Response to glucose load   In the fasting state, the liver produces glucose to meet basal energy requirements, a process that is primarily mediated by glucagon.[3] Insulin levels are low at this time, and the glucose released from the liver is primarily taken up by the brain (and to a lesser degree by the red cells and the renal medulla), tissues that do not require insulin for glucose utilization.[6]

The subsequent ingestion of glucose leads to a rise in the plasma glucose concentration, which increases the secretion of insulin and reduces that of glucagon (which also falls because of the suppressive effect of insulin).[18,21] Arterial blood enters the core of each islet, delivering substrates and information first to the beta cells, and then to the alpha and delta cells.[22] Thus, insulin released in response to a glucose load directly and appropriately suppresses glucagon release.

The degree of postprandial hyperglycemia is often minimized by concurrent fat-induced release of cholecystokinin.[23] This hormone delays gastric emptying, thereby slowing the rate of glucose absorption.

In normal subjects, the glucose-induced changes in insulin and glucagon secretion produce two major changes: a 50 to 70 percent inhibition of hepatic glucose production and the peripheral utilization of the 70 percent of the glucose load that is not taken up by the liver.[24,25] The net effect is that the plasma glucose concentration returns to baseline levels within several hours.

Response to hypoglycemia   These hormonal changes are reversed with hypoglycemia, as the secretion of insulin falls whereas that of glucagon rises.[6,26,27] The enhanced release of glucagon, which promotes both glycogenolysis and gluconeogenesis in the liver,[1,3] appears to be mediated by several factors, including the fall in insulin secretion, the decline in the plasma glucose concentration itself, and possibly a concurrent rise in epinephrine release.[28,29] In addition, glucose-sensing neurons in multiple brain areas appear to promote the release of glucagon and other counterregulatory hormones.[30] These include epinephrine and, if the hypoglycemia is prolonged, cortisol and growth hormone,[6,27] via both hepatic and peripheral effects (Fig. 25-1).[31-33]

Although less important than glucagon, other counterregulatory hormones that act in response to hypoglycemia are epinephrine, cortisol, and growth hormone:[27]

- Epinephrine, acting via β-adrenergic receptors, has hepatic effects similar to those of glucagon. It also increases the delivery of gluconeogenic substrates from the periphery, inhibits glucose utilization by several tissues, and via α_2-receptors, inhibits insulin secretion.
- Cortisol and growth hormone contribute to increased glucose utilization only if the hypoglycemia is severe and persists for several hours. These hormones limit glucose utilization and enhance hepatic glucose production.

Studies in which hypoglycemia is induced by insulin infusion have demonstrated that glucagon and epinephrine are of primary importance, as either hormone alone is sufficient to protect against an excessive fall in the plasma glucose concentration.[6,27,28] Epinephrine also has a second major effect, producing symptoms such as sweating, tremor, and tachycardia that provide an early warning signal to the patient to ingest glucose to prevent progressive neuroglycopenia.

Severe hypoglycemia can ensue if the ability to increase the secretion of these hormones is impaired, because of both diminished glucose generation and the lack of early warning symptoms.[6,34] This is of particular importance in diabetics, who may have such a combined hormonal defect resulting from concurrent pancreatic alpha cell dysfunction and autonomic neuropathy, respectively.[6,34] It is unclear why diabetics are unable to increase plasma glucagon levels in response to hypoglycemia, since they are able to respond to other stimuli such as amino acid ingestion.[26] One possible mechanism is the absence of the normal reduction in insulin secretion that in nondiabetic subjects is partially responsible for the hypoglycemia-induced rise in glucagon release.[29]

As a result, intensive insulin therapy to correct the hyperglycemia and possibly prevent diabetic microvascular complications[35] is associated with a much greater risk of symptomatic hypoglycemic episodes in patients with defective counterregulation.[34] This increase in risk is often enhanced by the attempt at strict glucose control that is associated with impairments in the threshold for the release of counterregulatory hormones and in the development of warning neurologic symptoms in response to hypoglycemia.[34,36,37] It has been suggested that these maladaptive changes result from recurrent episodes of hypoglycemia that are frequently induced by intensive insulin therapy. The combination of strict glycemic control plus prevention of hypoglycemia restores both the hormonal and the neurologic responses to or toward normal.[37]

In normal subjects, the following thresholds have been identified in the response to hypoglycemia:[26,27,38]

- Insulin secretion begins to fall when the plasma glucose concentration falls below 80 mg/dL.
- The release of glucagon and epinephrine rises when the plasma glucose concentration falls below 65 to 70 mg/dL.
- Growth hormone and cortisol secretion are enhanced at a plasma glucose concentration below 60 mg/dL.

These hormonal responses begin well before overt neuroglycopenia is seen.[27] Early cognitive dysfunction is noted in normals at a plasma glucose concentration of approximately *50 to 55 mg/dL*,[6,26,38-40] while more severe symptoms (such as lethargy and seizures) require a plasma glucose concentration below 45 to 50 mg/dL.[27] In comparison, the threshold for symptoms in poorly controlled diabetics may be higher, averaging about 80 mg/dL.[40] Chronic hyperglycemia may be responsible for this change by downregulating glucose transporters in the brain, thereby allowing neuroglycopenia to occur at a higher plasma glucose concentration.[41]

Hyperglycemia

Hyperglycemia generally requires the presence of insulin deficiency with or without insulin resistance, conditions that most often occur in patients with diabetes mellitus.[5,42,43] In addition to its direct effects on glucose metabolism, the lack of insulin also contributes to the development of hyperglycemia by promoting the secretion of glucagon and, to a lesser degree, catecholamines and growth hormone.[3,33,44-46] How these secondary changes occur is incompletely understood.

A characteristic sequence is seen with increasing severity of the disease. The plasma glucose concentration is initially *normal in the fasting state*, since low insulin secretion is appropriate in this setting. However, the insulin response to a glucose load is impaired (because of diminished secretion in type 1 and diminished sensitivity and secretion in type 2 diabetes), resulting in *postprandial hyperglycemia.*[5,47] This abnormality is mostly due to decreased peripheral glucose utilization in skeletal muscle.[47] In comparison, hepatic glucose production is at first appropriately suppressed, as a result of two factors: (1) The liver is perfused by the portal vein, which has a much higher insulin concentration than arterial blood,[48] and the hepatic effect requires only half as much insulin as the stimulation of peripheral glucose uptake.[7]

More severe insulin deficiency is also associated with *fasting hyperglycemia* due to increased hepatic glucose production.[5,24,49] This problem is primarily due to enhanced gluconeogenesis, with the contribution of glycogenolysis being limited by rapid depletion of glycogen stores.[24,49] The increase in glucose production in this setting is in part derived from alanine released from skeletal muscle; thus, fasting hyperglycemia may represent a catabolic state with loss of lean body mass. For example, hepatic glucose production in patients with poorly controlled diabetes (fasting plasma glucose concentration greater than 250 mg/dL) rises to a level *more than twice that seen in normal fasting subjects, despite the presence of hyperglycemia.*[5,24,49] The magnitude of this abnormality becomes more apparent when it is noted that even a minimal rise in the plasma glucose concentration in normal subjects increases insulin secretion and suppresses hepatic glucose production by 70 percent or more.[24,25]

Role of glucagon   In addition to the importance of insulin deficiency and/or resistance, the elevation in hepatic gluconeogenesis in uncontrolled diabetes is strongly dependent upon the hypersecretion of glucagon.[1,4] As described above, glucagon promotes gluconeogenesis by decreasing the formation of fructose 2,6-bisphosphate, thereby enhancing the conversion of fructose 1,6-bisphosphate into glucose (Fig. 25-2).[1,4,19] This effect interacts synergistically with insulin deficiency, since the latter increases the delivery of gluconeogenetic precursors (alanine and glycerol) to the liver.

The importance of glucagon in this setting can be illustrated by the observation that fasting hyperglycemia in insulin-deficient subjects can be markedly attenuated if glucagon release is prevented, either by infusing somatostatin or by the presence of a somatostatin-producing tumor.[3,50] However, *excess glucagon alone does not lead to marked hyperglycemia*, since its effects are readily counteracted by normal insulin secretion.[51] Patients with glucagon-secreting tumors, for example, typically have mild hyperglycemia that is easily controlled by diet, oral agents, or insulin and is not associated with diabetic ketoacidosis.

The increases in epinephrine and growth hormone release induced by insulin deficiency[46] can also contribute to the development of hyperglycemia.[31,33] These hormones enhance gluconeogenesis, diminish peripheral glucose uptake, and increase the delivery of alanine and glycerol to the liver (Fig. 25-1).[31-33] In addition, the release of epinephrine and cortisol are further increased by stress.[33] This may explain why acute problems such as infection or volume depletion are the most common precipitating factors in patients with diabetic ketoacidosis or non-ketotic hyperglycemia.[52,53]

Ketoacidosis

When decreased insulin effect impairs glucose utilization (as with fasting or diabetes mellitus), ketones are produced by the liver from free fatty acids to supply an alternative source of energy.[2,54] This adaptation also conserves body protein stores.[54] If ketones were not available, there would be a greater requirement for gluconeogenesis, much of which is derived from alanine that is released from skeletal muscle proteins.[55]

Two basic steps are required for ketogenesis to occur (Fig. 25-3).[1,2,4] First, lipolysis must be increased to *enhance the delivery of free fatty acids to the liver.* This is achieved by hormonal changes that are similar to those responsible for hyperglycemia—insulin deficiency[56] and, to a lesser degree, epinephrine, norepinephrine, growth hormone, and cortisol.[33,57,58]

Second, *hepatic metabolism must be altered* to allow ketone formation to occur. Excess fatty acids alone are insufficient, since they can be metabolized in the cytosol into triglycerides.[1,2] The rate-limiting step in hepatic ketogenesis is the entry of fatty acyl CoA into the mitochondria, a process regulated by the cytosolic enzyme *carnitine palmitoyl transferase* (CPT; Fig. 25-3). The activity of this enzyme appears to *vary inversely with the level of malonyl CoA,*[2,4,59] which may bind the regulatory subunit of CPT.[4] In the fed state, malonyl CoA is relatively abundant, CPT activity is low, and ketone synthesis will not occur even if free fatty acids are available.

These changes are reversed in poorly controlled diabetes, as malonyl CoA levels are low, CPT activity is increased, and ketogenesis can occur. *Glucagon excess* appears to play a major role in this hepatic response, lowering malonyl CoA production both by diminishing the availability of pyruvate for acetyl CoA formation (since the production of pyruvate from glucose is impaired; Fig. 25-2)[4] and by decreasing the activity of acetyl CoA carboxylase, the enzyme that converts acetyl CoA into malonyl CoA (Fig. 25-3).[2,4,60] In comparison, insulin has a relatively minor intrahepatic effect,[56,61] and epinephrine does not appear to stimulate hepatic ketogenesis, even at high concentrations.[57]

Acetoacetic acid is the initial ketone formed. It may then be reduced to β-hydroxybutyric acid or nonenzymatically decarboxylated to acetone.[62] Acetone is chemically neutral, but the other ketones are organic acids, and their accumulation will lead to metabolic acidosis. The degree of ketoacid accumulation is limited in fasting, usually to less than 12 meq/L.[63,64] This limitation may be mediated in part by ketone-induced stimulation of insulin release,[65] thereby decreasing the availability of free fatty acids. In contrast, severe metabolic acidosis can occur in insulin-deficient patients with diabetes mellitus, since this secondary increase in insulin secretion does not occur.[66,67]

It has been proposed that diminished ketone utilization may contribute to the acidemia in poorly controlled diabetes.[68] The importance of this problem is uncertain, however, as ketone utilization in diabetics is similar to that in fasting, at least until plasma ketone levels exceed 12 meq/L.[64]

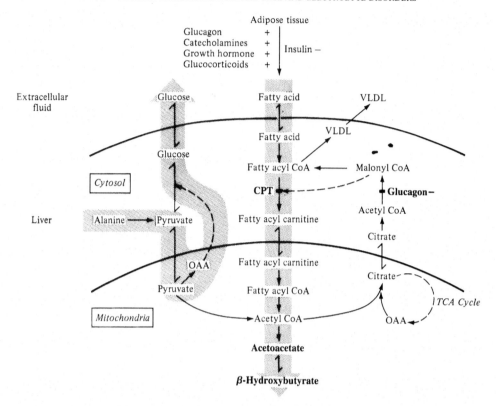

Figure 25-3 Summary of hepatic fatty acid and carbohydrate metabolism in uncontrolled diabetes mellitus, a low-insulin, high-glucagon state. In this setting, two changes occur: Free fatty acid delivery to the liver is enhanced, mostly because of insulin deficiency, and malonyl CoA levels in the hepatocyte are low. The latter effect is largely mediated by glucagon, which diminishes both acetyl CoA formation (since pyruvate synthesis from glucose is diminished; Fig. 25-2) and the activity of acetyl CoA carboxylase, which normally converts acetyl CoA into malonyl CoA. The net effect is enhanced activity of carnitine palmitoyl transferase (CPT), because of removal of the inhibitory action of malonyl CoA. As a result, the increased quantity of free fatty acids presented to the hepatocyte is able to enter the mitochondria and be metabolized to ketones. The metabolic pathways are different in the fed state, since glucagon secretion is reduced, pyruvate and malonyl CoA are abundant, and CPT activity is low. In this setting, any free fatty acids delivered to the liver will remain in the cytosol and be converted to very low density lipoprotein (VLDL) triglycerides. (*Adapted from Cahill GF Jr*, Kidney Int *20:461, 1982. Reprinted by permission from* Kidney International.)

Hypovolemia

Hypovolemia is an almost invariable finding with marked hyperglycemia and is primarily induced by the associated glucosuria. As the filtered load of glucose (glomerular filtration rate, or GFR, times plasma glucose concentration) rises, it eventually exceeds tubular reabsorptive capacity (see Chap. 3). As a result, glucose remains in the tubular lumen and acts as an osmotic diuretic, increasing the urinary loss of electrolytes and water.[66] In severely hyperglycemic patients, the fluid loss may reach 8 to 10 liters (almost 25 percent of the total body water) and produce circulatory insufficiency.[69]

In addition to producing volume depletion, the osmotic diuresis is also associated with water loss in excess of Na^+ plus K^+.[70] This will further elevate the plasma osmolality,[52,71] frequently contributing to the development of neurologic dysfunction (see "Symptoms," below).

Renal Insufficiency

Hypovolemia also reduces renal function. This may be an extremely important change, since the kidney can modify many of the metabolic abnormalities of diabetic ketoacidosis (Table 25-1). The maintenance of relatively normal renal function is in one sense beneficial, because both the hyperglycemia and the acidemia can be minimized by excretion of some of the excess glucose and acid in the urine. For example, urinary β-hydroxybutyrate (the major ketoacid anion) can buffer secreted H^+ ions to form β-hydroxybutyric acid or can be excreted with NH_4^+ (another source of acid excretion). In one study of patients with diabetic ketoacidosis, ketone production averaged 51 meq/h, while net acid excretion with the ketoacid anions averaged 15 meq/h.[72] Thus, 30 percent of the generated ketoacids were excreted in the urine, limiting the severity of the metabolic acidosis. (A second protective mechanism is the conversion of acetoacetic acid to acetone, which neutralizes another 15 to 25 percent of the acid load.)[62,72]

On the other hand, loss of β-hydroxybutyrate with either Na^+ or K^+ is in part detrimental. In most cases, *ketoacidosis is in part self-correcting*, since insulin-induced metabolism of the excess ketoacid anions results in the regeneration of HCO_3^-.[67,73] However, the degree to which this will occur is diminished if these anions are lost in the urine.[67] Volume and K^+ depletion will also be exacerbated by the ketonuria.

Normal renal function in patients with diabetic ketoacidosis is detrimental for a second reason: It maximizes the osmotic diuresis. This relationship can be illustrated by the response of patients with advanced underlying renal disease (including those already on dialysis) to uncontrolled diabetes.[71,74,75] The plasma glucose concentration can exceed 1000 to 1500 mg/dL in this setting, because the excess

Table 25-1   Effects of intact renal function in diabetic ketoacidosis

Beneficial	Detrimental
Excretion of some excess glucose	Volume depletion
	Exacerbation of hyperosmolality
Excretion of some excess acid, as β-hydroxybutyric acid or NH_4^+ salt of β-hydroxybutyrate (or to a lesser degree, acetoacetate)	Loss of Na^+ and K^+ salts of β-hydroxybutyrate, leading to volume and K^+ depletion and to loss of potential HCO_3^-
K^+ loss protects against initial hyperkalemia	K^+ loss contributes to marked K^+ depletion

glucose cannot be excreted. Despite this severe hyperglycemia, volume depletion and marked hyperosmolality are not usually seen because of the lack of a glucose osmotic diuresis. As a result, neurologic symptoms are often absent[71] unless there has been a very rapid rise in the plasma concentration.[74,76]

The kidney also plays an important role in K^+ balance in hyperglycemic patients. The triad of enhanced distal flow (due to the osmotic diuresis), ketonuria, and hypovolemia-induced hyperaldosteronism leads to increased urinary K^+ losses, which are largely responsible for the often marked K^+ deficit seen in these patients (see "Treatment," below).[42,69] In one sense, however, this effect is *protective*. At presentation, patients with diabetic ketoacidosis or nonketotic hyperglycemia are often hyperkalemic,[69] both because of the rise in P_{osm} (which pulls water and K^+ out of the cells) and because of insulin deficiency (which impairs K^+ entry into the cells; see Chap. 12).[77,78] The degree to which this occurs is limited to the concurrent K^+ depletion. In dialysis patients, on the other hand, there is no renal K^+ loss, and severe hyperglycemia can lead to life-threatening hyperkalemia (plasma K^+ concentration above 8 to 9 meq/L).[79]

Plasma Sodium Concentration

Variable changes in the plasma sodium concentration occur with hyperglycemia. Since glucose penetrates cells slowly, an increase in the plasma glucose concentration raises the effective P_{osm} and causes water to move from the cells into the extracellular fluid (ECF; see Fig. 22-1e).

Physiologic calculations suggest that the plasma sodium concentration should fall by 1 meq/L for every 62-mg/dL rise in the plasma concentration of glucose.[80] However, this standard correction factor was not verified experimentally. In an attempt to address this issue, hyperglycemia was induced in six healthy subjects by the administration of somatostatin (to block endogenous insulin secretion) and a hypertonic dextrose solution.[81] A nonlinear relationship was observed between the changes in the glucose and sodium concentrations. The $1:62$ ratio applied when the plasma glucose concentration was less than 400 mg/dL. At higher glucose concentrations, there was a greater reduction in the plasma sodium concentration. An overall ratio of $1:42$ (a 2.4-meq/L reduction in the plasma sodium concentration for every 100-mg/dL elevation in the plasma glucose) provided a better estimate of this association than the usual $1:62$ ratio.

If, for example, the plasma glucose concentration is 1000 mg/dL (930 mg/dL greater than normal), then the plasma Na^+ concentration should fall approximately 22 meq/L, from 140 to 118 meq/L. The effective P_{osm} in this setting can be estimated from (see page 247)

$$\text{Effective } P_{osm} \cong 2 \times \text{plasma } [Na^+] + \frac{[\text{glucose}]}{18}$$

$$\cong 292 \, \text{mosmol/kg}$$

This again demonstrates that hyperglycemia alone, as might occur in a diabetic dialysis patient, does not produce marked hyperosmolality ($P_{osm} \geq 330$ mosmol/

kg), since the rise in the P_{osm} is in part counteracted by water movement out of the cells.[71,75,76] However, dialysis patients are typically volume-expanded between dialyses, and the osmotic shift of water out of the cells can precipitate pulmonary edema in some cases.[74]

In many patients, however, the plasma Na^+ concentration differs from the value predicted from the degree of hyperglycemia. Most commonly, the plasma Na^+ concentration and therefore the effective P_{osm} are higher than expected due to the free-water loss induced by the osmotic diuresis.[69] On the other hand, the measured plasma Na^+ concentration may be artifactually reduced in patients with marked hyperlipidemia. The presence of lactescent serum should alert the physician to this possibility, which can be confirmed by measurement of the P_{osm} (see page 713). The latter will be substantially higher than predicted from the plasma Na^+, glucose, and urea concentrations.

ETIOLOGY

There are two major symptomatic hyperglycemia syndromes in humans: *diabetic ketoacidosis* (DKA) and *nonketotic hyperglycemia* (NKH).[42,69,82] These disorders are most often due to type 1 or type 2 diabetes mellitus, but they can also occur after the use of certain drugs or after total pancreatectomy (see below).

The factors responsible for the absence of ketoacidosis in NKH are incompletely understood. One proposed factor is differential sensitivity of fat and glucose metabolism to the effects of insulin. Studies in humans indicate that the concentration of insulin necessary to suppress lipolysis is only *one-tenth* that required to promote glucose utilization.[83] Consequently, with moderate insulin deficiency, there might be enough insulin available to block lipolysis but not enough to enhance glucose utilization. The result will be hyperglycemia without ketoacidosis, since even high levels of glucagon will not produce ketoacidosis if free fatty acid delivery is not increased. On the other hand, lipolysis will be enhanced with more severe insulin deficiency, and ketoacidosis will accompany the rise in the plasma glucose concentration.

Consistent with this model are the findings by some observers that patients with DKA tend to have higher plasma free fatty acid concentrations and lower plasma insulin concentrations than those with NKH.[69,84,85] In addition, DKA tends to occur in patients with type 1 (insulin-dependent) diabetes mellitus, who produce little or no endogenous insulin. In contrast, NKH is found primarily in older patients (average age 60 to 65) in whom insulin levels are reduced but not absent, and in whom there is either no history or one of mild, type 2 (non-insulin-dependent) diabetes mellitus.[53,82,86]

However, some observers have been unable to demonstrate these differences in the plasma insulin concentration,[87,88] and DKA can occur in patients with type 2 diabetes.[89] It is possible that these conflicting results represent an inconsistent relationship between insulin secretion and plasma insulin concentrations, and that measurement of C-peptide (rather than insulin) is a more accurate reflection of hepatic insulin delivery.[85] Alternatively, ketone formation in DKA may be due to more efficient hepatic synthesis (rather than increased free fatty acid delivery), possibly resulting from an increase in the glucagon/insulin ratio in the portal vein.

Regardless of the mechanism, it should be emphasized that DKA and NKH are not distinct disorders. They are best considered as part of a spectrum of findings in patients with insulin deficiency.[85]

Both DKA and NKH are usually precipitated by various stresses (infection, hypovolemia, surgery, emotional trauma), which act in part by increasing the secretion of catecholamines, glucagon, and cortisol.[53,69,82] Omission of insulin or oral hypoglycemic therapy or failure to augment insulin dosage when the plasma glucose concentration is poorly controlled is less often responsible. NKH can also be induced in diabetics by glucose loading, as occurs with peritoneal dialysis.[71] This complication is more common when hypertonic glucose solutions (such as 4.25% glucose) are used and can be prevented by careful monitoring of the plasma glucose concentration and by the addition of insulin to the dialysis fluid.[90]

Both DKA and NKH can also be induced in patients who do not have primary diabetes mellitus. As examples, DKA can be induced by total pancreatectomy,[91] while NKH can result from marked glucose loading in acutely ill stressed patients[92,93] or from the administration of dextrose in water to replace the high urine output in diabetes insipidus.[94] In the latter setting, the amount of glucose infused may be so large that it exceeds the normal maximum metabolic capacity.

SYMPTOMS

The patient with hyperglycemia may suffer from symptoms due to hyperosmolality, volume depletion, and, in DKA, metabolic acidosis. The severity of these symptoms is generally proportional to both the degree and the duration of the hyperglycemia. In some patients, however, these findings may be masked by the symptoms associated with the acute illness that precipitated the hyperglycemic state.

The earliest complaints associated with hyperglycemia are polyuria, polydipsia, and weight loss. This characteristic triad is due to the combination of the glucose osmotic diuresis and hypovolemia. In more severely affected patients, focal or generalized neurologic abnormalities may be seen, including lethargy, twitching, obtundation, motor or sensory defects, seizures, and coma.[69,95,96]

These symptoms and the response of the brain are similar to those seen when hyperosmolality is due to hypernatremia (see Chap. 24).[95] The increase in P_{osm} initially causes water movement out of the cells, leading to cellular dehydration, most importantly in the brain. Within 4 to 6 h, however, brain cell volume begins to rise toward normal as a result of the generation of *new osmoles* that pull water back into the cells.[95]

The mechanisms underlying this response have been best studied with hypernatremia. Initially, there is movement of Na^+ and K^+ into the brain, in part from newly formed cerebrospinal fluid.[95,97] If this were the only adaptation, however, the alterations in cell cation concentration could have deleterious effects on the activity of cell proteins.[98] This is prevented by the generation of solutes called *osmolytes* (or idiogenic osmoles), which do not interfere with protein function as their concentration rises.[98,99] Within the brain, inositol and the amino acids glutamine and glutamate appear to constitute a major part of the protective response to an elevation in the plasma Na^+ concentration.[100,101] New solutes are also generated in hyperglycemic states,[95] but it has not yet been determined if they are similar to those induced by hypernatremia.

Despite the relative preservation of brain volume, the severity of neurologic symptoms in DKA and NKH is roughly proportional to the degree of hyperosmolality.[96] Thus, coma is not usually seen unless the effective P_{osm} (equal to the measured P_{osm} minus the BUN/2.8, since urea is an ineffective osmole) is greater than 320 to 330 mosmol/kg.[75,96] In NKH, for example, the plasma glucose concentration frequently exceeds 1000 mg/dL, the effective plasma osmolality may reach 380 mosmol/kg, and neurologic abnormalities (including coma in 25 to 50 percent of cases) are often the reason that the patient is brought to medical care.[1,69,86,96] This degree of hyperosmolality occurs less often in DKA, where the plasma glucose concentration is generally below 800 mg/dL.[1,69]

The more severe hyperglycemia in NKH may reflect at least two factors. First, patients with NKH are older and frequently have impaired renal function. In contrast, DKA occurs primarily in young patients with type 1 diabetes mellitus who have a GFR that, in the first 5 years of the disease, may be as much as 50 percent above normal.[102] As a result, these patients generally have a much greater capacity to excrete glucose than those with NKH—a mechanism that will limit the degree of hyperglycemia. Second, patients with DKA may present early with the symptoms of metabolic acidosis (such as shortness of breath), rather than late with those of hyperosmolality.

The symptoms and signs produced by hypovolemia and metabolic acidosis are discussed in Chaps. 14 and 19. Circulatory insufficiency with hypotension or shock is not uncommon in NKH or DKA as a result of the marked fluid losses and, in the latter disorder, possibly severe acidemia, since the arterial pH is often below 7.10.[66,67]

In addition to those symptoms that are present at initial evaluation, neurologic deterioration and cerebral edema may develop in selected cases after fluid repletion and insulin therapy have been instituted (see "Treatment," below).[103,104]

DIAGNOSIS

The history and physical examination may provide important clues to the presence of uncontrolled diabetes mellitus. Hyperglycemia, for example, should be suspected in any patient complaining of polyuria, polydipsia, and weight loss. The findings of hyperventilation and the fruity odor of acetone on the patient's breath suggest that ketoacidosis is also present. In addition, hyperglycemia (and hypoglycemia) must be included in the differential diagnosis of any comatose patient.

Once suspected, the diagnosis can be easily confirmed by measuring the plasma glucose concentration directly or by using reagent sticks. Tablets or reagent sticks can also be used to detect glucosuria, ketonuria, and ketonemia. If serum or plasma that is undiluted or diluted 1 : 1 with normal saline has a 4+ reaction for ketones, then at least some degree of ketoacidosis can be assumed to be present. However, the nitroprusside tablets used in this test *react with aceto-acetate and acetone but not with β-hydroxybutyrate*. The ratio of β-hydroxybuty-rate to acetoacetate is about 3 : 1 in DKA but may be as high as 8 : 1 with alcoholic ketoacidosis or when there is coexistent lactic acidosis.[105] In the latter disorder, for example, the altered redox state that promotes conversion of pyruvate to lactate also favors the reduction of acetoacetate to β-hydroxybutyrate.

Thus, nitroprusside can underestimate the severity of the ketoacidosis. An indirect way around this problem is to add a few drops of hydrogen peroxide to the urinary specimen. This will convert β-hydroxybutyrate to acetoacetate, which will then be detectable by nitroprusside.[106] An alternative is to directly measure β-hydroxybutyrate in the blood; the KetoSite system (GDS Diagnostics, Elkhart, IN) is one method by which this can be performed.

A different problem in diagnosis arises with sulfhydryl drugs, such as capto-pril and penicillamine. These drugs can interact with the nitroprusside reagent to produce a false-positive ketone test.[107] Thus, a positive nitroprusside test for ketonuria or ketonemia cannot be reliably interpreted in patients treated with captopril. In this setting, the diagnosis of DKA must be made on clinical grounds (otherwise unexplained high anion gap metabolic acidosis in a patient with uncontrolled diabetes) or by direct measurement of β-hydroxybutyrate.

The presence of ketoacidosis should also be suspected in any patient with a high anion gap metabolic acidosis. As described on page 586, there is a variable relationship between the rise in the anion gap and the fall in the plasma HCO_3^- concentration in DKA. In particular, the loss of the Na^+ and K^+ salt of β-hydro-xybutyrate (or acetoacetate) will *lower the anion gap without affecting H^+ excretion or, therefore, the severity of the acidosis.*[73,108] Thus, patients who maintain relatively normal renal function may have marked ketonuria and can present with the combination of severe metabolic acidosis and an only mildly elevated anion gap. Furthermore, a true normal anion gap (or hyperchloremic) metabolic acidosis commonly occurs after therapy with insulin is begun. In this setting, the excess anion gap disappears as the ketones are metabolized, but some degree of acidemia will persist because of the loss of potential HCO_3^- when the ketoacid anions were excreted in the urine.[73,108]

A more complicated acid-base disorder can be seen in those patients who also have marked vomiting or have been treated with diuretics. The concurrent metabolic alkalosis in this setting will partially or even completely counteract the ketoacidosis, and the extracellular pH will depend upon the relative severity of the two disorders.[109] Even if the patient is initially alkalemic, the high anion gap and the presence of hyperglycemia should suggest the possibility of underlying ketoacidosis.

Although uncontrolled diabetes mellitus may be suggested by many of the above findings, hypoglycemic therapy with insulin should not be begun until the presence of hyperglycemia has been demonstrated. The *isolated finding of glucosuria or ketonemia does not necessarily mean that hyperglycemia is present, and the administration of insulin to such a patient may be dangerous.*[110] Diabetics, particularly those on insulin, can be in coma because of a low rather than an elevated plasma glucose concentration. If the patient has not emptied his or her bladder for several hours, the urine may still contain glucose, reflecting a period of hyperglycemia that may have existed several hours previously. The administration of insulin in this setting will further reduce the plasma glucose concentration and can produce neurologic deterioration and death.

Whenever there is a question as to the presence of hypoglycemia or hyperglycemia, it is always safer to give glucose (50 mL of 50% glucose intravenously) immediately after blood has been drawn for measurement of the plasma glucose concentration. This will dramatically improve the status of the hypoglycemic patient but will not be harmful to the patient with hyperglycemia.

In addition to diabetes mellitus, alcoholism (when accompanied by decreased carbohydrate intake) can also produce severe ketoacidosis (see page 600).[111,112] In this condition, the plasma glucose concentration is less than 250 mg/dL and may be less than 100 mg/dL. Other causes of a high anion gap metabolic acidosis that must be excluded in an alcoholic are methanol and ethylene glycol intoxication (see pages 607–610).[113]

The treatment of alcoholic ketoacidosis is the administration of glucose, which will suppress the secretion of glucagon and stimulate that of insulin, thereby diminishing both lipolysis and hepatic ketogenesis. Since the plasma glucose concentration frequently is normal, the administration of exogenous insulin is not indicated, since it can precipitate severe hypoglycemia.

TREATMENT

Therapy must be directed toward each of the metabolic disturbances that may be present in the hyperglycemic patient: hyperosmolality, ketoacidosis, hypovolemia, and potassium and phosphate depletion.[1,42] Since absolute or relative insulin deficiency is responsible for most of these problems, the administration of insulin and volume repletion are the mainstays of therapy. To assess the effect of treatment, the plasma glucose concentration should be measured every 2 h and the plasma electrolytes and arterial pH every 2 to 4 h until the patient is out of danger.

Insulin

Insulin acts to correct the hyperglycemia, to diminish ketone production (by diminishing both lipolysis and glucagon secretion), and perhaps to augment ketone utilization. The major effect of insulin on glucose metabolism is to diminish hepatic glucose production (gluconeogenesis), with enhanced peripheral utilization (which requires a higher concentration of insulin[7] being quantitatively less important.[49,114] The net effect is that the plasma glucose concentration usually *falls at a maximum rate of 65 to 125 mg/dL/h.*[114-117]

Although more rapid correction is not necessarily desirable, this response seems to reflect significant *insulin resistance*. Normal subjects, for example, can be made hyperglycemic (plasma glucose concentration about 650 mg/dL) by the combination of somatostatin (to block insulin release) and glucose.[81,117] The subsequent administration of insulin can lower the plasma glucose level by up to 500 mg/dL/h, a difference that cannot be explained by more rapid urinary glucose excretion.[117] The mechanism of insulin resistance in diabetic patients is probably multifactorial and includes primary tissue resistance in type 2 diabetes,[5] the initially high levels of glucagon, and possibly hyperosmolality itself.[118] The normal subjects had acute hyperglycemia, little time for an osmotic diuresis, and therefore a lower P_{osm} than is typically seen in DKA or NKH.

The effect of insulin on adipose tissue requires a much lower concentration than that required for glucose utilization;[83] as a result, any dose of insulin that corrects the hyperglycemia also will normalize ketone metabolism. Subsequent utilization of the excess ketones will tend to reverse the metabolic acidosis, since metabolism of the ketoacid anions results in the regeneration of HCO_3^-.[66] Although this occurs relatively rapidly over the first 5 to 10 h, acetone is cleared more slowly (in part via the lungs) and may remain in the blood for more than 36 h.[119] Thus, the persistence of ketonemia and ketonuria is not necessarily indicative of failure of insulin therapy.

Most patients with DKA or severe NKH are treated with a low-dose regular insulin regimen in which the total amount of insulin administration is usually between 40 and 100 units.[114-116,120,121] Insulin requirements do not appear to be substantially different in DKA and NKH.[69] A loading dose of 15 to 20 units should be given initially, followed by 8 to 15 units/h until the biochemical abnormalities are under reasonable control. Higher doses (such as 50 to 100 units/2 h) can be used but do not usually lower the plasma glucose concentration more rapidly.[115,116,120] Although diabetics are frequently insulin-resistant,[117] the equivalent effectiveness of the low- and high-dose regimens suggests that both doses saturate the cell membrane receptors and that the insulin resistance is generally due to a postreceptor defect.[1,5] Some patients, however, do not respond to low-dose insulin; in this setting, the dose must be increased to a level adequate to control the plasma glucose concentration.

Regular insulin can be given by the intravenous, subcutaneous, or intramuscular route; these appear to be equally effective in correcting the hyperglycemia and ketoacidosis.[121] Hospitalized patients are usually treated initially with intravenous insulin. A relatively concentrated solution should be used to minimize insulin absorption onto the glass and plastic tubing. If, for example, 40 units of regular insulin is added to 100 mL of isotonic saline, an infusion at 20 to 30 mL/h will deliver 8 to 12 units/h of insulin to the patient.

In patients who are markedly hypovolemic, insulin therapy is generally *withheld* for 30 to 60 min until 1 to 2 liters of fluid can be given. Insulin drives glucose and, because of the ensuing fall in P_{osm}, water into the cells. As a result, insulin can exacerbate the degree of extracellular volume depletion if it is given before fluid replacement has been begun.

Fluids

The average fluid loss is 3 to 6 liters in DKA, but it can reach 8 to 10 liters in NKH.[1,69] With each liter of water, only about 70 meq of monovalent cation (Na^+ and K^+) is lost. This reflects the enhanced water loss relative to solute induced by the glucose osmotic diuresis. Fluid repletion is generally begun with *isotonic saline*. This solution will replace the fluid losses, correct the extracellular volume depletion more rapidly than half-isotonic saline, lower the P_{osm} (since it is still hypotonic to the patient), and reduce the plasma glucose concentration by as much as 35 to 70 mg/dL/h.[122] The last effect results both from hemodilution and from increased urinary glucose losses as renal function is improved.

The optimal rate at which isotonic saline should be administered is dependent upon the clinical state of the patient. For example, fluids should be infused as quickly as possible in patients who are in shock. In comparison, patients who do not have an extreme volume deficit may be effectively repleted at a rate of 500 mL/h for the first 4 h followed by 250 mL/h for the next 4 h.[123] More rapid administration is not necessary and may actually delay correction of the acidemia, in part by a dilution-induced reduction in the plasma HCO_3^- concentration.[123]

The increase in renal perfusion leads to reductions in the blood urea nitrogen (BUN) and plasma creatinine concentration. Although the plasma creatinine concentration generally varies inversely with the GFR, this value may be misleading in DKA, since acetoacetate is a noncreatinine chromogen that is *measured as creatinine* in the standard colorimetric assay. As a result, the plasma creatinine concentration may be falsely elevated by as much as 2 mg/dL or more, leading to a marked underestimation of the glomerular filtration rate.[124] Metabolism of the acetoacetate following the administration of insulin will rapidly lower the measured plasma creatinine concentration toward its true value.

Although begun on isotonic saline, most patients are switched at some point to half-isotonic saline to replace the free-water loss induced by the osmotic diuresis. When this should occur, however, is uncertain, because of concern about the possible development of cerebral edema.

Cerebral edema is an unusual complication of therapy that occurs within 24 h after treatment has been initiated.[103,104,125] Headache is the earliest clinical manifestation; more severe neurologic symptoms (including brain herniation and death) can occur in up to 3 percent of children, particularly those treated with relatively dilute fluids.[125] Almost all cases occur in patients under the age of 20, as symptomatic cerebral edema appears to be a rare complication in adults.[103] However, *subclinical* brain swelling is much more common than symptomatic disease, as evidenced by computed tomography (CT) scanning and by an increase in cerebrospinal fluid pressure.[104,126,127]

The mechanisms responsible for cerebral edema are incompletely understood. The combination of insulin and fluids can lower the plasma glucose concentration by a maximum of 200 mg/dL/h or 11 mosmol/kg/h if there is no compensatory rise in the plasma Na^+ concentration as a result of the concurrent administration of relatively dilute fluids. This rapid reduction in the P_{osm} could, as in hypernatremia (see page 762), promote osmotic water movement into the brain.[104,125] Studies in an animal model suggest a primary role for a rapid fall in the plasma glucose concentration with no contribution from ketoacidosis.[128] Other factors also may be important, including a hyperglycemia-induced increase in blood-brain permeability[129] and perhaps acute dilutional hypoalbuminemia.[130]

Studies in diabetic animals with marked hyperglycemia suggest that insulin itself may play a role in the genesis of cerebral edema.[131] Lowering the plasma glucose concentration below 250 to 330 mg/dL with insulin can result in the generation of new (idiogenic) osmoles within the brain cells. This increase in brain cell osmolality can draw water into the brain and produce cerebral edema. The importance of insulin in this phenomenon is suggested by the absence of new osmole formation when the plasma glucose concentration is reduced without insulin via peritoneal dialysis.[131] This model is not entirely applicable to humans, however, since cerebral edema has been described at a time when more marked hyperglycemia is still present.[103]

In summary, it is likely that rapid reduction in the plasma glucose concentration and P_{osm} contribute to the common development of mild cerebral edema.[104,125,128] It is not clear, however, why only a small number of patients develop severe neurologic symptoms.[103]

The optimal regimen for safe fluid repletion is uncertain. Nevertheless, the following recommendations seem prudent:[104,125]

- Fluid repletion should be begun with isotonic saline, which is administered at the rate described above until tissue perfusion is adequate, as evidenced from the systemic blood pressure, urine output (once glucosuria has disappeared), and physical examination. At this point, the patient is out of danger, and complete correction should occur slowly over several days.

- Therapy with regular insulin should be discontinued and dextrose-containing saline solutions should be used when the plasma glucose concentration falls below 300 mg/dL.[69] Further insulin can be given as necessary. It is important to remember that persistent ketonemia or ketonuria frequently reflects the slower clearance of acetone and not persistent ketoacidosis.[119]

- Half-isotonic saline can be used once the phase of rapid fluid repletion has been completed, since slow administration of this dilute fluid will not lead to a rapid reduction in P_{osm}. It must be emphasized, however, that marked K^+ depletion is also typically present and that K^+ repletion is usually begun when the plasma K^+ concentration is ≤ 4.5 meq/L (see below). K^+ is as osmotically active as Na^+ (see page 687); as a result, the addition of 40 meq of KCl to each liter of isotonic saline now represents a hypertonic solution with an effective osmolality of almost 400 mosmol/kg (Na^+ plus K^+ concentration of 194 meq/L). Thus, K^+ should be given in half-isotonic (or even quarter-isotonic) saline unless the patient is still markedly hypovolemic.

- Patients should be observed for possible signs of cerebral edema, such as severe headache, incontinence, or decreased mental status. Early treatment with hypertonic mannitol in this setting may prevent irreversible neurologic damage.[103]

Bicarbonate

The indications for HCO_3^- therapy in the treatment of ketoacidosis are unclear. In general, insulin leads to partial correction of this problem, since metabolism of the ketoacid anions that have not been lost in the urine results in the regeneration of HCO_3^-.[66,67] Thus, several controlled trials in small numbers of patients have been unable to demonstrate that the use of $NaHCO_3$ leads to any clinical benefit or any important difference in the rate of rise in the plasma HCO_3^- concentration.[132,133] In addition, alkali therapy may increase hepatic ketone production, slowing the rate of recovery from the ketosis.[134]

These findings, however, do not address the issue that there may be selected patients who may benefit from cautious alkali therapy.[73,135] These include patients with severe acidemia (arterial pH < 7.0 to 7.1), in whom decreased cardiac contractility and peripheral vasodilatation can further impair tissue perfusion (see Chap. 19),[135] and patients with a relatively normal anion gap due to excretion of ketoacid anions in the urine.[73] In the latter setting, the quantity of HCO_3^- that can be generated from organic anion metabolism is minimized. As a result, there will be a normal anion gap acidosis during the correction phase (see page 586), and restoration of acid-base balance in the absence of alkali therapy will be a slow process, requiring renal excretion of the excess acid as NH_4^+.[73] The aim of HCO_3^- administration in patients with one or both of these indications is to raise the arterial pH above 7.15 to 7.20, a level at which the patient should be out of danger.

In addition, $NaHCO_3$ should also be given to patients with potentially life-threatening hyperkalemia. Bicarbonate drives K^+ into the cells, thereby lowering the plasma K^+ concentration (see Chap. 28).

Potassium

Most patients with DKA or NKH are markedly K^+-depleted. The average K^+ deficit is 3 to 5 meq/kg, but it can exceed 10 meq/kg in some patients.[42] Several factors contribute to this problem, including vomiting, increased urinary losses due to the osmotic diuresis and to ketoacid anion excretion, and the loss of K^+ from the cells due to glycogenolysis and proteolysis.[42,136]

Despite the K^+ deficit, the plasma K^+ concentration is usually normal or, in about one-third of patients, elevated.[42,69,136] This paradoxical finding results from a transcellular shift as K^+ moves from the cells into the extracellular fluid. Two factors appear to be of primary importance in this process:[136] insulin deficiency (since insulin normally promotes K^+ uptake by the cells)[137] and, more importantly, hyperosmolality (see Fig. 12-7).[77,78,138] The elevation in P_{osm} results in the osmotic movement of water out of the cells. This can promote parallel K^+ movement into the extracellular fluid via two mechanisms:

- The loss of cell water raises the cell K^+ concentration, thereby promoting passive K^+ diffusion through K^+ *channels* in the cell membrane.
- The frictional forces between solvent (water) and solute can result in K^+ being carried along with water through the *water pores* in the cell membrane. This phenomenon, called solvent drag, is independent of the electrochemical gradient for K^+.

In comparison, acidemia itself does not seem to play a major role, since organic acids are much less likely to influence the internal distribution of K^+ (see page 379).[136,139] Thus, hyperkalemia is as prevalent in NKH, where the pH is relatively normal, as it is in DKA.[69]

Although masked initially, the K^+ depletion becomes rapidly apparent as insulin therapy drives K^+ into the cells (both directly and by reversing the hyperglycemia). To prevent the development of potentially severe hypokalemia, 20 to 40 meq/L of KCl should be added to the intravenous infusions once the plasma K^+ concentration falls below 4.5 meq/L.

The need for K^+ repletion is more urgent in those patients who are *hypokalemic prior to therapy*. In this setting, K^+ replacement must be begun immediately, since insulin and fluids alone can produce a potentially dangerous reduction in the plasma K^+ concentration. The rate of K^+ administration is variable, with doses of up to 20 to 40 meq/h being required if serious cardiac arrhythmias are present. These higher doses are generally safer if they can be given orally. Careful monitoring of the plasma K^+ concentration and the electrocardiogram is important to determine the efficacy of therapy (see Chap. 27).

Phosphate

Cellular phosphate depletion with an initially elevated plasma phosphate concentration is another common finding in DKA or NKH.[42,66,140] The loss of phosphate is primarily related to decreased intake and to increased urinary losses, resulting from the osmotic diuresis, the direct effect of acidemia, and the rise in the plasma phosphate concentration.[42,140] The dissociation between phosphate stores and the plasma phosphate concentration again reflects a transcellular shift of phosphate out of the cells. Both the osmotic water shift induced by the rise in P_{osm} and the direct effect of an organic acidosis (by an unknown mechanism) may contribute to this response.[140,141]

Like the rise in the plasma K^+ concentration, the hyperphosphatemia is also rapidly corrected with insulin therapy. In one study, for example, the mean plasma phosphate concentration fell from 9.2 mg/dL on admission to 2.8 mg/dL at 12 h.[140] Furthermore, values as low as 1.0 mg/dL may be seen in selected patients with severe phosphate depletion.[66,142]

Despite these findings, the routine use of phosphate supplements in DKA or NKH has not been shown to improve morbidity or the rate of correction of the electrolyte disturbances.[143,144] In addition to lack of efficacy, phosphate administration is not without risk, since hyperphosphatemia and hypocalcemia may ensue.[145] It seems prudent, therefore, to reserve phosphate administration for the occasional patient who develops a severe, symptomatic reduction in the plasma phosphate concentration.

PROBLEMS

25-1 A 68-year-old woman with adequately controlled diabetes mellitus and previously normal renal function presents with fever, dysuria, nausea, recurrent vomiting, flank pain, and polyuria that have become progressively more severe over 4 days. The physical examination reveals a temperature of 39.6°C, reduced skin turgor, estimated jugular venous pressure below 5 cmH$_2$O, postural hypotension, and marked tenderness over the right costovertebral angle. The urine shows pyuria and bacteriuria, and a diagnosis of acute pyelonephritis is made. Other laboratory data reveal the following:

Plasma [glucose]	=	570 mg/dL	BUN	=	32 mg/dL
[Na$^+$]	=	135 meq/L	[Creatinine]	=	4.0 mg/dL
[K$^+$]	=	2.6 meq/L	Serum ketones	=	4$^+$, diluted 1:1
[Cl$^-$]	=	87 meq/L	Arterial pH	=	7.36
[HCO$_3^-$]	=	20 meq/L	P$_{CO_2}$	=	37 mmHg

The electrocardiogram shows prominent U waves in the precordial leads and occasional multifocal premature ventricular beats.

(a) What is the acid-base disturbance on admission?
(b) What factors account for the elevations in the BUN and plasma creatinine concentration?
(c) What would be your initial therapeutic regimen?

25-2 A 25-year-old woman with type 1, insulin-dependent diabetes is admitted to the hospital with a soft-tissue infection of the palate. The initial laboratory data include the following:

$$\text{Plasma [glucose]} = 147 \text{ mg/dL}$$

$$[\text{Na}^+] = 140 \text{ meq/L}$$

$$[\text{K}^+] = 3.8 \text{ meq/L}$$

$$[\text{Cl}^-] = 110 \text{ meq/L}$$

$$[\text{HCO}_3^-] = 23 \text{ meq/L}$$

The patient eats sparingly because of pain on swallowing. To minimize the risk of hypoglycemia, her insulin is withheld. Repeat blood tests are obtained 36 h later:

Plasma [glucose]	=	270 mg/dL	Anion gap	= 15 meq/L
$[Na^+]$	=	135 meq/L	Serum ketones	= 4^+, diluted 1:1
$[K^+]$	=	5.0 meq/L	Arterial pH	= 7.32
$[Cl^-]$	=	105 meq/L	P_{CO_2}	= 30 mmHg
$[HCO_3^-]$	=	15 meq/L		

A diagnosis of diabetic ketoacidosis is made.

(a) Why is the anion gap only slightly elevated despite the presence of ketoacidosis?

(b) How would you treat the patient at this time?

REFERENCES

1. Foster DW, McGarry JD. The metabolic derangements and treatment of diabetic ketoacidosis. *N Engl J Med* 309:159, 1983.
2. Cahill GF Jr. Ketosis. *Kidney Int* 20:416, 1981.
3. Unger RH, Orci L. Glucagon and the A cell: Physiology and pathophysiology. *N Engl J Med* 304:1518,1575, 1981.
4. Foster DW. From glycogen to ketones—and back. *Diabetes* 33:1188, 1984.
5. DeFronzo RA. The triumvirate: B-cell, muscle, liver. A collusion responsible for NIDDM. *Diabetes* 37:667, 1988.
6. Gerich JE. Glucose counterregulation and its impact on diabetes mellitus. *Diabetes* 37:1608, 1988.
7. Rizza RA, Mandarino LJ, Gerich JE. Dose-response characteristics for the effect of insulin on production and utilization of glucose in man. *Am J Physiol* 240:E630, 1981.
8. Yasuda K, Yamada Y, Inagaki N, et al. Expression of GLUT1 and GLUT2 glucose transporter isoforms in rats islets of Langerhans and their regulation by glucose. *Diabetes* 41:76, 1992.
9. Liang Y, Cushman SM, Whitesell RR, Matschinsky FM. GLUT1 is adequate for glucose uptake in GLUT2-deficient insulin-releasing beta cells. *Horm Metab Res* 29:255, 1997.
10. Matschinsky F, Linag Y, Kesavan P, et al. Glucokinase as pancreatic beta-cell glucose sensor and diabetes gene. *J Clin Invest* 92:2092, 1993.
11. Grupe A, Hultgren B, Ryan A, et al. Transgenic knockouts reveal a critical requirement for pancreatic beta cell glucokinase in maintaining glucose homeostasis. *Cell* 83:69, 1995.
12. Terauchi Y, Sakura H, Yasuda K, et al. Pancreatic beta-cell specific targeted disruption of glucokinase gene: Diabetes mellitus due to defective insulin secretion to glucose. *J Biol Chem* 270:30253, 1995.
13. Froguel P, Zonali H, Vionnet N, et al. Familial hyperglycemia due to mutations in glucokinase: Definition of a subtype of diabetes mellitus. *N Engl J Med* 328:697, 1993.
14. Aguilar-Bryan L, Nichols CG, Wechsler SW, et al. Cloning the β cell high-affinity sulfonylurea receptor: A regulator of insulin secretion. *Science* 268:423, 1995.
15. Bressler R, Johnson DG. Pharmacological regulation of blood glucose levels in non-insulin-dependent diabetes mellitus. *Arch Intern Med* 157:836, 1997.
16. Kane C, Shepherd RM, Squires PE, et al. Loss of functional K-ATP channels in pancreatic β-cells causes persistent hyperinsulinemic hypoglycemia of infancy. *Nat Med* 2:1344, 1996.
17. Kahn BB, Flier JS. Regulation of glucose-transporter gene expression in vitro and in vivo. *Diabetes Care* 15:548, 1990.
18. Phillippe J. Insulin regulation of the glucagon gene is mediated by an insulin-responsive DNA element. *Proc Natl Acad Sci U S A* 88:7224, 1991.
19. Pilkis SJ, El-Maghrabi MR, Claus TH. Fructose-2,6-bisphosphate in control of hepatic gluconeogenesis: From metabolites to molecular genetics. *Diabetes Care* 15:582, 1990.
20. Chen L, Komiya I, Inman L, et al. Effects of hypoglycemia and prolonged fasting on insulin and glucagon gene expression: Studies with in situ hybridization. *J Clin Invest* 84:711, 1989.

21. Cryer P, Gerich J. Glucose counterregulation, hypoglycemia, and intensive insulin therapy in diabetes mellitus. *N Engl J Med* 313:232, 1985.
22. Stagner JI, Samols E. The vascular order of islet cellular perfusion in the human pancreas. *Diabetes* 41:93, 1992.
23. Liddle RA, Rushakoff RJ, Morita ET, et al. Physiologic role for cholecystokinin in reducing post-prandial hyperglycemia in humans. *J Clin Invest* 81:1675, 1988.
24. Pehling G, Tessari P, Gerich JE, et al. Abnormal meal carbohydrate disposition in insulin-dependent diabetes: Relative contributions of endogenous glucose production and initial splanchnic uptake and effect of intensive insulin therapy. *J Clin Invest* 74:985, 1984.
25. Ferrannini E, Bjorkman O, Reichard GA Jr, et al. The disposal of an oral glucose load in healthy subjects. *Diabetes* 34:580, 1985.
26. Amiel S. Glucose counter-regulation in health and disease: Current concepts in hypoglycaemia recognition and response. *Q J Med* 80:707, 1991.
27. Cryer PE. Glucose counterregulation: Prevention and correction of hypoglycemia in humans. *Am J Physiol* 264:E149, 1993.
28. Bolli G, De Feo P, Perrierlo G, et al. Mechanisms of glucagon secretion during insulin-induced hypoglycemia in man: Role of the beta cell and arterial hyperinsulinemia. *J Clin Invest* 73:917, 1984.
29. Weir GC, Bonner-Weir S. Islets of Langerhans: The puzzle of interislet interactions and their relevance to diabetes. *J Clin Invest* 85:983, 1990.
30. Borg MA, Sherwin RS, Borg WP, et al. Local ventromedial hypothalamus glucose perfusion blocks counterregulation during systemic hypoglycemia in awake rats. *J Clin Invest* 99:361, 1997.
31. Eigler N, Sacca L, Sherwin RS. Synergistic interactions of physiologic increments of glucagon, epinephrine, and cortisol in the dog: A model for stress-induced hyperglycemia. *J Clin Invest* 63:114, 1979.
32. Sacca L, Vigorito C, Cicala M, et al. Role of gluconeogenesis in epinephrine-stimulated hepatic glucose production in humans. *Am J Physiol* 245:E294, 1983.
33. Press M, Tamborlane W, Sherwin RS. Importance of raised growth hormone levels in mediating the metabolic derangements of diabetes. *N Engl J Med* 310:810, 1984.
34. Clarke WL, Gonder-Frederick LA, Richards FE, Cryer PE. Multifactorial origin of hypoglycemic symptom unawareness in IDDM: Association with defective glucose counterregulation and better glycemic control. *Diabetes* 40:680, 1991.
35. The Diabetes Control and Complications Trial Research Group. The effect of intensive treatment of diabetes on the development and progression of long-term complications in insulin-dependent diabetes mellitus. *N Engl J Med* 329:977, 1993.
36. Amiel SA, Tamborlane WV, Simonson DC, Sherwin RS. Defective glucose counterregulation after strict glycemic control of insulin-dependent diabetes mellitus. *N Engl J Med* 316:1376, 1987.
37. Fanelli CG, Epitano L, Rambatti AM, et al. Meticulous prevention of hypoglycemia normalizes the glycemic thresholds and magnitude of most neuroendocrine responses to, symptoms of, and cognitive function during hypoglycemia in intensively treated patients with short-term IDDM. *Diabetes* 42:1683, 1993.
38. Schwartz NS, Clutter WE, Shah SD, Cryer PE. Glycemic thresholds for activation of glucose counterregulatory systems are higher than the threshold for symptoms. *J Clin Invest* 79:777, 1987.
39. De Feo P, Gallai V, Mazzotta G, et al. Modest decrements in plasma glucose concentration cause early impairment in cognitive function and later activation of glucose counterregulation in the absence of hypoglycemic symptoms in normal man. *J Clin Invest* 82:436, 1988.
40. Boyle PJ, Schwartz NS, Shah SD, et al. Plasma glucose concentrations at the onset of hypoglycemic symptoms in patients with poorly controlled diabetes and in nondiabetics. *N Engl J Med* 318:1487, 1988.
41. Matthaie S, Horuk R, Olefsky JM. Blood-brain glucose transfer in diabetes mellitus. Decreased number of glucose transporters at blood-brain barrier. *Diabetes* 35:1181, 1986.

42. Kreisberg RA. Diabetic ketoacidosis: New concepts and trends in pathogenesis and treatment. *Ann Intern Med* 88:681, 1978.

43. Eriksson J, Franssila-Kallunki A, Ekstrand A, et al. Early metabolic defects in persons at increased risk for non-insulin-dependent diabetes mellitus. *N Engl J Med* 321:337, 1989.

44. Felig P, Sherwin RS. Glucagon and blood glucose: Insights from artificial pancreas studies. *Ann Intern Med* 92:856, 1980.

45. Raskin P, Pietri A, Unger R. Changes in glucagon levels after four to five weeks of glucoregulation by portable insulin infusion pumps. *Diabetes* 28:1033, 1979.

46. Tamborlane WV, Sherwin RS, Koivisto V, et al. Normalization of the growth hormone and catecholamine response to exercise in juvenile-onset diabetic subjects treated with a portable insulin infusion pump. *Diabetes* 28:785, 1979.

47. Sacca L, Orofino G, Petrone A, Vigorito C. Differential roles of splanchnic and peripheral tissues in the pathogenesis of impaired glucose tolerance. *J Clin Invest* 73:1683, 1984.

48. Blackard WG, Nelson NC. Portal and peripheral vein immunoreactive insulin concentrations before and after glucose. *Diabetes* 19:302, 1970.

49. Luzi L, Barrett EJ, Groop LC, et al. Metabolic effects of low-dose insulin therapy on glucose metabolism in diabetic ketoacidosis. *Diabetes* 37:1470, 1988.

50. Unger RH. Somatostatinoma. *N Engl J Med* 296:998, 1977.

51. Sherwin RS, Fisher M, Hendler R, Felig P. Hyperglucagonemia and blood glucose regulation in normal, obese, and diabetic subjects. *N Engl J Med* 294:455, 1976.

52. Schade DS, Eaton RP. Prevention of diabetic ketoacidosis. *JAMA* 242:2455, 1979.

53. Gerich JE, Martin MM, Recant L. Clinical and metabolic characteristics of hyperosmolar nonketotic coma. *Diabetes* 20:228, 1971.

54. Cahill G. Starvation in man. *N Engl J Med* 282:668, 1970.

55. Chiasson JL, Atkinson RL, Cherrington AD, et al. Effects of fasting on gluconeogenesis from alanine in diabetic man. *Diabetes* 28:56, 1979.

56. Miles JM, Haymond MW, Nissen SL, Gerich JE. Effects of free fatty acid availability, glucagon excess, and insulin deficiency on ketone body production in postabsorptive man. *J Clin Invest* 71:1554, 1983.

57. Bahnsen M, Burrin JM, Johnston DG, et al. Mechanisms of catecholamine effects of ketogenesis. *Am J Physiol* 247:E173, 1984.

58. Schade DS, Eaton RP. The regulation of plasma ketone body concentration by counterregulatory hormones in man: I. Effects of norepinephrine in diabetic man. *Diabetes* 26:989, 1977.

59. McGarry JD, Mannaerts GP, Foster DW. A possible role for malonyl-CoA in the regulation of hepatic fatty acid oxidation and ketogenesis. *J Clin Invest* 60:265, 1977.

60. Cook GA, Nielson RC, Hawkins RA, et al. Effect of glucagon on hepatic malonyl coenzyme A concentration and on lipid synthesis. *J Biol Chem* 252:4421, 1977.

61. Keller U, Gerber PG, Stauffacher W. Fatty-acid independent inhibition of hepatic ketone body production by insulin in humans. *Am J Physiol* 254:E694, 1988.

62. Owen OE, Trapp VE, Skutches CL, et al. Acetone metabolism during diabetic ketoacidosis. *Diabetes* 31:242, 1982.

63. Reichard GA Jr, Owen OE, Haff AC, et al. Ketone body production and oxidation in fasting obese humans. *J Clin Invest* 53:508, 1974.

64. Ferry F, Balasse EO. Ketone body production and disposal in diabetic ketosis: A comparison with fasting ketosis. *Diabetes* 34:326, 1985.

65. Miles JM, Haymond MW, Gerich JE. Suppression of glucose production and stimulation of insulin secretion by physiological concentrations of ketone bodies in man. *J Clin Endocrinol Metab* 52:34, 1981.

66. Seldin DW, Tarail R. Metabolism of glucose and electrolytes in diabetic acidosis. *J Clin Invest* 29:552, 1950.

67. Adrogué HJ, Wilson H, Boyd AE, et al. Plasma acid-base patterns in diabetic ketoacidosis. *N Engl J Med* 307:1603, 1982.

68. Sherwin RS, Hendler RG, Felig P. Effect of diabetes mellitus and insulin on the turnover and metabolic response to ketones in man. *Diabetes* 25:776, 1976.

69. Arieff AI, Carroll HJ. Nonketotic hyperosmolar coma with hyperglycemia: Clinical features, pathophysiology, renal function, acid-base balance, plasma-cerebrospinal fluid equilibria and the effects of therapy in 37 cases. *Medicine* 51:73, 1972.

70. Seely JF, Dirks JH. Micropuncture study of hypertonic mannitol diuresis in the proximal and distal tubule of the dog kidney. *J Clin Invest* 48:2330, 1969.

71. Al-Kudsi RR, Daugirdas JT, Ing TS, et al. Extreme hyperglycemia in dialysis patients. *Clin Nephrol* 17:228, 1982.

72. Owen OE, Licht JH, Sapir DG. Renal function and effects of partial rehydration during diabetic ketoacidosis. *Diabetes* 30:510, 1981.

73. Adrogué HJ, Eknoyan G, Suki WK. Diabetic ketoacidosis: Role of the kidney in the acid-base homeostasis re-evaluated. *Kidney Int* 25:591, 1984.

74. Tzamaloukas AH, Levinstone AR, Gardner KD Jr. Hyperglycemia in advanced renal failure: Sodium and water metabolism. *Nephron* 31:40, 1982.

75. Popli S, Leehey DJ, Daugirdas JT, et al. Asymptomatic, nonketotic severe hyperglycemia with hyponatremia. *Arch Intern Med* 150:1962, 1990.

76. Daugirdas JT, Kronfol NO, Tzalaloukas AH, Ing TS. Hyperosmolar coma: Cellular dehydration and the serum sodium concentration. *Ann Intern Med* 110:855, 1989.

77. Nicolis GL, Kahn T, Sanchez A, Gabrilove JL. Glucose-induced hyperkalemia in diabetic subjects. *Arch Intern Med* 141:49, 1981.

78. Viberti GC. Glucose-induced hyperkalaemia: A hazard for diabetics? *Lancet* 1:690, 1978.

79. Montoliu J, Revert L. Lethal hyperkalemia associated with severe hyperglycemia in diabetic patients with renal failure. *Am J Kidney Dis* 5:47, 1985.

80. Katz M. Hyperglycemia-induced hyponatremia: Calculation of expected serum sodium depression (letter). *N Engl J Med* 289:843, 1973.

81. Hillier TA, Abbott RD, Barrett EJ. Hyponatremia: Evaluating the correction factor for hyperglycemia. *Am J Med* 106:399, 1999.

82. Flulop M. The treatment of severely uncontrolled diabetes mellitus. *Adv Intern Med* 25:327, 1984.

83. Zierler KL, Rabinowitz D. Effect of very small concentrations of insulin on forearm metabolism. Persistence of its action on potassium and free fatty acids without its effects on glucose. *J Clin Invest* 43:950, 1964.

84. Johnson RD, Conn JC, Dykman CJ, et al. Mechanisms and management of hyperosmolar coma without ketoacidosis in the diabetic. *Diabetes* 18:111, 1969.

85. Malchoff CD, Pohl SL, Kaiser DL, Carey RM. Determinants of glucose and ketoacid concentrations in acutely hyperglycemic diabetic patients. *Am J Med* 77:275, 1984.

86. Khardori R, Soler MG. Hyperosmolar hyperglycemic nonketotic syndrome: Report of 22 cases and brief review. *Am J Med* 77:899, 1984.

87. Joffe BI, Seftel HC, Goldberg R, et al. Factors in the pathogenesis of experimental nonketotic and ketoacidotic diabetic stupor. *Diabetes* 22:653, 1973.

88. Joffe BI, Goldberg RB, Krut LH, Seftel HC. Pathogenesis of nonketotic hyperosmolar diabetic coma. *Lancet* 1:1069, 1975.

89. Westphal SA. The occurrence of diabetic ketoacidosis in non-insulin-dependent diabetes and newly diagnosed diabetic adults. *Am J Med* 101:19, 1996.

90. Amair P, Khanna R, Leibel B, et al. Continuous ambulatory peritoneal dialysis in diabetics with end-stage renal disease. *N Engl J Med* 306:625, 1982.

91. Barnes AJ, Bloom SR, Alberti KGMM, et al. Ketoacidosis in pancreatectomized man. *N Engl J Med* 296:1250, 1977.

92. Wyrick WJ, Rea WJ, McClelland RM. Rare complications with intravenous hyperosmotic alimentation. *JAMA* 211:1697, 1970.

93. Rosenberg SA, Brief DK, Kinney J, et al. The syndrome of dehydration, coma, and severe hyperglycemia without ketosis in patients convalescing from burns. *N Engl J Med* 272:931, 1965.

94. Freidenberg GR, Kosnik EJ, Sotos JF. Hyperglycemic coma after suprasellar surgery. *N Engl J Med* 303:863, 1980.

95. Pollock AS, Arieff AI. Abnormalities of cell volume regulation and their functional consequences. *Am J Physiol* 239:F195, 1980.
96. Fulop M, Tannenbaum H, Dreyer N. Ketotic hyperosmolar coma. *Lancet* 2:635, 1973.
97. Pullen RGL, DePasquale M, Cserr HF. Bulk flow of cerebrospinal fluid into brain in response to acute hyperosmolality. *Am J Physiol* 253:F538, 1987.
98. Somero GN. Protons, osmolytes, and fitness of internal milieu for protein function. *Am J Physiol* 251:R197, 1986.
99. Strange K. Regulation of solute and water balance and cell volume in the central nervous system. *J Am Soc Nephrol* 3:12, 1992.
100. Heilig CW, Stromski ME, Blumenfeld JB, et al. Characterization of the major brain osmolytes that accumulate in salt-loaded rats. *Am J Physiol* 257:F1108, 1989.
101. Lien Y-HH, Shapiro JI, Chan L. Effect of hypernatremia on organic brain osmoles. *J Clin Invest* 85:1427, 1990.
102. Bank N. Mechanisms of diabetic hyperfiltration. *Kidney Int* 40:792, 1991.
103. Rosenbloom AL. Intracerebral crisis during treatment of diabetic ketoacidosis. *Diabetes Care* 13:22, 1990.
104. Durr JA, Hoffman WH, Sklar AH, et al. Correlates of brain edema in uncontrolled IDDM. *Diabetes* 41:627, 1992.
105. Marliss EB, Ohman JL Jr, Aoki TT, Kozak GP. Altered redox state obscuring ketoacidosis in diabetic patients with lactic acidosis. *N Engl J Med* 283:978, 1970.
106. Narins RG, Jones ERS, Stom MC, et al. Diagnostic strategies in disorders of fluid, electrolyte and acid-base homeostasis. *Am J Med* 72:496, 1982.
107. Csako G, Elin RJ. Unrecognized false-positive ketones from drugs containing free-sulfhydryl groups (letter). *JAMA* 269:1634, 1993.
108. Oh MS, Carroll HJ, Uribarri J. Mechanism of normochloremic and hyperchloremic acidemia in diabetic ketoacidosis. *Nephron* 54:1, 1990.
109. Cronin JW, Kroop SF, Diamond J, Rolla AR. Alkalemia in diabetic ketoacidosis. *Am J Med* 77:192, 1984.
110. Felig P. Diabetic ketoacidosis. *N Engl J Med* 290:1360, 1974.
111. Wrenn KD, Slovis CM, Minion GE, Rutkowski R. The syndrome of alcoholic ketoacidosis. *Am J Med* 91:119, 1991.
112. Miller PD, Heinig RE, Waterhouse C. Treatment of alcoholic acidosis. The role of dextrose and phosphorus. *Arch Intern Med* 138:67, 1978.
113. Hojer J. Severe metabolic acidosis in the alcoholic: Differential diagnosis and management. *Hum Exp Toxicol* 15:482, 1996.
114. Brown PM, Tompkins CV, Juul S, Sonksen PH. Mechanism of action of insulin in diabetic patients: A dose-related effect on glucose production and utilisation. *Br Med J* 1:1239, 1978.
115. Genuth SM. Constant intravenous insulin infusion in diabetic ketoacidosis. *JAMA* 223:1348, 1973.
116. Padilla AJ, Loeb JN. "Low dose" versus "high dose" insulin regimens in the management of uncontrolled diabetes: A survey. *Am J Med* 63:843, 1977.
117. Rosenthal NR, Barrett EJ. An assessment of insulin action in hyperosmolar hyperglycemic nonketotic diabetic patients. *J Clin Endocrinol Metab* 60:607, 1985.
118. Bratusch-Marrain PR, DeFronzo RA. Impairment of insulin-mediated glucose metabolism by hyperosmolality in man. *Diabetes* 32:1028, 1983.
119. Sulway MJ, Malins JM. Acetone in diabetic ketoacidosis. *Lancet* 2:736, 1970.
120. Soler NG, Wright AD, Fitzgerald MG, Malins JM. Comparative study of different insulin regimens in management of diabetic ketoacidosis. *Lancet* 2:1221, 1975.
121. Fisher JN, Shahshahani MM, Kitabshi AE. Diabetic ketoacidosis: Low-dose insulin therapy by various routes. *N Engl J Med* 297:238, 1977.
122. Page MM, Alberti KGMM, Greenwood R, et al. Treatment of diabetic coma with continuous lose-dose insulin infusion. *Br Med J* 2:687, 1974.
123. Adrogué HJ, Barrero J, Eknoyan G. Salutary effects of modest fluid replacement in the treatment of adults with diabetic ketoacidosis: Use in patients without extreme fluid deficit. *JAMA* 262:2108, 1989.

124. Molitch ME, Rodman E, Hirsch CA, Dubinsky E. Spurious creatinine elevations in ketoacidosis. *Ann Intern Med* 93:2800, 1980.
125. Harris GD, Fiordalisi I, Harris WL, et al. Minimizing the risk of brain herniation during treatment of diabetic ketoacidosis: A retrospective and prospective study. *J Pediatr* 117:22, 1990.
126. Krane EJ, Rockoff MA, Wallman JK, Wolfsdorf JH. Subclinical brain swelling in children during treatment of diabetic ketoacidosis. *N Engl J Med* 312:1147, 1985.
127. Clements RS Jr, Blumenthal SA, Morrison AD, Winegrad AI. Increased cerebrospinal-fluid pressure during treatment of diabetic ketosis. *Lancet* 2:671, 1971.
128. Silver SM, Clark EC, Schroeder BM, Sterns RH. Pathogenesis of cerebral edema after treatment of diabetic ketoacidosis. *Kidney Int* 51:1237, 1997.
129. Winegrad AI, Kern EFO, Simmons DA. Cerebral edema in diabetic ketoacidosis. *N Engl J Med* 312:1185, 1985.
130. Fein IA, Rackow EC, Sprung CL, Goodman R. Relation of colloid osmotic pressure to arterial hypoxemia and cerebral edema during crystalloid volume loading of patients with diabetic ketoacidosis. *Ann Intern Med* 96:570, 1982.
131. Arieff AI, Kleeman CR. Studies on mechanisms of cerebral edema in diabetic comas. *J Clin Invest* 52:571, 1973.
132. Morris LR, Murphy MB, Kitabachi AE. Bicarbonate therapy in diabetic ketoacidosis. *Ann Intern Med* 105:836, 1986.
133. Hale PJ, Crase J, Nattrass M. Metabolic effects of bicarbonate in the treatment of diabetic ketoacidosis. *Br Med J* 289:1035, 1984.
134. Okuda Y, Adrogué HJ, Field JB, et al. Counterproductive effects of sodium bicarbonate in diabetic ketoacidosis. *J Clin Endocrinol Metab* 81:314, 1996.
135. Narins RG, Cohen JJ. Bicarbonate therapy for organic acidosis: The case for its continued use. *Ann Intern Med* 106:615, 1987.
136. Adrogué HJ, Lederer ED, Suki WN, Eknoyan G. Determinants of plasma potassium levels in diabetic ketoacidosis. *Medicine* 65:163, 1986.
137. Cox M, Sterns RH, Singer I. The defense against hyperkalemia: The roles of insulin and aldosterone. *N Engl J Med* 299:525, 1978.
138. Goldfarb S, Cox M, Singer I, Goldberg M. Acute hyperkalemia induced by hyperglycemia: Hormonal mechanisms. *Ann Intern Med* 84:426, 1976.
139. Adrogué HJ, Madias NE. Changes in plasma potassium concentration during acute acid-base disturbances. *Am J Med* 71:456, 1981.
140. Kebler R, McDonald FD, Cadnapaphornchai P. Dynamic changes in serum phosphorus levels in diabetic ketoacidosis. *Am J Med* 79:571, 1985.
141. O'Connor LR, Klein KL, Bethane JE. Hyperphosphatemia in lactic acidosis. *N Engl J Med* 297:707, 1977.
142. Knochel JP. The pathophysiology and clinical characteristics of severe hypophosphatemia. *Arch Intern Med* 137:203, 1977.
143. Keller U, Berger W. Prevention of hypophosphatemia by phosphate infusion during treatment of diabetic ketoacidosis and hyperosmolar coma. *Diabetes* 29:87, 1980.
144. Wilson HK, Kever SP, Lea AS, et al. Phosphate therapy in diabetic ketoacidosis. *Arch Intern Med* 142:517, 1982.
145. Winter RJ, Harris CJ, Phillips LS, Green OC. Diabetic ketoacidosis: Induction of hypocalcemia and hypomagnesemia by phosphate therapy. *Am J Med* 67:897, 1979.

TWENTY-SIX

INTRODUCTION TO DISORDERS
OF POTASSIUM BALANCE

The maintenance of K^+ balance is essential for a variety of cellular and neuromuscular functions. This chapter will review the physiologic effects of K^+ and the factors governing K^+ homeostasis, topics that are generally discussed in greater detail in Chap. 12. The application of these principles to the common clinical problems of K^+ depletion and K^+ excess will then be presented in Chaps. 27 and 28.

PHYSIOLOGIC EFFECTS OF POTASSIUM

The total body K^+ stores in a normal adult are approximately 3000 to 4000 meq (50 to 55 meq/kg body weight). Roughly 98 percent of the body K^+ is located in the cells; this is in contrast to Na^+, which is primarily limited to the extracellular fluid. The localization of Na^+ and K^+ to the different fluid compartments is maintained by the Na^+-K^+-ATPase pump in the cell membrane, which transports Na^+ out of and K^+ into the cells in a $3:2$ ratio.[1,2] The net effect is that the K^+ concentration is about 140 meq/L in the cells but only 4 to 5 meq/L in the extracellular fluid (including the plasma).

Cell Function

Potassium plays an important role in cell function and in neuromuscular transmission. In the cells, K^+ participates in the regulation of such processes as protein and glycogen synthesis.[3] As a result, conditions of K^+ imbalance are associated with a variety of signs and symptoms. For example, patients with chronic K^+ depletion may complain of polyuria and polydipsia (increased urine output and thirst). These problems, which are reversed with K^+ repletion, are primarily due to diminished urinary concentrating ability, resulting from decreased tubular responsiveness to antidiuretic hormone.[4,5]

Resting Membrane Potential

In addition to the importance of the *absolute* amount of K^+ present, the *ratio* of the K^+ concentration in the cells to that in the extracellular fluid is the major determinant of the resting membrane potential (E_m) across the cell membrane. This relationship can be expressed by the following formula:

$$E_m = -61 \log \frac{r[K^+]_c + 0.01[Na^+]_c}{r[K^+]_e + 0.01[Na^+]_e} \tag{26-1}$$

where r is the $3:2$ active transport ratio of the Na^+-K^+-ATPase pump, 0.01 is the relative membrane permeability of Na^+ to K^+, and the subscripts c and e refer to the cellular and extracellular concentrations, respectively.[6]

If the normal concentrations for K^+ and Na^+ are substituted in Eq. (26-1) (see Table 1-5),

$$E_m = -61 \log \frac{3/2 \, (140) + 0.01 \, (12)}{3/2 \, (4.4) + 0.01 \, (145)}$$

$$= -86 \text{ mV} \quad \text{(cell interior negative)}$$

This resting potential is generated largely by the diffusion of K^+ out of the cell down its concentration gradient; Na^+ diffusion in the opposite direction is much less prominent because of the lower membrane permeability to Na^+. The loss of positively charged K^+ ions makes the interior of the cell electrically negative with respect to the extracellular fluid. The steady state described in Eq. (26-1) is reached when this cell negative potential (which tends to hold K^+ within the cell) is of the same magnitude as the concentration gradient that promotes K^+ diffusion out of the cell.

It is the resting membrane potential that sets the stage for the generation of the *action potential* that is essential for normal neural and muscular function.[7,8] During excitation, the steady state is altered, because the release of acetylcholine at synapses and motor end plates produces an increase in the number of open voltage-sensitive Na^+ channels (in which clusters of positively charged amino acid residues constitute the site of voltage activation).[9,10] The ensuing progressive increase in net Na^+ permeability has three consequences:[8,9,11]

- Na^+ diffuses into the cell down its concentration gradient.
- This Na^+ movement causes the membrane potential to be depolarized, i.e., it declines toward zero.
- Depolarization results in the opening of voltage-sensitive K^+ channels;[12] both the increased K^+ permeability and decreased cell interior electronegativity promote K^+ movement out of the cell.

The net effect depends upon the *degree of depolarization*. When the depolarizing stimulus is relatively small, there is only a minor increment in Na^+ permeability. As a result, the initial Na^+ movement into the cell is followed by a period in which K^+ exit exceeds further Na^+ entry, because of the greater K^+ permeability. This flux of K^+ raises the membrane potential back toward its baseline value, and generation of an action potential does not occur.

The *threshold potential* (E_t) is that potential at which the Na^+ permeability is sufficiently enhanced so that the *rate of Na^+ entry continues to exceed that of K^+ exit*. This induces a self-perpetuating cycle characterized by more depolarization (since the continued entry of Na^+ makes the cell interior less electronegative), a further increase in Na^+ permeability (up to 1000 times the basal value, as depolarization directly leads to continued activation of voltage-sensitive Na^+ channels), more Na^+ entry, more depolarization, etc.[8,9,11] The net effect is the generation of an action potential, in which the cell interior ultimately becomes *electropositive* as a result of the massive influx of Na^+. The propagation of these changes to adjacent cells is responsible for the transmission of neural impulses and the initiation of muscle contraction.

The action potential is followed by *repolarization and recovery*.[8] During repolarization, the permeability to Na^+ returns to its low baseline value, whereas that to K^+ is slightly increased because of activation of voltage-sensitive K^+ channels.[7,9] In this setting, the high cell K^+ concentration, high K^+ permeability, and favorable electrical gradient (cell interior now positive) all favor the passive movement of K^+ out of the cell, returning the potential to its negative resting level. In the recovery phase, the Na^+-K^+-ATPase pump extrudes the Na^+ that entered the cell during depolarization and pumps in the K^+ that left the cell during repolarization, resulting in the normalization of cell composition.

It should be noted that the quantity of ions that must cross the cell membrane to produce these changes is extremely small. The generation of a resting potential of 86 mV, for example, requires the separation of only 10^{-7} meq of K^+ per cm^2 of membrane, or about one one-hundred-thousandth of the intracellular K^+ pool.[13]

Membrane excitability   The excitability (or irritability) of neuromuscular tissue is defined as the difference between the resting and threshold potentials ($E_m - E_t$). Thus, any factor that alters either of these potentials affects excitability. In particular, small changes in the extracellular K^+ concentration (which is much lower than that in the cells) can produce relatively large changes in the $[K^+]_c/[K^+]_e$ ratio and consequently in the resting membrane potential.[14,15]

However, the effect of alterations in the plasma K^+ concentration on membrane excitability cannot be directly predicted from the $[K^+]_c/[K^+]_e$ ratio. As an example, an elevation in the plasma potassium concentration will decrease this ratio and partially depolarize the cell membrane (that is, make the resting potential less electronegative). This change will initially increase membrane excitability, since less of a depolarizing stimulus is required to generate an action potential. However, the later effect that is seen in patients is different. Persistent depolarization *inactivates Na$^+$ channels* in the cell membrane, thereby producing a net reduction in membrane excitability that may be manifested clinically by impaired cardiac conduction and/or muscle weakness or paralysis.[7]

Similarly, hypokalemia will induce initial hyperpolarization of the cell membrane (resting potential more electronegative), lowering membrane excitability. This change will remove the normal state of inactivation of Na^+ channels, thereby increasing neuromuscular excitability.[7] In the heart, these effects of hyperkalemia and hypokalemia can produce characteristic changes in the electrocardiogram and potentially fatal arrhythmias (see Chaps. 27 and 28).

The clinical manifestations of alterations in the plasma K^+ concentration are variable. One patient may have severe muscle weakness with a plasma K^+ concentration of 1.8 meq/L, whereas another may be relatively asymptomatic at the same level. At least two factors appear to be responsible for this individual variation.

The effect of hypokalemia (or hyperkalemia) is dependent upon the degree to which there is a similar change in cell K^+ concentration, thereby minimizing the alteration in the $[K^+]_c/[K^+]_e$ ratio. In particular, *transcellular shifts of K^+ are more likely to produce symptoms than changes in external balance*. In hypokalemic periodic paralysis, for example, extracellular K^+ acutely moves into the cells. Thus, the $[K^+]_c$ rises slightly, whereas the $[K^+]_e$ falls, resulting in a relatively large change in the $[K^+]_c/[K^+]_e$ ratio and the frequent development of muscle weakness or paralysis (see Chap. 27). The findings are different with K^+ depletion due to gastrointestinal or renal losses. In this setting, the fall in the plasma K^+ concentration creates a gradient that promotes passive K^+ movement out of the cells not the extracellular fluid.[16] As a result, the K^+ concentration is diminished in both compartments, leading to a smaller change in the $[K^+]_c/[K^+]_e$ ratio and therefore a lesser likelihood of symptoms. Similar principles apply to the risk of symptomatic hyperkalemia.

Membrane excitability is determined by factors other than K^+, including the plasma Ca^{2+} concentration and pH. The effect of Ca^{2+} becomes clinically important because it can counteract the membrane effects of hyperkalemia. How this occurs is not well understood, but the administration of calcium salts is the most rapid modality for reversing the neuromuscular and cardiac symptoms of severe hyperkalemia (see Chap. 28). Membrane excitability is also influenced by changes in the extracellular pH, being directly increased by alkalemia and decreased by acidemia. Thus, metabolic acidosis will tend to counteract the membrane effects of hypocalcemia, since each abnormality has a different effect on membrane excitability.

In summary, the degree to which an increase or decrease in the plasma K^+ concentration affects neuromuscular excitability is dependent upon a variety of factors. These include the mechanism of change (alteration in external balance versus transcellular shift) and the extracellular Ca^{2+} concentration and pH. As a result, the severity of symptoms does not necessarily correlate with the magnitude of the change in the plasma K^+ concentration. Since the electrocardiogram and muscle strength reflect the *functional consequences* of K^+ excess or depletion, monitoring of these parameters as well as the plasma K^+ concentration is essential in the management of patients with severe K^+ imbalance.

REGULATION OF POTASSIUM BALANCE

The maintenance of K^+ balance involves two functions: (1) the normal distribution of K^+ between the cells and extracellular fluid and (2) the renal excretion of the K^+ added to the extracellular fluid from dietary intake and endogenous cellular breakdown.

Distribution between Extracellular Fluid and Cells

Regulation of the internal distribution of K^+ must be extremely efficient, since the movement of as little as 1.5 to 2 percent of the cell K^+ into the extracellular fluid can result in a potentially fatal increase in the plasma K^+ concentration to as high as 8 meq/L or more. In the basal state, normal K^+ distribution is achieved primarily by the Na^+-K^+-ATPase pump.[1] In addition, the ability of K^+ to move between the cells and the extracellular fluid is also important.[16,17] As an example, K^+ enters the cells after a K^+ load. The importance of this response can be appreciated from a few simple calculations. Suppose a normal 70-kg man drinks three glasses of orange juice containing 40 meq of K^+. If this K^+ remained in the extracellular fluid (the extracellular volume being approximately 17 liters), there would be a potentially dangerous 2.4-meq/L increase in the plasma K^+ concentration. This is prevented by the rapid entry of most of the K^+ load into the cells,[16] followed, within 6 to 8 h, by the urinary excretion of the excess K^+.[17,18]

The physiologic and pathologic factors that influence the distribution of K^+ are listed in Table 26-1. The role of these factors in hypokalemic and hyperkalemic states will be discussed in the following two chapters. Nevertheless, it is useful at this time to briefly review the physiologic roles of catecholamines and insulin (both of which increase the activity of the Na^+-K^+-ATPase pump) and of the plasma K^+ concentration itself.[1]

Catecholamines and insulin   Catecholamines and insulin can affect K^+ distribution, as both β_2-adrenergic stimuli (due mostly to epinephrine) and insulin promote the cellular uptake of K^+ by skeletal muscle and liver.[17,20-23] These actions are primarily mediated by a hormone-induced increase in activity of the Na^+-K^+-ATPase pump.[1,23,24] The adrenergic effect may also be in part indirect, since, when

Table 26-1   Factors influencing the distribution of K$^+$ between the cells and the extracellular fluid

Physiologic
  Na$^+$-K$^+$-ATPase
  Catecholamines
  Insulin
  Plasma K$^+$ concentration
  Exercise
Pathologic
  Chronic diseases
  Extracellular pH
  Hyperosmolality
  Rate of cell breakdown

epinephrine levels are elevated, there is often a concurrent rise in insulin release, due both to a direct β_2-adrenergic effect on the pancreas and to the stimulation of glycolysis, leading to a rise in the plasma glucose concentration.[25]

The physiologic importance of catecholamines and insulin has been demonstrated by the response to the administration of β-adrenergic blockers or somatostatin (which impairs insulin secretion). In these settings, the increment in the plasma K$^+$ concentration after a K$^+$ load is greater and more prolonged than in normal subjects (see Fig. 12-2).[22,26,27] On the other hand, glucose-induced insulin release in normal subjects limits the degree of hyperkalemia following a glucose- and K$^+$-containing meal (see Fig. 12-4).[28]

It appears that it is the *basal levels* of epinephrine and insulin that enhance K$^+$ uptake, since a physiologic K$^+$ load (with a rise in the plasma K$^+$ concentration of less than 1 meq/L) produces little or no change in the plasma levels of these hormones.[20,29] It is possible, however, that there may be some release of insulin into the portal vein, thereby promoting hepatic K$^+$ uptake without increasing the peripheral plasma insulin concentration.[30]

If, on the other hand, the availability of epinephrine or insulin is increased (as with a glucose load for insulin), there will be a further tendency for K$^+$ to move into the cells.[26,31] This effect lasts for only several hours, because other factors (perhaps the plasma K$^+$ concentration itself) then cause K$^+$ to move back into the extracellular fluid.[31] This transient action of insulin is useful clinically, since the administration of insulin (with glucose to prevent hypoglycemia) is an important component of therapy in patients with severe hyperkalemia.

In summary, the primary physiologic effect of epinephrine and insulin is to *facilitate the disposition of an acute K$^+$ load, not to regulate the baseline plasma K$^+$ concentration.* Although a deficiency of these hormones may cause mild hyperkalemia,[22] this effect is transient, since the excess K$^+$ can reenter the cells or be excreted in the urine. As a result, the fasting plasma K$^+$ concentration is typically normal in patients treated with β-adrenergic blockers and in patients with diabetes mellitus who are given enough insulin to prevent marked hyperglycemia.[20,26]

Plasma potassium concentration   The combination of insulin deficiency and β-adrenergic blockade impairs but does not prevent the intracellular movement of K^+, indicating that other factors must also be involved.[32] One of these is probably the plasma K^+ concentration itself, which will rise after a K^+ load, thereby promoting the passive movement of some of the excess K^+ into the cells. Conversely, K^+ will leave the cells when hypokalemia is due to gastrointestinal or renal losses, an effect that will minimize the fall in the plasma K^+ concentration.

As a result, the plasma K^+ concentration usually varies directly with body K^+ stores, decreasing with K^+ depletion and increasing with K^+ retention. In general, a reduction in the plasma K^+ concentration from 4.0 to 3.0 meq/L is associated with a 200- to 400-meq deficit in total body K^+.[16] On the other hand, an elevation in the plasma K^+ concentration from 4.0 to 5.0 meq/L is usually associated with the retention of 100 to 200 meq of K^+.[16]

There are some exceptions to this rule, which occur with disorders that affect K^+ distribution. As examples, K^+ movement out of the cells is induced by insulin deficiency and hyperosmolality in uncontrolled diabetes mellitus, some forms of metabolic acidosis, severe exercise, and excess tissue breakdown. In these settings, hyperkalemia may occur even though total body K^+ stores are normal or even reduced.

These problems are discussed in detail in the next two chapters. It is important, however, to note that the effect of exercise can interfere with the routine measurement of the plasma K^+ concentration. After a tourniquet is applied to obtain a blood sample, the patient is frequently instructed to repeatedly clench and unclench his or her fist in an attempt to increase local blood flow and make the veins more prominent. This can result in K^+ movement out of the cells and an elevation in the plasma K^+ concentration of as much as 1 to 2 meq/L, leading to erroneous evaluation of the state of K^+ balance.[33]

Renal Excretion

Although small amounts of K^+ are lost each day in the feces and sweat, the urine is the major route by which the K^+ derived from the diet and endogenous cellular breakdown is eliminated from the body. The primary event in urinary K^+ excretion is the *secretion* of K^+ from the tubular cell into the lumen in the distal nephron, particularly in the *principal cells in the cortical and outer medullary collecting tubule* (see Chap. 12).[34-36] Although a substantial amount of K^+ is filtered, almost all of this is reabsorbed prior to the distal secretory sites. The amount of K^+ secreted varies appropriately with the state of K^+ balance: It is enhanced by a K^+ load and reduced by a low-K^+ diet. In addition, net distal reabsorption rather than secretion can occur in states of K^+ depletion.[34,36]

The secretion of K^+ from the cell into the lumen is primarily passive and is therefore a function of luminal membrane permeability and the concentration and electrical gradients across the luminal membrane.[34,35] *Aldosterone* and the *plasma* K^+ *concentration*, acting in concert, are the major physiologic determinants of K^+ secretion, as they vary directly with the state of K^+ balance (Fig. 26-1). The flow rate to the distal nephron and the lumen-negative potential difference generated by Na^+ reabsorption are also important, but they generally play a *permissive rather than a regulatory role* in that they do not necessarily change with alterations in K^+ balance.

Aldosterone and the plasma K^+ concentration   After a K^+ load, the small increase in the plasma K^+ concentration stimulates the release of aldosterone,[37] and both of these then promote distal K^+ secretion (see Fig. 12-10).[38-41] Aldosterone appears to enhance each of the major steps involved in distal K^+ secretion: (1) It makes the lumen more electronegative by promoting Na^+ reabsorption (this is the earliest change); (2) the subsequent transport of this Na^+ out of the cell by the Na^+-K^+-ATPase pump also results in K^+ movement into the cell, thereby raising the cell K^+ concentration; and (3) aldosterone increases the number of open K^+ channels in the luminal membrane, an additional change that facilitates K^+ secretion.[38-40] The importance of aldosterone in maintaining K^+ homeostasis can be illustrated by the response to spironolactone: This competitive inhibitor of aldosterone produces a variable increase in the plasma potassium concentration as a result of a reduction in potassium excretion.[42]

The small elevation in the plasma K^+ concentration after a K^+ load potentiates the effect of aldosterone.[41] Studies in adrenalectomized animals have demonstrated that K^+ loading alone replicates all of the changes in principal cell function

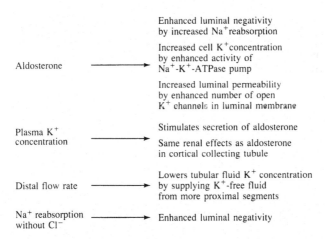

Figure 26-1   Major factors influencing K^+ secretion in the distal nephron, particularly the principal cells in the cortical collecting tubule. Aldosterone and the plasma K^+ concentration are the most important physiologic regulators of this process, both increasing with a K^+ load and falling with K^+ depletion. In the latter setting, increased active K^+ reabsorption in the intercalated cells in the cortical and outer medullary collecting tubules also contributes to the appropriate decline in K^+ excretion.

induced by aldosterone, resulting in both Na^+ reabsorption and K^+ secretion.[43,44] How these changes occur is not known. They are, however, less prominent than those seen in the intact animal, in which a K^+ load is appropriately accompanied by a rise in aldosterone secretion.[45]

Potassium depletion These changes in distal function are reversed with a low-K^+ diet or K^+ depletion.[34-36,46] Both the reduction in the plasma K^+ concentration and the associated decrease in aldosterone secretion lead to a marked decline in distal K^+ secretion. The ensuing fall in K^+ excretion is also due in part to *active K^+ reabsorption*.[47] This process appears to be mediated by H^+-K^+-ATPase pumps in the luminal membrane of the intercalated cells in the cortical and outer medullary collecting tubules.[47-50] The net effect is that urinary K^+ excretion can be reduced to 15 to 25 meq/day with a moderate K^+ deficit and to as low as 5 to 15 meq/day with marked K^+ depletion.[51]

Distal flow rate The distal flow rate affects K^+ secretion in a different manner, by influencing the *tubular fluid K^+ concentration not that of the cell*. The secretion of K^+ raises the tubular fluid K^+ concentration, thereby limiting the concentration gradient for further diffusion out of the cell. Increasing distal flow minimizes this effect, since the secreted K^+ is washed away and replaced with relatively K^+-free fluid delivered out of the loop of Henle (see Fig. 12-11).[52,53] Distal Na^+ delivery is also enhanced in this setting, and the associated increase in Na^+ reabsorption can contribute to the flow dependence of K^+ secretion.[54]

The distal flow rate plays an important role in both normal and disease states. In particular, it *allows aldosterone to regulate Na^+ balance and antidiuretic hormone (ADH) to regulate water balance without interfering with that of K^+*. In hypovolemic states such as congestive heart failure, enhanced secretion of aldosterone and ADH contribute to the retention of Na^+ and H_2O. These patients (if untreated) are not usually hypokalemic, however, since the associated increases in proximal Na^+ reabsorption and ADH-induced water reabsorption combine to reduce distal flow, thereby counteracting the direct stimulatory effects of aldosterone and ADH on K^+ secretion.[55-57] Conversely, an elevation in K^+ secretion does not occur in normal subjects if the distal flow rate is enhanced by high Na^+ intake.[58,59] In this setting, the ensuing volume expansion suppresses the secretion of aldosterone, allowing the excess Na^+ to be excreted without wasting K^+.

In comparison, inappropriate K^+ loss and hypokalemia will occur if distal flow is enhanced while aldosterone secretion is normal or elevated. This sequence may follow the administration of Na^+ to a patient with an aldosterone-producing adenoma (in whom aldosterone secretion is not suppressible by volume expansion)[59,60] or the use of a loop or thiazide-type diuretic.[61,62] In the latter setting, flow to the secretory site is increased because tubular reabsorption is impaired in the loop of Henle or the distal tubule (see Chap. 15); this is frequently accompanied by hyperaldosteronism and high ADH levels due to the diuretic-induced volume loss and often to the underlying disease, such as heart failure or cirrhosis.

Sodium reabsorption and the transepithelial potential difference   Since K^+ is a charged particle, its secretion is also affected by the transepithelial potential difference across the tubular cell. The normal potential difference in the K^+-secreting cells in the cortical collecting tubule is approximately -35 to -50 mV (lumen negative); this potential is generated by the reabsorption of Na^+ (which is positively charged) from the lumen into the peritubular capillary (see Fig. 12-12). This luminal negativity favors K^+ secretion into the lumen.[63]

The importance of Na^+ transport in this process can be illustrated by the response to the diuretic amiloride.[61,62,64] This drug impairs the entry of luminal Na^+ into the cells of the distal nephron by decreasing the number of open Na^+ channels in the luminal membrane.[65] The net effect is diminished Na^+ reabsorption, a reduction in the transepithelial potential difference, and a marked fall in K^+ secretion. Since amiloride has no known direct effect on K^+ handling, it is likely that the decrease in the potential difference is responsible for the decline in K^+ secretion.[64]

This stimulatory effect of Na^+ transport can, as noted above, contribute to the flow dependence of K^+ secretion.[54] This effect is most prominent if Na^+ is delivered to the distal nephron with an *anion other than Cl^- that is non-reabsorbable*.[63] For example, a volume-depleted subject has a strong stimulus to Na^+ reabsorption in the cortical collecting tubule that is mediated by aldosterone. Under normal conditions, the potential generated by Na^+ transport in this segment is in part dissipated by the reabsorption of Cl^-. However, if Na^+ is given with a nonreabsorbable anion such as SO_4^{2-}, there will be an increase in both the potential difference and K^+ secretion.[63,66]

Hypokalemia and Hyperkalemia

In summary, K^+ enters the body by dietary ingestion (normal K^+ intake is 40 to 120 meq/day) or intravenous infusion, is stored primarily in the cells, and is excreted in the urine and to a lesser degree in the feces and sweat (Fig. 26-2). An alteration in the plasma K^+ concentration must involve a change in one or more of these processes. For example, hypokalemia can be produced by increased K^+ entry into cells or by increased losses. Decreased dietary intake can contribute to these disorders; it will not, however, cause K^+ depletion in normal subjects unless intake is severely restricted, since the kidney can reduce K^+ losses to less than 15 to 25 meq/day.[51] As the tubular fluid K^+ concentration is lowered, more efficient K^+ conservation (to less than 5 meq/L, as with Na^+) may be prevented by

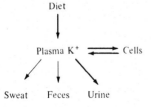

Figure 26-2   Schematic illustration of the factors involved in K^+ homeostasis.

leakage (down a favorable concentration gradient) from the cell into the lumen through a relatively nonselective cation channel in the luminal membrane of the inner medullary collecting duct.[67]

Conversely, hyperkalemia is most often due acutely to enhanced release of K^+ from cells or chronically to decreased urinary excretion. Unless given acutely, increased intake alone will not lead to hyperkalemia if adrenal and renal function are intact, since the excess K^+ will be excreted in the urine (a phenomenon called *potassium adaptation*; see page 889).[45,68,69] Normal subjects, for example, can slowly increase K^+ intake and excretion to over 400 meq/day (normal equals 40 to 120 meq/day) with only a small rise in the plasma K^+ concentration (see Fig. 26-3).[70]

PROBLEMS

26-1 A patient with recurrent diarrhea complains of severe muscle weakness. There is no history, e.g., carpopedal spasm, or physical findings, e.g., Trousseau's or Chvostek's sign, consistent with hypocalcemia. The electrocardiogram reveals ST-segment and T-wave changes with premature

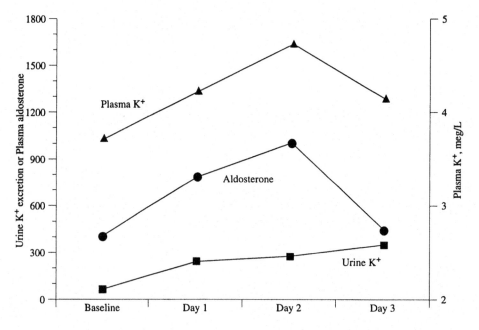

Figure 26-3 Response to increasing K^+ intake to 400 meq/day in normal subjects. Urinary K^+ excretion rises to this level within 2 days and is then maintained. This response is initially driven by elevations in the plasma K^+ and aldosterone concentrations. By day 20, the efficiency of K^+ secretion has increased, resulting in a lesser elevation in the plasma K^+ concentration (to 4.2 meq/L) and normalization of the plasma aldosterone concentration. (*Adapted from Rabelink TJ, Koomans HA, Hené RJ, Dorhout Mees EJ*, Kidney Int *38:942, 1990. Reprinted by permission from* Kidney International.)

ventricular beats, which are felt to be compatible with hypokalemia. The following laboratory data are obtained:

$$\text{Plasma } [Na^+] = 140 \, meq/L$$

$$[K^+] = 1.3 \, meq/L$$

$$[Cl^-] = 117 \, meq/L$$

$$[HCO_3^-] = 10 \, meq/L$$

$$[\text{Albumin}] = 4.1 \, g/dL \quad (\text{normal} = 3.5\text{--}5.0 \, g/dL)$$

$$[Ca^{2+}] = 6.3 \, mg/dL \quad (\text{normal} = 8.8\text{--}10.5 \, mg/dL)$$

$$\text{Arterial pH} = 7.26$$

$$P_{CO_2} = 23 \, mmHg$$

(a) What effect would correction of the metabolic acidosis have on the plasma K^+ concentration?

(b) Would correction by hypocalcemia be part of your initial therapeutic regimen?

REFERENCES

1. Clausen T, Everts ME. Regulation of the Na,K-pump in skeletal muscle. *Kidney Int* 35:1, 1989.
2. Sweadner K, Goldin SM. Active transport of sodium and potassium ions: Mechanism, function, and regulation. *N Engl J Med* 302:777, 1980.
3. Knochel JP. Neuromuscular manifestations of electrolyte disorders. *Am J Med* 72:521, 1982.
4. Rubini M. Water excretion in potassium-deficient man. *J Clin Invest* 40:2215, 1961.
5. Marples D, Prokiaer J, Dorup J, et al. Hypokalemia-induced downregulation of aquaporin-2 water channel expression in rat kidney medullary and cortex. *J Clin Invest* 97:1960, 1996.
6. DeVoe RD, Maloney PC. Principles of cell homeostasis, in Mountcastle VB (ed): *Medical Physiology*, 14th ed. St Louis, Mosby, 1980.
7. Berne RM, Levy MN. *Cardiovascular Physiology*, 4th ed. St Louis, Mosby, 1981, pp. 7–17.
8. Kuffler S, Nicholls JG. *From Neuron to Brain*, Saunderland, MA, Sinauer, 1976, chap 6.
9. Catterall WA. Structure and function of voltage-sensitive ion channels. *Science* 242:50, 1988.
10. Stuhmer W, Conti F, Suzuki H, et al. Structural parts involved in activation and inactivation of the sodium channel. *Nature* 339:597, 1989.
11. Gilly WF, Armstrong CM. Threshold channels—A novel type of sodium channel in squid giant axon. *Nature* 309:448, 1984.
12. Miller C. 1990: Annus mirabilus of potassium channels. *Science* 252:1092, 1991.
13. Wright E, Schulman G. Principles of epithelial transport, in Maxwell MH, Kleeman CR, Narins RG (eds): *Clinical Disorders of Fluid and Electrolyte Metabolism*, 4th ed. New York, McGraw-Hill, 1987.
14. Adrian RH. The effect of internal and external potassium concentration on the membrane potential of frog muscle. *J Physiol (Lond)* 133:631, 1956.
15. Shanes AM. Electrochemical aspects of physiological and pharmacological action in excitable cells: Part II. The action potential and excitation. *Pharmacol Rev* 10:165, 1958.
16. Sterns RH, Cox M, Feig PU, Singer I. Internal potassium balance and the control of the plasma potassium concentration. *Medicine* 60:339, 1981.
17. Brown RS. Extrarenal potassium homeostasis. *Kidney Int* 30:116, 1986.
18. Winkler AW, Hoff HE, Smith PK. The toxicity of orally administered potassium salts in renal insufficiency. *J Clin Invest* 20:119, 1941.
19. DeFronzo R, Taufield P, Black H, et al. Impaired renal tubular potassium secretion in sickle cell disease. *Ann Intern Med* 90:310, 1979.

20. DeFronzo RA, Bia M, Birkhead G. Epinephrine and potassium homeostasis. *Kidney Int* 20:83, 1981.
21. Brown MJ, Brown DC, Murphy MB. Hypokalemia from beta$_2$-receptor stimulation by circulating epinephrine. *N Engl J Med* 309:1414, 1983.
22. DeFronzo RA, Sherwin RS, Dillingham M, et al. Influence of basal insulin and glucagon secretion on potassium and sodium metabolism: Studies with somatostatin in normal dogs and in normal and diabetic human beings. *J Clin Invest* 61:472, 1978.
23. Ferrannini E, Taddei S, Santoro D, et al. Independent stimulation of glucose metabolism and Na$^+$-K$^+$ exchange by insulin in the human forearm. *Am J Physiol* 255:E953, 1988.
24. Clausen T, Flatman JA. Effect of insulin and epinephrine on Na$^+$-K$^+$-ATPase and glucose transport in soleus muscle. *Am J Physiol* 252:E492, 1987.
25. Schnack C, Podolsky A, Watzke H, et al. Effect of somatostatin and oral potassium administration on terbutaline-induced hypokalemia. *Am Rev Respir Dis* 139:176, 1989.
26. Rosa RM, Silva P, Young JB, et al. Adrenergic modulation of extrarenal potassium disposal. *N Engl J Med* 302:431, 1980.
27. Williams ME, Gervino EV, Rosa RM, et al. Catecholamine modulation of rapid potassium shifts during exercise. *N Engl J Med* 312:823, 1985.
28. Allon M, Dansby L, Shanklin N. Glucose modulation of the disposal of an acute potassium load in patients with end-stage renal disease. *Am J Med* 94:475, 1993.
29. Dluhy RG, Axelrod L, Williams GH. Serum immunoreactive insulin and growth hormone response to potassium infusion in normal man. *J Appl Physiol* 33:22, 1972.
30. Kurtzman NA, Gonzalez J, DeFronzo RA, Giebisch G. A patient with hyperkalemia and metabolic acidosis. *Am J Kidney Dis* 15:333, 1990.
31. Minaker KL, Rowe JW. Potassium homeostasis during hyperinsulinemia: Effect of insulin level, β-blockade, and age. *Am J Physiol* 242:E373, 1982.
32. DeFronzo RA, Lee R, Jones A, Bia M. Effect of insulinopenia and adrenal hormone deficiency on acute potassium tolerance. *Kidney Int* 17:586, 1980.
33. Don BR, Sebastian A, Cheitlin M, et al. Pseudohyperkalemia caused by fist clenching during phlebotomy. *N Engl J Med* 322:1290, 1990.
34. Giebisch G, Wang W. Potassium transport: From clearance to channels and pumps. *Kidney Int* 49:1624, 1996.
35. Stanton BA. Renal potassium transport: Morphological and functional adaptations. *Am J Physiol* 257:R989, 1989.
36. Stanton BA, Biemesderfer D, Wade JB, Giebisch G. Structural and functional study of the rat distal nephron: Effects of potassium adaptation and depletion. *Kidney Int* 19:36, 1981.
37. Himathongam T, Dluhy R, Williams GH. Potassium-aldosterone-renin interrelationship. *J Clin Endocrinol Metab* 41:153, 1975.
38. Muto S, Muto S, Giebisch G. Na-dependent effects of DOCA on cellular transport properties of CCDs from ADX rabbits. *Am J Physiol* 253:F753, 1987.
39. Rabinowitz L. Aldosterone and potassium homeostasis. *Kidney Int* 49:1738, 1996.
40. Young DB. Quantitative analysis of aldosterone's role in potassium regulation. *Am J Physiol* 255:F811, 1988.
41. Young DB. Paulsen AW. Interrelated effects of aldosterone and plasma potassium on potassium excretion. *Am J Physiol* 244:F28, 1983.
42. Rose BD. Diuretics. *Kidney Int* 39:336, 1991.
43. Muto S, Sansom S, Giebisch G. Effects of a high potassium diet on electrical properties of cortical collecting ducts from adrenalectomized rabbits. *J Clin Invest* 81:376, 1988.
44. Garg LC, Narang N. Renal adaptation to potassium in the adrenalectomized rabbit: Role of distal tubular sodium-potassium adenosine triphosphatase. *J Clin Invest* 76:1065, 1985.
45. Stanton B, Pan L, Deetjen H, et al. Independent effects of aldosterone and potassium on induction of potassium adaptation in rat kidney. *J Clin Invest* 79:198, 1987.
46. Linas SL, Peterson LN, Anderson RJ, et al. Mechanism of renal potassium conservation in the rat. *Kidney Int* 15:601, 1979.
47. Okusa MD, Unwin RJ, Velazquez H, et al. Active potassium absorption by the renal distal tubule. *Am J Physiol* 262:F488, 1992.

48. Garg LC. Respective roles of H-ATPase and H-K-ATPase in ion transport in the kidney. *J Am Soc Nephrol* 2:949, 1991.
49. Kraut JA, Hiura J, Besancon M, et al. Effect of hypokalemia on the abundance of HK alpha 1 and HK alpha 2 protein in the rat kidney. *Am J Physiol* 272:F744, 1997.
50. Codina J, Delmas-Mata J, DuBose TD. Expression of HK2 protein is increased selectiviely in renal medulla by chronic hypokalemia. *Am J Physiol* 275:F433, 1998.
51. Squires RD, Huth EJ. Experimental potassium depletion in normal human subjects: I. Relation of ionic intakes to the renal conservation of potassium. *J Clin Invest* 38:1134, 1959.
52. Khuri RM, Wiederholt M, Strieder N, Giebisch G. Effects of flow rate and potassium intake on distal tubular potassium transfer. *Am J Physiol* 228:1249, 1975.
53. Good DW, Wright FW. Luminal influences on potassium secretion: Sodium concentration and fluid flow rate. *Am J Physiol* 236:F192, 1979.
54. Malnic G, Berliner RW, Giebisch G. Flow dependence of potassium secretion in cortical distal tubules of the rat. *Am J Physiol* 256:F932, 1989.
55. Seldin D, Welt L, Cort J. The role of sodium salts and adrenal steroids in the production of hypokalemic alkalosis. *Yale J Biol Med* 29:229, 1956.
56. Field MJ, Stanton BA, Giebisch G. Influence of ADH on renal potassium handling: A micropuncture and microperfusion study. *Kidney Int* 25:502, 1984.
57. Cassola AC, Giebisch G, Wong W. Vasopressin increases density of apical low-conductance K^+ channels in rat CCD. *Am J Physiol* 264:F502, 1993.
58. Young DB, McCaa RE. Role of the renin-angiotensin system in potassium control. *Am J Physiol* 238:R359, 1980.
59. George JM, Wright L, Bell NJ, Bartter FC. The syndrome of primary aldosteronism. *Am J Med* 48:343, 1970.
60. Young DB, Jackson TE, Tipayamontri U, Scott RC. Effects of sodium intake on steady-state potassium excretion. *Am J Physiol* 246:F772, 1984.
61. Duarte CG, Chomety F, Giebisch G. Effect of amiloride, ouabain, and furosemide on distal tubular function in the rat. *Am J Physiol* 221:632, 1971.
62. Hropot M, Fowler N, Karlmark B, Giebisch G. Tubular action of diuretics: Distal effects on electrolyte transport and acidification. *Kidney Int* 28:477, 1985.
63. Giebisch G, Malnic G, Klose RM, Windhager EE. Effect of ionic substitutions on distal potential differences in rat kidney. *Am J Physiol* 211:560, 1966.
64. Garcia-Filho E, Malnic G, Giebisch G. Effects of changes in electrical potential difference on tubular potassium transport. *Am J Physiol* 238:F235, 1980.
65. Kleyman TR, Cragoe EJ Jr. The mechanism of action of amiloride. *Semin Nephrol* 8:242, 1988.
66. Schwartz WB, Jenson RL, Relman AS. Acidification of the urine and increased ammonium excretion without change in acid-base equilibrium: Sodium reabsorption as a stimulus to the acidifying process. *J Clin Invest* 34:673, 1955.
67. Light DB, McCann FV, Keller TM, Stanton BA. Amiloride-sensitive cation channel in apical membrane of inner medullary collecting duct. *Am J Physiol* 255:F278, 1988.
68. Hayslett JP, Binder HJ. Mechanism of potassium adaptation. *Am J Physiol* 243:F103, 1982.
69. Jackson CA. Rapid renal potassium adaptation in rats. *Am J Physiol* 263:F1098, 1992.
70. Rabelink TJ, Koomans HA, Hené RJ, Dorhout Mees EJ. Early and late adjustment to potassium loading in humans. *Kidney Int* 38:942, 1990.

HYPOKALEMIA

The introduction to disorders of potassium balance presented in Chap. 26 should be read before proceeding with this discussion.

ETIOLOGY

Potassium enters the body by dietary intake or intravenous infusion, is primarily stored in the cells, and is then excreted in the urine and, to a lesser degree, in the stool and in sweat. An abnormality in any one or more of these processes can lead to hypokalemia (Table 27-1). This section will review the causes of K^+ depletion as well as some aspects of the diagnosis and treatment of certain disorders. The general principles involved in the approach to the hypokalemic patient will be discussed separately later in the chapter.

Table 27-1   Etiology of hypokalemia

Decreased net intake
   A. Low dietary intake or K^+-free intravenous fluids
   B. Clay ingestion
Increased entry into cells, leading to transient hypokalemia
   A. Elevation in extracellular pH
   B. Increased availability of insulin
   C. Elevated β-adrenergic activity:[a] stress, coronary ischemia, delirium tremens, administration of β-adrenergic agonists for asthma or heart failure
   D. Period paralysis—hypokalemic form
   E. Treatment of megaloblastic anemias with vitamin B_{12} or folic acid, or of neutropenia with GM–CSF (granulocyte-macrophage colony-stimulating factor)
   F. Pseudohypokalemia
   G. Hypothermia
   H. Chloroquine intoxication
Increased gastrointestinal losses[a]
Increased urinary losses
   A. Loop and thiazide-type diuretics[a]
   B. Mineralcorticoid excess (see Table 27-2)
   C. Liddle's syndrome
   D. Bartter's or Gitelman's syndrome
   E. Increased flow to the distal nephron
        1. Loop and thiazide-type diuretics
        2. Salt-wasting nephropathies
   F. Sodium reabsorption with a nonreabsorbable anion
        1. Vomiting or nasogastric suction[a]
        2. Metabolic acidosis
        3. Penicillin derivatives
   G. Amphotericin B
   H. Hypomagnesemia[a]
   I. Polyuria
   J. L-dopa
Increased sweat losses
Dialysis
Potassium depletion without hypokalemia

[a] Most common causes.

Decreased Net Intake

The normal range of dietary K^+ intake is approximately 40 to 120 meq/day, with most of this K^+ then being excreted in the urine. If intake is diminished, urinary K^+ excretion can be appropriately reduced to a minimum of 5 to 25 meq/day.[1,2] This renal adaptation is associated with reabsorption rather than secretion of K^+ in the cortical and outer medullary collecting tubules. As described in Chap. 12, distal K^+ secretion occurs in the principal cells in these segments under the influence of aldosterone; active K^+ reabsorption, on the other hand, occurs in the intercalated cells and is mediated by H^+-K^+-ATPase pumps in the luminal membrane that reabsorb K^+ and secrete H^+; the activity of these pumps is increased by hypokalemia.[3-7]

The renal response to K^+ depletion is sufficiently effective that a low-K^+ diet (or a low K^+ content of intravenous feedings) will not lead to significant K^+ losses unless intake is severely limited. Since K^+ is present in meat, fruit, and some vegetables, marked K^+ restriction is difficult to sustain and is a rare cause of hypokalemia in otherwise normal subjects. However, reduced intake can contribute to other causes of K^+ depletion. For example, poor people living in rural areas may have an average K^+ intake of only 25 meq/day, in part because of the relatively high cost of K^+-containing foods.[8] These patients are more likely to become hypokalemic if treated with diuretics for hypertension. Similarly, the hypocaloric liquid protein diets used for rapid weight loss can lead to K^+ depletion unless K^+ supplements are given.[9]

Net K^+ intake can also be limited by chronic clay ingestion, a not uncommon practice in some rural areas in the southeastern United States.[10] The clay appears to bind dietary K^+ and iron directly, diminishing their ability to be absorbed. Hypokalemia and iron-deficiency anemia may ensue if the ingestion is continued for a prolonged period.*

Increased Entry into Cells

Translocation of K^+ from the extracellular fluid into the cells can occur in a variety of conditions, leading to a transient reduction in the plasma K^+ concentration that can become clinically important.

Elevation in extracellular pH   Alkalemia, either metabolic or respiratory, can promote K^+ entry into the cells. In alkalemic states, H^+ ions are released from the cellular buffers and move into the extracellular fluid to minimize the elevation in pH. To preserve electroneutrality, extracellular K^+ (and Na^+) enter the cells.[12,13] In general, the plasma K^+ concentration falls less than 0.4 meq/L per 0.1-unit increase in extracellular pH;[13] as a result, the degree of hypokalemia induced by the alkalemia is typically mild.

A similar reduction in the plasma K^+ concentration can occur when $NaHCO_3$ is administered to correct a metabolic acidosis. In this setting, both the elevation in pH and a direct effect of the increased plasma HCO_3^- concentration appear to contribute to the movement of K^+ into the cells.[14]

Although the effect of alkalemia alone is relatively small, *hypokalemia is a common finding in metabolic alkalosis.* Perhaps the major reason for this association is that the causative factor (diuretics, vomiting, hyperaldosteronism) induces both K^+ and H^+ loss. In addition, the development of hypokalemia may play an

---

* The effect of clay on K^+ balance varies with the type of clay ingested. Red clay, for example, contains a relatively large amount of K^+, and its ingestion can lead to hyperkalemia in patients with advanced renal failure.[11]

important role in the genesis and maintenance of the metabolic alkalosis (see Chap. 18). In patients with primary hyperaldosteronism, for example, metabolic alkalosis does not occur if hypokalemia is prevented by KCl replacement.[15]

At least three factors may contribute to this effect of K^+:

- A fall in the plasma K^+ concentration leads to a transcellular shift induced by K^+ movement out of the cells to replete extracellular stores. Electroneutrality is maintained in this setting by Na^+ and H^+ entry into the cells, leading to an *intracellular acidosis* and an *extracellular alkalosis*.[16,17] Hypokalemia then contributes to *maintenance* of the metabolic alkalosis by increasing H^+ secretion and HCO_3^- reabsorption by the tubular cells, thereby preventing excretion of the excess HCO_3^-.[18-20] This response probably reflects the intracellular acidosis,[21] which is a potent stimulus to H^+ secretion (see Chap. 11).

- Hypokalemia and aldosterone appear to have a potentiating effect on distal hydrogen secretion and therefore on the development and maintenance of metabolic alkalosis by stimulating the H^+-K^+-ATPase and H^+-ATPase pumps, respectively.[22] It is of interest in this regard that many of the causes of hypokalemia (such as vomiting, diuretic therapy, and primary hyperaldosteronism) are associated with both a reduction in the plasma K^+ concentration and increased aldosterone release.

- The lower K^+ concentration in the luminal fluid in hypokalemia may result in increased NH_4^+ attachment to the K^+ site on the Na^+-K^+-$2Cl^-$ carrier in the thick ascending limb of the loop of Henle. As a result, loop NH_4^+ reabsorption and subsequent medullary recycling of NH_3 are enhanced, thereby raising the efficiency of NH_3 secretion into the medullary collecting tubule and increasing net acid excretion (see page 341). Although this hypothesis is unproven for hypokalemia, the reverse effect—decreased loop NH_4^+ reabsorption, recycling, and urinary NH_4^+ excretion—has been demonstrated with hyperkalemia.[23,24]

Increased availability of insulin Insulin promotes the entry of K^+ into skeletal muscle and hepatic cells,[25,26] apparently by increasing the activity of the Na^+-K^+-ATPase pump.[27,28] The major setting in which this leads to hypokalemia is during the treatment of severe hyperglycemia due to uncontrolled diabetes mellitus. These patients are markedly K^+-depleted, but the initial plasma K^+ concentration is usually normal or elevated because the combination of insulin deficiency and hyperosmolality promotes the movement of intracellular K^+ into the extracellular fluid (see Chap. 25).[29] These abnormalities are corrected by insulin, which then unmasks the underlying K^+ depletion.

Mild hypokalemia can also be induced by a carbohydrate load or by the administration of exogenous insulin.[26,30,31] This effect can become important if intravenous KCl is given in dextrose-containing solutions as part of the therapy for hypokalemia. In this setting, there may be a transient further reduction in the plasma K^+ concentration and the possible induction of ventricular arrhythmias.[30]

Elevated β-adrenergic activity   Catecholamines promote K^+ entry into the cells, a response that is mediated by the β_2-adrenergic receptors[32,33] and that also involves increased activity of the Na^+-K^+-ATPase pump.[28] As a result, transient hypokalemia can be induced when epinephrine release is enhanced by hypoglycemia or by the stress of an acute illness.[31,34] For example, diuretic therapy in mild hypertension is often associated with mild hypokalemia (see below); however, stress-induced release of epinephrine (e.g., during an episode of coronary ischemia) can result in a potentially dangerous further reduction in the plasma K^+ concentration to below 2.8 meq/L (Fig. 27-1).[35] The now severe hypokalemia may promote the development of serious ventricular arrhythmias.[36]

Hypokalemia that presumably reflects stress-induced epinephrine release has been described in a variety of other conditions, including post–cardiopulmonary resuscitation, delirium tremens, acute head trauma, and theophylline intoxication, particularly if acute.[37-40] A similar effect, in which the plasma K^+ concentration can acutely fall by 0.5 to 1 meq/L, can also be induced by the administration of a β-adrenergic agonist (such as albuterol, terbutaline, dobutamine, or ritodrine) to treat asthma, heart failure, and other disorders.[41-44] In heart failure, for example, a rapid 0.4-meq/L fall in the plasma K^+ concentration following the administration of dobutamine may cause an exacerbation of ventricular arrhythmias.[43]

On the other hand, β-adrenergic agonists have been used to *treat hyperkalemia* in patients with advanced renal failure, since they can transiently lower the plasma K^+ concentration until the excess K^+ can be removed by a cation exchange resin or dialysis (see Chap. 28).[45]

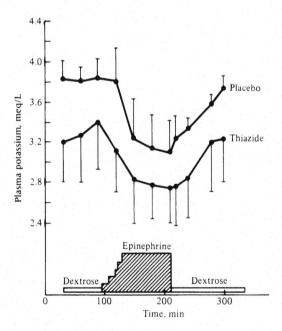

Figure 27-1 Plasma K^+ concentration during an infusion of epinephrine (in physiologic doses) in six patients pretreated with a placebo or a thiazide diuretic for 7 days. The plasma K^+ concentration fell in both groups but reached potentially dangerous levels in the diuretic-treated patients who had mild baseline hypokalemia. (*From Struthers AD, Whitesmith R, Reid JL, Lancet 1:1358, 1983, with permission.*)

The effect of epinephrine on K^+ balance can be prevented by nonselective β-adrenergic blockers, such as propranolol.[46] In comparison, β_1-selective agents such as atenolol are relatively ineffective,[46] since the epinephrine-induced K^+ shift is mediated by the β_2 receptors.[33] Although it protects the plasma K^+ concentration, propranolol may be associated with some risk in the presence of excess epinephrine, because the β_2-mediated vasodilator response is also inhibited. As a result, the concurrent α-adrenergic vasoconstriction is now unopposed, leading to a rise in diastolic pressure that can exceed 20 mmHg.[46]

Periodic paralysis   Periodic paralysis is a rare disorder characterized by recurrent episodes of muscle weakness or paralysis, which can be fatal if the respiratory muscles are involved.[47] The severity of individual attacks is variable, ranging from weakness in a single muscle group to diffuse paralysis.

Hypokalemic, hyperkalemic, and normokalemic forms have been described.[47,48] The hypokalemic form may be familial with autosomal dominant inheritance or may be acquired as a result of thyrotoxicosis (particularly in Chinese males).[49-53] In either disorder, episodes can be precipitated by rest after exercise, a carbohydrate meal, stress, or the administration of insulin or epinephrine.* These attacks are associated with the sudden movement of K^+ into the cells, resulting in an acute reduction in the plasma K^+ concentration (which is normal between attacks) to as low as 1.5 to 2.5 meq/L. The hypokalemia is often accompanied by hypophosphatemia and hypomagnesemia.[54] If the condition is untreated, muscle strength returns after 6 to 48 h as K^+ moves back into the extracellular fluid.

The pathogenesis of familial disease is now better understood. The abnormal gene in most cases is located on chromosome 1q; the defect is in the α_1 subunit of the dihydropyridine-sensitive calcium channel in skeletal muscle.[55,56] How a defect in the calcium channel might lead to episodic potassium movement into the cells is not known. Intracellular calcium is increased in these patients, so the defect in the receptor may promote increased calcium entry into the cells.[55] However, the mechanism may not involve calcium movement; the dihydropyridine-sensitive calcium channel also acts as a voltage sensor for excitation-contraction coupling,[57] and the defect in hypokalemic periodic paralysis is associated with a reduced sarcolemmal ATP-sensitive potassium current.[58] In vitro studies have shown that blockade of L-type calcium channels does not prevent membrane depolarization induced by insulin in muscle fibers from patients with hypokalemic periodic paralysis.[59]

In thyrotoxicosis, there is an increased sensitivity to catecholamines, and the administration of β-adrenergic blockers can minimize the severity and number of attacks and, in some cases, the fall in the plasma K^+ concentration.[50,51] These findings suggest an important role for increased sympathetic activity, although

---

* Most of these provocative factors, such as a carbohydrate meal or stress, will also lower the plasma K^+ concentration in normal subjects, but the effect is much less pronounced and symptoms do not occur.

how it leads to the exaggerated fall in the plasma K^+ concentration is uncertain.[48]

In addition, thyroid hormone increases Na-K-ATPase activity (thereby tending to drive potassium into cells), and thyrotoxic patients with periodic paralysis have higher sodium pump activity than those without paralytic episodes.[60] Excess thyroid hormone may therefore predispose to paralytic episodes by increasing the susceptibility to the hypokalemic action of epinephrine or insulin.[52] It is also possible that Asians who are susceptible to thyrotoxic periodic paralysis have a mutated calcium channel, which in the euthyroid state is not sufficient to produce symptoms.[47]

The diagnosis of hypokalemic periodic paralysis should be suspected from the history (including a possible familial incidence), the severity of the hypokalemia in the absence of any obvious cause, and the rapid normalization of the plasma K^+ concentration and relief of symptoms following the administration of K^+. Thyroid function studies should be obtained in patients with a negative family history.

A similar acute form of paralysis can be induced by barium poisoning, which usually results from contaminated foods.[48] In this disorder, barium blocks the K^+ channels in the cell membrane that normally allow cellular K^+ to diffuse into the extracellular fluid. Patients undergoing radiographic procedures are not at risk for this problem, since the barium sulfate used in gastrointestinal studies is not absorbed into the systemic circulation.

Treatment   Treatment of the acute episode in hypokalemic periodic paralysis involves the oral administration of 60 to 120 meq of KCl. This should lead to increased muscle strength within 15 to 20 min. If no improvement is observed, another 60 meq can be given. The presence of hypokalemia must be confirmed *prior* to the initiation of therapy, since K^+ administration can exacerbate both the hyperkalemic and normokalemic forms (see Chap. 28).[48,59] Furthermore, excess potassium administration during an acute episode may lead to posttreatment hyperkalemia as potassium moves back out of the cells.[52,54]

Prevention of hypokalemic episodes consists of the restoration of euthyroidism in thyrotoxic patients and the administration of a β-adrenergic blocker in either familial or thyrotoxic periodic paralysis. β-blockers can minimize the number and severity of attacks and, in most cases, limit the fall in the plasma potassium concentration.[52] A nonselective β-blocker (such as propranolol) should be given; β_1-selective agents are less likely to inhibit the β_2-receptor-mediated hypokalemic effect of epinephrine and may therefore be less likely to prevent paralytic episodes.[47]

Other modalities that may be effective for prevention include K^+ supplementation, K^+-sparing diuretics, a low-carbohydrate diet, and the carbonic anhydrase inhibitor acetazolamide.[48,52-62]

Treatment of anemia or neutropenia   An acute increase in hematopoietic cell production by the bone marrow is associated with K^+ uptake by the new cells, which may be of sufficient magnitude to induce hypokalemia. As an example, the administration of folic acid or vitamin B_{12} to patients with megaloblastic anemia frequently leads to a reduction in the plasma K^+ concentration to 3.0 meq/L or below, with the possible development of cardiac arrhythmias; this response is most pronounced within the first 48 h, when red cell and platelet production are at their peak.[63] In comparison, a significant fall in the plasma K^+ concentration is unusual with other anemias (such as that due to iron deficiency), since treatment of these disorders results in a much slower rate of new cell production.

Marked hypokalemia can also be induced by the administration of granulocyte-macrophage colony-stimulating factor (GM–CSF) to correct neutropenia. Those patients who have a marked increase in white cell production may have a plasma K^+ concentration that falls below 2 meq/L.[64]

The plasma K^+ concentration may also fall below 3.0 meq/L following multiple transfusions with frozen, washed red cells.[65] These cells, but not those stored in acid-citrate-dextran, lose up to 50 percent of their K^+ during storage. In the recipient, K^+ rapidly moves into the cells to repair the deficit.

Pseudohypokalemia Metabolically active cells can take up K^+ after blood has been drawn. In this setting, which has been described in cases of acute myeloid leukemia associated with a very high white cell count, the patient may have a relatively normal plasma K^+ concentration, but the measured value may be below 1.0 meq/L (without any symptoms) if the blood is first allowed to stand for a prolonged period at room temperature.[66] This problem can be avoided if the plasma or serum is rapidly separated from the cells or if the blood is stored at 4°C.

Hypothermia Accidental or induced hypothermia can lower the plasma K^+ concentration to below 3.0 meq/L, apparently as a result of K^+ entry into the cells.[67,68] This effect is readily reversible during rewarming and may be associated with "overshoot" *hyper*kalemia, particularly if K^+ has been given during the period of hypothermia.[67] Furthermore, patients who are essentially dead following accidental hypothermia may present with a plasma K^+ concentration above 10 to 20 meq/L as a result of irreversible tissue necrosis.[68]

Chloroquine intoxication Hypokalemia, with the plasma potassium concentration falling below 2.0 meq/L in severe cases, is a common finding in acute chloroquine intoxication.[69] This effect is presumably mediated by potassium movement into the cells and can be exacerbated by the administration of epinephrine to help treat the intoxication.

Increased Gastrointestinal Losses

In normal subjects, approximately 3 to 6 liters of gastric, pancreatic, biliary, and intestinal secretions is released into the gastrointestinal lumen each day. Almost all these fluids are then reabsorbed, as only 100 to 200 mL of water and 5 to 10 meq of K^+ are lost in the stool. Since each of these secretions contains K^+, the loss of any of them (because of decreased absorption or increased secretion) can lead to K^+

depletion. This can be seen with vomiting (although urinary losses are generally more important in this setting; see below), diarrhea, intestinal fistulas or tube drainage, or the loss of colonic secretions from a villous adenoma or from chronic laxative abuse.[70-76]

Hypokalemia is most common when the losses occur over a prolonged period, as with a villous adenoma, or are acute and massive.[77] In cholera, for example, daily stool losses may average 8 liters of water, 1000 meq of Na^+, and 130 meq of K^+.[71] Similarly, daily fluid losses in excess of 6 liters and K^+ losses in excess of 300 meq have been reported in patients with the VIPoma syndrome (severe, watery diarrhea and histamine-fast achlorhydria, usually but not always due to a vasoactive intestinal peptide–producing non-β-cell islet cell tumor).[72-74]

In many cases, however, increased fecal losses cannot explain all of the potassium deficit. Normal subjects ingest an average of about 80 meq of potassium per day. Urinary potassium excretion should fall below 15 to 25 meq/day in the presence of a potassium deficit.[1,2] Thus, fecal losses (normally about 10 meq/day) must exceed 55 to 65 meq/day to directly induce hypokalemia. Many patients who become hypokalemic have a lower level of fecal potassium excretion, indicating that other factors (such as decreased intake and perhaps hyperaldosteronism-induced urinary potassium excretion) must also play a contributory role.[77]

Increased Urinary Losses

Urinary K^+ excretion is primarily determined by K^+ secretion in the distal nephron, particularly the cortical collecting tubule (see Chap. 12). Inappropriate urinary K^+ loss leading to hypokalemia is most often due to conditions associated with mineralocorticoid excess and/or increased urinary flow of water and Na^+ to the distal secretory site (Table 27-1).

Loop and thiazide-type diuretics Hypokalemia is a relatively common problem with the loop and thiazide-type diuretics. When hydrochlorothiazide is used to treat essential hypertension, for example, the incidence of hypokalemia is dose-related, with the fall in the plasma potassium concentration averaging about 0.5 meq/L with 50 mg per day.[78,79] Chlorthalidone, which is longer-acting, has a greater kaliuretic effect, lowering the plasma potassium concentration by 0.8 to 0.9 meq/L at a 50-mg/day dose.[78]

Two factors appear to be responsible for the increase in K^+ excretion with these agents: (1) increased flow to the distal secretory site, as a result of inhibition of NaCl and water reabsorption in the loop of Henle or distal tubule, and (2) enhanced secretion of aldosterone, as a result of both the underlying disease (heart failure or cirrhosis) and the induction of volume depletion.[80,81] In addition, diuretic-induced hypomagnesemia (see below) and, with loop diuretics, decreased K^+ reabsorption by the Na^+-K^+-$2Cl^-$ carrier in the loop of Henle (see Fig. 4-2) also may promote K^+ loss in the urine.

The degree of K^+ loss is dose-dependent. This is an important issue in many patients with mild to moderate essential hypertension, in whom diuretic-induced hypokalemia has become a less frequent problem since the demonstration that low-dose thiazide therapy (e.g. 12.5 mg of hydrochlorothiazide or its equivalent) frequently produces an antihypertensive effect similar to that of higher doses with only a minimal reduction in the plasma K^+ concentration (Fig. 27-2).[82,83]

If the diuretic dose and dietary intake are relatively constant, then all of the K^+ loss will occur during the first 2 weeks of therapy (see page 453).[84] At this time, a *new steady state is reached in which K^+ intake and output are again equal.* Although the diuretic continues to promote K^+ wasting, this effect is counteracted by the combination of a decrease in distal flow (induced by the associated hypovolemia) and the direct K^+-sparing effect of hypokalemia (see "Symptoms," below).[1,2]

Treatment   Diuretic-induced hypokalemia has been associated with an increased incidence of arrhythmias,[85] and diuretic therapy in both hypertension and heart failure has been associated with an increased incidence of arrhythmic death that can be prevented by a K^+-sparing diuretic (such as spironolactone) and may therefore be due to K^+ depletion.[86-89] For these reasons, even mild diuretic-induced hypokalemia is usually treated, and some physicians try to maintain the plasma K^+ concentration above 4 meq/L in patients with heart failure. This can be achieved either with KCl supplements (usually requiring 40 meq/day to raise the plasma K^+ concentration by about 0.5 meq/L)[79] or with a K^+-sparing diuretic, which can also partially correct diuretic-induced magnesium depletion by diminishing magnesium excretion.[79]

Correction of hypokalemia may have an additional advantage in hypertensive patients, further lowering the blood pressure by 5 to 10 mmHg in some cases.[90,91] How this occurs is not well understood, but increased Na^+ excretion may contribute.

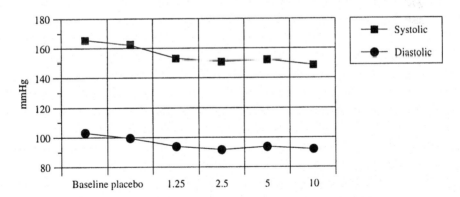

Figure 27-2   Antihypertensive response to bendrofluazide in relation to dose (multiply to 10 to get equivalent doses of hydrochlorothiazide). The initial dose of 1.25 mg lowers the blood pressure in comparison to placebo; however, higher doses produced little further antihypertensive response. Each treatment group contained approximately 52 patients. (*Data from Carlsen JE, Kober L, Torp-Pedersen C, Johannsen P, Br Med J 300:975, 1990, with permission.*)

Mineralocorticoid excess Aldosterone, the primary endogenous mineralocorticoid, stimulates the reabsorption of Na^+ and the secretion of K^+ and H^+ (see Chap. 6). Consequently, the excessive secretion of aldosterone (or any other mineralocorticoid) an lead to hypokalemia and metabolic alkalosis.[92-95] Edema, however, does not usually occur in otherwise normal subjects, since the initial Na^+ retention is followed by a spontaneous natriuresis, a phenomenon referred to as *aldosterone escape*. Both the ensuing rise in systemic blood pressure and enhanced secretion of atrial natriuretic peptide contribute to this increase in Na^+ excretion (see page 185).

For hypokalemia to occur, there must be adequate delivery of Na^+ and water to the distal nephron. When distal flow is reduced because of effective circulating volume depletion, K^+ secretion may be relatively unchanged despite the presence of hyperaldosteronism.[96] Thus, patients with uncomplicated heart failure or cirrhosis typically have a normal plasma K^+ concentration. However, hypokalemia may rapidly ensue if distal delivery is enhanced by the administration of diuretics.

Primary mineralocorticoid excess occurs in a variety of uncommon conditions (Table 27-2).[92-95] In addition to hypokalemia and metabolic alkalosis, these disorders are also associated with hypertension and mild hypernatremia. Volume expansion initiates the elevation in blood pressure[97] and also accounts for the rise in the plasma Na^+ concentration (to about 145 meq/L) by causing an upward resetting of the osmostat (see page 759).[98]

Primary hyperaldosteronism The autonomous hypersecretion of aldosterone may result from a unilateral adrenal adenoma or carcinoma or from bilateral hyperplasia.[92-95] An adenoma is responsible for about 65 percent of cases, with

Table 27-2 Causes of primary mineralocorticoid excess

Primary hyperaldosteronism
  A. Adenoma
  B. Hyperplasia
  C. Carcinoma
Cushing's disease (some cases)
Chronic ingestion of exogenous mineralocorticoid
  A. Fludrocortisone
Hyperreninism
  A. Renal artery stenosis
  B. Renin-secreting tumor
Glucocorticoid-remediable hyperaldosteronism
Hypersecretion of deoxycorticosterone or other mineralocorticoid
  A. CYP17 (17α-hydroxylase) deficiency
  B. CYP11B1 (11β-hydroxylase) deficiency
  C. Normal levels of cortisol with chronic licorice ingestion or the syndrome of apparent mineralocorticoid excess

hyperplasia accounting for most of the remaining patients. Because of the mild hypervolemia, the plasma renin activity is typically (but not always) reduced in these disorders.[92] Hyperplasia is generally a milder disease, with less hypersecretion of aldosterone and less hypokalemia.

The factors responsible for adrenal hyperplasia are not well understood.[94] Increased sensitivity of the adrenal zona glomerulosa to angiotensin II may be a contributing factor. This relationship could explain the characteristic rise in the plasma aldosterone concentration between an 8 A.M. supin sample and a noon upright sample, since assumption of the upright posture leads to pooling of blood in the lower extremities, mild effective volume depletion, and activation of the renin-angiotensin system. In comparison, there is usually no change or a slight decrease in aldosterone levels during the day in patients with an adrenal adenoma, a difference that has been used to distinguish between these conditions.

In another rare form of adrenal hyperplasia with autosomal dominant inheritance, the hypersecretion of aldosterone is reversed by the administration of a glucocorticoid such as dexamethasone.[99,100] Normal subjects synthesize aldosterone in the zona glomerulosa, but not in the adrenocorticotropic hormone (ACTH)–sensitive zona fasciculata, which lacks the enzymes required to add the necessary aldehyde to corticosterone at the 18-carbon position (Fig. 27-3).

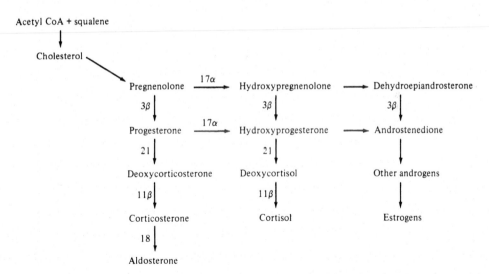

Figure 27-3   Schematic pathways of adrenal steroid biosynthesis. The numbers at the arrows refer to specific enzymes: 17α equals 17α-hydroxylase; 3β equals 3β-hydroxysteroid dehydrogenase; 21 equals 21-hydroxylase; 11β equals 11β-hydroxylase; 18 refers to a two-step process resulting in the addition of an aldehyde at the 18-carbon position. The last reactions occur only in the zona glomerulosa, which is the site of aldosterone secretion. A deficiency in any of these enzymes can lead to abnormal mineralocorticoid (as well as glucocorticoid and androgen) production.

Glucocorticoid-suppressible hyperaldosteronism appears to result from a *chimeric gene* on chromosome 8 containing the regulatory subunit of 11β-hydroxylase (the enzyme that converts deoxycortisol into cortisol) and the coding sequences for aldosterone synthase (the enzyme responsible for the addition at an 18-aldehyde).[99] The presence of the 11β-hydroxylase portion both locates the ensuing enzyme in the zona fasciculata and makes it ACTH-responsive. Thus, the normal levels of ACTH required for cortisol secretion lead to hypersecretion of aldosterone; this problem can be corrected by the exogenous administration of glucocorticoid, which will diminish ACTH release.

There is a second form of autosomal dominant familial hyperaldosteronism that is not reversed by glucocorticoid therapy. The pathogenesis of this disorder is not understood.[101]

Cushing's syndrome (glucocorticoid excess)   Cortisol, the most active glucocorticoid, is synthesized in the zona fasciculata under the influence of ACTH. Cortisol binds as avidly as aldosterone to the mineralocorticoid receptor; nevertheless, cortisol normally has weak mineralocorticoid activity because it is inactivated to cortisone at the aldosterone-sensitive cells in the collecting tubules (see "Licorice and the Syndrome of Apparent Mineralocorticoid Excess," below).[102,103] However, some patients with Cushing's syndrome develop hypokalemia and metabolic alkalosis. This is most likely to occur in patients with ectopic ACTH production who markedly oversecrete cortisol. In this setting, the rate of delivery of cortisol may exceed its rate of inactivation, thereby allowing it to act as a mineralocorticoid.[104] In addition, increased secretion of other ACTH-dependent mineralocorticoids (such as deoxycorticosterone and corticosterone) may play a contributory role.[105,106]

Hypercortisolism can result from hypersecretion of ACTH (due to a pituitary adenoma or a nonendocrine ACTH-producing tumor), from primary adrenal diseases (adenoma or carcinoma), or from exogenous glucocorticoid therapy.[107,108] The degree of hypokalemia is directly related to the level of cortisol secretion, being most severe in those states with the highest hormone production, namely, adrenal carcinoma and nonendocrine tumors.[106] Although Cushing's syndrome can also be seen with chronic therapy with oral prednisone or dexamethasone, these compounds have little mineralocorticoid activity and are less likely to produce hypokalemia or hypertension.

In contrast to primary hyperaldosteronism, the hypertension in Cushing's syndrome is not directly related to Na^+ retention and volume expansion.[97,109] As a result, the plasma renin activity is generally normal or increased, not reduced as with aldosterone excess.[93,109] Why the blood pressure rises in this disorder is not well understood.[109,110]

The complete approach to the diagnosis and therapy of Cushing's syndrome is beyond the scope of this discussion.[108,111,112] Reviewed briefly, patients generally have the classic cushingoid features, particularly central obesity, ecchymoses, and muscle weakness. There are three stages in the diagnostic evaluation of patients suspected to have Cushing's syndrome.

- Determining whether hypercortisolism is present, usually by measuring daily urinary cortisol excretion or the plasma cortisol concentration after the administration of low-dose dexamethasone.[111]
- Determining whether the hypercortisolism is ACTH-independent or ACTH-dependent; i.e., does the patient have primary adrenal disease or an ACTH-secreting tumor? This can usually be determined by measurement of plasma ACTH.[112]
- Determining the source of the excess ACTH in ACTH-dependent hyper-cortisolism; i.e., does the patient have an ACTH-secreting pituitary adenoma (Cushing's disease) or an ACTH-secreting nonpituitary tumor (ectopic ACTH syndrome)? The high-dose dexamethasone suppression test is usually the first test performed.[112]

Treatment generally consists of removal of a unilateral adrenal lesion or transsphenoidal microsurgery for pituitary disease.[113,114]

Congenital adrenal hyperplasia Deoxycorticosterone (DOC) and corticosterone are synthesized in the adrenal cortex and possess significant mineralocorticoid activity. The secretion of these hormones is regulated by ACTH, not angiotensin II and the plasma K^+ concentration, which are the primary determinants of aldosterone release (see Chap. 6). When cortisol production is reduced because of an adrenal enzyme deficiency, the secretion of ACTH and therefore of DOC and corticosterone will be persistently elevated unless the affected enzyme is required for their synthesis. This sequence can be seen in two forms of congenital adrenal hyperplasia, CYP11B1 (11β-hydroxylase) and CYP17 (17α-hydroxylase) deficiency (Fig. 27-3).[115] The latter is nonvirilizing, since androgen production is also dependent upon 17-hydroxylation.

Glucocorticoid and K^+ balance can be restored in these disorders by the administration of cortisol, which lowers ACTH, DOC, and corticosterone secretion to normal. There is, however, a risk of inducing Na^+-wasting and *hyper-kalemia* with this regimen, since the enzyme deficiencies also impair the synthesis of aldosterone (Fig. 27-3).[115] As a result, mineralocorticoid replacement with fludrocortisone may also be required.

A syndrome similar to that seen with CYP11B1 deficiency—hypersecretion of ACTH, DOC, corticosterone, and adrenal androgens—can also occur in the rare disorder known as familial glucocorticoid resistance.[116] This condition appears to result from an inherited abnormality in the glucocorticoid receptor, preventing it from binding to cortisol.[117] The net effect is adrenal stimulation due to high ACTH levels even though the plasma cortisol concentration is elevated.

Licorice and the syndrome of apparent mineralocorticoid excess Subjects who chronically ingest large amounts of licorice (or licorice-containing chewing tobacco or gum) can develop a reversible syndrome that is clinically similar to primary hyperaldosteronism.[118,119] A steroid in licorice, glycyrrhetinic acid, has slight mineralocorticoid activity; more importantly, this compound also impairs the action of the enzyme 11β-hydroxysteroid dehydrogenase, which converts cortisol to cortisone in aldosterone target tissues such as the collecting tubules in the kidney.[102,121]

As noted above, cortisol binds to the mineralocorticoid receptor with an avidity equal to that of aldosterone and circulates in a much higher concentration; thus, cortisol would inappropriately function as the primary mineralocorticoid were it not converted locally by 11β-hydroxysteroid dehydrogenase and other enzymes to *inactive* metabolites such as cortisone.[102,103] This conversion is impaired with licorice-induced inhibition of 11β-hydroxysteroid dehydrogenase, thereby allowing cortisol to activate the mineralocorticoid receptors and produce a clinical picture of primary hyperaldosteronism.[103,119] One major difference is that endogenous aldosterone secretion is appropriately suppressed in this setting.[102,103]

A similar pathophysiology occurs in the *syndrome of apparent mineralocorticoid excess*. This disorder is characterized by mutations in the 11β-hydroxysteroid dehydrogenase gene that once again allow cortisol to act as the major endogenous mineralocorticoid.[122,123] Therapy usually includes spironolactone (which competes for the mineralocorticoid receptor), potassium supplements, and a low-salt diet. In theory, the administration of dexamethasone (which has little activity at the mineralocorticoid receptor) should reverse the hypokalemia by diminishing the secretion of ACTH and therefore cortisol. However, preliminary clinical observations suggest that dexamethasone is only occasionally effective.[124]

Hyperreninism Primary hypersecretion of renin can result in a syndrome that mimics the clinical findings of primary hyperaldosteronism, except for the *elevated plasma renin activity*. This may occur with rare, renin-secreting tumors of the juxtaglomerular apparatus[125-127] or, more commonly, with renovascular hypertension (renal artery stenosis, malignant hypertension, vasculitis, scleroderma), in which renal ischemia induces nonsuppressible renin release.

Renal arteriography usually establishes the correct diagnosis, although small renin-secreting tumors may be missed.[126] Selective venography or renal vein renin sampling may be necessary in this setting, in which the findings of hypertension, hypokalemia, *increased* plasma renin activity, and normal renal arteries are suggestive of a renin-secreting tumor or possibly surreptitious diuretic use in a patient with underlying essential hypertension.

Other mineralocorticoids On rare occasions, the hypersecretion of other mineralocorticoids can lead to hypokalemia and hypertension. Included in this group are patients with DOC-producing adenomas[93,128] and, as described above, congenital adrenal hyperplasia due to CYP11B1 or CYP17 deficiency. Nonaldosterone mineralocorticoid excess can also be induced by the administration of fludrocortisone, a synthetic mineralocorticoid used in the treatment of hypoaldosteronism and also present in some nasal sprays.[129]

Liddle's syndrome A clinical picture similar to that of primary hyperaldosteronism, although independent of mineralocorticoids, is seen in Liddle's syndrome.

This is a rare autosomal dominant condition characterized by a mutation in the collecting tubule Na^+ channel, producing a primary *gain of function* with enhanced Na^+ reabsorption.[130,131] It is distinguished from true primary hyperaldosteronism by the combination of low renin and low aldosterone levels.

Therapy consists of the administration of amiloride or triamterene, K^+-sparing diuretics that directly close the sodium channels.[132] The mineralocorticoid antagonist spironolactone is ineffective, since the increase in Na^+ channel activity is not mediated by aldosterone.

Bartter's and Gitelman's syndromes Bartter's and Gitelman's syndromes are rare disorders that present with hypokalemia and metabolic alkalosis but, in contrast to primary hyperaldosteronism, no hypertension.[133-135] The pathogenesis of these disorders is similar to that seen with loop and thiazide-type diuretics, since there is a primary reduction in NaCl transport in the loop of Henle and the distal tubule, respectively.

The genetic defect in Bartter's syndrome involves the transporters in the thick ascending limb of the loop of Henle. The process of active sodium chloride transport in this segment is mediated at the luminal membrane by the loop diuretic–sensitive Na^+-K^+-$2Cl^-$ cotransporter, which results in sodium chloride entry into the tubular cells, and by potassium channels, which permit reabsorbed potassium to leak back into the lumen for continued Na^+-K^+-$2Cl^-$ cotransport (see Fig. 4-2).[136] At the basolateral membrane, chloride channels permit the chloride that has entered the cell to exit and be returned to the systemic circulation. Bartter's syndrome can result from a defect in the gene for any one of these three transporters, illustrating the requirement for their integrated function in loop transport.[137-139]

The genetic defect in Gitelman's syndrome is a mutation in the gene coding for the thiazide-sensitive Na-Cl cotransporter in the distal tubule.[140] A defect in this transporter can account for both the magnesium wasting and the often marked decrease in calcium excretion (the opposite of the hypercalciuria seen in Bartter's syndrome).[140] Gitelman's syndrome is often inherited, and both autosomal recessive and dominant forms have been described.[141]

Bartter's syndrome generally presents early in life (before the age of 6). The tendency to sodium wasting leads to hyperreninemia, hyperaldosteronism, and hypokalemic alkalosis.[133,142] Increased secretion of vasodilator prostaglandins (prostaglandin E and prostacyclin) is also present in this condition and may partially explain why the blood pressure remains normal.[142]

Other common findings are growth and mental retardation, polyuria, polydipsia, decreased concentrating ability, hypercalciuria,[143] and a plasma magnesium concentration that is normal or only mildly reduced. These urinary findings are compatible with the defect in the medullary portion of the thick ascending limb. This segment plays a central role in creating the counter-current gradient required for urinary concentration, and both calcium and magnesium are passively reabsorbed at this site down gradients created by sodium chloride transport (see Chaps. 3 and 4).

Gitelman's syndrome is a more benign condition than Bartter's syndrome. It is usually diagnosed incidentally in late childhood or even adulthood.[134,143] Affected patients may present with tetany or are discovered incidentally when they are found to have hypokalemia, metabolic alkalosis, and hypomagnesemia.[144] Other typical findings are hyperaldosteronism, hyperreninemia, and hypocalciuria;[143] concentrating ability is maintained, indicating intact function in the medullary thick limb.

The diagnosis of Bartter's or Gitelman's syndrome is basically one of exclusion.[133,134] Surreptitious diuretic use (which can usually be detected by a urine assay for diuretics) or vomiting can replicate most of the biochemical and hormonal findings,[145-147] although the urine Cl^- concentration should be low in the latter condition.[147]

Since the tubular defect cannot be corrected, treatment in these disorders is aimed at minimizing the effects of the secondary increases in aldosterone and prostaglandin secretion. The combination of a nonsteroidal anti-inflammatory drug (NSAID) and a potassium-sparing diuretic (such as spironolactone or amiloride, often in higher than usual doses of up to 300 and 40 mg/day, respectively, to more completely block distal potassium secretion) can raise the plasma potassium concentration toward normal, largely reverse the metabolic alkalosis, and partially correct the hypomagnesemia.[137,148-150]

A similar response can be induced by the use of an angiotensin converting enzyme inhibitor, which diminishes the production of angiotensin II and aldosterone.[151,152] The acute reduction in angiotensin II levels in this setting can lead to symptomatic hypotension in some cases. This problem is often transient (lasting only 3 to 4 days) and can be minimized by the initial use of low doses.

Most patients also require oral potassium and magnesium supplementation, since drug therapy is usually incompletely effective. However, the restoration of normal magnesium and potassium balance is often difficult to achieve. Diarrhea frequently limits the dose of magnesium given, and the magnesium that is absorbed tends to be excreted in the urine. Persistent hypomagnesemia can contribute to urinary potassium loss, making correction of the hypokalemia more difficult.

Increased flow to the distal nephron   Increased flow of water and Na^+ to the collecting tubules and possible K^+ wasting occurs in those states in which proximal, loop, or distal tubule NaCl reabsorption is decreased (Table 27-1). As described above with diuretics and Bartter's and Gitelman's syndromes, the initial Na^+ wasting leads to a secondary rise in aldosterone release, further contributing to the tendency to hypokalemia.

Salt-wasting nephropathies   In a variety of renal diseases, particularly tubulointerstitial disorders such as chronic interstitial nephritis (as with Sjögren's syndrome or lupus) or urinary tract obstruction, Na^+ and water reabsorption are impaired, leading to increased Na^+ delivery to the K^+ secretory site and secondary hyperaldosteronism. As a result, increased K^+ secretion and hypokalemia can occur in a manner similar to that induced by diuretics or Bartter's syndrome.[153-156]*

This mechanism may also account for the development of hypokalemia in hypercalcemic states, since calcium-induced tubular damage may impair Na^+ reabsorption.[159] Similarly, lysozyme-induced tubular injury may be at least in part responsible for the K^+ wasting and relatively marked hypokalemia that may be associated with leukemia, particularly acute monocytic or myelomonocytic leukemia.[160-162] K^+ entry into the metabolically active leukemic cells may also contribute to the fall in the plasma K^+ concentration in this disorder.[161]

Sodium reabsorption with a nonreabsorbable anion   The ability of increased distal delivery to enhance K^+ secretion is augmented if Na^+ is presented to the distal secretory site with a nonreabsorbable anion other than Cl^-. In this setting, the lumen-negative electrical gradient created by Na^+ reabsorption is increased, since it cannot be dissipated by Cl^-; the net effect is enhanced secretion of K^+ and H^+.

Examples in which the distal delivery of relatively large quantities of a nonreabsorbable anion can induce hypokalemia include HCO_3^- with vomiting or type 2 renal tubular acidosis (see below), β-hydroxybutyrate in diabetic ketoacidosis, hippurate following toluene use (glue-sniffing), or a penicillin derivative in patients receiving high-dose penicillin therapy.[163-165] As an example, the plasma potassium concentration has been reported to be below 2 meq/L in approximately one-fourth of patients with toluene-induced metabolic acidosis.[165]

The effect of nonreabsorbable anions is likely to be most prominent when there is concurrent volume depletion. In this setting, the decrease in distal Cl^- delivery and the enhanced secretion of aldosterone both promote K^+ secretion.[164] There is also evidence that anions differ in their ability to enhance K^+ secretion. In humans, for example, HCO_3^- (following the administration of a carbonic anhydrase inhibitor to diminish proximal HCO_3^- reabsorption) has a greater effect than sulfate (induced by the ingestion of sulfur-containing amino acids).[164] How this might occur is not known.

Vomiting or nasogastric suction   Hypokalemia is a common finding with persistent loss of gastric secretions. Although some K^+ is present in this fluid (about 5 to 10 meq/L), most of the K^+ deficit is initially due to urinary losses.[70] The mechanism by which this occurs is as follows. Gastric juice contains a high concentration of HCl. Thus, its removal leads to elevations in the plasma HCO_3^- concentration and the filtered HCO_3^- load [glomerular filtration rate (GFR) times plasma HCO_3^- concentration], as well as hypovolemia and secondary hyperaldosteronism. The excess filtered HCO_3^- initially exceeds reabsorptive capacity, which cannot increase acutely. As a result, $NaHCO_3$ and water delivery to the distal nephron are

---

* Na^+-wasting states can also lead to *hyper*kalemia if they are associated with hypoaldosteronism (see Chap. 28) or reduced renal perfusion due to lack of replacement of urinary Na^+ losses.[157,158]

enhanced; the ensuing reabsorption of some of this Na^+ in the cortical collecting tubule is accompanied by increased K^+ secretion, since HCO_3^- acts as a nonreabsorbable anion.

This K^+-wasting state is generally transient. Within 48 to 72 h, proximal Na^+ and HCO_3^- reabsorption rise in response to the hypovolemia, less HCO_3^- is delivered distally, and K^+ excretion falls (see page 566).[70] Further K^+ loss at this time is primarily due to continued removal of gastric secretions.

Metabolic acidosis Increased urinary K^+ loss also occurs in several forms of metabolic acidosis, generally by mechanisms similar to that in vomiting.[166]* In diabetic ketoacidosis, for example, increased quantities of Na^+ and water (due to the glucose osmotic diuresis) are presented to the distal nephron with β-hydroxybutyrate and acetoacetate.[29] In type 2 (proximal) renal tubular acidosis, on the other hand, Na^+ is delivered with HCO_3^- because of a primary reduction in proximal HCO_3^- transport.[167] This effect is most prominent after the institution of alkali therapy, which raises the filtered HCO_3^- load far above proximal reabsorptive capacity (see Fig. 19-7).

A somewhat different mechanism is operative in type 1 (distal) renal tubular acidosis. In this condition, distal H^+ secretion is reduced. As a result, Na^+ reabsorption must occur in exchange for K^+ if Na^+ balance is to be maintained (see page 616).[167] Severe K^+ depletion with a plasma K^+ concentration below 2.0 meq/L may occur in this disorder. Although renal tubular acidosis is a rare condition, one of the more common causes in adults is Sjögren's syndrome.[168] In some patients with this disorder, the renal manifestations can precede the characteristic extrarenal findings by several years or more.[168]

In addition to these factors, distal flow may be directly increased in metabolic acidosis. Approximately one-third of proximal Na^+ reabsorption is passive, occurring down gradients created primarily by HCO_3^- reabsorption (see Chap. 3). In metabolic acidosis, less HCO_3^- is reabsorbed proximally (since less is filtered), thereby decreasing passive NaCl and water transport and augmenting distal delivery.[169]

Amphotericin B Hypokalemia due to increased urinary losses occurs in up to half of patients treated with amphotericin B.[170,171] Increased membrane permeability due to an interaction of amphotericin with membrane sterols probably plays an important role in this complication.[172] This defect can promote distal K^+ secretion both by increasing the K^+ permeability of the luminal membrane and, via the mechanism described above, by the concurrent type 1 renal tubular acidosis that is often present.[170] The latter problem is probably related to increased membrane permeability to H^+ ions or the H_2CO_3, thereby allowing secreted acid to back-diffuse out of the tubular lumen.

---

* Despite the K^+ depletion, the plasma K^+ concentration may be normal or even elevated because acidemia promotes K^+ movement out of the cells (see page 379).[13]

Hypomagnesemia Hypomagnesemia is a relatively common finding in hypokalemic patients, being found in up to 40 percent of cases.[173,174] In some patients, the underlying abnormality, such as cisplatin toxicity or primary hyperaldosteronism, impairs both K^+ and magnesium reabsorption by the kidney.[175,176]

In addition, hypomagnesemia from any cause can lead to K^+ depletion (due to both urinary and fecal losses) and hypokalemia.[173,177] The mechanism responsible for the inappropriate kaliuresis is not well understood, although decreased reabsorption in the loop of Henle and perhaps the cortical collecting tubule may be responsible.[178,179]

Hypocalcemia, due to both diminished secretion of parathyroid hormone and skeletal resistance to its effect, is also commonly present in hypomagnesemic patients.[180-183] If otherwise unexplained, this combination of hypokalemia and hypocalcemia is highly suggestive of underlying magnesium depletion.[177]

Correction of the hypokalemia generally requires the restoration of magnesium balance.[173,174,177] Simply giving K^+ alone is usually ineffective, as the exogenous K^+ is excreted in the urine rather than being taken up by the cells.[169,170] Magnesium repletion should preferably begin with oral magnesium chloride or magnesium lactate in patients who are markedly K^+ depleted. Magnesium sulfate should initially be avoided, since it can initially increase urinary K^+ losses as the sulfate acts as a nonreabsorbable anion.[184]

Poluria A marked increase in urine volume can induce K^+ loss by an unusual mechanism. Normal subjects can lower the urine K^+ concentration to a minimum of 5 to 15 meq/L in the presence of K^+ depletion.[1] Although this generally leads to adequate K^+ conservation, the obligatory K^+ loss can exceed 50 to 150 meq/day if the urine output is 10 L/day or more. This degree of K^+ loss is most likely to occur with primary polydipsia.[185] Although a similar degree of polyuria can occur in central diabetes insipidus, these patients usually seek medical care soon after the polyuria has begun.

L-Dopa Increased urinary loss and mild hypokalemia can be induced by the administration of L-dopa.[186] The mechanism by which this occurs is uncertain, although local dopamine formation may be important.

Increased Sweat Losses

Only small amounts of K^+ are normally lost in the sweat each day, since the volume is low and the K^+ concentration is only 5 to 10 meq/L. However, substantial K^+ losses can occur when sweat production is chronically increased. For example, 10 L/day or more may be produced in subjects exercising in a hot climate.[187] Unless intake is appropriately increased, K^+ depletion may occur, a change that can predispose to the development of rhabdomyolysis (see below). Urinary losses also contribute to this problem, since aldosterone secretion is enhanced by both exercise (via catecholamine-induced renin secretion) and volume loss and is not immediately suppressed when Na^+ is ingested to restore normovolemia.[187,188]

Dialysis

Patients on chronic dialysis are typically dialyzed against a low-K^+ concentration to remove dietary K^+. Patients on chronic peritoneal dialysis, for example, may lose 30 meq of K^+ per day. This loss is generally well tolerated, but it can lead to K^+ depletion if intake is reduced or there are concurrent gastrointestinal losses.[189] Approximately 10 to 35 percent of patients on continuous peritoneal dialysis require potassium supplements.[190]

A somewhat different mechanism may be operative in patients with underlying K^+ depletion in whom severe acidemia results in the movement of K^+ out of the cells and therefore a relatively normal baseline plasma K^+ concentration. In this setting, acute hemodialysis can rapidly correct the acidemia, resulting in K^+ entry into cells and a potentially large fall in the plasma K^+ concentration even though little or no K^+ has been lost by dialysis.[191]

Potassium Depletion without Hypokalemia

In most conditions, the plasma K^+ concentration varies directly with body K^+ stores. Thus, hypokalemia is generally associated with K^+ depletion, as a 200- to 400-meq K^+ deficit is required to lower the plasma K^+ concentration from 4 to 3 meq/L.[192] However, this relationship is disturbed in disorders that affect the distribution of K^+ between the cells and the extracellular fluid. As noted above, an elevation in arterial pH, increased availability of insulin, and periodic paralysis are all associated with K^+ movement into the cells and hypokalemia without K^+ depletion. Conversely, acidemia can mask underlying K^+ depletion by maintaining a normal plasma K^+ concentration.[13,191]

Another example of this dissociation occurs in a variety of chronic diseases, such as heart failure, renal failure, cirrhosis, and malnutrition. Patients with these disorders may have a normal plasma K^+ concentration despite a 10 to 15 percent fall in body K^+ stores.[193-195] The preferential loss of K^+ from the cells is associated with an increase in the cell Na^+ concentration and a reduction in the magnitude of the resting membrane potential, suggesting impaired function of the Na^+-K^+-ATPase pump in the cell membrane.[195-197]

The clinical significance of these changes, which cannot be detected by routine laboratory tests, is not well understood. These patients do not have the symptoms or signs of hypokalemia, since the plasma K^+ concentration is normal (the K^+ that had been in the cells being excreted in the urine). Normalization of balance will occur only with reversal of the underlying disease.[193] K^+ supplements alone are ineffective, as they are excreted in the urine, not taken up by the cells.[193,194]

SYMPTOMS

A variety of abnormalities may be associated with K^+ depletion (Table 27-3). Although the severity of these changes is generally related to the degree of hypokalemia, there is substantial individual variability. Marked symptoms are unusual unless the plasma K^+ concentration is below 2.5 to 3.0 meq/L, but in susceptible patients even mild reductions in the plasma K^+ concentration can predispose to potential fatal arrhythmias.

Muscle Weakness

Hypokalemia can induce muscle weakness and paralysis. The mechanism by which this occurs is complex. Initially, hypokalemia increases the ratio of the K^+ concentration in the cell to that in the extracellular fluid, thereby hyperpolarizing the cell membrane (i.e., making the resting potential more cell-interior negative) according to the following equation:

$$E_m = -61 \log \frac{r[K^+]_c + 0.01[Na^+]_c}{r[K^+]_e + 0.01[Na^+]_e} \tag{27-1}$$

where E_m is the resting membrane potential, r is the $3:2$ active transport ratio of the Na^+-K^+-ATPase pump, 0.01 is the relative membrane permeability of Na^+ to K^+, and the subscripts c and e refer to the cellular and extracellular concentrations, respectively.[195]

As a result of these relationships, membrane excitability should be reduced, since the resting potential is now further away from the threshold that must be reached before an action potential can be generated. However, the initial hyperpolarization (greater electronegativity) of the cell membrane removes the normal state of inactivation of sodium channels; the ensuing increase in Na^+ permeability *enhances neuromuscular excitability*, as less of an exciting stimulus is now required to generate an action potential.[198] These changes may be manifested clinically by muscle weakness and cardiac arrhythmias.

Table 27-3   Abnormalities induced by hypokalemia

Muscle weakness or paralysis (including intestinal ileus)
Cardiac arrhythmias, especially with digitalis, coronary ischemia, or perhaps left ventricular hypertrophy
Rhabdomyolysis
Renal dysfunction
   A. Impaired concentrating ability, leading to polyuria and polydipsia
   B. Increased ammonia production (can induce hepatic coma in cirrhosis)
   C. Impaired urinary acidification
   D. Increased bicarbonate reabsorption
   E. Renal insufficiency
   F. Abnormal NaCl reabsorption
Hyperglycemia

Muscle weakness usually does not begin until the plasma K^+ concentration is less than 2.5 meq/L. There is, however, variability in this relationship because of the effects of the plasma Ca^{2+} concentration, the extracellular pH, and the rapidity and manner in which hypokalemia develops (see page 825). As an example, patients with chronic K^+ loss may be relatively asymptomatic because part of the K^+ lost from the extracellular fluid is replaced by K^+ movement out of the cells.[192] The deficit in both compartments *minimizes the change in the ratio of the K^+ concentrations* and, therefore, in the resting potential and membrane excitability. In contrast, acute K^+ entry into cells (as occurs in periodic paralysis) can lead to marked weakness or paralysis,[48] in part because the cell K^+ concentration has increased, resulting in a much larger change in the concentration ratio.

The pattern of muscle weakness is relatively characteristic.[199] The lower extremities are most commonly involved first, particularly the quadriceps. In more severe cases, the muscles of the trunk, of the upper extremities, and eventually of respiration become affected, and death may ensue from respiratory failure. The cranial nerves, in comparison, are rarely involved.

Cramps, paresthesias, tetany, muscle tenderness, and atrophy also may occur.[195] In addition, involvement of smooth muscles in the gastrointestinal tract can produce a paralytic ileus and the symptoms of abdominal distention, anorexia, nausea, vomiting, and constipation.

Cardiac Arrhythmias

A variety of cardiac arrhythmias can be induced by hypokalemia. These include premature atrial and ventricular beats, sinus bradycardia, paroxysmal atrial or junctional tachycardia, atrioventricular block, and even ventricular tachycardia or fibrillation.[200-203]

The mechanism by which arrhythmias occur in this setting is incompletely understood.[200,201] Hypokalemia directly *enhances automaticity* (perhaps via the increase in excitability noted above) and also *delays ventricular repolarization*. The primary event during the latter process is K^+ movement out of the cells; this occurs passively down the favorable electrochemical gradient (cell interior now positive) that is created during depolarization (see page 823).[200] The rate of repolarization is therefore in part dependent upon the K^+ permeability of the cell membrane, which appears to vary directly with the plasma K^+ concentration.[200,201,204] Thus, hypokalemia reduces K^+ permeability and consequently slows the rate of repolarization.

This delay in ventricular repolarization is important clinically, because it prolongs the duration of the relative refractory period. This change predisposes to *reentrant arrhythmias*, since the ensuing impulse is blocked from going down the normal conductive pathway.[200] As a result, the impulse travels down adjacent, slower pathways, eventually leading to depolarization of the blocked area in a retrograde manner and the establishment of a reentrant pathway.

As described above, diuretic therapy in both hypertension (particularly if there is left ventricular hypertrophy) and heart failure has been associated with an increased incidence of arrhythmic death that can be prevented by a K^+-sparing diuretic (such as spironolactone) and may therefore be due to K^+ depletion.[86-89,205] A possible contributing factor in some patients is stress-induced release of epinephrine, which can further lower the plasma K^+ concentration (Fig. 27-1).

Other risk factors are coronary ischemia[203] and digitalis therapy.[206-208] Digitalis-induced arrhythmias typically occur with toxic plasma levels if K^+ balance is normal, but can be seen with normal drug levels when hypokalemia is present.[208] Diuretic-induced hypokalemia and hypomagnesemia should be particularly avoided in patients who are also treated with drugs that prolong the QT interval, since this combination can predispose to polymorphic ventricular tachycardia and torsade de pointes.[88]

Electrocardiographic changes   The electrocardiogram is a reflection of the electrical events in the heart. The P wave represents atrial depolarization, the QRS complex represents ventricular depolarization, and the ST segment and T and U waves represent ventricular and Purkinje fiber repolarization, respectively.[198,200,209] The atrial repolarization wave is lost in the QRS complex.

In addition to arrhythmias, hypokalemia produces characteristic changes in the electrocardiogram that are primarily due to *delayed ventricular repolarization.*[201] There is depression of the ST segment, a decrease in the amplitude of the T wave, and an increase in the amplitude of U waves, which occur at the end of the T wave and are often seen in the lateral precordial leads V_4 to V_6 (Fig. 27-4). With more severe K^+ depletion, increased amplitude and width of the P wave, prolongation of the PR interval, and widening of the QRS complex may occur.[201] These changes begin to be seen when the plasma K^+ concentration is less than 3.0 meq/L and are present in approximately 90 percent of patients with a plasma K^+ concentration under 2.7 meq/L.[201,210] They are rapidly reversible with K^+ repletion.

Rhabdomyolysis

Muscle cramps, rhabdomyolysis, and myoglobinuria, possibly leading to renal failure, may be seen in patients with severe K^+ depletion (plasma K^+ concentra-

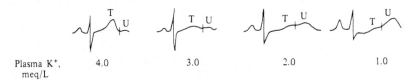

| Plasma K^+, meq/L | 4.0 | 3.0 | 2.0 | 1.0 |

Figure 27-4   Electrocardiogram in hypokalemia. As the plasma K^+ concentration falls, the initial changes are ST-segment depression, decreased amplitude of the T wave, and increased height of the U wave. With more severe hypokalemia, the P-wave amplitude is increased, as is the duration of the QRS complex. The approximate relationship between these changes and the plasma K^+ concentration is indicated, although there is substantial interpatient variability. (*Adapted from Surawicz B*, Am Heart J 73:814, 1967, with permission.)

tion less than 2.5 meq/L).[167,211-213] The role of K^+ in the regulation of skeletal muscle blood flow appears to play an important role in the development of this problem.[214] During exercise, there is normally an appropriate increase in muscle perfusion to meet enhanced energy demands. This hyperemic response is mediated in part by the release of K^+ from skeletal muscle cells. The ensuing local elevation in the K^+ concentration causes vasodilation, which enhances blood flow. However, the cellular release of K^+ is impaired by K^+ depletion. As a result, there is a lesser increase in blood flow, possibly resulting in cramps, ischemic necrosis, and rhabdomyolysis.[214] In addition to hypoperfusion, hypokalemia-induced impairment in muscle metabolism may contribute to the muscle dysfunction.[211]

Renal Dysfunction

K^+ depletion can interfere with a variety of renal functions (see Table 27-3).[199,215,216] Each of these changes is usually reversible with K^+ repletion. One important function that is maintained, however, is the ability to conserve K^+,[215] an adaptive response mediated both by decreased secretion and by enhanced active reabsorption (via a H^+-K^+-ATPase) in the collecting tubules (see page 393)[3,4,5-7] The increase in active reabsorption and reversible resistance to the kaliuretic action of aldosterone permit appropriate K^+ conservation even though aldosterone secretion may be enhanced due to concurrent hypovolemia (for example, as a result of gastrointestinal losses or diuretic therapy).[217]

Thus, patients with *extrarenal causes of K^+ depletion should excrete less than 25 meq of K^+ per day* in the urine.[1,2] This response may be important in the differential diagnosis of K^+ depletion of uncertain etiology (see "Diagnosis," below).

Impaired urinary concentration Polyuria and polydipsia are not uncommon in patients with chronic hypokalemia.[218] These symptoms may be due both to a primary stimulation of thirst and to diminished urinary concentrating ability.[219] The latter change is associated with diminished collecting tubule responsiveness to ADH. How this occurs is incompletely understood, but decreased expression of aquaporin-2, the ADH-sensitive water channel, may play at least a contributory role.[220] Hypokalemia may also impair countercurrent function by interfering with NaCl transport in the thick ascending limb.[221,222]

In general, the maximum urine osmolality (which in normal subjects is 900 to 1400 mosmol/kg) remains above 300 mosmol/kg with K^+ depletion (Fig. 27-5). This is in contrast to values that may be below 150 mosmol/kg in patients with central diabetes insipidus or congenital nephrogenic diabetes insipidus (see Chap. 24). Consequently, the degree of polyuria is typically mild with hypokalemia, as the urine output usually remains below 3 L/day.

The concentrating defect is both dose- and time-related.[218] The maximum urine osmolality begins to fall when the K^+ deficit exceeds 200 meq and reaches its minimum at a deficit of 400 meq, a level at which the plasma K^+ concentration should be below 3.0 meq/L. The fall in the urine osmolality occurs slowly over 2 to 3 weeks, presumably reflecting the gradual impairment in cell function (Fig. 27-5).

Ammonia production and urinary acidification   Hypokalemia results in an increase in NH_3 and NH_4^+ production by the renal tubular cells.[223] These compounds then enter both the tubular lumen and the peritubular capillary, resulting in increases in urinary NH_4^+ excretion and in the NH_3 concentration in the renal vein.[223-225]

This effect may be related in part to a transcellular cation exchange. K^+ tends to move out of the cells with hypokalemia in an attempt to replete the diminished extracellular stores.[192] Electroneutrality is maintained in this setting in part by H^+ entry into the cells.[16,17] The ensuing *intracellular acidosis*[21] can then stimulate NH_4^+ production and H^+ secretion,[226] a mechanism similar to that thought to be responsible for the appropriate increase in NH_4^+ excretion seen with metabolic acidosis (see Chap. 11).

These changes in renal function may be clinically important in patients with severe hepatic disease, in whom hypokalemia can precipitate hepatic coma.[225,227] In addition to the increase in NH_3 production, the commonly associated metabolic alkalosis may also contribute to this problem by driving the reaction

$$NH_3 + H^+ \quad \leftrightarrow \quad NH_4^+ \tag{27-2}$$

to the left. The relative increase in the concentration of nonpolar and therefore lipid-soluble NH_3 promotes the entry of NH_3 (and possibly other toxic amines) into the brain. Correction of these electrolyte disturbances with KCl may reverse the encephalopathy without any other therapy.[225,227]

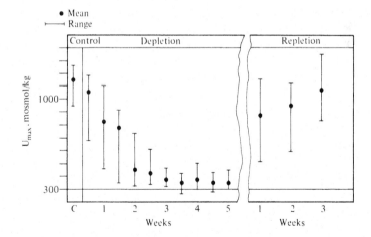

Figure 27-5   Impaired ability to maximally concentrate the urine (U_{max}) in patients with progressive potassium depletion. The average K^+ deficit was 350 meq, or about 10 percent of the total body K^+. (*From Rubin M, J Clin Invest 40:2215, 1961, by copyright permission of the American Society for Clinical Investigation.*)

The hypokalemia-induced increase in NH_3 excretion also can *raise the urine pH* by driving Eq. (27-2) to the right. In patients with concurrent metabolic acidosis due to diarrhea or laxative abuse, the relatively alkaline urine falsely suggests the presence of renal tubular acidosis. These possibilities can be distinguished by measurement of the *urine anion gap*, which is negative with hypokalemia alone, since NH_4^+ excretion is appropriately increased, but positive in renal tubular acidosis (see page 589).

Bicarbonate reabsorption   The increases in the cell H^+ concentration and H^+ secretion induced by hypokalemia also promote HCO_3^- reabsorption (see Fig. 11-16).[19,20,228] This effect can contribute to the perpetuation of a concurrent metabolic alkalosis, since it prevents excretion of the excess HCO_3^- in the urine (see Chap. 18).[18]

Nephropathy of potassium depletion   In humans, K^+ depletion produces a characteristic vacuolar lesion in the epithelial cells of the proximal tubule and occasionally the distal tubule.[215,216] This lesion occurs primarily with chronic K^+ depletion and generally requires at least 1 month to develop. Interstitial fibrosis, tubular atrophy, and cyst formation, particularly in the renal medulla, also may be seen.[229,230]

The pathogenesis of the tubulointerstitial lesions is not well understood. An intriguing hypothesis that has been documented in experimental animals is that the hypokalemia-induced elevation in NH_3 production (via the fall in intracellular pH) results in local NH_3 accumulation in the interstitium.[231] This NH_3 can directly activate the complement system, which may then produce tubular injury. It has also been proposed that the intracellular acidosis or perhaps the increase in ammonia formation may be a stimulus to the cellular proliferation that is required for cyst formation.[232]

Regardless of the mechanism, the vacuolar changes are reversed within weeks to months after $K+$ repletion. However, the secondary changes of interstitial fibrosis and tubular dilatation may be irreversible. Although the glomerular filtration rate may be reduced when the patient is hypokalemic, it usually improves after the restoration of normal K^+ balance.[215] However, persistent renal insufficiency following chronic K^+ depletion can occur, primarily in patients with advanced tubulointerstitial disease.[233]

NaCl reabsorption   Hypokalemia has a dual effect on Na^+ excretion, impairing both the ability to excrete a Na^+ load and the ability to conserve Na^+ maximally. As an example, a low-K^+ diet can increase tubular Na^+ reabsorption, apparently via an effect in the proximal tubule or loop of Henle.[223,234] This effect can, in patients on a high-Na^+ diet, lead to Na^+ retention and a small rise in systemic blood pressure.[90,235] It is unclear, however, whether the volume expansion is directly responsible for the hypertensive response. K^+ supplementation can lower the blood pressure by an average of 5 to 7 mmHg in patients with essential hypertension.[91,236] This hypotensive effective of K^+ is not seen in subjects who are on a low-Na$^+$ diet, suggesting that the hemodynamic effects of K$^+$ are at least in part related to changes in Na$^+$ balance.[237]

On the other hand, the ability to lower the urine concentration of NaCl to below 15 meq/L in the presence of volume depletion may also be impaired by moderate-to-severe hypokalemia.[216,238] Diminished Cl$^-$ reabsorption in the loop of Henle and collecting tubules has been demonstrated in this setting, although the mechanism by which it occurs is unclear.[221,239,240]

DIAGNOSIS

The cause of hypokalemia can usually be determined from the history, which may reveal complaints of vomiting or diarrhea, the use of diuretics, or recurrent acute episodes of muscle weakness in periodic paralysis. When the diagnosis is not readily apparent, the most likely diagnoses are *surreptitious* vomiting, diarrhea, or diuretic use or one of the causes of primary mineralocorticoid excess. In this setting, measurement of *urinary K$^+$ excretion* and assessment of *acid-base status* may be helpful.

Urinary Potassium Excretion

As described above, hypokalemic patients with extrarenal losses (or diuretic therapy after the drug effect has worn off) should excrete less than 25 meq/day of K$^+$ in the urine,[1,2] values above this level suggest at least a contribution from urinary K$^+$ wasting (see Fig. 27-5). The efficiency of K$^+$ conservation (minimum concentration 5 to 15 meq/L) is less than that for Na$^+$ (minimum concentration less than 5 meq/L).[1,2] This phenomenon may be related to leakage (down a favorable concentration gradient) of cellular K$^+$ into the lumen through a relatively nonselective cation channel in the luminal membrane of the inner medullary collecting duct.[241]

Random measurement of the urine K$^+$ concentration is simpler to perform, but may be less accurate than a 24-h collection. It is likely that extrarenal losses are present if the random urine K$^+$ concentration is below 15 meq/L (unless the patient is markedly polyuric[185]). Somewhat higher values, however, do not necessarily imply K$^+$ wasting. For example, a patient appropriately excreting 20 meq/day will have a seemingly high urine K$^+$ concentration of 50 meq/L if the daily urine volume is only 400 mL. This is most likely to occur with volume depletion; although secondary hyperaldosteronism is commonly present, its effect is counteracted by the associated reduction in distal flow.[96]

Hypovolemia (as evidenced by urine Na$^+$ concentration below 25 meq/L) can also diminish the degree of kaliuresis in patients with primary mineralocorticoid excess. In this setting, the response to volume repletion may be helpful. K$^+$ excretion will not change significantly in patients with extrarenal losses, because the ensuing increase in distal flow will be balanced by a reduction in aldosterone

Table 27-4 Acid-base disorders in hypokalemia

Metabolic acidosis may be seen	Metabolic alkalosis may be seen
Loss of lower intestinal secretions (diarrhea, laxative abuse)	Diuretic therapy
Ketoacidosis	Vomiting or nasogastric suction
Renal tubular acidosis	Mineralocorticoid excess
Salt-wasting nephropathies	Penicillin derivatives

release; in contrast, K^+ excretion may rise markedly in primary hyperaldosteronism, where aldosterone secretion is nonsuppressible.[242]

Acid-Base Status

Some hypokalemic states are associated with acid-base disturbances that may aid in establishing the correct diagnosis (Table 27-4). In a patient with *metabolic acidosis and urinary K^+ wasting*, for example, diabetic ketoacidosis, renal tubular acidosis (in which the urine pH is generally above 5.3; see Chap. 19), and salt-wasting nephropathy (in which renal insufficiency is typically present and accounts for the acidemia) should be excluded. If these disorders are not present and urinary K^+ excretion is low, then surreptitious diarrhea, perhaps due to laxative abuse, is likely to be present.[76]

In contrast, the combination of *hypokalemia and metabolic alkalosis* is usually due to diuretic use, vomiting (both of which may be surreptitious), or, less often, one of the causes of mineralocorticoid excess or one of the rare genetic disorders (Liddle's, Bartter's, or Gitelman's syndrome). The first two conditions are often associated with volume depletion. Thus, the findings of decreased skin turgor, flat neck veins, and postural hypotension are suggestive of one of these problems, since primary mineralocorticoid excess leads to mild volume expansion.

The urine Cl^- concentration also may be helpful,* since a value below 25 meq/L is strongly suggestive of vomiting or diuretic therapy (after the drug effect has dissipated). If, on the other hand, the urine Cl^- concentration exceeds 40 meq/L, a urinary assay for diuretics should be obtained.[145] If this is negative and the patient is *normotensive*, then Bartter's or Gitelman's syndrome may be present. If, however, the patient is *hypertensive*, the evaluation outlined in Fig. 27-6 should be initiated (see "Primary Hyperaldosteronism," below).

Clinical Examples

The following case histories illustrate how this approach can be utilized in patients in whom the cause of the hypokalemia is uncertain.

---

* The urine Cl^- concentration is often a more accurate indicator of volume status than the urine Na^+ concentration in patients with metabolic alkalosis (see page 565). The need to excrete the excess HCO_3^- in this disorder can lead to the loss of $NaHCO_3$ and a relatively high urine Na^+ concentration, despite the presence of volume depletion. The urine Cl^- concentration, in comparison, will be appropriately reduced.

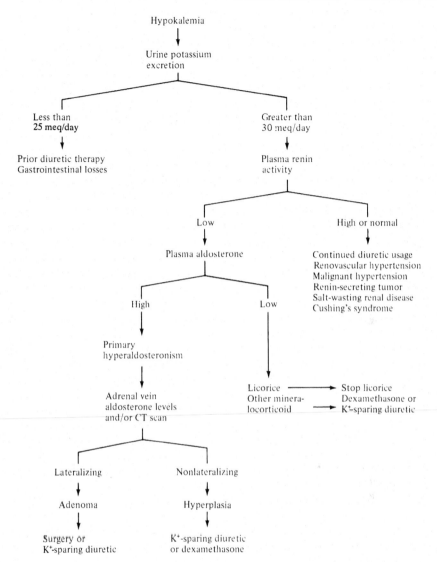

Figure 27-6   Stepwise approach to the evaluation of hypokalemia in hypertensive patients.

Case History 27-1   A 36-year-old woman is started on diuretics twice weekly for mild pedal edema. During a routine follow-up, she is noted to be hypertensive (duration unknown). Also noted are an estimated jugular venous pressure below $5\,cmH_2O$ and a moderate decrease in skin turgor. The following laboratory tests are obtained:

Plasma [Na$^+$]	=	136 meq/L	Arterial pH	=	7.47
[K$^+$]	=	3.0 meq/L	Urine [Na$^+$]	=	60 meq/L
[Cl$^-$]	=	98 meq/L	[K$^+$]	=	45 meq/L
[HCO$_3^-$]	=	29 meq/L	[Cl$^-$]	=	48 meqL

The patient is initially given 2 liters of isotonic saline over 12 h; the repeat urine Na$^+$ concentration is now 20 meq/L.

Comment The combination of hypertension, hypokalemia, hyperkaliuria, and metabolic alkalosis suggests the possible diagnosis of primary hyper-aldosteronism due, for example, to an adrenal adenoma. Diuretic therapy can produce a similar picture in a patient with essential hypertension, but drug intake seemed to be too infrequent in this case. However, the physical findings and the slight degree of hyponatremia point to the presence of volume depletion. Furthermore, the fall in the urine Na$^+$ concentration after saline administration is best explained by attenuation of the diuretic effect, thereby unmasking persistent hypovolemia. In comparison, a saline load in primary hyperaldosteronism should produce a marked and appropriate rise in Na$^+$ excretion.

Case History 27-2 A 22-year-old woman complains of persistent weakness, but denies all other symptoms. The physical examination is unremarkable, with the blood pressure being normal. The following laboratory data are obtained:

Plasma [Na$^+$]	=	136 meq/L	Arterial pH	=	7.30
[K$^+$]	=	2.7 meq/L	Urine [Na$^+$]	=	7 meq/L
[Cl$^-$]	=	108 meq/L	[K$^+$]	=	12 meq/L
[HCO$_3^-$]	=	17 meq/L			

Comment The low urine K$^+$ concentration suggests extrarenal losses. Although the patient denies vomiting or diarrhea, the low urine Na$^+$ concentration indicates that she is volume-depleted and must have some unadmitted source of fluid loss. The presence of metabolic acidosis points toward diarrhea, perhaps induced by laxative abuse.

Primary Hyperaldosteronism

Primary mineralocorticoid excess should be suspected in any patient with hyper-tension and unexplained hypokalemia, although renovascular hypertension and diuretic therapy are more common causes of this problem.[93,243] Normokalemic hyperaldosteronism does occur and may be more common than currently sus-pected. In one study, for example, more than 50 percent of recently diagnosed cases were not hypokalemic at presentation.[244] Similar findings have been found in the glucocorticoid-remediable hyperaldosteronism.[100] Aldosterone release in the latter disorder is primarily under the influence of ACTH. With the normal circadian rhythm of ACTH release, aldosterone secretion should be above normal for only part of the day, which may explain the lesser tendency to hypokalemia.

Despite these observations, it is not at present feasible to screen every hypertensive patient for the presence of primary hyperaldosteronism. However, at the least, screening should be performed in all patients with otherwise unexplained hypokalemia and in those with severe or resistant hypertension.[131] It has been suggested that use of the random plasma aldosterone-to-renin ratio described below may permit screening of many if not most hypertensive patients.

Even more rare are those patients with primary hyperaldosteronism who are hypokalemic but normotensive.[245] In this setting, the unexplained persistent reduction in the plasma K^+ concentration warrants evaluation for mineralocorticoid excess.

The following approach is recommended for the evaluation of the hypertensive patient with unexplained hypokalemia and metabolic alkalosis (Fig. 27-6).[94]

- *24-h urine collection*—A 24-h urine collection for K^+ will differentiate inappropriate urinary losses (greater than 25 to 30 meq/day) from extrarenal or previous urinary losses. Diuretics, which can directly increase K^+ excretion, must be discontinued prior to the collection. It is also important that the patient not be volume-depleted (as evidenced by a urine Na^+ concentration below 25 meq/L), since the associated decrease in distal delivery can lower K^+ excretion even in patients with hyperaldosteronism.

    On the other hand, the degree of K^+ wasting, and therefore the diagnostic accuracy, can be increased by a high-Na^+ diet, as the combination of augmented distal flow and hypersecretion of aldosterone enhances K^+ secretion.[242,246] A high-Na^+ diet can also be given to patients with a borderline plasma K^+ concentration, since *Na^+-induced hypokalemia is strongly indicative of nonsuppressible hyperaldosteronism.*[92,242] In comparison, increased K^+ loss and hypokalemia are not induced in normal subjects by Na^+ loading, because the ensuing volume expansion inhibits the secretion of renin and therefore of aldosterone.[242,246]

- *Plasma renin activity*—The plasma renin activity should be measured in those patients with persistent hypokalemia and an inappropriately high rate of K^+ excretion.[92-94] An elevated value is most often due to renovascular or malignant hypertension, diuretic usage, or a rare renin-secreting tumor. A low value is highly suggestive of some form of mineralocorticoid excess (or Liddle's syndrome in which there is a primary increase in collecting tubule Na^+ function[131,247]); the mild volume expansion in these disorders suppresses renin release. The plasma renin activity is typically normal in Cushing's syndrome, which is usually accompanied by a cushingoid appearance.[109]

- *Aldosterone secretion*—The triad of hypokalemia, urinary potassium wasting, and a low plasma renin activity is highly suggestive of mineralocorticoid excess. The disorders that can cause this problem can be differentiated from one another by measuring the plasma aldosterone concentration or the urinary excretion of aldosterone metabolites.[92-95] A low plasma level indicates the overproduction of a nonaldosterone mineralocorticoid.[93] Examples described above include severe Cushing's syndrome, some forms of congenital adrenal hyperplasia, DOC-producing tumors [which usually can be detected by computed tomography (CT) scanning or magnetic resonance imaging], the ingestion of licorice or the syndrome of apparent mineralocorticoid excess, the use of the synthetic mineralocorticoid fludrocortisone, and Liddle's syndrome.

On the other hand, a clearly high plasma aldosterone concentration (greater than 30 ng/dL or 24-h urinary aldosterone excretion (above 15 μg/day) points toward one of the causes of hyperaldosteronism.[243] The diagnostic accuracy of this measurement can be increased by attempting to *suppress endogenous aldosterone production* via the administration of 2 liters of isotonic saline intravenously over 4 h (while recumbent).[92,94,248] The plasma aldosterone concentration in normal subjects should fall to 6 ng/dL or below, whereas values above 10 ng/dL are consistent with primary hyperaldosteronism.[248] Levels between 6 and 10 ng/dL are nondiagnostic; in this setting, a more prolonged suppression test (in which the plasma aldosterone concentration should fall to less than 6 ng/dL) should be performed using a high-Na^+ diet plus 0.6 to 1.2 mg/day of fludrocortisone (a synthetic mineralocorticoid) for 3 days.[92,248]

Potentially confounding variables should be eliminated to prevent possible misinterpretation of these tests. Thus, the plasma aldosterone concentration should be measured with the patient recumbent, off K^+ supplements (both standing and K^+ loading can increase aldosterone secretion), and relatively normokalemic (since hypokalemia can reduce aldosterone release).[249]

- *Plasma aldosterone to renin ratio*—The presence of high plasma aldosterone levels (PA) and low plasma renin activity (PRA) in primary hyperaldosteronism has led to the suggestion that the PA/PRA ratio can be used as an effective screening test for primary hyperaldosteronism.[244,250] The mean value for the ratio in normal subjects and patients with essential hypertension is 4 to 5, versus more than 30 to 50 in most patients with primary hyperaldosteronism.[250,251]

Optimal performance of this test requires eliminating other factors that can affect renin and aldosterone. These include correction of hypokalemia with potassium chloride and the cessation of therapy with diuretics, calcium channel blockers, and high-dose beta-blockers.

In one study, for example, blood was drawn at 8 A.M. after 2 h of ambulation. The combination of a plasma aldosterone concentration above 20 ng/dL and a PA/PRA ratio above 30 (with the PRA expressed in units of ng/mL/h) had a sensitivity and specificity of 90 percent for the diagnosis of primary hyperaldosteronism.[250] In a selected population in which the incidence of primary hyperaldosteronism was 20 percent, the positive and negative predictive values for these findings were 70 and 98 percent. The mean value for the PA/PRA ratio in normotensive controls and patients with essential hypertension is 4 to 5.

It has also been suggested that the PA/PRA ratio can be used to screen normokalemic patients who otherwise would not be detected.[244] The cost-effectiveness of screening all hypertensive patients for primary hyperaldosteronism is uncertain, but screening is probably indicated in patients with severe or resistant hypertension.[244] Unfortunately, it is more difficult to discontinue antihypertensive medications in these cases. Another, less important limitation is that the ratio will not detect patients in whom excess mineralocorticoid activity is not due to aldosterone.

- *Adenoma versus hyperplasia*—Once the diagnosis of primary nonsuppressible hyperaldosteronism has been established, a *unilateral adenoma or carcinoma must be distinguished from bilateral hyperplasia* because of the differing therapies required: surgery with a unilateral tumor and medical therapy with bilateral hyperplasia (see below).[92-95,251] In general, hyperplasia is a less severe disease, with a lower rate of aldosterone secretion and a lesser degree of hypokalemia. There is, however, substantial overlap.

A variety of indirect tests have been utilized to make this distinction, but the correct diagnosis can be most accurately made by CT scanning or magnetic resonance imaging, or, if necessary, by measurement of adrenal vein aldosterone concentrations (a test that should be performed only by a radiologist experienced with this procedure).[44,244,252-254] The radiologic tests may identify a unilateral adrenal mass, which is indicative of an adenoma or rarely a carcinoma, with a sensitivity of 67 to 85 percent. However, the absence of a mass is not diagnostic of hyperplasia, since small tumors (less than 10 mm in diameter) can be missed in 15 to 25 percent of cases.[252,253] Furthermore, the finding of bilateral nodules may reflect a unilateral aldosteronoma plus a contralateral nonfunctioning nodule rather than adrenal hyperplasia.[253]

The net effect is that CT scanning alone may be inaccurate; in one study of 22 patients with a unilateral adenoma, for example, five were incorrectly diagnosed as having bilateral disease.[253] Thus, the presence of bilateral lesions on CT scan should be followed by measurement of adrenal vein aldosterone levels or iodocholesterol scanning to determine whether the hypersecretion of aldosterone is coming from one or both adrenal glands.[253,254] Although not widely available, scintillation scanning with ^{131}I-iodocholesterol (a precursor of aldosterone) may be even more accurate than CT scanning in detecting a unilateral lesion.[93,255]

The rationale for measuring adrenal vein aldosterone concentrations is that a unilateral adenoma is associated with a marked (usually greater than tenfold) increase in adrenal vein aldosterone concentration on the side of the tumor, whereas there is little difference between the two sides with bilateral hyperplasia.[256-258] The test is best performed before and 15 min after the administration of ACTH, which acutely stimulates aldosterone release and increases the difference between the two sides when an adrenal adenoma is present.[256] To be certain that the samples are from the adrenal veins, cortisol should also be measured in the same samples; the serum cortisol concentration should be roughly the same in both adrenal veins, but much higher than in a peripheral vein sample.

Adrenal vein sampling may be most useful when there is no adrenal abnormality on CT, or when both adrenal glands are abnormal but asymmetric. In one report, six of fifteen patients with normal or minimal adrenal thickening and four of nine with bilateral adrenal masses on CT had a unilateral source of aldosterone by adrenal venous sampling.[248]

TREATMENT

The initial step in the treatment of hypokalemia must be the assessment of the physiologic effects of the K^+ deficit. As described above, there is a wide variation in the degree to which a given reduction in the plasma K^+ concentration will produce symptoms. Thus, monitoring of the electrocardiogram and muscle strength, which *reflect the functional consequences of K^+ depletion*, is an essential part of the management of patients with severe hypokalemia.

As with other electrolyte disorders, the first aim of therapy is to get the patient out of danger, not to immediately correct the entire K^+ deficit. The potential risk of the overly rapid administration of K^+ is illustrated in Fig. 27-7. In this patient,

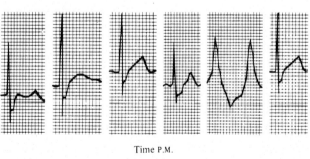

Time P.M.

(a) 12:10   (b) 12:18   (c) 12:22   (d) 12:24   (e) 12:25   (f) 12:30

Figure 27-7 Electrocardiogram (ECG) during the intravenous administration of 80 meq of K^+ over 15 min. (a) Initial ECG shows the typical changes of hypokalemia, with flat T wave and prominent U wave. (b) After 45 meq, the T wave is returning. (c) After 65 meq, the T wave is normal. (d and e) After 80 meq, signs of hyperkalemia appear: peaked T wave and widening of the QRS complex. (f) Slowing of K^+ infusion is associated with return of the tracing to normal. (*From Seftel HC, Kew MC, Diabetes 15:694, 1966, with permission.*)

who had hypokalemia and flaccid paralysis, the intravenous infusion of 80 meq of K^+ over 15 min resulted in a change in the electrocardiogram from one typical of hypokalemia to one characteristic of severe hyperkalemia.

Potassium Deficit

The potassium deficit can only be approximated, since there is no definite correlation between the plasma K^+ concentration and body K^+ stores. In general, a reduction in the plasma K^+ concentration from 4.0 to 3.0 meq/L requires the loss of 200 to 400 meq of K^+.[192,259] An additional 200- to 400-meq deficit will lower the plasma K^+ concentration to 2.0 meq/L. However, continued K^+ losses may not produce much more hypokalemia, as the release of K^+ from the cells is usually able to maintain the plasma K^+ concentration near 2.0 meq/L.[259]

These estimates of the K^+ deficit assume that there is a normal distribution of K^+ between the cells and the extracellular fluid. In patients with periodic paralysis, for example, body K^+ stores are normal, since the hypokalemia is due entirely to K^+ movement into the cells. In this setting, K^+ is given to normalize the plasma K^+ concentration, not to repair a K^+ deficit.

The effects of the extracellular pH and the plasma osmolality are also important in evaluating the potassium status of the patient. In particular, acidemia (in renal failure or renal tubular acidosis) or hyperosmolality (in diabetic ketoacidosis) frequently raises the plasma K^+ concentration and masks the severity of the K^+ depletion. This has important therapeutic implications, because correction of the acidemia or hyperglycemia can lead to marked hypokalemia.[29,191]

Use of Potassium Chloride

A variety of potassium preparations are available for oral and intravenous use, including the Cl^-, HCO_3^-,* phosphate, and gluconate salts. There are two major advantages to the use of KCl in K^+-depleted patients. First, metabolic alkalosis is commonly associated with hypokalemia. These patients tend to be Cl^- depleted as well (due, for example, to diuretics or vomiting), and the *administration of Cl^- is essential for correction of both the alkalosis and the K^+ deficit*. Other K^+ salts are less effective in inducing positive K^+ balance and may increase the severity of the alkalemia (since the anions are nonreabsorbable and therefore promote K^+ and H^+ loss; see page 568).[260,261]

Second, the $[K^+]_c/[K^+]_e$ ratio (the main determinant of the resting membrane potential) is affected primarily by changes in $[K^+]_e$ since the extracellular K^+ concentration is so much lower than that in the cells. Consequently, the aim of therapy is to rapidly increase the plasma (and extracellular) K^+ concentration in a severely hypokalemic patient with muscle weakness, arrhythmias, or advanced electrocardiographic changes. If equal doses of KCl and $KHCO_3$ are given,

---

*Acetate and citrate salts are also available. These organic anions are rapidly metabolized into HCO_3^- in the body.

there will be a significantly greater increase in the plasma K^+ concentration with KCl than with $KHCO_3$ (Fig. 27-8). This difference is probably related to the ability of HCO_3^- to enter the cells in comparison to that of Cl^-, which is mostly limited to the extracellular fluid.[262] As a result, K^+ follows HCO_3^- into the cells to maintain electroneutrality,* producing a lesser increase in the plasma K^+ concentration.

Although $KHCO_3$ is not as effective as KCl in metabolic alkalosis or severe hypokalemia, it may be the preferred K^+ salt in certain patients with mild degrees of hypokalemia and metabolic acidosis. For example, patients with renal tubular acidosis tend to waste K^+ in the urine and become K^+-depleted (see Chap. 19). In this setting, chronic therapy with $KHCO_3$ (or K^+ citrate, which is more palatable) tends to correct both the K^+ depletion and the acidemia.

Oral   KCl can be given orally in crystalline form (salt substitutes), as a liquid, or in a slow-release tablet or capsule. Slow-release preparations are generally better tolerated than the poorly palatable KCl solutions. However, these tablets or capsules can in rare cases lead to ulcerative or stenotic lesions in the gastrointestinal tract as a result of the local accumulation of high concentrations of K^+.[263,264] Salt substitute (which contains between 50 and 65 meq per level teaspoon) may be the ideal form of oral therapy, being safe, well tolerated, and much cheaper than the other preparations.[265]

In comparison, the traditional therapy of treating chronic hypokalemia (most often due to diuretics) with K^+-rich foods such as orange juice or bananas is less desirable. These foods contain phosphate and citrate rather than chloride and are therefore less likely to correct the hypokalemia and metabolic alkalosis.[260,266] In

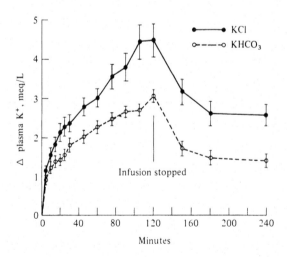

Figure 27-8   Changes in plasma K^+ concentration of potassium-depleted dogs during infusion with KCl and $KHCO_3$. (*From Villamil MF, DeLand EC, Henney P, Maloney JV Jr, Am J Physiol 229:161, 1975, with permission.*)

---

* Rather than HCO_3^- entering into the cells, intracellular H^+ ions may be released into the extracellular fluid to buffer the excess HCO_3^- ions. In either case, K^+ will tend to move into the cells to maintain electroneutrality.

addition, fruit ingestion involves an increase in caloric intake in excess of 350 kcal/day. This is a particular disadvantage with obese patients with hypertension, in whom weight reduction may lower the systemic blood pressure.[267]

Intravenous In patients who are unable to eat, K^+ must be given intravenously. The standard intravenous KCl solution contains 2 meq each of K^+ and Cl^- per milliliter. In most circumstances, 20 to 40 meq of K^+ (10 to 20 mL) is added to each liter of dextrose or saline solution. However, the addition of this quantity of K^+ to 1 liter of a dextrose solution may lead to a transient *reduction in the plasma K^+ concentration of 0.2 to 1.4 meq/L*, particularly when only 20 meq/L is added.[30] This effect is presumably due to enhanced insulin secretion stimulated by the infusion of glucose.

Although normal subjects can tolerate this decrease in the plasma K^+ concentration, arrhythmias may be precipitated in patients who are hypokalemic or taking digitalis.[30] Consequently, K^+ supplementation should be given in a non-dextrose-containing solution, usually in a concentration of 40 meq/L. In general, no more than 60 meq/L should be given through a peripheral vein, since higher concentrations of K^+ are very irritating, resulting in pain and sclerosis of the vein.

Rate of Potassium Repletion

The majority of patients have mild to moderate hypokalemia, with the plasma K^+ concentration ranging between 3.0 and 3.5 meq/L. This degree of K^+ depletion is usually well tolerated in the absence of digitalis therapy[206-208] or severe hepatic disease.[225,227] Treatment is not urgent in this setting and must be directed toward both repair of the K^+ deficit and prevention of further K^+ loss by correcting the underlying disorder (such as diarrhea). These patients can usually be treated with oral KCl at an initial dose of 60 to 80 meq/day. However, larger amounts will be required if there is continued K^+ loss. In primary hyperaldosteronism, for example, oral K^+ therapy is of minor benefit, and a K^+-sparing diuretic is required to maintain a normal plasma K^+ concentration.[268-270]

In the occasional patient with severe symptoms or marked hypokalemia, K^+ must be given more rapidly. This is more easily done orally, as the plasma K^+ concentration will acutely rise by as much as 1.0 to 1.5 meq/L after 40 to 60 meq and by 2.5 to 3.5 meq/L after 135 to 160 meq.[271,272] These maximum effects, however, are *transient*, since most of the administered K^+ will enter the cells to repair the cell deficit.[273] As a result, the plasma K^+ concentration must be carefully monitored and more K^+ given as necessary. A patient with a plasma K^+ concentration of 2.0 meq/L, for example, may have a total K^+ deficit of as much as 400 to 800 meq.[192]

Large doses of K^+ are much more difficult to give intravenously, since the limit of 60 meq/L means that a large volume of fluid also must be given. This tendency to fluid overload is enhanced by the preferential use of saline-containing solutions (such as one-quarter-isotonic saline) because of the desire to avoid dextrose administration.[30] Despite these obstacles, some patients must be treated intravenously.

In general, intravenous K^+ is administered at a *maximum rate of 10 to 20 meq/h,* although as much as 40 to 100 meq/h has been given to patients with paralysis or life-threatening arrhythmias.[274-276] In the latter setting, solutions containing as much as 200 meq of K^+ per liter (as with 20 meq in 100 mL of isotonic saline) have been used.[277,278] These solutions are best tolerated if given into a large vein (such as the femoral vein); infusions through a central venous line should probably be avoided (although they have been safely used[278]), since the local increase in the K^+ concentration might, in some cases, have deleterious effects on cardiac conduction.

The necessity for such aggressive therapy has been reported primarily in patients with diabetic ketoacidosis who are hypokalemic at presentation (see Chap. 25).[275,276] In this setting, the administration of insulin and the ensuing reduction in the plasma glucose concentration will drive K^+ into the cells, further reducing the plasma K^+ concentration if KCl is withheld. Since the average fluid deficit in these patients is 3 to 6 liters, rapid K^+ replacement can be achieved by adding 60 meq of K^+ to each liter of fluid. This example again illustrates that the factors that influence the internal distribution of K^+ (plasma osmolality, availability of insulin) must be taken into account when evaluating the hypokalemic patient.

It must be emphasized that the rapid administration of K^+ is *potentially dangerous even in severely K^+-depleted patients* and should be used only in life-threatening situations. A rate in excess of 80 meq/h can result in the electrocardiographic changes of hyperkalemia (Fig. 27-7) or complete heart block.[279] Thus, continuous monitoring of the electrocardiogram is essential in this setting. In addition, the concentrated solutions should contain only a limited amount of K^+ per container (as with 20 meq in 100 mL of isotonic saline) to avoid the accidental administration of very large quantities of K^+.[278]

Primary Hyperaldosteronism

The mode of therapy in primary hyperaldosteronism varies with the underlying disease. Surgery is the preferred treatment in patients with an adenoma or carcinoma, since unilateral adrenalectomy, which can be performed laparoscopically,[280] results in a fall in blood pressure, a marked reduction in aldosterone secretion, and correction of the hypokalemia in virtually all patients.[281-284] However, a lesser degree of hypertension persists in as many as 40 percent of cases.[282-284]

Surgery (subtotal adrenalectomy) is much less successful with adrenal hyperplasia, as only a minority of patients have a clinically important hypotensive response.[93,94,281] The reasons for the failure of surgery to control the blood pressure are incompletely understood. In some patients, the development of secondary nephrosclerosis after many years of uncontrolled hypertension may play a contributory role.[282,283] An alternative explanation is that adrenal hyperplasia may be a *variant of essential hypertension* in which increased sensitivity of the adrenal cortex to angiotensin II leads to the elevation in aldosterone release and hypokalemia, which is typically milder than in patients with an adenoma.[92]

As a result of these observations, *surgery should be considered only in patients with a unilateral tumor*, as determined by measurement of adrenal vein aldosterone concentrations or CT scanning. In patients who are not surgical candidates or who have hyperplasia, a K^+-sparing diuretic (spironolactone, triamterene, or amiloride) can lower the blood pressure and correct the hypokalemia.[268-270,285] These responses can be sustained over the long term.[285]

Amiloride (10 to 40 mg/day) may be the best tolerated, since it can be given once daily and avoids the gastrointestinal and endocrine side effects (menstrual irregularities, gynecomastia, and hypogonadism) associated with spironolactone.[268] If the hypertension persists in patients with bilateral hyperplasia, administration of an angiotensin converting enzyme inhibitor may be beneficial, perhaps reflecting the role of angiotensin II as an aldosterone secretagogue in this disorder.

A K^+-sparing diuretic is also indicated in the syndrome of apparent mineralocorticoid excess (in which cortisol is the major endogenous mineralocorticoid) and in Liddle's syndrome. In the latter disorder, either amiloride or triamterene should be given to close the Na^+ channels in the collecting tubule; spironolactone is relatively ineffective, since the increase in Na^+ channel activity is not mediated by aldosterone.[132]

In comparison, dexamethasone or another glucocorticoid is the treatment of choice in those patients with bilateral hyperplasia in whom aldosterone secretion appears to be mediated by ACTH (e.g., CYP11B1- or CYP17-deficient forms of congenital adrenal hyperplasia or glucocorticoid-remediable hyperaldosteronism). The last disorder should be suspected when children with a positive family history of hypertension (often in young adults) are affected.[100] The dexamethasone dose should be the lowest required to correct the hypokalemia and hypertension. Signs or symptoms of glucocorticoid excess should not occur.

PROBLEMS

27-1 A 22-year-old woman complains of easy fatigability and weakness. She has no other complaints. The physical examination is unremarkable, including a normal blood pressure. The following laboratory data are obtained:

$$Plasma\ [Na^+] = 141\ meq/L$$

$$[K^+] = 2.1\ meq/L$$

$$[Cl^-] = 85\ meq/L$$

$$[HCO_3^-] = 45\ meq/L$$

$$Urine\ [Na+] = 80\ meq/day$$

$$[K^+] = 170\ meq/day$$

(a) What is the differential diagnosis?
(b) What test would you order next?

27-2 A patient is noted to have a plasma K^+ concentration of 2.7 meq/L. Match the other laboratory changes that are present with the likely diagnosis.

(a)	Plasma $[HCO_3^-]$	=	27 meq/L	1.	Renal tubular acidosis
	Arterial pH	=	7.43		
	Urine $[K^+]$	=	10 meq/L		
	U_{osm}	=	102 mosmol/kg	2.	Hypomagnesemia
(b)	Plasma $[HCO_3^-]$	=	27 meq/L		
	$[Ca^{2+}]$	=	7.3 mg/dL		
	[Albumin]	=	4.1 g/dL	3.	Primary polydipsia
	Arterial pH	=	7.46		
	Urine $[K^+]$	=	45 meq/day		
(c)	Plasma $[HCO_3^-]$	=	14 meq/L	4.	Laxative abuse
	Arterial pH	=	7.28		
	Urine $[K^+]$	=	52 meq/day		
	Urine pH	=	6.0		
	Urine anion gap	=	+25	5.	Primary hyperaldosteronism
(d)	Plasma $[HCO_3^-]$	=	14 meq/L		
	Arterial pH	=	7.28		
	Urine $[K^+]$	=	18 meq/day	6.	Vomiting
	Urine pH	=	4.9		
	Urine anion gap	=	-27		

REFERENCES

1. Womersley RA, Darragh JH. Potassium and sodium restriction in the normal human. *J Clin Invest* 34:456, 1955.
2. Squires RD, Huth EJ. Experimental potassium depletion in normal human subjects: I. Relation of ionic intakes to the renal conservation of potassium. *J Clin Invest* 38:1134, 1959.
3. Garg LC. Respective roles of H-ATPase and H-K-ATPase in ion transport in the kidney. *J Am Soc Nephrol* 2:949, 1991.
4. Okusa MD, Unwin RJ, Velazquez H, et al. Active potassium absorption by the renal distal tubule. *Am J Physiol* 262:F488, 1992.
5. Linas SL, Peterson LN, Anderson RJ, et al. Mechanism of renal potassium conservation in the rat. *Kidney Int* 15:601, 1979.
6. Stetson DL, Wade JB, Giebisch G. Morphologic alterations in the rat medullary collecting duct following potassium depletion. *Kidney Int* 17:45, 1980.
7. Kraut JA, Hiura J, Besancon M, et al. Effect of hypokalemia on the abundance of HK alpha 1 and HK alpha 2 protein in the rat kidney. *Am J Physiol* 272:F744, 1997.
8. Langford HG. Dietary potassium and hypertension: Epidemiologic data. *Ann Intern Med* 98(part 2):770, 1983.
9. Amatruda JM, Biddle TL, Patton ML, Lockwood DH. Vigorous supplementation of a hypocaloric diet prevents cardiac arrhythmias and mineral depletion. *Am J Med* 74:1016, 1983.
10. Gonzalez JJ, Owens JW, Ungaro PC, et al. Clay ingestion: A rare cause of hypokalemia. *Ann Intern Med* 97:65, 1982.
11. Gelfand MC, Zarate A, Knepshield JH. Geophagia: A cause of life-threatening hyperkalemia in patients with chronic renal failure. *JAMA* 234:738, 1975.

12. Giebisch GE, Berger L, Pitts RF. The extrarenal response to acute acid-base disturbances of respiratory origin. *J Clin Invest* 34:231, 1955.

13. Adrogué HJ, Madias NE. Changes in plasma potassium concentration during acute acid-base disturbances. *Am J Med* 71:456, 1981.

14. Fraley DS, Adler S. Correction of hyperkalemia by bicarbonate despite constant blood pH. *Kidney Int* 12:354, 1977.

15. Kassirer JP, London AM, Goldman DM, Schwartz WB. On the pathogenesis of metabolic alkalosis in hyperaldosteronism. *Am J Med* 49:306, 1970.

16. Cooke RE, Segar W, Cheek DB, et al. The extrarenal correction of alkalosis associated with potassium deficiency. *J Clin Invest* 31:798, 1952.

17. Orloff J, Kennedy T Jr, Berliner RW. The effect of potassium in nephrectomized rats with hypokalemic alkalosis. *J Clin Invest* 32:538, 1953.

18. Sabatini S, Kurtzman NA. The maintenance of metabolic alkalosis: Factors which decrease HCO_3^- excretion. *Kidney Int* 25:357, 1984.

19. Capasso G, Kinne R, Malnic G, Giebisch G. Renal bicarbonate reabsorption in the rat: I. Effects of hypokalemia and carbonic anhydrase. *J Clin Invest* 78:1558, 1986.

20. Capasso G, Jaeger P, Giebisch G, et al. Renal bicarbonate reabsorption in the rat: II. Distal tubule load dependence and effect of hypokalemia. *J Clin Invest* 80:409, 1987.

21. Adam WR, Koretsky AP, Weiner MW. ^{31}P-NMR in vivo measurement of renal intracellular pH: Effects of acidosis and potassium depletion in rats. *Am J Physiol* 251:F904, 1986.

22. Elam-Ong S, Kurtzman NA, Sabatini S. Regulation of collecting tubule adenosine triphosphatases by aldosterone and potassium. *J Clin Invest* 91:2385, 1993.

23. DuBose TD Jr, Good DW. Effects of chronic hyperkalemia on renal production and proximal tubular transport of ammonium in rats. *Am J Physiol* 260:F680, 1991.

24. DuBose TD Jr, Good DW. Chronic hyperkalemia impairs ammonium transport and accumulation in the inner medulla of the rat. *J Clin Invest* 90:1443, 1992.

25. Zierler KL, Rabinowitz D. Effect of very small concentrations of insulin on forearm metabolism: Persistence of its action on potassium and free fatty acids without its effects on glucose. *J Clin Invest* 43:950, 1964.

26. Minaker KL, Rowe JW. Potassium homeostasis during hyperinsulinemia: Effect of insulin level, β-blockade, and age. *Am J Physiol* 242:E373, 1982.

27. Ferrannini E, Taddei S, Santoro D, et al. Independent stimulation of glucose metabolism and Na^+-K^+ exchange by insulin in the human forearm. *Am J Physiol* 255:E953, 1988.

28. Clausen T, Everts ME. Regulation of the Na,K-pump in skeletal muscle. *Kidney Int* 35:1, 1989.

29. Adrogué HJ, Lederer ED, Suki WN, Eknoyan G. Determinants of plasma potassium levels in diabetic ketoacidosis. *Medicine* 65:163, 1986.

30. Kunin AS, Surawicz B, Sims EAH. Decrease in serum potassium concentration and appearance of cardiac arrythmias during infusion of potassium with glucose in potassium-depleted patients. *N Engl J Med* 266:228, 1962.

31. Petersen K-G, Schluter KJ, Kerp L. Regulation of serum potassium during insulin-induced hypoglycemia. *Diabetes* 31:615, 1982.

32. DeFronzo RA, Bia M, Birkhead G. Epinephrine and potassium homeostasis. *Kidney Int* 20:83, 1981.

33. Brown MJ, Brown DC, Murphy MB. Hypokalemia from beta$_2$-receptor stimulation by circulating epinephrine. *N Engl J Med* 309:1414, 1983.

34. Morgan DB, Young RM. Acute transient hypokalemia: New interpretation of a common event. *Lancet* 2:751, 1982.

35. Struthers AD, Whitesmith R, Reid JL. Prior thiazide treatment increases adrenaline-induced hypokalemia. *Lancet* 1:1358, 1983.

36. Grimm RH Jr. The drug treatment of mild hypertension in the Multiple Risk Factor Intervention Trial: A review. *Drugs* 31(suppl 1):13, 1986.

37. Salerno DM. Postresuscitation hypokalemia in a patient with a normal prearrest serum potassium level. *Ann Intern Med* 108:836, 1988.

38. Wadstein J, Skude G. Does hypokalaemia precede delirium tremens? *Lancet* 2:549, 1978.

39. Conci F, Procaccio F, Boselli L. Hypokalemia from beta$_2$-receptor stimulation by epinephrine (letter). *N Engl J Med* 310:1329, 1984.

40. Shannon M, Lovejoy FH Jr. Hypokalemia after theophylline intoxication: The effects of acute vs chronic poisoning. *Arch Intern Med* 149:2725, 1989.

41. Lipworth BJ, McDevitt DG, Struthers AD. Prior treatment with diuretic augments the hypokalemic and electrocardiographic effects of inhaled albuterol. *Am J Med* 86:653, 1989.

42. Wong CS, Pavord ID, Williams J, et al. Bronchodilator, cardiovascular, and hypokalaemic effects of fenoterol, salbutamol, and terbutaline in asthma. *Lancet* 336:1396, 1990.

43. Goldenberg IF, Olivari MT, Levine TB, Cohn JN. Effect of dobutamine on plasma potassium in congestive heart failure secondary to idiopathic or ischemic cardiomyopathy. *Am J Cardiol* 63:843, 1989.

44. Braden GL, von Oeyen PT, Germain MJ, et al. Ritodrine- and terbutaline-induced hypokalemia in preterm labor: Mechanisms and consequences. *Kidney Int* 51:1867, 1997.

45. Montoliu J, Lens KL, Revert L. Potassium lowering effect of albuterol for hyperkalemia in renal failure. *Arch Intern Med* 147:713, 1987.

46. Reid JL, White KF, Struthers AD. Epinephrine-induced hypokalemia: The role of beta adrenoceptors. *Am J Cardiol* 57:23F, 1986.

47. Fontaine B, Lapie P, Plassart E, et al. Periodic paralysis and voltage-gated ion channels. *Kidney Int* 49:9, 1996.

48. Layzer RB. Periodic paralysis and the sodium-potassium pump. *Ann Neurol* 11:547, 1982.

49. McFadzean AJS, Yeung R. Periodic paralysis complicating thyrotoxicosis in Chinese. *Br Med J* 1:451, 1967.

50. Conway MJ, Seibel JA, Eaton RP. Thyrotoxicosis and periodic paralysis: Improvement with beta blockade. *Ann Intern Med* 81:332, 1974.

51. Yeung RTT, Tse TF. Thyrotoxic periodic paralysis: Effect of propranolol. *Am J Med* 57:584, 1974.

52. Ober KP. Thyrotoxic periodic paralysis in the United States: Report of seven cases and review of the literature. *Medicine (Baltimore)* 71:109, 1992.

53. Ko GT, Chow CC, Yeung VT, et al. Thyrotoxic periodic paralysis in a Chinese population. *Q J Med* 89:463, 1996.

54. Manoukian MA, Foote JA, Crapo LM. Clinical and metabolic features of thyrotoxic periodic paralysis in 24 episodes. *Arch Intern Med* 159:601, 1999.

55. Ptacek LJ, Tawil R, Griggs RC, et al. Dihydropyridine receptor mutations cause hypokalemic period paralysis. *Cell* 77:863, 1994.

56. Sillen A, Sorensen T, Kantola I, et al. Identification of mutations in the CACNL1A3 gene in 13 families of Scandinavian origin having hypokalemic periodic paralysis and evidence of a founder effect in Danish families. *Am J Med Genet* 69:102, 1997.

57. Tanabe T, Beam KG, Powell JA, Numa S. Restoration of excitation-contraction coupling and slow calcium current in dysgenic muscle by dihydropyridine receptor complementary DNA. *Nature* 336:134, 1988.

58. Tricarico D, Servidei S, Tonali P, et al. Impairment of skeletal muscle adenosine triphosphate-sensitive K^+ channels in patients with hypokalemic periodic paralysis. *J Clin Invest* 103:675, 1999.

59. Ruff RL. Insulin acts in hypokalemic periodic paralysis by reducing inward rectifier K^+ current. *Neurology* 53:1556, 1999.

60. Chan A, Shinde R, Cockram CS, Swaminathan R. In vivo and in vitro sodium pump activity in subjects with thyrotoxic periodic paralysis. *Br Med J* 303:1096, 1991.

61. Resnick JS, Engel WL, Griggs RC, Stam AC. Acetazolamide prophylaxis in hypokalemic periodic paralysis. *N Engl J Med* 278:582, 1968.

62. Riggs JE, Griggs RC, Moxley RT III. Dissociation of glucose and potassium arterial-venous differences across the forearm by acetazolamide: A possible relationship to acetazolamide's beneficial effect in hypokalemic periodic paralysis. *Arch Neurol* 41:35, 1984.

63. Lawson DH, Murray RM, Parker JLW. Early mortality in the megaloblastic anaemias. *Q J Med* 41:1, 1972.

64. Viens P, Thyss A, Garnier G, et al. GM-CSF treatment of hypokalemia (letter). *Ann Intern Med* 111:236, 1989.
65. Rao TLK, Mathru M, Salem MR, El-Etr AA. Serum potassium levels following transfusion of frozen erythrocytes. *Anesthesiology* 52:170, 1980.
66. Adams PC, Woodhouse KW, Adela M, Parnham A. Exaggerated hypokalemia in acute myeloid leukaemia. *Br Med J* 282:1034, 1981.
67. Koht AL, Cerullo LJ, Land PC, Linde HW. Serum potassium levels during prolonged hypothermia. *Anesthesiology* 51(suppl):S203, 1979.
68. Schaller M-D, Fischer AP, Perret CH. Hyperkalemia: A prognostic factor during acute severe hypothermia. *JAMA* 264:1842, 1990.
69. Clemessy JL, Favier C, Borron SW, et al. Hypokalaemia related to acute chloroquine ingestion. *Lancet* 346:877, 1995.
70. Kassirer JP, Schwartz WB. The response of normal man to selective depletion of hydrochloric acid: Factors in the genesis of persistent gastric alkalosis. *Am J Med* 40:10, 1966.
71. Watten RH, Morgan FM, Songkhla YN, et al. Water and electrolyte studies in cholera. *J Clin Invest* 38:1879, 1959.
72. Krejs GJ. VIPoma syndrome. *Am J Med* 82(suppl 5B):37, 1987.
73. Grier JF. WDHA (watery diarrhea, hypokalemia, achlorhydria) syndrome: Clinical features, diagnosis and treatment. *South Med J* 88:22, 1995.
74. McArthur KE, Anderson DS, Durbin TE, et al. Clonidine and lidamidine to inhibit watery diarrhea in a patient with lung cancer. *Ann Intern Med* 96:323, 1980.
75. Older J, Older P, Colker J, Brown R. Secretory villous adenomas that cause depletion syndromes. *Arch Intern Med* 159:879, 1999.
76. Schwartz WB, Relman AS. Metabolic and renal studies in chronic potassium depletion resulting from overuse of laxatives. *J Clin Invest* 32:538, 1953.
77. Agarwal R, Afzalpurkar R, Fordtran JS. Pathophysiology of potassium absorption and secretion by the human intestine. *Gastroenterology* 107:548, 1994.
78. Siegel D, Hulley SB, Black DM, et al. Diuretics, serum and intracellular electrolyte levels, and arrhythmias in hypertensive men. *JAMA* 267:1083, 1992.
79. Schnaper HW, Freis ED, Friedman RG, et al. Potassium restoration in hypertensive patients made hypokalemic by hydrochlorothiazide. *Arch Intern Med* 149:2677, 1989.
80. Hropot M, Fowler N, Karlmark B, Giebisch G. Tubular action of diuretics: Distal effects of electrolyte transport and acidification. *Kidney Int* 28:477, 1985.
81. Duarte CG, Chomety F, Giebisch G. Effect of amiloride, ouabain, and furosemide on distal tubular function in the rat. *Am J Physiol* 221:632, 1971.
82. Carlsen JE, Kober L, Torp-Pedersen C, Johannsen P. Relation between dose of bendrofluazide, antihypertensive effect, and adverse biochemical effects. *Br Med J* 300:975, 1990.
83. Johnston GD, Wilson R, McDermott BJ, et al. Low-dose cyclopenthiazide in the treatment of hypertension: A one-year community-based study. *Q J Med* 78:135, 1991.
84. Maronde R, Milgrom M, Vlachakis ND, Chan L. Response of thiazide-induced hypokalemia to amiloride. *JAMA* 249:237, 1983.
85. Kuller LH, Hulley SB, Cohen JD, Neaton J. Unexpected effects of treating hypertension in men with electrocardiographic abnormalities: A critical analysis. *Circulation* 73:114, 1986.
86. Siscovick DS, Raghunathan TE, Psaty BM, et al. Diuretic therapy for hypertension and the risk of primary cardiac arrest. *N Engl J Med* 330:1852, 1994.
87. Pitt B, Zannad F, Remme WJ, et al, for the Randomized Aldactone Evaluation Study Investigators. The effect of spironolactone on morbidity and mortality in patients with severe heart failure. *N Engl J Med* 341:709, 1999.
88. Hoes AW, Grobbee DE, Lubsen JL, et al. Diuretics, beta blockers, and the risk for sudden cardiac death in hypertensive patients. *Ann Intern Med* 123:481, 1995.
89. Cooper HA, Dries DL, Davis CE, et al. Diuretics and risk of arrhythmic death in patients with left ventricular dysfunction. *Circulation* 100:1311, 1999.
90. Kaplan NM, Carnegie A, Raskin P, et al. Potassium supplementation in hypertensive patients with diuretic-induced hypokalemia. *N Engl J Med* 312:746, 1985.

91. Whelton PK, He J, Cutler JA, et al. Effects of oral potassium on blood pressure: Meta-analysis of randomized controlled clinical trials. *JAMA* 277:1624, 1997.
92. Bravo EL, Tarazi RC, Dustan HP, et al. The changing clinical spectrum of primary aldosteronism. *Am J Med* 74:641, 1983.
93. Biglieri EG. Spectrum of mineralocorticoid hypertension. *Hypertension* 17:251, 1991.
94. Rose BD, Kaplan NM. Approach to the patient with hypertension and hypokalemia, in Rose BD (ed): *UpToDate in Medicine*. Wellesley, MA, UpToDate, 2000.
95. Stewart PM. Mineralocorticoid hypertension. *Lancet* 353:1341, 1999.
96. Seldin D, Welt L, Cort J. The role of sodium salts and adrenal steroids in the production of hypokalemic alkalosis. *Yale J Biol Med* 29:229, 1956.
97. Haack D, Mohring J, Mohring B, et al. Comparative study on development of corticosterone and DOCA hypertension in rats. *Am J Physiol* 233:F403, 1978.
98. Robertson GL, Aycinena P, Zerbe RL. Neurogenic disorders of osmoregulation. *Am J Med* 72:339, 1982.
99. Lifton RP, Dluhy RG, Powers M, et al. Hereditary hypertension caused by chimaeric gene duplications and ectopic expression of aldosterone synthase. *Nat Genet* 2:66, 1992.
100. Rich GM, Ulick S, Cook S, et al. Glucocorticoid-remediable aldosteronism in a large kindred: Clinical spectrum and diagnosis using a characteristic biochemical phenotype. *Ann Intern Med* 116:813, 1992.
101. Torpy DJ, Gordon RD, Lin JP, et al. Familial hyperaldosteronism type II: Description of a large kindred and exclusion of the aldosterone synthase (CYP11B2) gene. *J Clin Endocrinol Metab* 83:3214, 1998.
102. Funder J. Enzymes and the regulation of sodium balance. *Kidney Int* 41(suppl 37):S-114, 1992.
103. Morris DJ, Souness GW. Protective and specificity-conferring mechanisms of mineralocorticoid action. *Am J Physiol* 263:F759, 1992.
104. Ulick S, Wang JZ, Blumenfeld JD, Pickering TG. Cortisol inactivation overload: A mechanism of mineralocorticoid hypertension in the ectopic adrenocorticotropin syndrome. *J Clin Endocrinol Metab* 74:963, 1992.
105. Biglieri EG, Slaton PE, Schambelan M, Kronfield SJ. Hypermineralocorticoidism. *Am J Med* 45:170, 1968.
106. Christy NP, Laragh JH. Pathogenesis of hypokalemic alkalosis in Cushing's syndrome. *N Engl J Med* 265:1083, 1961.
107. Orth DN. Causes and pathophysiology of Cushing's syndrome, in Rose BD (ed): *UpToDate in Medicine*. Wellesley, MA, UpToDate, 2000.
108. Findling JW. The Cushing syndromes: An enlarging clinical spectrum. *N Engl J Med* 321:1677, 1989.
109. Whitworth JA. Adrenocorticotropin and steroid-induced hypertension in humans. *Kidney Int* 41(suppl 37):S-34, 1992.
110. Saruta T, Suzuki H, Handa M, et al. Multiple factors contribute to the pathogenesis of hypertension in Cushing's syndrome. *J Clin Endocrinol Metab* 62:275, 1986.
111. Orth DN. Establishing the diagnosis of Cushing's syndrome, in Rose BD (ed): *UpToDate in Medicine*. Wellesley, MA, UpToDate, 2000.
112. Orth DN. Establishing the cause of Cushing's syndrome, in Rose BD (ed): *UpToDate in Medicine*. Wellesley, MA, UpToDate, 2000.
113. Orth DN. Overview of the treatment of Cushing's syndrome, in Rose BD (ed): *UpToDate in Medicine*. Wellesley, MA, UpToDate, 2000.
114. Jeffcoate WJ. Treating Cushing's disease. *Br Med J* 296:227, 1988.
115. White PC, New MI, Dupont B. Congenital adrenal hyperplasia. *N Engl J Med* 316:1519, 1987.
116. Lamberts SW, Koper JW, Biemond P, et al. Cortisol receptor resistance: The variability of its clinical presentation and response to treatment. *J Clin Endocrinol Metab* 74:313, 1992.
117. Hurley DM, Accili D, Stratakis CA, et al. Point mutation of a single amino acid substitution in the hormone binding domain of the glucocorticoid receptor in familial glucocorticoid resistance. *J Clin Invest* 87:680, 1991.

118. Blachley JD, Knochel JP. Tobacco chewer's hypokalemia: Licorice revisited. *N Engl J Med* 302:784, 1980.

119. Farese RV Jr, Biglieri EG, Schackleton CHL, et al. Licorice-induced hypermineralocorticoidism. *N Engl J Med* 325:1223, 1991.

120. de Klerk GJ, Nieuwenhuis MG, Beutler JJ. Hypokalemia and hypertension associated with the use of liquorice flavoured chewing gum. *Br Med J* 314:731, 1997.

121. Kenouch S, Coutry N, Farman N, Bonvalet J-P. Multiple patterns of 11β-hydroxysteroid dehydrogenase catalytic activity along the mammalian nephron. *Kidney Int* 42:56, 1992.

122. Mune T, Rogerson FM, Nikkila H, et al. Human hypertension caused by mutations in the kidney isozyme of 11β-hydroxysteroid dehydrogenase. *Nat Genet* 10:394, 1995.

123. Dave-Sharma S, Wilson RC, Harbison MD, et al. Examination of genotype and phenotype relationships in 14 patients with apparent mineralocorticoid excess. *J Clin Endocrinol Metab* 83:2244, 1998.

124. White PC, Mune T, Agarwal AK. 11β-hydroxysteroid dehydrogenase and the syndrome of apparent mineralocorticoid excess. *Endocr Rev* 18:135, 1997.

125. Conn JW, Cohen EL, Lucas CP, et al. Primary reninism. *Arch Intern Med* 130:682, 1972.

126. Baruch D, Corvol P, Alhenc-Gelas F, et al. Diagnosis and treatment of renin-secreting tumors: Report of three cases. *Hypertension* 6:760, 1984.

127. Haab F, Duclos JM, Guyenne T, et al. Renin secreting tumors: Diagnosis, conservative therapeutic approach, and long-term results. *J Urol* 153:1781, 1995.

128. Kondo K, Saruta T, Saito I, et al. Benign desoxycorticosterone-producing adrenal tumor. *JAMA* 236:1042, 1976.

129. Mantero F, Armanini D, Opocher G, et al. Mineralocorticoid hypertension due to a nasal spray containing α-fluroprednisolone. *Am J Med* 71:352, 1981.

130. Shimkets RA, Warnock DG, Bositis CM, et al. Liddle''s syndrome: Heritable human hypertension caused by mutations in the beta subunit of the epithelial sodium channel. *Cell* 79:407, 1994.

131. Snyder PM, Price MP, McDonald FJ, et al. Mechanisms by which Liddle's syndrome mutations increase activity of a human epithelial Na^+ channel. *Cell* 83:969, 1995.

132. Botero-Velez M, Curtis JJ, Warnock DG. Brief report: Liddle's syndrome revisited: A disorder of sodium reabsorption in the distal tubule. *N Engl J Med* 330:178, 1994.

133. Stein JH. The pathogenetic spectrum of Bartter's syndrome. *Kidney Int* 28:85, 1985.

134. Monnens L, Bindels R, Grunfeld JP. Gitelman syndrome comes of age (editorial). *Nephrol Dial Transplant* 13:1617, 1998.

135. Cruz DN, Simon DB, Farhi A, et al. Reduced blood pressure in Gitelman's syndrome: A study of a large extended kindred (abstract). *J Am Soc Nephrol* 9:322A, 1998.

136. Gamba G. Molecular biology of distal nephron sodium transport mechanisms. *Kidney Int* 56:1606, 1999.

137. Simon DB, Karent FE, Hamdan JM, et al. Bartter's syndrome, hypokalaemic alkalosis with hypercalciuria, is cased by mutations in the Na-K-2Cl cotransporter NKCCC2. *Nat Genet* 13:183, 1996.

138. Simon DB, Karet FE, Rodriguez-Soriano J, et al. Genetic heterogeneity of Bartter's syndrome revealed by mutations in the K^+ channel, ROMK. *Nat Genet* 14:152, 1996.

139. Simon DB, Bindra RS, Mansfield TA, et al. Mutations in the chloride channel gene, CLCNKB, cause Bartter's syndrome type III. *Nat Genet* 17:171, 1997.

140. Simon DB, Nelson-Williams C, Bia MJ, et al. Gitelman's variant of Bartter's syndrome, inherited hypokalemic alkalosis, is caused by mutations in the thiazide-sensitive sodium-chloride cotransporter. *Nat Genet* 12:24, 1996.

141. Bettinelli A, Bianchetti MG, Borella P, et al. Genetic heterogeneity in tubular hypomagnesemia-hypokalemia with hypocalciuria (Gitelman's syndrome). *Kidney Int* 47:547, 1995.

142. Dunn MJ. Prostaglandins and Bartter's syndrome. *Kidney Int* 19:86, 1981.

143. Bettinelli A, Bianchetti MG, Girardin E, et al. Use of calcium excretion values to distinguish two forms of primary renal tubular hypokalemic alkalosis: Bartter and Gitelman syndrome. *J Pediatr* 120:38, 1992.

144. Simon DB, Cruz DN, Lu Y, Lifton RP. Genotype-phenotype correlation of NCCT mutations and Gitelman's syndrome (abstract). *J Am Soc Nephrol* 9:111A, 1998.

145. Jamison RL, Ross JC, Kempson RL, et al. Surreptitious diuretic ingestion and pseudo-Bartter's syndrome. *Am J Med* 73:142, 1982.

146. Sasaki S, Okumura M, Kawasaki T, et al. Indomethacin and atrial natriuretic peptide in pseudo-Bartter's syndrome. *N Engl J Med* 316:167, 1987.

147. Veldhuis JD, Bardin CW, Demers LM. Metabolic mimicry of Bartter's syndrome by covert vomiting: Utility of urinary chloride determinations. *Am J Med* 66:361, 1979.

148. Vinci JM, Gill JR Jr, Bowden RE, et al. The kallikrein-kinin system in Bartter's syndrome and its response to prostaglandin synthetase inhibition. *J Clin Invest* 61:1671, 1978.

149. Griffing GT, Komanicky P, Aurecchia SA, et al. Amiloride in Bartter's syndrome. *Clin Pharmacol Ther* 31:713, 1982.

150. Colussi G, Rombola G, De Ferrari ME, et al. Correction of hypokalemia with antialdosterone therapy in Gitelman's syndrome. *Am J Nephrol* 14:127, 1994.

151. Hene RJ, Koomans HA, Dorhout Mees EJ, et al. Correction of hypokalemia in Bartter's syndrome by enalapril. *Am J Kidney Dis* 9:200, 1987.

152. Morales JM, Ruilope LM, Praga M, et al. Long-term enalapril therapy in Bartter's syndrome. *Nephron* 48:327, 1988.

153. Wrong OM, Feest TG, MacIver AG. Immune-related potassium-losing interstitial nephritis: A comparison with distal renal tubular acidosis. *Q J Med* 86:513, 1993.

154. Bricker NS, Shwayri ES, Reardon JB, et al. An abnormality in renal function resulting from urinary tract obstruction. *Am J Med* 23:554, 1957.

155. Potter WZ, Trygstad CW, Helmer OM, et al. Familial hypokalemia associated with renal interstitial fibrosis. *Am J Med* 57:971, 1974.

156. Gullner H-G, Bartter FC, Gill Jr, et al. A sibship with hypokalemic alkalosis and renal proximal tubulopathy. *Arch Intern Med* 143:1534, 1983.

157. Uribarri J, Oh MS, Carroll HJ. Salt-losing nephropathy: Clinical presentation and mechanisms. *Am J Nephrol* 3:193, 1983.

158. Popovtzer MM, Katz FH, Pinggera WF, et al. Hyperkalemia in salt-wasting nephropathy: Study of the mechanism. *Arch Intern Med* 132:203, 1973.

159. Aldinger KA, Samaan NA. Hypokalemia with hypercalcemia: Prevalence and significance in treatment. *Ann Intern Med* 87:571, 1977.

160. Muggia FM, Heinemann HO, Farhangi M, Osserman EF. Lysozymuria and renal tubular dysfunction in monocytic and myelomonocytic leukemia. *Am J Med* 47:351, 1969.

161. Mir MA, Brabin B, Tang OT, et al. Hypokalaemia in acute myeloid leukaemia. *Ann Intern Med* 82:54, 1975.

162. Evans JJ, Bosdech MJ. Hypokalemia in nonblastic chronic myelogenous leukemia. *Arch Intern Med* 141:786, 1981.

163. Lipner HT, Ruzany F, Dasgupta M, et al. The behavior of carbenicillin as a nonreabsorbable anion. *J Lab Clin Med* 86:183, 1975.

164. Carlisle EJF, Donnelly SM, Ethier JH, et al. Modulation of the secretion of potassium by accompanying anions in humans. *Kidney Int* 39:1206, 1991.

165. Carlisle EJF, Donnelly SM, Vasuvattakul S, et al. Glue-sniffing and distal renal tubular acidosis: Sticking to the facts. *J Am Soc Nephrol* 1:1019, 1991.

166. Gennari FJ, Cohen JJ. Role of the kidney in potassium homeostasis: Lessons from acid-base disturbances. *Kidney Int* 8:1, 1975.

167. Sebastian A, McSherry E, Morris RC Jr. Renal potassium wasting in renal tubular acidosis (RTA): Its occurrence in types 1 and 2 RTA despite sustained correction of systemic acidosis. *J Clin Invest* 50:667, 1971.

168. Pun K-K, Wong C-K, Tsui E-L, et al. Hypokalemic periodic paralysis due to the Sjogren's syndrome in Chinese patients. *Ann Intern Med* 110:405, 1989.

169. Cogan MG, Rector FC. Proximal reabsorption during metabolic acidosis in the rat. *Am J Physiol* 242:F499, 1982.

170. Douglas JB, Healy JK. Nephrotoxic effects of amphotericin B, including renal tubular acidosis. *Am J Med* 46:154, 1979.
171. Berns JS, Cohen RM, Stumacher RJ, Rudnick MR. Renal aspects of therapy for human immunodeficiency virus and associated opportunistic infections. *J Am Soc Nephrol* 1:1061, 1991.
172. Cheng J-T, Witty RT, Robinson RR, Yarger WE. Amphotericin B nephrotoxicity: Increased renal assistance and tubule permeability. *Kidney Int* 22:626, 1982.
173. Whang R, Oei TO, Aidawa JK, et al. Magnesium and potassium interrelationships. Experimental and clinical. *Acta Med Scand* 647: (suppl):139, 1981.
174. Whang R, Whang DD, Ryan MP. Refractory potassium depletion. A consequence of magnesium deficiency. *Arch Intern Med* 152:40, 1992.
175. Dirks JH. The kidney and magnesium regulation. *Kidney Int* 23:771, 1983.
176. Schilsky RL, Anderson T. Hypomagnesemia and renal magnesium wasting in patients receiving cisplatin. *Ann Intern Med* 90:929, 1979.
177. Shils ME. Experimental human magnesium depletion. *Medicine* 48:61, 1969.
178. Nichols CG, Ho K, Hebert S. Mg^{2+}-dependent inward rectification of ROMK1 channels expressed in *Xenopus* oocytes. *J Physiol (Lond)* 476:339, 1994.
179. Kelepouris E. Cystosolic Mg^{2+} modulates whole cell K^+ and Cl^- currents in cortical thick ascending limb (TAL) cells of rabbit kidney. *Kidney Int* 37:564, 1990.
180. Rude RK, Oldham SB, Sharp CF Jr, Singer FR. Parathyroid hormone secretion in magnesium deficiency. *J Clin Endocrinol Metab* 47:800, 1978.
181. Estep H, Shaw WA, Watlington C, et al. Hypocalcemia due to hypomagnesemia and reversible parathyroid hormone unresponsiveness. *J Clin Endocrinol Metab* 29:842, 1969.
182. Freitag JJ, Martin KJ, Conrades MB, et al. Skeletal resistance to parathyroid hormone in magnesium deficiency: Studies in isolated perfused bone. *J Clin Invest* 64:1238, 1979.
183. Fatemi S, Ryzen E, Flores J, et al. Effect of experimental human magnesium depletion on parathyroid hormone secretion and 1,25-dihydroxyvitamin D metabolism. *J Clin Endocrinol Metab* 73:1067, 1991.
184. Farkas RA, McAllister CT, Blachley JD. Effect of magnesium salt anions on potassium balance in normal and magnesium depleted rats. *J Lab Clin Med* 110:412, 1987.
185. Hariprasad MK, Eisinger RP, Nadler IM, et al. Hyponatremia in psychogenic polydipsia. *Arch Intern Med* 140:1639, 1980.
186. Granerus A-K, Jagenburg R, Svanborg A. Kaliuretic effect of L-dopa treatment in Parkinsonian patients. *Acta Med Scand* 201:291, 1977.
187. Knochel JP, Dotin LN, Hamburger RJ. Pathophysiology of intense physical conditioning in hot climate: I. Mechanism of potassium depletion. *J Clin Invest* 51:242, 1972.
188. Kosunen KJ, Pakarinen AJ. Plasma renin, angiotensin II, and plasma and urinary aldosterone in running exercise. *J Appl Physiol* 41:26, 1976.
189. Rostand SG. Profound hypokalemia in continuous ambulatory peritoneal dialysis. *Arch Intern Med* 143:377, 1983.
190. Khan AN, Bernardini J, Johnston JR, Piraino B. Hypokalemia in peritoneal dialysis patients (letter). *Peri Dial Int* 16:652, 1996.
191. Wiegand CF, Davin TD, Raij L, Kjellstrand CM. Severe hypokalemia induced by hemodialysis. *Arch Intern Med* 141:167, 1981.
192. Sterns RH, Cox M, Feig PU, Singer I. Internal potassium balance and the control of the plasma potassium concentration. *Medicine* 60:339, 1981.
193. Nagant de Deuxchaisnes C, Collet RA, Busset R, Mach RS. Exchangeable potassium in wasting, amyotrophy, heart disease, and cirrhosis of the liver. *Lancet* 1:681, 1961.
194. Casey TH, Summerskill WHJ, Orvis AL. Body and serum potassium in liver disease: I. Relationship to hepatic function and associated factors. *Gastroenterology* 48:198, 1965.
195. Bilbrey GL, Carter NW, White MG, et al. Potassium deficiency in chronic renal failure. *Kidney Int* 4:423, 1973.
196. Edmondson RPS, Thomas RD, Hilton RJ, et al. Leucocyte electrolytes in cardiac and non-cardiac patients receiving diuretics. *Lancet* 1:12, 1974.

197. Cunningham JN Jr, Carter NW, Rector FC Jr, Seldin DW. Resting transmembrane potential difference of skeletal muscle in normal subjects and severely ill patients. *J Clin Invest* 50:49, 1971.
198. Berne RM, Levy MN. *Cardiovascular Physiology*, 4th ed. St Louis, Mosby, 1981, pp. 7–17.
199. Epstein FH. Signs and symptoms of electrolyte disorders, in Maxwell MH, Kleeman CR (eds): *Clinical Disorders of Fluid and Electrolyte Metabolism*, 3rd ed. New York, McGraw-Hill, 1980, pp.
200. Helfant RH. Hypokalemia and arrhythmias. *Am J Med* 80(suppl 4A):13, 1986.
201. Surawicz B. Relationship between electrocardiogram and electrolytes. *Am Heart J* 73:814, 1967.
202. Hollifield JW, Slaton PE. Thiazide diuretics, hypokalemia and cardiac arrhythmias. *Acta Med Scand* 209(suppl 647):67, 1981.
203. Nordrehaug JE, von der Lippe G. Hypokalemia and ventricular fibrillation in acute myocardial infarction. *Br Heart J* 50:525, 1983.
204. Weidmann S. Membrane excitation in cardiac muscle. *Circulation* 24:499, 1961.
205. McLenachan JM, Henderson E, Morris KI, Dargie HJ. Ventricular arrhythmias in patients with hypertensive left ventricular hypertrophy. *N Engl J Med* 317:787, 1987.
206. Davidson S, Surawicz B. Incidence of supraventricular and ventricular ectopic beats and rhythms and of atrioventricular conduction disturbances in patients with hypopotassemia. *Circulation* 34(suppl 3):85, 1966.
207. Lown B, Salzberg H, Enselberg CD, Weston RE. Interrelationship between potassium metabolism and digitalis toxicity in heart failure. *Proc Soc Exp Biol Med* 76:797, 1951.
208. Shapiro W, Taubert K. Hypokalaemia and digoxin-induced arrhythmias. *Lancet* 2:604, 1975.
209. Editorial. U-waves. *Lancet* 2:776, 1983.
210. Dreifus LS, Pick A. A clinical correlative study of the electrocardiogram in electrolyte imbalance. *Circulation* 14:815, 1956.
211. Knochel JP. Neuromuscular manifestation of electrolyte disorders. *Am J Med* 72:521, 1982.
212. Gross EG, Dexter JD, Roth RG. Hypokalemic myopathy with myoglobinuria associated with licorice ingestion. *N Engl J Med* 274:602, 1966.
213. Dominic JA, Koch M, Guthrie GP, Galla JH. Primary aldosteronism presenting as myoglobinuric acute renal failure. *Arch Intern Med* 138:1433, 1978.
214. Knochel JP, Schlein EM. On the mechanism of rhabdomyolysis in potassium depletion. *J Clin Invest* 51:1750, 1972.
215. Relman AS, Schwartz WB. The nephropathy of potassium depletion: A clinical and pathological entity. *N Engl J Med* 255:195, 1956.
216. Schwartz WB, Relman AS. Effects of electrolyte disorders on renal structure and function. *N Engl J Med* 276:383, 452, 1967.
217. Mujais SK, Chen Y, Nora NA. Discordant aspects of aldosterone resistance in potassium depletion. *Am J Physiol* 262:F972, 1992.
218. Rubini M. Water excretion in potassium-deficient man. *J Clin Invest* 40:2215, 1961.
219. Berl T, Linas SL, Aisenbrey GA, Anderson RJ. On the mechanism of polyuria in potassium depletion: The role of polydipsia. *J Clin Invest* 60:620, 1977.
220. Marples D, Prokiaer J, Dorup J, et al. Hypokalemia-induced downregulation of aquaporin-2 water channel expression in rat kidney medullary and cortex. *J Clin Invest* 97:1960, 1996.
221. Luke RG, Wright FS, Fowler N, et al. Effects of potassium depletion on renal tubular chloride transport in the rat. *Kidney Int* 14:414, 1978.
222. Bennett CM. Urine concentration and dilution in hypokalemic and hypercalcemic dogs. *J Clin Invest* 49:1447, 1970.
223. Tannen RL. Relationship of renal ammonia production and potassium homeostasis. *Kidney Int* 11:453, 1977.
224. Baertl JM, Sancelta SM, Gabuzda GJ. Relation of acute potassium depletion to renal ammonium metabolism in patients with cirrhosis. *J Clin Invest* 42:696, 1963.
225. Gabuzda GJ, Hall PW III. Relation of potassium depletion to renal ammonium metabolism and hepatic coma. *Medicine* 45:481, 1966.

226. Jaeger P, Karlmark B, Giebisch G. Ammonia transport in rat cortical tubule. Relationship to potassium metabolism. *Am J Physiol* 245:F593, 1983.
227. Artz SA, Paes IC, Faloon WW. Hypokalemia-induced hepatic coma in cirrhosis: Occurrence despite neomycin therapy. *Gastroenterology* 51:1046, 1966.
228. Fuller GR, MacLeod MB, Pitts RF. Influence of administration of potassium salts on the renal tubular reabsorption of bicarbonate. *Am J Physiol* 182:111, 1955.
229. Torres VE, Young WF Jr, Offord KP, Hattery RR. Association of hypokalemia, aldosteronism, and renal cysts. *N Engl J Med* 322:345, 1990.
230. Menahem SA, Perry GJ, Dowling J, Thomson NM. Hypokalaemia-induced acute renal failure. *Nephrol Dial Transplant* 14:2216, 1999.
231. Tolins JP, Hostetter MK, Hostetter TH. Hypokalemic nephropathy in the rat: Role of ammonia in chronic tubular injury. *J Clin Invest* 79:1447, 1987.
232. Alpern RJ, Toto RD. Hypokalemic nephropathy—A clue to cystogenesis. *N Engl J Med* 322:398, 1990.
233. Riemenschneider T, Bohle A. Morphologic aspects of low-potassium and low-sodium nephropathy. *Clin Nephrol* 19:271, 1983.
234. Friedberg CE, van Burren M, Bijlsma JA, Koomans HA. Insulin increases sodium reabsorption in diluting segment in humans: Evidence for indirect mediation through hypokalemia. *Kidney Int* 40:251, 1991.
235. Krishna GG, Kapoor SC. Potassium depletion exacerbates essential hypertension. *Ann Intern Med* 115:77, 1991.
236. Capuccio F, MacGregor FA. Does potassium supplementation lower blood pressure? A meta-analysis of published trials. *J Hypertens* 9:465, 1991.
237. Grimm RH Jr, Neaton JD, Elmer PJ, et al. The influence of oral potassium chloride on blood pressure in hypertensive men on a low-sodium diet. *N Engl J Med* 322:569, 1990.
238. Garella S, Chazan JA, Cohen JJ. Saline-resistant metabolic alkalosis or "chloride-wasting nephropathy." *Ann Intern Med* 73:31, 1970.
239. Luke RG, Booker BB, Galla JH. Effect of potassium depletion on chloride transport in the loop of Henle in the rat. *Am J Physiol* 248:F682, 1985.
240. Hulter HN, Sigala JF, Sebastian A. K$^+$ deprivation potentiates the renal alkalosis-producing effect of mineralocorticoid. *Am J Physiol* 235:F298, 1978.
241. Light DB, McCann FV, Keller TM, Stanton BA. Amiloride-sensitive cation channel in apical membrane of inner medullary collecting duct. *Am J Physiol* 255:F278, 1988.
242. George JM, Wright L, Bell NH, Bartter FC. The syndrome of primary aldosteronism. *Am J Med* 48:343, 1970.
243. Ganguly A. Primary aldosteronism. *N Engl J Med* 339:1828, 1998.
244. Gordon RD. Mineralocorticoid hypertension. *Lancet* 344:240, 1994.
245. Kono T, Ikeda F, Oseko F, et al. Normotensive primary aldosteronism: Report of a case. *J Clin Endocrinol Metab* 52:1009, 1981.
246. Young DB. Quantitative analysis of aldosterone's role in potassium regulation. *Am J Physiol* 255:F811, 1988.
247. Nakada T, Koike H, Akiya T, et al. Liddle's syndrome, an uncommon form of hyporeninemic hypoaldosteronism: Functional and histopathological studies. *J Urol* 137:636, 1987.
248. Holland OB, Brown H, Kuhnert L, et al. Further evaluation of saline infusion for the diagnosis of primary aldosteronism. *Hypertension* 6:717, 1984.
249. Kaplan NM. Hypokalemia in the hypertensive patient: With observations on the incidence of primary aldosteronism. *Ann Intern Med* 66:1079, 1967.
250. Weinberger MH, Fineberg NS. The diagnosis of primary aldosteronism and separation of two major subtypes. *Arch Intern Med* 153:2125, 1993.
251. Blumenfeld JD, Sealey JE, Schlussel Y, et al. Diagnosis and treatment of primary hyperaldosteronism. *Ann Intern Med* 121:877, 1994.
252. Radin DR, Manoogian C, Nadler JL. Diagnosis of primary hyperaldosteronism: Importance of correlating CT findings with endocrinologic studies. *AJR* 158:553, 1992.

253. Doppman JL, McGill JR, Miller DL, et al. Distinction between hyperaldosteronism due to bilateral hyperplasia and unilateral aldosteronism: Reliability of CT. *Radiology* 184:677, 1992.
254. Gleason PE, Weinberger MH, Pratt JH, et al. Evaluation of diagnostic tests in the differential diagnosis of primary aldosteronism: Unilateral adenoma versus bilateral micronodular hyperplasia. *J Urol* 150:1365, 1993.
255. Gross MD, Shapiro B, Grekin RJ, et al. Scintigraphic localization of adrenal lesions in primary aldosteronism. *Am J Med* 77:839, 1984.
256. Doppman JL, Gill JR Jr. Hyperaldosteronism: Sampling the renal veins. *Radiology* 198:309, 1996.
257. Sheaves R, Goldin J, Reznek RH, et al. Relative value of computed tomography scanning and venous sampling in establishing the cause of primary hyperaldosteronism. *Eur J Endocrinol* 134:308, 1996.
258. Young WF Jr, Stanson AW, Grant CS, et al. Primary aldosteronism: Adrenal venous sampling. *Surgery* 120:913, 1996.
259. Scribner BH, Burnell JM. Interpretation of the serum potassium concentration. *Metabolism* 5:468, 1956.
260. Schwartz WB, van Ypersele de Strihou CE, Kassirer JP. Role of anions in metabolic alkalosis and potassium deficiency. *N Engl J Med* 279:630, 1968.
261. Bleich HL, Tannen RL, Schwartz WB. The induction of metabolic alkalosis by correction of potassium deficiency. *J Clin Invest* 45:573, 1966.
262. Villamil MF, DeLand EC, Henney RP, Maloney JV. Anion effects on cation movements during correction of potassium depletion. *Am J Physiol* 229:161, 1975.
263. Weiss SM, Rutenberg HL, Paskin DL, Zaren HA. Gut lesions due to slow-release KCl tablets. *N Engl J Med* 296:111, 1977.
264. Aselton PJ, Jick H. Short-term follow-up study of war matrix potassium chloride in relation to gastrointestinal bleeding. *Lancet* 1:184, 1983.
265. Sopko JA, Freeman RM. Salt substitutes as a source of potassium. *JAMA* 238:608, 1977.
266. Kopyt N, Dalal F, Narins RG. Renal retention of potassium in fruit (letter). *N Engl J Med* 313:582, 1985.
267. Wassertheil-Smoller S, Blaufox MD, Oberman AS, et al. The trial of antihypertensive interventions and management (TAIM) study: Adequate weight loss, alone and combined with drug therapy in treatment of mild hypertension. *Arch Intern Med* 152:131, 1992.
268. Griffing GT, Cole AG, Aurecchia SA, et al. Amiloride in primary hyperaldosteronism. *Clin Pharmacol Ther* 31:56, 1982.
269. Brown JJ, Davies DL, Ferriss JB, et al. Comparison of surgery and prolonged spironolactone therapy in patients with hypertension, aldosterone excess, and low plasma renin. *Br Med J* 2:729, 1972.
270. Ganguly A, Weinberger MH. Triamterene-thiazide combination: Alternative therapy for primary aldosteronism. *Clin Pharmacol Ther* 30:246, 1981.
271. Keith NM, Osterberg AE, Burchell HB. Some effects of potassium salts in man. *Ann Intern Med* 16:879, 1942.
272. Nicolis GL, Kahn T, Sanchez A, Gabrilove JL. Glucose-induced hyperkalemia in diabetic subjects. *Arch Intern Med* 141:49, 1981.
273. Sterns RH, Feig PU, Pring M, et al. Disposition of intravenous potassium in anuric man: A kinetic analysis. *Kidney Int* 15:651, 1979.
274. Pullen H, Doig A, Lambie AT. Intensive intravenous potassium replacement therapy. *Lancet* 2:809, 1967.
275. Seftel HC, Kew MC. Early and intensive potassium replacement in diabetic acidosis. *Diabetes* 15:694, 1966.
276. Abramson E, Arky R. Diabetic acidosis with initial hypokalemia. *JAMA* 196:401, 1966.
277. Clementsen HJ. Potassium therapy: A break with tradition. *Lancet* 2:175, 1962.
278. Kruse JA, Carlson RW. Rapid correction of hypokalemia using concentrated intravenous potassium chloride infusions. *Arch Intern Med* 150:613, 1990.
279. Swales JD. Hypokalemia and the electrocardiogram. *Lancet* 2:1365, 1964.

280. Takeda M, Go H, Watanabe R, et al. Retroperitoneal laparoscopic adrenalectomy for functioning adrenal tumors: Comparison with conventional transperitoneal lararoscopic adrenalectomy. *J Urol* 157:19, 1997.
281. Biglieri EG, Schambelan M, Slaton PE, Stockigt JR. The intercurrent hypertension of primary aldosteronism. *Circ Res* 27(suppl 1):195, 1970.
282. O'Neil LW, Kissane JM, Hartcroft PM. The kidney in endocrine hypertension. *Arch Surg* 100:498, 1970.
283. Milsom SR, Espiner EA, Nicholls MG, et al. The blood pressure response to unilateral adrenalectomy in primary hyperaldosteronism. *Q J Med* 61:1141, 1986.
284. Celen O, O'Brien MJ, Melby JC, Beazley RM. Factors influencing outcome of surgery for primary aldosteronism. *Arch Surg* 131:646, 1996.
285. Ghose RP, Hall PM, Bravo EL. Medical management of aldosterone-producing adenomas. *Ann Intern Med* 131:105, 1999.

TWENTY-EIGHT

HYPERKALEMIA

The introduction to disorders of K^+ balance presented in Chap. 26 should be read before proceeding with this discussion.

DEFENSE AGAINST HYPERKALEMIA

Hyperkalemia is a rare occurrence in normal subjects, because the body is extremely effective in preventing excess K^+ accumulation in the extracellular fluid. For example, a 40-meq K^+ load could acutely raise the plasma K^+ concentration by 2.4 meq/L or more if it were distributed only through the normal extracellular volume of 15 to 17 L. However, the increment in the plasma K^+ concentration is often less than 1.0 meq/L in this setting,[1] because of an adaptive response consisting of two steps (see Chap. 12):

- Initial uptake of most of the excess K^+ by the cells, mediated primarily by insulin, the β_2-adrenergic receptors (both of which increase the activity of the Na^+-K^+-ATPase pump), and K^+ itself.[2-5]

- The subsequent urinary excretion of most of the excess K^+ within 6 to 8 h.[6,7] The small elevation in the plasma K^+ concentration is responsible for this appropriate increase in K^+ excretion, both directly and by increasing the release of aldosterone.[8-12]

In addition to these acute changes, the ability to tolerate a K^+ load is increased by the chronic ingestion of a high-K^+ diet. As a result, normal subjects can maintain K^+ balance as intake is *slowly* increased from the normal level of about 80 meq/day up to 400 meq/day or more.[13,14] This ability to handle what might be a lethal K^+ load if given acutely is called *K^+ adaptation*. This phenomenon is due primarily to more rapid K^+ excretion in the urine (see Fig. 12-13).[15] Two other factors, both of which are stimulated by aldosterone, also may play a contributory role: a possible increase in K^+ entry into the cells[16,17] and enhanced gastrointestinal losses due to colonic secretion of K^+.[18]

The facilitated kaliuresis during adaptation is due to *enhanced K^+ secretion throughout the late distal nephron*, including the short connecting segment and the principal cells in the cortical and outer medullary collecting tubules.[19-21] Both increased secretion of aldosterone and a small elevation in the plasma K^+ concentration are required for the complete expression of this response.[20,21] They act in part by enhancing Na^+-K^+-ATPase activity in these segments,[22,23] either directly or by increasing the entry of luminal Na^+ into the cell.[11,12] The elevation in pump activity, which is associated with a marked increase in the area of the basolateral membrane (the site at which the Na^+-K^+-ATPase pumps are inserted),[15] augments K^+ movement from the peritubular capillary into the tubular cells, thereby increasing the size of the K^+ transport pool and promoting passive K^+ secretion into the tubular lumen.

Potassium adaptation begins after a single K^+-containing meal[24] and then increases in efficiency with continued K^+ intake. The efficacy of adaptation in humans can be illustrated by the response to chronic K^+ loading (400 meq/day) in normal subjects.[14] The plasma K^+ concentration rose from 3.8 to 4.8 meq/L and the plasma aldosterone levels increased 2.5-fold in the first 2 days (Fig. 28-1). By 20 days, however, both the plasma K^+ concentration (4.2 meq/L) and the plasma aldosterone concentration had partially returned toward baseline levels, even though urinary K^+ excretion remained very high.

The increased efficiency of K^+ secretion at this time may have been related to the hyperkalemia-induced rise in Na^+-K^+-ATPase activity in the K^+ secreting cells.[22,23] Indirect evidence in support of this hypothesis in the above study of K^+ loading was the observation that discontinuing the K^+ load led to transient Na^+ retention that could have reflected the time required for distal Na^+-K^+-ATPase activity to fall back to normal.[14]

The major clinical example of K^+ adaptation is *chronic renal failure*. In this disorder, the combination of a constant K^+ intake and fewer functioning nephrons requires an increase in K^+ excretion per nephron.[25,26] This response allows relative normokalemia to be maintained even in advanced renal failure as long as intake is not excessive, the urine output and therefore distal flow rate are adequate, and aldosterone secretion can be appropriately enhanced.[27,28]

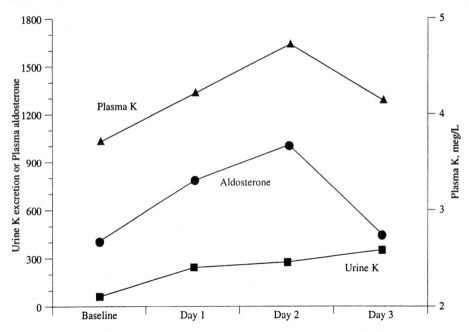

Figure 28-1   Response to increasing K^+ intake to 400 meq/day in normal subjects. Urinary K^+ excretion rises to this level within 2 days and is then maintained. This response is initially driven by elevations in the plasma K^+ and aldosterone concentrations. By day 20, the efficiency of K^+ secretion has increased, resulting in a lesser elevation in the plasma K^+ concentration (to 4.2 meq/L) and normalization of the plasma aldosterone concentration. (*Adapted from Rabelink TJ, Koomans HA, Hené RJ, Dorhut Mees EJ*, Kidney Int *38:942, 1990. Reprinted by permission from* Kidney International.)

Studies in experimental animals with renal failure have shown that Na^+-K^+-ATPase activity in the distal nephron is elevated, an expected correlate of enhanced K^+ secretion per nephron.[29] However, this elevation in pump activity is seen only when K^+ intake is normal, not when intake is *restricted in proportion to the fall in GFR*, a situation in which increased K^+ excretion per nephron is not required.[29] This finding suggests that the rise in Na^+-K^+-ATPase activity is appropriate and specific, not incidentally induced by renal insufficiency.

K^+ adaptation in renal failure is also associated with aldosterone-induced increases in Na^+-K^+-ATPase activity and K^+ secretion in the colon.[30] This response becomes physiologically important in patients with end-stage renal failure on chronic dialysis, in whom enhanced fecal losses may account for the excretion of as much as 30 to 50 percent of dietary K^+ intake.[31]

ETIOLOGY

Potassium enters the body by oral intake or intravenous infusion, is stored in the cells, and is then excreted primarily in the urine. Thus, an abnormality in any one or more of these processes can lead to hyperkalemia (Table 28-1). It should be noted, however, that *chronic hyperkalemia is always associated with an impairment in urinary K^+ excretion* (due primarily to hypoaldosteronism or diminished distal flow), since the elevation in the plasma K^+ concentration would not persist if excretory capacity were normal (Fig. 28-1).

This section will review the major causes of hyperkalemia, some of which are drug-related,[32,33] as well as the diagnosis and treatment of specific disorders. The general principles involved in the approach to the hyperkalemic patient will be considered separately later in the chapter.

Increased Intake

In normal subjects, an acute K^+ load produces a dose-dependent elevation in the plasma K^+ concentration.[1] For example, 135 to 160 meq of oral K^+ can transiently raise the plasma K^+ concentration by 2.5 to 3.5 meq/L, a change that generally is well tolerated.[7] Ingesting more than 160 meq, however, can produce a potentially fatal increase in the plasma K^+ concentration to above 8.0 meq/L, even in patients with normal renal function.[34]

Table 28-1   Etiology of hyperkalemia

Increased intake[a]
  A. Oral
  B. Intravenous
Movement from cells into extracellular fluid
  A. Pseudohyperkalemia[a]
  B. Metabolic acidosis
  C. Insulin deficiency and hyperosmolality in uncontrolled diabetes mellitus;[a] also acute hyperosmolality due to hypernatremia or the administration of hypertonic mannitol
  D. Tissue catabolism[a]
  E. β-Adrenergic blockade
  F. Severe exercise
  G. Digitalis overdose
  H. Periodic paralysis—hyperkalemic form
  I. Cardiac surgery
  J. Succinylcholine
  K. Arginine
Decreased urinary excretion
  A. Renal failure[a]
  B. Effective circulating volume depletion[a]
  C. Hypoaldosteronism[a] (see Table 28-2)
  D. Type 1 renal tubular acidosis—hyperkalemic form
  E. Selective potassium secretory defect

  [a] Most common causes.

Severe hyperkalemia is more likely to occur with a rapid intravenous infusion or in infants because of their small size. Severe hyperkalemia and even cardiac arrest have been reported in infants after the administration of potassium penicillin as an intravenous bolus,[35] the accidental ingestion of a KCl-containing salt substitute,[36] or the use of stored blood for exchange transfusions.[37] K^+ is gradually released from the red cells of stored blood, resulting in an extracellular K^+ concentration that by 21 days can reach 30 meq/L in whole blood and 90 meq/L in packed cells.[38,39] The risk of K^+ overload can be minimized by selecting only blood collected less than 5 days prior to transfusion and by washing any unit of blood immediately before infusion to remove extracellular potassium.

Hyperkalemia is more common when K^+ is given to patients with any of the causes of impaired K^+ excretion listed in Table 28-1. In this setting, a K^+ load that would normally be well tolerated can lead to substantial elevations in the plasma K^+ concentration. In addition to dietary intake, other sources of K^+ include K^+ supplements, salt substitute,[40,41] low Na^+ soups,[42] and red clay (clay ingestion is relatively frequent in certain rural areas in the southeastern United States).[43]

Movement from Cells into Extracellular Fluid

A transcellular shift of K^+ out of the cells is a relatively common cause of acute hyperkalemia (Table 28-1). In these disorders, the rise in the plasma K^+ concentration is too rapid to be corrected by excretion of the excess K^+ in the urine.

Pseudohyperkalemia Pseudohyperkalemia refers to those conditions in which the elevation in the measured K^+ concentration is due to K^+ movement out of the cells *during or after* the drawing of the blood specimen. The major cause of this problem is mechanical trauma during venipuncture, resulting in the release of K^+ from red cells. Since hemoglobin is also released in this setting, the serum will have a characteristic red tint. Repeated clenching and unclenching of the fist after the tourniquet has been applied (in an attempt to make the veins more apparent) may play a contributory role, artifactually raising the plasma K^+ concentration by as much as 1 to 2 meq/L as the exercise causes K^+ to be released from the cells (see "Severe Exercise," below).[44]

Another cause of pseudohyperkalemia results from measurement of the serum (the extracellular fluid separated from the red cells *after* clotting has occurred) rather than the plasma K^+ concentration. In normal subjects, a small amount of K^+ moves out of white cells and platelets during coagulation. Consequently, the measured serum K^+ concentration exceeds the true level in the plasma by 0.1 to as much as 0.5 meq/L, a difference that is clinically unimportant.[45,46] However, much more K^+ may be released in patients with marked leukocytosis or thrombocytosis (white cell or platelet count greater than 100,000/mm^3 or 400,000/mm^3, respectively). In these conditions, there may be a spurious elevation in the serum K^+ concentration to as high as 9 meq/L.[46-49] With thrombocytosis, for example, the serum K^+ concentration rises by approximately 0.15 meq/L for every 100,000/mm^3 elevation in the platelet count.[46]

A rare familial condition has also been described in which K^+ leaks out of abnormally permeable red cells.[50,51] True hyperkalemia does not occur in vivo, since the excess K^+ is excreted in the urine. Familial pseudohyperkalemia maps to the same gene locus as hereditary xerocytosis, a genetic disorder characterized by the presence in the peripheral smear of erythrocytes that are hyperchromic because of marked cellular dehydration; the gene product has not been identified.[52]

The presence of pseudohyperkalemia should be suspected when there is no apparent cause for the elevation in the plasma K^+ concentration and when there are no changes in muscle strength or the electrocardiogram, since the true K^+ concentration is normal. Careful venipuncture to avoid hemolysis and measurement of the plasma (not the serum) K^+ concentration usually establish the correct diagnosis. In the familial disorder, in vitro K^+ leakage can be prevented by rapid centrifugation to separate the red cells from the plasma.

Metabolic acidosis   Metabolic acidosis (other than organic acidoses such as lactic acidosis or ketoacidosis) results in K^+ movement out of the cells (see page 379); this transcellular shift is obligated by the need to maintain electroneutrality, as some of the excess H^+ ions are buffered intracellularly.[53] The rise in the plasma K^+ concentration is variable, ranging from 0.2 to 1.7 meq/L for every 0.1-unit reduction in the arterial pH.[53]

The net effect depends upon both the severity of the acidemia and the state of K^+ balance. Patients with marked acidemia and relatively normal K^+ stores may become hyperkalemic. In comparison, the plasma K^+ concentration may be normal or reduced if there is concurrent K^+ depletion due, for example, to diarrhea or renal tubular acidosis.[54,55] It should be appreciated, however, that the plasma K^+ concentration in this setting is still *higher than it should be* (in relation to body K^+ stores) and that correction of the acidemia will lead to hypokalemia unless K^+ supplements are also administered.

Insulin deficiency and hyperglycemia   Hyperkalemia due to K^+ movement out of the cells is a common finding in patients with diabetic ketoacidosis or nonketotic hyperglycemia, even though total body K^+ stores are almost invariably depleted (see Chap. 25).[56,57] Insulin deficiency (but probably not acidemia[53]) may contribute to this response, since insulin normally promotes K^+ entry into the cells.[58] However, the associated hyperglycemia and hyperosmolality appear to play a more important role.[1,59,60] This can be illustrated by the response to glucose administration (Fig. 28-2). In normal subjects, the ensuing release of insulin minimizes the rise in the plasma glucose concentration and produces a mild degree of *hypo*kalemia. In comparison, there is no increase in insulin secretion in insulin-dependent diabetics, resulting in both hyperglycemia and hyperkalemia.

The elevation in the plasma osmolality in this setting pulls water and K^+ out of the cells.[61,62] Two factors contribute to this response. First, the loss of water raises the K^+ concentration in the cells, thereby creating a favorable gradient for passive K^+ exit through *potassium channels* in the cell membrane. Second, the

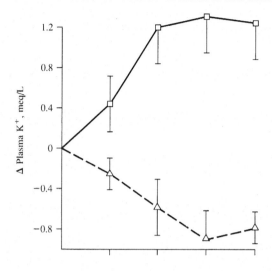

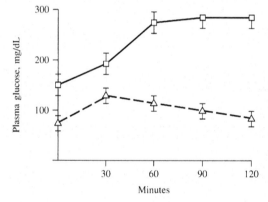

Figure 28-2   Effect of glucose infusion on the plasma K^+ and glucose concentrations in normal subjects (triangles) and in diabetics (squares). The plasma K^+ concentration falls in normals due to the release of insulin but rises in diabetics because of the development of hyperglycemia and hyperosmolality. (*From Nicolis GL, Kahn T, Sanchez A, Gabrilove JL*, Arch Intern Med *141:49, 1981. Copyright, 1981, American Medical Association.*)

frictional forces between the solvent (water) and the solute can result in K^+ being carried along with water through the *water channels* in the cell membrane. This phenomenon of solvent drag is independent of the electrochemical gradient for K^+ diffusion. (A similar translocation of K^+ out of the cells can occur when acute hyperosmolality is induced by hypernatremia or the administration of hypertonic mannitol.[62,63])

Although hyperkalemia at presentation is common in uncontrolled diabetes, the severity of this problem is limited by the concurrent renal and gastrointestinal K^+ losses.[56,57] In comparison, fatal hyperkalemia (with the plasma K^+ concentration exceeding 8 to 9 meq/L) can be induced by hyperglycemia in dialysis patients, who are less likely to become K^+-depleted because they do not have a glucose osmotic diuresis.[64]

Several other factors also may promote the development of hyperkalemia in diabetic patients, even if they are relatively well controlled. These include renal failure due to diabetic nephropathy, hyporeninemic hypoaldosteronism (see below), and decreased sympathetic activity due either to diabetic autonomic neuropathy or to the use of β-adrenergic blockers to treat hypertension.

Insulin deficiency also may contribute to the rise in the plasma K^+ concentration following the administration of somatostatin, which is available for clinical use as an intravenous infusion. The elevation in the plasma K^+ concentration averages 0.6 meq/L in normal subjects[58] but can reach 1.5 meq/L in patients with end-stage renal disease who may already be hyperkalemic prior to the infusion.[65] In this setting, potentially serious hyperkalemia can ensue.

Tissue catabolism   When the rate of tissue breakdown is increased, large amounts of K^+ may be released into the extracellular fluid; hyperkalemia can occur, particularly if renal failure is present. Clinical examples of hypercatabolism include trauma,[66] the administration of cytotoxic agents to patients with malignant lymphomas, leukemias, and occasionally solid tumors (called the tumor lysis syndrome);[67,68] massive hemolysis;[69] or the condition found in patients who are essentially dead following severe accidental hypothermia.[70] In the last setting, marked irreversible tissue necrosis can result in a plasma K^+ concentration above 10 to 20 meq/L. Since proteins (metabolized in part into urea), phosphates, and nucleic acids (metabolized into uric acid) are also released from the cells in catabolic states, increases in the blood urea nitrogen (BUN) and plasma phosphate and uric acid concentrations are also typically found.

β-Adrenergic blockade β-Adrenergic blockers interfere with the β_2-adrenergic facilitation of K^+ entry into cells (see Fig. 12-2).[71-73] In most cases, this effect is associated with only a minor elevation in the plasma K^+ concentration of less than 0.5 meq/L,[2] since the excess extracellular K^+ can be excreted in the urine. True hyperkalemia is rare[74] unless it is associated with a superimposed problem, such as a marked K^+ load, severe exercise, hypoaldosteronism, end-stage renal failure, or cardiac surgery (see below).[73,75-78] A relatively β_1-selective adrenergic blocker (such as atenolol) is safer in these settings.[79]

Severe exercise   Potassium is normally released from muscle cells during exercise. This response may in part reflect a delay between K^+ exit during depolarization and subsequent reuptake by the Na^+-K^+-ATPase pump.[2,4] With severe exercise, however, an additional factor may become important. Muscle cells have ATP-dependent K^+ channels that are inhibited by ATP. Thus, a reduction in ATP levels with marked exercise can open up more channels, thereby promoting K^+ release from the cells.[80]

The movement of K^+ out of the cells during exercise has a physiologic function. The *local* elevation in the plasma K^+ concentration has a vasodilatory effect that contributes to the enhanced blood flow (and therefore energy delivery) to the exercising muscle.[80,81]

The elevation in the *systemic* plasma K^+ concentration is less pronounced than the local rise and is directly related to the degree of exercise: 0.3 to 0.4 meq/L with slow walking,[82] 0.7 to 1.2 meq/L with moderate exertion (including prolonged aerobic exercise, as with marathon running),[73,75,83,84]* and as much as 2.0 meq/L with possible electrocardiographic alterations following severe exercise to exhaustion, which is often accompanied by lactic acidosis.[76,85,86] These changes are reversed after several minutes of rest and may be associated with a mild rebound hypokalemia of 0.4 to 0.5 meq/L below the baseline level.[83,86]

Exercise-induced hyperkalemia is attenuated by prior physical conditioning.[87] Conditioning enhances cellular Na^+-K^+-ATPase activity, an adaptation that may be responsible for the lesser release of K^+ during acute exercise.[4,87]

Although the rise in the plasma K^+ concentration is generally well tolerated, hyperkalemia may be in part responsible for some of the cases of sudden death that occur during exercise.[88] This may be more likely to occur if there is an additional abnormality in K^+ handling, such as rhabdomyolysis during a marathon race.[89] The plasma K^+ concentration can also approach 8.0 meq/L with severe exercise in patients taking a β-adrenergic blocker.[76] In addition to the effect of hyperkalemia, the postexercise mild hypokalemia may be arrhythmogenic, particularly in patients with underlying coronary heart disease.[85]

Digitalis overdose   The Na^+-K^+-ATPase pump in the cell membrane is inhibited in a dose-dependent manner by digitalis.[90] Thus, the administration of digitalis tends to increase the plasma K^+ concentration as a result of the release of K^+ from the cells. When digitalis is used in therapeutic doses, this effect is relatively small, although there may be some impairment in the ability to handle a large K^+ load.[91] However, severe hyperkalemia (plasma K^+ concentration up to 13 meq/L) has resulted from the ingestion of massive amounts of digitalis following a suicide attempt.[92,93]

Hyperkalemic periodic paralysis   The hyperkalemic form of periodic paralysis is a familial disorder with autosomal dominant inheritance that is characterized by recurrent attacks of muscle weakness or paralysis.[94-96] Most patients with this disorder also have myotonic symptoms, particularly in the cold. Episodes are precipitated by rest after exercise or the ingestion of K^+; they are associated with an elevation in the plasma K^+ concentration that is due either to K^+ release from the cells or to an inability of ingested K^+ to enter the cells.[94-97] The degree of hyperkalemia is frequently mild (less than 5.5 meq/L), although the plasma K^+ concentration can exceed 7 meq/L in some patients.[95] Attacks are also associated with a fall in the plasma Na^+ concentration and a rise in the plasma protein concentration; these findings suggest that Na^+ and water enter the cell as K^+ leaves.[97]

---

*A similar effect can be caused by repeated fist clenching during blood drawing.[44] This is an artifact of blood drawing, however, since it is limited to that forearm.

The primary abnormality in this condition in at least some families appears to be a point mutation in the skeletal muscle cell Na^+ channel gene.[96,98,99] This is associated with sustained Na^+ currents,[100] and the activity of this channel may be further increased by a slight elevation in the plasma K^+ concentration.[99] The ensuing entry of Na^+ into the cell will depolarize the cell membrane, thereby favoring K^+ diffusion out of the cells (since the concentration in the cell is so much higher than that in the extracellular fluid) and the development of hypokalemia.

The diagnosis of periodic paralysis should be suspected from the personal and family history of *recurrent* episodes of muscle weakness and the elevated plasma K^+ concentration during an attack. In contrast to hypokalemic periodic paralysis, in which the muscle weakness may be profound and last for up to 48 h, episodes are usually mild in the hyperkalemic form, with a duration of less than 1 to 2 h.[94] The diagnosis can be confirmed by the induction of muscle weakness and hyperkalemia after a relatively small oral K^+ load (0.5 to 1.0 meq/kg).[94-97]

Treatment is aimed at correcting the hyperkalemia and then attempting to prevent further episodes. Albuterol, a β-adrenergic agonist used to treat bronchoconstriction, may be particularly effective in reversing the acute symptoms by driving K^+ into the cells.[101] Modalities used chronically include limiting exercise (if this precipitates attacks), ingestion of a low-K^+, high-carbohydrate diet (carbohydrates promote K^+ entry into cells via increased insulin secretion), and inducing mild K^+ depletion with a thiazide diuretic or a mineralocorticoid (such as fludrocortisone).[94] The addition of the carbonic anhydrase inhibitor acetazolamide may also be beneficial, perhaps by increasing urinary K^+ excretion (see Chap. 15).[94,102]

Cardiac surgery Patients on cardiac bypass may develop a mild elevation in the plasma K^+ concentration as normal circulation is restored,[103] particularly if they have been taking a β-adrenergic blocker.[78] Two factors may contribute to this problem: (1) washout of ischemic areas that were underperfused during bypass and (2) rewarming (since the surgery is performed under hypothermic conditions). The induction of hypothermia causes K^+ to move into the cells by an unknown mechanism;[104,105] reversal of this effect with rewarming may be associated with "overshoot" hyperkalemia, particularly if K^+ has been given during the period of hypothermia.[104]

Succinylcholine Succinylcholine is a muscle relaxant used in general anesthesia. It acts by depolarizing the cell membrane, i.e., it reduces the magnitude of the resting membrane potential. Since the cell interior becomes less electronegative, this favors the movement of positively charged K^+ ions out of the cells into the extracellular fluid. In normal subjects, the result is a small rise in the plasma K^+ concentration of 0.5 meq/L or less.[106] However, in patients with burns, extensive trauma, tetanus, or neuromuscular diseases, succinylcholine can induce an increase in the plasma K^+ concentration of as much as 6 meq/L, leading to cardiac arrhythmias and even cardiac arrest.[106,107] Although it is unclear why these patients are at such high risk, the increase in the plasma K^+ concentration (which usually occurs within 5 min) can be minimized by the prior administration of tubocurarine.[106]

Arginine Arginine hydrochloride is metabolized in part to hydrochloric acid and has been used in the treatment of refractory metabolic alkalosis. Marked hyperkalemia is a potential complication with this drug and is presumably due to the movement of K^+ out of cells as cationic arginine enters the cells.[108,109] This effect may be more pronounced in HIV-infected patients.[110]

Decreased Urinary Excretion

Potassium excretion is normally so efficient that even a massive chronic increase in K^+ intake will not produce hyperkalemia in normal subjects (Fig. 28-1).[14] Thus, for hyperkalemia to persist, urinary K^+ excretory capacity must be reduced. There are three major causes of this problem: renal failure, effective circulating volume depletion, and hypoaldosteronism.

Renal failure As described above, K^+ balance is maintained in renal failure by increased excretion per functioning nephron.[25-27,111] This adaptation, which is mediated in part by aldosterone and enhanced Na^+-K^+-ATPase activity,[28,29] is effective as long as the urine output remains adequate. However, the ability to excrete K^+ falls once oliguria develops, primarily as a result of the decrease in flow to the distal secretory site.[27,112] In this setting, some of the K^+ derived from dietary intake is likely to be retained, resulting in a persistent elevation in the plasma K^+ concentration.[113]

When hyperkalemia develop in a nonoliguric patient, some other factor is usually superimposed, such as enhanced tissue breakdown, hypoaldosteronism (see below), or increased K^+ intake. As an example, patients with renal failure who are in balance on a regular diet may have an exaggerated rise in the plasma K^+ concentration following a K^+ load.[7,26,27,114] Despite a low absolute rate of K^+ excretion in this setting, the rate divided by the GFR (an index of K^+ excretion per functioning nephron) is similar to that in normal subjects given a K^+ load.[26] This finding suggests that the retention of K^+ in renal failure is due to *too few nephrons, not to a specific defect in K^+ secretion.*[27,114]

In addition to the diminished kaliuresis, K^+ entry into the cells is also impaired in renal failure.[113,115] This is manifested by a low cell K^+ concentration in the basal state (despite a normal or elevated plasma level)[116] and diminished cellular uptake of K^+ after a K^+ load (Fig. 28-3).[117,118,119] Decreased Na^+-K^+-ATPase activity (presumably due to retained uremic toxins that impair the transcription of mRNA for the α_1 isoform of the Na^+-K^+-ATPase pump in skeletal muscle)[120]* and possibly metabolic acidosis[53,54] are primarily responsible for the altered distribution of K^+ in this setting.

---

* One exception to the generalized reduction in Na^+-K^+-ATPase activity in uremia occurs in the renal cortical collecting tubule. Na^+-K^+-ATPase activity is increased and enhanced in these cells because of the need to increase K^+ secretion per nephron.[29]

Although insulin resistance is also present in renal failure, this defect is limited to the hypoglycemic response. The ability of insulin to promote K^+ entry into the cells appears to be preserved and therefore does not contribute to the tendency to hyperkalemia.[121,122]

There is, however, an abnormality in the relationship between carbohydrate and potassium metabolism in advanced renal failure, since fasting can lead to a modest elevation in the plasma K^+ concentration (averaging 1 meq/L after 36 h) in patients requiring maintenance dialysis.[123,124] Decreased insulin release induced by fasting appears to be of primary importance, since the hyperkalemia can be prevented or reversed by the administration of insulin plus glucose or, to a lesser degree, the administration of glucose alone.[119,124] On the other hand, the degree of hyperkalemia following a dietary K^+ load is minimized by concurrent glucose intake, which stimulates endogenous insulin secretion.[119]

Effective circulating volume depletion   Effective circulating volume depletion can be produced by fluid loss from the body, sequestration into a noncirculating space, or diminished tissue perfusion in heart failure or cirrhosis (see Chap. 8). K^+ depletion is often present in these disorders as a result of the loss of K^+-containing fluids, either as a primary event or secondary to the use of diuretics in heart failure.

However, the ability to handle a K^+ load is impaired by hypovolemia, an effect that can lead to an elevation in the plasma K^+ concentration in some patients. Reductions in urinary excretion and perhaps K^+ entry into cells contribute to this problem.[125,126] Volume depletion may be associated with both a low glomerular filtration rate and enhanced proximal Na^+ and water reabsorption. The net effect is an often marked decrease in distal fluid delivery, thereby diminishing K^+ secretion despite the hypovolemia-induced secondary hyperaldosteronism. Why cell entry of the excess K^+ is impaired in this setting is not understood.[17]

A clinical example of the effect of volume depletion may be seen in renal failure. One of the changes that can occur in this disorder is an inability to maximally conserve Na^+.[127,128] In most patients, the obligatory Na^+ loss is relatively small and not clinically important on a regular diet.[128] If, however, intake is decreased or extrarenal losses are enhanced, volume depletion will ensue. The resultant fall in renal perfusion can then lead to reduced K^+ excretion and hyperkalemia.[129]

The same sequence may be seen in severe congestive heart failure, which is associated with a reduction in renal perfusion. Life-threatening hyperkalemia can be seen in this setting, particularly in patients also taking KCl supplements.[130] The routine administration of angiotensin converting enzyme inhibitors in these patients also contributes to the tendency to hyperkalemia by impairing the synthesis of angiotensin II and therefore the release of aldosterone.[131]

A similar problem can occasionally occur in patients with relatively normal renal function, as illustrated by the following case history.

Case History 28-1   A 63-year-old woman complains of a diarrheal illness lasting for 4 to 5 days. During this time, her weight has dropped 3 kg, she has noted a marked reduction in urine output, and her intake has been limited primarily to fluids (particularly orange juice) and fruits. The physical examination reveals postural hypotension and decreased skin turgor. The laboratory data include the following:

Plasma [Na$^+$]	=	130 meq/L	BUN	=	31 mg/dL
[K$^+$]	=	6.7 meq/L	[Creatinine]	=	1.2 mg/dL
[Cl$^-$]	=	98 meq/L	Urine [Na$^+$]	=	12 meq/L
[HCO$_3^-$]	=	21 meq/L	[K$^+$]	=	62 meq/L

Comment The history, physical findings, and low urine Na$^+$ concentration are indicative of volume depletion. Although the urine K$^+$ concentration appears to be appropriately elevated, it is likely that the urine volume is below 500 mL/day and therefore that daily K$^+$ excretion is less than 30 meq. The combination of decreased urinary excretion and the relatively high K$^+$ intake (orange juice and fruits) is responsible for the hyperkalemia.

Hypoaldosteronism Hypoaldosteronism can be induced by a variety of conditions that interfere with either the production or the effect of aldosterone (Table 28-2). The most common causes are hyporeninemic hypoaldosteronism and K$^+$-sparing diuretics in adults, and adrenal enzyme deficiencies (particularly 21-hydroxylase deficiency) in children. Adrenal insufficiency, perhaps due to cytomegalo-

Table 28-2 Causes of hypoaldosteronism

Associated with decreased activity of the renin-angiotensin system
- A. Hyporeninemic hypoaldosteronism with mild to moderate renal insufficiency
- B. Nonsteroidal anti-inflammatory drugs, with the possible exception of sulindac
- C. Converting enzyme inhibitors
- D. Cyclosporine
- E. Acquired immune deficiency syndrome
- F. Hypervolemia in chronic dialysis patients

Primary decrease in adrenal synthesis
- A. Low cortisol levels
  - 1. Primary adrenal insufficiency
  - 2. Congenital adrenal hyperplasia—primarily 21-hydroxylase deficiency
- B. Normal cortisol levels
  - 1. Heparin
  - 2. Isolated hypoaldosteronism
  - 3. Post–removal of adrenal adenoma

Aldosterone resistance
- A. Potassium-sparing diuretics (including high-dose trimethoprim in AIDS)
- B. Cyclosporine
- C. Pseudohypoaldosteronism

virus, *Mycobacterium avium-intracellulare*, or HIV itself, is also a recognized find-ing in patients with AIDS,[132,133] although the administration of high-dose tri-methoprim to treat *Pneumocystis carinii* pneumonia also may contribute to the rise in the plasma K^+ concentration in these patients (see below).

In addition to hyperkalemia, varying degrees of Na^+ wasting and metabolic acidosis are present in hypoaldosteronism, since aldosterone normally promotes Na^+ reabsorption and H^+ as well as K^+ secretion (see Chap. 6).[134-136] The meta-bolic acidosis (called type 4 renal tubular acidosis; see Chap. 19) is also due in part to the hyperkalemia, as evidenced by correction of the acidemia when the plasma K^+ concentration is normalized.[137,138] This effect of hyperkalemia may be in part due to a transcellular action exchange; as some of the excess K^+ enters the cells (through K^+ channels in the cell membrane), electroneutrality is maintained in part by H^+ movement into the cells (perhaps via Na^+-H^+ exchange).[139,140] The ensuing *intracellular alkalosis* might then reduce both HCO_3^- reabsorption (see Fig. 11-14) and NH_4^+ secretion by the renal tubular cells.[138,139,141] As a result, there would be a reduction in net acid excretion, thereby leading to retention of some of the daily acid load and the subsequent development of metabolic acidosis.

Most NH_4^+ production occurs in the proximal tubule. Thus, a hyperkalemia-induced reduction in NH_4^+ excretion should be a proximal event if diminished production were the primary problem. In one experiment, however, hyperkalemia diminished NH_4^+ excretion but not its delivery out of the proximal tubule, suggest-ing that more distal segments must be involved.[142] One possibility is that the increased K^+ concentration in the luminal fluid competitively inhibits NH_4^+ attachment to the K^+ site on the Na^+-K^+-$2Cl^-$ carrier in the thick ascending limb of the loop of Henle (see Fig. 4-2); as a result, loop NH_4^+ reabsorption and subsequent medullary recycling would be impaired, thereby reducing the efficiency of NH_3 accumulation in the medullary interstitium and its subsequent secretion into the medullary collecting tubule (see page 341).[142,143]

Hyporeninemic hypoaldosteronism   In the absence of an obvious cause (oliguric renal failure, K^+ supplements, K^+-sparing diuretics, angiotensin converting enzyme inhibitors), the syndrome of hyporeninemic hypoaldosteronism appears to account for 50 to 75 percent of cases of initially unexplained hyperkalemia in adults.[134,144] This disorder has the following characteristics[134,145]:

- Most patients have mild to moderate renal insufficiency with a creatinine clearance of 20 to 75 mL/min.
- Approximately 50 percent have diabetes mellitus, with chronic interstitial nephritis accounting for most of the remaining cases.
- Roughly 85 percent have a reduced plasma renin activity.
- Patients typically present with asymptomatic hyperkalemia.

The hypoaldosteronism in this setting appears to be multifactorial.[134,145] The low renin levels can clearly contribute, since angiotensin II is, with K^+, the major physiologic stimulus to aldosterone secretion. On the other hand, several observations suggest that there may also be an *intraadrenal* defect. These include a normal plasma renin activity in some patients,[134,146] an inability of infused angiotensin II to stimulate aldosterone secretion,[147,148] and the demonstration that nephrectomized patients (who have no renin) still have normal aldosterone production that is directly stimulated by the associated rise in the plasma K^+ concentration.[149]

Studies in diabetic animals have demonstrated an impaired zona glomerulosa cell response to angiotensin II that is due to a postreceptor defect.[150] How this might occur is not known, but it appears to be relatively specific, since the increase in aldosterone release following ACTH is not diminished.

The presence of *renal insufficiency* is also an important determinant of the propensity to hyperkalemia. Although decreased aldosterone release can impair urinary K^+ excretion, patients with normal renal function can compensate because a small rise in the plasma K^+ concentration directly enhances distal K^+ secretion (see Fig. 12-10).[9] In diabetes mellitus, for example, hypoaldosteronism may occur relatively early, but hyperkalemia is not seen until the additional insult of renal insufficiency is superimposed.[148,151,152]

How these renal and adrenal changes might occur is incompletely understood. One possibility is that a *defect in prostaglandin production* might be involved,[153] since prostaglandins promote renin secretion (see Chap. 2) and appear to facilitate aldosterone release by angiotensin II.[154] Furthermore, nonsteroidal anti-inflammatory drugs (NSAID, which inhibit prostaglandin synthesis) can induce hyporeninemic hypoaldosteronism.[155,156] The rise in the plasma K^+ concentration is variable, averaging only 0.2 meq/L in patients with normal renal function, but occasionally exceeding 1 meq/L when renal insufficiency is superimposed.[157]

Another hypothesis suggests that hypervolemia associated with renal disease may be the primary event. Volume expansion leads to *enhanced release of atrial natriuretic peptide*, a hormone that can then directly suppress the renal release of renin and potassium-induced adrenal release of aldosterone (see Chap. 6).[158] Hyporeninemia, hypoaldosteronism, and high levels of atrial natriuretic peptide are, for example, common in patients with acute glomerulonephritis (such as postinfectious glomerulonephritis) and chronic renal disease, and prior to dialysis in patients with end-stage renal failure.[159,160] These changes can lead to hyperkalemia in selected patients with glomerulonephritis.[160] Removal of the excess fluid or recovery from the glomerular injury reverses these hormonal changes, resulting in the normalization of K^+ balance.

Volume expansion may also explain in part the propensity of diabetics to develop this disorder. This increased filtered load of glucose imposed by hyperglycemia directly enhances proximal Na^+ reabsorption by the Na^+-glucose cotransporter in the luminal membrane (see page 90). In addition, a defect in the conversion of the precursor prorenin (or inactive renin) into active renin has been demonstrated both in diabetics[161,162] and in other patients with renal disease and hypoaldosteronism.[163] How this abnormality might occur is unclear, although direct damage to the renin-producing juxtaglomerular cells may be involved.

Diabetes also may directly impair adrenal function, as evidenced by decreased release of aldosterone in response to angiotensin II.[148] This defect may be related to atrophy of the zona glomerulosa, possibly as a result of removal of the normal trophic effect of insulin on these cells.[164]

A syndrome similar to hyporeninemic hypoaldosteronism may be also seen in several other settings. These include the use of angiotensin converting enzyme inhibitors (which impair the conversion of angiotensin I into angiotensin II),[165,166]* the acquired immune deficiency syndrome,[167] and the administration of cyclosporine.[168,169] Renal transplant recipients treated with cyclosporine, for example, have higher plasma K^+ concentrations than those treated with prednisone and azathioprine. In addition to decreased aldosterone release, there is also evidence that cyclosporine impairs tubular K^+ secretion.[169,170]

How these renal and extrarenal effects occur is not well understood. In vitro studies suggest that cyclosporine can diminish Na^+-K^+-ATPase activity in the K^+ secretory cells in the cortical and outer medullary collecting tubules but not in most other nephron segments.[170] Such a defect would diminish K^+ accumulation in the tubular cells and therefore the size of the K^+ secretory pool. There is also evidence that cyclosporine directly impairs the secretory process by inhibiting the luminal K^+ channels through which K^+ is secreted.[171] The applicability of these findings to the development of hyperkalemia in humans is uncertain.

The decrease in aldosterone release with angiotensin converting enzyme (ACE) inhibitors may be due to two factors: a reduced concentration of circulating angiotensin II and diminished *intraadrenal* angiotensin II, which may mediate part or most of the stimulatory effect of hyperkalemia.[172,173] As with other causes of hypoaldosteronism, the rise in the plasma K^+ concentration after ACE inhibition is generally less than 0.5 meq/L if renal function is normal.[165] However, potentially dangerous hyperkalemia can occur in patients who have renal insufficiency and a high normal or elevated baseline plasma K^+ concentration or in patients who are also taking a K^+-sparing diuretic or K^+ supplements.[165,166] This interaction has become a more important concern, since both angiotensin converting enzyme inhibitors and the K^+-sparing diuretic spironolactone are given to many patients with heart failure because they improve survival.[174]

The hyperkalemia observed with HIV-infected patients is often multifactorial.[175] In addition to adrenal insufficiency, which may be infectious in origin,[132,133] other factors include drugs (trimethoprim, pentamidine; see below) and a diminished response to aldosterone.[176]

Primary adrenal insufficiency   Patients with primary adrenal insufficiency (or bilateral adrenalectomy) have diminished glucocorticoid as well as mineralocorticoid secretion. Autoimmune destruction of the steroid-producing cells in the adrenal cortex and AIDS are the most common causes of this problem in adults.[175,177] One major antigen against which the autoantibodies are directed in

---

* The plasma renin activity is typically increased, not reduced, with these agents, since angiotensin II normally decreases renin release by feedback inhibition.

autoimmune disease in adults appears to be the enzyme CYP21A2 (21-hydro-xylase).[178,179] This enzyme converts progesterone into deoxycorticosterone in the zona glumerulosa and 17-hydroxyprogesterone into deoxycortisol in the zona fasciculata. Other antibody targets CYP11A1 (side-chain cleavage enzyme) and CYP17 (17α-hydroxylase).[179]

The hormonal and electrolyte findings are different in patients with pituitary disease who have secondary hypoadrenalism. In this setting, aldosterone secretion is relatively normal, since adrenocorticotropic hormone (ACTH) does not have a major role in the regulation of aldosterone release (see page 182).[180,181] As a result, these patients do not become hyperkalemic.

Adrenal enzyme deficiencies   The pathways involved in adrenal steroid synthesis are illustrated in Fig. 28-3. In addition to aldosterone, deoxycorticosterone (DOC) and corticosterone also have mineralocorticoid activity. Their secretion, however, is determined primarily by ACTH—not, as with aldosterone, by angiotensin II or the plasma K^+ concentration.[180-182] Signs of mineralocorticoid deficiency may be seen with reduced activity of enzymes involved in steps *prior to the formation of DOC* (3β-hydroxysteroid dehydrogenase and CYP21A2) or in the *conversion of corticosterone to aldosterone.*[182]* The two steps involved in the latter conversion are mediated by a single multifunctional cytochrome P450 enzyme called CYP11B2 (aldosterone synthase or corticosterone methyl oxidase).[183,184] The activity of this enzyme is normally suppressed in the zona fasciculata,[185,186] preventing aldosterone secretion from being inappropriately regulated by ACTH.

Deficiencies in the enzymes prior to DOC formation may be associated with concurrent abnormalities in cortisol and androgen production.[182,183,188] On the other hand, children with a defect in aldosterone synthase have isolated hypoaldosteronism.[186,189] Congenital isolated hypoaldosteronism is a rare inherited disorder that is transmitted as an autosomal recessive trait. Affected infants have recurrent dehydration, salt wasting, and failure to thrive.[183,188]

Treatment varies with the type of enzyme deficiency. Mineralocorticoid replacement is sufficient in patients with isolated hypoaldosteronism, whereas those with the more common CYP21A2 deficiency require replacement of both glucocorticoid and mineralocorticoid.[190]

The response to glucocorticoid replacement (usually with hydrocortisone or dexamethasone) should be assessed by measuring serum 17-hydroxyprogesterone (which accumulates in untreated patients), androstenedione or testosterone (in girls and prepubertal boys to assess for virilization), growth velocity, and the rate of skeletal maturation. The goal is to use the lowest effective dose to prevent chronic glucocorticoid excess.

Mineralocorticoid is usually given as fludrocortisone, in a dose sufficient to restore normal serum sodium and potassium concentrations and to lower the

---

*Although CYP11B1 (11β-hydroxylase) deficiency also decreases aldosterone production by impairing the conversion of DOC to corticosterone, there is a build-up of DOC, leading to signs of mineralocorticoid excess (hypertension and hypokalemia), not mineralocorticoid deficiency.[180,187]

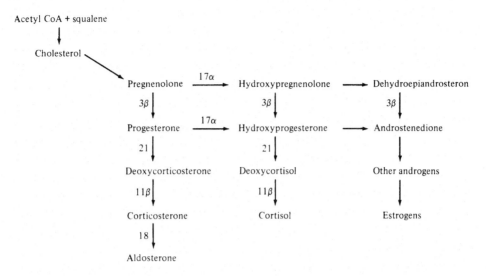

Figure 28-3 Schematic pathways of adrenal steroid biosynthesis. The numbers at the arrows refer to specific enzymes: 17α equals 17α-hydroxylase; 3β equals 3β-hydroxysteroid dehydrogenase; 21 equals 21-hydroxylase; 11β equals 11β-hydroxylase; 18 refers to a two-step process resulting in the addition of an aldehyde at the 18-carbon position. The last reactions occur only in the zona glomerulosa, which is the site of aldosterone secretion. A deficiency in any of these enzymes can lead to abnormal mineralocorticoid (as well as glucocorticoid and androgen) production.

plasma renin activity to normal; excessive dosing can induce hypertension, hypokalemia, and possibly impaired growth.

Heparin Heparin therapy reduces aldosterone secretion by a direct action on the adrenal gland.[191,192] It is not clear, however, whether this represents an effect of heparin itself or of its preservative chlorbutol.[193] Regardless of the mechanism, even low-dose heparin can lead to a 75 percent reduction in plasma aldosterone levels within 4 to 7 days.[194] Hyperkalemia, however, is seen only if some superimposed problem is present, such as renal insufficiency.[191,195] The aldosterone deficiency in this setting is readily reversible with discontinuation of the drug.

Post-removal of adrenal adenoma In patients with primary *hyper*aldosteronism due to an adrenal adenoma, the chronic overproduction of aldosterone suppresses the normal tissue in the zona glomerulosa. As a result, surgical removal of the tumor leads to a transient period of hypoaldosteronism that can last up to 6 months or more.[196,197]

Potassium-sparing diuretics The K^+-sparing diuretics impair distal K^+ secretion—spironolactone by antagonizing the effect of aldosterone, and amiloride and triamterene by directly closing the Na^+ channel in the luminal membrane of the collecting tubular cell (see Chap. 15). As a result, the use of any of these drugs can produce hyperkalemia, particularly in patients who have renal insufficiency or who are taking K^+ supplements, an angiotensin converting enzyme inhibitor, or a NSAID.[41,198]

Two antibiotics—trimethoprim (usually given as trimethoprim-sulfamethoxazole) and pentamidine—can also cause hyperkalemia by closing the sodium channels.[199-204] Trimethoprim-induced hyperkalemia is dose-dependent, being primarily seen at the very high doses used in patients with AIDS.[199-201] However, trimethoprim can raise the plasma potassium concentration even when used in conventional doses, particularly in the elderly.[202,203,205] One study performed a prospective chart review of 80 patients who did not have renal insufficiency or another cause of altered potassium homeostasis who were treated for at least 5 days with conventional doses of trimethoprim-sulfamethoxazole.[202] There was a mean rise in the plasma potassium concentration of 1.2 meq/L, from 3.9 to 5.1 meq/L; 21 percent of patients had a plasma potassium concentration $\geq$ 5.5 meq/L. The peak effect was at 4 to 5 days. Patients with mild renal insufficiency may be at risk for more severe hyperkalemia.[203]

Pseudohypoaldosteronism   Reduced aldosterone effect can be induced by either genetic or acquired end-organ resistance (called pseudohypoaldosteronism). This disorder is associated with volume depletion, Na^+ wasting, hyperkalemia, and markedly elevated levels of renin and aldosterone, findings similar to those with aldosterone resistance induced by K^+-sparing diuretics.[206,207]

The acquired form of pseudohypoaldosteronism is limited to the kidney and is seen primarily with tubulointerstitial diseases such as urinary tract obstruction, chronic pyelonephritis, acute interstitial nephritis, and amyloidosis.[208-211] It is presumed that tubular injury is responsible for the diminished response to aldosterone in these disorders.

There are two rare genetic forms of pseudohypoaldosteronism: type 1 and type 2. *Type 1 pseudohypoaldosteronism* consists of two different disorders with different modes of inheritance, clinical manifestations, course, and pathogenesis[212,213]:

- Autosomal recessive, in which the defect is permanent and all aldosterone target organs are involved (including the kidney, colon, and salivary glands)
- Autosomal dominant or sporadic, in which the defect may improve with age and, in some cases, involves only the kidney

The autosomal recessive form is due to a defect in the collecting tubule sodium channel, making it relatively unresponsive to aldosterone,[213,214] while the defect in the autosomal dominant or sporadic form often involves the gene for the mineralocorticoid receptor.[215]

The clinical presentation of type 1 pseudohypoaldosteronism in children is similar to that with the more common CYP21A2 deficiency. However, the normal serum concentrations of 17-hydroxyprogesterone and cortisol and the elevated serum concentration of aldosterone usually allow the diagnosis of pseudohypoaldosteronism to be established.

Initial therapy of type 1 pseudohypoaldosteronism consists of a high-salt diet, which prevents volume depletion and, by enhancing sodium delivery to the potassium secretory site in the collecting tubules, increases potassium excretion and lowers the plasma potassium concentration. High-dose fludrocortisone [1 to 2 mg/day (versus 0.05 to 0.1 mg/day in adrenal insufficiency)] or carbenoxolone may be beneficial if a high salt intake is ineffective or not well tolerated.[216] Carbenoxolone prevents the inactivation of cortisol to cortisone, thereby allowing cortisol (which circulates in much higher concentrations than aldosterone) to act as a mineralocorticoid. Infants should be followed carefully, since the aldosterone resistance often resolves within the first few years.[217]

Patients with *type 2 pseudohypoaldosteronism* (Gordon's syndrome) present with hyperkalemia but no other signs of hypoaldosteronism. Rather than being volume-depleted due to salt wasting, these patients present with hypertension, normal renal function, and low or low normal plasma renin activity and aldosterone concentrations.[218-220] The defect, which is probably transmitted as an autosomal dominant trait, may be in a gene located on chromosome 1, 12, and/or 17.[221,221a]

Although the abnormal gene product has not been identified, the primary defect in this disorder may be enhanced distal chloride reabsorption.[218,220] As a result, sodium is reabsorbed distally with chloride, not in exchange for potassium and hydrogen. The net effect is hyperkalemia, volume expansion, and hypertension, which secondarily suppress renin secretion. Many of these abnormalities can be corrected by a thiazide diuretic, suggesting that the primary defect in this condition may be increased activity of the thiazide-sensitive sodium-chloride cotransporter in the luminal membrane of the cells in the distal tubule and adjacent connecting segment.[220]

Type 1 renal tubular acidosis—hyperkalemic form Type 1 (distal) renal tubular acidosis (RTA) is an uncommon disorder characterized by impaired distal H^+ secretion, resulting in metabolic acidosis with an inappropriately high urine pH above 5.3 (see Chap. 19). *Hypo*kalemia frequently occurs in this disorder, in part because the decrease in H^+ secretion requires that Na^+ reabsorption occur in exchange for K^{+}.[55] However, hyperkalemia may be seen when the underlying mechanism is a primary decrease in distal Na^+ reabsorption.[222] The relative inability to reabsorb cationic Na^+ impairs the generation of the lumen-negative potential difference that promotes both H^+ and K^+ secretion.[222]

Hyperkalemic RTA most often occurs in patients with obstructive uropathy (in which decreased Na^+-K^+-ATPase activity may account for the reductions in Na^+ reabsorption and K^+ secretion)[223-225] and sickle cell disease.[6,226] These disorders, however, may also be associated with hyporeninemic hypoaldosteronism,[223,226] a condition that is treated differently from RTA.

The distinction between RTA and hypoaldosteronism can be established by measuring the plasma aldosterone concentration, which is normal in RTA, and the urine pH, which in the presence of metabolic acidosis is appropriately below 5.3 in most patients with aldosterone deficiency.[226,227] However, the separation between these disorders is not necessarily so clear. Some patients appear to have two different defects: an impairment in the H^+-ATPase pump, which is responsible for the RTA, and hypoaldosteronism or aldosterone resistance induced by tubular injury, which is responsible for the hyperkalemia.[228]

Treatment of hyperkalemia in type 1 RTA consists of alkali therapy (often given as Na^+ citrate, which is better tolerated than $NaHCO_3$), a low-K^+ diet, and, if necessary, a diuretic to increase flow to the K^+ secretory site.

Selective potassium secretory defect   In some patients, hyperkalemia occurs with inappropriately low urinary K^+ excretion, normal renin and aldosterone levels, and no Na^+ wasting. This rare syndrome of an apparently selective defect in K^+ secretion that does not respond to exogenous mineralocorticoid has been described with sickle cell anemia, renal transplant rejection, and lupus nephritis.[6,229,230]* The lack of Na^+ wasting and a normal antinatriuretic response to exogenous mineralocorticoid indicate that the underlying abnormality in these patients is not simple aldosterone resistance.

The pathogenesis of this defect is not understood, but a process similar to hyperkalemic RTA may be involved. About one-half of patients have a metabolic acidosis that, in at least in some cases, is associated with an elevated urine pH.[229,230] Alternatively, selective impairment of K^+ secretion may be the sole abnormality, since hyperkalemia can induce metabolic acidosis by, as described above, reducing NH_4^+ and therefore net acid excretion.[138-141]

The diagnosis of a selective K^+ secretory defect is made by exclusion. This disorder can be differentiated from one of the causes of hypoaldosteronism by demonstrating that aldosterone levels are normal and that the administration of fludrocortisone leads to a reduction in Na^+ excretion without affecting that of K^+.[6,230] This distinction is important therapeutically, since therapy consists of a high-Na^+, low-K^+ diet plus a diuretic, not mineralocorticoid replacement. Thiazides may be more effective than a loop diuretic in this setting;[230] why this might occur is uncertain, unless there is specific inhibition of increased distal NaCl reabsorption.

SYMPTOMS

The changes induced by hyperkalemia are essentially limited to muscle weakness and abnormal cardiac conduction, which can lead to potentially fatal arrhythmias. However, patients may also complain of symptoms related to the underlying disease, such as polyuria and polydipsia in uncontrolled diabetes

---

* Most hyperkalemic patients with lupus nephritis have either hyporeninemic hypoaldosteronism or advanced renal failure, not an isolated defect in K^+ excretion.[231]

mellitus or salt wasting, weight loss, and failure to thrive in infants with hypoaldosteronism.

Muscle Weakness

The muscle weakness associated with hyperkalemia appears to result from changes in neuromuscular conduction. The increase in the plasma K^+ concentration reduces the ratio of the intracellular K^+ concentration to that in the extracellular fluid, resulting in a decrease in the magnitude of the resting membrane potential (see Chap. 26). Although this should increase membrane excitability (since less of a depolarizing stimulus is required to generate an action potential), the effect seen in patients is different. Persistent depolarization *inactivates sodium channels* in the cell membrane, thereby producing a net *decrease* in membrane excitability[232] that may be manifested clinically by muscle weakness or paralysis and/or impaired cardiac conduction.

Muscle weakness typically does not develop until the plasma K^+ concentration exceeds 8 meq/L.[233-235] However, patients with periodic paralysis may become symptomatic at a plasma K^+ concentration below 5.5 meq/L,[95] probably because abnormal membrane function is the primary defect in this disorder.

Muscle weakness most often begins in the lower extremities and ascends to the trunk and upper extremities.[233] The respiratory muscles and those supplied by the cranial nerves are usually spared.

Cardiac Arrhythmias

Disturbances in cardiac conduction, which can lead to ventricular fibrillation or standstill, pose the greatest danger to the patient with hyperkalemia.[233,236] Consequently, monitoring of the electrocardiogram (ECG) is an essential part of the management of this disorder. As the plasma K^+ concentration rises, there is a characteristic sequence of changes in the ECG that is due to the effects of hyperkalemia on atrial and ventricular depolarization (represented by the P wave and QRS complex, respectively) and repolarization (represented by the T wave for ventricular repolarization, with the atrial repolarization wave being lost in the QRS complex).[236-239]

The earliest changes are peaked, narrow T waves and a shortened QT interval, which reflect abnormally *rapid repolarization* (Fig. 28-4).* On occasion, this may be confused with the tall T waves seen with myocardial ischemia. However, the QT interval is usually normal or prolonged during ischemic episodes.[236]

---

* The primary event during repolarization is K^+ movement into the cells; this occurs passively down the favorable electrochemical gradient (cell interior now positive) that is created during depolarization (see page 823). The rate of repolarization is therefore in part dependent upon the K^+ permeability of the cell membrane, which appears to vary directly with the plasma K^+ concentration.[236,238] Thus, hyperkalemia increases K^+ permeability and consequently augments the rate of repolarization.

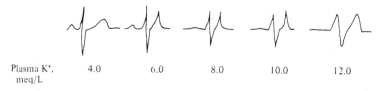

| Plasma K⁺, meq/L | 4.0 | 6.0 | 8.0 | 10.0 | 12.0 |

Figure 28-4   Electrocardiogram in hyperkalemia. The initial change is peaking and narrowing of the T wave with a short QT interval. With more severe hyperkalemia, widening of the QRS complex, decreased amplitude and eventual loss of the P wave, and a sine-wave pattern as the QRS complex merges with the T wave may be seen. The approximate relationship between these changes and the plasma K⁺ concentration is indicated, although there is a large interpatient variability. (*Adapted from Surawicz B*, Am Heart J *73:814, 1967, with permission.*)

The alteration in T-wave configuration typically becomes prominent when the plasma K^+ concentration exceeds 6 meq/L. At a plasma K^+ concentration above 7 to 8 meq/L, further changes in the electrocardiogram occur that are primarily due to *delayed depolarization.*[236]* The result is prolongation of the PR interval, widening of the QRS complex with no change in configuration (the electrocardiographic manifestation of slowed ventricular depolarization), and decreased amplitude, widening, and eventual loss of the P wave (Fig. 28-5). The final change is a sine-wave pattern as the widened QRS complex merges with the T wave, followed by ventricular fibrillation or standstill.

The tendency to severe arrhythmias also may be related in part to heterogeneous changes in myocardial conduction, as the epicardium is more prominently affected than the endocardium.[239] Despite these changes in conduction, the contractility of cardiac muscle seems to be unaffected by hyperkalemia.[242]

The approximate relationship between the degree of hyperkalemia and the ECG changes is depicted in Fig. 28-4. This relationship, however, is variable; in rare cases, the ECG may be normal or near normal despite a marked elevation in the plasma K^+ concentration to above 9 meq/L, a level that is usually life-threatening.[243]

The lack of predictability of the electrocardiographic changes in hyperkalemia is largely due to the influence of other factors that can affect cardiac conduction. As examples, the cardiac toxicity of hyperkalemia is enhanced by hypocalcemia,[244] hyponatremia,[245] acidemia,[246] and a rapid elevation in the plasma K^+ concentration (see "Treatment," below).[237,247] Thus, patients with renal failure may be particularly sensitive to hyperkalemia, since hypocalcemia (due to phosphate retention and vitamin D deficiency), metabolic acidosis (due to reduced NH_4^+ excretion), and hyponatremia (due to water retention) all may be present (see Chaps. 6, 19, and 23). On the other hand, hypernatremia and hypercalcemia

---

* Depolarization is mostly due to a marked elevation in the Na^+ permeability of the cell membrane, resulting in the rapid entry of Na^+ into the cell.[232,240,241] As described above, the fall in resting potential induced by hyperkalemia inactivates membrane Na^+ channels, thereby slowing the rate of depolarization.

counteract the membrane changes of hyperkalemia, thereby minimizing the cardiac risk.[243]

DIAGNOSIS

The initial evaluation of the hyperkalemic patient should include: a complete history (including questions about dietary intake and a history of kidney disease, diabetes mellitus, the use of K^+-sparing diuretics, or recurrent episodes of muscle weakness), physical examination (looking for muscle weakness or the signs of volume depletion or edema), an electrocardiogram, and measurement of arterial pH and the blood urea nitrogen (BUN), plasma creatinine, glucose, Na^+, and Ca^{2+} concentrations.

With this information, the approach to diagnosis can be simplified by considering separately the three groups of conditions associated with hyperkalemia: increased intake, K^+ release from the cells, and reduced urinary K^+ excretion. As described above, increased intake is the sole cause of hyperkalemia only when a massive load has been given acutely; it may, however, play an important contributory role in patients with underlying renal disease or hypoaldosteronism. Thus, a careful dietary history should be obtained, looking for the intake of K^+-rich foods and for the possible use of salt substitute or K^+ supplements.

The diagnosis of one of the disorders associated with K^+ release from the cells (Table 28-1) can usually be made from the history or laboratory data, as, for example, with marked hyperglycemia. *Pseudohyperkalemia* should be suspected if there is no apparent cause for the elevation in the plasma K^+ concentration or if there are no electrocardiographic changes at a plasma K^+ concentration greater than 6.5 to 7.0 meq/L. Once hemolysis during venipuncture has been excluded (by drawing blood without a tourniquet or clenching of the fist), the diagnosis of one of the other forms of pseudohyperkalemia can be confirmed by the findings of a normal plasma (not serum) K^+ concentration and a marked elevation in either the white blood cell or platelet count.

If none of these disorders is present or if the patient has persistent hyperkalemia, then decreased urinary K^+ excretion must be contributing to the rise in the plasma K^+ concentration. The kidney is so efficient in excreting K^+ that normal excretory function will prevent the persistence of hyperkalemia (see Fig. 28-1).[14] Measuring the urine K^+ concentration is generally *not helpful*, since the value must be *inappropriately low to permit perpetuation of the hyperkalemia*; however, calculation of the transtubular K^+ gradient permits estimation of the degree of aldosterone effect (see below).

Severe renal failure is a common cause of hyperkalemia. It is characterized by marked elevations in the BUN and plasma creatinine concentration or, in patients with acute renal failure, a progressive increase in these parameters. Hyperkalemia is more likely to occur if there is also an increased K^+ load. As an example, approximately 50 percent of patients with posttraumatic renal failure, in whom tissue catabolism is enhanced, develop a plasma K^+ concentration above 7 meq/L unless early therapy is instituted.[66]

Effective volume depletion as a cause of hyperkalemia can usually be excluded by the history (possibly including vomiting, diarrhea, heart failure) and physical examination. True volume depletion may be associated with decreased skin turgor, an estimated jugular venous pressure below 5 cmH$_2$O, tachycardia, and a postural fall in blood pressure (see Chap. 14). In contrast, heart failure is typically associated with peripheral and/or pulmonary edema, and cirrhosis with prominent ascites. If underlying renal function is normal, the urine Na^+ concentration should be less than 25 meq/L in these disorders, as Na^+ reabsorption is enhanced in an attempt to restore normovolemia.

Hypoaldosteronism

If renal function is normal or only moderately impaired and no other etiology of chronic hyperkalemia is apparent, the patient should be evaluated for one of the causes of hypoaldosteronism.

The age of the patient is an important determinant of the cause of hypoaldosteronism. In adults, hyporeninemic hypoaldosteronism and primary adrenal insufficiency are most common. The latter diagnosis should be suspected clinically if signs of cortisol deficiency are present, such as salt craving, fasting hypoglycemia, or hyperpigmentation of the skin and mucous membranes (due to the hypersecretion of ACTH). In comparison, enzyme deficiencies and type 1 pseudohypoaldosteronism begin in infancy or childhood.

Na^+ wasting may be relatively severe in children with hypoaldosteronism, who typically present with volume depletion, hyperkalemia, hyponatremia, metabolic acidosis, and an elevated urine Na^+ concentration. In comparison, adults with this disorder typically have less severe aldosterone deficiency and tend to present with asymptomatic hyperkalemia.[134] Sodium wasting and volume depletion are not typically seen in the absence of concurrent hypocortisolism due to primary adrenal insufficiency.[134] Other factors, such as angiotensin II, norepinephrine, and a mild reduction in blood pressure, can combine to maintain relatively normal Na^+ balance in this setting, despite the reduced levels of aldosterone (see Chap. 8). What is generally lost, however, is the ability to conserve Na^+ maximally. A urine Na^+ concentration below 10 to 15 meq/L is unusual, because this gradient is attained at the aldosterone-sensitive sites in the cortical and inner medullary collecting tubules.

The evaluation for hypoaldosteronism should begin with discontinuation of any potential offending drug, such as a NSAID, angiotensin converting enzyme inhibitor, K^+-sparing diuretic, or heparin. If these agents are not being used, measurement of the *morning* plasma renin activity and aldosterone and cortisol concentrations should establish the correct diagnosis (Table 28-3). To minimize the incidence of confusing borderline values, the patient should be given 20 to 40 mg of furosemide at 6 P.M. and 6 A.M. before the blood specimen is obtained. This

Table 28-3 Plasma renin activity, aldosterone and cortisol levels, and response to mineralocorticoid therapy in major causes of idiopathic hypoaldosteronism

Disorder	Plasma renin activity	Plasma aldosterone	Plasma cortisol	Response to aldosterone
Hyporeninism	↓–nl	↓	nl	nl
Primary adrenal insufficiency	↑	↓	↓	nl
Enzyme deficiencies				
Congenital adrenal hyperplasia	↑	↓	↓	nl
Isolated hypoaldosteronism	↑	↓	nl	nl
Pseudohypoaldosteronism	↑	↑	nl	0–↓

regimen enhances aldosterone secretion (via stimulation of renin) in normal subjects, but not in patients with hypoaldosteronism.[134]

An indirect way to estimate the effect of aldosterone would be to measure the tubular fluid K^+ concentration at the end of the cortical collecting tubule, after most of K^+ secretion has occurred. This can be estimated clinically if the following assumptions are correct: The urine osmolality at this site is similar to that of the plasma, since equilibration with the isosmotic interstitium will occur in the presence of ADH (see Chap. 4), and little or no K^+ secretion or reabsorption takes place in the medullary collecting tubule. In this setting, the K^+ concentration will rise in the medulla because of the loss of water; this can be accounted for by dividing the urine K^+ concentration by the (U_{osm}/P_{osm}). Thus the *transtubular K^+ gradient* (TTKG) is equal to[248]

$$TTKG = \frac{[U_{K^+} \div U_{osm}/P_{osm}]}{P_{K^+}}$$

This estimation is relatively accurate as long as the urine is not dilute and the urine Na^+ concentration is above 25 meq/L, so that Na^+ delivery is not limiting.[248]

The TTKG in normal subjects on a regular diet is 8 to 9 and rises to above 11 with a K^+ load, indicating increased K^+ secretion.[249] Thus, a value below 7 and particularly below 5 in a hyperkalemic patient is highly suggestive of hypoaldosteronism. If, for example, the U_{K^+} is 30 meq/L, the P_{K^+} is 6.5 meq/L, and the U_{osm} and P_{osm} are 560 mosmol/kg and 280 mosmol/kg, respectively, then

$$TTKG = \frac{30 \div 560/280}{6.5}$$

$$= 2.3$$

This low value is consistent with hypoaldosteronism.

TREATMENT

The treatment of hyperkalemia varies with the severity of the electrolyte disturbance.[68,250] As described above, severe symptoms usually do not occur until the plasma K^+ concentration is above 7.5 meq/L.[233,234] There is, however, substantial interpatient variability, since factors such as the plasma Ca^{2+} concentration and acid-base balance can modify the toxicity of hyperkalemia.[244,246] As a result, it is essential to monitor the ECG and muscle strength, which are the *functional consequences* of hyperkalemia, as well as the plasma K^+ concentration.

A plasma K^+ concentration above 8 meq/L, severe muscle weakness, or marked electrocardiographic changes (Fig. 28-5) are potentially life-threatening and require *immediate* treatment with almost all of the modalities in Table 28-4. In comparison, an asymptomatic elevation in the plasma K^+ concentration of 6.5 meq/L can be treated *solely with a cation exchange resin*, since rapid therapy is not necessary.

Reversing the effects of hyperkalemia can be achieved by direct antagonism of its membrane actions and by lowering the plasma K^+ concentration, either by driving K^+ into the cells (which will increase the $[K^+]_c/[K^+]_e$ ratio toward normal) or by removing K^+ from the body (Table 28-4).[115] In addition, further K^+ intake should be limited. Commonly ignored sources of K^+ are salt substitutes, stored blood, and K^+ penicillin, which contains 1.6 meq of K^+ per million units of penicillin.

Calcium

The severe symptoms of hyperkalemia are due to decreased membrane excitability resulting from inactivation of membrane Na^+ channels.[232] Via a mechanism that is not well understood, calcium antagonizes this effect of K^+, restoring membrane excitability toward normal.[251] Conversely, a decrease in the plasma Ca^{2+} concentration enhances the toxicity of hyperkalemia.[244]

Table 28-4   Treatment of hyperkalemia

Antagonism of membrane actions
  A. Calcium
  B. Hypertonic Na^+ solution (if hyponatremic)
Increased K^+ entry into the cells
  A. Glucose and insulin
  B. $NaHCO_3$
  C. β_2-Adrenergic agonists
  D. Hypertonic Na^+ solution (if hyponatremic)
Removal of the excess K^+
  A. Diuretics
  B. Cation-exchange resin (Kayexalate)
  C. Hemodialysis or peritoneal dialysis

The protective effect of Ca^{2+} administration begins within minutes but is relatively short-lived. Thus, Ca^{2+} is used only in patients with severe K^+ intoxication, who cannot wait the 30 to 60 min before glucose and insulin begin to act.

The usual dose is 10 mL (1 ampul) of a 10% calcium gluconate solution infused slowly over 2 to 3 min under electrocardiographic monitoring.* This dose can be repeated after 5 min if the electrocardiographic changes persist. Ca^{2+} should be used only when absolutely necessary (as with loss of P waves or widening of the QRS complex) in patients taking digitalis, because hypercalcemia, like hypokalemia, can precipitate digitalis toxicity.

Insulin and Glucose

Increasing the availability of insulin lowers the plasma K^+ concentration by driving K^+ into cells.[58,124,252] This effect is mediated by increased activity of the Na^+-K^+-ATPase pump, particularly the $\alpha(+)$ or α_2 isoform in skeletal muscle.[253-255]

Plasma insulin levels can be increased by administering insulin (10 units of regular insulin with 30 to 50 g of glucose to prevent hypoglycemia) or by enhancing endogenous insulin release by infusing glucose alone (50 mL of a 50 percent glucose solution given intravenously). This regimen usually lowers the plasma K^+ concentration by 0.5 to 1.5 meq/L, an effect that begins within 1 h and may last for many hours.[115] Plasma insulin levels are higher and the reduction in the plasma K^+ concentration more pronounced with the insulin-glucose combination.[124] However, insulin-glucose can cause symptomatic hypoglycemia unless an adequate amount of glucose is given both initially and as an ongoing dextrose infusion to prevent a late reduction in the plasma glucose concentration.[115,256]

Insulin alone may be sufficient in diabetic patients who are already hyperglycemic, while insulin-glucose can be given if the plasma glucose concentration is near normal. Care must be taken to avoid an elevation in the plasma glucose concentration, since the ensuing elevation in the plasma osmolality can exacerbate the hyperkalemia (see Fig. 28-2).

At least in end-stage renal failure, insulin and glucose more predictably lower the plasma K^+ concentration than either $NaHCO_3$ or a β_2-adrenergic agonist.[115,124,257] Although renal failure is associated with resistance to the hypoglycemic effect of insulin, the ability of insulin to increase Na^+-K^+-ATPase activity and therefore to promote K^+ entry into the cells is preserved.[121,122]

Sodium Bicarbonate

Whereas metabolic acidosis can result in the release of K^+ from the cells, raising the pH with $NaHCO_3$ drives K^+ into the cells.[53] In addition to the pH change, the elevation in the plasma HCO_3^- concentration appears to directly contribute to this

---

* Ca^{2+} should not be given in HCO_3^--containing solutions, since this combination can result in the precipitation of the insoluble salt $CaCO_3$.

effect (by an unknown mechanism).[258] Consequently, the infusion of $NaHCO_3$ will lower the plasma K^+ concentration and alleviate the signs of hyperkalemia, particularly in a patient with metabolic acidosis.[258,259] This effect begins within 30 to 60 min and may persist for many hours.

There is, however, a limitation to the administration of sodium bicarbonate. Most patients with severe hyperkalemia have advanced renal failure, which prevents excretion of the excess potassium. When used as monotherapy in this setting, sodium bicarbonate generally produces *little acute reduction* in the plasma potassium concentration.[113,257,260,261] The plasma K^+ concentration generally falls by no more than 0.5 meq/L in the first 6 h, half of which is due to dilution from the administered fluid. However, most of the patients in these studies had little or no metabolic acidosis; a potassium-lowering effect would be expected in patients with moderate to severe acidemia.

The usual dose is 44 to 50 meq of $NaHCO_3$ infused slowly over 5 min; this dose can be repeated within 30 min, if necessary. Alternatively, $NaHCO_3$ can be added to a glucose and saline solution.

Administration of a hypertonic bicarbonate solution may have an additional advantage in hyponatremic patients, since raising the plasma Na^+ concentration can reverse the electrocardiographic effects of hyperkalemia.[245,262] Both an increase in the rate of membrane depolarization and a fall in the plasma potassium concentration by dilution may contribute to this effect.[262]

β_2-Adrenergic Agonists

Like insulin, the β_2-adrenergic receptors drive K^+ into the cells[71-73] by increasing Na^+-K^+-ATPase activity.[4] One consequence of this relationship is that epinephrine released during a stress response can cause transient hypokalemia in a variety of clinical settings (see Chap. 27). There is less information on the use of β_2-agonists to treat hyperkalemia, but preliminary results suggest that albuterol (10 to 20 mg by nebulizer in 4 mL of saline over 10 min or 0.5 mg intravenously) can lower the plasma K^+ concentration by 0.5 to 1.5 meq/L.[113,263,264] The peak effect is seen within 30 min with intravenous infusion, but is delayed for 90 min with nasal inhalation.[264] Tachycardia and precipitation of angina pectoris are potential side effects; as a result, these agents should be avoided in patients with active coronary disease.

As with sodium bicarbonate, there is a limitation to the use of epinephrine in advanced renal failure, since there is a blunted hypokalemic response in this setting.[124,265] This relative resistance appears to reflect an increased sensitivity to the α-adrenergic actions of epinephrine; the α-receptors act to drive K^+ out of the cells (see page 375), thereby counteracting the reverse effect of β_2 stimulation.[265] β-adrenergic responsiveness is generally preserved, although four of ten patients in one study had less than a 0.5-meq/L fall in the plasma potassium concentration after the administration of albuterol.[266]

Thus, albuterol is the adrenergic agent of choice for severe hyperkalemia in end-stage renal disease. It should be given in combination with insulin plus glucose to maximize the reduction in the plasma potassium concentration.[266]

The effects of insulin, $NaHCO_3$ and β_2 agonists are transient, as the K^+ that is driven into the cells reenters the extracellular fluid after several hours. Thus, these measures are usually followed by diuretics, cation-exchange resins, or dialysis to remove the excess K^+ from the body. In addition, a cation-exchange resin alone may be sufficient in a patient with mild, asymptomatic hyperkalemia.

Diuretics

Loop or thiazide-type diuretics increase urinary K^+ excretion primarily by enhancing the flow rate to the K^+ secretory site in the distal nephron (see Chap. 15). These agents are not widely used in the treatment of acute hyperkalemia, since patients with this problem often have impaired renal function and are unlikely to respond to diuretic therapy with a significant rise in K^+ excretion. Diuretics are, however, useful in chronic hyperkalemia due to hypoaldosteronism,[267] heart failure (where they will also treat the fluid overload), or a selective K^+ secretory defect.[230]

Cation-Exchange Resin

The major cation-exchange resin available is sodium polystyrene sulfonate (Kayexalate), prepared in the sodium phase. In the gut, this resin takes up K^+ (and, to lesser degrees, Ca^{2+} and Mg^{2+}) and releases Na^+. Each gram of resin may bind as much as 1 meq of K^+ and release 1 to 2 meq of Na^+.[268,269]

When administered orally, 20 g of resin should be given with 100 mL of a 20% sorbitol solution to prevent constipation. This can be repeated every 4 to 6 h as necessary. Lower doses (5 g, two or three times a day) are generally well tolerated and can be used to treat chronic hyperkalemia that cannot be controlled by other means.

In patients who cannot take oral fluids, the resin can be given as a retention enema. In this situation, 50 g of resin is mixed with 50 mL of 70% sorbitol plus 100 to 150 mL of tap water and kept in the colon for at least 30 to 60 min and preferably 2 to 3 h. The colon should then be irrigated with a non-sodium-containing solution to prevent possible colonic mucosal injury.[270] Each enema can lower the plasma K^+ concentration by as much as 0.5 to 1.0 meq/L. The enemas can be repeated every 2 to 4 h if necessary.

The major side effects of sodium polystyrene sulfonate are nausea, constipation, hypokalemia (due to excessive use), and retention of the Na^+ that has been exchanged for K^+. In patients with oliguric renal failure or those with cardiac disease, for example, enough Na^+ may be retained to precipitate pulmonary edema.[268]

Intestinal necrosis is a potential complication, leading to severe abdominal pain and a usual requirement for surgery. The risk appears to be greatest, approaching 1 percent of cases, when the resin is given with sorbitol within the first week after surgery.[271-273] At least two factors are thought to increase the susceptibility to intestinal necrosis in this setting:

- Decreased colonic motility, due to postoperative ileus and/or the administration of opiates, increases the duration of drug contact with the intestinal mucosa.
- Hypertonic sorbitol may directly damage the intestinal mucosa.

It has been suggested that cleansing enemas given before and after resin enemas may be protective by preventing drug retention in the intestinal lumen.[272]

Dialysis

In almost all patients, the conservative measures described above will reverse hyperkalemia. However, when these measures are ineffective or severe hyperkalemia is present, either hemodialysis or peritoneal dialysis can be used. Hemodialysis is preferred, because the rate of K^+ removal is many times faster than with peritoneal dialysis.[274] Dialysis is particularly important in patients with acute renal failure who are hypercatabolic, as cell breakdown can result in the release of large quantities of K^+ into the extracellular fluid.[66]

Summary

One report found the following mean changes in the plasma K^+ concentration at 1 h after the institution of each particular therapy in hyperkalemic patients with end-stage renal disease[257]:

- No change with sodium bicarbonate in patients with little or no metabolic acidosis; thus, the main indication for bicarbonate therapy is the presence of moderate to severe acidemia.
- A 0.3-meq/L reduction with epinephrine; a greater response, similar to that with insulin and glucose, is typically seen with albuterol, which has no α-adrenergic activity.
- A 0.85-meq/L reduction with insulin and glucose.
- A 1.3-meq/L reduction with hemodialysis.

Hyporeninemic Hypoaldosteronism

The proper therapy of hyporeninemic hypoaldosteronism, the most common cause of unexplained hyperkalemia in adults, varies with the underlying etiology. If it is drug-induced, the offending agent should be discontinued, if possible.

Fludrocortisone, a synthetic mineralocorticoid, is in theory the mainstay of therapy in hyporeninemic hypoaldosteronism, since it corrects the mineralocorticoid deficiency. As much as 0.2 to 1.0 mg/day may be required (in comparison to 0.05 to 0.10 mg/day in primary adrenal insufficiency).[134,137] This supraphysiologic dose probably reflects aldosterone resistance induced by the underlying renal disease.

Although it can restore K^+ balance, fludrocortisone is *not used* in most patients because it can exacerbate preexistent hypertension or edema induced by the underlying renal insufficiency. Control of the hyperkalemia can usually be achieved by the combination of a low-K^+ diet plus a loop of thiazide-type diuretic to increase urinary K^+ losses.[134,267]

PROBLEMS

28-1 A 62-year-old man with mild chronic renal failure (plasma creatinine concentration equals 2.1 mg/dL) and normokalemia is started on a low-sodium diet for hypertension. Two weeks later, he notices that he is unable to lift himself out of a chair. On physical examination, slightly decreased skin turgor and marked proximal muscle weakness are found. The ECG reveals peaked T waves and some widening of the P wave and QRS complex. The following blood test results are obtained:

$$\text{Plasma } [Na^+] = 130 \, \text{meq/L}$$
$$[K^+] = 9.8 \, \text{meq/L}$$
$$[Cl^-] = 98 \, \text{meq/L}$$
$$[HCO_3^-] = 17 \, \text{meq/L}$$
$$[\text{Creatinine}] = 2.7 \, \text{mg/dL}$$
$$\text{Arterial pH} = 7.32$$

(a) What are the most likely factors responsible for the elevation in the plasma K^+ concentration?
(b) How do you know this is not pseudohyperkalemia?
(c) How would you treat the hyperkalemia?
(d) If the plasma K^+ concentration were only 6.4 meq/L and there were no changes in muscle strength or the ECG, how would you lower the plasma K^+ concentration?

28-2 A 54-year-old man with no prior medical history complains of chronic fatigue. The positive physical findings include a blood pressure of 100/60 and increased skin pigmentation. The skin turgor is relatively normal. The laboratory data are as follows:

Plasma $[Na^+]$	= 130 meq/L	BUN	=	28 mg/dL
$[K^+]$	= 6.8 meq/L	[Creatinine]	=	1.2 mg/dL
$[Cl^-]$	= 100 meq/L	Urine $[Na^+]$	=	50 meq/L
$[HCO_3^-]$	= 20 meq/L	$[K^+]$	=	34 meq/L
[Glucose]	= 90 mg/dL	U_{osm}	=	550 mosmol/kg

The electrocardiogram shows mild peaking of the T waves in the precordial leads. An infusion of glucose and insulin in appropriate proportions results in an episode of hypoglycemia.

(a) Is the urine K^+ concentration of 34 meq/L helpful in determining the correct diagnosis?
(b) What is the most likely diagnosis?
(c) How would you treat this patient?

REFERENCES

1. Nicolis GL, Kahn T, Sanchez A, Gabrilove JL. Glucose-induced hyperkalemia in diabetic subjects. *Arch Intern Med* 141:49, 1981.
2. Sterns RH, Cox M, Feig PU, Singer I. Internal potassium balance and the control of the plasma potassium concentration. *Medicine* 60:339, 1981.
3. Brown RS. Extrarenal potassium homeostasis. *Kidney Int* 30:116, 1986.
4. Clausen T, Everts ME. Regulation of the Na,K-pump in skeletal muscle. *Kidney Int* 35:1, 1989.
5. DeFronzo RA, Lee R, Jones A, Bia M. Effect of insulinopenia and adrenal hormone deficiency on acute potassium tolerance. *Kidney Int* 17:586, 1980.
6. DeFronzo R, Taufield P, Black H, et al. Impaired renal tubular potassium secretion in sickle cell disease. *Ann Intern Med* 90:310, 1979.
7. Winkler AW, Hoff HE, Smith PK. The toxicity of orally administered potassium salts in renal insufficiency. *J Clin Invest* 20:119, 1941.
8. Rabinowitz L. Aldosterone and potassium homeostasis. *Kidney Int* 49:1738, 1996.
9. Young DB, Paulsen AW. Interrelated effects of aldosterone and plasma potassium on potassium excretion. *Am J Physiol* 244:F28, 1983.
10. Young DB. Quantitative analysis of aldosterone's role in potassium regulation. *Am J Physiol* 255:F811, 1988.
11. Sansom S, Muto S, Giebisch G. Na-dependent effects of DOCA on cellular transport properties of CCDs from ADX rabbits. *Am J Physiol* 253:F753, 1987.
12. Muto S, Sansom S, Giebisch G. Effects of a high potassium diet on electrical properties of cortical collecting ducts from adrenalectomized rabbits. *J Clin Invest* 81:376, 1988.
13. Talbott JH, Schwab RS. Recent advances in the biochemistry and therapeusis of potassium salts. *N Engl J Med* 222:585, 1940.
14. Rabelink TJ, Koomans HA, Hené RJ, Dorhout Mees EJ. Early and late adjustment to potassium loading in humans. *Kidney Int* 38:942, 1990.
15. Stanton BA. Renal potassium transport: Morphological and functional adaptations. *Am J Physiol* 257:R989, 1989.
16. Alexander EA, Levinsky NG. An extrarenal mechanism of potassium adaptation. *J Clin Invest* 47:740, 1968.
17. Spital A, Sterns RH. Paradoxical potassium depletion: A renal mechanism for extrarenal potassium adaptation. *Kidney Int* 30:532, 1986.
18. Foster ES, Jones WJ, Hayslett JP, Binder HJ. Role of aldosterone and dietary potassium in potassium adaptation in the distal colon of the rat. *Gastroenterology* 88:1985, 1985.
19. Stanton BA, Biemesderfer D, Wade JB, Giebisch G. Structural and functional study of the rat distal nephron: Effects of potassium adaptation and depletion. *Kidney Int* 19:36, 1981.
20. Stanton B, Pan L, Deetjen H, et al. Independent effects of aldosterone and potassium on induction of potassium adaptation in rat kidney. *J Clin Invest* 79:198, 1987.
21. Kashgarian M, Ardito T, Hirsch DJ, Hayslett JP. Response of collecting tubule cells to aldosterone and potassium loading. *Am J Physiol* 253:F8, 1987.
22. Garg LC, Narang N. Renal adaptation to potassium in the adrenalectomized rabbit: Role of distal tubular sodium-potassium adenosine triphosphatase. *J Clin Invest* 76:1065, 1985.
23. Doucet A, Katz AI. Renal potassium adaptation: Na-K-ATPase activity along the nephron after chronic potassium loading. *Am J Physiol* 238:F380, 1980.
24. Jackson CA. Rapid renal potassium adaptation in rats. *Am J Physiol* 2634:F1098, 1992.
25. Schultze RG, Taggart DD, Shapiro H, et al. On the adaptation in potassium excretion associated with nephron reduction in the dog. *J Clin Invest* 50:1061, 1971.
26. Bourgoignie JJ, Kaplan M, Pincus J, et al. Renal handling of potassium in dogs with chronic renal insufficiency. *Kidney Int* 20:482, 1981.
27. Gonick HC, Kleeman CR, Rubini ME, Maxwell MH. Functional impairment in chronic renal disease: III. Studies of potassium excretion. *Am J Med Sci* 261:281, 1971.

28. Schrier RW, Regal EM. Physiological role of aldosterone in sodium, water and potassium metabolism in chronic renal disease. *Kidney Int* 1:156, 1972.
29. Schon DA, Silva P, Hayslett JP. Mechanism of potassium excretion in renal insufficiency. *Am J Physiol* 227:1323, 1974.
30. Bastl C, Hayslett JP, Binder HJ. Increased large intestinal secretion of potassium in renal insufficiency. *Kidney Int* 12:9, 1977.
31. Hayes CP Jr, Robinson RR. Fecal potassium excretion in patients on chronic intermittent hemodialysis. *Trans Am Soc Artif Intern Organs* 11:242, 1965.
32. Ponce SP, Hennings AC, Madias NE, Harrington JT. Drug-induced hyperkalemia. *Medicine* 64:357, 1985.
33. Rimmer JM, Horn JF, Gennari FJ. Hyperkalemia as a complication of drug therapy. *Arch Intern Med* 147:867, 1987.
34. Illingworth RN, Proudfoot AT. Rapid poisoning with slow-release potassium. *Br Med J* 2:485, 1980.
35. Moss MH, Rasen AR. Potassium toxicity due to intravenous penicillin therapy. *Pediatrics* 29:1032, 1962.
36. Kallen RJ, Rieger CHL, Cohen HS, et al. Near-fatal hyperkalemia due to ingestion of salt substitute by an adult. *JAMA* 235:2125, 1976.
37. Scanlon JW, Krakaur R. Hyperkalemia following exchange transfusion. *J Pediatr* 96:108, 1980.
38. Simon GE, Bove JR. The potassium load from blood transfusion. *Postgrad Med* 49:61, 1971.
39. LeVeen HH, Posternack HS, Lustrin I, et al. Hemorrhage and transfusion as the major cause of cardiac arrest. *JAMA* 173:770, 1960.
40. Lawson DH. Adverse reactions to potassium chloride. *Q J Med* 43:433, 1974.
41. Greenblatt DJ, Koch-Wesser J. Adverse reactions to spironolactone. *JAMA* 225:40, 1973.
42. Bay WH, Hartman JA. High potassium in low sodium soups (letter). *N Engl J Med* 308:1166, 1983.
43. Gelfand MC, Zarate A, Knepshield JH. Geophagia: A cause of life-threatening hyperkalemia in patients with chronic renal failure. *JAMA* 234:738, 1975.
44. Don BR, Sebastian A, Cheitlin M, et al. Pseudohyperkalemia caused by fist clenching during phlebotomy. *N Engl J Med* 322:1290, 1990.
45. Hyman D, Kaplan NM. The difference between serum and plasma potassium (letter). *N Engl J Med* 313:642, 1985.
46. Graber M, Subramani K, Copish D, Schwab A. Thrombocytosis elevates serum potassium. *Am J Kidney Dis* 12:116, 1988.
47. Chumbley LC. Pseudohyperkalemia in acute myelocytic leukemia. *JAMA* 211:1007, 1970.
48. Bronson WR, DeVita VT, Carbone PP, Cotlove E. Pseudohyperkalemia due to release of potassium from white blood cells during clotting. *N Engl J Med* 274:369, 1966.
49. Hartmann RC, Auditore JV, Jackson DP. Studies on thrombocytosis· I Hyperkalemia due to release of potassium from platelets during coagulation. *J Clin Invest* 37:699, 1958.
50. Stewart GW, Fyffe JA, Corrall RJM. Familial pseudohyperkalemia: A new syndrome. *Lancet* 2:175, 1979.
51. James DR, Stansbie D. Familial pseudohyperkalemia: Inhibition of erythrocyte K efflux at 4°C by quinine. *Clin Sci* 73:557, 1987.
52. Iolacson A, Stewart GW, Ajetunmob S, et al. Familial pseudohyperkalemia maps to the same locus as dehydrated hereditary stomatocytosis (hereditary xerocytosis). *Blood* 93:3120, 1999.
53. Adrogué HJ, Madias NE. Changes in plasma potassium concentration during acute acid-base disturbances. *Am J Med* 71:456, 1981.
54. Magner PO, Robinson L, Halperin RM, et al. The plasma potassium concentration in metabolic acidosis: A re-evaluation. *Am J Kidney Dis* 11:220, 1988.
55. Sebastian A, McSherry E, Morris RC Jr. Renal potassium wasting in renal tubular acidosis (RTA): Its occurrence in types 1 and 2 RTA despite sustained correction of systemic acidosis. *J Clin Invest* 50:667, 1971.

56. Adrogué HJ, Lederer ED, Suki WN, Eknoyan G. Determinants of plasma potassium levels in diabetic ketoacidosis. *Medicine* 65:163, 1986.
57. Arieff AI, Carroll HJ. Nonketotic hyperosmolar coma with hyperglycemia: Clinical features, pathophysiology, renal function, acid-base balance, plasma-cerebrospinal fluid equilibria and the effects of therapy in 37 cases. *Medicine* 51:73, 1972.
58. DeFronzo RA, Sherwin RS, Dillingham M, et al. Influence of basal insulin and glucagon secretion on potassium and sodium metabolism: Studies with somatostatin in normal dogs and in normal and diabetic human beings. *J Clin Invest* 61:472, 1978.
59. Viberti GC. Glucose-induced hyperkalemia: A hazard for diabetics? *Lancet* 1:690, 1978.
60. Goldfarb S, Cox M, Singer I, Goldberg M. Acute hyperkalemia induced by hyperglycemia: Hormonal mechanisms. *Ann Intern Med* 84:426, 1976.
61. Makoff DL, Da Silva JA, Rosenbaum BJ, et al. Hypertonic expansion: Acid-base and electrolyte changes. *Am J Physiol* 218:1201, 1970.
62. Conte G, Dal Canton A, Imperatore P, et al. Acute increase in plasma osmolality as a cause of hyperkalemia in patients with renal failure. *Kidney Int* 38:301, 1990.
63. Aviram A, Pfau A, Czackes JW, Ullman TD. Hyperosmolality with hyponatremia caused by inappropriate administration of mannitol. *Am J Med* 42:648, 1967.
64. Montoliu J, Revert L. Lethal hyperkalemia associated with severe hyperglycemia in diabetic patients with renal failure. *Am J Kidney Dis* 5:47, 1985.
65. Sharma AM, Thiede H, Keller F. Somatostatin-induced hyperkalemia in a patient on maintenance hemodialysis. *Nephron* 59:445, 1991.
66. Lordon RE, Burton JR. Post-traumatic renal failure in military personnel in Southeast Asia. *Am J Med* 53:137, 1972.
67. Arseneau JC, Bagley CM, Anderson T, Canellos GP. Hyperkalemia, a sequel to chemo-therapy of Burkitt's lymphoma. *Lancet* 1:10, 1973.
68. Kalemkerian GP, Darwish B, Varterasian ML. Tumor lysis syndrome in small cell carcinoma and other solid tumors. *Am J Med* 103:363, 1997.
69. Fortner RW, Nowakowski A, Carter CB, et al. Death due to overheated dialysate during dialysis. *Ann Intern Med* 73:443, 1970.
70. Schaller M-D, Fischer AP, Perret CH. Hyperkalemia: A prognostic factor during acute severe hypothermia. *JAMA* 264:1842, 1990.
71. Rosa RM, Silva P, Young JB, et al. Adrenergic modulation of extrarenal potassium disposal. *N Engl J Med* 302:431, 1980.
72. Brown MJ, Brown DC, Murphy MB. Hypokalemia from beta$_2$-receptor stimulation by circulating epinephrine. *N Engl J Med* 309:1414, 1983.
73. Williams ME, Gervino EV, Rosa RM, et al. Catecholamine modulation of rapid potassium shifts during exercise. *N Engl J Med* 312:823, 1985.
74. Swenson ER. Severe hyperkalemia as a complication of timolol, a topically applied beta-adrenergic antagonist. *Arch Intern Med* 146:1220, 1986.
75. Carlsson E, Fellenius E, Lundborg P, Svensson L. β-adrenoceptor blockers, plasma potassium, and exercise (letter). *Lancet* 2:424, 1978.
76. Lim M, Linton RAF, Wolff CB, Band DM. Propranolol, exercise and arterial plasma potassium. *Lancet* 2:591, 1981.
77. Arthur S, Greenberg A. Hyperkalemia associated with intravenous labetolol for acute hypertension in renal transplant recipients. *Clin Nephrol* 33:269, 1990.
78. Bethune DW, McKay R. Paradoxical changes in serum-potassium during cardiopulmonary bypass in association with non-cardioselective beta blockade. *Lancet* 2:380, 1978.
79. Castellino P, Bia MJ, DeFronzo RA. Adrenergic modulation of potassium metabolism in uremia. *Kidney Int* 37:793, 1990.
80. Daut J, Maier-Rudolph W, von Beckerath N, et al. Hypoxic dilation of coronary arteries is mediated by ATP-sensitive potassium channels. *Science* 247:1341, 1990.
81. Knochel JP, Schlein EM. On the mechanism of rhabdomyolysis in potassium depletion. *J Clin Invest* 51:1750, 1972.

82. Sessard J, Vincent M, Annat G, Bizollon CA. A kinetic study of plasma renin and aldosterone during changes of posture in man. *J Clin Endocrinol Metab* 42:20, 1976.
83. Struthers AD, Quigley C, Brown MJ. Rapid changes in plasma potassium during a game of squash. *Clin Sci* 74:397, 1988.
84. Rose LI, Carroll DR, Lowe SL, et al. Serum electrolyte changes after marathon running. *J Appl Physiol* 29:449, 1970.
85. Thomson A, Kelly DT. Exercise stress-induced changes in systemic arterial potassium in angina pectoris. *Am J Cardiol* 63:1435, 1989.
86. Lindringer M, Heigenhauser GJF, McKelvie RS, Jones NL. Blood ion regulation during repeated maximal exercise and recovery in humans. *Am J Physiol* 262:R126, 1992.
87. Knochel JP, Blachley JD, Johnson JH, Carter NW. Muscle cell electrical hyperpolarization and reduced exercise hyperkalemia in physically conditioned dogs. *J Clin Invest* 75:740, 1985.
88. Ledingham IMA, MacVicar S, Watt I, Weston GA. Early resuscitation after marathon collapse. *Lancet* 2:1096, 1982.
89. McKechnie JK, Leary WP, Joubert SM. Some electrocardiographic and biochemical changes recorded in marathon runners. *S Afr Med J* 41:722: 1967.
90. Smith TW. Digitalis: Mechanisms of action and clinical use. *N Engl J Med* 318:358, 1988.
91. Lown B, Black H, Moore FD. Digitalis, electrolytes and the surgical patient. *Am J Cardiol* 6:309, 1960.
92. Asplund J, Edhag O, Morgenson L, et al. Four cases of massive digitalis poisoning. *Acta Med Scand* 189:293, 1971.
93. Reza MJ, Kovick RB, Shine KI, Pearce ML. Massive intravenous digoxin overdosage. *N Engl J Med* 291:777, 1974.
94. Griggs RC, Ptacek LJ. Mutations of sodium channels in periodic paralysis: Can they explain the disease and predict treatment? *Neurology* 52:1309, 1999.
95. Gamstorp I, Hauge M, Helweg-Larsen HF, Mjones H. Adynamia episodica hereditaria: A disease clinically resembling familial periodic paralysis but characterized by increasing serum potassium during the paralytic attacks. *Am J Med* 23:385, 1957.
96. Fontaine B, Lapie P, Plassart E, et al. Periodic paralysis and voltage-gated ion channels. *Kidney Int* 49:9, 1996.
97. Clausen T, Wang P, Orskov H, Kristen O. Hyperkalemic periodic paralysis: Relationship between changes in plasma water, electrolytes, insulin, and catecholamines during attacks. *Scand J Clin Lab Invest* 40:211, 1980.
98. Rojas CV, Wang J, Schwartz LS, et al. A met-to-val mutation in the skeletal muscle Na^+ channel α-subunit in hyperkalemic periodic paralysis. *Nature* 354:387, 1992.
99. Fontaine B, Khurana TS, Hoffman EP, et al. Hyperkalemic periodic paralysis and the adult muscle sodium channel α-subunit gene. *Science* 250:1000, 1990.
100. Rojas CV, Neely A, Velasco-Loyden G, et al. Hyperkalemic periodic paralysis M1592V mutation modifies activation in human skeletal muscle Na^+ channel. *Am J Physiol* 276:C259, 1999.
101. Wang P, Clausen T. Treatment of attacks in hyperkalaemic familial periodic paralysis by inhalation of salbutamol. *Lancet* 1:221, 1976.
102. Streeten DH, Dalakos TG, Fellerman H. Studies on hyperkalemic periodic paralysis: Evidence of changes in plasma Na and Cl and induction of paralysis by adrenal glucocorticoids. *J Clin Invest* 50:142, 1971.
103. Lim M, Linton RAF, Band DM. Rise in plasma potassium during rewarming in open-heart surgery. *Lancet* 1:241, 1983.
104. Koht AL, Cerullo LJ, Land PC, Linde HW. Serum potassium levels during prolonged hypothermia. *Anesthesiology* 51(suppl): S203, 1979.
105. Bruining HA, Boelhouwer RU. Acute transient hypokalemia and body temperature (letter). *Lancet* 2:1283, 1982.
106. Birch AA, Mitchell GD, Playford GA, Lang CA. Changes in serum potassium response to succinylcholine following trauma. *JAMA* 210:490, 1969.

107. Cooperman LH. Succinylcholine-induced hyperkalemia in neuro-muscular disease. *JAMA* 213:1867, 1970.
108. Hertz P, Richardson JA. Arginine-induced hyperkalemia in renal failure patients. *Arch Intern Med* 130:778, 1972.
109. Bushinsky DA, Gennari FJ. Life-threatening hyperkalemia induced by arginine. *Ann Intern Med* 89:632, 1978.
110. Caramelo C, Bello E, Ruiz E, et al. Hyperkalemia in patients infected with the human immunodeficiency virus: Involvement of a systemic mechanism. *Kidney Int* 56:198, 1999.
111. Allon M. Hyperkalemia in end-stage renal disease: Mechanisms and management. *J Am Soc Nephrol* 6:1134, 1995.
112. Elkinton JR, Tarail R, Peters JP. Transfers of potassium in renal insufficiency. *J Clin Invest* 28:378, 1949.
113. Allon M. Treatment and prevention of hyperkalemia in end-stage renal disease. *Am J Kidney Dis* 43:1197, 1993.
114. Kleeman CR, Okun R, Heller RJ. The renal regulation of potassium in patients with chronic renal failure and the effect of diuretics on the excretion of these ions. *Ann N Y Acad Sci* 139:520, 1966.
115. Salem MM, Rosa RM, Batlle DC. Extrarenal potassium tolerance in chronic renal failure: Implications for the treatment of acute hyperkalemia. *Am J Kidney Dis* 18:421, 1991.
116. Bilbrey GL, Carter NW, White MG, et al. Potassium deficiency in chronic renal failure. *Kidney Int* 4:423, 1973.
117. Kahn T, Kaji M, Nicolis G, et al. Factors related to potassium transport in chronic stable renal disease in man. *Clin Sci* 54:661, 1978.
118. Bia MJ, DeFronzo RA. Extrarenal potassium homeostasis. *Am J Physiol* 240:F257, 1981.
119. Allon M, Dansby L, Shanklin N. Glucose modulation of the disposal of an acute potassium load in patients with end-stage renal disease. *Am J Med* 94:475, 1993.
120. Bonilla S, Goecke A, Bozzo S, et al. Effect of chronic renal failure on Na,K-ATPase $\alpha1$ and $\alpha2$ mRNA transcription in rat skeletal muscle. *J Clin Invest* 88:2137, 1991.
121. Alvestrand A, Wahren J, Smith D, DeFronzo RA. Insulin-mediated potassium uptake is normal in uremic and healthy subjects. *Am J Physiol* 246:E174, 1984.
122. Goecke IA, Bonilla S, Marusic ET, Alvo M. Enhanced insulin sensitivity in extrarenal potassium handling in uremic rats. *Kidney Int* 39:39, 1991.
123. Gifford JD, Rutsky EA, Kirk KA, McDaniel HG. Control of serum potassium during fasting in patients with end-stage renal disease. *Kidney Int* 35:90, 1989.
124. Allon M, Takeshian A, Shanklin N. Effect of insulin-plus-glucose infusion with or without epinephrine on fasting hyperkalemia. *Kidney Int* 43:212, 1993.
125. Anderson HM, Laragh JH. Renal excretion of potassium in normal and sodium depleted dogs. *J Clin Invest* 37:323, 1958.
126. Malnic G, Klose RM, Giebisch G. Micropuncture study of distal tubular potassium and sodium transport in rat nephron. *Am J Physiol* 211:529, 1966.
127. Danovitch GM, Bourgoignie JJ, Bricker NS. Reversibility of the "salt-losing" tendency of chronic renal failure. *N Engl J Med* 296:15, 1977.
128. Coleman AJ, Arias M, Carter NW, et al. The mechanism of salt-wasting in chronic renal disease. *J Clin Invest* 45:1116, 1966.
129. Popovtzer MM, Katz FH, Pinggera WF, et al. Hyperkalemia in salt-wasting nephropathy: Study of the mechanism. *Arch Intern Med* 132:203, 1973.
130. Chakko SC, Frutchey J, Gheorghiade M. Life-threatening hyperkalemia in severe heart failure. *Am Heart J* 117:1083, 1989.
131. Oster JR, Materson BJ. Renal and electrolyte complications of congestive heart failure and effects of treatment with angiotensin-converting enzyme inhibitors. *Arch Intern Med* 152:704, 1992.
132. Glasgow BJ, Steinsapir KD, Anders K, Layfield LJ. Adrenal pathology in the acquired immune deficiency syndrome. *Am J Clin Pathol* 84:594, 1985.

133. Freda PU, Wardlaw SL, Brudney K, Goland RS. Clinical case seminar: Primary adrenal insufficiency in patients with the acquired immunodeficiency syndrome: A report of five cases. *J Clin Endocrinol Metab* 79:1540, 1994.
134. DeFronzo RA. Hyperkalemia and hyporeninemic hypoaldosteronism. *Kidney Int* 17:118, 1980.
135. DuBose TD Jr, Caflisch CR. Effective of selective aldosterone deficiency on acidification in nephron segments of the rat inner medulla. *J Clin Invest* 82:1624, 1988.
136. Gabow PA, Moore S, Schrier RW. Spironolactone-induced hyperchloremic acidosis in cirrhosis. *Ann Intern Med* 90:338, 1979.
137. Sebastian A, Schambelan M, Lindenfeld S, Morris RC Jr. Amelioration of metabolic acidosis with fluorocortisone therapy in hyporeninemic hypoaldosteronism. *N Engl J Med* 297:576, 1977.
138. Szylman P, Better OS, Chaimowitz C, Rosler A. Role of hyperkalemia in the metabolic acidosis of isolated hypoaldosteronism. *N Engl J Med* 294:361, 1976.
139. Jaeger P, Karlmark B, Giebisch G. Ammonia transport in rat cortical tubule: Relationship to potassium metabolism. *Am J Physiol* 245:F593, 1983.
140. Altenberg GA, Aristimuno PC, Amorena CE, Taquini AC. Amiloride prevents the metabolic acidosis of a KCl load in nephrectomized rats. *Clin Sci* 76:649, 1989.
141. Fuller GR, MacLeod MB, Pitts RF. Influence of administration of potassium salts on the renal tubular reabsorption of bicarbonate. *Am J Physiol* 182:111, 1955.
142. DuBose TD Jr, Good DW. Effects of chronic hyperkalemia on renal production and proximal tubular transport of ammonium in rats. *Am J Physiol* 260:F680, 1991.
143. DuBose TD Jr, Good DW. Chronic hyperkalemia impairs ammonium transport and accumulation in the inner medulla of the rat. *J Clin Invest* 90:1443, 1992.
144. Schambelan M, Sebastian A, Biglieri E. Prevalence, pathogenesis, and functional significance of aldosterone deficiency in hyperkalemia patients with chronic renal insufficiency. *Kidney Int* 17:89, 1980.
145. Kokko JP. Primary acquired hypoaldosteronism. *Kidney Int* 27:690, 1985.
146. Williams FA JR, Schamberlan M, Biglieri EG, Carey RM. Acquired primary hypoaldosteronism due to an isolated zona glomerulosa defect. *N Engl J Med* 309:1623, 1983.
147. Tuck ML, Mayes DM. Mineralocorticoid biosynthesis in patients with hyporeninemic hypoaldosteronism. *J Clin Endocrinol Metab* 50:341, 1980.
148. Kogishi T, Morimoto S, Uchida K. Unresponsiveness of plasma mineralocorticoids to angiotensin II in diabetic patients with asymptomatic normoreninemic hypoaldosteronism. *J Lab Clin Med* 105:195, 1985.
149. Bayard F, Cooke C, Tiller D, et al. The regulation of aldosterone secretion in anephric man. *J Clin Invest* 50:1585, 1971.
150. Azukizawa S, Kaneko M, Nakano S, et al. Angiotensin II receptor and postreceptor events in adrenal zona glomerulosa cells from streptozotocin-induced diabetic rats with hypoaldosteronism. *Endocrinology* 129:2729, 1991.
151. Perez GO, Lespier L, Jacobi J, et al. Hyporeninemia and hypoaldosteronism in diabetes mellitus. *Arch Intern Med* 137:852, 1977.
152. Beretta-Piccoli C, Weidmann P, Keusch G. Responsiveness of plasma renin and aldosterone in diabetes mellitus. *Kidney Int* 20:259, 1981.
153. Nadler JL, Lee FO, Hsueh W, Horton R. Evidence of prostacyclin deficiency in the syndrome of hyporeninemic hypoaldosteronism. *N Engl J Med* 314:1015, 1986.
154. Campbell WB, Gomez-Sanchez CE, Adams BV, et al. Attenuation of angiotensin II- and III-induced aldosterone released by prostaglandin synthesis inhibitors. *J Clin Invest* 64:1552, 1979.
155. Tan SY, Shapiro R, Franco R, et al. Indomethacin-induced prostaglandin inhibition with hyperkalemia: A reversible cause of hyporeninemic hypoaldosteronism. *Ann Intern Med* 90:783, 1979.
156. Ruilope LM, Robles RG, Paya C, et al. Effects of long-term treatment with indomethacin on renal function. *Hypertension* 8:677, 1986.
157. Zimran A, Dramer M, Plaskin M, Hershko C. Incidence of hyperkalaemia induced by indomethacin in a hospital population. *Br Med J* 291:107, 1985.

158. Clark BA, Brown RS, Epstein FH. Effect of atrial natriuretic peptide on potassium-stimulated aldosterone secretion: Potential relevance to hypoaldosteronism in man. *J Clin Endocrinol Metab* 75:399, 1992.
159. Rodriguez-Iturbe B, Colic D, Parra G, Gutkowska J. Atrial natriuretic factor in the acute nephritic and nephrotic syndromes. *Kidney Int* 38:512, 1990.
160. Don BR, Schambelan M. Hyperkalemia in acute glomerulonephritis due to transient hyporeninemic hypoaldosteronism. *Kidney Int* 38:1159, 1990.
161. Hsueh WA, Carlson EJ, Leutscher JA, Grislis G. Activation and characterization of inactive big renin in plasma of patients with diabetic nephropathy and unusual active renin. *J Clin Endocrinol Metab* 51:535, 1980.
162. Bryer-Ash M, Fraze EB, Luetscher JA. Plasma renin and prorenin (inactive renin) in diabetes mellitus: Effects of intravenous furosemide. *J Clin Endocrinol Metab* 66:454, 1988.
163. Sowers JR, Beck FW, Waters BK, et al. Studies of renin activation and aldosterone and 18-hydroxycorticosterone synthesis in hyporeninemic hypoaldosteronism. *J Clin Endocrinol Metab* 61:60, 1985.
164. Rebuffat P, Belloni AS, Malendowicz LK, et al. Zona glomerulosa atrophy and function in streptozotocin-induced diabetic rats. *Endocrinology* 123:949, 1988.
165. Textor SC, Bravo EL, Fouad FM, Tarazi RC. Hyperkalemia in azotemic patients during angiotensin-converting enzyme inhibition and aldosterone reduction with captopril. *Am J Med* 73:719, 1982.
166. Burnakis TG, Mioduch HJ. Combined therapy with captopril and potassium supplementation: A potential for hyperkalemia. *Arch Intern Med* 144:2371, 1984.
167. Kalin MF, Poretsky L, Seres DS, Zumoff B. Hyporeninemic hypoaldosteronism associated with AIDS. *Am J Med* 82:1035, 1987.
168. Bantle JP, Nath KA, Sutherland DER, et al. Effect of cyclosporine on the renin-angiotensin system and potassium excretion in renal transplant recipients. *Arch Intern Med* 145:505, 1985.
169. Kamel KS, Ethier JH, Quaggin S, et al. Studies to determine the basis for hyperkalemia in recipients of a renal transplant who are treated with cyclosporine. *J Am Soc Nephrol* 2:1279, 1992.
170. Tumlin JA, Sands JM. Nephron segment-specific inhibition of Na^+-K^+-ATPase activity by cyclosporin A. *Kidney Int* 43:246, 1993.
171. Ling BN, Eaton DC. Cyclosporin A inhibits apical secretory K^+ channels in rabbit cortical collecting tubule principal cells. *Kidney Int* 44:974, 1993.
172. Kifor I, Moore TJ, Fallo F, et al. Potassium-stimulated angiotensin release from superfused adrenal capsules and enzymatically digested cells of the zona glomerulosa. *Endocrinology* 129:823, 1991.
173. Pratt J. Role of angiotensin II in potassium-mediated stimulation of aldosterone secretion in the dog. *J Clin Invest* 70:667, 1982.
174. Pitt B, Zannad F, Remme WJ, et al, for the Randomized Aldactone Evaluation Study Investigators. The effect of spironolactone on morbidity and mortality in patients with severe heart failure. *N Engl J Med* 341:709, 1999.
175. Glassock RJ, Cohen AH, Danovitch G, Parsa KP. Human immunodeficiency virus (HIV) infection and the kidney. *Ann Intern Med* 112:35, 1990.
176. Caramelo C, Bello E, Ruiz E, et al. Hyperkalemia in patients infected with the human immunodeficiency virus: Involvement of systemic mechanism. *Kidney Int* 56:198, 1999.
177. Orth DN. Causes of primary adrenal insufficiency (Addison's disease), in Rose BD (ed): *UpToDate in Medicine*. Wellesley, MA, UpToDate, 2000.
178. Song YH, Connor EL, Muir A, et al. Autoantibody epitope mapping of the 21-hydroxylase antigen in autoimmune Addison's disease. *J Clin Endocrinol Metab* 78:1108, 1994.
179. Chen S, Sawicka J, Betterle C, et al. Autoantibodies to steroidogenic enzymes in autoimmune polyglandular syndrome, Addison's disease, and premature ovarian failure. *J Clin Endocrinol Metab* 81:1871, 1996.
180. White PC, New MI, Dupont B. Congenital adrenal hyperplasia. *N Engl J Med* 316:1519, 1987.

181. Ganong WF, Coultan L, Alpert AB, Less TC. ACTH and the regulation of adrenocortical secretion. *N Engl J Med* 290:1006, 1974.
182. Kovacs WJ, Orth DN. Adrenal steroid biosynthesis and congenital adrenal hyperplasia, in Rose BD (ed): *UpToDate in Medicine*. Wellesley, MA, UpToDate, 2000.
183. White PC. Disorders of aldosterone biosynthesis and action. *N Engl J Med* 331:250, 1994.
184. Taymans SE, Pack S, Pak E, et al. Human CYP11B2 (aldosterone synthase) maps to chromosome 8q24.3. *J Clin Endocrinol Metab* 83:1033, 1998.
185. Shibata H, Ogishima T, Mitani F, et al. Regulation of aldosterone synthase cytochrome P450 in rat adrenals by angiotensin II and potassium. *Endocrinology* 128:2534, 1991.
186. Ulick S, Wang JZ, Morton DH. The biochemical phenotypes of two inborn errors in the biosynthesis of aldosterone. *J Clin Endocrinol Metab* 74:1415, 1992.
187. Kovacs WJ, Orth DN. Congenital adrenal hyperplasia due to CYP11B1 (11-beta-hydroxylase) deficiency, in Rose BD (ed): *UpToDate in Medicine*. Wellesley, MA, UpToDate, 2000.
188. Shizuta Y, Kawamoto T, Mitsuuchi Y, et al. Inborn errors of aldosterone biosynthesis in humans. *Steroids* 60:15, 1995.
189. Veldhuis JD, Melby JC. Isolated aldosterone deficiency in man: Acquired and inborn errors in the biosynthesis or action of aldosterone. *Endocr Rev* 2:495, 1986.
190. Kovacs WJ, Orth DN. Congenital adrenal hyperplasia due to CYP21A2 (21-hydroxylase) deficiency, in Rose BD (ed): *UpToDate in Medicine*. Wellesley, MA, UpToDate, 2000.
191. O'Kelly R, Magee F, McKenna TJ. Routine heparin therapy inhibits adrenal aldosterone production. *J Clin Endocrinol Metab* 56:108, 1983.
192. Oster JR, Singer I, Fishman LM. Heparin-induced aldosterone suppression and hyperkalemia. *Am J Med* 98:575, 1995.
193. Sequeira SJ, McKenna TJ. Chlorbutol, a new inhibitor of aldosterone biosynthesis identified during examination of heparin effect on aldosterone production. *J Clin Endocrinol Metab* 63:780, 1986.
194. Sherman RA, Ruddy MC. Suppression of aldosterone production by low-dose heparin. *Am J Nephrol* 6:165, 1986.
195. Phelps KR, Oh MS, Carroll HJ. Heparin-induced hyperkalemia: Report of a case. *Nephron* 25:254, 1980.
196. Biglieri EG, Slaton PE Jr, Silen WS, et al. Postoperative studies of adrenal function in primary aldosteronism. *J Clin Endocrinol Metab* 26:553, 1966.
197. Bravo EL, Dustan HP, Tarazi RC. Selective hypoaldosteronism despite prolonged pre- and postoperative hyperreninemia in primary aldosteronism. *J Clin Endocrinol Metab* 41:611, 1975.
198. Hollenberg NK, Mickiewicz C. Hyperkalemia in diabetes mellitus: Effect of a triamterene-hydroxhlorothiazide combination. *Arch Intern Med* 149:1327, 1989.
199. Choi M, Fernandez PC, Patnaik A, et al. Brief report: Trimethoprim-induced hyperkalemia in a patient with AIDS. *N Engl J Med* 328:703, 1993.
200. Greenberg S, Reiser IW, Chou SY, Porush JG. Trimethoprim-sulfamethoxazole induces reversible hyperkalemia. *Ann Intern Med* 119:291, 1993.
201. Velazquez H, Perazella M, Wright FS, Ellison DH. Renal mechanism of trimethoprim-induced hyperkalemia. *Ann Intern Med* 119:296, 1993.
202. Alappan R, Perazella MA, Buller GK. Hyperkalemia in hospitalized patients treated with trimethoprim-sulfamethoxazole. *Ann Intern Med* 124:316, 1996.
203. Perzella MA, Mahnensmith RL. Trimethoprim-sulfamethoxazole: Hyperkalemia is an important complication regardless of dose. *Clin Nephrol* 46:187, 1996.
204. Kleyman TR, Roberts C, Ling BN. A mechanism for pentamidine-induced hyperkalemia: Inhibition of distal nephron sodium transport. *Ann Intern Med* 122:103, 1995.
205. Marinella MA. Trimethoprim-induced hyperkalemia: An analysis of reported cases. *Gerontology* 45:209, 1999.
206. Oberfield SE, Levine LS, Carey RM, et al. Pseudohypoaldosteronism: Multiple target organ unresponsiveness to mineralocorticoid hormones. *J Clin Endocrinol Metab* 48:228, 1979.

207. Kuhnle U, Nielsen MD, Teitze H-U, et al. Pseudohypoaldosteronism in eight families: Different forms of inheritance are evidence for various genetic defects. *J Clin Endocrinol Metab* 70:638, 1990.

208. Rodriguez-Soriano J, Vallo A, Oliveros R, Castillo G. Transient pseudohypoaldosteronism secondary to obstructive uropathy in infancy. *J Pediatr* 103:375, 1983.

209. Daughaday WH, Rendleman D. Severe symptomatic hyperkalemia in an adrenalectomized woman due to enhanced mineralocorticoid requirement. *Ann Intern Med* 66:1197, 1967.

210. Cogan MC, Arieff AI. Sodium wasting, acidosis and hyperkalemia induced by methicillin interstitial nephritis: Evidence for selective distal tubular dysfunction. *Am J Med* 64:500, 1978.

211. Luke RG, Allison ME, Davidson JF, Duquid WP. Hyperkalemia and renal tubularacidosis due to renal amyloidosis. *Ann Intern Med* 70:1211, 1969.

212. Hanukoglu A. Type I pseudohypoaldosteronism includes two clinically and genetically distinct entities with either renal or multiple target organ defects. *J Clin Endocrinol Metab* 73:936, 1991.

213. Rose BD. Genetic disorders of the renal sodium channel: Liddle's syndrome and pseudohypoaldosteronism, in Rose BD (ed): *UpToDate in Medicine*. Wellesley, MA, UpToDate, 2000.

214. Chang SS, Grunder S, Hanukoglu A, et al. Mutations in the subunits of the epithelial sodium channel cause salt wasting with hyperkalemic acidosis, pseudohypoaldosteronism type 1. *Nat Genet* 12:248, 1996.

215. Geller DS, Rodriguez-Soriano J, Boado AV, et al. Mutations in the mineralocorticoid receptor gene cause autosomal dominant pseudohypoaldosteronism type I. *Nat Genet* 19:279, 1998.

216. Arai K, Tsigos C, Suzuki Y, et al. Physiological and molecular aspects of mineralocorticoid action in pseudohypoaldosteronism: A responsiveness test and therapy. *J Clin Endocrinol Metab* 79:1019, 1994.

217. Proesmans W, Geussens H, Corbeel L, Eeckels R. Pseudohypoaldosteronism. *Am J Dis Child* 126:510, 1973.

218. Schambelan M, Sebastian A, Rector FC Jr. Mineralocorticoid-resistant renal hyperkalemia without salt-wasting (type II pseudohypoaldosteronism): Role of increased renal chloride reabsorption. *Kidney Int* 19:716, 1981.

219. Gordon RD. Syndrome of hypertension and hyperkalemia with normal glomerular filtration rate. *Hypertension* 8:93, 1986.

220. Take C, Ikeda K, Kurasawa T, Kurokawa K. Increased chloride reabsorption as an inherited renal tubular defect in familial type II pseudohypoaldosteronism. *N Engl J Med* 324:472, 1991.

221. Mansfield TA, Simon DB, Farfel Z, et al. Multilocus linkage of familial hyperkalaemia and hypertension, pseudohypoaldosteronism type II, to chromosomes 1q31-42 and 17p11-q21. *Nat Genet* 16:202, 1997.

221a. Disse-Nicodeme S, Achard, JM, Desitter I, et al. A new locus on chromosome 12p13.3 for pseudohypoaldosteronism type II, an autosomal dominant form of hypertension. *Am J Human Genetics* 67:302, 2000.

222. Batlle DC. Segmental characterization of defects in collecting tubule acidification. *Kidney Int* 30:546, 1986.

223. Batlle DC, Arruda JAL, Kurtzman NA. Hyperkalemic distal renal tubular acidosis associated with obstructive uropathy. *N Engl J Med* 304:373, 1981.

224. Sabatini S, Kurtzman NA. Enzyme activity in obstructive uropathy: Basis for salt wastage and the acidification defect. *Kidney Int* 37:79, 1990.

225. Kimura H, Mujais SK. Cortical collecting duct Na-K pump in obstructive uropathy. *Am J Physiol* 258:F1320, 1990.

226. Batlle DC, Itsarayoungyuen K, Arruda JAL, Kurtzman NA. Hyperkalemic hyperchloremic metabolic acidosis in sickle cell hemoglobinopathies. *Am J Med* 72:188, 1982.

227. Batlle DC, Hizon M, Cohen E, et al. The use of the urine anion gap in the diagnosis of hyperchloremic metabolic acidosis. *N Engl J Med* 318:594, 1988.

228. Schlueter W, Keilani T, Hizon M, et al. On the mechanism of impaired distal acidification in hyperkalemic renal tubular acidosis: Evaluation with amiloride and bumetanide. *J Am Soc Nephrol* 3:953, 1992.

229. DeFronzo RA, Cooke CR, Goldberg M, et al. Impaired renal tubular potassium secretion in systemic lupus erythematosus. *Ann Intern Med* 86:268, 1977.

230. De Fronzo RA, Goldberg M, Cooke CR, et al. Investigations into mechanisms of hyperkalemia following renal transplantation. *Kidney Int* 11:357, 1977.

231. Lee FO, Quismorio FP, Troum OM. Mechanisms of hyperkalemia in systemic lupus erythematosus. *Arch Intern Med* 148:397, 1988.

232. Berne RM, Levy MN. *Cardiovascular Physiology*, 4th ed. St Louis, Mosby, 1981, pp. 7–17.

233. Epstein FH. Signs and symptoms of electrolyte disorders, in Maxwell MH, Kleeman CR (eds): *Clinical Disorders of Fluid and Electrolyte Metabolism*, 3rd ed. New York, McGraw-Hill, 1980.

234. Finch CA, Sawyer CG, Flynn JM. Clinical syndrome of potassium intoxication. *Am J Med* 1:337, 1946.

235. Bele H, Hayes WL, Vosburgh J. Hyperkalemic paralysis due to adrenal insufficiency. *Arch Intern Med* 115:418, 1965.

236. Surawicz B. Relationship between electrocardiogram and electrolytes. *Am Heart J* 73:814, 1967.

237. Surawicz B, Chlebus H, Mazzoleni A. Hemodynamic and electrocardiographic effects of hyperpotassemia: Differences in response to slow and rapid increases in concentration of plasma K. *Am Heart J* 73:647, 1967.

238. Weidmann S. Membrane excitation in cardiac muscle. *Circulation* 24:499, 1961.

239. Sutton PMI, Taggart P, Spear DW, et al. Monophasic action potential recordings in response to graded hyperkalemia in dogs. *Am J Physiol* 256:H956, 1989.

240. Kuffler S, Nicholls JG. *From Neuron to Brain*. Saunderland, MA, Sinauer, 1976, chap. 6.

241. Catterall WA. Structure and function of voltage-sensitive ion channels. *Science* 242:50, 1988.

242. Goodyer AVN, Goodkind MJ, Stanley EJ. The effects of abnormal concentrations of the serum electrolytes on left ventricular function in the intact animal. *Am Heart J* 67:779, 1964.

243. Szerlip H, Weiss J, Singer I. Profound hyperkalemia without electrocardiographic changes. *Am J Kidney Dis* 7:461, 1986.

244. Braun HA, Van Horne R, Bettinger C, Bellet S. The influence of hypocalcemia induced by sodium ethylenediamine acetate on the toxicity of potassium: an experimental study. *J Lab Clin Med* 46:544, 1955.

245. Garcia-Palmieri MR. Reversal of hyperkalemic cardiotoxicity with hypertonic saline. *Am Heart J* 64:483, 1962.

246. Abrams WB, Lewis DW, Bellet S. The effect of acidosis and alkalosis on the plasma potassium concentration and the electrocardiogram in normal and potassium depleted dogs. *Am J Med Sci* 222:506, 1951.

247. Surawicz B, Gettes LS. Two mechanisms of cardiac arrest produced by potassium. *Circ Res* 12:415, 1963.

248. West ML, Marsden PA, Richardson RM, et al. New clinical approach to evaluate disorders of potassium excretion. *Miner Electrolyte Metab* 12:234, 1986.

249. Ethier JH, Kamel KS, Magner PO, et al. The transtubular potassium concentration in patients with hypokalemia and hyperkalemia. *Am J Kidney Dis* 15:309, 1990.

250. Weiner ID, Wingo CS. Hyperkalemia: A potential silent killer. *J Am Soc Nephrol* 9:1535, 1998.

251. Winkler AW, Hoff HE, Smith PK. Factors affecting the toxicity of potassium. *Am J Physiol* 127:430, 1939.

252. Zierler KL, Rabinowitz D. Effect of very small concentrations of insulin on forearm metabolism: Persistence of its action on potassium and free fatty acids without its effects on glucose. *J Clin Invest* 43:950, 1964.

253. Ferrannini E, Taddei S, Santoro D, et al. Independent stimulation of glucose metabolism and Na^+-K^+ exchange by insulin in the human forearm. *Am J Physiol* 255:E953, 1988.

254. Clausen T, Flatman JA. Effect of insulin and epinephrine on Na^+-K^+-ATPase and glucose transport in soleus muscle. *Am J Physiol* 252:E492, 1987.
255. Lytton J, Lin JC, Guidotti G. Identification of two molecular forms of (Na^+-K^+)-ATPase in rat adipocytes. Relation to insulin stimulation of the enzyme. *J Biol Chem* 260:1177, 1985.
256. Fischer KF, Lees JA, Newman JH. Hypoglycemia in hospitalized patients: Causes and outcomes. *N Engl J Med* 315:1245, 1986.
257. Blumberg A, Weidmann P, Shaw S, Gnadinger M. Effect of various therapeutic approaches on plasma potassium and major regulating factors in terminal renal failure. *Am J Med* 85:507, 1988.
258. Fraley DS, Adler S. Correction of hyperkalemia by bicarbonate despite constant blood pH. *Kidney Int* 12:354, 1977.
259. Schwartz KC, Cohen BD, Lubash GD, Rubin AL. Severe acidosis and hyperpotassemia treated with sodium bicarbonate infusion. *Circulation* 19:215, 1959.
260. Blumberg A, Weidmann P, Ferrari P. Effect of prolonged bicarbonate administration on plasma potassium in terminal renal failure. *Kidney Int* 41:369, 1992.
261. Allon MA, Shanklin N. Effect of bicarbonate administration of plasma potassium in dialysis patients: Interactions with insulin and albuterol. *Am J Kidney Dis* 28:508, 1996.
262. Ballantyne F III, Davis LD, Reynolds EW Jr. Cellular basis for reversal of hyperkalemic electrocardiographic changes by sodium. *Am J Physiol* 229:935, 1975.
263. Montoliu J, Lens KL, Revert L. Potassium lowering effect of albuterol for hyperkalemia in renal failure. *Arch Intern Med* 147:713, 1987.
264. Liou HH, Chiang SS, Wu SC, et al. Hypokalemic effects of intravenous infusion or nebulization of salbutamol in patients with chronic renal failure: Comparative study. *Am J Kidney Dis* 23:266, 1994.
265. Allon M, Shanklin N. Adrenergic modulation of extrarenal potassium disposal in men with end-stage renal disease. *Kidney Int* 40:1103, 1991.
266. Allon M, Copkney C. Albuterol and insulin for treatment of hyperkalemia in hemodialysis patients. *Kidney Int* 38:869, 1990.
267. Sebastian A, Schambelan M. Amelioration of type 4 renal tubular acidosis in chronic renal failure with furosemide. *Kidney Int* 12:534, 1977.
268. Berlyne GM, Janab K, Manc MB. Dangers of resonium A in the treatment of hyperkalaemia in renal failure. *Lancet* 1:167, 1966.
269. Steinmetz PR, Kiley JE. Hyperkalemia in renal failure: The effectiveness of treatment depends on the gastrointestinal tract as a locus of exchange. *JAMA* 175:689, 1961.
270. Burnett RJ. Sodium polystyrene-sorbitol enemas (letter). *Ann Intern Med* 112:311, 1990.
271. Gerstman BB, Kirkman R, Platt R. Intestinal necrosis associated with postoperative orally administered sodium polystyrene sulfonate in sorbitol. *Am J Kidney Dis* 20:159, 1992.
272. Shephard KU. Cleansing enemas after sodium polystyrene sulfonate enemas (letter). *Ann Intern Med* 112:711, 1990.
273. Emmett D, Emmett M, Borejdo J, et al. Na polystyrene sulfonate resin/hypertonic sorbitol enema toxicity (abstract). *J Am Soc Nephrol* 6:439, 1995.
274. Nolph KD, Popovich RP, Ghods AJ, Twardowski Z. Determinants of low clearances of small solutes during peritoneal dialysis. *Kidney Int* 13:117, 1978.

TWENTY-NINE

ANSWERS TO THE PROBLEMS

CHAPTER 1

1-1 Excretion equals filtration minus net reabsorption. This simple relationship is often overlooked clinically. Acute renal failure, for example, is characterized by a low glomerular filtration rate. An increase in urine output in this setting is usually assumed to represent an elevation in filtration and therefore improved renal function. However, a decrease in reabsorption with no change in filtration also can account for the increase in output. These possibilities can be distinguished by following the plasma creatinine concentration, an indirect reflection of the glomerular filtration rate (see Chap. 2). If filtration has risen to an important degree, more creatinine will be filtered and excreted, resulting in a reduction in the plasma creatinine concentration toward baseline. In contrast, this parameter will remain stable or continue to rise if there has only been less reabsorption.

CHAPTER 2

2-1 The glomerular filtration rate cannot be estimated from the plasma creatinine concentration in this setting, since the patient is not in a steady state.

2-2 The administration of dopamine will
(*a*) Increase renal blood flow by diminishing renal vascular resistance.
(*b*) Produce no change or a lesser increase in glomerular filtration rate, since dilatation of the efferent arteriole will tend to lower the intraglomerular pressure, thereby counteracting the effects of afferent dilatation and enhanced flow.

(c) Reduce the filtration fraction, because less of the plasma delivered to the glomeruli is now filtered.

(d) Lower the albumin concentration in the peritubular capillary, since a lower filtration results in less hemoconcentration of the fluid leaving the glomeruli. This response may in part explain the ability of dopamine to decrease proximal Na^+ reabsorption (see page 208).

2.3 (a) By preferentially dilating the efferent arteriole, an angiotensin converting enzyme inhibitor will tend to lower the intraglomerular pressure. In comparison, dilatation of the afferent arteriole by other antihypertensive agents allows more of the systemic pressure to be transmitted to the glomeruli, thereby maintaining the intraglomerular pressure despite the reduction in systemic pressure.

(b) Intraglomerular "hypertension" has been thought to be an important mediator of secondary glomerular injury in a variety of slowly progressive renal diseases, including diabetic nephropathy. Thus, the reduction in intraglomerular pressure with a converting enzyme inhibitor might be beneficial in the long term.[1]

2-4 (a) The creatinine clearance can be estimated from

$$C_{cr}, mL/min = \frac{U_{cr} \times V}{P_{cr}}$$

$$= \frac{125 \, mg/dL}{3.5 \, mg/dL} \times \frac{800 \, mL/day}{1440 \, min/day}$$

$$= 20 \, mL/min$$

(b) The total creatinine excretion is 1000 mg or 12.5 mg/kg/day. This probably represents an incomplete collection (and therefore an underestimate of the creatinine clearance), since a normal man should excrete 20 to 25 mg/kg/day. On the other hand, the creatinine clearance itself (even when performed under optimal conditions) overestimates the true glomerular filtration rate in patients with renal disease, as a result of increased creatinine secretion by the organic cation secretory pump in the proximal tubule.

CHAPTER 3

3-1 Because of the phenomenon of glomerulotubular balance, an increase in the glomerular filtration rate without change in volume will

(a) Have no effect on fractional Na^+ reabsorption.

(b) Increase absolute Na^+ reabsorption, since a constant fraction of a larger load is being reabsorbed.

3-2 Because of diminished activity of the Na^+-H^+ antiporter, parathyroid hormone should

(a) Decrease proximal HCO_3^- reabsorption, which is largely mediated by the Na^+-H^+ exchanger (see Chap. 10).

(*b*) Reduce both the passive and active transport of Cl^-. In normal subjects, the former process results from the favorable concentration gradient generated by the preferential reabsorption of HCO_3^- in the early proximal tubule, and the latter process is mediated in part by a Cl^--formate$^-$ exchanger that operates in parallel with the Na^+-H^+ antiporter.

(*c*) Diminish proximal water reabsorption, which passively follows the osmotic gradient established by NaCl and NaHCO$_3$ transport.

3-3   (*a*) Volume depletion leads to enhanced proximal Na^+ and water reabsorption. The increased removal of water raises the tubular fluid urea concentration, resulting in enhanced passive urea reabsorption, a fall in urea excretion, and a rise in the BUN.

(*b*) The glomerular filtration rate is probably normal or near normal, since the plasma creatinine concentration is unchanged.

(*c*) Both increased urate reabsorption (promoted by enhanced Na^+ reabsorption) and reduced secretion (due to competition from the ketoacid anions) lead to a fall in urate excretion and hyperuricemia.

3-4   (*a*) The decrease in the plasma HCO_3^- concentration leads to reductions in the filtered HCO_3^- load and therefore proximal HCO_3^- reabsorption. This will be associated with a fall in proximal NaCl reabsorption, since HCO_3^- reabsorption by Na^+-H^+ exchange promotes both passive and active Cl^- transport (the latter in part via the Cl^--formate$^-$ exchanger that operates in parallel with the Na^+-H^+ antiporter).

(*b*) Proximal citrate reabsorption will be increased; the fall in pH associated with metabolic acidosis appears to act in part by converting filtered citrate^{3-} into the more easily reabsorbed citrate^{2-}.

(*c*) Stone formation is increased in distal renal tubular acidosis (see page 618). Several factors contribute to this complication, including the high urine pH (which promotes calcium phosphate precipitation) and the reduction in citrate excretion (since citrate is normally a potent inhibitor of calcium stone formation by forming a nondissociable but solute complex with calcium). Bone buffering of the excess acid also may play a role by increasing calcium release from bone and subsequent urinary calcium excretion.

CHAPTER 4

4-1   NaCl reabsorption without water in the medullary ascending limb and urea movement from the medullary collecting tubule into the interstitium are the two major factors in the generation of the medullary osmotic gradient. The vasa recta capillaries also play an important role by minimizing the removal of the excess solute.

4-2   NaCl reabsorption without water in the medullary ascending limb has two effects: (1) the medullary interstitium becomes hyperosmotic, and (2) the tubular fluid becomes dilute. Thus, this step plays a central role in both concentration and dilution.

NaCl reabsorption without water in the cortical ascending limb and distal tubule further lowers the urine osmolality and contributes to urinary dilution. Since cortical blood flow is so high, however, the cortical interstitium does not become hyperosmotic and urinary concentration is not directly affected.

4-3   (*a*) Concentrating ability will be increased as a result of the enhanced accumulation of interstitial solute.

(*b*) Reabsorption throughout the thick ascending limb is flow-dependent, being limited by the maximum tubular fluid-to-plasma concentration gradient for Na^+ that can be achieved. It may be, for example, that the minimum tubular fluid Na^+ concentration that can be achieved by the end of the cortical thick ascending limb is about 75 meq/L. Thus, increased NaCl reabsorption in the medullary aspect will lead to decreased reabsorption in the cortical aspect, since the limiting gradient cannot be exceeded. The net effect is that ADH has redistributed some NaCl transport from the cortex in the medulla; thus, concentrating ability is increased with no change in total Na^+ reabsorption.

4-4   From the answers to Prob. 4-2, a diuretic that inhibits both concentration and dilution acts in the medullary thick ascending limb. In comparison, a diuretic that impairs dilution but does not affect concentration probably acts in the cortical ascending limb or the distal tubule. Thus, the effects of diuretics on concentration and dilution are one of the methods that have been used to determine their sites of action within the nephron (see Chap. 15).

4-5   The tubular fluid leaving the proximal tubule is isosmotic to plasma. In the descending limb, osmotic equilibration with the concentrated interstitium leads to water reabsorption. Thus, any factor that decreases medullary tonicity will also reduce descending limb water transport. This occurs with an osmotic diuresis, because the associated increase in medullary blood flow washes out some of the medullary solute. A similar effect should occur in central diabetes insipidus, since the absence of ADH will diminish interstitial urea accumulation (Figs. 4-10 and 4-11).

4-6   Urea generation and subsequent excretion are diminished on a low-protein diet. Thus, less urea will accumulate in the interstitium, resulting in a mild decrease in concentrating ability.[2]

CHAPTER 6

6-1   Renin secretion is reduced by an autonomous adrenal adenoma, probably because of the volume expansion induced by the initial Na^+ and water retention. In comparison, renin release is enhanced by volume depletion, and the increased formation of angiotensin II is responsible for the secondary hyperaldosteronism.

6-2   The secretion of ADH is stimulated by a rise in the effective P_{osm}. Since urea is an ineffective osmole, an elevation in the BUN does not increase the effective P_{osm} or ADH release.

6-3   The loss of water in the urine will initially raise the P_{osm}, resulting in a potent stimulus to thirst. As a result, patients who lack ADH remain in near-normal water balance despite urinary losses that can exceed 10 L/day.

6-4   The major stimuli to renal calcitriol synthesis are parathyroid hormone and hypophosphatemia. Thus, ingestion of a high-phosphate diet and hypoparathyroidism (either primary or induced by a high-calcium diet) will lower calcitriol production. Phosphate retention is also largely responsible for the initial fall in calcitriol levels in patients with renal insufficiency. This can be reversed, however, if phosphate intake is restricted, thereby diminishing phosphate levels and allowing calcitriol secretion to increase toward normal.

6-5   (*a*) A Na^+ load without water will cause both volume expansion and an elevation in the plasma Na^+ concentration and P_{osm}. As a result, ANP and ADH levels will rise and aldosterone secretion will fall (see page 278 for a review of the differences between volume regulation and osmoregulation).
   (*b*) A water load will be rapidly excreted, since the ensuing fall in P_{osm} will diminish ADH release, resulting in the excretion of a dilute urine. This process is so efficient that ANP and aldosterone secretion will not change.
   (*c*) Isotonic saline will expand volume without affecting osmolality. Thus, ANP will rise, aldosterone will fall, and ADH will be unaffected.
   (*d*) Isosmotic volume loss will enhance the secretion of aldosterone and ADH (the latter via the aortic and cardiac volume receptors) and diminish the release of ANP.

6-6   Hypercalciuria may transiently lower the plasma Ca^{2+} concentration. However, this will stimulate the secretion of PTH, which then restores normocalcemia by increasing both bone resorption and, via enhanced calcitriol synthesis, intestinal CA^{2+} absorption. In the new steady state, the increment in Ca^{2+} excretion will be balanced by more efficient Ca^{2+} absorption.

6-7   Aldosterone does not raise the plasma Na^+ concentration because there will be equivalent retention of water in the collecting tubules if ADH is present. If ADH is absent, the ensuing small elevation in the plasma Na^+ concentration will stimulate both ADH release and thirst, also leading to water retention.

6-8   Renal prostaglandins play an important role in maintaining renal perfusion in conditions in which there are high levels of the vasoconstrictors angiotensin II and norepinephrine. This can occur with a low-salt diet, heart failure, or volume depletion due to severe vomiting (*a*, *d*, and *e*). In these settings, a nonsteroidal anti-inflammatory drug can induce renal ischemia and a fall in the glomerular filtration rate.

CHAPTER 7

7-1 The plasma Na^+ concentration is the primary determinant of the P_{osm}, since Na^+ salts are the major extracellular osmoles. There is, however, no predictable relationship between the plasma Na^+ concentration and the extracellular volume: The latter is determined by the total amounts of Na^+ and water present, whereas the former is determined by the *ratio* between the amounts of solute ($Na^+ + K^+$) and water that are present.

7-2 The addition of glucose to the extracellular fluid, as in uncontrolled diabetes mellitus, will (*a*) raise the P_{osm} and (*b*) cause water to move out of the cells, thereby increasing the extracellular volume, reducing the intracellular volume, and lowering the plasma Na^+ concentration (by dilution).

7-3 The P_{osm} can be calculated from

$$P_{osm} \cong 2 \times \text{plasma } [Na^+] + \frac{BUN}{2.8} + \frac{[glucose]}{18}$$

$$290 \cong 250 + \frac{28}{2.8} + \frac{[glucose]}{18}$$

$$[\text{Glucose}] \cong 540 \, \text{mg/dL}$$

7.4 (*a*) An increase in arterial blood pressure will have little direct effect on the plasma volume, because of autoregulation of the capillary hydraulic pressure by the precapillary sphincter.

(*b*) A decrease in venous pressure will reduce capillary hydraulic pressure, thereby promoting the movement of interstitial fluid into the capillary and plasma volume expansion.

(*c*) A mild reduction in the plasma albumin concentration should have little effect on the plasma volume. The transcapillary oncotic pressure gradient will remain relatively stable in this setting as a result of a parallel decline in the interstitial oncotic pressure. Both washout of interstitial proteins by increased lymphatic flow and diminished albumin movement across the capillary wall (due to the hypoalbuminemia) will contribute to this response.

CHAPTER 8

8-1 (*a*) An acute myocardial infarction will initially diminish the effective circulating volume (because of the fall in cardiac output) and therefore urinary Na^+ excretion, without affecting either the plasma volume or total extracellular volume.

(*b*) A high-Na^+ diet will expand the plasma, extracellular, and effective circulating volumes and increase urinary Na^+ excretion.

(*c*) The retention of ingested water will also expand the plasma, extracellular, and effective circulating volumes and increase urinary Na^+ excretion.

8-2   Diuretic-induced hypovolemia enhances the release of renin. The ensuing increase in the formation of angiotensin II will tend to raise the blood pressure, thereby minimizing the hypotensive effect of the diuretic.[3]

8-3   (*d*) The rate of urinary Na^+ excretion is generally the best estimate of the effective circulating volume, since it reflects the physiologic assessment of the kidney's systemic hemodynamics. A low rate of Na^+ excretion (urine Na^+ concentration below 25 meq/L in the absence of marked polyuria) is generally diagnostic of volume depletion unless there is selective renal ischemia due to bilateral renal artery stenosis or acute glomerular disease. The cardiac output, plasma volume, and systemic blood pressure are less accurate. For example, a fall in blood pressure may be prevented by the compensatory rise in sympathetic tone. On the other hand, the cardiac output may be misleadingly elevated if there are arteriovenous fistulas or vasodilatation, as occurs in hepatic cirrhosis.

8-4   In the steady state, Na^+ intake and excretion are equal even in a patient on diuretic therapy. In this setting, the natriuretic effect of the diuretic is counteracted by enhanced Na^+ reabsorption, which may be induced by the compensatory increases in angiotensin II, aldosterone, and norepinephrine production. The new steady state is generally attained within 2 weeks, as long as diuretic dose and dietary Na^+ intake remain relatively constant (see page 453).

8-5   (*a*) Isotonic saline will expand volume without affecting osmolality. Thus, ANP will rise, aldosterone will fall, and ADH will be unaffected. The net effect is that the excess Na^+ will appropriately be excreted in a relatively isosmotic urine.

(*b*) A water load will be rapidly excreted, as the ensuing fall in P_{osm} will diminish ADH release. This will lead to a fall in U_{osm} with little change in the rate of Na^+ excretion (although the urine Na^+ concentration will fall by dilution).

(*c*) A Na^+ load without water will cause both volume expansion and an elevation in the plasma Na^+ concentration and P_{osm}, thereby activating both the volume regulatory and osmoregulatory systems. As a result, ANP and ADH levels will rise and aldosterone secretion will fall. In this setting, both the urine Na^+ concentration and U_{osm} will be elevated, allowing the excretion of the excess Na^+ with little water loss.

(*d*) Half-isotonic saline will cause volume expansion and hypoosmolality. Therefore, ANP and Na^+ excretion will rise, while aldosterone, ADH, and the U_{osm} will fall. The net effect is that the excess Na^+ will appropriately be excreted in a dilute urine.

CHAPTER 9

9-1   The loss of isosmotic diarrheal fluid will (*a*) reduce the effective circulating volume, (*b*) diminish urinary Na^+ excretion, (*c* and *d*) have no direct effect on the P_{osm} or the plasma Na^+ concentration, and (*e* and *f*) increase ADH release and therefore the U_{osm}. The ingestion of water in this setting will result in water retention (because of the high ADH levels) and hyponatremia.

9-2 The $Na^+ + K^+$ concentration in the fluid that is lost is less than that in the plasma in this example. As a result, water is being lost in excess of effective solute. Since the plasma Na^+ concentration is generally determined by

$$\text{Plasma } [Na^+] \cong \frac{Na_e^+ + K_e^+}{TBW}$$

the plasma Na^+ concentration will rise.

9-3 There is no predictable relationship between the plasma Na^+ concentration (which is regulated by the osmoregulatory pathway) and urinary Na^+ excretion (which is determined by changes in the effective circulating volume).

9-4 Two factors contribute to the inability to excrete water normally in volume depletion: increased release of ADH and reduced fluid delivery to the diluting segment in the ascending limb of the loop of Henle because of enhanced proximal Na^+ and water reabsorption.

9-5 The minimum U_{osm} is unaffected by beer drinking. However, the C_{H_2O} is also dependent upon the rate of solute excretion. Since Na^+, K^+, and urea excretion are low in a subject ingesting only beer, solute excretion will also be low. Suppose, for example, that the U_{osm} can be lowered to 75 mosmol/kg and that the P_{osm} is 300 mosmol/kg. The maximum urine output in this setting will be 10 liters in a normal subject excreting 750 mosmol of solute per day, but only 3 liters in a beer drinker excreting 225 mosmol of solute. The respective C_{H_2O} will be as follows:

$$C_{H_2O} = V\left(1 - \frac{U_{osm}}{P_{osm}}\right)$$

$$= 10\left(1 - \frac{75}{300}\right)$$

$$= 7.5 \text{ liters in a normal subject}$$

$$C_{H_2O} = 3\left(1 - \frac{U_{osm}}{P_{osm}}\right)$$

$$= 2.25 \text{ liters in a beer drinker}$$

9.6 (a) Although the U_{osm} is the same in both examples, there are important differences in the rate of electrolyte-free water reabsorption:

$$T^e_{C_{H_2O}} = V\left[\left(\frac{U_{Na^+} + K^+}{P_{Na^+}}\right) - 1\right]$$

In the patient with the syndrome of inappropriate ADH secretion,

$$T^e_{C_{H_2O}} = 1\left[\left(\frac{130}{130}\right) - 1\right]$$

$$= 0$$

Thus, there is no electrolyte free water reabsorption in this setting. In comparison, in the patient with heart failure,

$$T^e_{C_{H_2O}} = 1\left[\left(\frac{60}{130}\right) - 1\right]$$

$$= -540\,\text{mL}$$

(*b*) At similar levels of water intake, the patient with heart failure will be less likely to retain water and become hyponatremic because the kidney is excreting 540 mL of free water each day (a minus value for free water reabsorption represents free water excretion).

CHAPTER 10

10-1 Buffers minimize changes in the free H^+ concentration by appropriately taking up $(H^+ + Buf^- \rightarrow HBuf)$ or releasing $(HBuf \rightarrow H^+ + Buf^-)$ H^+ ions. The efficacy of a buffer is determined by the quantity of buffer present and the relation of the pK_a of the buffer to the pH of the solution. In addition, the ability to excrete CO_2 increases the effectiveness of the HCO_3^--CO_2 buffer system.

10-2 The fall in the plasma HCO_3^- concentration is due to the different rates with which the administered HCO_3^- enters the different fluid compartments. The added HCO_3^- is initially limited to the vascular space, resulting in a large increase in the plasma HCO_3^- concentration. The HCO_3^- then equilibrates throughout the total extracellular fluid (within 15 min) and subsequently with the cell buffers (a process that reaches completion within 2 to 4 h). Both of these processes reduce the plasma HCO_3^- concentration toward the baseline level. As discussed in Chap. 11, acid-base balance is restored in this setting by the excretion of the excess HCO_3^- in the urine.

This time-related effect of exogenous HCO_3^- becomes clinically important when HCO_3^- is given to treat metabolic acidosis (see Chap. 19). The increment in the plasma HCO_3^- concentration and therefore in the extracellular pH will be greater if measured within 15 min than after equilibration with the cell buffers has occurred at 2 to 4 h. Thus, it should not be assumed that early measurements (which will overestimate the true elevation in the plasma HCO_3^- concentration) represent the steady-state condition.

10-3 The quantity of available extracellular and intracellular buffers will determine how much of a reduction in pH will occur. Buffering capacity is best estimated from the initial plasma HCO_3^- concentration. Patients with a low baseline level due to preexisting metabolic acidosis are more prone to a major reduction in pH following an acid load.

CHAPTER 11

11-1 The primary adaptive response of the kidney to an acid load is increased NH_4^+ production and excretion. As a result, reduced titratable acid excretion will have little effect on acid-base balance, since enhanced NH_4^+ excretion can compensate for this defect. In comparison, the ability to augment titratable acid excretion is limited. Thus, a marked decline in NH_4^+ excretion (as occurs in advanced renal failure) will lead to H^+ retention and metabolic acidosis.

11-2 The buffering of HCl and H_2SO_4 by $NaHCO_3$ results in the respective generation of NaCl and Na_2SO_4. When the NaCl is presented to the distal nephron, the reabsorption of Na^+ will be followed by that of Cl^-. In comparison, SO_4^{2-} is a nonreabsorbable anion; thus, the distal reabsorption of Na^+ creates a greater lumen-negative potential difference that promotes the luminal accumulation of H^+. The relatively low luminal Cl^- concentration in this setting also may contribute by generating a more favorable gradient for Cl^- to be cosecreted with H^+. The net effect is increased acid excretion and therefore a lesser degree of metabolic acidosis when H_2SO_4 is given.[4]

11-3 (*a*) Net acid excretion is equal to the following:

$$\text{Net acid excretion} = NH_4^+ + \text{titratable acidity} - HCO_3^-$$

$$= 80 \text{ meq/day in the normal subject}$$

$$= 215 \text{ meq/day in the patient with metabolic acidosis}$$

(*b*) In comparison, total H^+ secretion is equal to

$$\text{Total acid excretion} = HCO_3^- \text{ reabsorption} + NH_4^+ + \text{titratable acidity}$$

$$= 4320 \ (180 \times 24) + 50 + 30$$

$$= 4400 \text{ meq/day in the normal subject}$$

$$= 1080 \ (180 \times 6) + 140 + 75$$

$$= 1295 \text{ meq/day in the patient with metabolic acidosis}$$

Note that net acid excretion is appropriately increased in metabolic acidosis even though total H^+ secretion is actually reduced as a result of the marked reduction in the filtered HCO_3^- load.

11-4 At a urine pH of 5.80 with 60 mmol of phosphate,

$$5.80 = 6.80 + \log \frac{x}{60 - x}$$

$$[HPO_4^{2-}] = x = 5.45 \text{ mmol}$$

$$[H_2PO_4^-] = 60 - x = 54.55 \text{ mmol}$$

In the filtrate, however, the initial pH was 7.40, similar to that in the plasma. Thus

$$7.40 = 6.80 + \log \frac{x}{60 - x}$$

$$[HPO_4^{2-}] = 48 \, mmol$$

$$[H_2PO_4^-] = 12 \, mmol$$

Thus, 42.55 mmol of HPO_4^{2-} (48 − 5.45) has been converted to $H_2PO_4^-$ by buffering; this is the quantity of titratable acidity excreted as $H_2PO_4^-$.

Titratable acidity is measured by the number of milliequivalents of NaOH that must be added to an acid urine to return the pH to 7.40. NH_4^+ excretion is not included in this titration, since the pK_a of the NH_3-NH_4^+ system is 9.0. Thus, raising the urine pH from 5.80 to 7.40 will have little effect on the NH_3/NH_4^+ ratio.

11-5 The metabolic alkalosis persists in this setting because both volume and Cl^- depletion enhance HCO_3^- reabsorption, thereby preventing the excretion of the excess HCO_3^- (see Chap. 18).

CHAPTER 12

12-1 Aldosterone deficiency initially decreases urinary K^+ excretion. The ensuing rise in the plasma K^+ concentration, however, is a direct stimulus to distal K^+ secretion, eventually leading to a new steady state in which intake and output are again equal (see Fig. 12-10).

12-2 Increasing Na^+ intake will enhance distal flow, resulting in augmented K^+ secretion and hypokalemia in patients with primary hyperaldosteronism.[5] K^+ wasting does not occur in normal subjects, because the high Na^+ diet suppresses the release of aldosterone.[5]

12-3 Urinary K^+ excretion should be helpful in this setting, being less than 25 meq/day with extrarenal losses (or with a diuretic when the drug effect has worn off) but above this level with renal K^+ wasting.

12-4 Spontaneous K^+ wasting and hypokalemia do not occur with effective volume depletion, because the decline in distal flow counteracts the stimulatory effect of secondary hyperaldosteronism. If, however, distal flow is augmented with a loop or thiazide-type diuretic, then urinary K^+ losses will increase and the plasma K^+ concentration may fall.

12-5 (*a, c,* and possibly *e*). A converting enzyme inhibitor diminishes the release of aldosterone; a β-adrenergic blocker impairs the entry of K^+ into the cells after a K^+ load; and glucose can, in diabetics, raise the plasma K^+ concentration by elevating both the plasma glucose concentration and plasma osmolality (see Fig. 12-7).

12-6 There will be little direct effect on K^+ excretion, since the stimulatory effect of the high distal flow is counteracted by removal of ADH, which normally promotes K^+ secretion. In some patients, however, K^+ wasting can occur because the urine K^+ concentration cannot be reduced below 5 to 10 meq/L. Thus, a urine output of 10 L/day can lead to obligatory K^+ losses of 50 to 100 meq/day.[6]

CHAPTER 14

14-1 (*a*) The shock state is probably due to the sequestration of fluid in the infarcted bowel.

(*b*) Fluid replacement should proceed with isotonic saline. Blood is not necessary initially, since the hematocrit of 53 percent suggests hemoconcentration due to loss of fluid from the vascular space.

(*c*) The high urine Na^+ concentration indicates that this is a Na^+ diuresis, not a water diuresis as in diabetes insipidus (see Chap. 24 for a discussion of the approach to the polyuric patient). In this patient who had a *positive* balance of 7 liters prior to surgery, it is likely that the diuresis represents an *appropriate* attempt to excrete the excess Na^+; true Na^+ wasting of this degree is extremely rare.

(*d*) The correct therapy is to administer replacement fluids (such as half-isotonic saline at 50 to 100 mL/h), while allowing the patient to develop negative fluid balance. If the diuresis is appropriate, it will cease spontaneously without the patient developing any of the signs of volume depletion, such as diminished skin turgor or hypotension.

14-2 For each liter of water lost, about 60 percent comes from the cells and 40 percent from the extracellular fluid. Although the water is initially lost from the extracellular fluid, the ensuing rise in the P_{osm} pulls a proportionate volume of water out of the cells. In comparison, each liter of isotonic Na^+ loss comes entirely from the extracellular fluid, producing a greater reduction in the extracellular volume and possibly also in the arterial blood pressure.

14-3 There is no role for the use of pure dextrose solutions in the treatment of hypovolemic shock, since only 40 percent of the fluid will remain in the extracellular space. In addition, the retention of free water can lead to symptomatic hyponatremia. Isotonic saline is the solution of choice; this applies even to patients who are hypernatremic, since isotonic saline will still be hypoosmotic to plasma, thereby tending to lower the plasma Na^+ concentration toward normal.

14-4 (*a*) Volume repletion is responsible for the increases in Na^+ excretion and urine output.

(*b*) The central venous pressure alone is not an adequate determinant of volume status, since the normal range is 1 to $8\,cmH_2O$. Thus, $3\,cmH_2O$ is normal in some subjects and low in others.

(*c*) The elevation in BUN on admission represents urea accumulation over 10 days as a result of reduced urea excretion. Although normovolemia was restored over 18 h, a longer period is required for the renal excretion of the excess urea.

14.5 (*a*) The patient is depleted of Na^+ and water (physical findings) and K^+. In addition, the hypernatremia indicates that water has been lost in excess of solute. Thus, the replacement fluid should be hypotonic and contain Na^+ and K^+; for example, quarter-isotonic saline to which 20 to 40 meq of K^+ per liter has been added. This solution can be safely given at an initial rate of 100 mL/h. (The formula for calculating the rate of correction of hypernatremia is derived on page 776.)

14-6 (*a*) Any definition of hypotension must be made in relation to the patient's baseline blood pressure. Although 110/70 appears normal, it is probably low in this patient with a past history of hypertension.

(*b*) Volume depletion from unreplaced insensible losses must be accompanied by a rise in the plasma Na^+ concentration, since relatively solute-free water has been lost. The normal plasma Na^+ concentration in this patient indicates that Na^+ and water have been lost in proportion and therefore that a source of Na^+ loss must be present. In this case, the history of hypertension and the concurrent hypokalemia and metabolic alkalosis suggest that diuretic therapy is the likely cause.

CHAPTER 15

15-1 1. (*c*) The thiazides are the treatment of choice for hypercalciuric stone disease, since they lower calcium excretion both by increasing distal Ca^{2+} reabsorption and, via volume depletion, by increasing proximal Na^+ and secondary Ca^{2+} reabsorption.

2. (*d*) Spironolactone is preferred in cirrhosis, occasionally being more effective than a loop diuretic (since it does not require secretion into the tubular lumen) and protecting against the development of hypokalemic alkalosis, which can precipitate hepatic coma in some cases.

3. (*a*) Acetazolamide will cause preferential loss of $NaHCO_3$, thereby correcting both the metabolic alkalosis and fluid overload.

4. (*b*) Loop diuretics directly increase Ca^{2+} excretion by diminishing passive Ca^{2+} reabsorption in the loop of Henle.

5. (*b*) A loop diuretic is also helpful in hyponatremic patients, who tend to have high ADH levels and therefore inappropriate water retention. By interfering with loop NaCl reabsorption, the medullary accumulation of solute and therefore concentrating ability and the degree of water retention are diminished.

15-2 (*a*) Hypoalbuminemia limits the degree of protein-binding, resulting in a wider extravascular distribution of the diuretic and therefore a slower rate of delivery to the kidney.

(*b*) Both angiotensin II and aldosterone enhance Na^+ reabsorption (in the proximal and collecting tubules, respectively), directly impairing the natriuretic response to the diuretic.

(*c*) Hypotension, via the pressure natriuresis phenomenon, increases Na^+ reabsorption, thereby counteracting the effect of the diuretic.

CHAPTER 16

16-1 (*a* and *d*) Tissue perfusion may fall after the appropriate use of diuretics in heart failure and cirrhosis. With mild hypoalbuminemia or renal failure, on the other hand, there is primary renal Na^+ retention, and removal of the excess fluid will lower the effective circulating volume from a high level down toward normal.

(*b*) A reduction in the effective circulating volume will lead sequentially to increased proximal Na^+ and water reabsorption, enhanced passive proximal urea reabsorption, and a rise in the BUN. The urine Na^+ concentration is already low (in the absence of diuretics) in most patients with heart failure and cirrhosis, and a small further reduction is hard to detect.

16-2 (*a*) The oliguria and azotemia are due to effective volume depletion resulting from either overdiuresis or a primary fall in cardiac output following the myocardial infarction.

(*b*) No. Patients with diastolic dysfunction have a normal ejection fraction but a low output due to impaired diastolic filling. Furthermore, a moderately reduced ejection fraction does not necessarily mean that cardiac output is reduced, since cardiac dilatation may allow a normal stroke volume to be maintained despite the impaired contractility.

(*c*) No. Primary left ventricular damage may be associated with normal right ventricular function. Remember that a low jugular venous pressure may be normal (normal range equals 1 to $8\,cmH_2O$).

(*d*) The extracellular volume in this previously healthy man was normal on admission and then must have declined after fluid removal with the diuretic.

(*e*) Therapy should be aimed at increasing the effective circulating volume toward normal. If there is no evidence of pulmonary congestion, overdiuresis may be the primary problem, and cautious liberalization of Na^+ intake may restore normal tissue perfusion. If this is ineffective or if pulmonary congestion is present, then treatment must be aimed at increasing cardiac function and therefore renal perfusion with vasodilators or digitalis.

CHAPTER 17

17-1 (*a*) 26 nanoeq/L ($40 \times 0.8 \times 0.8$)

(*b*) The H^+ concentration is 63 nanoeq/L at a pH of 7.20 ($40 \times 1.25 \times 1.25$) and 80 nanoeq/L at a pH of 7.10 (63×1.25). Thus, the H^+ concentration at a pH of 7.15 is 72 nanoeq/L [$63 + 0.5 \times (80 - 63)$].

(*c*) The H^+ concentration at a pH of 7.30 is 50 nanoeq/L (40×1.25). Thus, at a pH of 7.24, the H^+ concentration is 59 nanoeq/L [$50 + 0.6 \times (63 - 50)$].

17-2 (*a*) Metabolic acidosis—low pH, low HCO_3^- concentration, compensatory reduction in P_{CO_2}.

(*b*) Chronic respiratory alkalosis—high pH, low P_{CO_2}, compensatory reduction in HCO_3^- concentration. Note that a low HCO_3^- concentration does not necessarily reflect a metabolic acidosis.

(*c*) Combined respiratory and metabolic acidosis—low pH, high P_{CO_2}, low HCO_3^- concentration.

(*d*) Metabolic alkalosis—high pH, high HCO_3^- concentration, compensatory elevation in P_{CO_2}.

17-3 (*a*) This patient has a pure metabolic acidosis.

(*b*) If the P_{CO_2} remains constant, the plasma HCO_3^- concentration must be raised to 5 meq/L to increase the pH to 7.20 (H^+ concentration equals 63 nanoeq/L):

$$63 = 24 \times \frac{13}{[HCO_3^-]}$$

$$[HCO_3^-] = 5 \, \text{meq/L}$$

(*c*) At a P_{CO_2} of 18 mmHg,

$$63 = 24 \times \frac{13}{[HCO_3^-]}$$

$$[HCO_3^-] = 6.9 \, \text{meq/L}$$

These examples illustrate that in patients who are able to hyperventilate in response to metabolic acidosis, only a small elevation in the plasma HCO_3^- concentration is initially required to get the patient out of danger.

CHAPTER 18

18-1 (*a*) The acute metabolic alkalosis is due to the citrate load from the multiple blood transfusions.

(*b*) The urine Na^+ should be less than 15 meq/L and the urine pH acid (due to maximum $NaHCO_3$ reabsorption), since effective volume depletion persists. It is possible, however, that HCO_3^- reabsorptive capacity may not be sufficiently increased to reabsorb all of the marked increment in the filtered HCO_3^- load. In this setting, the urine Na^+ concentration and pH may be elevated because of the obligatory $NaHCO_3$ excretion. A low urine Cl^- concentration will still be present, because the patient remains hypovolemic.

(*c*) Acetazolamide is the preferred therapy, both to remove the excess fluid and to cause a preferential $NaHCO_3$ diuresis. Saline loading is not indicated, since it will result in a marked increase in ascites formation.

18-2 (*a*) This patient is both volume- and K^+-depleted. Thus, treatment should consist of half-isotonic saline to which 40 meq of K^+ (as KCl) should be added.

(*b*) Correction of volume and Cl^- depletion will allow the excess HCO_3^- to be excreted. Thus, the anion gap between the high urine ($Na^+ + K^+$) concentration and low urine Cl^- concentration is due primarily to HCO_3^-. If, for example, the urine pH is 7.8 (H^+ concentration equals 16 nanoeq/L) and the urine P_{CO_2} is 46 mmHg (similar to the renal venous P_{CO_2}), then

$$[H^+] = 24 \times \frac{P_{CO_2}}{[HCO_3^-]}$$

$$16 = 24 \times \frac{46}{[HCO_3^-]}$$

$$[HCO_3^-] = 69 \, meq/L$$

Note that the urine Cl^- concentration is still low in this patient, indicating the need for further fluid and Cl^- replacement; the urine Na^+ concentration is not an accurate estimate of volume status in this setting because the excretion of HCO_3^- obligates Na^+ loss.

18-3 (*a*) The differential diagnosis of unexplained hypokalemia, urinary K^+ wasting, and metabolic alkalosis includes surreptitious diuretic use or vomiting (during the phase of HCO_3^- excretion in which both Na^+ and K^+ excretion are increased; see page 565) or some form of primary hyperaldosteronism. The normal blood pressure in this patient excludes all of the causes of the last condition other than Bartter's syndrome.

(*b*) The urine Cl^- concentration should be measured next. A value below 25 meq/L is highly suggestive of vomiting (which was present in this case), whereas a higher value is consistent with diuretic use or Bartter's syndrome. The last two conditions can usually be distinguished by a urinary assay for diuretics.

CHAPTER 19

19-1 (*a*) No. The extracellular pH has not been measured, so the patient may have chronic respiratory alkalosis with an appropriate compensatory reduction in the plasma HCO_3^- concentration.

(*b*) Yes. Although the pH is relatively well maintained, this occurs only by marked hyperventilation (P_{CO_2} equals 14 mmHg) that is probably symptomatic. The administration of $NaHCO_3$ will partially correct the acidemia and therefore the stimulus to ventilation.

19-2 (*a*) This patient has a combined respiratory and high anion gap metabolic acidosis, most likely due to seizure-induced lactic acidosis.

(*b*) No. Cessation of the seizure will allow the excess lactate to be metabolized back to HCO_3^-. ·

(*c*) There is likely to be no change, since neither lactic acidosis nor its correction seems to affect the internal distribution of K^+.

19-3 (*a*) 3. Type 1 RTA in adults is associated with a progressive but slow decline in the plasma HCO_3^- concentration as some of the dietary H^+ load is retained each day.

(*b*) 2. Type 1 RTA in infants is associated with a more rapid fall in the plasma HCO_3^- concentration because the higher urine pH also obligates a fixed degree of HCO_3^- loss.

(*c*) 1. The plasma HCO_3^- concentration falls rapidly in type 2 RTA and then stabilizes once the reduced level of HCO_3^- reabsorptive capacity has been reached.

At a near-normal plasma HCO_3^- concentration following HCO_3^- administration, these disorders can be distinguished by calculating the fractional excretion of HCO_3^-: less than 3 percent in type 1 RTA in adults, 5 to 10 percent in infantile type 1 RTA, and greater than 15 percent in type 2 RTA (see Fig. 19-6).

19-4 (*a*) 2. Hypoaldosteronism is associated with hyperkalemia, an acid urine pH, but a positive urine anion gap, since hyperkalemia impairs NH_4^+ production and excretion.

(*b*) 1. Diarrhea can lead to hypokalemia, which raises both NH_3 production and excretion, thereby elevating the urine pH. This disorder can be distinguished from RTA since NH_4^+ excretion is appropriately increased, as evidenced by the negative urine anion gap.

(*c*) 3. The high urine pH and positive urine anion gap are suggestive of type 1 RTA. The degree of metabolic acidosis is more severe than is typically seen with type 2 RTA, which can induce all of the other findings in this example.

19-5 (*a*) This patient has a mixed metabolic and respiratory acidosis, since a P_{CO_2} of 40 mmHg is inappropriately high in a patient with a plasma HCO_3^- concentration of 9 meq/L. The expected value is about 22 mmHg, since the P_{CO_2} normally falls by about 1.2 mmHg for every 1 meq/L reduction in the plasma HCO_3^- concentration.

(*b*) The H^+ concentration at a pH of 7.20 is 63 meq/L. Thus,

$$[H^+] = 24 \times \frac{P_{CO_2}}{[HCO_3^-]}$$

$$63 = 24 \times \frac{40}{[HCO_3^-]}$$

$$[HCO_3^-] = 15 \, meq/L$$

(*c*) At this degree of acidemia, the initial distribution of the excess acid is 50 to 70 percent of lean body weight. Thus,

$$HCO_3^- \text{ deficit} = 0.6 \times 80 \times (15 - 9)$$

$$= 288 \, meq$$

(*d*) The above formula is dependent upon the presence of a steady state. Since this patient is losing 1 liter of diarrheal fluid per hour, there is continuing HCO_3^- loss that is not being replaced.

(e) Body K^+ stores are probably markedly reduced. This is masked as the marked acidemia promotes K^+ movement out of the cells, thereby accounting for the initially normal plasma K^+ concentration.

19-6 (a) The metabolic acidosis in renal failure is primarily due to reduced NH_4^+ excretion, which prevents the urinary excretion of all of dietary acid load.

(b) The second arterial pH was measured only 30 min after the administration of $NaHCO_3$, before equilibration with the intracellular buffers had occurred. Thus, the later reductions in the plasma HCO_3^- concentration and pH probably reflected the effect of intracellular buffering; in addition, continued acid retention also may have played a contributory role.

CHAPTER 20

20-1 It is easiest to answer this problem by first determining the acid-base disorders represented by the three sets of blood values:

(a) The low pH and high P_{CO_2} indicate a respiratory acidosis. The P_{CO_2} is 25 mmHg above normal; in chronic respiratory acidosis, this should be associated with a plasma HCO_3^- concentration of approximately 33 meq/L (3.5 meq/L increase in the plasma HCO_3^- concentration for each 10 mmHg elevation in the P_{CO_2}). Thus, the HCO_3^- concentration of 37 meq/L represents a superimposed metabolic alkalosis.

(b) At a P_{CO_2} of 60 mmHg, the plasma HCO_3^- concentration should be roughly 26 meq/L in acute respiratory acidosis (1 meq/L increase per 10 mmHg elevation in the P_{CO_2}) and 31 meq/L in chronic respiratory acidosis. Therefore, the measured HCO_3^- concentration of 26 meq/L can reflect either uncomplicated acute respiratory acidosis *or* chronic respiratory acidosis with a superimposed metabolic acidosis (which lowers the HCO_3^- concentration from 31 to 26 meq/L).

(c) Uncomplicated chronic respiratory acidosis *or* acute respiratory acidosis with a superimposed metabolic alkalosis (raising the HCO_3^- concentration from 26 to 32 meq/L).

The correct diagnosis can be made only by correlating the history with the laboratory values:

1. Chronic bronchitis plus diarrhea suggests chronic respiratory acidosis with a superimposed metabolic acidosis, or (b).
2. Marked obesity suggest chronic hypercapnia, or (c).
3. Severe acute asthma suggests acute respiratory acidosis, or (b).
4. Chronic bronchitis plus diuretic therapy suggests chronic respiratory acidosis with superimposed metabolic alkalosis, or (a).

20-2 (a) From the history and laboratory values, the probable diagnosis is acute superimposed upon chronic respiratory acidosis (see Fig. 20-6).

(*b*) Patients with chronic hypercapnia rely on the hypoxemic drive to ventilation. This is removed by the administration of oxygen, resulting in further hypoventilation and a rise in the P_{CO_2}.

(*c*) The patient cannot tolerate the administration of oxygen, nor can he tolerate the P_{O_2} on 30 mmHg of room air. Thus, some form of mechanical ventilation and probably endotracheal intubation are required.

(*d*) Rapid normalization of the P_{CO_2} will lead to a posthypercapnic alkalosis, since the elevated plasma HCO_3^- concentration will persist.

(*e*) Correction of the posthypercapnic alkalosis requires the urinary excretion of the excess HCO_3^- as $NaHCO_3$. In the presence of volume depletion (low urine Na^+ concentration), however, HCO_3^- excretion will not occur until normovolemia is restored.

20-3 (*a*) Metabolic alkalosis, with the elevated P_{CO_2} reflecting the appropriate respiratory compensation.

(*b*) The (A-a) O_2 gradient is 13 mmHg, making underlying lung disease and chronic hypercapnia unlikely.

$$(\text{A-a}) \ O_2 \ \text{gradient} = P_{I_{O_2}} - 1.25 Pa_{CO_2} - Pa_{O_2}$$

$$= 150 - 64 - 73$$

$$= 13 \, \text{mmHg}$$

CHAPTER 22

22-1 (*a*) The P_{osm} can be calculated from

$$\text{Calculated } P_{osm} = 2 \times \text{plasma } [Na^+] + \frac{BUN}{2.8} + \frac{[\text{glucose}]}{18}$$

$$= 250 + 50 + 6$$

$$= 306 \, \text{mosmol/kg}$$

(*b*) No. The effective P_{osm} is actually reduced at 256 mosmol/kg, since the contribution of the ineffective osmole urea must be excluded.

22-1 (*a*) The administration of isotonic fluids to a patient who can excrete only an isosmotic urine will lead to hyperosmolality and a rise in the plasma Na^+ concentration, since no free water is given to replace insensible losses from the skin and respiratory tract.

(*b*) Half-isotonic saline plus 77 meq/L of KCl is also an isosmotic fluid and therefore will have the same osmotic effect as isotonic saline. At first glance, it may seem that the addition to the extracellular fluid of a solution with a Na^+ concentration less than that of the plasma (and extracellular fluid) should lower the plasma Na^+ concentration. However, not all of this fluid remains in the extracellular space. This can be appreciated if each liter of the added fluid is viewed as having two components: 500 mL of isotonic NaCl, which stays in the extracellular fluid, and 500 mL of isotonic KCl, which must either enter the cells or be excreted in the urine to prevent fatal hyperkalemia.

Thus, the osmotic effect of this solution is similar to that of isotonic saline. In comparison, the administration of half-isotonic saline alone will lower the P_{osm} and the plasma Na^+ concentration, since it is a hypotonic fluid. These concepts are clinically important, since the osmotic contribution of K^+ in intravenous fluids is frequently ignored.

CHAPTER 23

23-1 All of these factors contributed to the hyponatremia. Hydrochlorothiazide induced volume depletion (physical findings plus low urine Na^+ concentration), which enhanced ADH release (high U_{osm} of 540 mosmol/kg), resulting in water retention and hyponatremia. The loss of K^+ also played a contributory role via a transcellular K^+-Na^+ exchange.

Therapy should include the administration of Na^+ and K^+ in a hypertonic solution, such as 40 meq of KCl added to each liter of isotonic saline. There is little justification for water restriction, since the patient is volume-depleted. In view of the metabolic alkalosis, KCl, not potassium citrate, is indicated (since citrate is metabolized into HCO_3^-). Half-isotonic saline should also be avoided, because it is a hypotonic solution that will further lower the plasma Na^+ concentration.

23-2 The hyponatremia in this patient is due to volume depletion, probably induced by diuretic therapy for hypertension. The physical findings suggestive of hypovolemia, hypokalemia, and high plasma HCO_3^- concentration are all compatible with this diagnosis.

Pseudohyponatremia due to mannitol is not present, since the measured P_{osm} is low and is similar to the calculated value [Calculated $P_{osm} = 2 \times 120 + (125/18) + (15/2.8) = 252$ mosmol/kg]. SIADH due to the stroke also cannot account for the hyponatremia; the hyponatremia must have *preceded* the stroke, since the patient subsequently received only 100 mL of water, a quantity that is insufficient to lower the plasma Na^+ concentration.

23-3 1. (*b*) This edematous patient is both water- and sodium-overloaded, and should be treated with both water and sodium restriction.

2. (*f*) The combination of marked hyponatremia and a very concentrated urine should be treated with hypertonic saline plus a loop diuretic (such as furosemide) to lower the U_{osm}.

3. (*d*) True volume depletion with mild hyponatremia is best treated with isotonic saline.

4. (*c*) No therapy is required for pseudohyponatremia (normal P_{osm}).

5. (*b*) This edematous patient, like the one with renal failure, is both water- and sodium-overloaded.

6. (*a* or *e*) Either water restriction alone or the use of hypertonic saline is reasonable in this patient with presumed SIADH and asymptomatic hyponatremia. A loop diuretic is not necessary, since the U_{osm} is only 290 mosmol/kg.

23-4 (*a*) The most likely diagnosis is SIADH due to the oat cell carcinoma.

(*b*) Hypertonic saline should be given initially in view of the marked hyponatremia and neurologic symptoms. The approximate Na^+ deficit that must be corrected to raise the plasma Na^+ concentration to a safe value of 120 meq/L can be estimated from

$$Na^+ \text{ deficit} = 0.6 \times 70 \times (120 - 105)$$

$$= 630 \text{ meq}$$

This requires approximately 1200 mL of 3% saline, which should be given at the rate of 40 mL/h over 30 h to raise the plasma Na^+ concentration by 0.5 meq/L/h. Furosemide will enhance the efficacy of this regimen by lowering U_{osm}, thereby increasing free-water excretion.

23-5 Volume depletion increases the proximal reabsorption of Na^+ and secondarily that of uric acid (see page 90). The result is an increase in the plasma uric acid concentration. In comparison, SIADH is associated with initial volume expansion, thereby increasing Na^+ and uric acid excretion. Thus, the plasma uric acid concentration is typically below 4 mg/dL in this disorder.[7]

CHAPTER 24

24-1 (*a*) Polydipsia and polyuria with a dilute urine is due either to primary polydipsia or to central or nephrogenic diabetes insipidus. Sarcoidosis can produce each of these conditions: the first two by hypothalamic infiltration and nephrogenic diabetes insipidus by hypercalcemia.[8] The only clue to the correct diagnosis is the low plasma Na^+ concentration and P_{osm}, suggesting water overload due to primary polydipsia.

(*b*) The diagnosis can be established by the water-restriction test followed by the administration of dDAVP or aqueous vasopressin after the maximum U_{osm} has been achieved or the P_{osm} reaches 295 mosmol/kg.

24-2 (*b* and *e*) Insensible water losses that were not replaced as a result of decreased thirst were the major factors responsible for the hypernatremia in this patient. The diarrhea also may have made a contribution, if it was an osmotic diarrhea in which the $(Na^+ + K^+)$ concentration in the diarrheal fluid was less than that in the plasma (see page 293). In this setting, water would be lost in excess of effective solute (thereby promoting the development of hypernatremia), even though the diarrheal fluid was isosmotic to plasma.

The low urine Na^+ concentration in this patient is indicative of volume depletion. There is no predictable relationship between the plasma Na^+ concentration (a measure of osmolality) and the urine Na^+ concentration (which varies with the effective circulating volume).

(*d*) The water deficit can be approximated from

$$\text{Water deficit} = 0.4 \times 50 \times \left(\frac{174}{140} - 1\right)$$

$$= 5 \text{ liters}$$

This deficit should be repaired gradually over 68 h (34 meq/L reduction in the plasma Na^+ concentration at a rate of 0.5 meq/L per h); thus, fluid should be given at the approximate rate of 75 mL/h. Continuing insensible losses of 40 mL/h must also be replaced, leading to a total of 115 mL/h of free water. In addition, this patient is also Na^+-depleted from diuretic therapy and diarrhea. Thus, initial fluid therapy should probably be given as quarter-isotonic saline. This fluid, however, is only three-quarters free water. Therefore, 150 mL/h [(4/3) × 115] must be given to provide the necessary free water.

24-3 (*a*) The diagnosis of central diabetes insipidus can be confirmed by the administration of dDAVP or aqueous vasopressin, which should raise the U_{osm} and lower the urine volume. There is no need to do the water-restriction test, since the P_{osm} is already 350 mosmol/kg.

(*b*) The water deficit can be estimated from

$$\text{Water deficit} = 0.5 \times 70 \times \left(\frac{168}{140} - 1\right)$$

$$= 7 \text{ liters}$$

(*c*) This deficit should be replaced gradually over 56 h at the rate of 125 mL/h. Another 50 mL/h should be added to replace continuing insensible losses. Thus, 175 mL/h can be given as dextrose in water. There is no history of Na^+ loss and therefore no requirement for saline administration.

(*d*) The late development of hyponatremia is probably due to SIADH. The administration of vasopressin tannate in oil results in nonsuppressible plasma ADH levels, which can lead to water retention if too much water is taken in.

CHAPTER 25

25-1 (*a*) The patient has both diabetic ketoacidosis and a superimposed metabolic alkalosis due to vomiting. Notice that the anion gap is 28 meq/L (16 meq/L above normal), which should be associated with a reduction in the plasma HCO_3^- concentration to about 10 meq/L. The substantially high value in this case is indicative of the underlying metabolic alkalosis.

(*b*) Dehydration undoubtedly is responsible for much of the decline in renal function. In addition, acetoacetate is measured as creatinine in the standard assay, resulting in a further apparent elevation in the plasma creatinine concentration.

(*c*) The major electrolyte problems in this patient are hypokalemia and volume depletion. The hyperglycemia and metabolic acidosis are relatively mild; immediate correction of these disturbances with insulin is not necessary and may be deleterious by driving K^+ into the cells, possibly inducing arrhythmias. Thus, the initial therapy should consist of isotonic or half-isotonic saline to which 40 meq/L of KCl is added. This regimen will correct the hypokalemia and volume depletion and will slowly ameliorate the hyperglycemia, both by dilution and by improving renal function, thereby enhancing glucose excretion.

The patient should also be started on antimicorbial therapy for presumed acute pyelonephritis. This infection was probably responsible for the loss of diabetic control.

25-2 (*a*) The acidemia is due to retention of H^+ ions from the ketoacids; the associated anions (β-hydroxybutyrate and acetoacetate) were presumably excreted in the urine, resulting in only a minor elevation in the anion gap.

(*b*) The patient should be given insulin with glucose. This will correct the ketoacidosis without the risk of hypoglycemia.

CHAPTER 26

26-1 (*a*) Correction of the acidemia will drive K^+ into the cells, further reducing the plasma K^+ concentration. In this setting, in which the acidemia is not severe, alkali therapy should be withheld until K^+ supplements have partially corrected the hypokalemia.

(*b*) Hypocalcemia *protects* against the effects of hypokalemia via an uncertain mechanism. Thus, treatment of the hypokalemia should precede correction of the hypocalcemia.

It should be noted that, for the same reasons, hypokalemia protects against the neuromuscular effects of hypocalcemia. Thus, increasing the plasma K^+ concentration in this setting may precipitate hypocalcemic tetany.[9] However, this risk is generally less serious than the potentially fatal cardiac arrhythmias that can be induced by severe hypokalemia.

CHAPTER 27

27-1 (*a*) The differential diagnosis of unexplained hypokalemia, urinary K^+ wasting, and metabolic alkalosis includes surreptitious diuretic use or vomiting (during the phase of HCO_3^- excretion in which both Na^+ and K^+ excretion are increased; see page 566) or some form of primary hyperaldosteronism. The normal blood pressure in this patient excludes all of the causes of the last condition other than Bartter's syndrome.

(*b*) These disorders can be distinguished by viewing this as a diagnostic problem of metabolic alkalosis and measuring the urine Cl^- concentration (see Chap. 18). A value below 25 meq/L is highly suggestive of vomiting (which was present in this case), whereas a higher value is consistent with diuretic use or Bartter's syndrome. The last two conditions can usually be distinguished by a urinary assay for diuretics.

27-2 (*a*) 3. The low U_{osm} is consistent with primary water overload, which shuts off ADH secretion. Although the urine K^+ concentration is appropriately reduced, the urine volume is probably very high, resulting in an inappropriately high absolute level of K^+ excretion.

(*b*) 2. The major clue suggesting hypomagnesemia is the presence of hypocalcemia.

(*c*) 1. Metabolic acidosis with a high urine pH and positive urine anion gap (see Chap. 19) is diagnostic of renal tubular acidosis.

(*d*) 4. Metabolic acidosis with a normally acid urine pH, an appropriately negative urine anion gap (reflecting the adaptive increase in NH_4^+ excretion), and a low urine K^+ concentration is compatible with extrarenal losses of K^+ and HCO_3^-, as occurs with laxative abuse.

CHAPTER 28

28-1 (*a*) The underlying renal insufficiency, superimposed volume depletion (due to Na^+ wasting after the acute institution of a low-Na^+ diet), and metabolic acidosis all may play a contributory role. However, many patients have these problems without life-threatening hyperkalemia. Therefore, the patient should be questioned about increased K^+ intake; this patient gave a history of using large quantities of KCl-containing salt substitute.

(*b*) By definition, pseudohyperkalemia produces no symptoms or signs of K^+ intoxication.

(*c*) The patient has both severe muscle weakness and electrocardiographic changes. Therefore, therapy should be initiated with calcium gluconate, followed by glucose, insulin, and $NaHCO_3$ to temporarily drive K^+ into the cells. For example 500 mL of 10% dextrose in saline plus 10 units of regular insulin plus 45 meq of $NaHCO_3$ infused over 30 min will lower the plasma K^+ concentration, raise the plasma Na^+ concentration, and produce volume expansion. Sodium polystyrene sulfonate should be given orally and repeated as necessary to remove the excess K^+. Dialysis should not be required, since the patient does not have severe renal failure.

(*d*) Mild asymptomatic hyperkalemia can be treated solely with sodium polystyrene sulfonate.

28-2 (*a*) By definition, patients with chronic hyperkalemic have a defect in renal K^+ excretion, since normal subjects would rapidly excrete the excess K^+ in the urine. Thus, the urine K^+ concentration of 34 meq/L is inappropriately low. The transtubular K^+ gradient (TTKG) can be calculated in this patient to assess the degree of aldosterone effect:

$$TTKG = \left[U_{K^+} \div \frac{U_{osm}}{P_{osm}} \right] \div P_{K^+}$$

$$= \left[34 \div \frac{550}{275} \right] \div 6.8$$

$$= 2.5$$

where 275 represents the calculated P_{osm}. The TTKG is low in this patient, a finding that is consistent with some form of mineralocorticoid deficiency or resistance.

(b) The findings of low blood pressure, increased skin pigmentation, a low TTKG, and hypoglycemia after the administration of glucose and insulin all point to the probable diagnosis of primary adrenal insufficiency.

(c) Acutely, sodium polystyrene sulfonate can be given to lower the plasma K^+ concentration. Chronically, both glucocorticoid and mineralocorticoid replacement will be required because of the persistent adrenal dysfunction.

REFERENCES

1. Jacobsen HR, Klahr S. Chronic renal failure: Pathophysiology; management. *Lancet* 338:419, 423, 1991.
2. Epstein FH, Kleeman CR, Pursel S, Hendrikx A. The effect of feeding protein and urea on the renal concentrating process. *J Clin Invest* 36:635, 1957.
3. Vaughan ED Jr, Carey RM, Peach MJ, et al. The renin response to diuretic therapy: A limitation of antihypertensive potential. *Circ Res* 42:376, 1978.
4. DeSousa RC, Harrington JT, Ricanati ES, et al. Renal regulation of acid-base equilibrium during administration of mineral acid. *J Clin Invest* 53:465, 1974.
5. George JM, Wright L, Bell NH, Bartter FC. The syndrome of primary aldosteronism. *Am J Med* 48:343, 1970.
6. Hariprasad MK, Eisinger RP, Nadler IM, et al. Hyponatremia in psychogenic polydipsia. *Arch Intern Med* 140:1639, 1980.
7. Beck LH. Hypouricemia in the syndrome of inappropriate secretion of antidiuretic hormone. *N Engl J Med* 301:528, 1979.
8. Stuart CA, Neelon FA, Lebovitz HE. Disordered control of thirst in hypothalamic-pituitary sarcoidosis. *N Engl J Med* 303:1078, 1980.
9. Engel FL, Martin SP, Taylor H. On the relation of potassium to the neurologic manifestations of hypocalcemic tetany. *Bull Johns Hopkins Hosp* 84:295, 1949.

SUMMARY OF EQUATIONS
AND FORMULAS

UNITS OF MEASUREMENT

$$\text{mmol/L} = \frac{\text{mg/dL} \times 10}{\text{molecular weight}}$$

$$\text{meq/L} = \text{mmol/L} \times \text{valence}$$

$$\text{mosmol/kg} = \text{n} \times \text{mmol/L}$$

where n = number of dissociable particles per molecules.

TUBULAR FUNCTION

Variations in tubular reabsorption are the major way in which the kidneys alter solute and water excretion. There are, however, *no absolute normal values* for the urine Na^+ or K^+ concentration, osmolality, or pH, since these parameters vary with intake. For example, the urine Na^+ concentration should be less than 10 to 15 meq/L with volume depletion but may exceed 100 meq/L after a Na^+ load. Similarly, the U_{osm} may fall below 100 mosmol/kg after a large water load but should exceed 800 mosmol/kg after water restriction has led to a rise in the plasma Na^+ concentration above 145 meq/L. Thus, a U_{osm} of 300 mosmol/kg is *inappropriately low* in the latter setting, suggesting either lack of or resistance to antidiuretic hormone.

ACID-BASE

$$pH = 6.10 + \log\frac{[HCO_3^-]}{0.03P_{CO_2}}$$

$$[H^+] = 24 \times \frac{P_{CO_2}}{[HCO_3^-]}$$

Plasma anion gap $= [Na^+] = ([Cl^-] + [HCO_3^-])$

Urine anion gap $= ([Na^+] + [K^+]) - [Cl^-]$

Conversion of pH into Hydrogen Concentration

pH of $7.40 = [H^+]$ of 40 nanoeq/L

For each 0.1-unit increase in pH, multiple $[H^+]$ by 0.8:

pH of $7.60 = 40 \times 0.8 \times 0.8$

$[H^+] = 26$ nanoeq/L

For each 0.1 unit fall in pH, multiply $[H^+]$ by 1.25:

pH of $7.30 = 40 \times 1.25$

$[H^+] = 50$ nanoeq/L

Renal and Respiratory Compensations in Acid-Base Disorders

Metabolic acidosis:

1.2-mmHg fall in P_{CO_2} per 1-meq/L decrease in plasma $[HCO_3^-]$

Metabolic alkalosis:

0.6-mmHg rise in P_{CO_2} per 1-meq/L elevation in plasma $[HCO_3^-]$

Respiratory acidosis:

Acute: 1-meq/L increase in plasma $[HCO_3^-]$ per 10-mmHg rise in P_{CO_2}
Chronic: 3.5-meq/L elevation in plasma $[HCO_3^-]$ per 10-mmHg increase in P_{CO_2}

Respiratory alkalosis:

Acute: 2-meq/L fall in plasma $[HCO_3^-]$ per 10-mmHg decrease in P_{CO_2}
Chronic: 4-meq/L reduction in plasma $[HCO_3^-]$ per 10-mmHg fall in P_{CO_2}

Estimation of Bicarbonate Deficit and Excess

In severe metabolic acidosis with a plasma HCO_3^- concentration below 10 meq/L:

$$HCO_3^- \text{ deficit (meq)} \cong 0.7 \times \text{lean body weight (kg)} \times (10 - \text{plasma } [HCO_3^-])$$

This formula applies only when the plasma HCO_3^- concentration is very low and the cell and bone buffers are responsible for almost all buffering of excess H^+ ions. Once the plasma HCO_3^- concentration is above 10 meq/L, however, there is more extracellular buffering and the apparent space of distribution of HCO_3^- falls to 0.5 times the lean body weight.

In metabolic alkalosis

$$HCO_3^- \text{ excess (meq)} \cong 0.5 \times \text{lean body weight} \times (\text{plasma } [HCO_3^-] - 24)$$

OSMOLALITY AND THE PLASMA SODIUM CONCENTRATION

$$P_{osm} \cong 2 \times \text{plasma } [Na^+] + \frac{[\text{glucose}]}{18} + \frac{BUN}{2.8}$$

$$\text{Effective } P_{osm} \cong 2 \times \text{plasma } [Na^+] + \frac{[\text{glucose}]}{18}$$

$$\text{Plasma } [Na^+] \cong \frac{Na_e^+ + K_e^+}{\text{total body water}}$$

Plasma Sodium Concentration in Hyperglycemia

For each 62-mg/dL increment in the plasma glucose concentration, there will be a reciprocal 1-meq/L reduction in the plasma Na^+ concentration because of the osmotic movement of water from the cells into the extracellular fluid. Thus, hyperglycemia results in a dissociation between the P_{osm} (which is increased) and the plasma Na^+ concentration (which may be reduced).

Hyponatremia

$$Na^+ \text{ deficit (meq)} \cong 0.6^* \times \text{lean body weight (kg)} \times (140 - \text{plasma } [Na^+])$$

This formula estimates the amount of Na^+ required to raise the plasma Na^+ concentration back up to 140 meq/L. It may not represent the total Na^+ deficit, however, since there may be an additional *isosmotic* Na^+ and water loss (due, for example, to diuretics or diarrhea).

---

* The percent of lean body weight (in kg) used to estimate the total body water in this and the following equation refers to men. In women, a 10 percent lower value should be used, for example, 0.5, not 0.6, times the lean body weight for the sodium deficit.

Hypernatremia

$$\text{Water deficit (liters)} \cong 0.5 \times \text{lean body weight (kg)} \times \left(\frac{\text{plasma } [Na^+]}{140} - 1\right)$$

MISCELLANEOUS

Alveolar-Arterial Oxygen Gradient

$$(\text{A} - \text{a}) \; O_2 \text{ gradient} = P_{I_{O_2}} (150 \text{ mmHg on room air}) - 1.25 \times Pa_{CO_2} - Pa_{O_2}$$

Plasma Calcium Concentration and Hypoalbuminemia

For every 1-g/dL fall in the plasma albumin concentration, there will be less bound Ca^{2+} leading to an 0.8 mg/dL reduction in the plasma Ca^{2+} concentration. This does not represent true hypocalcemia, however, since there is no change in the physiologically important free (or ionized) Ca^{2+} concentration.

INDEX

Page numbers in *italic* indicate figures, those followed by "t" indicate tables.